Concise Veterinary Dictionary

General Editor

Robert S. Hine BSc, MSc
Market House Books Ltd.

Consultant Editors

Professor Christopher M. Brown BVSc, PhD, MRCVS, Dip.ACVIM
Department of Large Animal Clinical Sciences, Michigan State University

D. A. Hogg BVMS, PhD, MRCVS
Department of Anatomy, University of Glasgow

Professor D. F. Kelly MA, PhD, BVSc, MRCVS, FRCPath
Department of Veterinary Pathology, University of Liverpool

Specialist Consultants

Parasitology: W. N. Beesley MSc, PhD
Poultry diseases: F. T. W. Jordan BSc, DSc, PhD, FRCVS, DPMP
Biochemistry: D. E. Kidder BSc, PhD, MIBiol, FRSC
Pharmacology: P Lees BPharm, PhD
Mycology: G. A. Pepin BSc
Bacteriology: Professor I. M. Smith MSc, PhD, MRCVS

Concise Veterinary Dictionary

Oxford New York

OXFORD UNIVERSITY PRESS

Melbourne Toronto

1988

Oxford University Press, Walton Street, Oxford OX2 6DP

Oxford New York Toronto
Delhi Bombay Calcutta Madras Karachi
Petaling Jaya Singapore Hong Kong Tokyo
Nairobi Dar es Salaam Cape Town
Melbourne Auckland

and associated companies in
Berlin Ibadan

Oxford is a trade mark of Oxford University Press

British Library Cataloguing in Publication Data
Concise veterinary dictionary.
1. Veterinary medicine—Encyclopaedias
636.089'03'21
ISBN 0-19-854208-9

Library of Congress Cataloging in Publication Data
(Data Available)

Text prepared and typeset by
Market House Books Ltd., Aylesbury
Printed in Great Britain by
Richard Clay Ltd
Bungay, Suffolk

Preface

This dictionary is an entirely new and up-to-date compilation covering all the major fields in veterinary science. It has been devised primarily for farmers, stockbreeders, agricultural and veterinary students, and veterinary assistants. However, it should also prove useful for practitioners themselves, at one end of the spectrum, and pet owners at the other. Research workers in the pharmaceutical industry and in other fields related to veterinary science will also find the book useful.

A wide range of topics is covered in the dictionary, including:

- animal husbandry
- biochemistry
- diagnostic techniques
- diseases of livestock and other domestic animals
- disease-causing organisms and their vectors
- drugs used to treat and prevent disease (including mode of action and side effects)
- endocrinology
- genetics
- histology
- immunology
- laws relating to animals and diseases (England and Wales and Federal US legislation)
- meat inspection
- physiology
- skeletal components and body organs
- stockbreeding
- surgical operations and instruments
- toxicology
- veterinary institutions and animal welfare bodies

The entries are free of jargon, and any scientific terms used in an entry are defined elsewhere in the book. An asterisk immediately preceding a word in an entry denotes that further information relevant to the entry can be found under the asterisked word. However, not every word that is defined in the book is necessarily given an asterisk when used in text. Some entries simply refer the reader to another entry, indicating either that they are synonyms or that—together with related terms—they are best explained in one of the dictionary's longer entries. Major synonyms are shown in brackets immediately after the entry headword; other synonyms are listed at the end of the entry.

1988   *Robert Hine*

Contributors

Norma C. Bailie BVMS, MS, MRCVS

Professor Kenneth P. Baker MA, MSc, PhD, FRCVS

Hugh Bassett MVB, MRCVS

Anthony Bate MA, VetMB, MRCVS, Barrister-at-Law

Terence C. Bate BVSc, LLB, MRCVS, Barrister-at-Law

Malcolm J. Bearley MA, VetMB, MRCVS

Margaret E. Cooper LLB

G. P. David BVSc, MRCVS

John Dixon MA, PhD, VetMB, MRCVS

Professor T. A. Douglas BSc, PhD, MRCVS

P. Dutt BSc

Carwyn, A. Ellis BSc

Roderick W. Else BVSc, PhD, MRCVS

Professor E. J. H. Ford DVSc, FRCVS, FRCPath

P. C. Garnsworthy BSc, PhD, MIBiol

John J. B. Gill BSc, PhD

D. E. Hall BSc, MIBiol, Dip.RCPath

John Hamilton DVM, PhD, BVMS, FRCPath, FRCVS

D. A. Hogg BVMS, PhD, MRCVS

Judith M. Hunt BVSc, PhD, MRCVS

R. P. Kitching BSc, BVetMed, MSc, PhD, MRCVS

D. G. Lewis DVR, FRCVS

Janet D. Littlewood MA, BVSc, MRCVS, DVR

James M. Morrison BSc, PhD

Raymond Nachreiner DVM, PhD

T. Nicholson BSc, BVetMed, MRCVS

Margaret A. Parry BSc, PhD

Professor Jack M. Payne BSc, PhD, FIBiol, FRSA, MRCVS

Catherine Payne-Johnson BVSc, FRCVS

Rosemary Prince MA

Kenneth Randall MA, MSc

Barbara E. Robinson PhD

T. G. Rowan BVSc, PhD, MRCVS

Elspeth W. Scott BVMS, MRCVS

J. W. Simpson SDA, BVMS, MPhil, MRCVS

Michael R. Slanker DVM, MS

Professor John Earle Smith PhD, MRCVS

Leslie Theobald BVSc, MRCVS

Ninetta M. Theobald BVSc, MRCVS

A. J. Trees BVMS, MRCVS, PhD

B. P. Viner BVetMed, MRCVS

Robert D. Walker MS, PhD

Andrew Wilson DVSM, MRCVS

Zerai Woldehiwet PhD, DVM, MRCVS

A

a- (an-) *Prefix denoting* absence of; lacking; not. Examples: *amorphic* (lacking definite form); *atoxic* (not poisonous).

ab- *Prefix denoting* away from. Example: *abembryonic* (away from or opposite the embryo).

abdomen The region of the trunk between the *thorax and tail. Separated from the thorax by the *diaphragm, the abdomen has muscular walls, generally lined with *peritoneum on their inner surface, which surround and protect the abdominal organs, such as the digestive organs (stomach, liver, intestine) and excretory organs (kidneys, bladder, etc.). In females, the reproductive organs – ovaries and uterus – are also contained in the abdomen.

abdomin- (abdomino-) *Combining form denoting* the abdomen. Example: *abdominothoracic* (relating to the abdomen and thorax).

abdominal catastrophe Any of various life-threatening conditions affecting the abdominal organs, principally the gastrointestinal tract. These include *intussusception, *volvulus, *torsion of the stomach, abomasum, mesentery, or spleen, and gastric or abomasal dilatation.

abducens nerve The sixth *cranial nerve (VI). It supplies the lateral rectus and retractor bulbi muscles of the eye.

abduct To move part of the body from the midline of the body or to move the digits away from the midline of the limb. *Compare* adduct.

abductor A muscle that performs abduction (*see* abduct).

abiotrophy An inherited pathological trait involving disordered function of an organ or system and giving rise to premature ageing. The disease may remain latent in the individual rather than becoming apparent. *Cerebellar abiotrophy* has been reported in Hereford calves and Arabian foals, which develop *ataxia at an age of 3–8 months; affected animals fail to exhibit a menace reflex, although examination reveals their sight to be intact. The onset of clinical signs is sudden, but progression thereafter may well be slow or even unapparent. Microscopic inspection of the affected areas shows degeneration of the neurones of the cerebellum.

abomasopexy Surgical fixation of the abomasum in a certain position. This can form part of the surgical treatment of left displacement of the abomasum in cattle. The displacement is corrected manually and the abomasal wall is then sutured to the parietal peritoneum. *See also* omentopexy; pyloropexy.

abomasum The fourth and final chamber of the ruminant stomach. It is filled from the *omasum and consists of a blind-ending fundus to the front, a middle body, and a pyloric region, which empties into the small intestine (duodenum) to the rear. The abomasum lies against the lower abdominal wall at the front of the abdomen, mainly to the right of the midline. It can undergo displacement to the left, especially in dairy cattle (*see* displaced abomasum). The abomasum is comparable to the stomach of single-stomached (monogastric) species. See illustration at stomach.

abortion The expulsion of a non-viable foetus before full term of *gestation. Abortion may occur at any time from early pregnancy onwards, but in cattle and mares it is defined

1

abscess

as expulsion before 271 and 300 days (in full gestation lengths of 280 and 335 days) respectively. The clinical signs may include a vaginal discharge, straining, membranes hanging from the vulva, and the passage of a recognizable or mummified foetus (*see* mummification). In grazing animals the foetus may be readily removed by predators. It is important to isolate the aborted animal from the rest of the flock or herd; if found, the foetus should be placed in a clean plastic bag since samples may be needed for veterinary analysis. Any contaminated bedding should be burnt. The veterinary surgeon should be informed so that an accurate diagnosis of the cause can be made, particularly as certain conditions are transmissible to man (e.g. brucellosis and toxoplasmosis; see below).

Abortion may be spontaneous or induced, and it may result from infectious or noninfectious causes. Infectious agents include bacteria, viruses, fungi, and protozoa, while noninfectious causes include nutritional deficiencies, ingestion of *mycotoxins or poisonous plants, hormonal imbalances, chromosomal abnormalities in the foetus, and physical or psychological stress. In **cattle**, infectious agents are responsible for a relatively small proportion of abortions; now that abortion due to *brucellosis is largely controlled (at least in the UK), the main bacteria involved are *Campylobacter foetus* (*see* campylobacteriosis of cattle), *Corynebacterium pyogenes*, and various species of *Leptospira* (*see* leptospirosis). *Mycotic abortion due to the ingestion of mouldy feedstuffs is also important. Nutritional deficiencies are a common cause of abortion in **sheep**, in addition to infectious agents, such as *Toxoplasma gondii* (*see* toxoplasmosis), *Campylobacter foetus* (*see* campylobacteriosis of sheep), and *Chlamydia* (*see* enzootic ovine abortion). In **pigs**, however, there are no

established infectious agents that commonly cause abortions; factors such as *vitamin A deficiency and various forms of stress are more likely to be responsible. The most important noninfectious cause of abortion in **mares** is twinning, as there is inadequate placental area to support two foetuses, but infectious agents, such as equine herpesvirus 1 and various bacteria, may be involved. In **dogs** and **cats**, most abortions are due to infections, such as *distemper (bitch) and *feline viral enteritis and toxoplasmosis (queen).

abscess A localized accumulation of pus surrounded by a fibrous capsule. The usual cause is infection by bacteria, including staphylococci, streptococci, *Escherichia coli*, and species of *Actinomyces*, *Actinobacillus*, *Corynebacterium*, *Pseudomonas*, and *Mycobacterium*. A number of pathogenic fungi and some protozoa also cause abscesses. The microorganisms enter from the outside via a wound or spread from infection elsewhere within the body. Bacteria may be conveyed from another lesion to the site of abscess formation in the bloodstream or lymphatic system or by the movement of some foreign body or parasite within the tissues. For example, tail abscesses are common in pigs, due to infection of injuries caused by fighting; these may spread into the spinal cord and vertebrae, causing spinal abscesses.

Acute abscesses form as a result of *inflammation and the accumulation of dead *neutrophils. Together with the dead tissue remains, the neutrophils form a zone of liquefactive necrosis, which becomes encapsulated. The fate of abscesses depends on the virulence of the causal organism, the location of the lesion in relation to the organ surface, and the resistance of the animal. Loss of local or general resistance is a frequent accompaniment to abscess formation. An abscess that ruptures to the body surface and discharges its pus usually heals, although an abscess may sometimes continue to discharge to the surface via a sinus. Rupture may occur into a body cavity or into the vascular system with consequent persistence and spread of the infection. Furthermore, abscesses may become chronic or dormant; dormant lesions eventually undergo caseation or calcification.

Acute abscesses are accompanied by the classical inflammatory signs of heat, swelling, redness, and pain. There may also be systemic signs, including fever. Local lymph nodes are often enlarged. These signs abate rapidly after rupture and evacuation of the abscess.

The usual treatment is by surgically opening and draining the abscess. Reinfection or incomplete drainage may lead to sinus formation, so two or more openings may enhance drainage. A dressing can be applied to the site to absorb residual discharge; this should be changed regularly and should not prevent drainage. Drainage tubes may be inserted in some cases. Local or parenteral administration of *antibiotics or sulphonamides to combat the infection may be withheld in selected cases in order not to impede the natural process of rupture and resolution. Heat in the form of *fomentations may assist this process. *Chronic abscesses* are most often associated with infections of *Mycobacterium tuberculosis* or species of *Actinomyces, Actinobacillus,* or *Staphylococcus*; if they occur as a sequel to an acute abscess they often become heavily fibrotic. Compared to acute lesions the pus is often thinner owing to the presence of much serum and fewer cells; it may, however, be thickened (inspissated), caseous, or calcified. Heat and reddening are not usually marked and systemic signs are generally less. Treatment depends on diagnosis of the cause and use of the correct antibiotic, sulphonamide, or other therapy. Tuberculous chronic abscesses may require the destruction of the animal (*see* tuberculosis).

Absidia A genus of saprophytic fungi, belonging to the order Mucorales of the class Zygomycetes, some of which can infect man or animals causing diseases called either *mucormyosis or *zygomycosis.

absorption 1. (in physiology) The transfer of substances, especially digested food (*see* digestion), from the lumen of the *alimentary tract to the blood or lymph. Little is absorbed from the mouth, although some drugs may be. Ethanol and some organic acids are absorbed from the stomach; in ruminants, most of the *volatile fatty acids produced in the rumen by microbial fermentation are absorbed through the walls of the rumen, reticulum, and omasum. In general, water, ions, and nutrients are absorbed chiefly through the wall of the small intestine, which is lined with minute finger-like projections (*see* villus) that greatly increase its surface area. Water and ions are also absorbed from the large intestine. Absorption may occur by simple diffusion, by facilitated diffusion (involving a carrier mechanism in the cell membrane), or by *active transport (including *pinocytosis). Fats are absorbed as fatty acids and glycerol separately, to be reconstituted in the mucosal cells and enter the lymphatic vessels as *chyle. Proteins are absorbed mainly as amino acids and peptides; intact proteins are absorbed in the newborn receiving *colostrum, but to a much lesser extent in adults. Carbohydrates are absorbed as simple sugars (monosaccharides), except in herbivores where fermentation in the large intestine produces volatile fatty acids, which are absorbed through the walls of the caecum and colon.

2. (in pharmacology) The process whereby drugs are transferred from the alimentary tract or site of injection/administration to the blood.

acanthosis Thickening of the epidermis of the skin as a result of increased cell division. It may result from natural causes, for example, at pressure points, or in chronic inflammation. Acanthotic skin feels thickened and roughened and is usually marked by hair loss. *See also* acanthosis nigricans.

acanthosis nigricans A skin disorder, particularly affecting areas where the skin is folded to allow for movement. The affected skin is black and much thickened with many fissures. The condition in humans may be associated with internal cancer, but this is not so in domestic animals. In dogs it may be associated with obesity or chronic irritation, although the cause cannot always be determined.

acapnia (hypocapnia) A condition in which the level of carbon dioxide in the blood is abnormally low. This is caused by hyperventilation, either voluntary overbreathing or, during anaesthesia, positive pressure ventilation under the control of the anaesthetist. The concentration of carbon dioxide in blood determines the rate of breathing by stimulating respiratory centres in the brain. Hence acapnia tends to suppress breathing.

acaricide An agent used to kill *mites and *ticks. Compounds active against mites include chlorinated hydrocarbons, organophosphorus compounds, pyrethroids, carbamates, rotenone, sulphur compounds, benzyl benzoate, and ivermectin. Protection against tick infestations requires a compound with persistent effects. Acaricidal compounds can be applied in dips, washes, sprays, powders,

pour-ons, or injected parenterally (*see* ivermectin).

acarid A member of the order Acarina (class *Arachnida), which comprises the tiny *mites and larger *ticks. Found worldwide in all habitats, they have an undivided globular body, four pairs of legs, and mouthparts variously modified for biting, sawing, piercing, and sucking. The eggs hatch into larvae with three pairs of legs, and these develop into sexually immature nymphs which resemble the adult. All ticks and some genera of mites are ectoparasites of livestock, poultry, pets, and humans, feeding on the blood and tissue fluids of their hosts. They are responsible for transmitting a large number of diseases.

accessory nerve The eleventh *cranial nerve (XI). It is formed by two roots, the cranial root from the brain and the spinal root from the cervical part of the spinal cord. The nerve divides just outside the skull into two branches. The internal branch joins the *vagus nerve, its fibres probably supplying the muscles of the larynx. The external branch supplies the brachiocephalic, sternocephalic, omotransversarius, and the trapezius muscles.

accommodation Adjustment of the shape of the lens to change the focus of the eye. When the ciliary muscle (*see* ciliary body) is relaxed, the zonular fibres attaching the ciliary processes to the lens are stretched, which causes the lens to be flattened. The eye is then able to focus on distant objects. To focus the eye on near objects the ciliary muscles contract and the tension in the ligaments is thus lowered, allowing the lens to become rounder. Contraction of the ciliary muscle is controlled by the parasympathetic nervous system.

accredited veterinarian (USA) A veterinarian practising in the USA who has been evaluated and approved by the Federal Government to be involved in the control and eradication of animal diseases.

acebutolol See beta blockers.

acepromazine See phenothiazines.

Acer poisoning See red maple poisoning.

acetabulum The cup-shaped socket of the hip joint that accommodates the head of the femur. It is formed from adjoining portions of the major bones of the pelvis – ilium, ischium, and pubis – and in the dog from the acetabular bone as well. Changes in the acetabulum occur in *hip dysplasia.

acetaminophen Paracetamol. *See* NSAID.

acetazolamide A *sulphonamide derivative that reduces the rate of formation of aqueous humour in the eye and is used occasionally in the treatment of *glaucoma to reduce intraocular pressure. It can be administered orally or injected intramuscularly, and causes an increase in urine volume and alkalinity with increased urinary sodium and potassium excretion. This results in metabolic *acidosis. Acetazolamide also reduces the rate of formation of cerebrospinal fluid and inhibits some epileptic seizures. It was also used as a diuretic but other drugs (e.g. *frusemide) are now preferred. The drug acts by inhibiting the enzyme carbonic anhydrase, which catalyses the dissociation of carbonic acid into carbon dioxide and water. The enzyme is active at many sites, including the kidney, eye, gastrointestinal tract, and central nervous system.

acetonaemia See ketosis.

acetone (propanone) A colourless flammable volatile compound. It is one of the *ketone bodies and is produced in animals with *ketosis. The sweet smell on the breath of highly ketotic individuals is caused by acetone, which sometimes also taints the milk of ketotic cows.

acetonuria See ketonuria.

acetylcholine The acetic acid ester of the organic base choline: the *neurotransmitter released at the synapses of parasympathetic nerves and at *neuromuscular junctions. After relaying a nerve impulse, acetylcholine is rapidly broken down by the enzyme *cholinesterase. *Parasympatholytic agents, such as *atropine, are *anticholinergic* – i.e. they prevent acetylcholine from functioning as a neurotransmitter. *Parasympathomimetic agents, such as *physostigmine, are *cholinergic* – i.e. they enhance or mimic the effects of acetylcholine. *See also* anticholinesterase.

acetylpromazine See phenothiazines.

acetylsalicylic acid Aspirin. *See* NSAID.

achalasia A condition in which smooth muscle fibres in the walls of the oesophagus fail to relax, thereby impeding the passage of food through the gut. Food is normally propelled by *peristalsis, which involves simultaneous contraction and relaxation of muscles in adjacent regions of the oesophagus. *Cricopharyngeal achalasia* in dogs is associated with failure of the cricopharyngeal muscle to relax and allow food to enter the upper oesophagus. Hence it causes difficulty in swallowing (dysphagia) and pharyngeal retching.

Achilles tendon

Achilles tendon *See* common calcaneal tendon.

achondroplasia An inherited condition in which affected individuals have short limbs and short wide heads. It is a form of *dwarfism due to defective development of cartilage (*see* chondrodysplasia), and has been reported in all species of domestic animal. It is the most economically important form of dwarfism in cattle; affected animals often have protruding lower jaws with the mandibular teeth extended 1–4 cm beyond the dental plate, resulting in grazing difficulties. The deformation of the bones of the head often causes obstruction of the respiratory tract, resulting in *dyspnoea. The condition seems to be chiefly *recessive, although *dominant forms have been described. Heterozygotes vary in their phenotype, many showing desirable 'beefy' characteristics, which has resulted in increased frequencies of the recessive allele. Detection of the heterozygote *carriers is imperative; endocrinological tests may be of use because of a possible link with *hypothyroidism. The best method of finding carriers is to mate them with known carriers of the gene. Similar recessive conditions have been reported in Telemark cattle in Norway; calves are stillborn or die soon after birth.

Achorion An obsolete genus of dermatophytic fungi; its species are now included in the genera *Trichophyton and *Microsporum.

acid A compound that yields hydrogen ions in solution and therefore has a *pH below 7. Acids are classified according to the number of displaceable hydrogens in each molecule and can be monobasic (one hydrogen), dibasic (two), or polybasic (more than two). *Strong acids* (e.g. sulphuric acid and hydrochloric acid) are almost completely dissociated in water,

whereas *weak acids* (e.g. acetic acid) are only partially dissociated. Acidic compounds are usually sour or sharp tasting. Strong acids are used as *disinfectants because of their ability to destroy microorganisms. However, when in contact with skin they cause burns. The acid should then be neutralized using a weak *alkali and the skin washed with copious amounts of water.

acidaemia A condition of abnormally high blood acidity. This may result from an increase in the concentation of acidic substances and/or a decrease in the level of alkaline substances in the blood. *See also* acidosis. *Compare* alkalaemia.

acid-base balance The regulation of the concentrations of acids and bases in blood and other body fluids so that the *pH remains within a physiologically acceptable range. This is achieved by the presence of natural *buffer systems, such as the bicarbonate and phosphate systems. These effectively mop up excess acids and bases and therefore prevent any large shifts in pH. The acid-base balance is also influenced by the selective removal of certain ions by the kidneys and the rate of removal of carbon dioxide from the lungs.

acid-fast Describing bacteria, spores, etc. which are not decolorized by acid after staining with dyes, for example carbol fuchsin and malachite green. This is due to the presence of a waxy coat to which the dye adheres tightly.

acidifying agent An agent used to increase the acidity of body fluids. *Urinary acidifiers* are used to decrease the pH of urine. These include ammonium chloride, sodium acid phosphate, ascorbic acid (vitamin C), methionine, and chlorethamine. Urinary acidification is used to improve the excretion of basic substances, enhance the activity of some antibiotics (e.g. penicillins), treat certain types of urinary calculi, and prevent the growth of some types of bacteria.

acidophilic 1. (in histology) Describing tissues, cells, or parts of cells that stain with acid dyes. **2.** (in bacteriology) Describing bacteria that grow well in acid media.

acidosis A condition in which the acidity of body fluids and tissues is abnormally great, i.e. when body *pH falls below the normal value of 7.4. A pH of below 7.0 is considered life threatening. There are two main types of acidosis. *Respiratory acidosis* occurs as a consequence of hypoventilation (decreased breathing), when carbon dioxide accumulates in the body as carbonic acid. *Metabolic acidosis* is caused by various changes in the body's metabolism. There may be depletion of electrolytes (salts), particularly bicarbonate ions, which act as a *buffer. This happens, for instance, in persistent diarrhoea. Altered carbohydrate metabolism, which occurs in *diabetes mellitus, produces an excess of organic acids. Disruption of the body's buffering mechanisms, which normally regulate acidity and are under the control of the kidney, may occur in cases of renal failure. Respiratory acidosis is treated by improving ventilation (breathing) to remove the excess carbon dioxide. Metabolic acidosis is corrected by administering bicarbonate. *Compare* alkalosis.

acinus (*pl.* **acini**) **1.** A small rounded saclike structure, lined by secretory cells, that lies at the end of the duct system of an exocrine gland. The term is sometimes used synonymously with *alveolus. **2.** (in the liver) The mass of liver tissue associated with the fine terminal branches of the portal vein, hepatic artery, and bile duct.

acne An infectious disease affecting the hair follicles of cats and dogs. Canine acne is most common in short-haired dogs, for example, boxers, bulldogs, and Doberman pinschers, usually between the ages of 3 months and 1 year, though it may persist throughout life. Feline acne occurs in adults and may persist throughout life. In both species, blackheads occur on the lips and chin – regions containing well developed *sebaceous glands. Papules, pustules, and itching (*pruritus) may develop subsequently with secondary bacterial infection. Poor hygiene contributes to the development of acne and affected areas should be kept clean and dry. Persistent cases may require antibiotic therapy. There is no evidence that the disease is comparable with human acne, which is caused by the effects of androgen hormones on the hair follicles and sebaceous glands. In horses, infection with *Corynebacterium pseudotuberculosis* in the areas of the harness contact is known as *contagious acne*. However, *Staphylococcus* species may also be isolated from the areas of folliculitis and furunculosis.

aconite poisoning A toxic condition arising from ingestion of monkshood, aconite, or wolfbane (*Aconitum napellus*), larkspur (*Delphinium* spp.), globe flower, columbine, or other plants containing aconitine or alkaloids with a similar action. The first clinical signs of poisoning are salivation, coughing, and laboured breathing. Incoordination is followed by convulsions and paralysis. Death occurs from respiratory paralysis. About 0.5 kg of monkshood is toxic for a horse and about 5 g for a dog. Affected animals should be removed from the plant source, kept warm, and given small doses of *physostigmine.

acoprosis Absence of faecal material within the intestine. This implies decreased food intake or gut stasis.

acorn poisoning A toxic condition caused by ingestion of acorns, the fruit of oak trees (*Quercus* spp.). The condition tends to occur in grazing cattle, horses, and sheep towards the end of hot dry summers when herbage is scarce but the acorn crop is prolific. In **cattle**, ingestion of acorns, particularly unripe ones, produces dullness, cessation of rumination, and constipation, which is followed in some instances by the onset of foul-smelling diarrhoea with blood-stained faeces. Toxic damage to the kidney interferes with the excretion of urea. In the **horse**, ingestion is followed by signs of flatulent *colic. Laparotomy reveals a stomach and small intestine distended by gas, and death is often due to gastric rupture. Horses and cattle should be given *liquid paraffin and a suspension of calcium hydroxide by stomach tube. The latter helps to neutralize the tannic acid (7–9% in acorns), which is believed to be the main cause of the toxicity. **Pigs** are able to eat considerable quantities of acorns with impunity. Ingestion of oak leaves and twigs will also cause toxicity.

acoustic Of or relating to sound or the sense of hearing.

acral lick dermatitis A raised thickened plaque seen on the limb of an adult dog usually just below the carpus or tarsus. The lesion apparently starts as an irritation, with prolonged licking and chewing resulting in chronic inflammation, which may extend over several square centimetres. The whole process may initially arise out of boredom. *See* dermatitis.

acriflavine A water-soluble acridine dye, bright orange in colour, that is used topically as an *antiseptic. Acriflavine maintains its activity in the presence of serum and thus is used for dressing burns and wounds. It is a *bacteriostat, with a fairly narrow spectrum of activity, mainly against Gram-positive organisms.

acro- *Prefix denoting* extremity; tip. Example: *acrohypothermy* (abnormal coldness of the extremities).

acrocentric A chromosome in which the *centromere is not situated centrally, being closer to one end.

acrochordon A small pedunculated tumour in the form of a skin tag, several millimetres in length, seen on the skin of old dogs, particularly on the trunk, axillae (armpits), and eyelids. They may be flesh-coloured, brown, or black, and can be removed surgically.

acromegaly A disease characterized by overgrowth of bone, connective tissue, and viscera, and caused by excessive secretion of *growth hormone after puberty has been reached; prior to puberty, excess growth hormone will cause gigantism. Chronic stimulation by *progestins will also result in acromegaly because of excess growth hormone release. Spontaneous acromegaly due to pituitary tumours has been reported, and it can result from tumours at any location in the body producing excess growth-hormone-releasing factor. *Somatomedin is also increased in animals with excessive growth hormone. The anti-insulin effects of growth hormone and somatomedin can cause secondary *diabetes mellitus. Therapy involves correcting the underlying cause.

acrosome The caplike structure on the front end of a spermatozoon. It breaks down just before fertilization, releasing a number of enzymes that assist penetration between the follicle cells and the *zona pellucida that surround the oocyte.

ACTH *See* adrenocorticotrophic hormone.

actin A protein, found in muscle, that plays an important role in the process of contraction (*see* striated muscle). Actin is also found within cells, as part of the cytoskeleton.

actinobacillosis (wooden tongue) A disease of cattle and, rarely, sheep characterized by hard swellings in the soft tissues of the head and neck and caused by the Gram-negative bacterium *Actinobacillus lignieresi*. The disease is sporadic but widely distributed. Infection enters via damage to the mucous membranes of the mouth, and affects chiefly the muzzle, lips, gums, hard and soft palates, and lymph nodes. The swelling is not normally painful, but may put pressure on neighbouring nerves or blood vessels and can result in respiratory embarrassment by obstructing the trachea. The tongue is affected in a small percentage of cases, causing its eventual hardening, thickening, and protrusion so that feeding is impaired. As the swelling increases in size its core is replaced with thick creamy or greyish pus, which eventually discharges to the exterior if the abscess is superficial. Other organs may be affected, e.g. oesophagus, liver, and stomachs. Treatment is with *streptomycin and organic *iodides. *See also* actinomycosis.

Actinobacillus A genus of nonmotile pleomorphic Gram-negative *bacteria distributed worldwide. Four species are known to cause diseases in domestic animals: *A. lignieresi* is a normal commensal of the mouth and rumen in sheep and cattle, but following abrasions and injury it causes multiple abscesses, usually in the neck, tongue, pharynx, and other soft tissues. The frequently diagnosed form of the disease is wooden tongue (*see* actinobacillosis). *A. equuli* causes septicaemia, kidney abscesses (*see* sleepy foal disease), and *joint-ill in young foals; *A. suis* causes *septicaemia and death in piglets; and *A. salpingitis* causes *salpingitis in fowls.

Actinomyces A genus of filamentous nonmotile anaerobic Gram-positive *bacteria. The organisms are strict parasites of the mouth and pharynx and cause disease when they gain entry to body tissue. *A. bovis* causes *actinomycosis, or lumpy jaw, which affects the jaw bones in cattle. It may also infect the mammary glands of pigs and some organs of dogs and cats. *A. israeli* causes human actinomycosis.

actinomycin Any of a group of polypeptide antibiotics produced by *Streptomyces bacteria. Actinomycins bind to double-helical DNA preventing transcription of DNA by RNA polymerases. This leads to inhibition of rapidly proliferating cells, and some members of the group, for example dactinomycin and cactinomycin, are potent antitumour agents. Both normal and neoplastic cell proliferation are affected and toxic side-effects of bone marrow suppression and gastric ulceration are commonly found. Actinomycins are administered by intravenous injection.

actinomycosis (lumpy jaw) A disease of cattle, dogs, pigs, and humans characterized by chronic *granulomatous lesions and caused by the Gram-positive bacterium *Actinomyces bovis* or related species (*A. viscosus* in dogs, *A. israeli* in man, and others). *A. bovis* is widespread and may be found in the mouths of healthy cattle. It penetrates the mucous membrane through minor abrasions or tooth cavities and enters the jaw bones or *turbinates. The infected bone becomes enlarged and honeycombed, typically seen as a painless hard swelling on the side of the jaw level with the molar teeth. A *sinus (fistula) may develop through which pus is discharged into the mouth or to the exterior. The yellowish pus within the swelling contains very small hard yellow 'sulphur granules'; these are the bacterial colonies. The bones of the face can be seriously distorted over a period of months or years and this eventually interferes with feeding. In dogs the organisms affect the soft tissues, and in pigs the mammary glands are affected. Treatment with organic *iodides, *penicillin, and radiotherapy has been attempted, usually without long-term success. *See also* actinobacillosis.

action potential The change in voltage that occurs across the membrane of a nerve or muscle cell when a *nerve impulse is triggered. It is due to the passage of charged particles across the membrane (*see* depolarization) and is an observable manifestation of the passage of an impulse.

active site The area on the surface of an *enzyme molecule to which the substrate(s) bind and where catalysis occurs.

active transport (in biochemistry) An energy-dependent process in which certain substances (including ions, some drugs, glucose, and amino acids) are able to cross cell membranes against a concentration gradient.

actomyosin A protein complex formed in muscle between actin and myosin during the process of contraction. *See* striated muscle.

Acuaria A genus of parasitic *nematodes containing *A. uncinata*, which is found in the oesophagus, gizzard, small intestine, and proventriculus of ducks, geese, swans, and other aquatic birds. The adults attach to the mucous membrane and form caseous nodules, which may obstruct the digestive tract. Affected birds become listless and emaciated and there is a high mortality. The intermediate host is the water flea, *Daphnia pulex*, eradication of which is probably the best current method of control.

acupuncture A traditional Chinese therapy in which thin metal needles are inserted into selected points in the skin. The needles are stimulated by rotation or by an electric current. Hypotheses suggest that this activates sensory nerves, causing the release from the pituitary and hypothalamus of *endorphins – the body's natural painkillers. More recently, similar effects have been obtained using a hand-held electrical acupuncture unit. This bears a short probe which delivers a small electric current without penetrating the skin. Acupuncture is used widely in the Far East for the relief of pain, both in human and veterinary medicine. Some veterinary practitioners in the West are now exploring its potential, particularly for pain relief following orthopaedic surgery.

acute 1. Describing a disease of rapid onset, severe signs, and brief duration. *Compare* chronic. **2.** Describing any intense sign, such as severe pain.

acute death syndrome (flip-over syndrome) A condition of growing broilers characterized by the occurrence of sudden fatal heart attacks. It is typically seen in the fastest growing birds not long before slaughter. Mortality can reach 0.5% and no definite cause has been established. It is often found along with *fatty liver/kidney syndrome, and an imbalance in the levels of potassium, sodium, and chloride has been suggested. However, current thinking suggests that the condition is closely linked with broiler *ascites, and is caused by heart abnormalities due to the high oxygen demand of modern strains of fast-growing broilers.

acute respiratory distress syndrome (ARDS) A condition of severe usually fatal respiratory embarrassment resulting from any acute disease of the lungs, such as viral and/or bacterial *pneumonia, *endotoxaemia and associated shock syndromes, aspiration pneumonia, chemical or drug toxicity (e.g. *paraquat poisoning), *disseminated intravascular coagulation, or *uraemia. Membranous deposits of *hyaline are characteristically found lining the alveoli and airways.

acyclovir An antiviral drug with activity against herpesviruses. It is a synthetic purine nucleoside, similar to guanosine; in infected cells it is converted to the triphosphate form, which is incorporated into viral DNA causing termination of DNA strand synthesis. Acyclovir is available in topical ointments, as an intravenous injection, and for oral administration. *Deoxyacyclovir*, a *prodrug, is also available for oral administration and is absorbed better than acyclovir from the gastrointestinal tract. Acyclovir has been used in the treatment of herpesvirus infections in animals, but it is expensive and frequent dosing is required. Toxicity with topical acyclovir is rare, but after intravenous infusion there may be renal toxicity, local phlebitis, and vomiting.

ad- *Prefix denoting* towards or near. Examples: *adaxial* (towards the main axis); *adoral* (towards or near the mouth).

adamantinoma *See* ameloblastoma.

Addison's disease *See* hypoadrenocorticism.

adduct To move part of the body towards the midline of the body or to move the digits towards the midline of the limb. *Compare* abduct.

adductor Any muscle that performs adduction (*see* adduct).

adductor muscles A large mass of muscles on the medial (inner) side of the thigh. Three muscles may occur – *adductor longus*, *adductor brevis*, and *adductor magnus*. They act to adduct the hip joint.

aden- (adeno-) *Prefix denoting* a gland or glands. Examples: *adenogenesis* (development of); *adenopathy* (disease of).

adenine One of the nitrogen-containing bases (*see* purine) that occurs in the nucleic acids DNA and RNA. *See also* ATP.

adenitis *Inflammation of a gland. The type of gland is denoted by the prefix. For example, *sialadenitis* is inflammation of a salivary gland; *lymphadenitis* is inflammation of a lymph gland. The cause is usually infection, often bacterial, in which case treatment with antibiotics will either kill the bacteria or prevent further multiplication.

adenocarcinoma *See* carcinoma.

adenohypophysis (*pl.* **adenohypophyses**) The anterior part of the *pituitary gland, consisting of the pars tuberalis, pars intermedia, and pars distalis.

adenoma A benign epithelial tumour derived from or showing some similarity to glandular tissue and often retaining some secretory function. Common examples in animals are polyps of the gastrointestinal tract, sebaceous adenomas of the skin, and adenomas of the endocrine glands, such as pituitary and thyroid adenomas. Varieties include *fibroadenomas*, where there is proliferation of connective tissue in addition to the glandular changes (seen in the mammary gland), and *cystadenomas*, where cells form secretory acini without excretory ducts resulting in the accumulation of secretion and the development of large cystic spaces.

Adenomas are generally slow-growing and well circumscribed. They do not infiltrate or metastasize but cause adjacent normal tissues to atrophy due to pressure and may replace essential tissue. Secretory endocrine adenomas can cause considerable clinical disturbance due to excess production of hormone, which is not subject to the normal feedback control. For example Cushing's syndrome (*see* hyperadrenocorticism) in dogs may be caused by increased production of ACTH due to a pituitary adenoma, and feminization may occur due to oestrogen secretion by Sertoli cell adenomas. Adenomas are amenable to surgical removal although in certain sites, such as the pituitary gland, the task will be difficult, if not impossible.

adenomatosis A proliferation of glandular tissue. The most significant conditions are *porcine intestinal adenomatosis* affecting pigs and occasionally other species and *pulmonary adenomatosis in sheep, a virus disease otherwise known as *jaagsiekte*. The porcine condition is caused by the bacterium *Campylobacter sputorum* subsp. *mucosalis*. This organism is found within cells lining the lower small intestine. It produces thickening of the bowel wall mucosa, seen post mortem as having a ridged appearance with haemorrhages on the crests of the folds. The disease affects young growing pigs, causing inappetence and

decreased weight gain. The condition can progress to necrotic *enteritis, regional *ileitis, or *haemorrhagic bowel syndrome – all involving other tissues in the small intestine. A proportion of affected animals recover spontaneously.

adenosine A molecule containing adenine and the sugar ribose: it occurs in ATP. *See also* nucleoside.

adenosine diphosphate (ADP) *See* ATP.

adenosine monophosphate *See* AMP.

adenosine triphosphate *See* ATP.

adenovirus A family of DNA *viruses that infect most animal species, usually causing relatively mild respiratory signs, although one member causes *canine viral hepatitis. They have a naked icosahedral *capsid with characteristic fibres projecting from the corners. Some are capable of transforming cells in culture (*see* oncogenic virus).

adenovirus infection (in layers) *See* egg-drop syndrome.

ADH *See* antidiuretic hormone.

adhesion The union of two normally separate surfaces by the development of fibrous connective tissue. They occur particularly in body cavities with membranous linings, such as the pleural and pericardial cavities of the chest, the abdomen, joint cavities, and the cranial cavity. Adhesions develop during the course of inflammatory disease. The normally smooth membrane becomes roughened and sticky. Flimsy fibrinous connections in the initial stages are replaced by tough fibrous tissue. Adhesions may interfere with organ function, for instance lung expansion during breathing or emptying and filling of the heart.

adipose tissue *Connective tissue packed with fat cells. It forms a variably thick layer under the skin and also occurs around the kidneys. It serves both as an insulating layer and as an energy store; food in excess of requirements is converted into fats and stored within these cells. Following castration or spaying animals have an increased tendency to deposit fat.

ad lib (ad libitum) The feeding of animals freely and continuously in accordance with their desires. Under ideal conditions, the amount consumed by animals fed ad lib will represent their *voluntary food intake. In practice ad lib feeding is often difficult to achieve because of restrictions to intake imposed by feeder design, competition for available feeder space, and general management practices. Ad lib feeding systems require less labour and are employed especially for rapidly growing stock where overconsumption of nutrients is unlikely. However, where excessive feed intake is possible ad lib systems lead to nutrient wastage (e.g. in gestating sows) or over-fat carcasses (e.g. in finishing pigs); feed intake is restricted in such cases.

ADP (adenosine diphosphate) *See* ATP.

adrenal cortical (adrenocortical) tumours Tumours affecting the cortex of the *adrenal gland. *Adrenocortical adenomas* are seen occasionally in older dogs and very rarely in horses, cattle, and sheep. They are often an incidental finding at post-mortem examination and are usually small brownish-yellow well-demarcated slow-growing tumours affecting only one of the two glands. Large adenomas up to several centimetres in

diameter may replace a large part of an affected gland. Some secrete cortisol, which causes atrophy of the other adrenal gland and, in the dog, leads to Cushing's syndrome (*see* hyperadrenocorticism).
Cortical carcinomas occur less frequently than adenomas and are seen especially in older dogs, and also in cattle. They are generally larger, yellow-red, and extensively invade surrounding tissues, including the vena cava and aorta, resulting in intra-abdominal haemorrhage and metastases to distant sites. They often affect both glands. Removal of the affected gland is feasible for cortical adenomas but carcinomas, because of their invasive nature, are difficult to remove and may already have metastasized at diagnosis.

adrenal glands (suprarenal glands) Paired endocrine glands, each of which is located adjacent (usually cranial and medial) to a kidney and contains four distinct zones – the *zona glomerulosa*, *zona fasciculata*, and *zona reticularis* of the cortex, and the inner medulla. The cortical zones all produce steroid hormones: the outer zona glomerulosa produces mineralocorticoids, such as *aldosterone, in response to angiotensin II. The zona fasciculata and zona reticularis produce glucocorticoids in response to adrenocorticotrophic hormone (*see* corticosteroid). In addition some sex hormones are secreted in low concentrations from the cortex. *Chromaffin cells of the medulla secrete the hormones *adrenaline and *noradrenaline in response to stimulation by the sympathetic nervous system. The adrenal glands have the capability of producing any naturally occurring steroid, and adrenal tumours can give rise to a wide variety of clinical signs – including Cushing's disease, masculinization of females, and feminization of males –

adrenaline

depending on the hormone(s) produced by the tumour.

adrenaline (epinephrine) A *catecholamine hormone secreted by chromaffin cells in the medulla of the adrenal gland. It also occurs in small quantities at sympathetic nerve endings, where it functions as a neurotransmitter (although the principal sympathetic neurotransmitter in the peripheral nervous system is the related substance *noradrenaline). Adrenaline is released from the adrenal gland into the bloodstream in response to sympathetic stimulation in excitement or stress to prepare the body for 'fright, flight, or fight', and has wide-ranging physiological effects. These include: increased heart rate and blood pressure; vasoconstriction of arterioles in the skin, mucous membranes, and abdominal organs; vasodilatation of arterioles in skeletal muscle and heart; relaxation of bronchioles in the lungs; inhibition of gastrointestinal secretion and motility; and dilatation of the pupil of the eye. Adrenaline also raises blood sugar levels by, for example, stimulating the breakdown of liver glycogen stores.
Adrenaline is used therapeutically in various situations. Being poorly absorbed from the gastrointestinal tract it is administered by intravenous or intramuscular injection, and has a very short duration of action (1–2 minutes). It is used to treat anaphylactic reactions, reducing the bronchoconstriction and counteracting the drop in blood pressure brought about by histamine release. It can also be injected into the heart after cardiac arrest to try to initiate a heartbeat. Adrenaline should not be used in animals anaesthetized with halothane or cyclopropane anaesthesia because these agents sensitize the heart to catecholamines and adrenaline can induce ventricular fibrillation. Adrenaline can be used locally as a *haemostatic and to cause vasocon-

striction in an area prior to surgery to reduce the risk of haemorrhage. In local anaesthetic solutions adrenaline may be incorporated to prolong their action.

adrenergic Describing nerve fibres that release *noradrenaline as a neurotransmitter. *Compare* cholinergic.

adrenoceptor agonist An agent that acts at *adrenergic receptors in the sympathetic nervous system. These include the catecholamines *adrenaline, *noradrenaline, and isoprenaline. Adrenaline acts at alpha (α) and beta (β) receptors, noradrenaline at α and β_1 receptors, and isoprenaline at β receptors. In veterinary therapy the most important such agents are those that act on the β_2 receptors in the smooth muscle of the bronchi, uterus, and skeletal muscle vasculature, for example *clenbuterol.

adrenoceptor antagonist An agent that blocks the action of adrenaline or noradrenaline at *adrenergic receptors in the sympathetic nervous system. Drugs are available with specific actions at α_1 and α_2 receptors or at β_1 and β_2 receptors (*see* alpha blocker; beta blocker).

adrenocorticotrophic hormone (ACTH; corticotrophin) A protein hormone, synthesized and stored in the adenohypophysis of the pituitary gland, that stimulates the adrenal gland to produce glucocorticoid hormones (*see* corticosteroid). The release of ACTH is controlled by ACTH-releasing hormone (ACTHRH or CRH), produced by the hypothalamus; glucocorticoids act on the hypothalamus and pituitary gland to decrease ACTHRH and ACTH production. However, stressors, such as fear, pain, and toxins, can override the negative feedback to cause increased ACTH release and glucocorticoid concentrations in the plasma.

adsorbent 1. An agent that can adsorb material onto its surface. Adsorbents are used in attempts to inactivate bacterial toxins in the gastrointestinal tract, draw debris and secretions from wounds, and prevent or impede the absorption of poisons from the digestive tract. For example, activated charcoal, *kaolin, or bismuth are adsorbents that may be administered to treat poisoning. **2.** Describing such an agent.

adventitia (tunica adventitia) 1. The outer, loose connective tissue covering of organs not covered by serous membrane. **2.** The outer coat of the wall of blood vessels, consisting of connective tissue and, in larger vessels, containing small blood vessels (*vasa vasorum) for the supply of the wall.

adventitious 1. Occurring in a place other than the usual one. **2.** Relating to the adventitia.

-aemia (*US* **-emia**) *Suffix denoting* a specified condition of the blood. Example: *hyperglycaemia* (excess sugar in the blood).

aer- (aero-) *Prefix denoting* air or gas. Examples: *aerogastria* (gas in the stomach); *aerogenesis* (production of gas).

aerobe Any organism, especially a microorganism, that requires the presence of free oxygen for life and growth. *See also* anaerobe; microaerophilic.

aerobic 1. Of or relating to *aerobes: requiring free oxygen for life and growth. **2.** Describing a type of cellular *respiration in which foodstuffs are completely oxidized by atmospheric oxygen, thereby yielding the maximum amount of chemical energy. **3.** Describing any reaction that requires oxygen.

aerosol A suspension of very small liquid or solid particles in a gas – usually air or oxygen. Drugs can be dispersed in a fine mist over a large area in aerosol form, and some antibiotics are available in aerosol cans for topical use. Using a *nebulizer*, liquid can be made into a fine spray; nebulization is used to produce a drug-containing aerosol for inhalation in the treatment of lung conditions.

aestivation A state of inactivity occurring in some animals, notably lungfish, during prolonged periods of drought or heat. Feeding, respiration, movement, and other bodily activities are all considerably slowed down.

aetiology (etiology) 1. The study or science of the causes of disease. **2.** The cause of a specific disease.

afferent 1. Designating neurones or nerves that convey impulses from sense organs and other receptors towards the central nervous system, i.e. sensory neurones or nerves. **2.** Designating blood vessels that convey blood towards a capillary network, e.g. afferent arterioles of a glomerulus in the kidney. **3.** Designating lymphatic vessels that convey lymph towards a lymph node. *Compare* efferent.

aflatoxicosis A toxic condition arising from the ingestion of aflatoxins, metabolites of the fungi *Aspergillus flavus* and *A. parasiticus*. Animal diets may contain aflatoxins when crops, particularly groundnuts (peanuts), cotton seed, and maize (corn), are contaminated with *A. flavus* and stored in damp warm conditions, which encourage fungal growth. Young pigs, calves, ducklings, turkey poults, fish,

15

African horse sickness

and guinea pigs are most susceptible; sheep and horses among the most resistant. The nature and severity of clinical signs are related to the amount of aflatoxins consumed, but a constant post-mortem finding is the presence of liver lesions – cellular necrosis, fibrosis, and bile duct proliferation resembling the condition produced in *ragwort poisoning. In guinea pigs aflatoxin produces exudative hepatitis, and in rats and ducklings, liver tumours are found. Prevention requires careful monitoring of feedstuffs to ensure that animal rations are free of aflatoxins. *See also* turkey X disease.

African horse sickness A noncontagious disease of horses and other equines characterized by fever, swelling of the head, and respiratory distress. It is caused by *orbiviruses, which are transmitted by midges and mosquitoes, hence outbreaks tend to be seasonal. The disease is endemic in Africa south of the Sahara, but periodically spreads into North Africa, southern Europe, the Middle East, and India. Following an incubation period of 4–9 days acute cases show a fever of over 41°C and death may occur within 12 hours due to the accumulation of fluid in the lungs. In less severe cases the fever is maintained at 40°C and there is a variable degree of swelling of the tissues of the head and sometimes the chest. Horses imported into the enzootic area are most susceptible, and mortality may exceed 90%, while indigenous horses may show only mild clinical signs. Mules, donkeys, and zebra are susceptible but develop few clinical signs. Control is by annual vaccination with a live polyvalent attenuated vaccine consisting of a mixture of the nine immunologically distinct types of orbivirus that cause the disease, backed up by control of the insect vectors. The virus has been isolated from dogs, which may act as reservoir

hosts for the disease. In the UK and elsewhere in the West African horse sickness is a *notifiable disease.

African swine fever (ASF) A peracute, acute, subacute, or chronic disease of pigs, characterized by fever, haemorrhages in the skin and lymphoid tissue, and death. The causal virus is a double-stranded DNA virus and was originally classified in the iridovirus family. However, it appears now to have more affinity with the *poxviruses. ASF is endemic in most of Africa south of the Sahara, where it is transmitted between wart hogs and soft ticks (*Ornithodoros moubata), which inhabit the wart hog burrows. Disease is seen in domestic pigs when the virus is transmitted directly by the bite of an infected tick, or when pigs are fed on food infected with ASF virus or come into contact with fomites (*see* fomes) contaminated with virus. ASF can be transmitted directly between domestic or feral pigs without an intermediate host. Following an incubation period (sometimes as short as 3–4 days) the animal develops fever (up to 42°C) accompanied by loss of appetite and incoordination. Death usually occurs 7–10 days later. Haemorrhages may be seen in the skin, particularly on the ears and ventral abdomen; coughing, diarrhoea, vomiting, and nasal and eye discharges may develop. The virus is present in all body fluids and discharges.

ASF has been enzootic in Spain and Portugal since 1960 and in Sardinia since 1978, infecting the Iberian species of soft tick, *O. erraticus*. The clinical signs caused by European strains of the virus are not as acute and mortality may be less than 50%. Pigs continue to transmit infection to susceptible pigs up to 1 month after recovery, and their meat can remain infectious for up to 4 months. Moreover, recovered pigs subjected to stress may start to re-excrete ASF virus. The antibodies produced by ASF-infected pigs are not neutralizing, thus making the development of a conventional vaccine against ASF unlikely. The only effective method of control is by slaughter of all infected and in-contact pigs, movement controls, and regulations prohibiting the feeding of uncooked swill to domestic pigs, particularly waste food collected from international airports or docks. ASF is a notifiable disease in the UK.

afterbirth The placenta, umbilical cord, and foetal membranes, colloquially known as 'cleansing', that are expelled following birth of the foetus. In species normally giving birth to two or more young, the afterbirths are shed following the delivery of individual foetuses.

agalactia A decrease in or absence of mammary secretion. The cause may be hereditary, infectious, hormonal, stress-related, or a combination of these factors. In many cases the cause is unknown. Agalactia is an important sign of *MMA (mastitis-metritis-agalactia) syndrome in sows. *See also* contagious agalactia; lactation.

agar A gelatinous *polysaccharide prepared from seaweeds of the genus *Gelidium* and used extensively in bacteriology as the solidifying base for culture media. The agar is supplemented with various constituents to make specific media for isolation and culture of various microorganisms. Agar can also be used orally for the treatment of constipation (e.g. sodium chromoglycate).

agar-gel immunodiffusion test A test used for identifying antigens or antibodies, particularly in blood serum. Small wells are cut into agar or agarose gel solidified onto a glass or plastic surface. Serum is placed in one well and diseased tissue or specif-

ically prepared virus or bacterial culture is placed in an adjacent well. The soluble antibodies and antigens diffuse in all directions through the gel. Where they meet, an insoluble precipitate may form between the two wells. Alternatively, either antigen or antibody can be incorporated in the gel and the test reagent placed in a well. As the test reagent diffuses away from the well a ring of precipitate is formed around the well. The line may be emphasized by staining with specific protein stains, such as Coomassie Blue. The test may be used to identify antigens by using specific antibodies or vice versa. It is particularly useful in the identification of animals that have been infected with certain viral diseases and consequently have antibodies to those viral antigens. Routine diagnosis of *bluetongue, *pox disease, and *rinderpest is performed using this test. The version employed in diagnosing *equine infectious anaemia is known as the Coggins test.

agenesis Absence of an organ, usually due to total failure of its development in the embryo.

agglutination The clumping of particles in liquid suspension. Agglutination may affect many kinds of biological particles, including bacteria and cells. *Antibodies can act as *agglutinins to bring about agglutination by binding specifically to suspended particles, which function as *antigens. Since antibody molecules have two binding sites, they are able to form bridges between the particles; if the concentrations of particle and antibody are equivalent, the agglutination process proceeds to the formation of a lattice in which the particles are bound by the antibody into regular three-dimensional arrangements. In vitro, this form of agglutination may be visible to the naked eye. Agglutination provides a method for the detection and estimation of antibody or antigen. For example, sera containing different known agglutinins can enable the identification of unknown bacteria. *See also* precipitation.

agglutinin Any *antibody capable of bringing about *agglutination.

agglutinogen Any *antigen that elicits in vivo the formation of *agglutinins.

aggressiveness A character trait that produces confrontational behaviour with other animals (of the same or of different species), with inanimate objects, or with humans. This trait is sometimes seen in particular breeds, or lines within a breed. It may be selected for in particular animals, for example in guard dogs. Within domestic situations a breakdown in the human–animal relationship may occur, with the animal seeking to dominate the owner.

aglossia An inherited condition in which the tongue is absent. A less severe form is *microglossia*, in which the tongue is much reduced in size. Aglossia is often associated with *agnathia or related conditions, and with *synotia. The condition is invariably lethal and is reported in all domestic animals.

agnathia A *recessive inherited disorder in which there is complete absence of the jaw. In some cases there may be rudimentary jaw bones and teeth. Related conditions are those involving an abnormally small jaw (*micrognathia*) or an abnormally short jaw (*brachygnathia*). Agnathia is lethal, with most affected animals being stillborn or dying soon after birth. It is seen in most species of domestic animals, and is often associated with *aglossia or microglossia.

air sacculitis Inflammation of the air sacs of birds. It may occur as part of various infectious respiratory diseases in poultry. The thin clear glistening walls of the air sacs become cloudy, opaque, and yellow. Later the sacs become filled with a caseous thick yellow pus, often in association with *E. coli* or mycoplasma infections.

air sacs The series of thin-walled sacs in the avian respiratory system. They communicate with parts of the bronchial system and are important in creating a continuous circulation of air through the *parabronchi of the lungs. They also give rise to extensions that invade parts of the skeleton producing pneumatization of the bones. In the domestic fowl the following sacs are present: *cervical* (single); *clavicular* (single); *cranial* and *caudal thoracics*; and *abdominal* (all paired).

akabane An insect-borne disease of cattle, sheep, and goats characterized by congenital deformities in their offspring and caused by a *bunyavirus. The disease is subclinical in young and adult animals but causes developmental abnormalities in the foetus if infection occurs during the last part of the first trimester of pregnancy (76–96 days gestation in cattle; 30–36 days gestation in sheep). Consequently, the disease is not seen in countries or areas where the virus is enzootic since all animals are infected before reaching reproductive age. However, on the fringes of an enzootic area, infection can sporadically spread into susceptible animals causing enzootics of congenital deformities of newborn animals. Akabane is enzootic in Africa, India, the tropical Far East, and northern Australia. A vaccine is being used in Japan to control the disease, but it has proved difficult to establish when best to attempt control measures.

alanine *See* amino acid.

albendazole *See* benzimidazoles.

albendazole sulphoxide *See* benzimidazoles.

albinism Absence of the body pigment *melanin, due to a defective or missing enzyme in the pigment's synthetic pathway. It is normally a *recessive autosomal inherited condition, and affected individuals are known as *albinos*. In turkeys it is associated with blindness, in dogs (and often cats) there is associated deafness, and in many species there is *photosensitization.

albino *See* albinism.

albumin (albumen) One of a group of globular proteins that are soluble in water but form insoluble coagulates when heated. *Serum albumins* constitute a class of blood plasma proteins, with functions including the binding of *fatty acids, *bilirubin, and some *hormones. They also help determine the osmotic pressure of blood and hence plasma volume. Depletion of albumins, for example in starvation, results in excessive water in the tissues (*oedema). Other albumins are found in *milk (lactalbumin), eggs (ovalbumin), etc., but these are not related to serum albumins.

albuminuria *See* proteinuria.

alcohol Any organic compound containing a hydroxyl (-OH) group, such as methyl alcohol (methanol), CH_3OH, and ethyl alcohol (ethanol), C_2H_5OH. The latter is the alcohol in alcoholic drinks and is produced by the fermentation of sugars and other carbohydrates by yeasts. 'Pure' alcohol contains not less than 94.9% by volume of ethyl alcohol and is obtained by distillation. Alcohols (in solution) are used externally on the skin as antiseptics and to remove oils and fats which are insoluble in water. They are also used to disinfect instruments and skin prior to surgery or injections.

Alcohol poisoning Alcohol may be ingested if an animal eats fermented vegetable material. It is rapidly absorbed into the bloodstream and metabolized in the tissues with very little excreted unchanged in urine. It causes blood vessels supplying the skin to dilate, which may lead to heat loss. But the main effect is depression of the central nervous system, manifested as reduced sensory perception, muscular incoordination, and, in severe cases, coma, respiratory paralysis, and death. Treatment can involve the use of stimulants, such as caffeine. Alcohol is metabolized fairly rapidly and animals usually recover within 24 hours.

aldosterone A steroid hormone, secreted by the zona glomerulosa of the *adrenal gland, that acts on the kidneys to regulate salt and water balance. It is the major mineralocorticoid hormone (*see* corticosteroid). Aldosterone is secreted in response to the hormone *angiotensin II, and acts on the distal renal tubules to promote sodium absorption, with consequent fluid retention.

Aleutian disease A disease of mink caused by a *parvovirus and characterized by loss of appetite, persistent diarrhoea, and wasting. Certain mink strains, bred for particular pelt colours, are unable to eliminate the Aleutian disease virus, resulting in chronic infection. The immune system of the infected mink nevertheless attempts to control the disease by producing high levels of ineffective antibody. The immune complexes which develop in the circulating blood cause severe and irreversible damage to the kidneys. Death occurs after a few months. Infected animals showing symptoms of the disease excrete large quantities of virus, and transmission occurs by contact with the virus in the environment or in utero from the mother. There is no vaccine available to date.

alexin An old term for *complement.

algal poisoning See blue-green alga poisoning.

-algia Suffix denoting pain. Example: neuralgia (pain in a nerve).

alimentary toxaemia See toxic fat syndrome.

alimentary tract The hollow, often tubular, organs of the digestive system extending from lips to anus. It is concerned with the intake and storage of food (ingestion), the breakdown and absorption of food (digestion), and the removal of waste products (egestion or defecation). The principal organs are the mouth, *pharynx, *oesophagus, *stomach, small intestine (*duodenum, *jejunum, and *ileum), large intestine (*caecum and ascending, transverse, and descending *colons), and the *rectum. Carnivores, such as dogs, have this basic arrangement (see intestine). Ruminants, such as the ox, sheep, and goat, have a highly specialized compartmented stomach consisting of *reticulum, *rumen, *omasum, and *abomasum. The reticulum and rumen allow storage of food material prior to its regurgitation and remastication, i.e. 'chewing the cud'. Additionally, breakdown of food material occurs in the rumen by microbial fermentation. Ruminants, other herbivorous species, for example the horse, and omnivores, such as the pig, also have specialization within the large intestine to promote the microbial breakdown of plant cellulose in their diet. In the horse, the caecum leads to the ascending colon (large colon), which

has the form of a long bent U-shaped loop. This connects via the transverse colon to an elongated descending colon (small colon), which continues as the rectum. In the ox, sheep, goat, and pig the caecum passes into a coiled ascending colon – the *spiral loop – continuous with the transverse colon.

In birds the lips, cheeks, and teeth are replaced by a horny beak. The oesophagus may have an enlargement, the *crop, which enables food storage. The stomach consists of two parts, the *proventriculus or glandular part, which produces digestive juices, and the *ventriculus (muscular part or gizzard), which has a mechanical grinding function. This leads to the small intestine. In some species, including the domestic fowl, the large intestine may have paired caeca, whereas in other species the caecum may be single or even absent, as in the budgerigar. The remainder of the large intestine constitutes the rectum, and this terminates by uniting with the urogenital tract in the *cloaca.

alkalaemia Abnormally high blood alkalinity. This may be caused by an increase in the concentration of alkaline substances and/or a decrease in that of acidic substances in the blood. See also alkalosis. Compare acidaemia.

alkali A compound that reacts with an acid to form water and a salt. Alkalis are generally hydroxides, carbonates, or bicarbonates of an alkali metal, and dissolve to give solutions with a high pH. Strong alkalis are used as disinfectants and can be combined with halogens, such as chlorine as in Chloros. They are often used for the disinfection of premises after a major disease outbreak. Caustic alkalis, such as sodium hydroxide, are occasionally used to erode warts or tumours. *Sodium bicarbonate is a weak alkali that is used as an alkalizing agent, for example to counteract acidosis in cases of grain poisoning, scours, and diabetes mellitus.

alkali disease *See* Astragalus poisoning.

alkalinizing agent (alkalizing agent) A compound used to increase alkalinity. Such agents are used to decrease acidity in the stomach or increase urinary pH, and include sodium bicarbonate and soluble citrates, acetates, or lactates.

alkaloid Any nitrogen-containing organic base obtained from plants. The names of alkaloids end in *-ine*. Many are poisonous but others are used therapeutically, for example *morphine, caffeine (*see* xanthine), quinidine, nicotine, *atropine, *physostigmine, and *pilocarpine.

alkalosis A condition in which the alkalinity of body fluids and tissues is abnormally high. This arises because of a failure of the mechanisms that usually maintain a balance between alkalis and acids in the blood (*see* acid-base balance). Alkalosis may be associated with loss of acid through vomiting or with excessive sodium bicarbonate administration.

allantois (*pl.* **allantoides**) One of the *foetal membranes. It develops as an outgrowth of the embryonic hindgut and progressively enlarges as it accumulates the foetal urine, resulting in its apposition to and fusion with the *chorion. Its outer (mesodermal) layer contains blood vessels, which run via the umbilical cord to the *placenta.

allele (allelomorph) One of two or more alternative forms of a *gene, only one of which can be present in a chromosome. Two alleles of a particular gene occupy the same relative positions on a pair of *homologous chromosomes. If the two alleles are

the same, the individual is *homozygous for the gene; if they are different it is *heterozygous. *See also* dominant.

allelomorph *See* allele.

allergen Any antigen capable of inducing *allergy.

allergic alveolitis (extrinsic allergic alveolitis) Inflammation of the alveoli of the lungs caused by *hypersensitivity to inhaled organic dusts. A common example is *bovine farmer's lung* in cattle, due to repeated exposure to dust from mouldy hay; the commonest sensitizing component is spores of the thermophilic actinomycete *Micropolyspora faeni*. (The corresponding condition in humans is called *farmer's lung.*) Sensitization may require several winters' exposure, clinical signs then appearing in older cattle when subsequently exposed to the dust. Onset may be rapid, with a substantial drop in milk yield, laboured breathing, and reduced appetite; or insidious, with coughing cows progressively losing weight and yield while remaining alert with a normal temperature. Affected animals usually show dermal hypersensitivity and circulating precipitating antibody reactions to antigens of *M. faeni*, but these are not diagnostic in themselves. There is an influx of inflammatory cells into the alveolar wall with alveolar distension and exudation and blockage in the bronchioles. *Emphysema is present in more advanced cases. Prevention entails avoiding the use of mouldy fodder, particularly hay that has overheated after being baled when damp. Adequate ventilation is also important. Anti-inflammatory treatment with corticosteroids and administration of atropine and antihistamines have been tried, but the results are difficult to evaluate. Once emphysema is marked, recovery is unlikely.

allergic contact dermatitis A relatively uncommon disease resulting from the allergic response of sensitized skin when in contact with a sensitizing agent (*see* allergy). Thus, those parts of the body regularly in contact with the floor or with collars or harnesses are most likely to be affected. For instance, in dogs the relatively hairless belly may be affected if it becomes sensitized to substances in floor coverings or soft furnishings. Similarly the neck in dogs or cats may show an allergic contact reaction to flea collars, and sensitized horses may develop allergic contact dermatitis at the contact points of harnesses or bridles. The condition can be caused by a wide range of both natural and synthetic substances: for example nickel, chromium, rubber additives, leather, dyestuffs, wool, and certain carpet cleaners.

There is a latent period following initial exposure to the agent during which time the body's immune system is programmed to react on subsequent exposures. The condition must therefore be distinguished from contact *dermatitis, in which irritant substances act immediately on first exposure. Signs are a rash of spots and fluid-filled vesicles with redness and itching. With repeated challenges the skin in the affected area becomes thickened and often darker. *Patch tests are used for diagnosis. The most effective therapy is removal of the causal allergen but this may be impracticable. *Antipruritic preparations and anti-inflammatory therapy may be prescribed (*see* antihistamine).

allergic dermatitis Inflammation of the skin due to an allergic reaction, which may result from the ingestion, injection, or inhalation of or contact with an allergen (*see* allergic contact dermatitis). Allergy to biting insects is particularly important and common in dogs and cats (e.g. flea hypersensitivity) and horses (*sweet itch).

Examples of other common allergens are beef (ingested) and house dust mites (inhaled). The intradermal test using a range of possible allergens aids the diagnosis of inhalant and contact allergies; it has no place in the diagnosis of food allergies.

allergy 1. A state of changed reactivity to a substance. Used in this sense, the term may apply to all the immunological phenomena. These include protective *immunity, *hypersensitivity, and *tolerance. It may apply to the body as a whole or to organs, tissues, or cells. **2.** Hypersensitivity to foods, pollen, and other naturally occurring materials, which is acquired following previous exposure to the same substance.

allograft A tissue or organ graft exchanged between unrelated members of the same species.

allometric growth The regular and systematic pattern of growth such that the mass or size of any organ or part of a body can be expressed in relation to the total mass or size of the entire organism according to the allometric equation: $Y = bx^{\alpha}$, where Y = mass of the organ, x = mass of the organism, α = growth coefficient of the organ, and b = a constant.

alopecia The absence of hair from areas where it is normally present. It may be localized or generalized, and can be caused by numerous infectious agents (viruses, bacteria, fungi), ectoparasites (e.g. as in *mange), poor nutrition, poisons, excessive friction, allergy, autoimmunity, endocrine imbalance, or heredity.

alpha blocker A drug that acts at alpha adrenergic receptors, thereby blocking the effects of adrenaline or noradrenaline. Alpha receptors are located postsynaptically in vascular smooth muscle (except skeletal muscle vasculature) and secretory glands, and alpha blockers have been used in the treatment of shock after blood volume replacement to induce vasodilatation and thereby prevent damage to small blood vessels and consequent irreversible shock. This type of drug also has limited use in the treatment of hypertension in man. Alpha blockers include the imidazolines (e.g. phentolamine), which act competitively at alpha receptors, and the haloalkylamines (e.g. phenoxybenzamine), which act noncompetitively and have a longer duration of action. The *phenothiazine tranquillizers also act as alpha blockers, and the resultant hypotension may be detrimental during anaesthesia. α_2 receptors are located presynaptically on noradrenergic nerves. They control the reuptake of the transmitter noradrenaline into the neurone. α_1 agonists include the sedation drugs, xylazine, detomidine, and medetomidine. Yohimbine is an α_2 blocker.

alphachloralose A powerful CNS-depressant drug formed by the condensation reaction of glucose and chloral. It is used as a rodenticide and to control bird numbers, especially wood pigeons. It induces anaesthesia and kills animals by reducing their body temperature. To be effective it should be used out of doors since chilling will not occur in centrally heated buildings.
Alphachloralose poisoning This can occur in dogs and cats if baited food or a contaminated carcass is eaten. It acts on the central nervous system causing depression in most cases but occasionally stimulation. Usually, affected animals become comatose and enter a state of deep anaesthesia, but hyperexcitability, aggression, and incoordination sometimes precede loss of consciousness. To treat animals in deep coma, respiratory stimulant drugs (e.g. doxaprom) can be used.

Metabolism of alphachloralose occurs, so the animal should recover fully providing it is kept warm and hydrated during the period of anaesthesia.

alphadolone *See* Saffan.

alphavirus A genus of the *togavirus family, formerly called *arbovirus A group.

alphaxalone *See* Saffan.

alpine laurel poisoning *See* Kalmia poisoning.

ALT (alanine aminotransferase) An *aminotransferase enzyme that catalyses the reaction: glutamate + pyruvate = α-ketoglutarate + alanine. Elevated plasma levels of this enzyme indicate damage to particular tisues that are rich in this enzyme. In the dog and cat, the enzyme is located almost exclusively in the liver, but in cattle and horses it is also found in striated muscle. Former name: **GPT (glutamate pyruvate transaminase).**

alula (alular digit) (*pl.* alulae) The most rudimentary *digit in the wing of a bird, otherwise known as the *bastard wing*.

alveld (elf fire) A disease of sheep in Norway that is believed to be due to the ingestion of bog asphodel (*Narthecium ossifragum*). It is thought that saponins contained in the plant interfere with biliary excretion and cause hepatogenous *photosensitization and *jaundice. Sheep should not be grazed on pastures containing bog asphodel.

alveolar abscess An abscess within the root cavity of a tooth. Important clinically in dogs and horses, alveolar abscesses develop following *periodontal disease when bacteria gain entrance to the bony tooth sockets. The organisms multiply within the confined cavity causing acute inflammation and pain. Other signs may include swelling of the affected side of the face, sometimes with a discharging sinus. In dogs this is known as a *malar abscess*, often involving the upper *carnassial tooth or fourth *premolar. In horses, depending on which tooth is affected, the abscess may drain into the nasal cavity, either directly or via the maxillary sinus, or may erupt on the face. The condition is treated by opening up the cavity to allow drainage, which usually involves removal of the tooth.

alveolar process The *process of the maxilla that bears tooth sockets.

alveolar sac The terminal part of an alveolar duct, which is surrounded by *alveoli.

alveolitis Inflammation of an *alveolus or alveoli, the microscopic terminal air sacs in the mammalian lung. Inflammation of the alveoli with thickening of the walls is seen in *allergic alveolitis (bovine farmer's lung). *Diffuse fibrosing alveolitis* is a condition of old cows and probably represents the end stage of bovine farmer's lung, or possibly of other conditions. The cow is thin but bright and eats well. There is increased depth and rate of breathing and abnormal respiratory sounds may be present. Eventually there may be signs of *heart failure. At postmortem examination the lungs are pale throughout and heavy (10–15 kg) and show replacement of the thin alveolar walls by fibrous tissue, which impedes gaseous exchange. There is no effective treatment.

alveolus (*pl.* **alveoli**) **1.** A blind-ending sac-like structure in the lung. Alveoli lie along the course of *alveolar ducts* and open into the duct cavity, which in turn communicates with respiratory *bronchioles. The walls of alveoli are formed of very thin squamous cells (type I *pneumocytes), with occasional taller cells (type II pneumocytes) believed to be responsible for the production of *surfactant. In the septa between alveoli lies a very dense blood capillary network. Thus carbon dioxide and oxygen are readily exchanged across the thin alveolar walls, which represent the blood/air barrier. In humans, total surface area of the alveoli is comparable to the size of a tennis court. **2.** A socket in the jaw bearing a tooth and its root after eruption is complete. **3.** Any small sac-like structure.

alveus A cavity, groove, or canal. The *alveus of hippocampus* is the thin covering of efferent nerve fibres (white matter) over the ventricular aspect of the hippocampus in the brain; many of the fibres converge to form the *fimbria.

Amanita poisoning A toxic condition resulting from the ingestion of toadstools produced by saprophytic fungi of the genus *Amanita*. The toadstools are characterized by having white gills and a broken membranous ring (volva) around the stalk; the caps are variously coloured. Poisonous species include the blusher (*A. rubescens*), Caesar's mushroom (*A. caesarea*), death cap (*A. phalloides*), destroying angel (*A. virosa*), fly agaric (*A. muscaria*), and panther amanita (*A. pantherina*). The toxic principles are muscimole, cyclopeptides, ibotenic acid, and others. Clinical signs are stimulation of the parasympathetic nervous system, severe inflammation of the intestinal tract, irreversible damage to liver and kidneys, convulsions, and death. Treatment is symptomatic.

Amaranthus poisoning A toxic condition arising from ingestion of the annual herbaceous plant, *A. retroflexus* (pigweed), which contains soluble oxalates, nitrates, and an unknown toxin. The latter can cause kidney damage in pigs and calves resulting in perirenal oedema and haemorrhage. The clinical signs are weakness, trembling, and incoordination, leading to complete paralysis of the hindlegs, coma, and death. Treatment is of the signs. Mature ruminants are also susceptible to nitrate and nitrite accumulation, which produces methaemoglobinaemia (*see* nitrate poisoning).

Amblyomma A genus of hard *ticks ectoparasitic on all domestic animals and man in Africa and Central and South America. Their bite produces sores and some species transmit the rickettsiae that cause *heartwater (in cattle) and *Q fever (in cattle, sheep, and goats), as well as some virus diseases, such as *Nairobi sheep disease and *tick paralysis.

ameloblastoma (adamantinoma) A benign tumour arising from the odontogenic epithelium (from which the teeth originate). Although relatively uncommon in domestic animals, this tumour is most frequent in dogs. It affects the lower mandible as a proliferative mass, disrupting the dental arcade and invading the underlying bone. Radical surgery is necessary to remove the whole tumour.

American hemp *See* Apocynum poisoning.

American Society for the Prevention of Cruelty to Animals (ASPCA) A nongovernmental organization, founded in 1866, dedicated to animal welfare and protection. It lobbies for animal protection legislation and its enforcement, maintains animal shelters, operates veterinary hospitals and animal clinics, and conducts wide-ranging educational and information programmes. Address: 441 E92nd St., New York, NY 10128.

American Veterinary Medical Association (AVMA) A national political and educational organization for the veterinary profession in the USA. The Association acts to promote and protect the interests of the profession and publishes *The Journal of the American Veterinary Medical Association* and the *American Journal of Veterinary Research*. It has approximately 46 000 members. HQ address: 930 North Meacham Road, Shaumburg, Illinois 60196-1074, USA.

amethocaine *See* local anaesthetic.

amicarbalide An antiprotozoal drug with activity against *Babesia* spp., the causal agents of *babesiosis. It has no activity against *Theileria parva*, the causal agent in *East coast fever. It is available for intramuscular, subcutaneous, or slow intravenous injection. When used to treat babesiosis there is an improvement in clinical condition but the parasites may not be completely eradicated, allowing the development of immunity. Two doses at 24-hour intervals are usually needed, and the antiprotozoal effect does not persist. Toxicity is low, but there can be salivation, hyperpnoea, and diarrhoea. After subcutaneous injection local swelling may develop. Tradename: **Diampron**.

amine One of a class of organic compounds derived by replacing one or more of the hydrogen atoms in ammonia by an organic group. *Primary amines* contain the amino group $(-NH_2)$ and include many biologically important molecules, such as the *amino acids, *catecholamines, and *polyamines.

amino acid Any of a group of water-soluble organic compounds that possess both an amino $(-NH_2)$ and a

amino acid

amino acid	abbreviation	formula
alanine	ala	$CH_3-\overset{H}{\underset{NH_2}{C}}-COOH$
*arginine	arg	$H_2N-\overset{NH}{C}-NH-CH_2-CH_2-\overset{H}{\underset{NH_2}{C}}-COOH$
asparagine	asn	$H_2N-\overset{O}{C}-CH_2-\overset{H}{\underset{NH_2}{C}}-COOH$
aspartic acid	asp	$HOOC-CH_2-\overset{H}{\underset{NH_2}{C}}-COOH$
cysteine	cys	$HS-CH_2-\overset{H}{\underset{NH_2}{C}}-COOH$
glutamic acid	glu	$HOOC-CH_2-CH_2-\overset{H}{\underset{NH_2}{C}}-COOH$
glutamine	gln	$H_2N-\overset{O}{C}-CH_2-CH_2-\overset{H}{\underset{NH_2}{C}}-COOH$
glycine	gly	$H-\overset{H}{\underset{NH_2}{C}}-COOH$
*histidine	his	$HC=C-CH_2-\overset{H}{\underset{NH_2}{C}}-COOH$ (imidazole ring)
*isoleucine	ile	$CH_3-CH_2-CH-\overset{H}{\underset{NH_2}{\underset{CH_3}{C}}}-COOH$
*leucine	leu	$\overset{H_3C}{\underset{H_3C}{}}CH-CH_2-\overset{H}{\underset{NH_2}{C}}-COOH$
*lysine	lys	$H_2N-CH_2-CH_2-CH_2-CH_2-\overset{H}{\underset{NH_2}{C}}-COOH$
*methionine	met	$CH_3-S-CH_2-CH_2-\overset{H}{\underset{NH_2}{C}}-COOH$
*phenylalanine	phe	$C_6H_5-CH_2-\overset{H}{\underset{NH_2}{C}}-COOH$
proline	pro	(pyrrolidine ring) $\overset{H}{\underset{N}{C}}-COOH$; 4-hydroxyproline
serine	ser	$HO-CH_2-\overset{H}{\underset{NH_2}{C}}-COOH$
*threonine	thr	$CH_3-\overset{OH}{CH}-\overset{H}{\underset{NH_2}{C}}-COOH$
*tryptophan	trp	(indole ring) $-CH_2-\overset{H}{\underset{NH_2}{C}}-COOH$
tyrosine	tyr	$HO-C_6H_4-CH_2-\overset{H}{\underset{NH_2}{C}}-COOH$
*valine	val	$\overset{H_3C}{\underset{H_3C}{}}CH-\overset{H}{\underset{NH_2}{C}}-COOH$

The amino acids occurring in proteins

* an essential amino acid

carboxyl (−COOH) group attached to the α-carbon atom. Amino acids have the general formula R−CH-(NH₂)COOH, where R may be hydrogen or an organic group and determines the properties of the particular amino acid. Amino acids occur both as free molecules and, when linked together by *peptide bonds, as structural units of *peptides, *polypeptides, and *proteins. Twenty different amino acids (see table) are found in proteins although any individual protein need not contain all 20. Some proteins contain other amino acids (e.g. *hydroxyproline, thyroxine) which are derived by modification of the constituent amino acids after the protein has been synthesized in the cells. Amino acids in proteins are L-isomers, but short peptides of microbial origin (e.g. certain antibiotics) contain D-isomers as well as certain amino acids not found in proteins.

In order to synthesize proteins, animals require a steady supply of amino acids. Some can be made in the body; however, the *essential amino acids cannot be synthesized in the body and must be supplied in the diet. Amino acids in excess of the amount required for protein synthesis are used for energy generation or other processes, since there is no mechanism for protein storage in animals. The metabolism of amino acids by *transamination and *deamination generates ammonia; this is converted to urea in mammals by the *urea cycle. In birds and terrestrial reptiles, *uric acid is the end-product of amino acid metabolism. The non-nitrogenous 'carbon skeleton' of the various amino acids is metabolized by the *Krebs cycle and other pathways. Those amino acids whose skeletons can give rise to glucose (see gluconeogenesis) are termed glucogenic; others, especially those with aliphatic alkyl groups, yield acetyl CoA (see coenzyme A) and so can be converted to *fat or *ketone bodies; hence they are sometimes termed ketogenic.

aminocyclitol Any of a group of antibiotics, similar in structure to the *aminoglycosides, that are mainly active against Gram-negative bacteria; some are also active against mycoplasmas. They are bacteriostatic, inhibiting bacterial protein synthesis at the ribosomes. Spectinomycin has good activity against the mycoplasmas infecting poultry and is used orally and also in an injectable form in poultry, pigs, and cattle. Apramycin is not active against mycoplasmas; being poorly absorbed after oral administration it is used to treat enteric infections in pigs.

aminoglycoside Any of a group of antibiotics that have similar bactericidal activity and chemical structure − all contain an aminocyclitol nucleus with two amino sugars attached. They act on bacterial ribosomes, inhibiting protein synthesis due to misreading of the genetic code by transfer RNA. The most important clinically are streptomycin, dihydrostreptomycin, neomycin, gentamicin, amikacin, and kanamycin. Their main spectrum of activity is against Gram-negative bacteria, but neomycin has some activity against Gram-positive organisms. Gentamicin and amikacin have even broader spectra. Aminoglycosides have a synergistic action with penicillins and cephalosporins, possibly because they are able to penetrate bacteria better after the cell wall has been damaged.

All members of this group are poorly absorbed from the alimentary tract. For systemic infections the antibiotic must be injected intramuscularly or intravenously. Some drugs are given by slow intravenous injection. Most of the drug is excreted in the active form. Resistance of microorganisms to aminoglycosides develops rapidly and prolonged therapy should be avoided. Streptomycin and dihydrostreptomycin are injected in combination with penicillins to broaden the spectrum of activity to include Gram-negative bacteria. Neomycin (which in purifed form is known as framycetin or framomycin) is used orally to treat enteric infections and used topically in ear and eye preparations. Gentamicin has good activity against *Pseudomonas* and *Klebsiella*, and can be injected intramuscularly to treat these infections.

Various forms of toxicity can occur. Damage to the *vestibulocochlear nerve and the sensory cells of the vestibular apparatus can cause ataxia, incoordination, and nystagmus. This is usually reversible if the drug is withdrawn. Ototoxicity with deafness also occurs and is irreversible. Dihydrostreptomycin is the most toxic but the others can also produce these effects. Cats may be especially sensitive and parenteral use of aminoglycosides in felines should be avoided. Another side-effect of parenteral aminoglycosides, especially neomycin and gentamicin, is acute necrosis of kidney tubules. Aminoglycosides also cause neuromuscular blocking, and high doses given parenterally may cause impaired respiration; this action is potentiated by anaesthetics.

aminonitrothiazole An antiprotozoal drug, slightly soluble in water. It is used therapeutically and prophylactically against *blackhead in turkeys, being active against both the parasite and the worm intermediate host. For maximum protection the drug must be used continuously and can be incorporated in feed or in the water. Unlimited fresh water must be provided to prevent toxic effects on the kidneys.

aminophylline *See* xanthine.

aminotransferase (**transaminase**) An enzyme that catalyses the transfer of an amino group from an *amino acid to a keto acid (e.g. α-ketoglutarate) to form a new amino acid and keto acid. The various enzymes in this class have different specificities towards the initial amino acid; all use pyridoxal phosphate as a cofactor.

amitosis Division of the nucleus of a cell by a process, not involving *mitosis, in which the nucleus is constricted into two.

amitraz A topical pesticide that is stable in aqueous solution and is used as a dip or wash for the control of ectoparasites. It has activity against lice, ticks, keds, and mange mites. In the UK it is available as a wash for the control of mange and lice in cattle and pigs. In sheep it is used as a dip to kill lice and keds, and gives protection against ticks for up to 3 weeks. It is also used to treat demodectic mange in dogs. It should not be used in horses. Compared with other ectoparasiticides (e.g. organophosphorus compounds) it is relatively nontoxic, but protective clothing should be worn when handling the compound. Amitraz is harmful to fish.

ammonia A colourless strong-smelling gas, chemical formula NH_3. It is given off by decaying plant and animal material. Ammonia fumes from soiled litter have been shown to decrease the performance of poultry and pigs. Larger quantities of ammonia are toxic and inhalation of concentrated ammonia can prove fatal. Increased levels of ammonia in the blood may be one of the agents causing CNS signs in liver disease. In ruminants fed excess urea, toxicity can occur if the liver is unable to metabolize the ammonia that is formed in the rumen and absorbed into the blood (*see* urea poisoning). Small quantities of ammonia act as a stimulant and were used in the past in smelling salts for reviving collapsed patients.

amnion (*pl.* **amnions** or **amnia**) One of the *foetal membranes. It forms initially over the dorsal surface of the embryo but soon expands so that the enclosed *amniotic cavity* containing the *amniotic fluid surrounds the foetus completely.

amniotic fluid The fluid contained within the amniotic cavity. It surrounds the growing foetus, protecting it from external pressure. The fluid is initially secreted from the *amnion and is later supplemented by urine from the foetal kidneys. Some of the fluid is swallowed by the foetus and absorbed through its intestine.

amoebic dysentery A disease, primarily of humans but also occasionally of other primates and, rarely, dogs and others, caused by the protozoan parasite *Entamoeba histolytica*. It is predominantly a disease of tropical regions, transmitted in water or on food, especially raw vegetables. The parasite invades the gut wall causing ulceration and dysentery and may spread in the bloodstream causing abscesses in other organs. Specific treatment is available.

amoxycillin *See* penicillin.

AMP (adenosine monophosphate) A *nucleotide molecule consisting of the purine base *adenine, the pentose sugar *ribose, and phosphate (which is normally bonded to the 5′ position of the ribose). *Cyclic AMP (cAMP)*, in which the phosphate is bound to both 3′ and 5′ positions, occurs widely in animal cells as an intermediate messenger in the action of certain hormones, such as adrenaline. It is also involved in controlling gene expression and cell division, in

immune responses, and in nervous transmission. *See also* ATP.

amphibolic Describing a metabolic pathway that is capable of functioning in both a *catabolic and an *anabolic fashion, for example the *Krebs cycle.

amphotericin B An antibiotic with antifungal properties. Chemically it is a large cyclic lactone, fairly insoluble in water. It binds to the fungal cell membrane causing altered permeability. Amphotericin B is available as a powder, which is reconstituted in water and injected intravenously; absorption from the gut is poor. It diffuses well throughout the body, except to the cerebrospinal fluid, and is used in the treatment of systemic yeast and other fungal infections, for example *candidiasis and *aspergillosis. Side-effects include vomiting, diarrhoea, and phlebitis at the injection site. Nephrotoxicity and depression of the bone marrow may occur with long-term therapy.

ampicillin *See* penicillin.

ampoule A small glass container, usually flat at the base and with a pointed end that is sealed to keep the contents sterile. It is used to hold a single dose of a vaccine or a small volume of drug.

amprolium hydrochloride *See* coccidiostat.

ampulla (*pl.* **ampullae**) An enlarged part of a tube or canal. Each *semicircular canal of the ear widens to form an ampulla at one end. The ampulla of the *uterine tube is the expanded thin-walled main part of the tube in which fertilization normally occurs.

amputation The surgical removal of a limb, part of a limb, or other structure. Amputation of limbs is indicated following severe irreparable injury, or if the limb is permanently paralysed and constitutes a nuisance. In cattle amputation of individual digits is required when incurable local infection may spread systematically and must be performed before the fetlock joint is involved if it is to be successful. Amputation is performed to remove accessory teats, or to permit surgical drainage from very grossly damaged mammary glands affected by necrotic mastitis. Penile amputation may be required where gross damage to the penis has resulted. Amputation of the urethral process in sheep is an initial procedure in the treatment of urolithiasis. *See also* dehorning.

amylase An *enzyme that catalyses the hydrolysis of α-1,4 glycosidic bonds in polysaccharides, such as amylose and glycogen, to yield maltose, glucose, etc. Amylases are found in saliva and pancreatic juice and also in certain plants (e.g. germinating barley).

amyloidosis Infiltration of the liver, kidneys, and other organs with amyloid, a waxy starchlike substance. It can be associated with an immune-based response and the deposition of amyloid protein on basement membranes. Amyloidosis is often accompanied by dysfunction or failure of the organ(s) involved. For example in cases of kidney involvement there is massive *proteinuria.

Amyloidosis is a common cause of loss in adult ducks, characterized by amyloid enlargement of the liver and spleen: there may be a variable degree of *ascites. The causes are uncertain but a higher incidence has been variously linked to stress, overcrowding, or the prevalence of some other chronic infectious condition.

amylopectin *See* starch.

amylose *See* starch.

anabolic 1. Describing a hormone that promotes metabolic processes leading to an increase in mass of skeletal muscle. **2.** (Also **biosynthetic**) Describing a metabolic pathway that leads to an increase in complexity of substances in the body, i.e. the processes of anabolism.

anaemia (erythropenia) An abnormally low amount of the oxygen-carrying pigment *haemoglobin in the blood. The degree of anaemia can be determined by measuring the haemoglobin concentration, the *packed cell volume, or the erythrocyte count (number of red blood cells per litre). The clinical signs include lethargy, poor exercise tolerance, and pale mucous membranes, and a cardiac murmur is sometimes audible due to lowered blood viscosity.

Anaemia has various causes. *Haemorrhagic anaemia* is the result of blood loss through bleeding. This may be caused by injury, chronic lesions, poisoning (e.g. by bracken or warfarin), blood-feeding parasites (e.g. liver fluke), haemophilia (rare in livestock), or platelet deficiency (*thrombocytopenia) and deficient blood clotting. *Haemolytic anaemia is due to destruction of the red blood cells (haemolysis). *Dyshaemopoietic anaemia* is due to the failure of red blood cell production as a result of mineral or vitamin deficiencies (e.g. iron deficiency in piglets; vitamin B_{12} and folic acid deficiencies – both rare), poisoning (e.g. bracken poisoning), radiation, or systemic illness (e.g. neoplasia, chronic renal failure). Treatment depends on the underlying cause. In severe cases blood transfusions can be carried out.

Anaemias can also be classified on the basis of the size of the red cells and the haemoglobin content. Normocytic normochromic anaemia (with normal size and normal haemoglobin concentration within the cell) occurs in cases of chronic bleeding and bone marrow depression. Macrocytic hypochromic anaemia (with enlarged cells and lowered haemoglobin concentration) is found in the autoimmune anaemias and vitamin B_{12} and folic acid deficiencies. Microcytic hypochromic anaemia occurs in iron deficiency.

anaerobe Any organism, especially a microorganism, that is able to live and grow in the absence of free oxygen. A *facultative anaerobe* is a microorganism that grows best in the presence of oxygen but is capable of some growth in its absence. An *obligate anaerobe* can grow only in the absence of free oxygen. *Compare* aerobe; microaerophilic.

anaerobic 1. Of or relating to *anaerobes. 2. Describing a type of cellular *respiration in which foodstuffs are partially oxidized with the release of chemical energy, in a process not involving molecular oxygen. *See also* fermentation. 3. Describing any reaction that does not require molecular oxygen.

anaesthesia The loss of feeling or sensation in all or part of the body. Anaesthesia of a part of the body may occur as a result of injury to or disease of a nerve. The term is usually applied, however, to the technique of reducing or abolishing a patient's sensation of pain to enable surgery to be performed. This is achieved by administering drugs by injection or inhalation or a combination of both (*see* anaesthetic).
General anaesthesia involves complete loss of consciousness and is employed for major surgical operations. Commonly, a hypnotic or narcotic drug is administered initially as a premedication to help ensure smooth induction and recovery. Induction of anaesthesia is achieved by injecting a soluble anaesthetic (e.g. barbiturate) intrave-

nously, and anaesthesia can be maintained by the inhalation of a volatile anaesthetic (*see* endotracheal anaesthesia) where prolonged anaesthesia is required. Animals should be allowed to recover from general anaesthesia in quiet surroundings so that they will remain recumbent until fully able to rise. Cattle should be supported in sternal recumbency to ensure that aspiration of saliva does not occur.
Local or *regional anaesthesia* abolishes pain from a specific part of the body without inducing unconsciousness, and without necessarily abolishing all sensation. Hence it is more properly referred to as *analgesia. It may be achieved by injection of a *local anaesthetic into the required area itself; into the tissues surrounding the area (*field block*); around the trunk of a nerve supplying the area (*see* nerve block); around the appropriate spinal nerves (*paravertebral anaesthesia*); or into the spinal canal (*see* spinal anaesthesia).

anaesthetic An agent that induces *anaesthesia. *General anaesthetics* and *dissociative anaesthetics* act on the central nervous system (CNS) producing unconsciousness and loss of sensation throughout the body. They are used for immobilization, muscle relaxation, and *analgesia during surgical procedures, and are administered by inhalation (*see* endotracheal anaesthesia) or injected intravenously, intramuscularly, intraperitoneally, or subcutaneously. In small animals and birds some agents can be given orally. Inhalational agents give greater control over the depth of anaesthesia. Apart from the *inhalational anaesthetics, agents used include *barbiturates, *Saffan, *ketamine, *metomidate, and *chloral hydrate. *Local anaesthetics produce loss of touch and pain sensation around the site of application.

anal Referring to the *anus.

analeptic A drug that stimulates the central nervous system, either by enhancing excitation or blocking inhibitory inputs. The main drugs used therapeutically are the xanthines (e.g. caffeine, theophylline), amphetamines, bemegride, doxapram, and nikethamide. They are used to stimulate respiration in neonates (especially lambs), and to treat overdosage with injectable anaesthetics.

analgesia A temporary absence of sensitivity to pain, usually produced by the administration of certain drugs (*analgesics).

analgesic A compound that causes pain relief without the loss of consciousness. *Narcotic analgesics* act on the central nervous system and induce drowsiness in some species (e.g. the dog). *Antipyretic analgesics* act both centrally and locally at the site of pain, as do local *anaesthetics. The narcotic analgesics, such as morphine, are used to treat severe pain after surgery or trauma and also prior to or during anaesthesia to reduce the amount of anaesthetic drug needed. When combined with a sedative or tranquillizer, narcotic analgesics can produce a state of neuroleptanalgesia sufficient to allow minor surgery to be carried out. Antipyretic analgesics, such as aspirin, are used mainly for the long-term treatment of less severe pain.

anal gland One of a pair of sac-like structures, each about 1 cm in diameter, that lie on either side of the anal canal in carnivores, between the internal and external anal *sphincters. Each has a duct which opens to the skin at the anal orifice (*see* anus). The glands secrete a foul-smelling liquid into the *paranal sinus*, which normally empties on defecation. Frequently the paranal sinuses become enlarged due to blockage and may become infected and painful. An infected sinus may occasionally rupture through the skin producing a fistula.

anamnesis (*pl.* **anamneses**) **1.** Clinical history. This is an important part of diagnosis, and details should include: age; sex; breed; previous ownership; length of time on premises; vaccinal status; grazing history; previous disease of the individual, related animals, and members of its group; present disease signs; and any treatment given. **2.** (in immunology) A secondary immunological response occurring when an animal is subsequently exposed to an antigen to which it has previously responded. Special *lymphocytes (memory T-lymphocytes) have an immunological memory and recognize the antigen. The result is a more exaggerated and sustained immunological response. This is why vaccines, particularly dead vaccines, are administered on several occasions to harness the anamnestic response and produce protective levels of antibody.

anaphase The third stage of *mitosis and of each division of *meiosis. In mitosis and anaphase II of meiosis the chromatids separate, becoming daughter chromosomes, and move apart along the spindle fibres towards opposite ends of the cell. In anaphase I of meiosis the pairs of homologous chromosomes separate from each other. *See* disjunction.

anaphrodisia A state of reduced libido induced by a drug or other substance (anaphrodisiac).

anaphylaxis **1.** *Hypersensitivity. **2.** A particular form of Type I hypersensitivity in which generalized damaging changes are induced by the release of *histamine. *Anaphylactic shock* is an extreme and generalized allergic reaction in which widespread histamine release causes bronchial constriction (and hence respiratory distress), dilatation of the veins, circulatory collapse, and possibly death.

anaplasia A loss of normal cell characteristics or differentiation. Malignant fast-growing lesions are described as anaplastic when they show complete loss of differentiation and no longer resemble the tissue of origin.

Anaplasma A genus of *rickettsiae in the family Anaplasmataceae, commonly found as obligate parasites within red blood cells or freely in the blood of various animals. They are transmitted by ticks. In blood smears the anaplasmas appear as minute deeply staining particles near the margin of the red cells. The genus includes three species that cause *anaplasmosis in domestic animals. *A. marginale* is characteristically located on the margin of the red cells (marginal bodies) of cattle. *A. centrale* causes a milder disease in cattle and the organisms reside in the centre of the red cells (central bodies). *A. ovis* affects sheep in the USA and Africa.

anaplasmosis (gallsickness) A disease of cattle and sheep caused by rickettsiae of the genus *Anaplasma. It occurs in tropical and subtropical regions and is transmitted by a variety of bloodsucking insects and ticks. It can also be transmitted by the transfer of infected blood in transfusions or via contaminated needles. The parasites destroy their host's red cells causing anaemia, fever, and, in severe cases, jaundice. The disease is of most importance in cattle. Animals that recover remain infected but immune for life. The disease may be treated with tetracycline antibiotics; vaccines are available.

anasarca The presence of excessive amounts of fluid (*oedema, or dropsy) in the tissues beneath the skin. Pits form when pressure is applied to the skin. The condition arises as a result of lowered plasma protein levels (*hypoproteinaemia), lymphatic obstruction, or increased venous pressure associated with *heart failure. It has also been reported as a specific condition in newborn Ayrshire calves. Fluid may be removed by administering *diuretic drugs, but effective treatment depends on correcting the underlying cause.

anastomosis 1. (in anatomy) A communication between two blood vessels without any intervening capillary network. *See* arteriovenous anastomosis. **2.** (in surgery) An artificial connection between two tubular organs or parts, especially between two normally separate parts of the intestine.

anatipestifer infection An infectious disease causing high mortality (up to 75%) in young ducklings, caused by the bacterium *Pasteurella anatipestifer*. It affects birds aged 2–6 weeks old, sometimes up to 8 weeks, and the appearance of clinical signs is normally triggered by poor husbandry or stress. The bacterium is probably passed on through the egg and can also be transmitted from bird to bird. In specific cases of stress, such as moving the birds, signs appear 3 days later, although in the most acute form, death occurs before the onset of clinical signs. Otherwise, typical signs are hunching of the head into the body or continual shaking of the head; there may be watery eyes, ruffled feathers, green diarrhoea with a pale-green stained vent, and a congested beak. Post-mortem examination reveals the liver and spleen to be enlarged and congested. Intramuscular injection with suitable antibiotics is the most effective treatment, but medication of the drinking water can be used. Prevention relies on good management, especially on minimizing stress. Feed or water medication has been used prophylactically, and a vaccine has been prepared and is on field trial. Other names: **duck septicaemia; infectious serositis; new duck disease**.

anatomy The study of the structure of the body. It may be concerned with a single species (e.g. human anatomy) or with the structural similarities and differences between species (comparative anatomy). The principal methods of study include dissection, microscopy, and radiography. Apart from gross anatomy (naked eye study, sometimes termed morphology), the discipline also involves *histology (study of tissues), *embryology (study of the development of the embryo, sometimes termed developmental anatomy), neuroanatomy (study of the nervous system), *cytology (study of cells), and applied (surgical) anatomy.

anatoxin *See* toxoid.

Ancylostoma A genus of parasitic nematodes (*see* hookworm) occurring in the small intestine of cats and dogs in tropical and subtropical areas. Small stocky worms, the adults attach to the mucous membrane and suck blood, causing a chronic and debilitating condition in their host. At post mortem the mucous membrane can be almost white from loss of blood. *A. caninum* and *A. braziliense* occur in dogs, and *A. tubaeforme* in cats. *A. braziliense* can infect humans and cause creeping eruption (larva migrans) beneath the skin. Eggs are passed in the faeces, where they develop into infective larvae. These infect another host either by ingestion, or by penetrating the skin and migrating to the lungs, where they are carried up the windpipe and swallowed. The larvae are vulnerable to desiccation, and infestation can be controlled by keeping housing well cleaned and drained. Infected animals can be treated with bephenium or benzimidazole compounds.

androgen Any of a group of steroid hormones with masculinizing and anabolic properties. The naturally occurring androgens, *testosterone, androstenedione, and dehydroepiandrosterone, are produced principally in the testis but also in the adrenal glands and ovary; they are responsible for the formation of secondary male sexual characteristics. Various synthetic androgens are also available for veterinary use. Those with androgenic properties are used to modify reproductive activity (*see* testosterone). Steroids with less androgenic activity but greater anabolic action (e.g. *trenbolone acetate, nandrolone, boldenone, and methandienone) are used therapeutically in, for example, pregnancy toxaemia, chronic disease, fracture repair, and after sugery. Their anabolic effects include improved protein utilization, increased appetite, calcium retention, and increased weight gain. Trenbolone has been used as a growth promoter but is now banned in EEC countries.

androstenedione *See* androgen.

anergy 1. (in immunology) Absence of reactivity to an *antigen. *General* or *cachectic anergy* may result from chronic disease or malnutrition. *Specific anergy* to a given antigen may be associated with clinical susceptibility to organisms bearing the antigen. Occasionally, specific anergy is accompanied by high resistance to the relevant microorganism. This may result, for instance, when a highly effective cellular immune response to an organism coincides with a negative, or anergic, antibody response. Anergy can follow from inactivation of antigen-specific lymphocyte clones or from T-lymphocyte dysregulation. In these cases the condition is identical to specific acquired tolerance. **2.** Lack of energy.

aneuploidy The state in which the complement of chromosomes carried by a nucleus or organism is not a whole multiple of the basic number (n) in the genome. Most aneuploid individuals are either $2n + 1$ (*see* trisomy) or $2n - 1$ (*see* monosomy); usually it is one of the sex chromosomes that is present in an abnormal number.

aneurin *See* vitamin B_1.

aneurysm Ballooning or dilatation of the wall of an artery, vein, or the heart as a result of weakening of the wall. This produces a sac, which is liable to rupture and cause massive haemorrhage. In the horse, aneurysms can develop in the root of the cranial mesenteric artery as a consequence of lesions caused by infestation with the parasitic nematodes *Strongylus vulgaris*. Aneurysms have also been described in the aorta.

angi- (angio-) *Prefix denoting* blood or lymph vessels. Examples: *angiectasis* (abnormal dilatation of); *angiopathy* (disease of); *angiotomy* (cutting of).

angiitis (angitis) Inflammation of a small vessel, usually a blood vessel or a lymphatic vessel (*see* lymphangitis). Angiitis may be associated with bacterial or viral infections, endotoxins, parasites, or immune complexes. Inflammatory cells are visible microscopically in and around the vessel wall, and the changes may activate clotting mechanisms resulting in *thrombosis and vascular occlusion. *Compare* arteritis; phlebitis.

angioedema *See* urticaria.

angiography *Radiography of blood vessels. This is undertaken after an injection of a radio-opaque substance into the artery (arteriography) or vein (venography), producing radiographs termed, respectively, *arteriograms* and *venograms*.

angioma A benign tumour of endothelial cells. *Haemangiomas* arise from blood vessels. They occur in all animal species and are particularly common in the dog, where they may be found in any tissue, although most occur in the skin and subcutaneous tissues. Haemangiomas appear as single ovoid red-black masses of varying size, moderately firm in consistency and well-circumscribed. Histologically, *cavernous* lesions consist of blood-filled vascular spaces lined by a single layer of well-differentiated endothelium and separated by broad connective-tissue septae. *Capillary* angiomas show a dense network of capillary-sized vessels in a stroma of well-formed collagen. Haemangiomas do not recur after complete surgical removal.
Lymphangiomas arise from lymphatic vessels and are rare benign tumours; they may be capillary, cavernous, or cystic. The latter two forms may progressively enlarge, divide along fascial planes, and prove difficult to excise.

angiosarcoma A malignant tumour of endothelial cells. *Haemangiosarcomas* arise from blood vessels and are commonest in the dog, although recorded in other species. In the dog, the common primary sites are spleen, right atrium of the heart, liver, and subcutaneous tissues. Characteristically the tumour is a reddish-black haemorrhagic lesion; it may become large in the spleen due to haemorrhage into its substance. Beneath the skin, the tumour forms a spongy poorly circumscribed haemorrhagic mass; in the heart its surface is covered by thrombus giving it a reddish-grey to yellow coloration. Haemangiosarcomas are highly malig-

Angiostrongylus

nant neoplasms that are inclined to metastasize early in the course of disease, especially to the lungs. Surgical excision is extremely difficult, if not impossible, with a high risk of local recurrence and metastatic disease.
Lymphangiosarcomas arise from lymphatic vessels and are rare in domestic animals. They are diffusely invasive and metastasize widely, and so have a poor prognosis.

Angiostrongylus A genus of parasitic *nematodes containing *A. cantonensis*, which is found in rodents, mainly in the Far East, but may also infect humans. The larvae migrate to the heart and may reach the brain via the carotid artery. They feed on the meninges and cause a condition called eosinophilic meningoencephalitis, which is characterized by granulomatous tissue surrounding the worms. The resultant vascular congestion can be fatal. The chief intermediate host is a snail, but freshwater prawns, oysters, and slugs may also be used. Humans may be infected by eating raw prawns or vegetables contaminated with the larvae.

angiotensin II A peptide hormone, comprising eight amino acids, that stimulates secretion of *aldosterone from the adrenal cortex. The precursor *angiotensinogen*, derived from the liver, is converted to the peptide *angiotensin I* by the enzyme *renin*, which is released from the kidney in response to decreased sodium, high potassium, or low oxygen tension of the blood perfusing the kidney. An enzyme from the lung found in the circulation removes two amino acids from angiotensin I to form angiotensin II. Angiotensin is also capable of causing constriction of blood vessels, thus raising blood pressure.

angleberry A benign tumour of the epidermis of the skin, seen in horses and cattle and associated with infec-

tion by *papovaviruses. The tumours may be single or multiple and can develop in hairy skin, on the teats, the genitalia, or the eyelid. They vary in size from a small nodule to a large fungoid mass; the lesion protrudes from the skin surface, is thickened, crusty, and pigmented, and is vulnerable to damage and liable to ulcerate and bleed. They often regress spontaneously. *See also* papilloma.

anidrosis (anhidrosis) The abnormal absence of sweating. This may be due to disease or a congenital abnormality, for example the absence of sweat glands, but in horses it is a common problem in hot humid climates. In such cases sweat glands are present, but have a reduced or absent response to stimuli to induce sweating. Signs include reduced performance and dry hair coat. Treatment is to keep the horse in an air-conditioned stall or return it to a temperate climate.

Animal and Plant Health Inspection Service (APHIS) *See* United States Department of Agriculture.

Animal Boarding Establishments Act (1963) (England and Wales) An Act of Parliament requiring that the keeper of an establishment for boarding cats and dogs must hold a licence (renewable annually) issued by the local authority. In granting or renewing a licence, the authority must judge that the animals will be properly housed, fed, watered, bedded, and exercised. There must also be protection against disease, fire, and other emergencies, and a register must be kept of all animals entering and leaving the establishment.

Animal Health Act (1981) (England and Wales) An Act of Parliament that provides for Orders for the control of animal diseases, including regulating the movement and importation of animals. *See also* notifiable disease.

Animals Act (1971) (England and Wales) An Act of Parliament that contains provision for the civil liability of keepers of dogs for injury done by their dogs to livestock, and for the owners of livestock for damage and expenses due to trespass by their livestock.

Animals (Scientific Procedures) Act (1986) (England and Wales) An Act of Parliament governing the protection of animals used for experimental or other scientific purposes. The Act prohibits regulated procedures being applied to an animal without personal and project licences. A regulated procedure includes any experimental or other scientific procedure, applied to a protected animal, that may have the effect of causing that animal pain, suffering, distress, or lasting harm. A personal licence is required by individual researchers, specifying procedures and types of animals they may use and limiting their authority according to their competence, training, experience, and general suitability. A project licence is needed for every specific programme of work; it defines permissible aims and methods of the project, keeping in balance the severity of the work and its potential benefit. Home Office inspectors have the duty of inspecting all designated establishments and work done under the Act, and of considering applications for licences and certificates.

Animal Welfare Act (USA) A federal Act that makes provisions for the humane treatment of animals in several areas, including animal fighting, transporting, exhibition, sale, and experimentation.

ankylosis A process whereby a joint ceases to be mobile and the bones gradually fuse across the joint space. It may arise from disease, injury, or surgical intervention and represents the final stage of a pathological process. The fusion is initially fibrous but eventually the joint surfaces are united by a bony bridge. At this stage the joint is no longer painful and instead of articulating behaves as a stiff rod.

anoestrus The absence of *oestrus or 'heat'. This is caused by reduced ovarian activity in which follicular growth, ovulation, and associated hormonal surges are diminished or suspended. *Seasonal anoestrus* occurs naturally in many species during the winter months, and in mares anoestrus extends from late summer to late winter. In contrast, sheep after giving birth in spring enter a period of anoestrus in response to the increasing daylength; this may last 4–5 months in some breeds. Cattle and pigs tend to be *polyoestrous and come into oestrus at any time of year. Following parturition there is in most species a period of minimal ovarian activity resulting in *lactational anoestrus*. In bitches, queens, and sows this lasts throughout lactation, although sows commonly show an anovulatory oestrus (i.e. one in which there is no ovulation) 3–7 days after farrowing. In ewes and mares, on the other hand, the oestrous cycle resumes during lactation.

Anoestrus may also result from certain pathological conditions, for example *ovarian cysts or *pyometra, malnutrition, or certain congenital abnormalities, for example *freemartins lack functional ovaries. Various methods have been tried to reduce the period of anoestrus and so increase animal productivity. For example in ewes, the use of intravaginal sponges containing *progesterone followed by an injection of *PMSG (pregnant mare's serum gonadotrophin) has successfully induced oestrus in midsummer.

Anopheles A genus of *mosquitoes found worldwide and distinguished by their habit of holding the body at an angle of about 45° to the surface when feeding; also, they usually have spotted wings. *Anopheles* spp. transmit the malarial parasite, *Plasmodium*, to humans and some species transmit the nematode worms, *Wuchereria bancrofti* and *Dirofilaria immitis*, that cause filariasis in humans and *dirofilariasis in dogs respectively.

Anoplocephala A genus of *tapeworms that are parasitic in the intestine of herbivorous mammals and birds. They are relatively short, about 5–8 cm long, with short and very broad proglottids. The intermediate host is an oribatid mite, which lives among grass, where it may be swallowed by a grazing herbivore. *A. perfoliata*, which lives in the large and small intestine of the horse, is not uncommon in Britain.

anorexia Complete loss of appetite. It occurs for various reasons, including lesions of the mouth, tongue, gums, and throat, which prevent the ingestion of food, or any condition causing stasis of the alimentary tract, such as indigestion or fever. Obstruction of the oesophagus or chronic *bloat also prevent eating. Other causes of anorexia include infestation of the gut with worm parasites and chronic debilitating diseases, such as tuberculosis. Anorexia is a clinical sign of certain vitamin deficiencies, such as *vitamin B_1 (thiamine) deficiency and *vitamin B_{12} deficiency. In ruminants anorexia can occur as a result of rumenal *acidosis, *milk fever, and *ketosis.

Although anorexia nervosa as seen in humans does not occur in other species, psychological problems can be involved. Companion animals may pine in the absence of their owners, or exotic (wild) species may refuse food when confined in unusual environments. Some animals refuse food because they prefer certain tastes. Treatment of anorexia involves remedying the cause. Various preparations can be used to stimulate alimentary activity, for example, drenches of ginger and nux vomica (containing small quantities of strychnine), and various *parasympathomimetic drugs. *Compare* inappetence.

anoxaemia A condition in which there is less than the normal concentration of oxygen in the blood. *See also* anoxia; hypoxia.

anoxia A condition in which there is an inadequate supply of oxygen to the body tissues. Tissues require oxygen for aerobic cellular respiration. Anoxia develops as a consequence of impaired blood supply or reduced oxygen-carrying capacity of the blood (due to e.g. shortage of blood, red blood cells, or haemoglobin, or to circulatory failure) or because of breathing problems (e.g. due to a congestive disorder of the lungs, such as pneumonia). Thus, treatment is of the cause. In severe cases, irreversible changes occur in the nervous system after more than 3 or 4 minutes of oxygen deprivation.

The newborn animal must cope with the transfer from a placental oxygen supply to its own respiration. Undue delay in this transfer leads to anoxia. Anoxic foals and calves suffer brain damage and various clinical syndromes occur. Premature foals, which are especially susceptible, may become 'barkers' or 'wanderers'. Similarly anoxic calves may suffer from the 'weak calf syndrome' and fail to thrive. Chronic anoxia can occur in animals moved from low to high altitudes, where the atmospheric oxygen tension is lower.

ant A small social insect belonging to the order Hymenoptera. Ants are found worldwide but are most common in tropical and subtropical regions. Apart from being a nuisance for livestock, some ant species are intermediate hosts for parasites. For example, in the UK, the ant species *Formica fusca* is an intermediate host for the sheep liver fluke, *Dicrocoelium dendriticum*, found only in western Scotland and North Wales.

antacid An agent that is used to counteract acidity in the stomach. The most widely used antacid compound is sodium bicarbonate, which can be incorporated into stomach powders, added to food, or made up in a drench.

antagonist 1. (in anatomy) A muscle whose action opposes that of another muscle (the *agonist* or *prime mover*). Antagonists relax to allow the agonists to contract. **2.** (in pharmacology) A drug or other substance with opposite action to that of another drug or natural body chemical, which it inhibits. Examples are the *antimetabolites.

ant- (anti-) *Prefix denoting* opposed to; counteracting; relieving. Examples: *antarthritic* (relieving arthritis); *antibacterial* (destroying or stopping the growth of bacteria).

ante- *Prefix denoting* before. Example: *antepartum* (before the onset of labour).

antebrachium (*pl.* **antebrachia**) The forearm; i.e. the region of the forelimb related to the radius and ulna.

antepartum Occurring before the onset of labour.

anterior Describing or relating to the front (or ventral) part of a body, limbs, or organ. In veterinary anatomy, due to the quadripedal form of the main species, the term is largely replaced by *ventral (i.e. towards the belly) and restricted to a few special cases, e.g. the anterior chamber of the eye.

anthelmintic An agent that kills helminth parasites. They can be subdivided according to their effectiveness against the different types of helminths: for example nematocides have activity against nematodes (roundworms); anticestodal compounds have activity against tapeworms; and antitrematodal (flukicidal) compounds are used to kill flukes. Anthelmintics are used in mammals, birds, and reptiles both to treat overt disease due to parasitic infestations, and as part of programmes to control parasite numbers and minimize subclinical disease and consequent economic losses. Ideally the drug should kill the parasites effectively without toxicity to the host, have a broad spectrum of activity with efficacy against adult and larval stages of the parasites, be easy to administer, persist in tissues long enough to kill the parasites yet not leave tissue residues, and be inexpensive. Anthelmintics can be administered orally as tablets, pastes, drenches, incorporated in feed or water, or given as slow-release or pulse-release boluses. Soluble preparations can be injected. A topical pour-on preparation (containing levamisole) is also available. Some parasites have developed resistance to various groups of anthelmintics.

Compounds with a broad spectrum of activity include the *benzimidazoles, *ivermectin, *levamisole, *nitroscanate, *pyrantel, *morantel, and *organophosphorus compounds. Other compounds with a narrower spectrum of activity include *piperazine, *diethylcarbamazine, bephenium, *bunamidine, *diamphenethide, clorsulon, *niclosamide, *oxyclozanide, *nitroxynil, brotianide, *rafoxanide, *praziquantel, phthalofyne, and thenium.

Anthisan Tradename for the *antihistamine mepyramine maleate. It is available for both topical and oral administration to treat allergic reactions, for example insect bites, *urticaria, or *photosensitization. The drug works best if given before histamine release occurs. The main side-effect is drowsiness due to depression of the central nervous system.

anthracosis The presence of small particles of carbon in a tissue or organ. This may be seen either as a prominent black deposit or as fine dark speckling. The carbon particles are usually inhaled from the atmosphere in urban environments. Consequently the main sites of deposition are the lungs and the lymph nodes draining the respiratory tract. The carbon is inert and in small amounts produces no significant effects.

anthraquinones A group of *purgative drugs, originally derived from plants (e.g. aloes, senna, and rhubarb) but now produced synthetically. The active principle is absorbed from the small intestine and metabolized to an anthraquinone, which is excreted into the large intestine, where it has an irritant effect. Purgation occurs several hours after dosing, depending on the volume of contents in the intestinal tract. Anthraquinones are active in all nonruminant species.

anthrax A contagious disease of warm-blooded animals characterized, in herbivores, by fever and sudden death and caused by the bacterium *Bacillus anthracis*. Cattle, sheep, and goats are most susceptible and are frequently found dead, causing confusion of diagnosis with lightning strike, snake bite, or acute poisoning. The disease is less acute, although usually fatal, in camels and horses, and is

seen as extensive swelling of the neck and ventral parts of the body. Pigs and dogs are more resistant and the disease causes swelling of the throat region or intestinal signs, such as diarrhoea or constipation. Scavenger animals tend to show fewer clinical signs of anthrax and many birds appear refractory to the disease, although anthrax can be a problem in captive birds, such as ranched ostriches.

The blood of animals that have died of anthrax contains large numbers of infectious organisms, which form spores when exposed to the air. This may occur when the carcasses are eaten by scavengers (e.g. dogs or vultures) or as carcasses ooze blood or other discharges; milk is also contaminated. Organisms within the carcass and not exposed to air die in 2–3 days. Spore formation is optimal at 37°C in moist conditions at pH 8.0 and will occur within 8 hours. The process stops below 20°C and above 40°C, below relative humidity of 60%, and below pH 6.0. The spores may be dispersed by water, wind, or scavengers, and may persist in the environment for many years. Also, biting flies may transmit the bacteria mechanically. Infection is usually associated with dry dusty conditions when the spores are widely disseminated, or with animals feeding or drinking in areas where animals have previously died of the disease; these areas may be very localized. Possible sources of infection include the effluent from tanneries and inadequately sterilized bone meal.

Animals suspected of having died from anthrax should not be autopsied. Diagnosis is by the demonstration of the organism in fixed blood smears taken from a superficial blood vessel. Care should be taken to inactivate any spores in the smear. Infected animals should be treated with high doses of penicillin, although this will not prevent death due to the toxin produced by the replicating bacteria. Contact animals should be vaccinated with a live spore vaccine, and a routine annual or six-monthly vaccination of other susceptible stock considered. Dead animals and their bedding should be cremated or buried as deep as possible, although spores from buried carcasses have been brought to the surface even after many years. Anthrax is a notifiable disease in the UK and North America.

The bacterium can be transmitted to humans by contact with animal hair, hides, or excrement and causes a potentially fatal disease, attacking either the lungs and causing pneumonia (*woolsorter's disease*), or the skin and producing severe ulceration (*malignant carbuncle* or *malignant pustule*). The administration of large doses of penicillin or tetracycline is usually effective. Other name: **splenic fever**.

anthropozoonosis *See* zoonosis.

antibacterial An agent that destroys or prevents the multiplication of bacteria. *See* antibiotic; antiseptic; disinfectant.

antibiotic A substance, produced by bacteria or fungi, that destroys or prevents the growth of other species of microorganisms (bacteria, fungi, or viruses). Many antibiotics are used to treat bacterial, fungal, and some viral infections in animals, including humans. *Penicillin, originally obtained from the mould *Penicillium notatum*, now from *P. chrysogenum*, was the first antibiotic to be introduced. Antibiotics can be extracted from a culture of microorganisms, but many are now synthesized. They are divided into groups according to their structure or source, and can also be classified according to the types and range of organisms killed. *Broad-spectrum antibiotics* have activity against a wide range of pathogens, including

both Gram-positive and Gram-negative bacteria. *Narrow-spectrum antibiotics* are active against specific groups of microorganisms. Antibiotics used in veterinary therapy include penicillins, *tetracyclines, *aminoglycosides, *macrolide antibiotics, *chloramphenicol, *polymyxins, *lincomycin, *nystatin, *amphotericin B, *griseofulvin, *natamycin, *imidazoles, *bacitracin, vancomycin, and *aminocyclitols. Some are used prophylactically as feed additives to prevent or control infections. Only antibiotics not generally used in human medicine should be employed for this purpose, because of the risk of increasing the incidence of resistant strains of microorganisms. The administration of antibiotics may alter the normal microbial populations at various sites in the body (e.g. intestine, lungs) by destroying one or more groups of harmless organisms. This may result in infections due to overgrowth of resistant organisms, and is more likely to occur with broad-spectrum antibiotics. Resistance may also develop in the organisms being treated (for instance, due to incorrect dosage), and some antibiotics may cause allergic reactions.

antibody Any of a group of serum proteins (*immunoglobulins*) that are produced by certain cells of the *lymphocyte series in response to the presence of *antigens. Antibodies bind specifically to molecules of the eliciting antigen but not to other antigens. This binding protects the body against invading organisms and other foreign antigens, and is fundamental to *immunity. It may also assist in the ingestion of antigenic matter by *phagocytes (*opsonization) and also activate *complement. Immunoglobulin molecules each comprise two parallel 'heavy' chains (of high molecular weight) and two 'light' chains, all united by disulphide bonds. The amino acid sequence in certain regions of both heavy and light chains is highly variable. These variable regions contribute to the three-dimensional structure of the two antigen-binding sites on each molecule, and confer specificity on the antibody.

There are several classes of antibodies, according to the nature of the invariable regions of their heavy chains. IgM antibodies have mu (μ) heavy chains; they are a polymerized form of antibody secreted during the early response to antigens. IgG antibodies, with gamma (γ) heavy chains, appear later in the immune response and are the most abundant immunoglobulin class in normal blood serum. IgA antibodies, with alpha (α) heavy chains, are secreted at mucous surfaces, especially in the alimentary and respiratory tracts. IgE, with epsilon (ε) heavy chains, has a special role in relation to *mast cells and in the mediation of Type I *hypersensitivity.

Maternal IgG antibody passes to the foetus across the placenta before birth in primates and rodents. In most herbivorous mammals, antibody transfer takes place in the first 2 days of life of the newborn, which absorbs the IgG and IgA antibodies across *colostrum across the gut mucosa.

Antibodies can be detected and estimated by means of the reactions they undergo with antigens in vitro (*see* agglutination; precipitation; complement fixation test; enzyme-linked immunosorbent assay). They are also now used in a wide range of assays and tests to label specific antigenic components (*see* monoclonal antibody).

anticholinesterase A drug that inhibits acetylcholinesterase, the enzyme present at nerve endings that degrades the neurotransmitter acetylcholine thereby liberating choline, which is taken up into the synaptic vesicles and reused. The inhibition of acetylcholinesterase leads to a build-

up of acetylcholine at the receptor site, causing continuous stimulation of the post-synaptic cell. The main effects of anticholinesterases are due to a build-up of acetylcholine at parasympathetic postganglionic synapses and neuromuscular junctions. This causes slowing of the heart, salivation, increased gastric and intestinal secretion, increased peristalsis, diarrhoea, bronchoconstriction, increased bronchial secretion, miosis, and skeletal muscle tremor followed by flaccidity. *Reversible anticholinesterases* include *edrophonium, *neostigmine, *physostigmine, pyridostigmine, ambenonium, and carbamate insecticides. *Irreversible anticholinesterases* include many *organophosphorus compounds. The binding of reversible anticholinesterases to the enzyme subsequently breaks down, allowing the release of acetylcholinesterase. Recovery from the action of irreversible anticholinesterases requires new acetylcholinesterase to be synthesized. *Parasympatholytic drugs, e.g. *atropine, act as antidotes to anticholinesterases.

anticoagulant An agent that prevents the coagulation (clotting) of blood. Anticoagulants are used to preserve blood in a liquid state for laboratory examination or to treat or prevent thrombosis or other conditions involving intravascular coagulation. The body's natural anticoagulant, *heparin, is also employed therapeutically; synthetic agents include *warfarin and *dicoumarol. *EDTA is used as an anticoagulant for blood samples taken for certain laboratory tests.

anticonvulsant Any drug that is used to control or prevent *fits. Anticonvulsants are used mainly in dogs but occasionally in cats and other species and are normally administered orally over long periods. The main drugs used are *phenytoin sodium, *phenobarbitone, *primidone, and *diazepam. Phenobarbitone is the drug of choice for maintenance therapy and diazepam is used to treat *status epilepticus*. All have a sedative effect. A combination of drugs may be necessary since the effectiveness of any single drug can change over a period of prolonged dosing. Metabolism of these drugs may be markedly slower in cats and phenobarbitone at a low dose rate or diazepam are the most suitable. For convulsions caused by tetanus or strychnine poisoning or for treatment during fits, diazepam administered intravenously should be used because of its rapid onset of action compared with phenobarbitone.

antidiuretic hormone (ADH) *See* vasopressin.

antidote A substance used to counteract the effects of a poison or other harmful agent. Some antidotes act directly on the poisonous agent making it ineffective, whereas others combat the action the poison produces, for example vitamin K in *warfarin poisoning. Unfortunately not all poisons have a suitable antidote.

antiemetic An agent used to prevent *vomiting. Vomiting is controlled by the vomiting centre in the medulla in the brain, which receives impulses from the chemoreceptor trigger zone in the medulla, from local receptors in the gastrointestinal tract, and from receptors in the labyrinths of the ear. Certain antiemetics act locally to reduce gastric irritation. These include *demulcents (e.g. dextrose and glycerin), which protect and lubricate the gastric mucosa, *antacids (e.g. sodium bicarbonate and magnesium oxide or carbonate), *kaolin, and *bismuth. *Local anaesthetics given orally (e.g. benzocaine and amethocaine) have been used to reduce local nerve stimulation in the gastric mucosa. Other antiemetics act on the central nervous system (CNS). These include the *parasympatholytic drugs (e.g. hyoscine and atropine), *phenothiazine tranquillizers (e.g. promethazine, chlorpromazine, promazine, and acetylpromazine), the dopamine agonist *metoclopramide, and the *antihistamines (e.g. diphenhydramine, dimenhydramine, and meclizine). Phenothiazines and antihistamines are used in dogs to prevent *travel sickness. Chlorbutol, which is used in humans and dogs to prevent travel sickness, has both a local effect on the gastric mucosa and acts as a depressant on the vomiting centre in the CNS.

antifoaming agent *See* antizymotic.

antifreeze poisoning *See* ethylene glycol poisoning.

antifungal An agent used to control fungal infections. Some antibiotics have activity against certain species of fungi, including the polyene macrolide antibiotics (*amphotericin B, *nystatin, and *natamycin), *imidazoles, and *griseofulvin. *Sodium iodide has also been used parenterally to treat fungal infections. A wider range of topical antifungal agents are available to treat localized infections affecting skin, ears, eyes, and mucous membranes. These are incorporated into washes, lotions, sprays, powders, and creams, and include benzoic acid, undecylenate, propionic acid, iodine preparations, copper sulphate, dichlorophen, salicylic acid, gentian violet, phenol, sulphur compounds, imidazoles, hydroxyquinolines, and polyene antibiotics.

antigen Any substance that is capable of being recognized by the immunocompetent body as foreign, such as invading organisms, toxins, nonself tissues, etc. This recognition gives rise to an immune response (*hypersensitivity or *antibody formation) and often some degree of acquired *resistance to the antigen. Antigens are always compounds of substantial molecular weight (over 5 KD). *See also* hapten; immunity.

antigenic variation The process by which a pathogenic organism, such as a virus, changes its antigenic appearance to the host cell or animal (*see* antigen). The variation may be caused by mutation or selection of a new strain of the virus or by some other mechanism. *See* influenzavirus.

antiglobulin An *antibody formed in response to and specific for *globulin antigens. Antiglobulins are usually induced when animals are injected with globulin from another species.

antihistamine A drug that inhibits the action of *histamine in the body and so reduces acute inflammation, especially in allergic reactions (H_1-receptor antagonists). Antihistamines blocking H_1 receptors have a structure resembling that of histamine and work by competing for histamine's normal receptor sites in tissues. Hence antihistamines are of value only if administered prior to histamine release or immediately an inflammatory reaction occurs. They are used to treat allergic reactions, for instance insect bites, urticaria, and photosensitization. In acute cases the antihistamine can be given intravenously although excitation of the central nervous system (CNS) may occur. Antihistamines acting on H_1 receptors have a structure similar to tranquillizers, hence their side-effects of drowsiness (at normal doses) or excitation (at high doses). Thus some, for example cyclizine (Marzine), are used to prevent travel sickness.

The main antihistamines are mepyramine maleate (*Anthisan), diphenhydramine hydrochloride (Piriton), tripelennamine hydrochloride (Vetibenzamine), promethazine (Phenergan), and cyclizine. Of these Piriton is the most potent, whereas Phenergan is longer acting with effects lasting up to 24 hours. Vetibenzamine has been used intravenously as a CNS stimulant in the *downer cow syndrome. Histamine is also involved in the control of gastric secretion, but the histamine receptors involved (H_2 receptors) are not affected by the above compounds. However, cimetidine (Tagamet) and metiamide are antihistamines that do act to reduce gastric acid secretion, and these H_2 antagonists can be used in dogs to treat gastric ulcers.

anti-inflammatory An agent that reduces *inflammation. The various groups of anti-inflammatory agents have activity against one or more of the mediators that initiate or maintain an inflammatory response. Some groups suppress only certain aspects of the inflammatory response. *Antihistamines act in the early stages of inflammation; *NSAIDs have activity against prostaglandin-mediated inflammation; and glucocorticoids (*see* corticosteroid) influence the entire inflammatory response. In cases of acute inflammation associated with *anaphylaxis, *adrenaline can be used to antagonize the actions of the inflammatory mediators. Many other agents, including gold salts, metalloproteins, plant products (e.g. cinchophen), *hyaluronic acid, and polysulphated glycosaminoglycans, are used in the treatment of chronic inflammatory conditions.

antimetabolite Any of a group of drugs used in the treatment of malignant diseases. They closely resemble certain molecules (metabolites) that are essential for the functioning and multiplication of cells and are incorporated into rapidly dividing tumour cells thereby leading to their death.

antimitotic An agent that causes disruption of cell division (mitosis). Antimitotics have a wide variety of mechanisms, with activity at specific phases during the cell cycle. Rapidly dividing cells, such as neoplastic cells, cells of the bone marrow, and gastrointestinal epithelial cells, are more susceptible to the effects of such agents. Examples of antimitotic drugs are *colchicine, 5-fluorouracil, cytosine arabinoside, *vincristine, vinblastine, and alkylating agents (e.g. *cyclophosphamide). These drugs are used in the treatment of cancer. Their side-effects are due to disruption of mitosis in areas of rapid cell division (e.g. the bone marrow and gastrointestinal tract), causing immunosuppression, vomiting, and diarrhoea. However, the immunosuppression can be used to prevent transplant rejection and in the treatment of immune-mediated diseases, such as rheumatoid arthritis, systemic lupus erythematosus, and autoimmune haemolytic anaemia.

antimony potassium tartrate A drug used to treat protozoan infections and first introduced in 1918. It inhibits phosphofructokinase, an enzyme in the *glycolysis pathway, but mammalian phosphofructokinase is much less sensitive to antimony compounds than the corresponding enzyme in protozoa. Absorption from the gut is poor and the drug is administered slowly intravenously. The drug binds to red blood cells and its excretion from the kidneys is very slow, taking several days. It has been used to treat *schistosomiasis, *trypanosomiasis, and other protozoan infections. Possible side-effects include coughing, pneumonia, joint pain, and cardiac and hepatic dysfunction. The drug is contraindicated in animals with hepatic, renal, or cardiac conditions.

antimycotic A drug used in the treatment of fungal infections. Some are used orally but others are more toxic and thus are applied topically. Griseofulvin, natamycin, nystatin, miconazole, and amphotericin B are the main drugs in veterinary use. Besides these a large number of other compounds are used topically (either singly or in mixtures) against fungi, including mercury preparations, iodine preparations, copper sulphate, sulphur, benzoic acid, salicylic acid, and crystal violet.

antioxidant A molecule which can inhibit the oxidation of other molecules. For example, in animal metabolism *vitamin E functions as a natural antioxidant, inhibiting the oxidation of unsaturated fatty acids in the body.

antiperistalsis A wave of muscular contraction in the alimentary tract that passes in the direction of the mouth. It occurs during regurgitation in ruminants (see rumination).

antipruritic A drug that reduces itching of the skin (*pruritus). Most have anti-inflammatory properties (e.g. *corticosteroids). Topical applications of cream or ointment containing various mixtures of anti-inflammatory drugs and local anaesthetics can be used.

antipyretic A drug that reduces *fever (pyrexia) by lowering body temperature. Such drugs include the antipyretic analgesic anti-inflammatory agents (see NSAID), *phenothiazines, and *quinidine. The application of cold water to the body surface also reduces body temperature, by evaporative cooling.

antiseptic A substance that is applied to living tissue to destroy pathogenic microorganisms or to prevent their growth. Antiseptics are used to clean wounds and in the preparation of the skin surface prior to surgery. An antiseptic should have a wide spectrum of activity against microorganisms, be nonirritant to living tissue, and retain its activity in the presence of exudates. Among the more commonly used antiseptics are *phenols, iodine- and chorine-containing compounds (e.g. *iodophors), *cationic detergents, *alcohols, *gentian violet, acridine dyes, chlorhexidine, hydrogen peroxide, benzoyl peroxide, and various acids.

antiserum (*pl.* **antisera**) Serum containing antibodies of known specificity. It may be injected to treat, or to give temporary protection (passive *immunity) against, specific diseases. In the laboratory, antisera are used to identify unknown microorganisms (*see* agglutination).

antisialic (antisialogogue) An agent that reduces the secretion of saliva, for example *atropine. Antisialics are used prior to anaesthesia when irritant inhalational anaesthetics, such as ether, are to be administered. They are less useful in ruminants, since they lead to formation of a thick viscid saliva, but secretion is not abolished.

antispasmodic *See* spasmolytic.

antitoxin An *antibody formed in response to and specific for a toxin antigen. Antitoxins precipitate the corresponding toxin, and may be protective if administered to an animal.

antitussive An agent that relieves or suppresses coughing. It may be a depressant drug that acts centrally on the cough centre in the brain (e.g. *codeine and *butorphanol) or an agent that reduces the irritation and inflammation in the pharyngeal region. Various cough mixtures are available incorporating soothing agents (e.g. *linctus). Reduction of viscosity of bronchial secretions using *bromhexine can also alleviate coughing.

antivenin **1.** An *antitoxin to a *venom. **2.** An antiserum containing such antitoxins.

antiviral agent An agent that prevents the multiplication of viruses and is used to treat viral infections. Viruses multiply using host-cell apparatus, hence antiviral agents have a tendency to be toxic to the host. They are mainly used in human medicine, although such drugs as *acyclovir, idoxuridine, ribavirin, amantadine, and rimantadine have some veterinary applications. *Interferons are the body's natural antiviral agents, and several drugs are used in human medicine to try to increase interferon levels. However, these drugs are toxic and are not used widely in animal treatment because of their expense. Species specific interferons will become available for veterinary usage in future.

antizymotic An agent that reduces fermentation and gas formation in the gastrointestinal tract or reduces the stability of foam and allows the release of gas. They are used in the control of *bloat in ruminants and, occasionally, to treat *colic in horses. Antizymotics that reduce the number of gas-producing organisms in the digestive tract include oil of *turpentine, linseed oil, *formalin, and antibiotics. Antifoaming agents, which are used especially to prevent and treat frothy bloat, include poloxalene, polymerized methyl silicone, polyethylene glycol, and various vegetable oils.

Polyoxypropylene-polyoxyethylene polymer series derivatives (PPD) give fast relief in cases of frothy bloat and protect against reformation for the next 12 hours. They can be used in dairy cattle because they are not excreted in the milk. Turpentine oil is liable to taint milk and should not be used in lactating cattle.

antrum A space or cavity. The *antrum folliculi* is the fluid-filled cavity within an ovarian *follicle. The *pyloric antrum* is the initial two-thirds of the pyloric part of the stomach, and is relatively wide and thin-walled.

ANTU (alpha naphthyl thiourea) A thiourea derivative that is used as a rodenticide. It is a tasteless, odourless, crystalline powder used in bait to kill rats. Toxicity varies with species, brown rats being more susceptible than black rats; poultry are not affected. It causes a massive increase in permeability of the lung capillaries with consequent fluid-filled lungs (pulmonary oedema) leading to lack of oxygen (anoxia) and death.
ANTU poisoning This is most commonly seen in dogs. If rat bait containing ANTU is consumed on an empty stomach, vomiting occurs and thus very little poison is absorbed. If the stomach is partly full the drug is retained longer and signs of pulmonary oedema, laboured breathing, and frothing at the mouth occur. There is no satisfactory treatment. Emetics and diuretics can be tried but once pulmonary oedema develops the prognosis is poor.

anuria Failure of urine production by the kidneys. This can occur in a variety of conditions producing sustained low blood pressure and consequent inadequate blood supply to the kidneys with a lowering of filtration pressure in the glomeruli. Anuria may also arise due to acute kidney damage by toxic substances or infection, or because of obstruction to the flow or urine from the kidneys, for example by calculi (*see* calculus), which increases the back pressure within the urinary system and eventually stops

glomerular filtration. Anuria is potentially life-threatening: toxic metabolites are not eliminated from the body and there is disturbance of electrolyte levels and the *acid-base balance. Treatment requires accurate diagnosis and resolution of the cause.

anus The terminal opening of the *alimentary tract through which faeces are discharged to the exterior from the final part of the alimentary canal (the *anal canal*). The anus is surrounded by the external and internal anal *sphincters, which close the orifice except during defecation. *See also* anal gland.

aorta (*pl.* **aortae** or **aortas**) The largest artery in the body, arising from the left ventricle of the heart and carrying oxygenated blood via its branches to all parts of the body. Its walls are thick and contain much elastic tissue. The first, ascending part of the aorta leads to the *aortic arch, which curves upward and backward to the descending part. The portion in front of the diaphragm is termed the *thoracic part* of the aorta while the portion behind the diaphragm is the *abdominal part*.

aortic arch That part of the *aorta that curves upward, backward, and slightly to the left of the midline. It gives rise to arteries supplying the head and neck (common carotid) and forelimb (subclavian). The wall of the aortic arch contains nerve endings that monitor blood pressure and thereby help to regulate this. Occasionally the aortic arch may be formed by abnormal persistence of a vessel on the right – *persistent right aortic arch*. This can lead to vascular constriction of the oesophagus resulting in difficulty in swallowing solid food.

aortic rupture Tearing of the *aorta, which results in a fatal haemorrhage.

Supravalvular aortic ruptures occur in horses as a result of a sudden increase in blood pressure. *Aortic ring ruptures* have been described in stallions, and a similar problem occurs in turkeys. The latter usually affects heavy turkeys, often the most rapidly growing birds, but may occur in younger birds as well as capons and laying hens. Most at risk are male turkeys aged 5–22 weeks, especially at 10–14 weeks, and the incidence varies from a few cases to 5% or more. There are no warning signs. The dead birds have pale heads from loss of blood due to internal haemorrhage, and occasionally there is blood seepage from the mouth. Usually it is the abdominal aorta that ruptures, filling the abdominal cavity with blood. The condition is associated with the turkey's naturally high blood pressure, in combination with *atherosclerosis. Degeneration of the blood vessels is more frequent in male birds and blood pressure peaks at about 22 weeks. A tranquillizer can be used in the feed to lower the birds' blood pressure.

aortic valve A valve in the heart guarding the opening from the left ventricle into the ascending part of the aorta. It consists of three half-moon-shaped flaps (*see* semilunar valve) and prevents blood returning to the ventricle from the aorta. Narrowing of the valve's orifice (aortic *stenosis) results in obstruction of blood flow into the aorta. Incompetence of the valve leads to regurgitation of blood into the left ventricle.

aortoiliac thrombosis A condition of horses in which a blood clot partially occludes the blood supply to one or both back legs. The horse is suddenly unwilling to exercise but recovers quickly. The affected limb is cool and has poor venous filling. Rectal examination may be helpful in diagnosis, and confirmation may be

possible with *ultrasonography. Treatment regimes include rest, Dextran 70, and sodium gluconate.

apex (*pl.* **apices**) The tip or summit of an organ. For example, an *apical abscess* surrounds the root of a tooth. The *apex beat* is felt on the chest wall when this is struck by the apex of the heart during *systole.

aphthous fever *See* foot-and-mouth disease.

aphthovirus A genus of the *picornavirus family containing the bovine *foot-and-mouth disease virus.

Apicomplexa A phylum of parasitic protozoa, formerly called Sporozoa, characterized by having complex structures at the cell apex (visible by electron microscopy). It includes important disease-causing parasites, such as *Plasmodium, *Babesia, *Theileria, *Toxoplasma, *Eimeria, and *Cryptosporidium.

aplasia Total or partial failure of development of an organ or tissue. *See also* agenesis.

apnoea Cessation of breathing. Respiration is stimulated by the medullary respiratory centre in the brainstem, and apnoea may occur as a result of general anaesthesia, particularly in aged, debilitated, or toxaemic animals. *Analeptic drugs, for example picrotoxin or Megimide, are used to stimulate breathing in such cases.

apocrine 1. Describing a method of *secretion in which large secretory droplets develop in the cytoplasm of the apex of the cell and are subsequently released from the cell along with the surrounding cytoplasm and the plasma membrane. **2.** Describing a gland whose cells perform apocrine secretion, such as sweat glands and mammary glands.

Apocynum poisoning A toxic condition arising from ingestion of various species of *Apocynum*, a genus of perennial herbaceous plants distributed throughout the USA and including the Indian hemp and dogbane. They contain cardiac glycosides and resinoids, which cause increased body temperature, sweating, anorexia, elevated pulse, discoloration of mucous membranes, gastrointestinal disorders, and death. Treatment is of the clinical signs.

apomorphine A derivative of *morphine used to stimulate vomiting. It is no longer available for veterinary use in the UK.

aponeurosis (*pl.* **aponeuroses**) A thin but strong sheet of fibrous tissue that acts as a *tendon in muscles that are flat and sheetlike and have a wide area of attachment.

apophysis A projection from a bone.

apoplexy A sudden neurological disturbance producing loss of consciousness, usually associated with intracranial haemorrhage. In animals injury is the most likely cause; 'strokes' are not commonly recognized.

appendix A small structure that joins another main structure. The *appendix epididymis* and *appendix testis* are abnormal persistent remnants of the embryonic mesonephric and paramesonephric ducts respectively and may occur near to the head of the *epididymis. The *vermiform appendix* of man is a short tube attached to the end of the caecum.

appetite The desire to find and ingest food, normally as a result of hunger. Appetite depends on the activity of the hunger and satiety centres in the *hypothalamus, although food intake is regulated by other factors as well (*see* voluntary food intake). Depraved appetite (*pica) may be shown by animals suffering certain diseases, especially nutritional deficiencies.

apricot *See* cherry laurel poisoning.

aqueduct A narrow fluid-filled canal. For example, the *cerebral aqueduct* (or *aqueduct of Sylvius*) connects the third and fourth ventricles of the brain. The *vestibular aqueduct* is a canal in the *temporal bone of the skull that carries the endolymphatic duct.

aqueous humour The clear watery fluid that fills the anterior and posterior chambers of the *eye. It is continually produced in the *ciliary processes and drains away through the angle between the cornea and sclera into the venous system. Increased pressure of aqueous humour leads to *glaucoma.

Arachnida A class of arthropods (*see* Arthropoda) which includes the ticks, mites, scorpions, and spiders. All arachnids have a body divided into two regions. The anterior cephalothorax (*prosoma*) bears two pairs of appendages used for grasping or piercing or for sensory purposes, and, in the adults, four pairs of legs. The posterior abdomen (*opisthosoma*) may bear various sensory or silk-spinning appendages. The eggs hatch into miniature adults and there is no pupal stage. Most are terrestrial and carnivorous but all *ticks and some *mites are parasites of livestock and pets.

arachnoid (arachnoid mater) The middle of the three membranes (*meninges) that surround the brain and spinal cord. The arachnoid is thin and finely textured with no blood supply of its own. Within it lies the *pia, to which it is attached by numerous fine strands across the intervening subarachnoid space, which contains *cerebrospinal fluid and blood vessels. Outside the arachnoid lies the *dura, from which it is separated by the potential subdural space. Numerous fine processes, the arachnoid villi, project from the arachnoid into venous sinuses of the dura to allow the cerebrospinal fluid to pass into the venous system.

arbovirus An obsolete term for an assorted group of viruses that are all transmitted by arthropods, particularly insects, hence *ar*(thropod) *bo*(rne) *virus*. Members of this group are now reclassified in the *togavirus, *bunyavirus, *reovirus, and *rhabdovirus families.

arch- (arche-, archi-, archo-) *Prefix denoting* first; beginning; primitive; ancestral. Example: *archinephron* (first-formed embryonic kidney).

archenteron The primitive gut: the cavity of the yolk sac from which the embryonic gut is formed.

area eradication A scheme for the gradual eradication of an enzootic animal disease from a country or region by successively eliminating it from selected areas. It requires a highly developed state veterinary service, cooperation from the livestock industry, and comprehensive and effective identification of animals and regulation of their movements. Initially, 'eradication areas' are selected in which the disease already has a low incidence, and effort is concentrated upon eliminating the remaining disease-carrying animals (reactors) from these areas. This is achieved by testing and slaughter or authorized sale of reactors outside the eradication area. Movement of animals into the area is restricted. When an area becomes disease-free or vitually so, surveillance continues while a similar regime is applied to other areas. When the whole country is within the scheme, the level of surveillance can be relaxed, but not discontinued entirely. Area eradication has been successfully used in the UK for the almost complete elimination of *tuberculosis and *brucellosis in cattle.

arecoline An alkaloid derived from betel nut that acts as a *parasympathomimetic agent. It was formerly used as a purgative and to treat tapeworm infestations in dogs but has now been replaced by safer drugs.

areolar tissue Loose *connective tissue consisting of a meshwork of collagen, elastic tissue, and reticular fibres interspersed with numerous connective tissue cells. It binds the skin to underlying muscles and forms a link between organs while allowing a high degree of movement.

Argas A genus of soft *ticks found worldwide, also known as fowl ticks or tampans. They are ectoparasites of birds, especially domestic fowls, but will also bite humans, horses, and cattle. The adults and nymphs feed at night while the host is asleep and are usually found in the host's nest; the larvae remain attached to the host for 5–10 days. The adults can survive for 5 years without feeding if no suitable host is available. A heavy infestation causes intense irritation, anaemia, and even death while moderate attacks lead to loss of condition and a reduction in egg production. In the tropics they also transmit protozoan parasites, causing fevers, as well as bacterial diseases, such as fowl *spirochaetosis.

Argemone *See* blood root poisoning.

arginine *See* amino acid; urea.

Arizona infection A disease of young turkeys caused by the bacterium *Salmonella arizona*. It is usually transmitted through the egg from infected breeder flocks, and can cause up to 50% mortality in poults during the first week of life. The clinical signs are of general ill-health with nervous signs, including huddling, diarrhoea with pasted vent, twisted neck, listlessness, convulsions, and paralysis. From 2 weeks the nervous signs are less severe but other signs, including blindness, are more frequent. Clinical signs and mortality are very rare in adult birds. Treatment with nitrofurans is generally successful, but should be followed by thorough cleaning and disinfection of the building once the flock has been cleared. Infected breeder flocks show no clinical signs and are best eliminated.

aromatic Describing an organic molecule that contains the ring-shaped benzene molecule in its structure or has chemical properties similar to benzene. Many biologically important molecules contain aromatic rings, including the *amino acids phenylalanine, tyrosine, and tryptophan, and the hormone *adrenaline.

arrhythmia Deviation from the normal rhythm (sinus rhythm) of the heart. The heart rhythm is normally controlled by the heart's natural pacemaker, the *sinoatrial node, which is located in the wall of the right atrium and controls the contractions of heart muscle via a specialized conducting network (*see* atrioventricular bundle; atrioventricular node) that transmits impulses from the walls of the atria to the ventricles. The system is designed to achieve optimum coordination of atrial and ventricular contractions and thus maximum mechanical efficiency. *Sinus arrhythmia* is a normal slight alteration of heart rhythm related to breathing: the heart quickens on inspiration and slows during expiration. Other arrhythmias

can have pathological significance and arise because of disturbances in the nerve impulses or the conducting network. They may be detected in the pulse or by listening to the heart but are best investigated by *electrocardiography. *Premature beats* occur when the ventricles beat prematurely. In *atrial fibrillation*, which occurs in dogs, horses, and cows, the atrial contractions are increased and ineffective. In dogs, this condition may develop in congestive *heart failure or in association with *cardiomyopathy. Treatment can include the administration of *cardiac glycosides, quinidine, disopyramide, or propranolol. In *heart block there is a failure of the conduction system or increased influence of the *vagus nerve producing slower and less forceful contractions. Ventricular *tachycardia involves an increase in the ventricular contraction rate due to ectopic activity, sometimes from foci of diseased muscle.

arsanilic acid An organic compound containing arsenic that is used in pig and poultry production as a growth promoter and to control disease. It is incorporated in pig feed to control *swine dysentery. Chronic poisoning can occur in pigs especially when fresh water is not readily available. Signs of toxicity are blindness, head tremor, staggering, incoordination, and eventually paralysis and death. Affected pigs recover if the drug is withdrawn and unlimited fresh water is provided. In any case, the drug should be withdrawn prior to slaughter to ensure that tissues are free of residues.

arsenic A greyish metallic element, some compounds of which are highly toxic to animals. The most common compound is the relatively insoluble arsenic trioxide (As_4O_6), although arsenites are used as slug bait and in weedkillers, sheep dips, grain dressings, and wood preservatives, and arsenates are used in sprays to control pests on fruit. Organic arsenic compounds are used in pig and poultry feeds as growth promoters and to prevent disease (*see* arsanilic acid). Absorption of arsenic compounds depends on their solubility and particle size: arsenites are absorbed rapidly whereas trioxides often pass out unchanged in the faeces. Absorption can occur through skin or wounds as well as the gut. Generally, compounds containing trivalent arsenic are more toxic than those with the pentavalent form, and organic arsenicals are less toxic than inorganic compounds.

Arsenic poisoning *Acute poisoning* usually occurs when an animal accidentally consumes arsenic. Also therapeutic doses of organic arsenicals may become toxic in debilitated or dehydrated patients. Signs of acute toxicity are salivation, thirst, vomiting, colic, haemorrhagic diarrhoea, low body temperature, collapse, and convulsions. Some cases show haemorrhagic dermatitis. *Chronic toxicity* is occasionally seen in animals grazing around smelting works where pastures may be contaminated by arsenic. Signs are a wasting disease with a dull coat and congested mucous membranes. Arsenic poisoning can be diagnosed by testing urine samples or samples taken post mortem from liver, kidney, hair, or hooves. *Emetics should be administered in cases of acute toxicity. *Demulcents can be used to coat the damaged gastrointestinal tract. Dimercaprol (British Anti-Lewisite) is given as an antidote. It is injected as a 5% solution although it is less useful against inorganic arsenicals.

arter- (arteri-, arterio-) *Prefix denoting* an artery. Examples: *arteriopathy* (disease of); *arteriorrhaphy* (suture of); *arteriovenous* (relating to arteries and veins).

arteriogram 1. A radiograph of an artery (*see* arteriography). **2.** The tracing of the wave form of an arterial pulse.

arteriography *Radiography of an artery. The radiograph (*arteriogram*) is is taken after injection of a radioopaque substance into the arterial system; the column of radio-opacity produced outlines the internal walls of the artery. Correct timing is of great importance.

arteriole A small branch of an artery leading into many smaller vessels – the *capillaries. Arterioles have a well-developed layer of smooth muscle in their walls under the influence of the sympathetic division of the autonomic nervous system. By their constriction and dilation they are the principal controllers of blood flow and pressure.

arteriovenous anastomosis A blood vessel that directly connects an arteriole and a venule, thereby bypassing the capillary network. The vessel wall contains smooth muscle under autonomic nervous control. When the vessel is dilated, blood passes directly to the venous system; when constricted it flows through the capillary network. Such anastomoses occur in various tissues, particularly in the skin, to control heat loss, and in erectile tissue. *Compare* glomus.

arteritis Inflammation of the wall of one or more arteries. This may occur as an extension of a local tissue disorder, especially suppurative or necrotizing inflammation caused by bacteria and fungi. It may also occur in *septicaemia and *viraemia, notably in cases of salmonellosis, swine fever, swine erysipelas, bovine malignant catarrhal fever, and equine viral arteritis. The condition is also found in association with Type III *hypersensitivity reactions and several parasitisms, including *Strongylus vulgaris* infestation, *dirofilariasis, and *schistosomiasis. The effects of arteritis depend on the extent and distribution of the inflammation within the vessel wall. Inflammation of small arteries may have few consequences, particularly if the endothelium is unaffected. Endothelial damage often leads to thrombosis with consequent infarction or embolism. The latter process is involved in producing the characteris-

tic skin lesions found in swine fever and swine erysipelas. Arteritis may be accompanied by oedema and haemorrhage; these are highly characteristic changes in equine viral arteritis.

Polyarteritis and *periarteritis nodosa* describe a form of arteritis often found in virus infections that lead to immunological disorder such as *Aleutian disease in mink. The lesions begin as oedema in the media and adventitia of the wall, and subse-

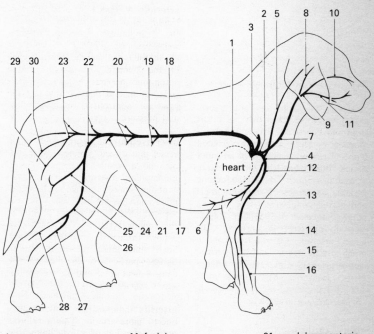

1 aorta	11 facial	21 caudal mesenteric
2 brachiocephalic trunk	12 axillary	22 external iliac
3 left subclavian	13 brachial	23 internal iliac
4 right subclavian	14 median	24 deep femoral
5 vertebral	15 ulnar	25 femoral
6 internal thoracic	16 radial	26 popliteal
7 common carotid	17 coeliac	27 cranial tibial
8 internal carotid	18 cranial mesenteric	28 caudal tibial
9 external carotid	19 renal	29 internal pudendal
10 maxillary	20 testicular or ovarian	30 caudal gluteal

Principal arteries of the dog

artery

quently develop through necrotic, exudative, and fibrotic stages. In the latter the vessel may show nodular enlargement due to the presence of many mononuclear cells.

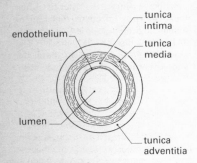

Transverse section through an artery

artery A blood vessel carrying blood from the heart. All except the *pulmonary artery carry oxygenated blood. Their walls consist of an inner tunica *intima lined by *endothelium, a middle tunica *media containing variable quantities of smooth muscle and elastic connective tissue, and an outer connective tissue layer (tunica *adventitia) (see illustration). The larger arteries, e.g. *aorta, contain much elastic tissue and are termed *elastic arteries*, while smaller arteries further from the heart contain more smooth muscle and are termed *muscular arteries* (see arteriole).

arthr- (arthro-) *Prefix denoting* a joint. Examples: *arthrology* (science of); *arthrosclerosis* (stiffening or hardening of).

arthritis (*pl.* **arthritides**) Inflammation of one or several joints. There are several types of arthritis. *Infective* or *septic arthritis* is caused by infectious agents, usually bacteria (see mycoplasmal arthritis). These may have pene-

trated the joint from the exterior or pre-existing local infection, or they may have been carried by the bloodstream. The affected joint is hot, swollen, and very painful. The synovial membrane becomes reddened and thickened, and proteolytic enzymes produced by the bacteria damage the articular cartilage. The lubricant properties of the synovial fluid are affected by inflammatory exudates, with increased amounts of protein, white blood cells, and cellular debris. In some cases the fluid may be purulent. Treatment usually involves the administration of antibiotics to control the infection. In some instances the joint cavity may be irrigated in an attempt to limit damage to the articular surface.

In **poultry**, arthritis is seen most commonly in the limb joints. In epizootic form it is caused by a reovirus or a mycoplasma, while sporadically it may be associated with *Staphylococcus*, *Salmonella*, *Pasteurella*, and *Aspergillus* species and coliform bacteria.

In *osteoarthritis* (more correctly known as *osteoarthrosis*) there is degeneration of the joint structures rather than infection. With increasing age the articular cartilage becomes less resilient and develops a felt-like appearance. Cracks and other defects arise, eventually leading to exposure of the underlying bone; the synovial membrane becomes inflamed. New bone forms around the joint margins. These changes result in joint stiffness and pain. Treatment includes the administration of *anti-inflammatory drugs and *analgesics. In *autoimmune arthritis*, the inflammation is associated with the production of antibodies against self antigens (see rheumatoid arthritis; systemic lupus erythematosus). Treatment is designed to suppress the inflammatory response. *See also* arthrosis; polyarthritis.

54

arthrodesis The surgical fusion of bones across a joint space. This is performed to eliminate movement of the joint, for example when the joint is very painful, highly unstable, or grossly deformed. *Compare* arthroplasty.

arthrography *Radiography of a joint cavity. The radiograph (*arthrogram*) is taken after injection of a radio-opaque substance into the joint space. A thorough knowledge of the joint anatomy is vital, particularly in complex joints (e.g. tarsus), which have communicating joint cavities.

arthrogryposis Congenital fixation of the limb joints. It has been recorded in many breeds of cattle and also in pigs and sheep. There are both genetic and environmental causes, resulting in *muscular dystrophy and consequent immobilization of the joints and spinal deformities. In Charolais cattle this condition is associated with *cleft palate, being known as the *syndrome of arthrogryposis and palatoschisis (SAP)*. It is caused by a *recessive allele, whose frequency in the population has increased due to associated fertility and longevity advantages in the heterozygote. When severe, SAP is lethal. It is suspected that arthrogryposis in the absence of cleft palate may also be inherited. Of the environmental causes, intrauterine infection with *akabane virus is important. The condition is often accompanied by *spina bifida and kyphoscoliosis (i.e. a combination of *kyphosis and *scoliosis).

arthropathy Any disease or disorder involving a joint.

arthroplasty Surgical construction of a new joint or surgical remodelling of a diseased joint. Excision of the head of the femur (*hip excision arthroplasty*) is employed in the management of severe hip pain, due to, for example,

Legge-Perthes disease, hip dysplasia, etc. Alteration of the shape of the hip socket (acetabulum) is a form of arthroplasty that can relieve pain by changing the apposition of the weight-bearing surfaces.

Arthropoda A phylum of invertebrates and the largest in the animal kingdom. Arthropods have a segmented body and a hard exoskeleton, so that growth can occur only by moulting. Each body segment has a pair of jointed appendages which can function variously as mouthparts, legs, wings, gills, sense organs, or reproductive organs. The phylum includes the crustaceans, arachnids, insects, centipedes, and millipedes. Many are of great veterinary importance, especially the *mites, *ticks, and insects (*see* Insecta).

arthroscopy The direct examination of the interior of a joint using a special optical instrument – an *arthroscope*. Arthroscopy permits the evaluation of many joint lesions and facilitates the taking of biopsies for histological examination and the removal of small bone fragments. The progress of arthritic cases can be monitored by repeated arthroscopic examination, thereby avoiding full-scale *arthrotomy. All arthroscopic examinations require aseptic conditions.

arthrosis 1. (in anatomy) A joint. **2.** Degenerative disease of a joint or joints, known colloquially as *arthritis (which refers nonspecifically to inflammation of a joint). Arthrosis is a problem of ageing and occurs in load-bearing joints. It may be a primary condition or develop secondarily after injury or in association with other joint abnormalities, such as *hip dysplasia or *osteochondritis. The normally smooth articular cartilage undergoes degeneration in a process known as *fibrillation*, becoming

arthrotomy

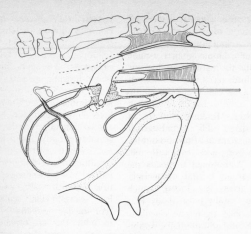

Artificial insemination in the cow. A hand is inserted into the rectum in order to position the cervix to receive the pipette or straw. The inseminate is deposited in the anterior cervix or body of the uterus.

discoloured and developing fissures and defects. Since mature cartilage cannot repair itself the lesions persist. The bone lying immediately beneath the defective tissue responds by increasing in density (*subchondral sclerosis*) and spurs of new bone (*periarticular osteophytes*) develop around the joint; these may be seen radiographically. The joint capsule becomes thickened due to proliferation of the synovial membrane and inflammatory changes. The affected joint is stiff and painful and shows a decreased range of movement. Heavy exercise exacerbates the condition. *Crepitus may be felt on palpation. Treatment is designed to alleviate the pain and reduce inflammation and may involve the administration of *analgesics and *anti-inflammatory drugs.

arthrotomy Surgical incision into a joint. It is performed for exploration of a diseased joint, to permit removal of loose portions of articular cartilage in cases of *osteochondritis, and to permit ligament repair or replacement of a ligament by a prosthesis.

articulation *See* joint.

artifact (artefact) (in microscopy) A structure seen in a tissue under a microscope that is not present in the living tissue. Artifacts, which are produced by faulty *fixation or staining of the tissue, may give a false impression that disease or abnormality is present in the tissue when it is not.

artificial insemination (AI) The introduction of spermatozoa into the uterus or vagina in the absence of copulation. The technique may be employed in all domestic species and exploits the fact that there are far more spermatozoa present in an ejaculate than are needed to fertilize one oocyte; thus it is possible to collect, dilute, and store *semen from genetically superior sires and use this for inseminating females. AI thus enables genetic improvement in a population to be made more rapidly and on a wider scale than would be possible with natural insemination. Other advantages of AI include a reduced risk of transmitting venereal diseases, and elimination of the need to feed and house a potentially dangerous breeding male. Disadvantages include the necessity for very good *oestrus detection and accurate timing of insemination, as well as a *conception rate that is usually slightly lower than natural service. Moreover, widespread use of few sires leads to *inbreeding and the attendant risk of undesirable traits being expressed. Once collected, the semen is examined to assess the concentration and viability of spermatozoa before being diluted, which increases the number of doses that can be obtained from one ejaculate. The diluent contains nutrients, antibiotics, and buffers, as well as a cryoprotectant (such as *glycerol) to protect the cells if they are to be frozen. Most semen is now stored in small plastic straws for freezing; each straw contains sufficient spermatozoa to ensure that enough viable cells remain after thawing.

In **cattle**, the widespread use of AI (around 70% of the UK dairy herd is currently inseminated) is due to the suitability of bovine semen for deep-freezing, which preserves its viability for an indefinite period. Semen is collected using an artificial vagina or occasionally by electroejaculation (*see* ejaculation), although this tends to produce an inferior sample. The use of AI in beef cattle has increased since the advent of *oestrus synchronization techniques has reduced the need for accurate heat detection. See illustration.

In **sheep**, semen is collected using an artificial vagina. Most inseminations use fresh semen since the intracervical insemination of thawed frozen semen gives poor results. Using a *laparoscope it is possible to inseminate successfully into the uterus using thawed frozen semen, but it is doubtful if this will become a commercial technique.

In **pigs**, only about 5% of the UK breeding herd currently uses AI because of the problem in trying to freeze boar semen satisfactorily. Thus, most pig AI involves the use of fresh semen, which has a shelf-life of only a few days; this means rapid processing and delivery before the semen's viability decreases. Collection involves the use of an artificial vagina.

In **horses**, AI is not widely used in the UK due to the fact that equine spermatozoa lose their fertilizing capacity very quickly at room temperature. Additionally, the long oestrus period in the mare makes it difficult to time insemination accurately. Moreover, the UK Thoroughbred Breeder's Association will not register a foal born to AI. Semen can be collected using an artificial vagina or a condom (in which case the stallion performs a natural service). In North America AI is widely used for many breeds of horse, particularly Quarter horses and standardbreds.

In **dogs and cats**, semen can be collected using an artificial vagina or by digital manipulation. Dog semen may be used fresh or frozen, but cat semen is best used fresh. *See also* insemination.

artificial respiration The maintenance of airflow into and out of the lungs by extraneous means of ventilation. This is required when the natural breathing reflexes are insufficient or absent, for example after drowning or poisoning or when the animal is undergoing an operation under general *anaesthesia. As a first-aid measure, intermittent pressure on the chest wall followed by withdrawal of the pressure to permit elastic recoil is often sufficient to provide pulmonary ventilation. The artificial respiration must be maintained until spontaneous breathing recommences. When breathing ceases under general anaesthesia induced by the endotracheal administration of gases, positive-pressure ventilation of the lungs can be achieved by intermittent pressure on the rebreathing bag. Following expansion of the chest wall, pressure on the bag should be released immediately to permit exhalation, otherwise serious circulatory obstruction may occur.

arytenoid cartilage One of a pair of cartilages of the *larynx that articulate with the *cricoid cartilage. Each has a ventral vocal process, to which is attached the vocal ligament, and a lateral muscular process.

Ascaris A genus of relatively large parasitic *nematodes that occur in most mammals, notably pigs, horses (*see* Parascaris), and humans, and in domestic fowls. For example, *A. lumbricoides*, the roundworm of humans, and *A. suum*, the roundworm of pigs, can reach a length of 20 cm. The adult worm inhabits the lumen of the small intestine. The life cycle is direct: after eggs are passed in the faeces, some larval development takes place within the egg; the larvae are ingested by the host and migrate to the liver and the lungs, subsequently passing up the trachea to be swallowed. In young **pigs** the passage of the larvae through the lungs can cause a serious form of pneumonia, characterized by coughing, distressed breathing ('thumps'), weakness, and general malaise. The migrating larvae of *A. suum* damage the liver in pigs, causing *milkspot liver. Heavy infestations can cause enteritis and even complete blockage of the gut. Control is by scrupulous cleanliness in housing and avoidance of contaminated areas. Ascarid eggs are resistant to disinfectant and can persist for many years. In affected animals the anthelmintics fenbendazole, thiabendazole, ivermectin, and dichlorvos are effective against adult worms.

ascites The accumulation of fluid within the abdominal cavity. The fluid, which is usually pale and watery, produces abdominal distension and discomfort. A fluid thrill (wave) may be felt on ballottement (tapping the abdomen). There are a number of causes. Ascites may develop in association with liver disease, particularly where the venous circulation is impeded resulting in hypertension (increased pressure) of the portal vein and consequent transudation of fluid into the abdomen. The lymphatic circulation may also be interrupted with similar effects. Reduced protein synthesis by the diseased liver leads to a lowering of plasma proteins and hence lowered plasma osmotic pressure, which prevents effective resorption of tissue fluid. Ascites may develop in other protein-losing conditions, such as *glomerulonephritis, renal *amyloidosis, or protein-losing *enteropathy. It may also occur in rightsided *heart failure as a result of increased venous pressure. The retention of sodium in heart failure may also contribute to the development of ascites. The fluid can be removed by *paracentesis (draining by needle) or *diuretic therapy, neither of which will correct the underlying cause.

In **poultry**, death due to ascites has become increasingly troublesome in commercial broiler flocks in recent years. It can affect birds from a few days old up to slaughter, with the heart, liver, and kidneys all showing enlargement. The underlying cause is thought to be high oxygen demand and increased blood circulation of modern fast-growing broilers, which can lead to strain and enlargement of the heart. A heart valve may fail, either completely – the probable cause of *acute death syndrome – or partially, leading to poor circulation and oedema. The cause of the oxygen deficit has been suggested as lung damage in early age, or poor ventilation, particularly since cases are more frequent in winter when attempts are made to conserve heat.

ascorbic acid *See* vitamin C.

-ase *Suffix denoting* an enzyme. Examples: *lactase*; *dehydrogenase*.

asepsis The complete absence of bacteria, fungi, viruses, or other microorganisms that can cause disease. Asepsis is the ideal state for performing surgical operations so that the risk of infection is minimized and rapid healing of the wound occurs. Aseptic procedures involve preparation of the operative site by removal of local hair, cleaning and defatting of the exposed skin surface, and repeated applications of suitable disinfectant solutions, and the use of sterile operation drapes. All surgical instruments must be efficiently sterilized (*see* sterilization) and the surgeon must carry out full hand preparation and gowning.

asparagine *See* amino acid.

aspartic acid (aspartate) *See* amino acid.

aspergillosis Invasion of the tissues or colonization of body cavities by saprophytic fungi of the genus *Aspergillus*, affecting especially the respiratory tract of birds and mammals. The most prevalent pathogen is *A. fumigatus*. Aspergillosis may involve any of a wide spectrum of diseases, according to the site and course of the infection. For example, progressive placental infection in cattle causes *mycotic abortion. Strictly, the term does not include diseases caused solely by an allergic reaction to inhaled *Aspergillus* spores. Rotting plant material is the main habitat of *A. fumigatus* and other pathogenic species. Mouldy bedding or fodder can release vast numbers of the spores, which tend to be ubiquitous in the environment. Prolonged exposure to high concentrations of spores may initiate infection; fewer spores may establish an *opportunistic infection in a host whose normal defence mechanisms have been impaired.

In **poultry**, a fatal respiratory infection follows the inhalation of *Aspergillus* spores, usually *A. fumigatus*. The spores are released from mouldy litter, feed, or nest-box lining. Turkeys and game birds are more susceptible than domestic fowls. The infection can occur as severe outbreaks among chicks or poults, or sporadic cases in older flocks. Eggs may become infected from mouldy nest-box material or due to poor storage; this can lead to reduced hatchability or outbreaks after hatching. The disease in young chicks is often called *brooder pneumonia*, and unsatisfactory brooding can be a contributory factor. Mortality may be 10–50%, with outbreaks occurring in the first 3 or 4 weeks. Sometimes there will be breathing difficulties or gasping, followed by death in 48 hours, but often the condition is so acute that no clinical signs are seen. In adults the breathing difficulties and gasping are the first signs, followed by weight loss and weakness in walking, and then usually death. There is no treatment and prevention depends upon management of litter and feed to minimize the presence of fungal spores.

Diagnosis is usually based upon the microscopic demonstration of septate hyphae in the affected tissue, in conjunction with clinical appraisal. Minimizing exposure is the most effective control measure. Specific treatment of most forms of aspergillosis in animals is seldom attempted and rarely successful, though surgical excision of infected tissue supplemented by antifungal therapy may be effective in, for example, canine nasal aspergillosis.

Some *Aspergillus* species can produce potent *mycotoxins, responsible for a range of diseases in animals consuming feed that contains them (*see* aflatoxicosis).

aspermia A lack or failure of formation of spermatozoa leading to *infertility. The condition may be temporary or permanent depending on the cause. A congenital failure to develop seminiferous tubules or germ cells will result in aspermia. The condition may also be caused by extreme changes in environmental temperature or by febrile disease.

asphyxia Suffocation: a life-threatening condition in which oxygen is prevented from reaching the tissues. This may be the result of obstruction or damage to the respiratory system or to a lack of oxygen in inspired air. Causes of respiratory obstruction include *choking and excess fluid in the airways (*see* pulmonary oedema).

aspiration 1. The withdrawal of fluid or gas from a body cavity, organ, or swelling using a needle, catheter, or cannula. Suction is often required. The procedure may be diagnostic to determine the type of fluid present or may be part of a treatment if the gas or fluid is interfering with normal bodily functions, for example when large volumes of fluid are present in the chest. Aseptic precautions are necessary. *See also* enterocentesis; paracentesis; pleurocentesis. **2.** The inhalation of fluids or solid particles into the air passages. *Aspiration pneumonia* is caused by inhalation of foreign material into the lungs.

aspirin *See* NSAID.

assay A test or trial to determine the strength of a solution, the proportion of a compound in a mixture, the potency of a drug, or the purity of a preparation. *See also* bioassay.

assimilation The process by which food substances are taken into the cells of the body after they have been digested and absorbed.

AST (aspartate aminotransferase) An *aminotransferase enzyme that catalyses the reaction: glutamate + oxaloacetate = α-ketoglutarate + aspartate. Elevated plasma levels of this enzyme indicate tissue damage, especially of cardiac muscle and liver. Former name: **GOT (glutamate oxaloacetate transaminase).**

astasia Inability to stand. The muscles show incoordination and perform jerky movements, and it is usually a sign of disease affecting the *cerebellum in the brain.

aster A star-shaped object in a cell that surrounds the *centrosome during mitosis and meiosis and is concerned with the formation of the *spindle.

asthenia Weakness or loss of strength. For example, *myasthenia gravis is a condition in which skeletal muscles become progressively weaker on exercise.

asthma An allergic disorder (*see* hypersensitivity) in which there is constriction of the bronchioles in the lungs resulting in periods of difficult breathing. The narrowing of the air passages is often accentuated by inflammatory epithelial thickening and mucus secretion. Asthma is classically a human condition, but truly analogous disorders probably occur in cattle, dogs, cats, and guinea pigs. As in humans, susceptibility may be genetically determined, and the hypersensitive reaction is also probably similar to that in humans, resulting from the release of *histamine and other inflammation-promoting substances from *mast cells sensitized to specific antigens (e.g. spores or pollen). Asthma may be suspected if the signs of respiratory distress are accompanied by blood eosinophilia. Treatment consists in removal of the causal antigen if it can be identified, and the suppression of the inflammatory response by *corticosteroids.

asthmaweed *See* Lobelia poisoning.

Astragalus poisoning Any of various toxic conditions arising from the ingestion of perennial herbaceous plants of the genus *Astragalus*. Certain members of this genus, and also members of the genus *Oxytropis*, are known as locoweed. They are found primarily in the western USA and contain a toxic principle, swainsonine, which causes depression, incoordination, abortion, and emaciation. Some animals show extreme nervousness and may become violent if stressed.

Other members of the *Astragalus* genus are selenium accumulators and cause a selenium toxicosis when consumed. Some plants may contain up to 3000 parts per million (ppm) of selenium; any plant containing more than 5 ppm is potentially toxic. The clinical signs for *acute toxicosis* are anorexia, depression, coma, and death due to respiratory or cardiac failure. The *chronic toxicosis* may take two forms. One is *blind staggers*, usually the result of ingestion of plants with selenium contents in the range 50–200 ppm. The animal wanders aimlessly but may have bouts of excitement. The condition progresses to cause weakness, dyspnoea, paralysis, and death from respiratory failure. The second and more chronic form is *alkali disease*, typically the result of consuming plants containing 5–50 ppm selenium. The animal may develop lameness with erosions of the articular surface, hoof deformities, and loss of the long hairs of the tail; death is usually from starvation. Lesions common to both chronic forms include gastrointestinal irritation, myocardial atrophy, degenerative changes in the kidneys and liver, and cirrhotic livers in long-standing cases. In all cases, treatment is of the clinical signs.

astringent A substance that causes cells to shrink by precipitating proteins on their surfaces, thus resulting in tissue contraction or stoppage of secretions or discharges. Lotions containing astringents, for example blue copper sulphate, zinc sulphate, dilute acids, or tannic acid, are used to harden and protect the skin.

astrocyte (astroglial cell) A type of cell with numerous sheet-like processes extending from its cell body, found throughout the central nervous system. It is one of the several different types of cell that make up the neuroglia. The cells have been ascribed the function of providing nutrients for neurones and possibly of taking part in information storage processes.

astrocytoma A tumour of the brain and spinal cord derived from non-nervous cells (*neuroglia). They occur in dogs and, occasionally, in other species. A well-differentiated astrocytoma is a slow-growing firm whitish mass, poorly defined at the margin where it merges with surrounding tissue. It consists of interwoven bundles of elongated fibrous *astrocytes. Larger and more malignant examples are prone to haemorrhage, oedema, necrosis, and cystic change. Astrocytomas are fast-growing, infiltrative, and destructive causing clinical signs related to dysfunction of the affected part of the brain and increased intracranial pressure. There is no effective treatment and prognosis is poor.

astrovirus A group of RNA *viruses that have not yet been systematically classified. They cause gastrointestinal infections in lambs and calves.

Asuntol Tradename for the organophosphate compound coumaphos. It is a pale-grey powder that is made up in water for dipping or spraying to control ectoparasites in sheep, cattle, and goats. Asuntol controls ticks, blowflies, lice, and keds and has a residual effect lasting for up to 20 weeks, depending on the parasite and climatic conditions. Signs of toxicity (due to inhibition of cholinesterase) are salivation, laboured breathing (dyspnoea), stiffness, diarrhoea, bradycardia, muscle tremor, and convulsions. *Atropine sulphate should be used to treat cases of toxicity. *See also* organophosphorus compounds.

asymptomatic Not showing any signs of disease, whether disease is present or not.

asystole A form of *cardiac arrest in which the heart stops beating completely. There is no detectable pulse, and the heart muscle is flaccid. Treatment includes direct cardiac massage, intravenous administration of calcium and bicarbonate, and intracardiac administration of isoprenaline or adrenaline (*see* artificial respiration). *Compare* fibrillation.

ataractic *See* tranquillizer.

ataxia Unsteady or irregular gait resulting from incoordination of the muscles, which can be caused by a variety of lesions throughout the nervous system.

atel- (atelo-) *Prefix denoting* imperfect or incomplete development. Examples: *atelencephaly* (of the brain); *atelocardia* (of the heart).

atelectasis (*pl.* **atelectases**) Failure of part of the lung to expand. Affected areas are not ventilated by respiratory movements and therefore cause reduced respiratory efficiency. In the newborn, atelectasis can occur if there is a deficiency of surfactant in the lung and will result in neonatal death. In adults areas of atelectasis result from pulmonary disease, often associated with bronchial obstruction. These atelectatic areas commonly become the site of secondary infection and lead to further complications.

atheroma Deposition of lipid material in the inner wall of the arteries. The deposits are composed of cholesterol, fatty acids, triglycerides, and phospholipids, and initially appear as yellow streaks before developing into plaques. They cause narrowing of the arterial lumen (*see* atherosclerosis). In humans atheroma is associated with high levels of saturated fats and cholesterol in the diet and also with hypertension. The disruption of the inner arterial surface predisposes to *thrombosis.

atherosclerosis Disease of the arteries in which fatty plaques develop in their inner walls, resulting in eventual hardening of the wall and narrowing of the lumen (*see* atheroma). This condition is of much greater importance in humans than in animals. In dogs it may occur in association with *hypothyroidism. The distortion of the vessel interferes with blood flow and there may be calcification of the lipid and increased fibrous tissue, so reducing elasticity of the vessel. It may also be a factor in *aortic rupture in turkeys.

atlas The first *cervical vertebra. It articulates with the skull, via the atlanto-occipital joint, and with the *axis, via the atlantoaxial joint. These joints allow free movement for nodding and shaking of the head respectively.

atony A state in which muscles are floppy, lacking their normal tone.

atopy An inherited predisposition for Type I *hypersensitivity. Atopic individuals tend to produce antibodies of the IgE class readily and in excessive amounts and, usually, in response to a wide variety of antigens. Any of the clinical signs associated with Type I hypersensitivity may occur. However, the best recognized atopic disorder occurs in **dogs**. They suffer an itchy dermatitis in response to antigens acquired by inhalation, ingestion, or direct skin contact. The most potent environmental allergen is that produced by the house dust mite, *Dermatophagoides pterynissinus.* In some individuals flea bites are directly antigenic. The lesion is a chronically irritant skin inflammation, often worsened by the animal scratching and biting the affected part. Other organs may exhibit signs of hypersensitivity, causing, for instance, concurrent conjunctivitis or rhinitis. In **cats** the skin is again commonly affected, the causative antigen most frequently being found in food. In all cases the best treatment is identification and removal of the antigen responsible. The *allergic state of an individual may be altered by injecting the antigen to change the predominant antibody type to a nonreaginic class; Type I hypersensitivity consequently wanes. Glucocorticoid therapy is an effective alternative.

atoxyl (sodium arsanilate) An organic arsenical used in the treatment of protozoal infections. It is a white powder that can be reconstituted in water and injected intravenously or intramuscularly. Atoxyl has been used to treat trypanosomiasis and as an in-feed growth promoter for pigs and poultry. However, toxicity can occur (*see* arsenic) and in many countries its use is restricted.

ATP (adenosine triphosphate) A nucleotide that is of fundamental importance as a carrier of chemical energy in all living organisms. It consists of adenine linked to D-ribose (i.e. adenosine); the D-ribose component bears three phosphate groups, linearly linked by covalent bonds. ATP drives most of an organism's energy-requiring reactions by yielding the high free-energy of its phosphate-phosphate (pyrophosphate) bonds. It is formed in the *mitochondria of cells under aerobic conditions by the oxidative phosphorylation of ADP (adenosine diphosphate), and also by transfer of phosphate to ADP from other energy-rich molecules, for example phosphoenolpyruvate; this latter is the only means of energy generation under anaerobic conditions (*see* respiration). *See also* AMP.

atresia 1. Congenital absence or abnormal narrowing of a body opening. Atresia of the alimentary tract can occur at most points along the tract. This causes blockage of the tract and marked abdominal distension soon after birth. Death normally occurs within days. Atresia of the anus (*atresia ani*) is quite common and is believed to be inherited. It can be surgically corrected in some cases. Inherited atresia of the ileum (*atresia ilei*) has been reported in cattle, and atresia of the colon (*atresia coli*) has been recorded in horses. **2.** The degeneration of an ovarian follicle at any stage during its maturation.

atri- (atrio-) *Prefix denoting* an atrium, especially the atrium of the heart. Example: *atrioventricular* (relating to the atria and ventricles of the heart).

atrioventricular bundle (AV bundle, bundle of His) A bundle of specialized heart muscle fibres that arises from the *atrioventricular node and passes through the fibrous tissue

atrioventricular node

between atria and ventricles to enter the interventricular septum, where it divides into two – the *left* and *right crura*. It transmits the impulse to contract from the atria to the ventricles such that the onset of ventricular contraction is delayed until the atrial contraction is completed.

atrioventricular node (AV node) A clump of specialized heart muscle in the septal wall of the right atrium. It receives impulses from the atrial muscle and transmits these via the *atrioventricular bundle to the ventricles.

atrioventricular valve (AV valve) A heart valve between an atrium and a ventricle that prevents backflow of blood into the atrium when the ventricle contracts. It is formed of either two (*bicuspid or mitral valve) or three (*tricuspid valve) pocket-like cusps, the margins of which are attached by *chordae tendineae to the papillary muscles of the ventricles. Disease of these valves can lead to incompetence and produces a systolic heart *murmur.

atrium (*pl.* **atria**) **1.** One of a pair of relatively thin-walled chambers of the *heart. The right atrium receives deoxygenated blood from the venae cavae and coronary sinus, and the left atrium receives oxygenated blood from the lungs via the pulmonary veins. Contractions of the atrial walls force blood to flow into the corresponding right and left *ventricles. *See also* auricle. **2.** Any of various anatomical chambers into which one or more cavities open. **3.** The *atrium ruminis* (cranial sac), which is part of the *rumen. **4.** One of the extensions of the *parabronchi in the avian lung.

atrophic myositis A condition seen in the dog in which there is wasting of the muscles on both sides of the head, particularly the temporal and masseter muscles, producing a foxlike

contour and causing difficulty in opening the mouth. The muscle fibres are smaller than usual with no evidence of regeneration, and there is increased fibrous tissue. The condition may develop from an earlier acute phase when the muscles are painful and swollen, or it may develop insidiously.

atrophic rhinitis A disease of the upper respiratory tract occurring in young pigs and characterized by sneezing, loss of the nasal turbinate bones, and ultimately distortion and shortening of the snout. An acute nasal inflammation may occur in young piglets (3–8 weeks old), particularly those bred from young gilts. Weaners show a subacute form. Various infective agents have been implicated, particularly the Gram-negative bacterium *Bordetella bronchoseptica* and toxigenic strains of *Pasteurella* species. Signs include sneezing, eye discharge, difficulty in breathing, and rubbing the snout, resulting in retarded growth and economic loss. Sectioning the snout from affected pigs shows loss of the scrolls of the turbinate bones inside the nasal cavity. In severe cases the turbinate bones disappear entirely. The nasal septum may also be lost. Once established in a herd, the disease can only be eradicated by complete herd dispersal and re-establishment with disease-free stock, although the use of *antibiotics in the feed will control the disease. Improved hygiene and ventilation, breeding from older sows, whose litters tend to be more protected, and buying in weaners from disease-free herds will all help reduce the incidence of the disease.

atrophy A decrease in size or wasting of a fully developed organ or tissue. It may be a natural process or the result of disease, and can involve decrease in the number or the size of the component cells. *Physiological* *atrophy* occurs in the thymus, which regresses as the young animal develops to maturity. *Disuse atrophy* occurs in skeletal muscle immobilized after a fracture. *Neurogenic atrophy* occurs, for instance, in the cricoarytenoideus muscle of dogs and horses following paralysis of the left recurrent laryngeal nerve. *Pressure atrophy* results from compression by a space-occupying lesion. *Endocrine atrophy* develops due to lack of endocrine stimulation producing a decrease in size of the target organs. *Brown atrophy* is seen in the liver in cases of starvation, and *senile atrophy*, for example of the brain or gonads, is associated with old age.

atropine An alkaloid, first obtained from *Atropa belladonna* (deadly nightshade), that acts as a *parasympatholytic. It can be injected subcutaneously, intramuscularly, or intravenously, administered orally, or used topically in the eye. Atropine is used as a premedicant before general anaesthesia to reduce salivary and bronchial secretions and reduce vagal reflexes (in ruminants salivary secretions from the parotid and submandibular glands may be reduced but viscosity is increased). It is also used as a spasmolytic to reduce gut motility; there is also reduced gastrointestinal secretion. Topical use of atropine in the eye causes *mydriasis and allows examination of the eye. It is used following *pilocarpine to break down adhesions in the eye. When administered systemically, atropine is hydrolysed in the liver and has activity for 3–6 hours. When used topically in the eye its effects last for several days. Atropine is the antidote in *anticholinesterase overdosage, for example in cases of organophosphorus poisoning.

The toxicity of atropine varies between species: rabbits metabolize the drug rapidly and are less susceptible than other species. Signs of toxicity include dryness of the oral cavity, thirst, mydriasis, tachycardia, and hyperpnoea. Severe toxicity involves stimulation of the central nervous system, with ataxia and convulsions then depressed respiration and death. To treat overdosage a reversible anticholinesterase compound, such as physostigmine, neostigmine, or edrophonium, should be used.

The alkaloid hyoscine (scopolamine) and the semisynthetic compound homatropine are similar parasympatholytic agents. Homatropine is used in ophthalmic preparations to cause mydriasis; it has a shorter duration of action than atropine. *See also* deadly nightshade poisoning.

attenuated strain *See* attenuation.

attenuation The reduction in virulence of a previously pathogenic organism. Attenuation of disease-producing organisms may occur naturally during the course of a disease outbreak. However, the term usually refers to the laboratory manipulation of a virulent organism to render it safe for use in a live *vaccine. Repeated passage of a virus through tissue culture or an abnormal host animal invariably changes the characteristics of the virus and may result in attenuation. However, the virus may go through cycles of increasing and decreasing virulence as it is passaged. *Rinderpest, *sheep pox, and *bluetongue vaccines are examples of attenuated viral vaccines. Some viruses, such as *foot-and-mouth disease virus, are too unstable to maintain their reduced virulence and are thus unsuitable for use as live vaccines.

Attested Area (England and Wales) An area, designated for the purposes of controlling diseases of cattle, in which the Minister is satisfied that any particular disease is, for practical purposes, nonexistent. *See also* Animal Health Act (1981).

audi- (audio-) *Prefix denoting* hearing or sound.

auditory Relating to the ear or to the sense of hearing.

auditory nerve *See* vestibulocochlear nerve.

auditory tube (Eustachian tube) The tube that connects the nasopharynx and the middle *ear thereby allowing the equalization of pressure on either side of the tympanic membrane. The tube is closed by the action of muscles attached to its wall, except during swallowing. In the horse a ventral diverticulum is present – the *guttural pouch.

Auerbach's plexus *See* myenteric plexus.

Aujeszky's disease A contagious disease of pigs characterized by abortion and nervous signs in young pigs and caused by *herpesvirus. It is endemic in most pig-rearing countries although in the UK its distribution is restricted. Transmission is usually by mouth. Pregnant sows infected with Aujeszky's virus abort or give birth to stillborn, mummified, or weak piglets (SMEDI) and may develop an associated uterine infection. Young pigs, under 3 weeks old, develop pneumonia and nervous signs and die. Older pigs develop few clinical signs but become persistently infected and can remain a potential source of infection to susceptible pigs. Cattle, dogs, foxes, rats, and cats may become infected and can develop an intense irritation at the site of entry of the virus, causing the animal to mutilate itself ('mad itch'). The disease is usually fatal in the abnormal hosts, kittens particularly may die of acute disease before developing other clinical

signs. Control in the UK (apart from Northern Ireland) is by slaughter of affected pigs. In Northern Ireland and elsewhere control is by vaccination; although this will not prevent infection, vaccination reduces the severity of clinical signs. Humans may rarely become infected with the virus. It is a *notifiable disease in the UK. Other name: **pseudorabies**.

aural Relating to the ear.

auricle 1. The visible portion of the external *ear, which receives sound waves and directs them into the external acoustic meatus. Consisting of skin-covered elastic cartilage, its shape is highly variable and characteristic of species and breed. Numerous muscles attach to the auricle allowing it to be directed towards the source of sound. **2.** Any earlike structure, such as the small blind-ending pouch in the wall of each *atrium of the heart. The term is also used incorrectly as a synonym for atrium.

auriscope An instrument for examining the *ear canals and eardrum (tympanic membrane). It consists of a light source and a tubular ear piece, which can be varied in size and length to suit the animal concerned. Small crocodile forceps may be inserted through the ear piece to grasp and remove foreign material. Auriscopes can be used in conscious animals but sedation may be required if the ear is painful; general anaesthesia may be necessary for large animals.

auscultation The process of listening to sounds produced by the body and transmitted to the surface. This may be achieved by the ear alone, in direct contact with the skin and hair, but is helped by use of a *stethoscope. Care must be taken to differentiate 'true sounds' from 'false sounds', for example those due to movement of the animal or sounds from the abdomen being transmitted to the chest. Auscultation of the heart can reveal abnormalities of rhythm (*see* arrhythmia; fibrillation; heart block) or abnormal cardiac sounds, such as occur in *pericarditis or *valvular disease. Auscultation of the respiratory system may show pulmonary diseases (*see* rale; rhonchus) or abnormalities involving the pleural cavity and auscultation of the abdomen can indicate over- or underactivity of the gut or the presence of an abnormally distended gut. *See also* percussion.

aut- (auto-) *Prefix denoting* self. Example: *autokinesis* (voluntary movement).

autoantibody An *antibody formed by the body in response to its own tissue. *See* autoimmune disease.

autoclave A piece of equipment designed for the sterilization of objects by steam under pressure. It consists of an insulated air-tight chamber in which surgical instruments, dressings, or other apparatus can be placed. Some autoclaves have a drying cycle which helps to remove the moisture from drapes and dressings after steam treatment. All materials to be sterilized must be exposed to the steam, not left in sealed or impervious packaging.

autoimmune disease Any disorder involving inflammation or destruction of tissues by the body's own immune system. Such disorders result from the activity of lymphocytes primed to act in response to 'self antigens'; *antibodies, *complement, *hypersensitivity reactions, and other immune mechanisms may be directed against 'self' tissues. Specific autoimmune diseases in the dog are well studied and include *canine autoimmune haemolytic anaemia, systemic *lupus erythematosus, some forms of idiopathic *thrombo-

cytopenia, autoimmune *thyroiditis, a number of skin inflammations, such as *pemphigus, and possibly *rheumatoid arthritis and polyarteritis nodosa. *Glomerulonephritis, caused by the deposition of antigen-antibody complexes in the kidney, occurs in many species. Other diseases of suggested autoimmune origin are ophthalmitis and *orchitis. Why autoimmunity develops is largely unknown. Treatment depends on the suppression of the immunological response, usually by *steroid therapy. *See also* bovine autoimmune haemolytic anaemia; equine autoimmune haemolytic anaemia.

autoinfection Reinfection of a host by larvae of a parasite already within the host. This can occur, for example, with the nematode *Trichinella spiralis*, which inhabits the small intestine of pigs, some carnivores, and humans. Larvae from the adult parasites invade the gut wall and are carried by the circulation to skeletal muscle, where they encyst.

autolysis The destruction of tissues or cells brought about by the actions of their own enzymes. *See* lysosome.

autonomic nervous system (ANS) The part of the *peripheral nervous system that innervates smooth muscle, cardiac muscle, and glandular tissue. It functions without direct voluntary control and consists of two divisions, the *sympathetic nervous system and the *parasympathetic nervous system. Most organs are innervated by both divisions, which tend then to have antagonistic actions.

autonomic polyganglionopathy *See* dysautonomia.

autoploidy The normal condition in cells or individuals, in which each cell has a chromosome set consisting of *homologous pairs, which allows cell division to occur in a normal manner.

autopsy (necropsy) The systematic external and internal examination of a dead animal in order to establish or confirm the cause of death. Samples of diseased or abnormal tissue may be removed for further more detailed examination and attempts may be made to isolate infectious organisms, such as bacteria or viruses. Analysis of serum or gut contents may reveal the presence of toxic chemicals or abnormal concentrations of metabolites.

autosome Any chromosome that is not a *sex chromosome and that occurs in pairs in diploid cells.

autovaccine A vaccine prepared from pathogenic organisms taken from a specified animal or group of animals and used to stimulate immunity in the same animal(s). For example, a preparation of wart material may be used to inoculate the bovine from which the wart was originally collected in order to stimulate an immune response sufficient to eliminate the remaining warts on the animal. The effectiveness of such vaccines is difficult to evaluate because *control animals are usually not available. Also the time taken to produce the autovaccine is probably frequently sufficient for the animal to make its own unaided recovery.

autumn house fly A non-biting *fly, *Musca autumnalis*, also known as the face fly. Adults may collect on tree trunks or walls in the sun and they often irritate grazing cattle and horses, feeding on secretions from the nostrils and eyes and discharges from small wounds. The autumn fly transmits an eyeworm of cattle and *New Forest disease. The eggs are laid in fresh cattle dung, on which the larvae feed.

aux- (auxo-) *Prefix denoting* increase; growth.

avermectin Any of a group of macrocyclic lactones, first isolated from the actinomycete bacterium *Streptomyces avermitilis*, with activity against helminth parasites. They include the commercially available anthelmintic *ivermectin.

avian contagious epithelioma *See* fowl pox.

avian diphtheria *See* fowl pox.

avian encephalomyelitis *See* infectious avian encephalomyelitis.

avian infectious laryngotracheitis (ILT) A highly infectious disease of domestic fowls, caused by a *herpesvirus and characterized by inflammation of the trachea and larynx, which becomes obstructed with blood and mucus. It is found in all ages but young adult layers are most frequently affected. Most other poultry and birds appear to be resistant, but pheasants are susceptible. The disease takes three forms – acute, subacute, and chronic (mild). The *acute form* begins with the rapid appearance of severe respiratory signs, although some birds may die without warning. Birds struggle for breath with heads stretched forward, make rasping and gurgling noises, cough up blood and mucus, and shake their heads. There may be a discharge from the eyes. Death from asphyxiation follows in a few days and mortality ranges from 10 to 70%. The *subacute form* develops more slowly and mortality ranges up to 30%. In the *chronic form* the signs can be very mild, with *conjunctivitis and lowered performance, some respiratory signs, and occasional deaths over several months, with mortality perhaps well under 1%. Postmortem examination reveals the lesions to be confined to the upper respiratory tract. There is no effective treatment and surviving birds become carriers, thus infected flocks may need to be culled. The virus is spread in the expectorated material, and can be physically transmitted on boots, vehicles, equipment, etc.; avoidance of this demands rigorous hygiene. Windborne transmission may be significant when large numbers of birds of different ages are housed on the same site. However, the virus has low survivability outside the bird and destocking for 2 months may be recommended after outbreaks. The disease is probably widespread in its mild form, but shows regional variations in incidence. An eye-drop vaccine is available. The acute form needs to be distinguished from other respiratory infections, especially *Newcastle disease. Post-mortem signs in the mild form may resemble avian diphtheria (see fowl pox).

avian influenza (fowl plague) A disease of poultry and other birds caused by various strains of influenzavirus (A group) and characterized by respiratory signs and general depression. Most avian species appear to be susceptible. The severity of the disease depends on the strain of virus involved, the species, age, and immune status of the host, and intercurrent infection. Mortality in domestic fowls and turkeys can be around 10%, but in the acute form, known as *fowl plague*, it can be far higher. The method of transmission is not fully understood but is believed to require close contact. Wild ducks are probably significant vectors for domestic flocks. In most countries, including the UK, avian influenza is a *notifiable disease.

avian leukosis The general name for a group of malignant diseases of domestic fowls, caused by the avian RNA tumour viruses. These chiefly affect adult birds and give rise to tumours of the internal organs and other parts of the body and/or *leukaemia. The three main forms are lymphoid, myeloid, and erythroid leukoses, while *osteopetrosis is a rarer form. The causative viruses are normally present in most individuals, but mortality is typically only 1–2% since nearly all birds have adequate resistance. This resistance is largely genetically determined, but is also influenced by the manner of infection: leukosis appears more often in birds that acquire the virus vertically (i.e. through the egg) than in those that are infected horizontally (i.e. from other birds), since the latter produce antibodies in response to the infection. The viruses cannot survive long outside the body, so for commercial flocks leukosis is essentially an egg-transmitted disease. In Britain the prevalence of the leukoses is relatively low in commercial breeding flocks. There is no treatment for infected birds.

Lymphoid leukosis, the most common form, affects birds aged over 6 months. A few weeks after the initial infection the virus gives rise to microscopic primary tumours in the *cloacal bursa (bursa of Fabricius). In all but a few birds these tumours regress after some months. However, in the remainder these primaries give rise to secondary tumours or metastasize to the major organs, mainly the liver – massively enlarged liver is characteristic of lymphoid leukosis. Tumours can also form elsewhere, commonly in the bursa, kidney, spleen, and gonads. *Erythroid leukosis* involves the proliferation of immature red blood cells, causing *erythroblastosis, true leukaemia, and anaemia. The liver and spleen assume a distinctive bright-red appearance. *Myeloid leukosis* takes two forms: a diffuse form, which results in an enlarged and granular liver and spleen; and a discrete form, which produces nodular tumours on these organs and elsewhere, including the kidneys and bones. *Compare* Marek's disease.

avian malaria Any of a group of infections of birds caused by related protozoa of the genera *Plasmodium*, *Leucocytozoon*, and *Haemoproteus*. These are of most significance in tropical areas, where a large number of domestic and wild bird species are affected. The life cycles of these parasites and the disease produced are broadly similar to human *malaria (see illustration). Diagnosis depends on the demonstration of parasites in stained blood smears. Prevention of the disease depends on control of the insect vectors, namely mosquitoes, blackflies, or midges.

avian malignant oedema (gangrenous dermatitis) A condition of chicks, particularly broilers, up to 7 weeks old, involving gangrene of the muscle tissue and also sometimes the skin. The affected tissue dies and varying amounts of gas may be produced, which can accumulate under the skin. Mortality can reach 50%. It is caused by *Clostridium septicum*, although other bacteria, such as *Staphylococcus*, may be involved. Infection often appears to follow in the wake of some other immunosuppressive disease, and to be encouraged by a high stocking density and poor hygiene. Infected birds should be culled to prevent cross-infection; antibiotic treatment is not particularly successful.

avian monocytosis (pullet disease) A disease, of unknown cause, that affects domestic fowls and turkeys and is marked by digestive disorders, lowered performance, and some mortality. Now rare, the disease is mostly encountered in summer, especially late summer, and usually affects pullets at point of lay or soon after. Outbreaks can spread rapidly through a flock, lasting for a week or two and

causing mortality of up to 10%. Signs include a drop in egg production, listlessness, reduced appetite, watery diarrhoea, and blue-purple coloration to the comb. Death may follow in a few days; initially some birds may die without showing signs. Post-mortem examination often shows distension of the crop with a mixture of food and more unusual material (i.e. evidence of *pica). There is enlargement or degeneration of the kidneys, which contain urate deposits (*see* gout); disruption of the ovarian follicles; and *monocytosis – a proliferation of large white blood cells. Among the suggested causes is the consumption of new-crop wheat. However, current thought favours a virus. There is no specific treatment, but antibiotics given in the feed or drinking water, particularly tetracyclines, can give a good response. A reduction in food intake may help, with a switch to wet mash and the omission of whole grains. Other names: **blue comb**; **contagious indigestion**; **new wheat poisoning**; **summer disease**.

avian mycoplasmosis Any of various diseases of birds caused by infection with species of *Mycoplasma*. *M. gallisepticum* infection, formerly known as chronic respiratory disease (CRD) or infectious sinusitis of turkeys, is of significant economic importance in domestic fowls and turkeys, and may also affect partridges, pheasants, pigeons, and other Columbiformes and Psittaciformes. It causes respiratory signs, including *tracheitis, with coughing, nasal discharge, and *air sacculitis. These lead to downgrading of carcasses, lowered egg production, reduced hatchability, and suboptimal feed conversion. Mild cases will be unnoticed; more severe attacks can be triggered by stress or by other infections, such as *infectious bronchitis. The pathogen can be transmited via the egg or from bird to bird, and infected birds are recog-

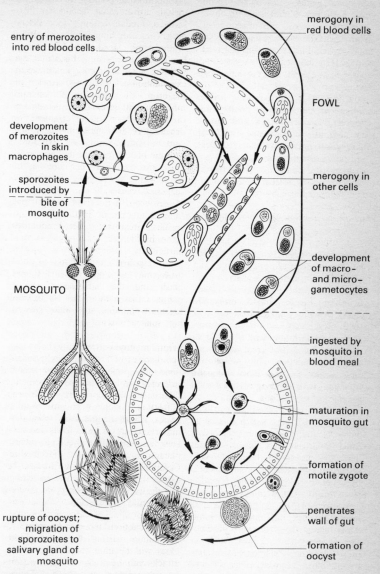

merogony in
red blood cells

entry of merozoites
into red blood cells

FOWL

development
of merozoites
in skin
macrophages

merogony in
other cells

sporozoites
introduced by
bite of
mosquito

MOSQUITO

development
of macro-
and micro-
gametocytes

ingested by
mosquito in
blood meal

maturation in
mosquito gut

formation of
motile zygote

penetrates
wall of gut

rupture of oocyst;
migration of
sporozoites to
salivary gland of
mosquito

formation of
oocyst

The life cycle of *Plasmodium gallinaceum*, the causal agent of avian malaria in
domestic fowls

nized by a blood test. Both vaccination and flock medication with antibiotics (tetracyclines, spiramycin, spectinomycin) reduce the worst effects but may not completely prevent egg infection. Hatching eggs are sometimes dipped in Tylosin for the latter purpose.

Infection with *M. synoviae* causes *infectious synotivitis of poultry, and upper respiratory disease and chronic air sacculitis in domestic fowls. *M. meleagridis* principally affects turkeys, causing primarily air sacculitis and poor growth, but also osteodystrophy, crooked necks, feather abnormalities, and reduced hatchability.

avian pasteurellosis (fowl cholera)
See cholera.

avian salmonellosis Any of various infectious diseases of poultry and other birds caused by bacteria of the genus *Salmonella*. *S. pullorum* causes *pullorum disease, and *S. gallinarum* causes *fowl typhoid. However, the term 'salmonellosis' is commonly applied to infection with the 200 or so other *Salmonella* serotypes occurring in poultry, of which *S. typhimurium* is the most frequent. Infection with these gives rise to a general septicaemia, and *S. typhimurium* can cause high mortality in chicks, ducklings, and poults up to 3 weeks old; many other serotypes cause relatively few losses. Deaths tend to increase if birds are kept under poor conditions or are affected by other diseases, especially coccidiosis. Clinical signs in chicks and poults are effectively the same as for pullorum disease, but ducklings sometimes show 'keel disease', whereby they keel over backwards and die after drinking. Salmonellosis commonly affects a wide range of wild and caged birds. The signs vary but diarrhoea is a regular feature. In poultry, older birds rarely show clinical signs but may become carri-

ers. Infected poultry carcasses and meat can transmit *Salmonella* infection to humans, causing food poisoning. Cross-contamination can occur in the poultry processing plant. *Salmonella* bacteria also occasionally find their way into duck eggs destined for consumption. Breeding stock can transmit the infection to offspring through contamination of the shell or, more rarely, ovarian transmission. Control relies on good hatchery practice. Another source of infection is contaminated feed. Litter, nest material, and equipment can also harbour salmonellae for months. Treatment of affected birds with nitrofurans is possible, but this does not prevent birds becoming carriers. In the UK, salmonellosis must be reported under the Zoonosis Order.

avian spirochaetosis An acute or subacute frequently lethal tick-borne *septicaemia of all common poultry species caused by the spirochaete bacterium *Borrelia anserinum* (*B. gallinarum*). It is of economic importance in tropical and subtropical regions, being transmitted by the common fowl tick (*Argas persicus*), and other tick species. These become infected while feeding on blood, and the infection passes, by transovarian infection, to the next generation of ticks. Affected birds show fever, diarrhoea, anorexia, and drowsiness. A single dose of penicillin generally effects a complete cure. Vaccines are available in some countries. Other control measures are tick eradication or the provision of tick-proof roosting quarters.

avian tuberculosis (going light) An infectious wasting disease of poultry and most other birds, caused by *Mycobacterium avium*. It is a common problem in traditional husbandry systems, where birds are kept for several years, but is rarely seen on modern intensive poultry units, where birds are kept for a year or two at the most. The most common route of infection is through contaminated ('fowl-sick') land or litter; infected birds excrete the bacteria in large amounts, and they can survive in the ground for up to 4 years. Thus infection is more likely under unhygienic conditions or where heavy densities of birds are kept on the same ground for a long period of time, as in small backyard runs or overstocked free-range units. Birds become unthrifty and egg output is depressed; they lose weight steadily until badly emaciated, despite normal eating; there is diarrhoea and a pale comb. The bacteria invade the intestines, liver, kidneys, bone marrow, and joints, the latter often resulting in lameness of one leg. Birds tend to squat with exhaustion. Occasional deaths can follow months after the onset of clinical signs. Some birds die suddenly without warning signs. There is no effective treatment. Control depends upon sound management and hygiene, with culling and safe disposal of infected birds.

Avicalm Tradename for metoserpate hydrochloride, an alkaloid sometimes used as a tranquillizer for poultry. It acts by depleting stores of noradrenaline and 5-hydroxytryptamine in both the central and peripheral nervous sytems, causing a slow fall in blood pressure. It is used in domestic fowls to prevent stress during transportation and handling. In turkeys it is used to reduce stress and lower the incidence of aortic rupture.

avitaminosis Lack of one or more *vitamins in the diet. The term is usually qualified by the name of the vitamin involved, for example, avitaminosis D.

AVMA *See* American Veterinary Medical Association.

avoparcin A glycopeptide antibiotic produced by a strain of the bacterium *Streptomyces candidus*. It is active against Gram-positive bacteria and is used in feed for pigs, cattle, and poultry as a growth promoter. Absorption from the gastrointestinal tract is extremely low and most of the drug is excreted unchanged in the faeces. Development of resistance by bacteria is not widespread and there is no cross-resistance with other antibiotics.

avulsion (evulsion) The tearing or forcible separation of part of a structure. For example, a tendon may be torn from the bone to which it attaches.

axilla (*pl.* **axillae**) The space between the forelimb and the trunk, corresponding to the armpit in humans. Below it is bounded by the *pectoral muscles, above by muscle attaching the scapula to the thoracic wall. The adjacent region of the body contains the axillary artery and vein and the *brachial plexus – the major blood vessels and nerves supplying the forelimb.

axillary nerve One of the nerves of the forelimb, extending from the *brachial plexus. It carries motor fibres to the flexor muscles of the shoulder and sensory fibres from part of the forelimb.

axis 1. An imaginary line through the body or one of its parts, for example, a limb or a joint, about which the body or part moves. **2.** The second cervical vertebra. It articulates with the *atlas at the atlantoaxial joint, allowing the head to rotate from side to side, and with the third cervical vertebra.

axolemma The cell membrane enclosing the axon of a *neurone.

axon A single long process of a *neurone that conducts nerve impulses away from the cell body. It may give rise to several collateral branches along its length and terminally divides into numerous fine short branches or telodendria (*see* telodendron). These make contact with other neurones or with muscles or gland cells. The axon is surrounded by other cells, for example, Schwann cells in the *peripheral nervous system; these may form a *myelin sheath, which is interrupted at intervals by gaps called *nodes of Ranvier.*

axoplasm The cytoplasm of the *axon. It contains many *neurofilaments and *microtubules but not the dark-staining *Nissl granules seen in the neurone cell body. These axoplasmic structures convey proteins produced in the cell body of the neurone to the peripheral parts of the axon.

azaperone A tranquillizer/sedative of the *butyrophenone group used in large animals, primarily pigs. It has a wide safety margin and few side-effects. In **pigs** the drug is injected intramuscularly at low dose rates as a tranquillizer to prevent aggressive behaviour after mixing groups of pigs. At higher doses azaperone can be used in combination with *metomidate to produce general anaesthesia. Pigs should not be disturbed while the drug is taking effect. Penile prolapse with possible risk of penile injury can be a complicating factor in entire males. In **horses** azaperone is injected intramuscularly as a sedative; intravenous use can produce excitement and ataxia.

azoospermia A lack of spermatozoa in the semen. This may involve a lack or failure of formation of spermatozoa (*see* aspermia) or may be produced by vasectomy. *See also* infertility.

azoturia A condition of horses in which they pass dark-coloured urine containing the muscle pigment myoglobin (*myoglobinuria). The condition varies in severity and develops when a horse is exercised, sometimes after a period of rest on heavy rations. The gluteal muscles and those of the upper hindlimb become rigid and swollen and the animal is distressed. The muscle damage results in the release of myoglobin, which is excreted in the urine. The pigment may precipitate in the kidney tubules causing renal failure. Blood levels of the muscle enzyme creatine phosphokinase are raised and there is necrosis of muscle fibres and inflammation. Treatment includes rest and the administration of anti-inflammatory drugs. In a mild form of the condition, known as *tying-up syndrome*, the animal may merely show stiffness and shortening of gait. Other names: **exertional rhabdomyolysis; set fast.**

B

Babesia A genus of protozoan parasites that live in the red blood cells of mammals and are transmitted by *ticks. Some species are responsible for the disease *babesiosis, which affects livestock and other domestic animals worldwide. Each species of *Babesia* is specific to a particular host species, but each host species may be affected by several different species of *Babesia*. The organisms range in size from 1 to 5 μm and vary from roughly circular to pear-shaped, often occurring in characteristic linked pairs. During the initial stages of infection, the parasites divide in red blood cells and invade nonparasitized cells until 10% or more of red blood cells are infected. In animals that

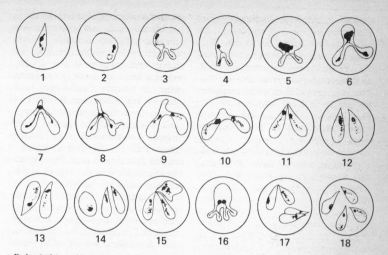

Babesia bigemina: stages in the parasite's multiplication in the red blood cells of cattle

recover, parasite numbers fall until they are no longer easily detected in the blood. They persist in low numbers in the circulation for the life of the host, evading the host's defences by exhibiting *antigenic variation. At this stage they usually cause no harm but are a potential source of infection for other animals. When ticks feed on the blood of an infected animal, the parasite multiplies in the tick and invades many of its tissues. It is transmitted via the salivary glands of either the same tick, or, in the case of a female, its larval offspring. See illustration.

There are several *Babesia* species responsible for disease in cattle, with different geographical distributions. *B. divergens* affects cattle in northwestern Europe and is transmitted by the sheep tick *Ixodes ricinus*. In tropical regions of Africa and South America, the major cause of babesiosis is *B. bigemina*, transmitted by *Boophilus* spp. *B. bovis* is another tropical species with a similar distribution and is the chief pathogenic species in Australia. *B. canis* parasitizes dogs in tropical regions (*see* canine babesiosis). Additionally, there are species of *Babesia* causing disease in horses (*see* equine babesiosis), sheep, pigs, and cats. *See also* Texas fever.

babesiosis A disease of mammals caused by protozoan parasites of the genus *Babesia* and transmitted by ticks. Of worldwide occurrence, this is a particularly important disease in tropical regions. The disease is characterized by fever, anaemia, and *haemoglobinuria and can be fatal. The discoloured urine gives the disease its colloquial name of redwater. Disease incidence is seasonal and related to tick activity. Babesia organisms are found in stained blood smears during the febrile phase but may be difficult to find in more advanced cases. Specific babesicidal drugs are available for therapy but supportive treatment, possibly including blood transfusions, may be necessary. Animals that recover remain infected and immune for life (*premunity). They may serve as a source of infection for ticks but are

bacillary haemoglobinuria

unlikely to suffer clinical disease again unless severely stressed, in which case relapses can occur. The disease is especially important in cattle. Young cattle (up to about 9 months of age) are much less susceptible to disease than older animals, for reasons not yet fully understood. This inverse age resistance persists much longer than antibodies passed from the dam.

In enzootic areas where there are high levels of infection in hosts and ticks, and where ticks are active and common for much of the year, disease is rare since young stock acquire infection and concurrent immunity at an age when they are unlikely to suffer disease. Problems arise when either susceptible animals are moved into areas where ticks are common or ticks become scarce or seasonally restricted in activity. In some parts of the world, vaccines are available, based on the injection of infected blood from donor animals. Elsewhere in tropical areas, dipping animals with *acaricides at suitable intervals controls tick numbers and hence the babesiosis. *See also* canine babesiosis; equine babesiosis. Other names: **piroplasmosis; Texas fever.**

bacillary haemoglobinuria An *enterotoxaemia, mainly of cattle, caused by the multiplication in necrotic liver foci of the bacterium *Clostridium novyi* (*Cl. oedematiens*) type D. The initiating factor is liver damage by migrating larvae of flukes, especially *Fasciola hepatica*. Severe or fatal forms show *haemoglobinuria and blood in the intestine, but some cases have no clinical signs. For control measures, *see* black disease.

bacillary white diarrhoea See pullorum disease.

Bacillus A genus of spore-forming aerobic Gram-positive *bacteria. Many of these rod-shaped bacteria are soil saprophytes and under normal conditions do not cause disease, with the notable exception of *B. anthracis*, which causes *anthrax in animals and humans. This is a large Gram-positive rod that forms long chains in culture. In tissues and blood of infected animals it occurs as single rods or short chains and is regularly encapsulated. Spores are formed in abundance only in the presence of air, therefore spores are rare in blood and infected tissues. The spores are very resistant to physical and chemical agents, and soils contaminated with spores can remain infective for decades. Factors and conditions that allow sporulation and subsequent vegetative multiplication, such as alkaline soil, high nitrogen levels, and decaying vegetation, increase the prevalence of disease.

bacillus (*pl.* **bacilli**) A rod-shaped bacterium (*see* bacteria).

bacitracin An antibiotic synthesized by the bacteria *Bacillus licheniformis* and *B. subtilis* var. *tracy* that has activity against Gram-positive bacteria. It inhibits the synthesis of certain components of the bacterial cell wall. Absorption from the gastrointestinal tract is poor and it is not used systemically because of toxicity to the kidneys. Its main use is as zinc bacitracin, which is added to pig and poultry feeds as a growth promoter. Resistance of bacteria to bacitracin is very slow to develop. It is also available for topical use in, for example, ear and eye infections and local skin infections.

back bleeding (oversticking) A condition occurring in carcasses when animals are bled inexpertly during slaughter and the blade of the knife is inserted too close to the entrance of the thorax. Blood penetrates into the thoracic cavity and sometimes under the pleura, necessitating washing and scraping. It is commonest in pigs because of their short neck.

backbone *See* vertebral column.

backcross 1. A mating between an offspring and its parent. The offspring of such a cross has a 0.5 probability of being *homozygous for any *allele carried by the parent. The term is used colloquially to mean the crossing of an animal with another whose *genotype is identical or nearly identical to one of its parents. This system is widely used in grading-up programmes where the offspring is the result of the cross between a desired type that exists in low numbers and an unrelated type. The animal thus bred is then crossed with another animal of the desired type and very closely related to its desired-type parent. The offspring is then crossed again with a desired type. This system of crossing, when carried on for a number of generations, will produce animals that are phenotypically identical and genotypically very nearly identical to the original desired type, thereby increasing the numbers of the desired type. **2.** To undertake such a mating.

back muscle necrosis *See* porcine stress syndrome.

baconer A meat pig that has reached the optimum slaughter weight for bacon, or one that is destined to do so. The final liveweight is usually 90 kg, which is determined by the requirements of the bacon-curing process and is reached from about 145 days of age.

bacteraemia The presence of bacteria in circulating blood without accompanying signs of disease, although the term is sometimes used to mean *septicaemia. Bacteraemia may occur transiently when bacteria enter the bloodstream from outside

the body and multiply before localizing in specific organs, or when bacteria enter the blood from foci of infection in other tissues. Continuous bacteraemia may occur when infection is widespread throughout the body (*see* septicaemia) or when certain organisms multiply in the blood components themselves.

bacteri- (bacterio-) *Prefix denoting* bacteria. Example: *bacteriolysis* (dissolution of).

bacteria (*sing.* **bacterium**) A group of unicellular microorganisms that lack a distinct nuclear membrane and have a cell wall of unique composition. They are widely distributed in nature either as free-living saprophytes or obligate parasites of animals, insects, and plants, in which they may or may not cause diseases. Pathogenic bacteria produce poisonous *toxins, which cause clinical signs in their hosts. Bacteria are usually classified according to their reaction to *Gram's stain, whether or not they can replicate in the presence of oxygen (*aerobic or *anaerobic), and on the basis of their shape. Bacterial cells may be spherical (coccus), rod-like (bacillus), spiral (spirillum), comma-shaped (vibrio), corkscrew-shaped (spirochaete), or filamentous. In some the bacterial cells can have more than one shape (*pleomorphism). Structurally, bacteria contain a cell wall, cytoplasmic membrane, and DNA forming a single coiled chromosome (see illustration). Some motile bacteria possess organs of locomotion (*flagella). Others have *fimbriae that enable them to attach to surfaces. Certain bacteria are enveloped by a slimy protective capsule, while others can be transformed into resting phases known as *endospores, which are very resistant to chemical and physical agents. In general, bacteria reproduce asexually by simple division of cells; incomplete separation of daughter cells leads to

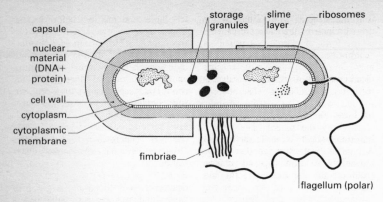

Generalized diagram of a bacterial cell

the formation of colonies. A few groups may reproduce sexually by *conjugation.

bactericide A substance that kills bacteria. Bactericides include *antibiotics, *antiseptics, and *disinfectants.

bacteriology The study of *bacteria, including those associated with disease in animals.

bacteriophage (phage) A *virus that infects a bacterium. Bacteriophages are either *virulent or *temperate.

bacteriostat A substance that prevents the growth and multiplication of bacteria but does not kill them. The use of such agents to treat infections depends on a competent host immune system to kill the organisms. Also, it is essential to maintain an effective concentration of the bacteriostat during the course of treatment or the organisms may recover and resume reproduction.

Bacteroides A genus of Gram-negative anaerobic *bacteria, commonly found as saprophytes in the gastrointestinal tract. *B. nodosus*, however, is an important cause of *foot rot in sheep and possibly also in goats and cattle (*see* foul-in-the-foot), usually in association with *Fusobacterium necrophorum*. Morphologically *B. nodosus* appears as a large curved or straight rod, both ends of which are enlarged. The organism survives better during prolonged wet and warm conditions.

Badgers Act (1973) (England and Wales) An Act of Parliament that prohibits the taking or killing, or attempted taking or killing, of badgers on land without prior written consent of the landowner.

balanitis Inflammation of the glans penis (in the male) or the clitoris (in the female). It is usually due to bacterial infection and may cause breeding problems. Involvement of the prepuce is common, resulting in *balanoposthitis*. Other names: **pizzle rot; sheath rot.** *See also* posthitis.

Balantidium A genus of *ciliate protozoa. The only species of veterinary significance is *B. coli*, a ubiquitous and common inhabitant of the lumen of the large intestine of pigs. It occurs less commonly in humans and primates, and, rarely, in dogs. *B. coli* is transmitted in faeces, either as the normal ciliated form or, more usually, in the form of cysts. It is usually a *commensal but on rare occasions it may invade the gut wall causing ulceration and diarrhoea or *dysentery.

baldness See alopecia.

ball-and-socket joint (enarthrosis) A type of *synovial joint that allows movement to occur in all planes. Examples are the shoulder joint and hip joint.

ballottement The technique of determining the presence of a solid object within a fluid-filled part of the body. A sharp short tap is given to the wall of the fluid-filled structure in an attempt to bounce the solid structure against the wall. Ballottement is used in pregnancy diagnosis, where the embryo or foetus is surrounded by fluid in the uterus. It can also be used in examination of the abdominal contents.

bandage A piece of material used to support an injured part of the body, to retain dressings, or to protect parts of the body from possible injury.

bar (of hoof) The parts of the wall of the equine *hoof that converge from the angles (heels) on either side of the frog.

barbiturate One of a group of drugs that cause depression of the central nervous system (CNS). All are derivatives of barbituric acid, which has no activity on the CNS. Barbiturates are used as intravenous anaesthetics, sedatives, and as agents for euthanasia and to control epilepsy. Members of the group are classified according to the rapidity of onset of action and length of activity (e.g. long-acting, medium-acting, short-acting, and ultra-short-acting). They all act chiefly to depress motor functions of the brain, possibly by interfering with transmitter release and oxidative processes. CNS depression can vary from mild sedation and hypnosis to general anaesthesia; increasing doses cause coma and death. Their action on sensory functions in the brain is less, and perception of pain is not affected until unconsciousness is reached, giving poor analgesia; at low doses *hyperaesthesia and hyperalgesia may occur.

Barbiturates cause some respiratory depression, but effects on the cardiovascular system are less, with minor hypotension and myocardial depression following high doses given rapidly intravenously. Muscle relaxation is quite good and tissue toxicity is low. Short- and ultra-short-acting barbiturates are given intravenously as the sodium salt in solution. Less irritant solutions can be given intraperitoneally. Long-acting barbiturates can be given orally. Metabolism varies among the different compounds. The N-methyl barbiturates and thiobarbiturates, which are highly lipid-soluble, become redistributed to fat and other tissues and are slowly metabolized. Other barbiturates undergo oxidation and the metabolites are excreted in the urine. The rate of metabolism is high in sheep and lower in dogs, cats, and horses.

Thiopentone (US thiopental) is an ultra-short-acting barbiturate administered intravenously to induce anaesthesia of short duration. The sodium salt is highly alkaline in solution, which is irritant and should only be given intravenously – subcutaneous injection causes skin sloughing. A 2.5% or 5% solution is used in small animals and a 10% solution in large animals. Induction of anaesthesia takes about 30 seconds and anaesthesia lasts about 10–15 minutes. The action is terminated by redistribution of thiopentone from the CNS into fat tissue; this may be incomplete in thin animals, e.g. greyhounds, and young animals with low fat reserves. Metabolism of the drug takes several days, and recovery is prolonged if additional injections are used to maintain anaesthesia. *Thiamylal* is similar to thiopentone but with slightly increased potency. It is not used in the UK but is the most commonly used short-acting barbiturate in North America.

Methohexitone (US *methohexital*) is an ultra-short-acting barbiturate used as an induction agent for anaesthesia. The sodium salt produces an alkaline solution, which is injected intravenously. Anaesthesia is induced within 30 seconds and lasts for 5–10 minutes. Recovery is due partly to redistribution of the drug from the CNS to fat, but mainly to metabolism of the drug, making it safer than thiopentone in young and thin animals. It is twice as potent as thiopentone and is used as a 2.5% solution in small animals. Respiratory depression is similar to that produced by thiopentone, and muscle twitching and convulsions are seen in some animals during induction and recovery.

Pentobarbitone (US *pentobarbital*) is a short-acting barbiturate used as an intravenous anaesthetic agent and for euthanasia. The sodium salt is less alkaline in solution than thiopentone sodium and is therefore less irritant, allowing intraperitoneal injection as well as intravenous injection. Induction of anaesthesia takes about 2 minutes after intravenous injection and 5 minutes after intraperitoneal injection. Anaesthesia lasts about 20 minutes in sheep and 30–90 minutes in dogs, cats, and horses. Recovery from anaesthesia is due to metabolism of the drug.

Quinalbarbitone (US *quinalbarbital*) and *butobarbitone* (US *butobarbital*) are intermediate-acting barbiturates, which are administered orally to produce sedation. This lasts 2–5 hours with quinalbarbitone, 10–15 hours with butobarbitone.

Phenobarbitone (US *phenobarbital*) is a long-acting barbiturate used as an anticonvulsant in the treatment of epileptiform convulsions. It is administered orally and acts for 12–24 hours. In treating epilepsy the dose should ideally produce CNS depression and control the fits while causing the minimum of sedation and ataxia. Combination therapy with, for example *phenytoin sodium, is used. Phenobarbitone is not used to treat status epilepticus because it acts too slowly.

Overdosage with barbiturates causes respiratory depression, which can lead to death. Maintenance of the patient using positive-pressure ventilation may allow redistribution or metabolism of the drug and produce recovery. *Analeptics can be administered to stimulate respiration in the treatment of overdosage. Rapid intravenous injection of high doses of barbiturates causes myocardial depression and heart failure can occur occasionally in poor risk patients. Overdosage with phenobarbitone causes ataxia followed by coma and respiratory depression. Other side-effects with phenobarbitone therapy include restlessness, polydipsia, polyphagia, and polyuria. Increased excretion of phenobarbitone can be induced by increasing the alkalinity of the urine by administering sodium bicarbonate intravenously. Barbiturates cause liver enzyme induction, which can increase the rate of metabolism of other drugs administered concurrently.

barium sulphate A white compound, insoluble in water, that is opaque to X-rays. It is given orally in a suspension or mixed with food to allow visualization of the oesophagus, stomach, and intestinal tract, during radiography.

barium sulphide A compound that is made up as a paste, often mixed with *barium sulphate, and applied to skin to remove hairs. It may irritate the skin.

bark eating A form of unusual appetite (or *pica) in which animals denude the bark from trees. The most common cause is mineral deficiency, especially of phosphorus or certain trace elements. Analysis of blood samples will detect the specific deficiency and enable appropriate dietary supplementation, although this may not correct the pica if the habit becomes a vice. The phenomenon also often occurs in early spring when horses or cattle run short of fodder and attempt to satisfy their hunger with any available semi-edible material. (Goats and deer may eat bark as part of their normal diet.)

barley beef (cereal beef) A system of rearing *beef cattle for meat production that uses barley or other cereals as the main feedstuff. The system was developed in the late 1950s to utilize surplus bull calves from dairy herds. The steers, or preferably bulls, should be either purebred Friesians or Friesian crosses sired by a large bull, such as a Charolais or South Devon. Early maturing breeds and heifers are unsuitable since they get fat before slaughter weight is reached. After weaning at about 5 weeks of age, the calves receive an all-concentrate ration containing 170 g kg^{-1} crude protein. From the age of 10–12 weeks (when they should weigh 100–120 kg) the animals are fed ad lib rolled barley supplemented with protein to give 140 g kg^{-1} crude protein. From about 6 months of age (when they weigh about 250 kg) the crude protein content of the diet can be reduced to 120 g kg^{-1}. Animals not bedded on straw must have access to some long roughage, either hay or straw, to reduce the incidence of *rumenitis and *bloat. Monensin sodium (see ionophore) can be included in the ration to improve feed conversion efficiency. See also beef cattle; bull beef; bull husbandry; calf husbandry.

barley poisoning See carbohydrate overload.

baroreceptor (pressoreceptor) A nerve ending within the wall of a blood vessel that is specialized to detect changes in *blood pressure. The main baroreceptors lie in the *carotid sinus, the arch of the *aorta, in other large blood vessels, and within the walls of the heart. Impulses from the baroreceptors are transmitted to centres within the medulla oblongata of the brain, and from here connections are made via the *autonomic nervous system to regulate heart rate and the resistance in the peripheral blood vessels.

bar pad (frog pad) A leather or synthetic pad that is fitted between a short shoe and the horse's foot to cover the posterior portion of the foot, the frog, bars, and the heels. It provides protection for a bruised sole and has antislip and anticoncussion properties.

Barr body A darkly staining body, found in the nucleus of many cells of female mammals, that constitutes the inactive X-chromosome. Abnormal individuals with three X-chromosomes possess two Barr bodies; those with four X-chromosomes have three Barr bodies. See also sex chromosome.

barrel heart See round heart disease.

barrow A North American term for a castrated male pig.

bar shoe A symmetrical horseshoe in which the open ends are joined by a 'bar'. When weight is borne by the foot, expansion at the heels is much decreased and the caudal part of the foot is supported.

Bartonella *See* Haemobartonella.

bartonellosis *See* haemobartonellosis.

basal cell tumour A tumour derived from the germinal cells of the stratum germinativum in the epidermis of the skin. They are common in dogs and cats but less so in other species. The growths are usually solitary, well-demarcated, and involve the dermis and lower layers of the epidermis. They may be found on the head, neck, and limbs; ulceration of the overlying skin is frequent. Basal cell tumours are composed of cords or nests of cells resembling the normal stratum germinativum. Various forms are described, the most common being solid, adenoid, cystic, and medusoid. Cystic forms are more common in the cat, as are tumours containing abundant melanin pigment. The tumours do not metastasize and rarely recur if excision has been complete.

basal ganglia (basal nuclei) Several large masses of grey matter lying deep in the *cerebrum of the brain. They include the *caudate nucleus*, *lentiform nucleus* (composed of the *putamen* and the *globus pallidus*), and the *claustrum*. Together with the intervening internal and external capsules of white matter they constitute the *corpus striatum. They have many connections, especially to the cerebral cortex and thalamus, and are involved in the control of muscular activity at a subconscious level.

basal lamina The dense layer of fine fibrillar material embedded in glycoprotein within a *basement membrane.

basal metabolic rate (BMR) The rate of energy metabolism required to maintain an animal at rest. BMR is measured in terms of heat production per unit time: it indicates the energy consumed in order to sustain such vital functions as heartbeat, breathing, nervous activity, active transport, and secretion. Different tissues have different metabolic rates (e.g. the BMR of brain tissue is much greater than that of bone tissue) and therefore the tissue composition of an animal determines its overall BMR. For any comparable group of animals (such as mammals) BMR is proportional to body weight according to the allometric equation (*see* allometric growth); small animals tend to have a higher metabolic rate per unit weight than large ones.

basement membrane A layer of dense amorphous material associated with many cell types (e.g. epithelia, capillary endothelium, muscle cells) that lie adjacent to connective tissue. It consists of a dense layer of fine fibrillar material (*basal lamina) supported by a layer of *reticular fibres, and may give support to the associated cells and control the diffusion of substances. Changes in its thickness are often associated with pathological conditions, for example *glomerulonephritis.

basidiobolomycosis Disease caused by a noncontagious infection with the fungus *Basidiobolus haptosporus*; a type of *entomophthoromycosis. It is primarily an infection of subcutaneous tissues, occurring sporadically in humans in tropical Africa, southeast Asia, and South America. Until recently it was not reported in animals, except once in horses in Indonesia. However, it is now well recognized as a cause of *equine phycomycosis in Australia, accounting for about 18% of cases studied. The disease is not readily distinguishable from *conidiobolomycosis, although the lesions are more common on the flanks, chest, head, and neck. Definitive diagnosis is by isolation of the fungus in culture from 'kunkers' (*see* equine phycomycosis). Surgical excision of lesions is the recommended treatment, supported by oral or intravenous administration of iodides.

basophil A variety of white blood cell (*see* leucocyte) of the granulocyte series whose granules stain with basic dyes. Basophils are closely related to *mast cells and probably have similar functions.

basophilia 1. A property of a microscopic structure whereby it shows an affinity for basic dyes. **2.** An increase in the number of certain white blood cells (*basophils) in the blood. *See* leucocytosis.

basophilic Readily stainable by basic dyes: showing *basophilia.

bathing The washing or wetting of animals to clean them, treat skin diseases, kill skin parasites, or reduce their body temperature. A specialized bath called a dip (*see* dipping) is used for sheep and sometimes cattle to control parasites; alternatively a *spray race may be used. Some forms of skin inflammation or diseases can be treated by bathing with an antiseptic shampoo. Animals are often bathed before exhibitions or sale to improve their appearance. Animals from temperate climates living in the tropics suffer severely from heat stress, and this can be relieved by the provision of showering facilities. The water temperature is immaterial since body heat is lost through the latent heat of evaporation.

battery systems Intensive husbandry systems in which the animals, usually laying hens, are housed in an array of wire cages. Birds are placed in the cages (usually four or so per cage) prior to the onset of sexual maturity for the duration of their laying period. The rows of cages are arranged in tiers, three or four high. Codes of welfare for poultry give minimum sizes for the cages. Eggs roll down the sloping cage floor to the front where they are collected, either manually or automatically. Food is administered automatically into troughs running the entire length of each row. Water is provided from a central supply through nipple drinkers installed within each cage.

Battery systems enable the requirements of birds to be met precisely, reduce problems associated with *cannibalism, enable a high degree of automation, and make best use of the available space. Currently (1987) approximately 90% of the eggs consumed in Great Britain are from battery systems. However, there is considerable public disquiet throughout Europe concerning their use with calls to ban such systems altogether. Alternatives include deep *litter or various free-range systems, but there are environmental and management problems associated with each. Also, increased egg prices would invariably result from their adoption (*see* poultry husbandry).

Battery systems have been used for rearing pigs, but not widely adopted.

BCG (bacille Calmette-Guérin) A *vaccine produced from an avirulent strain of *Mycobacterium tuberculosis* and used in human medicine to give immunity against *tuberculosis. It has been used to immunize cats and dogs at risk from a tuberculin-infected owner, and has also been assessed as an immunostimulant in the treatment of chronic diseases, such as *equine sarcoid or *demodectic mange in dogs.

bedding Material provided for animals to lie on. Bedding should be comfortable, insulate the animal against heat loss through the floor, protect bony projections of the animal's body against injury from a hard floor, and absorb dung and urine thus keeping the animal cleaner. A variety of materials are used, the choice depending mainly on price and availability. The most satisfactory bedding material for all classes of livestock is wheat *straw. Oat straw may also be used when available but barley straw is not advisable for dairy cows or pigs as the awns tend to irritate the udder and soft skin of other regions. Sawdust, shavings, and sand are particularly useful for dairy cows housed in *cubicles, although sawdust has been associated with coliform *mastitis. Special rubber mats are available as a substitute for bedding in cow cubicles. In all cases, bedding material should be kept dry and fresh material provided regularly. *See also* litter.

beef cattle Cattle reared specifically for beef production. In the UK, more than half the cattle used for beef production originate from dairy herds, i.e. culled breeding bulls, culled dairy cows, purebred calves, or crossbred calves sired by a bull of a recognized beef breed, especially the Hereford, Charolais, Limousin, Simmental, or Aberdeen Angus. These breeds have the advantage of colour-marking their progeny, thereby clearly demonstrating to buyers their beef breeding. The remaining beef cattle come from specialized beef breeding herds (*see* suckler herd). Because Friesians and Holsteins are the predominant dairy breeds, most crossbred calves have one of these as a dam breed. However, Holstein crosses are less suitable for beef production since they take longer to reach slaughter condition than a Friesian cross unless fed a ration with a higher energy concentration. Unfortunately, the two crosses are virtually indistinguishable in the

market. *See also* barley beef; bull beef; cattle husbandry.

beet-top poisoning *See* oxalate poisoning.

bemegride An *analeptic drug used occasionally as a stimulant in cases of barbiturate overdosage.

Benadryl Tradename for *diphenhydramine.

Bence-Jones protein A type of protein derived from immunoglobulins and found in the urine of animals with multiple *myeloma and certain other cancers.

benethamine penicillin *See* penicillin.

benign 1. Describing a tumour that does not invade and destroy the tissue in which it originates or spread to distant sites in the body, i.e. a tumour that is not cancerous. **2.** Describing any disorder or condition that does not produce harmful effects. *Compare* malignant.

benzalkonium chloride *See* cationic detergent.

benzamine lactate One of the ester-type group of local *anaesthetics. It is used mainly in eye operations. Other names: **eucaine; betacaine.**

benzathine penicillin *See* penicillin.

benzene hexachloride (BHC) An *organochlorine compound, more correctly named hexachlorocyclohexane (HCH), that is used as an insecticide. It has five isomers with differing toxicities, of which gamma BHC (also known as lindane) is the most frequently used. BHC acts as a contact poison for insects, although the knock-down effect takes several minutes. It is used to kill lice, fleas, and mites on poultry, pigs, horses, and cattle. In small animals BHC is used to control fleas, lice, and mange mites. Activity against sarcoptic mange mites is good but efficacy against *Demodex* spp. is poor. It is available as a dusting powder, spray, a powder for making up suspensions for bathing animals, in skin creams, and in ear drops. The concentration of BHC is typically 0.1–0.2% in these products. Cats and young animals should be treated using dusting powders to reduce the risk of toxicity; excess powder should be brushed out of the coat 15–30 minutes after treatment to reduce the risk of ingestion of BHC during grooming.

Acute BHC toxicity produces excitability, convulsions, paralysis, and death. The administration of pentobarbitone or diazepam can control nervous signs. Chronic toxicity is more likely with the beta isomer, which is more persistent in tissues. Signs of chronic toxicity include muscle tremors, convulsions, depression, respiratory failure, and death. Convulsions have a slow onset but gradually become more frequent. Recovery on removal of the source of BHC can take several weeks, with intermittent convulsions. BHC was formerly used in sheep dips and sprays to control external parasites, such as sheep scab. It is no longer used for this because of the persistence of organochlorine compounds in tissues and the risk of toxicity. *See also* organochlorine poisoning.

benzene hexachloride (BHC) poisoning *See* organochlorine poisoning.

benzimidazoles A group of related anthelmintics with the same basic benzimidazole structure. Differences in the chemical groups attached to this structure influence the efficacy and pharmacokinetics (solubility and rate of metabolism). The more mod-

ern broad-spectrum compounds all contain a carbamate group, and differences in efficacy are due solely to drug kinetics. The benzimidazoles are thought to act by preventing the formation of microtubules in the parasites; these are necessary to allow transport of nutrients and waste products. There is also inhibition of enzymes, and the parasites become deficient in energy and die, although this process can take several days. The benzimidazoles are poorly soluble in water and lipids, and are available as suspensions for oral drenching or intraruminal injection – in slow-release and pulse-release ruminal boluses or in tablet form.

Thiabendazole, the first benzimidazole to be introduced (in 1961), is the only member to also have antifungal properties (it is used in seed dressings and to spray fruit bushes). It has good efficacy against adult gastrointestinal nematodes but efficacy against larvae and lungworms is poor, with no activity against inhibited larvae in the gastrointestinal mucosa. It is inexpensive and can be used for routine worming in all species. *Cambendazole* has similar activity to thiabendazole and is used in pigs. *Thiophanate*, a benzimidazole prodrug, is metabolized to a compound with similar activity to thiabendazole. The drugs *parbendazole*, *oxibendazole*, *mebandazole*, and *flubendazole* have good efficacy against gastrointestinal parasites and some activity against lungworms. Activity against inhibited larvae is poor.

The modern benzimidazoles – *fenbendazole*, *oxfendazole*, and *albendazole* – all have good efficacy against gastrointestinal nematodes and flukes, lungworms, and inhibited larvae; albendazole at higher doses has activity against adult liver flukes. These drugs are used in sheep, cattle, goats, pigs, horses, small animals, and game birds. In horses there is good efficacy against strongylids and *Oxy-*

benzocaine

uris but poorer efficacy against stomach worms (e.g. *Habronema* and *Trichostrongylus axei*); activity against *Strongyloides westeri* and *Parascaris* in foals may be variable. In cats and dogs these agents are effective against roundworms, hookworms, and tapeworms. Daily dosing for five consecutive days is required to obtain expulsion of the parasites in these small animals. *Triclabendazole* has anticestodal activity and also good efficacy against adult liver flukes and larval stages down to less than 3 weeks of age; it has no activity against gastrointestinal nematodes and lungworms. It is used to remove all stages of flukes in sheep, cattle, goats, and occasionally horses.

After oral administration some of the more potent benzimidazoles are metabolized in the liver to the sulphoxide derivative, which also has anthelmintic activity: fenbendazole is metabolized to oxfendazole, and albendazole forms albendazole sulphoxide; febantel is metabolized to fenbendazole then to oxfendazole; netobimin forms albendazole then albendazole sulphoxide. Further metabolism to the sulphone abolishes anthelmintic activity.

The modern benzimidazoles are unlikely to cause toxicity, and even the more soluble compounds require excessive overdosing (up to 20 times the normal dose) to cause toxicity, which is more likely in small animals. Signs of toxicity are inappetence, haemorrhagic gastroenteritis, shock, and death. Cambendazole has been withdrawn from use in sheep after anaphylactoid reactions. The benzimidazoles influence the development of the mitotic spindle during cell division and have been found to have a teratogenic effect if excessive doses are given at certain periods during gestation (e.g. day 17 in sheep). Some sheep and horse parasites (including *Trichostrongylus*, *Haemonchus contortus*, *Ostertagia circumcinta*, and small strongylids) have become resistant to benzimidazoles, with cross-resistance between members of the group.

benzocaine A local anaesthetic in the form of a white powder, very insoluble in water, that is used in dusting powders to relieve pain in wounds and mucosal surfaces. Chemical name: **ethyl aminobenzoate.**

benzoic acid (benzenecarboxylic acid) A white crystalline compound with antiseptic properties that was formerly given orally to treat urinary infections since it is excreted as hippuric acid thus making the urine acidic. It has also been used with salicylic acid as a topical antifungal to treat skin conditions, such as ringworm.
Benzoic acid poisoning Benzoic acid can be used as a food preservative and cases of poisoning have been recorded in cats fed on preserved meat containing excessive amounts. Clinical signs are muscle tremors, incoordination, increased sensitivity to touch, and apparent blindness followed by convulsions and death.

benzyl benzoate A volatile oil that is used in an emulsion as a dressing in the treatment of parasitic skin diseases, for instance *sarcoptic mange in horses and sarcoptic and *otodectic mange in small animals. If applied frequently or over a large area toxicity may occur. Cats are particularly susceptible and should not be given the drug. Signs of toxicity are vomiting, diarrhoea, nervous excitability, and depression of the heart and breathing rate. Sedation with short-acting *barbiturates may be used to treat cases of poisoning.

benzylpenicillin *See* penicillin.

beri-beri A disorder resulting from *vitamin B_1 (thiamine) deficiency.

Clinical signs include inappetence, emaciation, muscular weakness, and progressive dysfunction of the nervous system leading to paralysis. Pigs and chickens may be affected, but because they commonly consume whole cereal grains, deficiency is rare. Signs of beri-beri are normally limited to humans eating restricted diets.

Bermuda grass photosensitization
A form of hepatogenous *photosensitization of cattle occurring sporadically in southern states of the USA. It is associated with the grazing of Bermuda grass (*Cynodon dactylon*) damaged by frost or drought and subsequently colonized by saprophytic fungi. However, the cause is unknown.

Bermuda grass staggers A nervous syndrome occurring sporadically in the USA among cattle ingesting Bermuda grass (*Cynodon dactylon*). It is clinically similar to *paspalum staggers but is not associated with a *Claviceps* infection; the cause is uncertain.

beta agonist Any of a group of drugs that act at beta adrenergic receptors in the sympathetic nervous system. Beta receptors can be divided into β_1 and β_2 subtypes, with β_1 receptors in the heart and β_2 receptors in smooth muscle of the bronchi, uterus, and skeletal muscle vasculature. The body's own beta agonists are the catecholamines *adrenaline and *noradrenaline, although noradrenaline acts mainly at β_1 receptors. Isoprenaline is a synthetic catecholamine that acts on all beta receptors, causing increased heart rate, relaxation of bronchial muscle, and vasodilatation in skeletal muscles. This drug was used to treat asthma in humans but it has a short duration of action and causes tachycardia and reduction in blood pressure. Now specific β_2 agonists are available. The main one used in veterinary therapy is *clenbuterol, although others, such as salbutamol, terbutaline, and orciprenaline, are available for human use. β_2 agonists are used to treat respiratory disease in horses and also to delay parturition or to cause uterine relaxation in the treatment of dystocia. These newer drugs are metabolized relatively slowly and are thus longer-acting (e.g. 6–8 hours).

beta blockers A group of drugs that selectively block beta (β) adrenergic receptors in the *sympathetic nervous system. Beta receptors can be subdivided into β_1 receptors, found in the heart, and β_2 receptors, occurring in the smooth muscle of the bronchi, uterus, and skeletal muscle blood vasculature. Propranolol was the first beta blocker to have widespread clinical use. It acts as a competitive antagonist at β_1 and β_2 receptors and is used in the treatment of heart conditions to lower the heart rate and improve cardiac filling and cardiac output. However, activity at β_2 receptors causes bronchoconstriction, which can be detrimental. Other nonselective beta blocking agents available (on the human market) are alprenolol, bunolol, nadolol, oxprenolol, penbutolol, pindolol, sotalol, and *timolol.

Selective β_1 blocking drugs have now been developed, which have activity on the heart but no effect at β_2 receptors. Practolol was the first of these, but toxicity with long-term use produced disruption to epithelial structures causing skin eruptions, peritoneal adhesions, and corneal damage. Other β_1 blockers are available on the human market, including metoprolol, atenolol, acebutolol, bevantolol, pafenolol, and tolamolol. These drugs are used in the treatment of cardiac disorders, such as canine cardiomyopathy, ventricular tachycardia, and other cardiac arrhythmias. They are of little use in the treatment of atrial fibrillation and should not be used in cases of advanced congestive cardiac failure until oedema fluid has been removed, since they may precipitate circulatory collapse and death. Butoxamine, a selective β_2 blocker, has little clinical use.

betamethasone *See* corticosteroid.

BHC *See* benzene hexachloride.

BHS (beta haemolytic streptococci) *See* Streptococcus.

bi- *Prefix denoting* two; double. Examples: *biciliate* (having two cilia); *binucleate* (having two nuclei).

bicarbonate of soda *See* sodium bicarbonate.

biceps brachii muscle A muscle located on the front of the upper forelimb. It originates on the supraglenoid tubercle of the *scapula and inserts to the *radius and *ulna. Its main action is to flex the elbow joint.

biceps femoris muscle A large long muscle lying in the caudal part of the thigh, consisting of two heads. In the **horse** it is fixed with part of the superficial gluteal muscle (*see* gluteus) to form the *gluteobiceps muscle*. The biceps femoris acts to extend the hip, stifle, and hock joints. If the limb is free it acts to flex the stifle joint.

bicuspid valve (mitral valve, left atrioventricular valve) The valve guarding the opening between the left atrium and left ventricle in the heart. It consists of two flaps or cusps. *See* atrioventricular valve.

bifurcation (in anatomy) The point at which division into two branches occurs, for example in blood vessels or in the trachea.

big head A condition of young stud rams characterized by *cellulitis and gelatinous oedema of the head region. It follows infection of wounds, sustained during fighting, with the bacterium *Clostridium novyi* (*Cl. oedematiens*) type A, and usually leads to rapid death from toxaemia. It occurs chiefly in Australia and South Africa. Antibiotic or hyperimmune serum therapy may be used for valuable animals.

bilateral (in anatomy) Relating to or affecting both sides of the body.

bile An alkaline secretion produced by the liver and conveyed to the *duodenum through the *bile duct system. The secretion may be stored and concentrated in the *gall-bladder when present. Bile neutralizes the acid digesta from the stomach, thereby providing the optimum pH for duodenal and pancreatic enzymes. It also contains the *bile acids, chiefly cholic acid and chenodeoxycholic acid, which are involved in the emulsification of fats thus aiding their digestion and absorption. The bile acids are largely reabsorbed from the *ileum and returned to the liver for resecretion, thereby conserving the body pool of bile acids.

Bile is also a route for the excretion of various substances, including bilirubin, a breakdown product of the haem nucleus of haemoglobin (*see* bile pigments). Hormones, drugs, and a variety of toxic materials are also eliminated from the circulation via bile. They are usually conjugated in the liver with glucuronic acid and so rendered inactive. Bile secretion is stimulated by a number of factors (*choleretics*), principally the bile acids. Also instrumental are peptide hormones, such as *secretin, and, to a a lesser extent, *cholecystokinin and *gastrin. Vagus nerve stimulation is also effective. Blockage of the bile duct, for example by calculi, will interfere with bile secretion and hence with digestion and detoxification.

bile acids The acids (or their sodium or potassium salts) that are present in *bile and play an important role in fat digestion in the small intestine. They are based on cholic acid and chenodeoxycholic (chenic) acid, which are synthesized in the liver from cholesterol and are conjugated with glycine or taurine to form the bile acids – glycocholic, taurocholic, glycochenic, and taurochenic acids. These conjugated forms are less susceptible to precipitation and more slowly absorbed from the proximal small intestine, thus increasing their effectiveness. A high proportion of both forms is reabsorbed and recycled to the liver for resecretion in the bile. The bile acids are effective emulsifying agents and assist the stabilization of fats as particles of 0.5–1.0 μm diameter. The conjugated acids also reduce the pH optimum of pancreatic *lipase thereby rendering it more effective in the small intestine, where it acts to hydrolyse fats. The bile acids form multimolecular aggregates (*micelles) with monoglycerides and fatty acids, thereby maintaining them

in a soluble form and aiding their diffusion towards the intestinal mucosa. The micelles split up at the intestinal surface and the fatty acids and bile acids are absorbed separately.

bile duct Any of the ducts that convey bile from the liver, especially the main duct which discharges bile into the duodenum. Bile is drained from the liver cells by many small ducts, the *bile canaliculi*; in many species these unite into right and left hepatic ducts, which join to form the common hepatic duct. This is joined by the cystic duct from the *gall-bladder, when present, to form the bile duct, which opens into the duodenum at the major duodenal papilla. In the dog a number of hepatic ducts join the bile duct in a variable manner. See illustration.

bile pigments A mixture of the pigments *bilirubin* and *biliverdin*, which are present in *bile and colour it variously yellow, green, or brown, depending on their relative proportions. They are excretory products produced by the degradation of haemoglobin and other haem-contain-

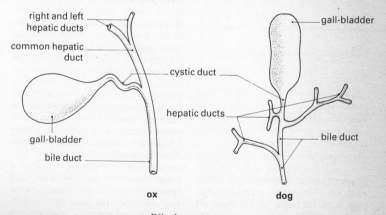

Bile duct system

ing proteins.

bile salts *See* bile acids.

bilharziasis *See* schistosomiasis.

biliary fever *See* equine babesiosis.

bilirubin *See* bile pigments.

bilirubinaemia An excess of the *bile pigment bilirubin in the blood. This causes the yellowing of tissues known as *jaundice. Bilirubin is a product of haemoglobin breakdown and is normally excreted in bile; only a small amount is usually present in blood. Where there is excessive breakdown of red blood cells, as in *haemolytic anaemia, the capacity of the liver to metabolize the bilirubin is exceeded and its level in the blood rises. This also occurs as a result of liver injury or in obstructive jaundice, in which there is obstruction of bile outflow.

biliuria The presence of bile salts or bile in the urine. This may occur in obstructive *jaundice. It can be detected by scattering a small amount of flowers of sulphur on the urine sample. Normally the sulphur grains will float, but if the bile salts are present they reduce the surface tension causing the sulphur grains to sink.

biliverdin *See* bile pigments.

binocular Relating to or involving the use of both eyes.

binocular vision The ability to focus both eyes on an object at the same time so that a single image is seen. This enables judgment of distance and depth. Binocular vision is best developed in hunting animals, such as carnivores, where the eyes are situated near the front of the head. In herbivores the eyes are more laterally located resulting in less binocular vision but a wider total visual field.

binovular twins Two conceptuses in the same pregnancy that originate from separate ova.

bio- *Prefix denoting* life or living organisms. Example: *biosynthesis* (formation of a compound within a living organism).

bioassay Estimation of the activity or potency of a drug or other substance by comparing its effects on living organisms with the effects of a preparation of known strength. Bioassays are used to determine the strength of preparations of hormones or other material of biological origin when other physical or chemical methods are not available.

biochemistry The study of the chemical processes and substances occurring in living things.

biology The study of living organisms – plants, animals, and microorganisms – including their structure and functioning and their relationships with one another and with the inanimate world.

biometry The measurement of living things and the processes associated with life, including the application of mathematics, particularly statistics, to problems in biology.

biopsy The removal of tissue from a living animal for examination in order to identify specific disease processes or to recover pathogens. Histological examination of biopsy material can distinguish between types of cancer and is valuable in deciding a prognosis. Also, the examination of biopsy material from organs enables the identification of degenerative changes due to disease. Biopsies are usually performed under local or general anaesthetic.

biotin A water-soluble *vitamin that serves in the body as an essential coenzyme for many carboxylation reactions in various enzyme systems, including those responsible for *gluconeogenesis and for the synthesis of fatty acids and proteins, for example *keratin. It is synthesized by microorganisms in the reticulorumen and intestines and is found in many plant and animal tissues. However, its synthesis by intestinal microorganisms may be suppressed by the administration of antibiotics. The vitamin's biological availability in most cereal products, except maize (corn), is low. Good sources are yeast, liver, meat, milk, green leafy crops, molasses, and soya-bean meal. Biotin is stable in most diets but is bound in an unavailable form by the protein avidin, which is found in raw egg white and injured epithelial tissues of fowl, and by streptavidin, a product of *Streptomyces* bacteria. Heat inactivates both avidin and streptavidin.

Biotin deficiency Pigs and poultry given inadequately supplemented cereal-based diets may show signs of deficiency. In pigs these include low growth rates, dry skin, dermatitis, loss of hair, and soft and cracking hooves; sows exhibit longer weaning-to-remating intervals and lower conception rates. In poultry deficiency signs include low hatchability of eggs, reduced viability of chicks, impaired growth rates, chondrodystrophy, foot-pad lesions, breast blisters, and *fatty liver and kidney syndrome. Cats and dogs given either antibiotics or fed large quantities of raw egg white may show signs of deficiency, including rough dry hair coats, alopecia, and dry scaly dermatitis. Horses, cattle, and sheep fed on large quantities of cereals may show deficiency signs, including soft and cracking hooves. In fish deficiency signs include loss of appetite, dark coloration, muscle atrophy, and anaemia. For diagnosis and treatment *see* vitamin. Other names: **vitamin B_8; vitamin H**.

biotype A group of individuals presumed to have the same genetic composition. The term is used colloquially to mean a group sharing the same physiological characters or reaction to an environment.

bipolar Having two poles or processes. In neurology, a neurone that has two processes extending in different directions from its cell body.

bird fancier's disease (pigeon fancier's disease) A respiratory condition of humans caused by a Type III *hypersensitivity response to the spores of moulds growing on bird droppings. The symptoms include cough and laboured breathing, and the condition is similar to farmer's lung (*see* allergic alveolitis).

bird import controls (Britain) Legislation governing the importation of live poultry, other birds, or hatching eggs into Great Britain, which stipulates that such importation is permitted only if a licence is held under the Importation of Birds, Poultry, and Hatching Eggs Order (1979).

bird louse A biting *louse (order Mallophaga). Most biting lice are ectoparasites of birds, such as the shaft louse (*Menopon gallinae*) that infests poultry, ducks, and pigeons, the poultry head louse (*Cuclotogaster heterographus*), and *Columbicola columbae* of pigeons. All cause intense irritation and have a large, often broad head with two large toothed biting mandibles for feeding on feathers or skin debris.

bird malaria *See* avian malaria.

birdsville disease A toxic condition occurring in horses grazing on pastures containing birdsville indigo (*Indigofera dominii*) in Australia. The plant contains the amino acid indospicine, which causes liver lesions and consequent loss of condition, drowsiness, laboured breathing, incoordination, dragging of the limbs, and discharges from the nose and eyes. Some protection to horses at risk is provided by supplementing their rations with a source of arginine, such as groundnut (peanut) meal or gelatine.

bismuth A white crystalline metal with a pinkish tinge. Its insoluble inorganic salts were formerly used as a contrast medium for radiography of the gastrointestinal tract, but have now been superseded by *barium sulphate.
Bismuth poisoning This can occur as a result of therapeutic administration of bismuth salts. Clinical signs are acute gastroenteritis leading to vomiting, diarrhoea, collapse, and death.

bitter almond poisoning *See* cherry laurel poisoning.

bittersweet poisoning *See* solanine poisoning.

bitterweed Any of various North American plants that can cause toxic conditions in animals. They include certain members of the genera *Helenium* (*see* Helenium poisoning), *Hymenoxus* (*see* Hymenoxus poisoning), and *Senecio* (*see* ragwort poisoning).

black disease An acute disease of sheep, cattle, and, more rarely, pigs and horses caused by toxins produced by the bacterium *Clostridium oedematiens* (*novyi*) type B infecting a damaged liver. In practice, black disease is usually associated with the liver damage due to *fascioliasis (liver fluke) although other forms of liver

damage may precipitate it. The toxaemia develops rapidly so that affected animals are most commonly found dead; when signs are seen in sheep they usually comprise depression, inability to follow the flock, and transient fever followed by subnormal temperature and recumbency. In cattle the course of the disease is longer but the signs are similar. In all species recovery is rare. Post-mortem examination of carcasses reveals rapid putrefaction and darkening of the inside of the hide, hence the name of the disease. The liver shows engorgement, haemorrhage, necrosis, and evidence of recent parasitism by liver flukes. Diagnosis is confirmed by the laboratory demonstration of pathogenic strains of *Cl. oedematiens* in the liver lesions. No treatment is available; control is by vaccination and treatment/prevention of fluke infestation. Other names: **bradsot; infectious necrotic hepatitis**. *See also* bacillary haemoglobinuria.

blackhead (histomoniasis) A disease of turkeys and, rarely, domestic fowls, distributed worldwide and caused by the protozoan parasite *Histomonas meleagridis*. Although the disease is rare in domestic fowls, these may serve as important reservoirs of infection for turkeys. Transmission of the disease is complex and indirect, involving a parasitic roundworm (*Heterakis*) and often also earthworms (*see* Histomonas). Consequently, most at risk are young free-range turkeys with access to ground where chickens are or have been, but intensively reared turkeys can also suffer the disease.
In turkeys the disease occurs in poults up to about 8–12 weeks of age; older birds are resistant and rarely suffer severe disease. The parasite multiplies in the large intestine, invades the bloodstream, and passes to the liver where it grows in colonies expanding radially and destroying the

liver tissue producing very characteristic circular areas of pale dead tissue. Affected birds become dull and depressed and pass typically soft sulphur-yellow droppings. Although the comb and wattle may become darkened this is neither a universal nor a unique feature, so the name 'blackhead' is something of a misnomer. Disease may be prevented in poults by the continuous feeding of appropriate drugs during the first few weeks of life. Similarly, outbreaks of disease can be treated with appropriate drugs in feed or water. Histomoniasis also occurs in other gallinaceous birds, such as peafowl and guinea fowl. Other name: **infectious enterohepatitis**.

blackleg (blackquarter) An acute infectious disease of cattle and sheep (and occasionally horses) caused by the bacterium *Clostridium chauvoei*. Although true blackleg is associated with cattle, particularly calves and yearlings aged between six months and two years, a similar syndrome is seen in sheep. The disease occurs in most parts of the world and is a soil-borne infection, entering the body by ingestion. The spores of the bacterium are taken up by macrophages in the alimentary tract and deposited in muscle, where they lie dormant until activated, often by damage to the muscles.

Affected animals are often found dead due to the speed at which the disease progresses. If observed prior to death the animals show signs of swelling in the upper part of the leg, which is hot at first but soon becomes cold and painless. This is accompanied by a high body temperature (41°C), rapid pulse rate, depression, and marked lameness. In sheep the disease is usually associated with wounds acquired at shearing, docking, or lambing.

When the disease occurs it usually affects a number of animals in the space of a few days and is usually fatal. Because the spores can survive for many years in the soil certain fields are often associated with the disease. Vaccination is the best form of prevention. *See also* malignant oedema.

blackquarter *See* blackleg.

blackspot A condition occurring in carcasses in which black spots of mould, about 5 mm in diameter, are scattered throughout exposed surfaces. It is caused by the fungus *Cladosporium harbarum* and is commonest in imported frozen lamb carcasses. The mould penetrates the tissues and is difficult to remove.

black tongue A nutritional disorder resulting from deficiency of *nicotinic acid, a B vitamin. It can occur in pigs, poultry, and dogs and resembles human 'pellagra'. Most livestock diets contain adequate supplies of the vitamin or its precursor, the amino acid, tryptophan. However, maize (corn) contains very little tryptophan and thus pigs and poultry fed on a predominantly maize diet may show deficiency because they cannot synthesize the vitamin. Low protein intake exacerbates the problem. Clinical signs include ill-thrift and diarrhoea with dehydration. The term 'black tongue' refers to the characteristic inflammation and ulceration of the mouth, which is accompanied by a foul odour and causes inappetence. Similar lesions occur throughout the digestive tract. The disease responds to nicotinic acid supplementation of the diet. This vitamin is customarily added to pig rations based on maize, so the problem should be rare.

black vomit A type of vomit characteristically associated with haemorrhage in the stomach. The blood pigment haemoglobin is precipitated by the hydrochloric acid in the gastric secretion to form fine black particles resembling coffee grains. The bleeding may be due to, for instance, ulceration, mucosal damage, trauma, or neoplasia.

bladder 1. (**urinary bladder**) A sac-shaped organ that has a wall of smooth muscle and stores the urine produced by the kidneys. Urine passes into the bladder through the *ureters; the release of urine from the bladder is controlled by sphincter-like activity at its junction with the *urethra. The organ is covered by peritoneum and held in place with the aid of three peritoneal folds – the single median ligament and the paired lateral ligaments. 2. Any of various hollow organs containing fluid, such as the *gall-bladder.

bladder tumours Any of various tumours that arise in the urinary bladder or associated structures. They occur mainly in cattle (in which they are associated with enzootic *haematuria), sheep, and older dogs and cats; other species show infrequent incidence. *Polyps and *carcinomas are the predominant types, although tumours of smooth and striated muscle and of connective and vascular tissues have been reported, especially in relation to enzootic haematuria. Most arise from the epithelium of the bladder, but origin from the renal pelvis, urethra, and ureter occasionally takes place.
Bladder polyps may be single or multiple well-circumscribed noninvasive lesions consisting of long fingers of loose connective tissue covered by epithelium. *Bladder carcinomas* are diffusely invasive and result in thickening of the bladder wall; they are often extensive when first diagnosed. In both types, ulceration with infection and haemorrhage may occur, leading to *dysuria and the presence of blood and pus in the urine. Infiltration through the bladder wall may

allow spread to adjacent fat deposits and organs, such as the urethra, ureter, or kidney, or to implantation into the peritoneal cavity. Regional lymph nodes are often involved, with blood-borne spread to the lungs and other organs occurring as a later development. Although such chemicals as β-naphthylamine can induce bladder tumours in dogs, the cause of spontaneous tumours is unclear. In cattle, enzootic haematuria is associated with the ingestion of bracken, and constituents of the plant may have a carcinogenic effect on the bladder wall (*see* bracken poisoning). The success of treatment for bladder tumours in dogs and cats is dependent upon the tumour type. Solitary neoplasms of connective tissue origin may be removed surgically and the prognosis may be fair to good. However, bladder carcinomas tend to be multifocal and invasive in nature and the results of attempted surgical excision are often poor. Cytotoxic *chemotherapy may be palliative. *See also* polypoid cystitis.

bladderworm The intermediate larval stage in the development of certain *tapeworms. Its host is always different from that of the adult tapeworm, hence it was originally regarded as a distinct species. A bladderworm is a large fluid-filled cyst in which one or more tapeworm heads are invaginated. There are three principal types: the *cysticercus and *coenurus of the genus *Taenia* and the *hydatid cyst of the genus *Echinococcus*.

-blast *Suffix denoting* a formative cell. Example: *osteoblast* (formative bone cell).

blastema Any zone of embryonic tissue that is still differentiating and growing into a particular organ. The term is usually applied to the tissue that develops into the kidneys and gonads.

blasto- *Prefix denoting* a germ cell or embryo. Example: *blastogenesis* (early development of an embryo).

blastocoele The fluid-filled cavity that develops within the *blastocyst. The cavity increases the surface area of the blastocyst and thus improves its ability to absorb nutrients and oxygen.

blastocyst An early stage of embryonic development that consists of a hollow ball of cells with a localized thickening (*embryonic disc*) that will develop into the actual embryo; the remainder of the blastocyst is composed of *trophoblast (see illustration). At first the blastocyst is unattached, but it soon becomes implanted on the wall of the uterus. *See* implantation.

blastomere Any of the cells produced by the *cleavage of the *zygote, during the earliest stages of embryonic development until the formation of the *blastocyst. Blastomeres divide repeatedly without overall growth and so decrease in size.

blastomycosis Disease caused by infection with the *dimorphic fungus *Blastomyces dermatitidis*, occurring in animals and humans. The disease is noncontagious and infection is acquired by inhalation of spores from the mycelial phase growing on rotting organic material in the environment. It is enzootic in some states of the USA, mostly in the southeast and Midwest, but extends into Canada. The old name of *North American blastomycosis* is belied by human cases reported from South America, Africa, and a number of other countries.
The disease is common in **dogs** in enzootic areas but rare among other species. Unlike *coccidioidomycosis and *histoplasmosis, asymptomatic self-limiting infection seems rare and

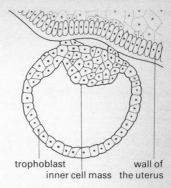

Section through a blastocyst

canine blastomycosis is a progressive disease. Initial signs of a cough and dyspnoea, sometimes with fever or debility, are followed by the appearance of cutaneous ulcers and subcutaneous abscesses. Skin lesions in dogs, unlike those in humans, usually indicate an advanced stage of the disease with dissemination to other organs, often including the eye. Diagnosis can be made by the demonstration, in tissues or exudate from lesions, of spherical yeast cells (8–30 μm in diameter) with thick doubly-refractile walls and budding on a characteristically broad base. Confirmation by culture requires the conversion of isolates between the yeast and mycelial phases to ensure correct identification. Most cases of canine blastomycosis are curable by vigorous treatment with *amphotericin B initially, sometimes followed by the less toxic but slower acting drug ketoconazole. The term was formerly used for infection by any of various yeasts.

'bleeder' horse Describing a racehorse that bleeds from the nostrils during or after a race. The blood originates from the lungs and its presence may be an indication of structural changes in the lungs and the competitive stresses of racing. Some blood may be swallowed. Bleeding during a race tends to reduce the animal's speed.

blenn- (blenno-) *Prefix denoting* mucus. Example: *blennorrhagia* (excessive production of).

blephar- (blepharo-) *Prefix denoting* the eyelid. Example: *blepharotomy* (incision into).

blepharitis Inflammation of the eyelid, particularly its margin. It may be associated with inflammation of the eye (as in conjunctivitis, keratitis, or inflammation of the cornea) or with inflammatory lesions of the skin around the eye. The margin of the eyelid is reddened and swollen, and there is an excess of tears (*epiphora) and an ocular discharge. Specific causes include bacterial infection, nearby ringworm lesions, mite infestation, allergy, injury, or neoplasia.

blepharospasm Spasm of the orbicularis oculi muscle – the superficial facial muscle that encircles the eye. This produces partial or complete closure of the eyelids. It is usually associated with painful lesions of the cornea, conjunctiva, or eyelid.

blindness Loss of vision. This may be partial or total, and may involve one or both eyes. Blindness can arise due to: defective transmission of light through the eye (involving the cornea, aqueous humour, lens, or vitreous humour); diseases of the retina, such as *progressive retinal atrophy or *collie eye anomaly; and disease of the visual pathway connecting the eye and the brain. Early loss of vision is not always appreciated, hence the changes might be quite advanced before blindness is diagnosed. The animal may bump into objects or show reluctance to go out at night.

Tests designed to investigate blindness are sometimes difficult to perform and interpret because of difficul-

ties in getting the patient to cooperate. The *pupillary light reflex* consists of shining a light in one eye; normally, the pupil of that eye should respond by contracting (the direct response) and the pupil of the other eye should also contract (the consensual response). This test depends on intact *oculomotor and *optic nerves. Furthermore, harmless light objects, such as a piece of cottonwool, directed at the eye should elicit reflex closing of a normal eye. This tests functioning of the optic nerve and *facial nerve. Examination of the different structures within the eye is performed using an *ophthalmoscope.

blind staggers *See* Astragalus poisoning.

blister beetle *See* Spanish fly.

bloat (ruminal tympany) A condition of ruminants, especially cattle and sheep, in which the rumen becomes overdistended due to a build-up of gas. The enlarged rumen exerts pressure on the diaphragm, heart, and lungs, making breathing difficult and eventually causing collapse and death. *Primary bloat* is a result of dietary factors that cause excessive gas production. Succulent pastures, especially those rich in young rapidly growing legumes (e.g. clover) are often involved, particularly in New Zealand. Foaming of the ruminal contents (*frothy bloat*) can be caused by certain plant components, such as proteins, pectins, saponins, and hemicelluloses. Bloat may also follow the ingestion of large amounts of easily fermentable carbohydrate (*see* carbohydrate overload). *Secondary bloat* is the result of impeded *eructation. The *oesophagus may become blocked, for example by potatoes or other food items. Swelling around the oesophagus caused by inflammation or *tumours may also cause the condition, while *carcinomas or *papillomas affecting the oesophageal groove can lead to disturbances of eructation. Bloat is a common sign in cases of vagus *indigestion or *traumatic reticulitis, in which the nerve supply to the rumen is affected.

Treatment of primary bloat consists of voiding the gas and relieving the pressure by inserting a *stomach tube into the rumen via the oesophagus or puncturing the rumen through the body wall by means of a *trocar. Antifoaming agents, such as mineral oil, are administered in cases of frothy bloat. Outbreaks of frothy bloat can be prevented by spraying strip-grazed pasture with vegetable oils or emulsified tallow. Treatment of secondary bloat depends upon removal of the basic cause.

blood A fluid body tissue that circulates through the *cardiovascular system, providing a vehicle for the transportation of an immense variety of substances between the various organs and tissues. It is composed of a liquid medium, *plasma, in which are suspended blood cells, categorized broadly as *leucocytes, *erythrocytes, and *platelets. Principally, the blood carries oxygen and absorbed nutrients to the body tissues, and transports carbon dioxide and nitrogenous wastes for excretion. In addition, it carries *hormones, and also cells and other components of the immune system (*see* immunity). The blood, moreover, has a prime role in maintaining the optimum working environment for tissues (*see* homeostasis).

blood corpuscle A blood cell. *See* erythrocyte; leucocyte.

blood count An estimate of the number of cells in a given sample or volume of blood. *See* cell count.

blood group *See* blood typing.

Normal resting blood pressure for various species

Species	Systolic/diastolic (mm Hg)
Horse	130/95
Ox	140/95
Sheep	140/90
Pig	140/80
Dog	120/70
Cat	140/90
Fowl	175/145

blood leucocyte differential *See* cell count.

blood poisoning The presence of bacterial toxins and/or large numbers of bacteria in the bloodstream causing serious illness. *See* bacteraemia; septicaemia.

blood pressure The pressure of blood within blood vessels, usually the arteries, i.e. arterial blood pressure. Pressure is highest during *systole, when the ventricles are contracting (*systolic pressure*), and lowest during *diastole, when the ventricles are relaxing (*diastolic pressure*). Normal resting blood pressures in various species are shown in the table. Muscular exertion, fear, and excitement all raise blood pressure. Severe haemorrhage or shock can result in abnormally low blood pressure (*hypotension) and various diseases can lead to an abnormally raised blood pressure (*hypertension). Blood pressure is adjusted by the sympathetic nervous system and hormonal control.

blood root poisoning A toxic condition due to ingestion of the North American herbaceous plant *Sanguinaria canadensis* (blood root). It contains several toxic isoquinoline alkaloids, which are also found in other genera of the poppy family: *Argemone* spp. (e.g. Mexican poppy,

blood spavin

prickly poppy); *Papaver* spp. (poppies); *Dicentra* spp. (e.g. golden eardrops, squirrel corn, steers head); *Corydalis* spp. (e.g. fitweed, golden corydalis); and *Chelidonium* spp. (celandines). The clinical signs of poisoning are vomiting, decreased heart rate and diminished strength of heart contractions, depressed central and peripheral nervous activity, dilated pupils, and respiratory difficulty. Treatment is symptomatic.

blood spavin A condition of horses in which there is swelling at the hock (*see* tarsus) due to distension of the saphenous vein.

blood splashing A condition of carcasses and offal characterized by small capillary haemorrhages scattered throughout the meat. The vast majority of cases occur after electrical stunning before the animal is bled. It occurs in all animals but is commonest in pigs and lambs, affecting the lungs, heart, mesentery, and muscles of the diaphragm, abdomen, and hind legs.

blood spot (in eggs) A small blood clot found occasionally in the albumen of eggs. It results from slight leakage of blood during ovulation (release of the yolk into the oviduct) and causes quality downgrading. Blood spots are detected by routine candling over a light source in packing stations.

blood transfusion *See* transfusion.

blood typing Any test that determines the presence or absence of certain inherited *antigens on the surface of the red blood cells. Such tests may be required in preparing blood for *transfusion, because the antigens of incompatible blood may, in some circumstances, be attacked by the recipient's antibodies with resultant destruction of the transfused red cells. Blood typing may also be used to investigate parentage. In each species there are several independent blood group systems. Each blood group may have from one to over 50 possible antigens (*isoantigens) although usually only one antigen for each blood group is expressed by any individual animal. The individual will thus recognize all other isoantigens in that blood group as foreign. Exposure of an individual to isoantigens leads to isoimmunization and the formation of isoantibodies, which destroy the incompatible blood cells.

Blood typing entails mixing samples of red cells with typing reagents – isoimmune sera containing specific isoantibodies, or *monoclonal antibodies. A reaction causes haemagglutination (clumping) of the red cells or, in the presence of *complement, *haemolysis. A positive result indicates the presence of the specific isoantigen. In some blood group systems the antigens are not freely available on the cell surface and are less reactive. The sensitivity of the typing reactions is then increased by using an *antiglobulin test or by prior treatment of the red cells with enzymes.

Where typing sera are not available, *cross-matching* of blood is a satisfactory way of ensuring compatibility. It is also a desirable precaution before transfusing animals with autoimmune haemolytic disorders. Cross-matching is a direct test for the presence of isoantibody against donor red cells and involves incubating batches of donor cells in samples of the patient's serum for 30 minutes at 4°C, room temperature, and 37°C. The incubated cells are then examined for evidence of haemolysis or agglutination. The control test is a similar incubation of donor cells in their own serum. As a subsidiary test the recipient's red cells are incubated in the donor's serum under an identical regime. A positive reaction in either the main or subsidiary test indicates incompatibility. However, administering incompatible donor serum carries much less risk than administering incompatible donor cells. In the horse, cross-matching should be done in the presence of complement to reveal the full activity of haemolytic isoantibodies.

Blood typing may be used to establish parentage, for example to identify the true sire of a dam's offspring. All the animals involved are typed and, if possible, other members of their progeny. The test can exclude certain putative parents but cannot positively prove parentage.

blowfly Any of various large robust flies found throughout the world near human and animal habitats. Blowflies may cause disease by visiting faeces and animal accommodation and subsequently alighting on food, and the larvae of several are parasites of humans and animals (*see* myiasis). Blowflies include the bluebottle (*Calliphora* spp.), which normally lays its eggs on meat, the *green-bottle fly, the *screw-worm flies, and the African *tumbu fly.

blue comb *See* avian monocytosis.

blue-green alga poisoning A toxic condition (toxicosis) due to ingestion of blue-green algae. Three genera – *Microcystis*, *Anabena*, and *Aphanizomenon* – are most commonly responsible; all have a worldwide distribution. Several factors must coincide to produce conditions in which toxicosis is possible, such as warm sunny weather, eutrophic (nutrient-rich) water producing algal bloom, and wind conditions to concentrate the algae, e.g. by the shore. The algae contain toxic polypeptides and alkaloids. There may be sudden death, due to respiratory paralysis as a result of a rapid-acting alkaloid neuromuscular toxin, or a less acute illness due to massive liver damage, haemorrhage, and shock caused by polypeptide toxins. Clinical signs may include abdominal pain, muscle tremors, dyspnoea, cyanosis, salivation, icterus, bloody faeces, photosensitization, prostration, convulsions, and death. Treatment with activated charcoal and heavy mineral oil, administered orally, and sodium thiosulphate, administered intravenously or orally, has been employed with some success.

bluetongue A noncontagious disease of sheep caused by *orbiviruses and characterized by fever and congestion of the membranes of the mouth and feet. It is endemic in Africa, the Middle East, Asia, northern Australia, and North and South America. This distribution reflects that of the midges responsible for transmitting the disease, and although these are mainly tropical and subtropical species, temperate midges transmit bluetongue in North America. Related species of midge in northern Europe are capable of transmitting bluetongue, but the disease is not established in this area. Outbreaks of clinical bluetongue are most common in sheep imported into enzootic areas and where infected insect vectors spread into previously clear areas. There are over 24 immunologically distinct types of bluetongue virus and previous infection with one type does not give immunity to the others. However, there is evidence that combined immunity to several types broadens the animal's immunity to cover types not previously encountered.

The incubation period is approximately 7 days, followed by fever and oral discomfort. A watery and later mucoid discharge develops from the mouth and nose, ulcers may develop in the mouth, and those on the lips become scabs. Lameness due to inflammation of the feet and degeneration of skeletal muscle may occur. Abortion and congenital deformities may also occur in pregnant animals. Mortality as high as 90% has been recorded. Symptomless infection in cattle, goats, camels, wild ungulates, and indigenous sheep can conceal the presence of bluetongue in enzootic areas. Control is by annual vaccination with live attenuated vaccines containing all the types of bluetongue virus present in the area. Bluetongue is a *notifiable disease in the UK, the USA, and Canada.

blue wool A form of *lumpy wool in which secondary infection with the bacterium *Pseudomonas indigofera* gives a blue pigmentation to the soiled wool.

B-lymphocyte See lymphocyte.

boar 1. An uncastrated male pig, whether used for meat production or breeding purposes. **2.** The wild boar, *Sus scrofa*. It is an ancestor of the domestic *pig and is still hunted in parts of Europe.

body temperature The heat of the body as measured by a clinical thermometer; in animals this is usually inserted into the rectum. Body temperature is monitored and controlled by the *hypothalamus. Normal body temperatures in domestic species are shown in the table. A rise in body

Normal body temperature for various species

Species	Average temperature	
	°C	°F
Horse	37.7	99.9
Ox	38.5	101.3
Sheep, goat	39.1	102.3
Pig	39.2	102.5
Dog	38.9	102.0
Cat	38.6	101.5
Fowl	41.7	107.1

temperature is an important clinical sign occurring in *fever. See also heat exhaustion; malignant hyperthermia; hypothermia.

bog asphodel poisoning See alveld; plochteach.

bog spavin Swelling of the joint capsule of the tibiotarsal joint of the equine hock (see tarsus) due to the presence of excess synovial fluid. The swelling is most pronounced on the inner (medial) anterior aspect, but also occurs behind the joint, on both sides. Causes are poor conformation, injury, and nutritional factors. Bog spavin does not usually cause lameness, unless due to a recent injury, and in young horses the condition may regress as the animal matures. Diagnosis depends on physical examination, no bone changes and treatment consists of rest and correcting any mineral or vitamin deficiencies. Anti-inflammatory drugs and pressure bandaging are sometimes used.

boil A painful red nodule-like skin lesion containing pus. The infection is usually caused by *Staphylococcus bacteria, which enter via a hair follicle or break in the skin. Local injury or lowered constitutional resistance may encourage the development of boils (see furunculosis). Surgical lancing may be necessary to release the pus, coupled with topical and, possibly, systemic antibiotics to treat the infection. Medical name: **furuncle**. Compare abscess.

bolus 1. (in physiology) A discrete mass of gut contents that is moved along the oesophagus or intestine, either by *peristalsis or by antiperistalsis (see rumination). **2.** (in pharmacology) A large pill. **3.** US (in medicine) A single rapid intravenous injection.

bone The hard extremely dense connective tissue that forms the skeleton of the body. It is composed of a matrix of collagen fibres impregnated with bone salts (chiefly calcium carbonate and calcium phosphate). *Compact bone* forms the outer shell of bones; it consists of a hard virtually solid mass made up of bony tissue arranged in concentric layers (*osteones). *Cancellous bone*, found beneath compact bone, consists of a meshwork of bony bars (*trabeculae*) with many interconnecting spaces containing marrow. See illustration.

Individual bones may be classed as long, short, flat, or irregular. The outer layer of a bone is called the *periosteum. The *medullary cavity* is lined with *endosteum and contains the marrow. Bones not only form the skeleton but also act as stores for mineral salts and play an important part in the formation of blood cells.

bone marrow (marrow) The tissue contained within the internal cavities of the bones. At birth, these cavities are filled entirely with blood-forming *myeloid tissue* (*red marrow*) but in later life the marrow in the limb bones is replaced by fat (*yellow marrow*). Samples of bone marrow may be obtained for examination by *aspiration through a stout needle or by *trephine biopsy. *See also* haemopoiesis.

bonemeal A ground mineral feedstuff produced as a by-product of the animal slaughter industry. It must be sterilized prior to incorporation into animal *diets to prevent the risk of transmitting infectious agents. It is a useful source of calcium and phosphorus.

bone pinning The surgical technique whereby the alignment of a fractured bone is maintained during healing by the insertion of stainless-steel pins. The simplest and most extensively

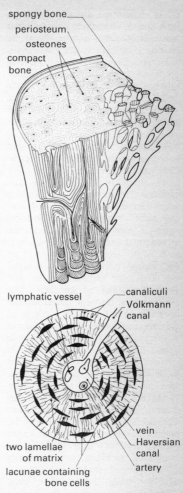

Section of the shaft of a long bone (above) with detail of a single osteone (below)

used is the round-section trocar pointed pin, which is placed lengthways in the medullary cavity of the bone across the fracture site. This is particularly successful where the bone is reasonably straight and where the fracture site tends to key together to

bone spavin

prevent rotational distortion. Slender hook-ended and sledgerunner-tipped pins (Rush pins) are employed to provide dynamic fixation of certain fractures, principally at the distal end of the femur. *Kirschner-Ehmer splints employ double-pin units drilled transversely through the bone above and below the fracture site and joined by externally positioned rods.

bone spavin *Arthritis of the equine hock (*see* tarsus). The condition principally affects the bones on the lower inner aspect of the hock, i.e. the proximal third metatarsal (canon bone) and the medial third and central tarsal bones. It is caused by injury or poor conformation resulting in abnormal stresses on the joint; animals with excessive angulation or with narrow hocks are most susceptible. The joint becomes painful and swollen resulting in lameness. The *spavin test* is used for diagnosis: the hock is held in flexion for a couple of minutes, then released and the animal allowed to move off; in cases of bone spavin the severity of the lameness is temporarily but markedly increased by this procedure. X-ray examination reveals a narrowing of the joint space of the two distal joints and the formation of *osteophytes. Progression of the condition leads to fusion of the bones (*ankylosis), which is no longer painful. A variety of treatments have been used, including rest, sectioning of the cunean tendon, neurectomy, and corrective shoeing. The most effective is *arthrodesis to produce ankylosis.

Boophilus A genus of hard *ticks found in the tropics and often known as cattle ticks, since they are chiefly ectoparasites of cattle, although they will infest other animals. They transmit the protozoan parasites responsible for *babesiosis, anaplasmosis, spirochaetosis, and some bacterial diseases.

booster A repeat dose of a *vaccine administered to further stimulate the immunity of the animal. Dead vaccines usually require a booster within 1 month of the initial vaccination in order to stimulate an immunity sufficient to last 6 months or a year. Thereafter a single booster vaccination every 6 months or annually is sufficient to maintain immunity for most agents. Live vaccines usually require only a single initial dose, with booster vaccinations given at intervals of 2 years or longer, depending on the particular vaccine.

boot Any of various devices that are used to cover the foot and lower leg of a horse to provide support, protection, or for veterinary use. Buckles or Velcro are used for fastenings. *Brushing boots* are designed to protect a foot from damage by the opposite foot (i.e. brushing), which can occur when the horse is in motion. They are made of leather, felt and leather, rubber, or synthetic materials, and can be lined for added protection, although this makes them heavy when wet. A *speedy-cut boot* is a tall brushing boot fitted to prevent damage from high brushing (often called 'speedy cutting'). A *Yorkshire boot* is a felt and tape boot used to protect the fetlock when lunging the horse or performing other work on the flat. It covers the fetlock and pastern. A *fetlock boot* is similar to the Yorkshire boot but covers the fetlock area only and is harder wearing. A felt *kicking boot* is used on the hind feet of mares to prevent injuries to a stallion when 'trying' or serving. There are also various designs of *veterinary boot* to provide support or protection to injuries, while a *poultice boot* is a rubber boot used to keep dirt away from dressings. It also insulates a poultice, helping to keep it warm.

borax A colourless solid, soluble in water, that has weak antiseptic properties. Both it and boric acid are used in eye drops, cough mixtures, and skin lotions. Boric acid should be used sparingly in topical application since local toxicity can occur. Signs are diarrhoea, anorexia, depression, coma, and death. Chemical name: **disodium tetraborate-10-water.**

borborygmus (*pl.* **borborygmi**) Audible sounds of intestinal movement usually associated with the presence of gas.

Border disease A disease of sheep and goats caused by a *pestivirus similar to that causing *bovine virus diarrhoea and characterized by abortion, congenital abnormalities, and persistently infected lambs. Infection causes no apparent symptoms in the young or adult animal. However, the virus can cross the placenta of the pregnant ewe or nanny goat, and depending on the stage of gestation, can cause abortion or neurological and skin lesions in the developing foetus. Lambs may be born with a covering of hair instead of wool and have an abnormal gait and persistent muscular spasms; these animals have been aptly described as 'hairy shakers'. Some lambs have few clinical signs but develop a tolerance to the virus so that they continually excrete the virus and are a source of infection to other susceptible animals; as adults they may repeatedly produce clinically affected lambs. There are no commercially available vaccines.

Bordetella A genus of Gram-negative *bacteria, occurring as short rods or coccobacilli. The genus includes *B. pertussis* and *B. parapertussis*, which cause whooping cough in young children, and *B. bronchiseptica*, a species of veterinary importance. It is an obligate parasite of the upper respiratory tract of pigs, dogs, and rodents and is a common secondary invader to respiratory viral infections, such as *distemper. It is also found in *kennel cough in dogs, *atrophic rhinitis in pigs, and *bronchitis in turkeys.

boric acid *See* borax.

borogluconate *See* calcium borogluconate.

Borrelia A genus of Gram-negative *spirochaete bacteria that cause relapsing fevers in humans and animals. They are transmitted by ticks, and wild rodents are common reservoirs of infection. The *Borrelia* are distinguished from the other spirochaetes by their ease of staining and by their coarse shallow and irregular spirals. *B. theileri* has been associated with febrile disease in cattle, sheep, and goats in Africa. *B. anserinum* (*B. gallinarum*) causes both goose *septicaemia and *avian spirochaetosis in many parts of the world. *B. burghdorferi* produces *Lyme disease, a tick-transmitted zoonosis which occurs in Britain and the USA.

bot fly Any of various *flies whose larvae are parasites of livestock or, occasionally, humans. They include the *horse bot, the *sheep nostril fly, the *horse nasal bot fly, and the *torsalo fly. *See also* warble fly.

botriomycosis A term formerly applied to chronic *abscess formation in horses associated with a staphylococcal infection (*see* Staphylococcus), which develops rather slowly and is liable to induce localized fibrous reactions. Such abscesses occur in the shoulder region in draught horses due to damage by the collar, and in the spermatic cord after castration (*see* scirrhous cord).

botulism A noncontagious disease of birds, reptiles, and mammals characterized by paralysis and death and

bougie

caused by toxins produced by certain strains of *Clostridium botulinum*. Spores of this bacterium can persist on pasture for a considerable period, and toxins are produced by the replicating bacteria, typically in decomposing organic material. Wound botulism may occur when wounds are infected with the bacteria, leading to the clinical signs. In cattle, outbreaks of botulism may be associated with phosphorus deficiency causing them to eat bones. In water fowl outbreaks of botulism may follow periods of drought associated with large amounts of rotting aquatic plants. Two to ten days after ingestion of the toxin animals show incoordinated movements and eventually become totally paralysed. Treatment is usually unsuccessful and control is by vaccination. *See also* limberneck.

bougie A slender flexible solid or hollow cylindrical instrument designed to be introduced into a tubular organ or duct, such as the oesophagus, rectum, or teat canal, to effect dilation, or to apply medication.

bovine atopic rhinitis A *hypersensitivity reaction involving nasal inflammation and occurring in certain strains of cattle. It is found sporadically in the summer months, usually in grazing cattle under 4 years old, and is probably caused by repeated exposure to grass pollen and mites. Affected animals show laboured breathing with a snorting respiratory sound. There is eye and nose discharge. Small hard white nodules are palpable in the nasal chambers. These are found to be inflammatory zones infiltrated with eosinophils, plasma cells, and mast cells, with thickening of the overlying epithelium. Control is possible by selective breeding of resistant strains of cattle.

bovine autoimmune haemolytic anaemia A disorder of newborn calves in which the red blood cells are destroyed by antibodies, resulting in anaemia. Although an *autoimmune disease, the condition does not occur spontaneously but may be accidentally induced by the use of vaccines derived from blood. A cow may react to such vaccines by producing anti-red-cell antibodies, which are passed to her calf in the colostrum and destroy the calf's red cells. The signs are *anaemia of variable severity occurring in the first 48 hours of life. In acute cases the calf will pass haemoglobin in the urine, which then acquires a brownish discoloration. Diagnosis is confirmed in the laboratory by detecting antibody attached to affected red cells. Treatment consists of fluid transfusion or blood transfusion using the blood of an unvaccinated cow. The disease can be predicted if the pregnant cow is found to have circulating antibodies to the sire's red cells. In this case, the newborn calf should be given the colostrum and milk of an unvaccinated cow and not permitted to suckle its own dam for the first 48 hours. *See also* equine autoimmune haemolytic anaemia. *Compare* canine autoimmune haemolytic anaemia.

bovine enzootic leukosis *See* enzootic bovine leukosis.

bovine farcy A chronic condition of cattle, occurring chiefly in Africa and Asia, characterized by superficial *lymphadenitis and *lymphangitis, with caseation and suppuration. Firm painless subcutaneous swellings appear, often first at the prescapular or precrural lymph nodes, enlarging slowly to considerable size and multiplying along the lymph vessels, which become prominent and cordlike. The lesions contain caseous pus, but do not rupture spontaneously. Spread to the lungs or other viscera may lead to a gross pathological appearance resembling *tuberculosis. *Nocardia* *farcinica* (a bacterium probably identical with *N. asteroides*) was originally described as the cause, but in at least some cases **Mycobacterium* species (termed *M. farcinogenes* and *M. senegalense*) are implicated. The bacteria enter through contamination of skin wounds with soil. Iodides are used in treatment. Other names: **bovine nocardiosis**; **mycotic lymphangitis**; **tropical actinomycosis**. *Compare* skin tuberculosis.

bovine farmer's lung *See* allergic alveolitis.

bovine herpes mamillitis A disease of cattle caused by a *herpesvirus and characterized by teat and udder lesions, especially in newly calved cattle. The disease is enzootic in the UK and is probably distributed worldwide. The seasonal incidence of herpes mamillitis suggests that it is mainly insect transmitted, but milking machine transmission is also possible. The incubation period is 3–10 days followed by swelling and irritation of the teats. Vesicles may develop but usually these are not seen and the skin ruptures releasing a clear discharge which quickly dries as a scab. Healing takes place within 3 weeks but more usually this is prevented by milking procedures or suckling calves. Lesions may spread to the mouths of calves or around the vulva of the affected cow. Secondary *mastitis may be a problem. Other name: **bovine ulcerative mamillitis**. *See also* pseudocowpox.

bovine infectious infertility *See* campylobacteriosis of cattle.

bovine infectious petechial fever (Ondiri disease) A tick-borne disease that affects cattle, sheep, goats, and wild ruminants in East Africa. It is caused by the rickettsia **Cytoecetes ondiri*, which is regarded as a strain of *C. phagocytophila*, the causative agent of *tick-borne fever in temperate climates. After an incubation period of 4–6 days, the animal develops fever followed by depletion of circulating white blood cells and extensive petechial haemorrhages in the mucosa. The organisms are found in abundance initially in the spleen but eventually in circulating leucocytes. Giemsa-stained blood smears are essential for diagnosis. Treatment with tetracyclines and gloxazone is usually effective.

bovine malignant catarrhal fever *See* malignant catarrhal fever.

bovine papilloma A wartlike growth on cattle caused by *papovaviruses. Depending on the strain of virus, papillomas may be found on the skin, teats, penis, or intestinal tract. They are usually benign but may develop into malignant carcinomas when they occur in association with other predisposing factors, such as bracken feeding. Autogenous vaccines can be prepared by grinding a sample of the papilloma with sterile saline, sand, and formaldehyde. However, the success of these vaccines is difficult to assess as spontaneous recovery from the infection is common, without any treatment.

bovine papular stomatitis An infectious disease of cattle caused by a parapoxvirus (*see* poxvirus) and characterized by spots and ulcers on the muzzle. It is distributed worldwide. Closely related strains of parapoxvirus cause *pseudocowpox. Transmission is by direct or indirect contact with infected cattle. The disease causes little discomfort and has no economic importance except that the lesions may be confused with those seen in *foot-and-mouth disease, *rinderpest, or *mucosal disease. The incubation period of 3–7 days is followed by the development of small white spots which become ulcers. Wart-like

bovine paralytic myoglobinuria

lesions may develop around the teeth. Although the primary lesions may heal within a few weeks, further lesions are frequent. Relapses are common, particularly when the animal is stressed, and infection is probably persistent. Control is not usually considered necessary. The virus can also infect humans.

bovine paralytic myoglobinuria A disease of cattle that is clinically similar to *azoturia in horses. It occurs in young stock soon after they are turned out after being housed through the winter. The condition is precipitated by unaccustomed exercise, sometimes accompanied by a dietary deficiency of vitamin E and/or selenium. Clinical signs include stiffness, recumbency, and *myoglobinuria. Some animals may be found dead, with no warning signs. Post-mortem findings include muscle degeneration and necrosis.

bovine pulmonary emphysema *See* fog fever.

bovine spongiform encephalopathy (BSE) A disease, apparently restricted to Friesian-Holstein cattle, involving the central nervous system and characterized by behavioural changes and impaired gait. The cause is unknown and the disease was unrecorded prior to scattered outbreaks in the UK in 1987. Animals between 3 and 8 years old have been affected. They show increasing nervousness and hesitancy, clumsy gait, particularly affecting the hind legs, and intermittent trotting. Collapse and death invariably follow. There is no treatment. Because of the apparent breed specificity, genetic factors may be involved.

bovine syncytial virus (bovine respiratory syncytial virus) *See* pneumovirus.

bovine ulcerative mamillitis *See* bovine herpes mamillitis.

bovine virus diarrhoea (BVD) An infectious disease of cattle characterized by abortion and persistent infection and caused by a *pestivirus. It has a worldwide distribution. *Border disease virus of sheep is similar to BVD virus. Initial infection of calves and adult cattle usually causes few signs, although nasal discharge, salivation, and diarrhoea together with small ulcers in the mouth may occur. The virus will cross the placenta of pregnant cows and, depending on the stage of gestation, can cause abortion, congenital abnormalities in newborn calves, or apparently normal calves that persistently carry the virus. These persistently infected calves fail to develop antibody to BVD virus and tend to be more susceptible to other infections. Infection with a second strain of the BVD virus can lead to *mucosal disease, an often fatal condition. Transmission of BVD is usually by contact with persistently infected animals; semen from these animals also contains BVD virus. Control is difficult because of the need to identify infected animals entering the herd. There are no safe and effective vaccines.

bowel *See* intestine.

bowel oedema *See* oedema disease.

bowie A disease of suckling lambs occurring in New Zealand and resembling rickets. Although of unknown cause it is probably a form of phosphorus deficiency. The characteristic feature is lateral curvature of the long bones of the forelimbs, sometimes progressing to severe deformity, with the sides of the feet becoming overworn giving rise to lameness. The lambs fail to thrive because their mobility is impaired. The disease differs from rickets in that vitamin D fails to effect a cure, although dietary phosphorus supplementation may be effective. Other name: **bentleg**.

bow-legs Bending of the limb bones to produce an abnormal bow-shaped contour. This may be due to differences in the rate of bone growth (*see* valgus vara) or to metabolic bone disease, such as *rickets, in which structurally weaker cartilage is not replaced by bone and so bends under pressure.

Bowman's capsule *See* glomerulus.

brachial Relating to the region of the forelimb extending from the shoulder joint to the elbow joint.

brachialis A muscle that is situated on the front of the upper forelimb and contracts to flex the elbow joint.

brachial paralysis Paralysis of the forelimb, commonly as a result of damage to the spinal cord or spinal nerve roots in the lower cervical region. The entire limb is paralysed and usually insensitive, and appears longer than normal because the elbow is dropped; the upper part (dorsum) of the foot is dragged on the ground. Recovery is comparatively rare or slow.

brachial plexus A network of nerves situated in the armpit region (*axilla) and comprising the last few cervical spinal nerves and first one or two thoracic spinal nerves. These give rise to the various nerves of the forelimb.

brachiocephalic A muscle that runs from the humerus to the skull and neck region. Its clavicular intersection represents the remnant of the clavicle.

brachium (*pl.* **brachia**) The arm; i.e. the region of the forelimb related to the humerus.

brachy- *Prefix denoting* shortness. Example: *brachydactylia* (shortness of the digits).

brachycephalic Describing a short wide skull or head, as in Pekingese dogs. *Compare* dolichocephalic; mesaticephalic.

bracken poisoning A toxic condition caused by ingestion of the bracken fern (*Pteridium aquilinum*), the male fern (*Dryopteris filix-mas*), or horsetail (*Equisetum* spp.). Bracken contains a number of substances with different toxic effects. One of these is the enzyme thiaminase. In **horses** and sometimes **pigs** that consume large amounts of bracken (3 kg per day for a horse) a deficiency of thiamine (vitamin B_1) arises. The horse becomes incoordinated and staggers when moving or stands with its back arched and feet spread out. Muscular tremors develop, recumbency occurs, and convulsions are followed by death. In the early stages the clinical signs may be reversed by daily injections of 100 mg of thiamine.

In adult **cattle**, illness may arise when animals are bedded on dry bracken, while grazing bracken-infested pasture, or some time after removal from access to bracken. Affected animals are depressed, develop diarrhoea, which is often blood-stained, and bleed from the nose, eyes, vulva, or rectum. The temperature is often high, and in calves there is sometimes oedema of the larynx, which causes 'roaring' breathing. Autopsy reveals widespread haemorrhages and pale bone marrow. *Thrombocytopenia and *leucopenia suggest that toxic action on the bone marrow produces a dyshaemopoietic *anaemia. In some areas of the world, prolonged access to bracken leads to the development of chronic *haematuria accompanied by the presence of tumours, both benign and malignant, in the bladder. Papillomas of the mouth and oesophagus of cattle in the west of Scotland have been associated with grazing on bracken-infested pasture. **Sheep** may develop intestinal tumours as well as a haemorrhagic syndrome similar to that in cattle. They also suffer from a form of retinal degeneration known as *bright blindness*.

Affected animals must be denied further access to the plant. Most attempts at therapy have been made in cattle. High temperatures are treated with injections of antibiotics. Butyl alcohol, a substance that stimulates bone marrow, has been used (daily subcutaneous injections of 1 g in 10 ml olive oil) but there are doubts about its efficacy. In cases with anaemia, blood transfusions may be of value. Large areas of hill grazing are infested with bracken and control is often difficult, but the selective herbicide Asulam is of some value.

brady- *Prefix denoting* slowness.

bradycardia Slowing of the heart rate. This may occur in healthy individuals with high vagal tone or be due to pathological changes, notably *heart block. Bradycardia may also develop when the potassium concentration in the blood is elevated, for instance in certain toxaemias, renal failure, and hypoadrenocorticism. It is also a feature of *hypothyroidism.

bradykinin A naturally occurring polypeptide consisting of nine amino acids. Bradykinin is a very powerful vasodilator and causes contraction of smooth muscle; it is formed in the blood under certain conditions and is thought to play an important role as a mediator of inflammation. *See* kinin.

brailing The confinement of a bird by means of a leather thong around the wings. It is most commonly applied to hawks, but may occasionally be used for game birds.

brain The enlarged and highly developed part of the central nervous system that lies in the cranium of the skull at the anterior end of the spinal cord and which is the main site of nervous control (see illustration). It is surrounded by three concentric protective membranes, the *meninges, and floats in *cerebrospinal fluid, which also fills the brain's internal cavities (*ventricles). The paired *cerebral hemispheres (which together form the *cerebrum) form a prominent mass overlying much of the rest of the brain. They are responsible for receiving and processing stimuli from the major sense organs, initiating responses in the form of voluntary muscle contractions, and storing information. Beneath and to the rear lies the *cerebellum, concerned with balance, muscle tone, and coordination. Involuntary muscle actions, such as those responsible for breathing and swallowing, are controlled by the *medulla oblongata, which is situated where the spinal cord enters the brain and which forms part of the *brainstem. Deep within the brain is the *hypothalamus, responsible for regulating thirst, hunger, and other physiological functions. Paired *cranial nerves arise from the brain to supply the eyes, ears, nose, and muscles of the head. The brain is divided into three anatomical regions: *forebrain (prosencephalon); *midbrain (mesencephalon); and *hindbrain (rhombencephalon).

brainstem The part of the brain comprising the *medulla oblongata, *pons, and *midbrain; it may also include the *diencephalon (see illustration). It is continuous with and resembles the spinal cord, and is connected to the *cerebrum and the *cerebellum.

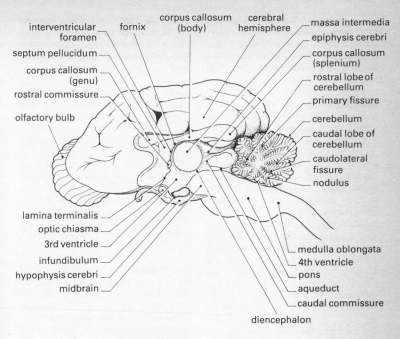

Mid-sagittal section of dog brain

brain tumours Any of various benign or malignant growths in the brain. They account for about 3% of all canine tumours, but are only infrequently reported in other domestic species. The clinical signs are those associated with any space-occupying lesion in the brain, and include seizures of varying intensity, behavioural changes, dementia, depression, head pressing, loss of vision, incoordination, and paresis. Treatment is rarely attempted in animals. Many types of brain tumour have been reported, and some are more common in certain species, for example, *astrocytoma (in dogs), glioblastoma (cattle, dogs and pigs), and *meningioma (cats and dogs). Brain tumours due to metastasis from tumours elsewhere in the body are most common in the dog, especially in cases of mammary adenocarcinoma (*see* mammary tumours), oral malignant *melanoma, haemangiosarcoma (*see* angiosarcoma), and *osteosarcoma.

Brambell Committee An advisory body, chaired by Professor F. W. R. Brambell, whose report, *The Welfare of Animals Kept Under Intensive Livestock Husbandry Systems* (1965), led to the Agriculture (Miscellaneous Provisions) Act (1968) and the publication of official *welfare codes for various livestock species.

bran A fibre-rich feedstuff and by-product of the milling industry consisting essentially of the seed coat (husk) of the wheat grain. It is not considered suitable for rapidly growing nonruminants but is used in diets for breeding sows and is often incorporated into diets for ruminants and horses. Dry bran tends to counteract scouring, but a *bran mash* made with boiling water acts as a laxative.

branding A method of permanently marking cattle or other animals for identification purposes. Branding with a hot iron has been superseded by *freeze branding*, which is much simpler and more humane: the hide is clipped, sprayed with alcohol, and a brand applied; this has been reduced to an extremely low temperature using liquid nitrogen. The low temperature kills the pigment cells of the hair follicles so that when the hair regrows it is white. Therefore, freeze branding is most effective on the black areas of Friesian cattle, less effective on red or brown cattle, and ineffective on white areas. A freeze-branded number is usually applied to the back of the leg or rump. Cattle can be freeze branded at any age but if they are done before 1 year old the brands may distort.

brassica poisoning A toxic condition that may arise in animals after ingesting plants of the genus *Brassica*, such as kale, rape, cabbage, turnips, and swedes, or the related mustards (*Sinapis* spp.) or charlock (*S. arvensis*). Cattle fed large amounts of kale for prolonged periods can develop both haemolytic anaemia and haemoglobinuria. The condition can be exacerbated by phosphate deficiency. The anaemia-producing agent in kale is S-methylcysteine sulphoxide, which gives rise to dimethyldisulphide by fermentation in the rumen. Affected animals should be removed from the kale, given iron tonics, and, in advanced cases, blood transfusion. Brassicas also contain a goitrogen – 1,5-vinyl-2-thioxazolidine. Heavy losses have occurred in lambs from kale-fed ewes; the lambs are

born with *goitre. Charlock and the mustards contain an irritant volatile oil which causes acute gastroenteritis with colic, severe diarrhoea, and rapid death. *See also* rape poisoning.

braxy A condition of young sheep involving acute infection of the abomasum with the bacterium *Clostridium septicum*, which causes local necrosis with blood-stained oedema and leads to a fatal septicaemia. The organism is a normal inhabitant of the intestine, but an accessory factor, such as the ingestion of frosted roots or grass, initiates its multiplication in the abomasal mucosa. Effective vaccines are available. The meat of braxy carcasses was once considered a delicacy.

breast blisters A condition of poultry in which blisters occur in the skin of the breast over the keel of the sternum. They are caused by pressure while resting or perching. False bursae develop containing serous fluid, and large abscesses may eventually occur.

breathing The alternation of active *inhalation* (*inspiration*) of air into the lungs through the mouth or nose with the more passive *exhalation* (*expiration*) of the air. During inhalation the *diaphragm and *intercostal muscles contract, which enlarges the chest cavity and draws air into the lungs. When these muscles relax the lungs contract forcing air out during exhalation. Breathing is part of *respiration and its frequency and character are very variable. It increases during exercise, in hot conditions, and in various diseases of the respiratory system. *See also* apnoea; dyspnoea; hyperpnoea; tachypnoea.

breed 1. A group of organisms that share various traits that, either individually or in their sum, distinguish the group from all other members of the species. When mated to each other, the members of a breed produce young identical to themselves for those characters that define the breed. *Compare* strain. **2.** *See* breeding (def. 1).

breeder A sexually mature domestic fowl of either sex that is used in the production of progeny for meat or egg production. *See* poultry husbandry.

breeding 1. The mating of animals to produce young, especially under controlled circumstances. **2.** A colloquial term for the ancestry of an animal.

Breeding of Dogs Act (1973) (England and Wales) An Act of Parliament that requires the licensing of canine breeding establishments by the local authority. A breeding establishment is defined as any premises (including a private dwelling) where more than two bitches are kept for the purpose of breeding for sale. Inspections may be made by an officer of the local authority or by a veterinary surgeon appointed by the local authority for the purpose. The local authority must consider the accommodation, feeding, watering, bedding, and exercising of the dogs on the premises, and whether there is adequate protection against the spread of disease or fire.

breeding value An estimate of the probable genetic effect on a population of a particular breeding individual (usually a sire). This can be expressed as twice the mean deviation from the population mean of a group of offspring resulting from matings between the particular individual and a random sample of animals from the population. A breeding value is applicable only to the population in which it was determined. *See also* performance testing; progeny testing.

brewers' grains (draff) A by-product of the brewing industry used as a feedstuff for cattle and sheep. It comprises insoluble residue left after the removal of the wort from fermented barley grains. Fresh brewers' grains, which contain 70–75% water, are sometimes fed but do not keep well and are usually ensiled (*see* silage), or dried to increase the dry matter content to 900 g/kg. Brewers' grains are extremely palatable to cattle and sheep and are particularly useful for dairy cows, which can be given up to 16 kg per day of fresh or ensiled grains. They have higher nutritive value (metabolizable energy 10 MJ/kg DM; crude protein 200 g/kg DM). Because of their high fibre content they are not normally fed to pigs or poultry. *Compare* distillers' grains.

bright blindness *See* bracken poisoning.

brisket disease *See* mountain sickness.

British Veterinary Association A nonstatutory association representing the veterinary profession at national and (by its Territorial Divisions) at regional levels. It has many affiliated organizations representing specialized sectors of the veterinary profession, such as the British Small Animal Veterinary Association, the British Equine Veterinary Association, the British Veterinary Zoological Society, and the British Laboratory Animals Veterinary Association. Address: 7 Mansfield Street, London, W1M 0AT.

broad ligament (of the uterus) The paired fold of *peritoneum that attaches the ovary (mesovarium), uterine tube (mesosalpinx), and the uterus (mesometrium) to the walls of the abdomen and pelvis. It carries blood vessels to these organs.

broiler A domestic fowl reared for meat production and destined for slaughter at 'broiler weight'. This is typically 2 kg liveweight, achieved at around 50 days of age, although this may vary with local market requirements. *See also* poultry husbandry.

broiler ascites *See* ascites.

broken heads (sheep head-fly disease) A condition affecting the head of sheep, caused by the nonbiting fly *Hydrotaea irritans*. Swarms of the flies feed on nose and eye secretions of the sheep, causing the sheep to rub their heads on fences or undergrowth, or scratch with their hindfeet. Injuries so caused are commoner in sheep with relatively less wool about the head.

broken hock Dislocation or dislocation and fracture of the central tarsal bone in the hock joint (*see* tarsus). It is most common in racing greyhounds in the offside leg, resulting from extreme compresive and shearing forces exerted on the bone when the dog extends and turns the leg at speed. Treatment is based on that normally given for *dislocation or *fracture; special measures may include replacement of the affected bone with a plastic prosthesis.

broken mouth A colloquial term applied to sheep that have lost some of their cheek teeth due to *periodontal disease. The animal may chew slowly and irregularly; sometimes local infection produces discrete swellings on the face. The condition seriously hampers eating and causes loss of weight. It is a common reason for culling sheep. However, some ewes may be moved from upland to lowland pastures where there is easier grazing and so prolong their breeding life.

broken wind (heaves) A respiratory condition of stabled horses characterized by coughing and poor exercise tolerance. It develops as an allergic response to the inhaled dust from mouldy hay and bedding. There is increased effort as the animal breathes out, with additional contraction of abdominal muscles producing a biphasic expiration. This can be abolished by administering *atropine. Hypertrophy of the rectus abdominis muscle produces an outwardly visible 'heaves' line. Pathological changes in the lung include excess mucus production, bronchospasm, and *bronchiolitis, eventually producing *emphysema. Exposure to moulds and dusts is reduced by bedding the animal on shavings or peat and dampening hay before feeding. Alternatively, complete diets containing chopped roughage can be fed. *Bronchodilators and *mucolytics will improve clinical signs. Inhalants of sodium cromoglycate can be given prophylactically to affected animals prior to encountering likely sources of the mould to prevent the onset of signs. Other name: **chronic obstructive pulmonary disease (COPD)**.

bromhexine An *expectorant (a mucolytic) that acts by decreasing the viscosity of mucus, thereby improving the flow of mucus through the airways. It is available as a solution for injection or as a powder for oral dosing, and may also be used in combination with antibacterial drugs to treat airway diseases.

bronch- (broncho-) *Prefix denoting* the bronchial tree. Examples: *bronchopulmonary* (relating to the bronchi and lungs); *bronchotomy* (incision into).

bronchiectasis Widening of the bronchi. Occasionally this is a congenital abnormality, but it usually develops as a sequel to *bronchitis, particularly in cattle. Whole segments of the airway may be affected; the widened bronchi contain mucopurulent exudate and there are structural changes in the bronchial wall.

bronchiole Any of several generations of air passages within the bronchial tree of the lungs, succeeding the larger *bronchi. They lack cartilage in their walls and have a simple epithelium which becomes progressively thinner. *Terminal bronchioles* form the furthest extensions of the bronchial tree and conduct air to the *respiratory bronchioles*, which have *alveoli opening through their walls. Each respiratory bronchiole terminates in a number of alveolar ducts.

bronchiolitis Inflammation of the bronchioles in the lungs. This may occur in respiratory infections and in some toxic or allergic states. There is damage to the lining epithelium, mucus production, and exudate formation. The narrow bronchioles may become blocked, thereby obstructing the passage of air into adjacent lung tissue leading to *atelectasis. In *bronchiolitis fibrosa obliterans* there is fibrous organization of the bronchiolar exudate.

bronchitis Inflammation of the bronchi. This can be due to extension of disease affecting the upper respiratory tract or disease affecting the lung. Bronchopneumonia involves inflammatory changes in both the conducting and respiratory systems of the lung (*see* pneumonia). Bronchitis has many causes and may be acute or chronic. Examples include acute bacterial respiratory infections (such as *kennel cough in dogs), viral infections (e.g. *infectious bronchitis in poultry), secondary bacterial infection of viral bronchopneumonias (as in *calf pneumonia), and *parasitic bronchitis in cattle caused by the lungworm *Dictyocaulus viviparus.*

Coughing is the principal sign; auscultation of the chest reveals abnormal respiratory sounds, and on X-ray examination the bronchial walls are found to be thickened. There is increased mucus production, and the airway is often blocked or partially blocked by an inflammatory exudate containing mucus, white blood cells, and sloughed epithelial cells. In chronic bronchitis the epithelium may be grossly thickened with a marked increase in the number of mucus-secreting glands. Treatment depends on the cause. Antibiotics and anthelmintics are used to control bacterial and parasitic infections respectively. Bronchodilators and mucolytic drugs are given to improve respiratory function.

bronchodilator An agent that causes relaxation of smooth muscle in the bronchi and bronchioles, allowing dilatation of the airways. Bronchodilators are used in the treatment of anaphylactic reactions and to treat respiratory diseases. The commonly used drugs are *xanthines, and drugs with activity at β_2 *adrenergic receptors in the smooth muscle, such as *adrenaline, *isoprenaline, and the specific β_2 agonist, *clenbuterol. For example, adrenaline is used to counteract the bronchoconstriction caused by histamine release in anaphylactic reactions, whereas for respiratory diseases the longer-acting compounds (e.g. clenbuterol or one of the xanthines) are used.

bronchopneumonia *See* pneumonia.

bronchus (*pl.* **bronchi**) Any of several generations of air passages within the bronchial tree of the lungs, succeeding the trachea (see illustration). In most species the trachea divides terminally into right and left *principal bronchi* for the corresponding lungs. These then divide into *lobar bronchi* for the lung lobes and are succeeded

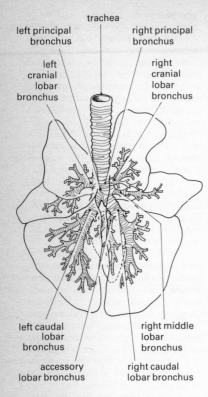

trachea

left principal bronchus

right principal bronchus

left cranial lobar bronchus

right cranial lobar bronchus

left caudal lobar bronchus

right middle lobar bronchus

accessory lobar bronchus

right caudal lobar bronchus

Bronchial tree of dog's lungs

by *segmental bronchi*, which supply units of each lobe (termed bronchopulmonary segments). In ruminants and the pig the bronchus for the right cranial lobe arises directly from the trachea and is termed the *tracheal bronchus*. Further generations of progressively smaller bronchi finally lead to *bronchioles. The walls of the bronchi contain cartilage plates, and are lined by mucous membrane, the epithelium of which becomes progressively thinner. The mucosal epithelium of larger bronchi contains glands.

brooder An apparatus for rearing birds after hatching. It provides optimum heat, light, food, water, and security to minimize post-hatching mortality. Designs range from tier brooders, consisting of trays arranged one above the other, to floor brooders, which are more common in poultry production.

brooder pneumonia *See* aspergillosis.

brown atrophy (lipofuscinosis) A condition of old cows in which a fine brownish-yellow pigment appears in the heart muscle. The heart is also smaller in size. It is more marked in chronic wasting diseases.

brown fat A type of *adipose tissue containing small fat cells with multiple small fat droplets in their cytoplasm. Brown fat tissue is particularly abundant in rodents and in newborn and hibernating animals, occurring in various parts of the body, including the axillary and neck regions. Compared to normal white fat, deposits of brown fat are more richly supplied with blood vessels and have a higher proportion of unsaturated fatty acids. They can also be more rapidly converted to heat energy, especially during arousal from hibernation and during cold stress in young animals. Since the deposits are strategically placed near major blood vessels, the heat they generate warms the blood returning to the heart.

Brucella A genus of Gram-negative nonmotile *bacteria occurring as small rods or coccobacilli. They are obligate parasites in a variety of animals. The genus includes five species of medical and veterinary importance causing febrile diseases, generally known as *brucellosis. *B. melitensis* is the cause of brucellosis in humans, sheep, and goats. The main reservoirs of infection for humans are goats, which serve as a natural habitat for the organisms. The disease is prevalent in southern Europe. *B. abortus* causes brucellosis in cattle but it can also affect humans and other animals. *B. suis* is an obligatory parasite of pigs that can cause brucellosis in pigs and humans, while *B. ovis* is an obligatory parasite of sheep, particularly in Asia and Australia. *B. canis* is an obligatory parasite of dogs that causes genitourinary infections.

brucellosis Any of several diseases caused by infection with bacteria of the genus *Brucella*. *B. abortus* causes a disease in cattle ('contagious abortion') characterized by abortion in late pregnancy, often with retention of the foetal membranes. In bulls *orchitis may occur. It is of major economic importance worldwide, particularly in dairy cattle. Infection with the organism is principally by contact with infected aborted foetuses or foetal membranes, resulting in chronic inflammation of the uterus. Abortion does not always occur and some infected cows run to full term. Infection of large numbers of animals in a herd is referred to as an *abortion storm*. Diagnosis depends upon laboratory isolation of the causative organism or the demonstration of anti-*Brucella* antibodies in the blood by the *agglutination test or *complement fixation test. Two types of vaccine are available, a live attenuated vaccine (strain or 'S' 19) and a killed vaccine (S 45/20). Neither provides total protection and abortion may still occur in vaccinated stock. In Britain the disease has recently been eradicated by a systematic programme of herd testing and slaughter of carriers (*see* area eradication).

B. ovis infection causes disease mainly in rams, although in New Zealand abortion in ewes is significant. In rams *orchitis and consequent infertility is the major sign. *B. suis* causes infertility and abortion in sows, *septicaemia in piglets, and orchitis in boars. The disease does not occur in Canada or Britain. *B. melitensis* causes disease in goats worldwide except in Britain and Scandinavia. In the UK, abortions due to *B. abortus* or *B. melitensis* must be reported under the *notifiable diseases legislation. *B. canis* causes abortion in bitches.

Humans are susceptible to *Brucella* infection (also known as Malta fever, Mediterranean fever, or undulant fever) through contact with an infected animal or by drinking nonpasteurized contaminated milk or cheese. Symptoms include headache, sickness, loss of appetite, and weakness, progressing to chronic fever and swelling of the lymph nodes. Prolonged administration of antibiotics and sulphonamides is effective; untreated the disease may persist for years.

Brugia A genus of threadlike parasitic nematodes (*see* filaria) found in the lymph nodes and vessels of cats, dogs, and primates. The lymphatics become blocked due to a fibrous reaction and cause enlargement of the skin and underlying connective tissues (elephantiasis in humans). *B. malayi* infects cats, dogs, and primates; *B. pahangi* infects only cats and dogs. Treatment consists in administering *diethylcarbamazine.

bruise (contusion) An area of skin discoloration due to the release of blood from ruptured underlying vessels following injury. As the blood is degraded, it produces the characteristic colours of the ageing bruise, changing from initial pinkness through purple to grey-black. The hair covering of domesticated animals usually conceals bruises but the accompanying *oedema may produce slight swelling in the skin. Bruising may be caused by ill-fitting harness or other gear. In horses, bruising of the sole of the hoof may result from poor shoeing techniques. Prolonged bruising as a result of constant rubbing can lead to *callosity. Bruising about the legs and wings of poultry carcasses is very common due to the methods employed in catching the live birds.

brush border *See* microvillus.

brush sampling A method of detecting the presence of *dermatophyte fungi in the hair coat or on the skin of clinically normal animals. Any brush free of fungal contamination and of appropriate size is used to thoroughly brush the animal. Spores and fragments of debris adhering to the brush are then transferred to a selective agar culture medium by gently pressing the bristles or spines into its surface. The subsequent growth of a dermatophyte in culture does not determine conclusively whether the animal was infected or merely contaminated, but indicates a need for closer and repeated examination to trace the source of the dermatophyte and exclude subclinical infection.

bryony poisoning A toxic condition due to the ingestion of white (or red) bryony (*Bryonia dioica*) or black bryony (*Tamus communis*). These plants contain irritant glycosides which cause diarrhoea, colic, convulsions, and death. The leaves of black bryony have silicaceous raphae (ridges), which cause mechanical irritation of the intestine when ingested and necrosis of the skin when applied externally.

bubo A localized inflamed swelling. In *bubonic plague in humans, such swellings develop in the lymph nodes, particularly in the groin and armpit.

bubonic plague An infectious disease, primarily of humans, caused by the bacterium *Yersinia pestis*, which also infects the large grey rat (*Rattus norvegicus*) and the black rat (*R. rattus*). The bacterium is transmitted from rats to humans by rat fleas (*Xenopsylla cheopis*; *Ceratophyllus fasciatus*), which leave the cooling carcasses of dead rats. Dogs and other domestic animals are occasionally affected. The uniquely characteristic sign is the bubo, a hardened subcutaneous lymph node. In another form, *pneumonic plague*, person-to-person infection occurs through coughing. The Black Death of the 14th century was a plague pandemic, likewise the London plague of 1665.

buccal 1. Relating to the mouth or the hollow part of the cheek. **2.** Describing the surface of a tooth adjacent to the cheek.

buccal cavity *See* oral cavity.

buccal glands Small salivary glands in the mucous membrane of the cheek, divided into dorsal and ventral groups. In carnivores the dorsal group are consolidated into the *zygomatic gland.

buccinator muscle The cheek muscle. Its contractions direct food from the *vestibule of the mouth between the teeth for mastication.

buccostomy An operation to create a permanent opening (*fistula) through the cheek to the oral cavity. It has been advocated to prevent *windsucking in horses.

buckwheat poisoning *See* photodynamic; photosensitization.

budding (virology) The process by which an enveloped *virus (*see* envelope) passes through the nuclear or cytoplasmic membrane of its host cell, acquiring part or all of its envelope as it does so.

buffalo fly *See* horn fly.

buffalo gnat A minute, black, hump-backed *fly, also known as the black-fly, found worldwide, usually near running water. The females are ecto-parasites of livestock and humans, feeding on their blood with a short, powerful, sucking proboscis. The eggs, laid on stones, twigs, etc., just below the surface of well-aerated running water, hatch into aquatic larvae which develop into aquatic air-breathing pupae. The adults are most active in the early morning and evening and may attack in swarms, causing cattle to stampede. Their bite is irritating and painful and blisters may develop. In Africa, they transmit the nema-tode responsible for human *onchocerciasis, while in Europe, North America, and Asia, they act as carriers of the protozoan, *Leuco-cytozoon*, which parasitizes geese, ducks, and turkeys; it may cause death in young birds. Insect repellents can be used on livestock; the imma-ture stages may be killed by adding a suitable insecticide to rivers or streams where they breed, although this should be strictly controlled because of pollution dangers to wild-life and drinking water.

buffalopox A mild disease of buffa-loes characterized by teat lesions and caused by an orthopoxvirus (*see* poxvirus). It appears on the teats of lactating buffaloes as pustular lesions, which rupture and become scabs. Healing may be delayed by milking procedures or suckling calves and mastitis is a frequent secondary prob-lem. Control is by isolation of affected animals.

buffer A solution that resists change in pH when an acid or alkali is added or when the solution is diluted. It consists of an acid-base conjugate pair. The two most effective buffer systems in the body are bicarbonate (H_2CO_3/HCO_3^-) and phosphate ($H_2PO_4^-/HPO_4^{2-}$) (*see* acid-base bal-ance).

bufotenine A thick creamy-white venom present in the skin of the common toad *Bufo vulgaris*. Poisoning is usually seen in dogs and cats dur-ing the summer months. Animals that have bitten a toad show distress, excessive salivation, and retching last-ing 8–12 hours. Vomiting occurs occasionally and inappetence may last for 48 hours. If a toad is ingested signs of toxicity occur 24 hours later, with abdominal pain, vomiting, inco-ordination, and occasionally death due to heart failure. Treatment with *steroids and *sedatives may help and recovery takes up to 6 days.

bulb 1. Any rounded structure or a rounded expansion at the end of an organ or part, for example the olfac-tory bulb or bulb of the penis. **2.** The *medulla oblongata.

bulbar 1. Relating to a *bulb. **2.** Relating to or affecting the *medulla oblongata. **3.** Relating to the eyeball.

bulbourethral glands (Cowper's glands) A pair of accessory male glands that produce a secretion which contributes to the *semen. They lie on either side of the pelvic part of the urethra, into which they open. They occur in the stallion, bull, boar (in which they are very large), and the cat but are lacking in the dog. In castrated animals they are very much reduced in size.

bull 1. An uncastrated male ox (*see* cattle). Bulls are used for meat pro-duction (*see* bull beef) or for breeding (*see* bull husbandry). **2.** The male of various other large mammals, such as elephant, whale, or seal.

bulla (*pl.* bullae) (in anatomy) A rounded bony prominence.

bull beef Beef produced from bulls specifically reared for meat production and slaughtered at 10–18 months of age. Compared to *steers, bulls produce leaner, heavier carcasses and show about 10% greater liveweight gain and food conversion efficiency. The behavioural problems associated with adult bulls (see bull husbandry) are largely avoided because of the early slaughter age. Stress in the animal immediately prior to slaughter can lead to undesirable dark-coloured meat during cutting. This problem can be overcome with modern lairage and slaughterhouse management techniques. Bull beef can also mean beef from breeding bulls slaughtered at the end of their useful life. Such meat is likely to be of poor quality and only suitable for processing.

bulldog calf An inherited disorder of cattle characterized by short nasal bones, a broad skull, and protrusion of the lower jaw. In severe cases there may be associated *hermaphroditism. It occurs in most breeds of cattle and, in Holstein and Guernsey breeds, is known to be controlled by an autosomal *recessive *allele. *Chondrodysplasia of the facial bones is often present. In Jersey cattle the disorder seems to be controlled by a *dominant allele; the heterozygotes are recognized by shortness of the limbs. The condition is normally non-lethal but can cause calving difficulties. Grazing is hampered due to misalignment of the jaw. Similar conditions occur in most species; some breeds of dog have 'pug-like' features as breed requirements.

bull husbandry All aspects of the rearing and management of bulls. Bulls reared for beef (see bull beef) should be kept in groups of less than 20 animals. New members should not be added to established groups, and groups should not be mixed.

Although bulls of beef breeds generally have a more docile temperament than dairy bulls, all bulls are potentially dangerous and should be treated with caution. In the UK, it is a legal requirement that bulls kept for breeding purposes should be housed in safe pens when not running with their cows. A bull pen normally consists of a covered box and an outside run to provide exercise space and, if possible, a view of the cows. There should be a water bowl and a manger that can be filled from outside the pen. The pen should be of robust construction with escape routes for stockpersons, and an arrangement for shutting the bull into either the box or the run, without entering the pen, so that the other area can be cleaned out. For ease of handling and safety, a breeding bull over the age of 6 months is usually fitted with a ring through the septum of its nose by which it can be led or restrained. Frequent handling is desirable in order to exercise the animal, keep his feet hard, and maintain docility. Bulls confined for long periods without work are more likely to have bad tempers. In feeding, the aim is to keep the bull fit without being fat. Good-quality forage alone may be adequate, with a small quantity of supplementary concentrates for an active animal.

A bull is generally considered ready to commence service from the age of 10–12 months. About 20 matings with heifers is sufficient in his first year, and no more than 4 matings per week in the second year. Overwork or excessive fatness will lead to infertility. The bull's health can have a lasting influence on the progeny of the herd. One of the problems associated with natural mating (rather than *artificial insemination) is the transmission of *genital vibriosis, so he should be treated against this. The feet are periodically checked and, if necessary, trimmed; tremendous pressure is exerted on the feet when mounting. *Lice may also be a problem and periodic de-lousing is recommended.

bullock *See* steer.

bumblefoot A condition affecting the feet of domestic fowls and turkeys, involving inflammation and lameness due to abscesses. It can affect one or both feet and is caused by entry of the bacterium *Staphylococcus aureus* via wounds and abrasions. Cases tend to occur as birds get older and heavier, especially broiler breeder males, and incidence is increased by unsuitable surfaces or perches that can damage the skin. Bumblefoot can affect other species of bird in certain circumstances; for instance, when birds with talons are given perches that are too narrow, or when wading birds are kept on concrete. Individual birds may be treated surgically, and antibiotics are also effective.

bunamidine An anthelmintic, available as bunamidine hydrochloride, given orally to treat infestations of certain tapeworms, especially *Taenia* spp. and *Dipylidium* spp.; efficacy against *Echinococcus* spp. is much poorer and repeat treatments at six-weekly intervals are necessary. The drug causes disintegration of the tapeworm segments. The animal should be starved prior to administration. Vomiting, especially if the tablet is crushed, and diarrhoea are seen frequently, and sudden death after treatment has been reported, possibly because the drug sensitizes the heart to the arrhythmogenic effect of *catecholamines. Preventing excitement in the animal after dosing may reduce the risk. Tradename: **Scholaban**.

bundle (fasciculus) A group of nerve or muscle fibres situated close together and running in the same direction, for example the atrioven-

tricular bundle or the cuneate fasciculus.

bunostomiasis Disease caused by *hookworms of the genus *Bunostomum* and affecting cattle (*B. phlebotomum*) and sheep and goats (*B. trigonocephalum*). The hookworms have a typical direct life cycle and the adults inhabit the small intestine. Eggs are passed 30–56 days after infestation is established. The larvae infect the final host by ingestion or by penetrating the skin. Treatment is with benzimidazoles or ivermectin.

bunt order The order of social dominance or rank in cattle. It is particularly important in herds of dairy cattle, where competition for space, food, and water can be strongest. Generally heifers are lower in the bunt order than older cows, but rank is often independent of age or size. Dominant cows can deprive weaker cows of water at a water trough or of feed at a trough or silage face. Therefore more than one watering point should be provided and an adequate width allowance given at feeding sites.

bunyavirus A family of RNA *viruses that have enveloped helical *capsids and contain segmented negative-strand RNA. The most notable veterinary example is the agent of *Nairobi sheep disease.

bupivacaine *See* local anaesthetic.

buprenorphine A semisynthetic opioid (*see* opiate) with partial agonist action on opiate receptors. It is used as an analgesic in dogs and horses. Its pharmacological activity is similar to *morphine but it is about 20 times more potent; its analgesic effect in dogs lasts for approximately 4–6 hours. Administration can be oral or by injection, either intramuscularly or slowly intravenously. Side-effects are similar to those obtained with morphine (*see* morphine). Reversal of the effects of buprenorphine, once they have developed, requires very high doses of an *opioid antagonist, such as naloxone. Buprenorphine is not a controlled drug because it does not have the addictive properties associated with morphine. It should not be used in cats. Tradename: **Temgesic**.

burdizzo An instrument used in the bloodless *castration of calves (and occasionally lambs). Similar to a pair of pliers but with long handles for better leverage, it crushes the blood supply to the testes, thereby resulting in their atrophy. The surfaces of the jaws are rounded and cannot quite come into contact, thus minimizing trauma to the skin. The *spermatic cord is felt through the neck of the scrotum and crushed in two places to ensure destruction of the blood vessels. To minimize pain the second crush should be below the first. The process is repeated with the second spermatic cord, care being taken that the crushes are not directly opposite each other but are staggered, since this reduces the risk of scrotal sac necrosis.

Bureau of Veterinary Medicine (USA) *See* Food and Drug Administration.

burn Tissue damage caused by such agents as heat, chemicals, electricity, sunlight, or nuclear radiation. For example, in small animals burns most usually result from contact with hot liquids or from infrared warming lamps being placed too close to the skin. The degree of injury varies from mild redness (erythema) to blistering or actual destruction of the skin with severe tissue loss. The nature of the damage in localized burns may not be apparent until after several days, when there may be extensive sloughing of the skin. Extensive damage can result in severe fluid loss with danger to life. In *first-degree burns* only the superficial layers of the epidermis are damaged with little cell destruction; the skin is reddened and there is pain but no blisters. Healing is rapid. *Second-degree burns* involve the epidermis and dermis to a variable degree without destruction of the deep dermis. There is blister formation and serum exudation with marked pain. Healing is slow, proceeding from the undamaged lower layers of the skin. In *third-degree burns* there is complete destruction of all layers of the skin and extreme pain; healing can only occur from the wound margins.

Treatment of mild burns is by immediate application of cold or iced water. Occlusive dressings, butter, or oil should not be applied because these insulate the burned tissue and prolong the tissue damage. When the skin is cool the surrounding hair should be clipped and removed and sterile dressings (e.g. 0.5% aqueous silver nitrate solution) applied with appropriate *antibiotic therapy. A tetanus antitoxin injection should be given. Skin grafts are essential if the burns are extensive. In severe cases burn shock resulting from fluid loss can cause death, and body fluid replacement is essential. Burns on the head may be associated with internal burns to the lungs as a result of inhalation of smoke.

bursa (*pl.* **bursae**) **1.** A small sac of fibrous tissue that is lined with synovial membrane and filled with fluid (synovia). Bursae occur where parts move over one another; they help to reduce friction. They are normally formed around joints and in places where ligaments and tendons pass over bones. However, they may be formed in other places in response to unusual pressure or friction. **2.** A compartment that is partially separated from a main cavity, for example the omental bursa, ovarian bursa, or cloacal bursa.

bursa of Fabricius *See* cloacal bursa.

bursitis Inflammation of a *bursa. It may arise in horses, cattle, and larger breeds of dog, usually in response to local trauma, and causes swelling and discomfort. Bursae occur at several sites in the body, such as the olecranon of the elbow and the calcaneus of the hock. Bursitis at these particular sites may lead to *capped elbow or capped hock. In *acquired bursitis*, a bursa that is not normally present forms as a result of repetitive trauma. Bursitis may also be associated with infection. Treatment involves eliminating the cause, usually repetitive local trauma, such as an improperly fitting saddle. Excess fluid can be drained from the site, pressure bandages applied, and in severe cases the synovial tissues removed surgically. *See also* infectious bursal disease.

buserelin *See* gonadorelin.

bush sickness A name used in North Island, New Zealand, for the clinical signs of *cobalt deficiency in cattle and sheep. Characteristic signs include ill-thrift, anaemia, and infertility. Deficiency of cobalt in the soil leads to inadequate levels in the herbage. The condition occurs in other parts of the world and is variously called 'pine', 'vanquish' or 'vinquish' in Scotland, 'nakurkitis' in Kenya, 'coast disease' in Tasmania, and 'salt-sickness' in Florida.

butacaine *See* local anaesthetic.

butobarbitone (*US* **butobarbital**) *See* barbiturate.

butorphanol An opioid drug, available as butorphanol tartrate, used as an *analgesic and *antitussive. In

horses it is used intravenously as an analgesic in cases of moderate to severe pain (e.g. colic). Possible side-effects are mild sedation and ataxia. Its analgesic effect lasts about 4 hours. In **dogs** butorphanol is used intramuscularly, subcutaneously, or orally as an antitussive in upper respiratory tract conditions where there is a nonproductive cough. There may be side-effects, such as ataxia, respiratory depression, sedation, and anorexia. If the drug causes severe respiratory depression its action can be reversed using an opioid antagonist, for example naloxone. Butorphanol should not be used in **cats**.

buttercup poisoning A toxic condition that can affect horses, cattle, and sheep following ingestion of one or more members of the buttercup family Ranunculaceae, which are often found in pastures. Plants involved include the celery-leaved buttercup or crowfoot (*Ranunculus sceleratus*), the meadow buttercup (*R. acris*), the bulbous buttercup (*R. bulbosus*), the creeping buttercup (*R. repens*), the lesser celandine (*R. ficaria*), and the marsh marigold or kingcup (*Caltha palustris*). The plants contain proto-anemonin, an irritant substance which, on ingestion, causes salivation, ulceration of the mouth, diarrhoea, and abdominal pain. In severe cases, there may be unsteady gait followed by convulsions and death. Treatment includes the use of demulcents and sedatives. Buttercup poisoning is not common in the UK although the plants are widespread, probably because they are not palatable and are only eaten in quantity when grass growth is poor in hot dry weather. Hay made from buttercup-infested pastures is innocuous because proto-anemonin polymerizes to the nontoxic anemonin during drying.

butterfat The fat present in milk. Cows' milk contains on average 3.6%

fat, goats' milk 4.5%, ewes' milk 7.4%, and sows' milk 8.5%. The triglycerides of milk fat contain both saturated and unsaturated fatty acids, the proportions varying with species. Within a species, butterfat content of milk varies with breed, age of animal, stage of lactation, and diet. For ruminants, adequate dietary roughage is essential to maintain butterfat levels in the milk.

butyric acid (butanoic acid) A *volatile fatty acid having four carbon atoms. It is one of the principal products of carbohydrate digestion in ruminants and is converted to β-hydroxybutyrate during its passage across the walls of the rumen and omasum into the blood. This in turn is metabolized in tissues via the *Krebs cycle to provide a source of energy.

butyrophenones A group of tranquillizers with similar structure and action. Like the *phenothiazines they act as antagonists at dopamine receptors in the central nervous system, and may have agonistic action at gamma-aminobutyric acid receptors. They cause depression of motor activity, muscle relaxation, hypotension, hypothermia, and reduced sensory perception. *Azaperone is used primarily in pigs, and some members (e.g. *fluanisone) are used with narcotic analgesics to produce *neuroleptanalgesia.

BVA *See* British Veterinary Association.

C

cab-horse disease Thickening of the forelegs just below the fetlock joint occurring especially in older horses that have been extensively worked on hard surfaces, such as metalled roads. The swelling results from *periostitis and *exostoses on the shaft of the first phalanx, or long pastern bone. The exostoses can cause lameness while they are forming, but not once they are fully formed because they involve neither the distal nor proximal joint. Hence they are classified as false *ringbones.

cadmium poisoning Toxicity due to ingestion of cadmium. An acute toxicity has occurred in pigs dosed with cadmium anthranilate to control ascariasis (*see* Ascaris). Diarrhoea and vomiting is followed by death. Chronic ingestion of cadmium, which may occur due to fallout in the vicinity of zinc smelters, causes anaemia by damaging the bone marrow. Overdosage of cadmium can be treated by the injection of sodium calcium edetate (sodium versenate), which chelates the cadmium and causes it to be excreted.

caecolith A calculus or concretion within the *caecum. Most common in horses or cattle, they are often formed around an ingested pebble or similar object and may become very large. *See* calculus.

caecum (*pl.* **caeca**) A blind-ending pouch that forms part of the large intestine. In mammals it is sited at the junction of the ileum and ascending colon (see illustration). The form varies greatly between species, being particularly large and comma-shaped in the horse with longitudinal bands of smooth muscle (taeniae) in the wall producing numerous small sacculations (haustra). In birds the caecum can be single, paired (e.g. domestic fowl), or even absent (e.g. budgerigar). When present it arises at the junction of the ileum and rectum. The caecum is important in herbivores, in which it contains a large

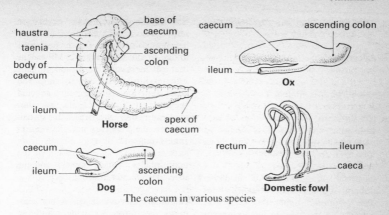

The caecum in various species

population of symbiotic bacteria that break down the cellulose in plant food. *See also* alimentary tract.

Caesarean section A surgical operation to deliver one or more foetuses through incisions made in the abdominal wall and uterus. In small animals this is a common procedure, usually performed under general anaesthesia via a midline abdominal incision. It may be required in cases of difficult birth (*dystocia) due to an oversized foetus(es) or uterine inertia. In farm animals the operation is generally performed under local anaesthesia, again in dystocia cases. In horses the operation is uncommon. The favoured approach in small animals and horses in the UK is a midline abdominal incision under general anaesthesia. In cattle and sheep a flank approach is usual. In all cases, operative delay prejudices the survival of the foetus(es) and, eventually, the life of the dam. This is true especially in the horse as placental separation during labour is rapid and consequently death of the foal before or shortly after surgery is common.

A Caesarean section is generally performed during the second stage of labour (*see* parturition) in cases of dystocia that will not respond to intrauterine manipulation. Elective

Caesarean sections may be undertaken during the first stage of labour or even before if there are strong indications that severe dystocia will occur. They are also performed to obtain *specific pathogen-free (gnotobiotic) neonates.

caffeine *See* xanthine.

cage layer fatigue A condition of laying hens housed in battery cages, involving paralysis of the legs and thin brittle bones. It is thought to be an extreme form of *osteoporosis, in which calcium from the bones is mobilized for eggshell production; it is aggravated by high rates of lay and lack of exercise. Affected birds fall over and soon die, some without any warning signs. A deficiency of calcium or phosphorus may be involved, but the condition can arise even with well-balanced rations. Supplementary *vitamin D_3 and phosphorus may be beneficial. Genetics may play a part.

calamine Zinc carbonate. *Calamine BP* is a mixture of zinc carbonate and ferric oxide that is used as a powder, lotion, or incorporated into a cream or ointment for topical application to soothe areas of inflamed skin. It has weak *astringent properties.

calc-

calc- (calci-, calco-) *Prefix denoting* calcium or calcium salts.

calcaneus One of the tarsal bones. *See* tarsus.

calciferol *See* vitamin D.

calcification The deposition of calcium salts in tissue. This occurs as part of the normal process of bone formation (*see* ossification).

calcined magnesite An insoluble mineral supplement, containing about 85% magnesium oxide, that is used as a source of magnesium in the prevention of hypomagnesaemic tetany (*see* hypomagnesaemia) in grazing animals, especially dairy cattle. It can be incorporated into fertilizer in an effort to increase the magnesium content of herbage, dusted onto pasture during periods of high risk, or incorporated in feed. The powdered form is more readily absorbed from the gastrointestinal tract than the granular form. Excessive intake can cause diarrhoea.

calcinosis A disease involving widespread calcification of the internal organs and soft tissues, usually caused by ingestion of certain poisonous plants of which *Solanum malacoxylon* (in Argentina and Brazil) and *Trisetum flavescens* (in Bavaria) are the best known. The leaves of these plants contain high concentrations of a toxic glycoside (1α,25-dihydroxycholecalciferol glycoside or a related vitamin D analogue). This highly potent form of vitamin D causes calcium levels in the blood to rise beyond normal (*hypercalcaemia). The disease also occurs when excess vitamin D is ingested or injected, and is also seen in dogs and other animals as a spontaneous condition of the skin. The hormone *calcitonin, secreted in response to the hypercalcaemia, starts the process of calcification of the body tissues. Signs are progressive and chronic. Walking becomes painful and the animals tend to 'graze on their knees'. Movement becomes increasingly stiff and animals suffer ill-thrift and body wasting. The heart function is especially affected because calcification seems to commence in the cardiovascular system beneath the endocardium. Prevention entails removal of the animals from affected pastures or eradication of the toxic plants. Other names: **enteque seco**; **Manchester wasting disease**.

calcinosis circumscripta A non-neoplastic condition occurring mainly in young dogs, particularly of the larger breeds. The lesion, seen as an opaque mass on radiography, is found beneath the skin surface, often over one of the limb joints, and is often confused with neoplastic lesions. It is gritty in consistency and contains numerous foci of chalky-white calcified debris surrounded by a foreign body-type reaction and embedded in a dense stroma of fibrous tissue. The cause is unknown but a genetic basis has been suggested. Surgical excision is generally curative but, if untreated, the overlying skin usually ulcerates to produce a chronically discharging sinus.

calcitonin (thyrocalcitonin) A protein hormone produced by cells of ultimobranchial origin, which are associated with the *thyroid gland in which they form its parafollicular (or C) cells. It lowers the concentration of calcium (and phosphate) in the blood, and thus works in opposition to *parathyroid hormone.

calcium A metallic element and one of the major minerals required by animals. Calcium (chiefly as calcium phosphate and calcium carbonate) is a major constituent of bones and teeth, which account for about 99% of total body calcium. Calcium ions serve as *cofactors for a range of enzymes involved in blood coagulation (clotting), the transmission of nerve impulses, and the contraction of muscles.

Mammalian blood plasma usually contains 80–120 mg calcium/litre, a concentration regulated by the hormones *parathyroid hormone and *calcitonin, as well as by *vitamin D. The skeleton acts as a calcium reservoir, from which the element can be mobilized when demand is high, for example during lactation or egg production, or when calcium intake or absorption is inadequate. For example, the availability of calcium in feedstuffs may be reduced by the presence of phytic acid (see phytin), which binds calcium. Also, a dietary excess of *phosphate may adversely influence calcium availability. A breakdown in the homeostatic mechanism controlling blood calcium is common at the end of pregnancy and beginning of lactation, when there are sudden demands for calcium. This causes *hypocalcaemia and a variety of clinical conditions, including *milk fever, *lambing sickness, *eclampsia, and *lactation tetany. Symbol Ca.

calcium borogluconate A calcium salt used widely in the treatment of hypocalcaemia (*milk fever in cattle, *lambing sickness in sheep, and *eclampsia in pigs and dogs). It is given in aqueous solution at a concentration of 20% or 40% w/v, subcutaneously or intravenously (slow intravenous infusion is used to minimize the risk of heart block or ventricular fibrillation). Calcium leaves the circulation rapidly, so that subcutaneous administration is used concurrently with intravenous infusion to maintain plasma concentrations.

calcium supplements Any of various calcium-rich feedstuffs that can be incorporated in the diet of farm animals. Calcium supplements are required by lactating animals and laying hens, where output of calcium exceeds intake. The commonest calcium supplements are ground limestone, steamed bone flour, and dicalcium phosphate. The ratio of calcium to phosphorus in the diet should be maintained in the range 1:1 to 2:1. Laying hens require a higher ratio and can be given calcium in the form of calcareous grit to appetite.

calculus (*pl. calculi*) A stone or concretion formed in a body tissue or organ. It may be composed of several different salts, most commonly magnesium ammonium phosphate, often termed *struvite*. The formation of calculi is a complex multifactoral process and may include any of the following: ingestion of a pebble or other foreign body on which the calculus forms; bacterial or viral infection; high concentrations of salts in body secretions; or changes in pH of body secretions. Calculi may form in many different sites; they are most common in the urinary tract (see urolithiasis) and biliary tract (see cholelithiasis). Other sites include the intestines (*enterolithiasis; see, e.g., caecolith) and prostate gland. Calculi may be present without causing any clinical signs, but if they interfere with organ function, most typically by obstruction of ducts, then clinical signs develop. Diagnosis is aided by radiographic examination of the tissue concerned. Treatment may require surgical removal of the calculus. *Dental calculus* is a mineral deposit that forms on the surface of teeth.

calf 1. A young ox, usually up to weaning age, but sometimes up to one year of age. *See* calf husbandry. **2.** The young of various large mammals, such as an elephant or whale.

calf diphtheria A disease of young cattle characterized by lesions in the mouth or larynx and caused by a bacterium, *Fusobacterium necrophorum* (*see* necrobacillosis). The organism gains entry to the mouth and larynx principally through damaged mucous membranes, caused, for instance, by erupting molar teeth. Mouth infections result in swelling of the cheek or cheeks, loss of appetite, raised body temperature, and the presence of foul-smelling dead tissue covering an ulcerated area of the cheek or gums. Such infections are more common in calves aged between 2 weeks and 3 months. The disease spreads through calves penned in unhygienic conditions, probably through bucket feeding, though not all calves are susceptible. Infections of the larynx, which may be fatal, are characterized by swelling of the throat, coughing, difficulty in breathing, and raised body temperature. These are more common in older calves and yearlings. Treatment involves the administration of *sulphonamides or broad-spectrum *antibiotics. The disease has no geographical limits but is more common in countries where animals are housed in winter or otherwise closely confined. Other name: **oral necrobacillosis**.

calf husbandry All aspects of the rearing and management of the *calf from birth until *weaning or until 12 weeks of age, when it is referred to as a reared calf. (For husbandry of the naturally reared calf, i.e. one suckling its mother, *see* suckler herd.) Whatever rearing system is used, it is vital that the calf receives adequate *colostrum during the first few hours of life. This provides antibodies and helps build up disease resistance. Artificial rearing systems provide the calf with whole milk or a cheaper milk substitute until weaning at 5–8 weeks of age. During this period, intake of *concentrates and *roughage steadily increases as the calf's rumen becomes fully functional. After weaning calves are fed exclusively on

the dry feed. Water is also provided from the outset. The milk or milk substitute can be given in buckets, either once or twice a day, warm or cold, or fed ad lib either cold, using acidified milk substitute, or warm from an automatic mixing and dispensing machine. Calves on bucket-rearing systems are usually housed in individual pens; this allows closer monitoring of individuals and also checks disease and bullying. Group pens are favoured for ad lib systems. Calves destined for intensive fattening systems are probably better reared on an ad lib system. The basic housing requirements are a clean dry bed, freedom from draughts, adequate ventilation to keep the relative humidity low, and adequate space and light (*see* housing). The common diseases of calves are *calf scours, *calf diphtheria, *navel ill, *pneumonia, *anthrax, and *blackleg. Lice (*see* louse) and *ringworm can affect the coat and skin, while *bloat is a common digestive disorder. Other problems include *cerebrocortical necrosis and lead poisoning. *See also* cattle husbandry.

calf pneumonia A respiratory disease of calves characterized by fever and respiratory distress and initiated by a variety of viruses. Primary respiratory disease can result from infection with *parainfluenzavirus, *infectious bovine rhinotracheitis virus, bovine respiratory syncytial virus (*see* pneumovirus), *adenovirus, or *rhinovirus. However, these infections do not usually result in serious or fatal disease unless associated with predisposing factors, such as poor ventilation, high humidity, or overcrowding. These stress factors appear to reduce the calves' ability to resist infection and allow the rapid development of secondary bacterial *pneumonia. Mixing of animals from different environments and inadequate colostrum intake by calves are also important factors. Therefore, calf pneumonia can be ascribed mainly to poor husbandry. *See* calf husbandry; housing.

calf scours Diarrhoea of young calves. It usually occurs in animals under 6 weeks of age and can be caused by a number of factors. Nutritional diarrhoea can result from feeding excessive amounts of milk or, where calves are fed on *milk substitutes, incorrectly mixed milk. A number of bacteria can cause diarrhoea, including *E. coli* (*see* enteric colibacillosis of calves), *Salmonella dublin*, *S. typhimurium*, *Campylobacter* species, and *Clostridium perfringens*. Of the viruses, *rotavirus is a common cause of calf scours while *coronavirus infection is relatively rare. Among the protozoa, parasites of the genus *Cryptosporidium* are more usually associated with calf scours than *Eimeria* spp. Calf scours is characterized by increased passage of soft or watery faeces, often leading to pasting of faeces around the hindquarters and base of the tail. There may be raised body temperature and loss of appetite. If not promptly treated, signs of dehydration, such as sunken eyes and loss of skin pliability, soon set in. Some clinical signs may indicate a particular pathogen. For instance, very yellow diarrhoea is often seen in rotavirus infection; *dysentery may be associated with *Salmonella* or *Clostridium* infection. However, identification of the causal agent often requires laboratory tests. Treatment initially consists of replacing milk feeds with a balanced solution of electrolytes (salts) and glucose to counteract dehydration. *Kaolin and chlorodyne may also be administered to alleviate the clinical signs. Calf scours can be prevented by a number of measures. Calves should be born under clean conditions and provided with adequate *colostrum within 8 hours of birth. Milk powder should be fed according to the manufacturer's instructions. A clean comfortable dry environment, free from draughts, helps minimize disease, and animals should be given daily health checks, with prompt isolation and treatment of affected animals. Calf houses should be cleaned and disinfected between batches. *See also* calf husbandry.

calicivirus A family of RNA *viruses similar to and formerly included with the *picornaviruses, but now classified as a separate family because of their different mode of replication. The most important veterinary examples are the agents of *vesicular exanthema of swine and feline calicivirus (*see* cat flu).

California fern *See* hemlock poisoning.

California hemlock A perennial herbaceous plant belonging to the genus *Cicuta* and containing the toxic alkaloid, cicutoxin. *See* hemlock water dropwort poisoning.

California mastitis test *See* cell count.

calkin A turned-down section of the outer heel of a horseshoe that provides a projection for better grip on the ground. They are used for the shoes of driving horses and hunters; when roughed they help to avoid slipping on ice.

calliper 1. An instrument with two prongs designed for measuring diameters; the most widespread verterinary use is for measuring the skin-fold thickness in *tuberculin testing. **2.** A form of splint that is applied to a limb so that body weight is borne by the splint rather than by the limb.

callosity (callus) Hardening and thickening of the skin due to prolonged friction. Calluses are usually found over pressure points, for example, on protuberances of the limb bones, and are particularly common in large breeds of dog. The areas are typically fairly prominent (2–4 cm in diameter), hairless, grey, and fissured, and are characteristically insensitive, though they may become infected with resulting pain. Calluses represent the normal protective hardening of the skin and should not be confused with *ringworm or *mange, which they can resemble superficially. Where pressure is persistent, a cyst or *bursa may develop beneath the callus.

callus *See* callosity.

calmodulin A calcium-binding protein that participates in many calcium-dependent enzyme-catalysed reactions. The Ca^{2+}-calmodulin complex binds to and thus activates an otherwise inactive enzyme.

calomel Mercurous chloride. It is a white powder, insoluble in water, and was formerly used as a purgative. It is still used topically as an antiseptic in ointment, although it is potentially toxic (*see* mercury).

calving The act of *parturition in cattle. Calving usually occurs at around 280 days after insemination, although this may range from 275 to 285 days, depending on breed. The udder enlarges considerably in the last 3–4 weeks of gestation as *colostrum starts to accumulate; this can usually be expressed a few days prior to calving. Approximately 24 hours before delivery, the pelvic ligaments slacken and a depression can be felt in the skin on either side of the tail head. The vulva swells and the animal exhibits concurrent increased restlessness and decreased appetite. In a field situation, the parturient cow usually seeks seclusion from the rest of the herd. The signs associated with the first stage of labour vary; heifers

may show indications of abdominal pain whereas cows frequently do not. This stage lasts for 6–9 hours. The second stage is shorter (about 3 hours) and straining is usually apparent. The chorioallantois (*see* allantois) protrudes through the vulva before rupturing, and the animal is usually recumbent by this stage. The majority of calves have an anterior *presentation and the umbilical cord generally ruptures at delivery. The dam smells the calf and may lick any membranes adhering to it. The placenta is expelled about 6 hours later and is frequently eaten by the dam. Due to the relatively large size of the foetus and its body proportions, *dystocia is common, particularly when the calf has a posterior presentation. Other common problems following calving are *hypocalcaemia (milk fever) and *retention of the placenta, which may in turn lead to *mastitis, *metritis, and *pyometra. To try to reduce the incidence of the latter three conditions, close attention should be paid to hygiene at calving. Occasionally, some of the above conditions may interact. Other conditions, such as obturator paralysis (*see* obturator nerve), may be present; this results in the *downer cow syndrome, whereby the animal becomes recumbent and is unable to regain its feet. US name: **freshening**. *See also* calf husbandry.

calving index (calving interval) The number of days between successive calvings for an individual cow, or the average interval for all cows in a herd. The optimum interval for both beef and dairy cows is 365 days; this maximizes returns from milk production and calf sales. In the UK the average calving index is about 395 days. Reasons for this extended interval include poor *conception rates, embryonic mortality, and *abortion. But the greatest factors are an over-prolonged interval between calving and service (*see* service period) and poor *oestrus detection. The average *gestation period of a cow is 281 days, so to achieve an average calving index of 365 days, cows should conceive 84 days after calving. Therefore, allowing for missed heats and returns to service, the target should be to serve each cow between 50 and 60 days after calving. In practice, cows are often not served until the first heat after 60 days, but cows can be served at the first heat after 50 days without lowering the conception rate.

calyx (*pl.* calyces) A cup-shaped part, especially any of the subdivisions of the *ureter within the *kidney. In the ox the ureter divides to form two *major calyces*, while in the pig these arise from the renal pelvis, the expanded commencement of the ureter. Major calyces subdivide into a number of *minor calyces*, each associated with one renal pyramid.

cambendazole *See* benzimidazoles.

Campylobacter A genus of Gram-negative microaerophilic *bacteria. They require reduced oxygen tension for growth and appear as curved rods, either singly or joined to form spirals. *C. fetus venerealis* (formerly called *Vibrio fetus*) causes abortions and infertility in cattle (*see* campylobacteriosis of cattle). *C. fetus fetus* causes abortions in sheep and occasionally in cattle (*see* campylobacteriosis of sheep). *C. jejuni* causes *winter dysentery in cattle and gastroenteritis in dogs, cats, and humans. Transmission is by ingestion of the bacteria. *C. sputorum mucosalis* is associated with *intestinal adenomatosis in pigs.
Campylobacter spp., particularly *C. jejuni*, are now the primary cause of foodborne enteric infections in humans. Disease is acute but rarely fatal, with symptoms, including headache, nausea, diarrhoea, and vomiting, lasting for 3–5 days. Contaminated

meat, milk, and water are possible sources of infection, although any warm-blooded animal is a potential carrier. Attention to routine hygiene, such as rinsing carcasses with chlorinated water, kills the organisms.

campylobacteriosis of cattle Infection of the genital tract of cattle by bacteria of the genus *Campylobacter. C. fetus venerealis* (formerly *Vibrio fetus*) is the usual cause of the condition generally known as *bovine infectious infertility*. The infection is transmitted venereally. Infected bulls show no signs of disease and their spermatozoa are normal, but the semen is infectious. Infected heifers or young cows conceive but return repeatedly to service at irregular intervals greater than the usual oestrous cycle (21 days), due to early death of the fertilized ovum or embryo and its subsequent absorption or unnoticed expulsion. The animal thus appears to be infertile. Later, when an individual cow has developed a degree of resistance, more extended pregnancy occurs and a dead foetus is aborted.
Diagnosis is possible by laboratory culture or serological testing of vaginal mucus samples, but in a newly infected herd the cause may not be suspected until one of the cows aborts, and the bacterium is recovered from its foetus. Antibiotic treatment gives varying results. Bulls kept at artificial insemination centres are stringently monitored for infection and, since the disease cannot pass from cow to cow, use of purchased semen leads to gradual disappearance of the disease from the herd.
C. fetus fetus (*see* campylobacteriosis of sheep) also causes infertility or sporadic abortions in cattle; the infection may or may not be venereally transmitted. It has been isolated from rare instances of subclinical mastitis in cows. Some cattle are symptomless intestinal carriers, and infection of humans may result in enteritis. Other

names: **infectious infertility**; **genital campylobacteriosis**; **'vibrionic abortion'**; **'vibrionic infertility'**.

campylobacteriosis of sheep ('vibrionic abortion') Bacterial infection of the ovine placenta and foetus involving either *Campylobacter fetus fetus* (formerly *Vibrio fetus intestinalis*) or, less often, *C. jejuni* (formerly *V. jejuni*), leading to abortion. Venereal transmission does not occur (*compare* campylobacteriosis of cattle) and infection is introduced into a flock by carriers, which are probably intestinal. Campylobacteriosis accounts for only a small proportion of outbreaks of ovine abortion in the UK. Its appearance in a flock generally results in numerous abortions (an 'abortion storm') in the first year. A solid immunity rapidly develops in infected animals. Thus, a procedure sometimes advocated is to retain ewes that have aborted within the flock, mixing them with nonpregnant females to allow the latter's immunity to build up before tupping. This perpetuates the infection within the flock, but generally controls clinical abortions; it is contraindicated when *enzootic ovine abortion is also present. Both species of *Campylobacter* are transmissible to humans, *C. jejuni* being the more important cause of human enteritis.

canal A tubular channel or passage, such as the alimentary canal or auditory canal.

canaliculus (*pl.* **canaliculi**) A small channel or canal. Canaliculi occur, for example, in compact bone, linking the small cavities (lacunae) that contain the bone cells. Bile canaliculi are minute channels within the liver that transport bile to the bile ducts.

cancellous Lattice-like: cancellous (spongy) bone consists of a meshwork of bars (trabeculae) enclosing marrow-filled spaces.

cancer Any *malignant tumour. The two main categories are the *carcinomas, derived from epithelial tissues, and the *sarcomas, derived from mesenchymal tissues, i.e. skeletal and connective tissue, the blood and vascular system, and the visceral (smooth) muscles. Cancers arise from the abnormal and uncontrolled division of cells that then invade and destroy the surrounding tissues. Spread of cancer cells (*metastasis) may occur, thus setting up secondary tumours at sites distant from the original (primary) tumour.

There are many causes, including genetic factors (*see* oncogene), viruses, chemical agents (*see* carcinogen), and radiation. For many cancers incidence increases with age of the animal. Treatment depends on the type of tumour, the site of the primary tumour, and the extent of spread.

Candida A genus of fungi containing several species associated with infections (*candidiasis) in animals. The most common pathogen of this genus is *C. albicans*.

candidiasis Any of the various primary or secondary diseases caused by mycelial yeasts of the genus *Candida*, most commonly *C. albicans*. *Candida* spp. occur in the environment, can grow extensively in some wet-stored cereals, and form part of the normal flora of many domestic animals. They inhabit the digestive tract especially but may also be found on the skin and mucosal surfaces of other tracts, which they sometimes invade causing disease, particularly in animals that are young or whose normal defences have been compromised by poor nutrition, broad-spectrum antimicrobial therapy, or immunosuppression. Infections are usually localized and lesions are characterized by a white pseudomembrane overlying the affected tissue. Species of *Candida* are among the commoner causes of *mycotic mastitis and are occasionally responsible for *mycotic abortion and, rarely, systemic infections leading to septicaemia, endocarditis, or meningitis.

In poultry, *C. albicans* infection of the mouth and crop occurs sporadically, and occasionally causes a serious epizootic disease, especially where hygiene is poor and the environment has been heavily contaminated. Turkey poults are particularly affected and outbreaks start when the birds are 1-2 weeks old. Mortality peaks at around 6 weeks, sometimes attaining 75%; surviving birds may be unthrifty. There are no definite clinical signs, but complications can include *coccidiosis, dermatitis, and signs of vitamin deficiency. Postmortem examination of the crop reveals raised whitish plaquelike lesions, sometimes confluent and ridged in a form commonly described as 'turkish towelling'. Management factors, such as poor nutrition, insanitary conditions, and overcrowding, have been implicated in outbreaks. Diagnosis is established by the demonstration of pseudohyphae or true hyphae along with budding yeast cells during direct microscopic or histological examination of specimens from infected tissue. Care must be taken to distinguish these from occasional commensal *Candida* organisms. *Nystatin administered in the feed can be used to treat candidiasis in poultry (and intestinal candidiasis in mammals). Contaminated poultry houses and equipment should be thoroughly disinfected. Other names: **bronchomycosis**; **candidosis**; **dermatocandidiasis**; **muguet**; **thrush**.

canicola fever *See* leptospirosis.

canine (dental anatomy) In most species, the tooth fourth from the midline in either jaw, giving a total of four. In ruminants they occur only in the lower jaw and in mares are often absent altogether. They are relatively large in carnivores, being used for the tearing of flesh. In male pigs, the canines form prominent tusks, which continue to grow throughout life. Canines are present in both the temporary and permanent sets of teeth.

canine adenovirus infection *See* canine viral hepatitis; kennel cough.

canine autoimmune haemolytic anaemia (AIHA) An *autoimmune disease of dogs in which the red blood cells are damaged or destroyed by the animal's own antibodies, resulting in *anaemia. The commonest form is an apparently spontaneous haemolysis, which can occur at any age. Haemolysis may take place within the blood vessels or in the spleen and may be acute or chronic. *Acute AIHA* presents as a haemolytic crisis with *packed cell volume below 10% and red cell count below 1.5 × 10^{12}/l. There is prostration and, in severe cases, jaundice and staining of the urine with haemoglobin. *Chronic AIHA* presents as a moderate to severe intolerance of exercise with frequent episodes of breathlessness and high pulse rate. In addition to haemolysis, permanent or intermittent inactivity of the bone marrow (dyshaemopoietic *anaemia) is common. Affected animals sometimes show spontaneous agglutination of their red cells when blood samples are examined by the naked eye. This is a strongly suggestive finding. There is frequently antibody and/or complement bound to the red cells, as revealed by a positive direct Coombs test. Red cells damaged by the autoimmune process assume a characteristic microscopic appearance, the *spherocyte.

Treatment is by steroids. Dexamethazone or prednisolone (*see* corticosteroid) are usually effective in controlling the condition when used in high doses. The disease tends to persist, however, and will frequently require maintenance doses to be continued over long periods. Relapses are common so that regular monitoring of recovered dogs is advisable. In some unresponsive cases, antimitotic drugs, such as *vincristine and *cyclophosphamide, have been used with effect, but caution is required since these agents will suppress bone marrow function. Blood transfusion is used as a life-saving measure but cross-matching for blood group compatibility is desirable. Furthermore, transfusion may suppress the natural processes of regeneration in the bone marrow. Splenectomy has been carried out when other treatments have failed, but its results are uncertain.

AIHA may also occur in newborn puppies as a result of antibodies acquired by the dam. Such antibodies are presumed to arise as a result of sensitization of the dam by paternal red cell antigens in the developing foetus. This mechanism is analogous to the one responsible for *equine autoimmune haemolytic anaemia, though the canine disorder is encountered much more rarely than the equine one. The *systemic lupus erythematosus syndrome may also give rise to AIHA.

canine babesiosis (piroplasmosis)

A disease of dogs occurring mainly in the tropics and caused by the protozoan parasites *Babesia canis* or *B. gibsoni*, which infect their host's red blood cells and are transmitted by the hard ticks *Rhipicephalus sanguineus*, *Dermacentor* spp., and others (*see* babesiosis). *B. canis* is $4-5\ \mu m$ long, pear-shaped, and occasionally occurring in linked pairs; *B. gibsoni* is smaller, roughly circular in shape, and rarely paired. The sometimes fatal disease may be acute or chronic and is characterized by fever, anaemia, jaundice, and perhaps *haemoglobinuria. A large variety of other clinical signs may also be pre-sent, including oedema, haemorrhage, and enteric, respiratory, and nervous signs. Unlike bovine babesiosis, in which young cattle are resistant to disease, canine babesiosis can occur in dogs of any age that are exposed to ticks. Diagnosis is confirmed by the finding of babesia organisms in stained blood smears, but in chronic disease these may be very difficult to find. Specific babesicidal drugs are available for use in dogs, and supportive treatment, including blood transfusions, may be useful. In enzootic areas, regular treatment of dogs with an *acaricide to prevent tick infestation may be worthwhile.

canine chronic active hepatitis (CAH)

A form of *hepatitis occurring in dogs and said to be the counterpart to CAH in humans. Affected dogs have a history of nonspecific hepatitis for a period of 6 months or more, with biopsy evidence of active hepatitis. The latter is crucial for diagnosis. Lesions consist of bridging necrosis (i.e. extension between portal triads or central vein region), piecemeal necrosis (i.e. necrosis of the periportal area of *hepatocytes at the outer border of a lobule), and active *cirrhosis with fibrosis. The inflammatory response consists of lymphocytes, plasma cells, and eosinophils in portal and periportal regions. In humans, grossly elevated serum aminotransferases are detected clinically; this is not always the case in dogs. The exact cause is not known; there may be an autoimmune reaction against the individual's own hepatocytes, but some authorities have suggested a genetic predisposition to CAH. Immunosuppressants, such as azathioprine and penicillamine to inhibit complex formation, are advocated for treatment.

canine eosinophilic gastroenteritis

A disease of dogs characterized by chronic vomiting and diarrhoea due to an infiltration of the tissues lining the bowel wall with *eosinophils – a type of white blood cell. While the exact cause of the condition is unknown, it is suspected that it may be of allergic origin, and can be treated with the long-term administration of *corticosteroids.

canine herpesvirus A member of the *herpesvirus family responsible for various infections in dogs. Although it causes only mild respiratory and genital infections in adult dogs, the virus may be transmitted to newborn puppies from the mother and contribute to the *fading puppy syndrome. There is as yet no cure or prevention for canine herpesvirus infection.

canine juvenile osteodystrophy A bone disease of dogs caused by calcium deficiency. The deficiency stimulates the parathyroid gland to secrete parathyroid hormone, which induces bone resorption to restore blood calcium levels. Eventually this softens the bones resulting in *osteodystrophy. A similar disorder occurs in other species, such as cats and certain primates. Growing animals are most severely affected because their need for calcium is greatest. The cause may be complex, but essentially comprises mineral imbalance that involves calcium deficiency or phosphorus excess leading to *hypocalcaemia. The disorder primarily affects puppies (or kittens) fed diets predominantly of meat and containing too little calcium but too much phosphorus. Unsupplemented meat diets are not adequate for these growing animals. Clinical signs include reluctance to move, lameness, and outward splaying of the paws. Palpation of the bones elicits pain. Softening of the jaw bones leads to loosening and loss of teeth. Tentative diagnosis can be confirmed by analysis of the diet and also by analysis of blood serum calcium, inorganic phosphorus, and alkaline phosphatase concentrations. Treatment involves dietary supplementation with calcium gluconate or lactate to achieve a calcium/phosphorus ratio of 2:1. Long-term prevention demands a diet with a calcium/phosphorus ratio of approximately 1.2:1.0. Other name: **nutritional secondary hyperparathyroidism**.

canine nasal mite A tiny *mite, *Pneumonyssus caninum*, that is an ectoparasite of dogs, living in the nasal passages and causing itching and a nasal discharge.

canine panosteitis A condition of dogs in which there is localized excessive production of bone (endostoses) along the length of one or more of the long bones. This results in pain and lameness. The cause is unknown, but the condition generally affects dogs aged between 5 months and 1 year and becomes self-limiting by around 20 months of age. The diagnosis may be confirmed radiographically. Palliative treatment with pain-killing drugs may be indicated in severe cases. Other name: **eosinophilic panosteitis**.

canine parvovirus A type of *parvovirus that causes a disease of dogs characterized by high mortality in young puppies and diarrhoea and vomiting in older dogs. The virus is closely related to *feline viral enteritis virus and the sudden widespread appearance of the disease in 1979 has led to the suggestion that it originated from an attenuated feline enteritis vaccine strain. In puppies below 8 weeks of age, but occasionally also in older dogs, the disease causes damage to the heart muscle, and a high percentage of affected puppies die of heart failure. Although mortality in young dogs (over 8 weeks of age) may be as high as 10%, in older dogs death is rare and enteritis is the main consequence. Puppies

canine staphylococcal dermatitis

may be protected by maternal antibody up to 16 weeks of age. Vaccination against canine parvovirus is usually started at 12 weeks of age but must be repeated at 16 weeks, when the development of immunity can take place without the interference of maternal antibody. Annual vaccination is recommended.

canine staphylococcal dermatitis A form of *dermatitis affecting dogs and caused by infection with *Staphylococcus epidermidis*. This bacterium is commonly found on normal skin, but is present in excessive numbers in this disease due to some factor compromising the normal skin defence mechanisms. This factor may be extrinsic, such as parasites or irritant chemicals, or intrinsic, such as a hormonal imbalance, an allergic reaction, or a physical abnormality (e.g. as seen in breeds of dogs with deeply folded skin). The clinical signs will depend on the depth of skin infection and the degree of secondary damage inflicted by the dog, but may include the formation of pustules, reddening, scaling, weeping from the surface of the skin, and loss of hair. The underlying cause of the infection should be identified and removed if possible. Oral antibiotics are usually given, sometimes together with a topical antibacterial preparation.

canine viral hepatitis A contagious disease of dogs and foxes characterized by *hepatitis, *nephritis, and fever and caused by canine *adenovirus. Transmission is by contact of susceptible animals with infected urine, or with equipment and locations contaminated with infected urine. The clinical signs may vary with the virulence of the virus strain and the age of the animal; they may be mild or inapparent, or there may be enlargement of the *lymph glands and tonsils, or even severe abdominal pain and death. Sometimes the dis-

ease remains chronic with persistent excretion of virus in the urine. Protection can be provided by vaccination with a dead or live attenuated vaccine.

'Blue eye' is a *keratitis caused by an immunologically mediated response which may follow vaccination with the live attenuated vaccine, resulting in cloudiness of the cornea. For this reason, an attenuated strain of the antigenically related canine adenovirus 2 is usually preferred. Other name: **Rubarth's disease**. *See also* kennel cough.

canker 1. A colloquial term for inflammation of the ear (otitis externa) of cats and dogs (*see* otitis). **2.** A colloquial term for decay and inflammation of the sole of the hoof associated with an offensive odour (*see* thrush).

cannibalism Any of various vices in which an animal attacks its own kind. Pecking vices are common in intensively housed poultry. Cannibalism usually follows *feather pecking, which denudes and may draw blood. Overcrowding may be a contributory factor, but attacks are often apparently unprovoked and may be sustained, with no retaliation from the victim. The attacker is likely to aim for exposed flesh, e.g. the cloaca of a laying hen, especially one with a prolapsed oviduct, or patches devoid of feather cover. Without intervention, the result is invariably death either by haemorrhage or shock. The risk of cannibalism may be reduced by lowering the light intensity in buildings, but this is not practicable under free-range conditions. Prevention can be achieved with a variety of practices, including *debeaking and *desnooding.

Cannibalism of newborns by the dam can occur in some species, especially pigs and dogs, following stress or, sometimes, for no apparent reason.

cannula (*pl.* **cannulas** or **cannulae**) A hollow tube of rigid material, generally used with a *trochar, that can be inserted into the body. The solid pointed trochar guides the cannula, which fits tightly around the trochar; once in place the trochar is removed allowing gas or fluid to escape through the cannula. The most common use is for the relief of acute *bloat in ruminants, especially cattle, when the trochar and cannula are inserted into the rumen.

cantharidin A toxic and irritant chemical derived from cantharides, a preparation of dead beetles, especially the blister beetle or Spanish fly, *Lytta vesicatoria*. It was formerly used as a blistering agent but is now considered too toxic for therapy. It may be present in some hays in North America, causing poisoning in horses.

canthoplasty *See* tarsorrhaphy.

canthus Either corner of the eye; the angle at which the upper and lower eyelids meet.

Capillaria A genus of *nematodes parasitizing domestic fowls, rodents, cats, and dogs. Domestic fowls are affected by two species, *C. annulata*, which is found in the crop or oesophagus, and *C. obsignata* and *C. caudinflata*, which are found in the intestine. *C. aerophila* occurs in the respiratory tract of cats, dogs, and foxes, while *C. hepatica* is found in the liver of rats and some other rodents. The life cycle is normally direct, but the eggs may be eaten by earthworms, in which case the eggs hatch but no larval development occurs. Heavy infestations may elicit an inflammatory reaction, which can lead to sloughing of the mucous membrane in the digestive tract. In **domestic fowls** affected birds have diarrhoea, become emaciated, and will often huddle together in a corner. The disease can be controlled by adding methyridine or *levamisole to the birds' drinking water.

capillary An extremely narrow blood or lymphatic vessel, approximately 5–20 μm in diameter. Capillaries form networks in most tissues; they are supplied with blood by arterioles and drained by venules. The vessel wall is a simple squamous endothelium, only one cell thick, which enables exchange of oxygen, carbon dioxide, water, salts, etc. between the blood and the tissues (see illustrations).

capitulum The small rounded end of a bone that articulates with another bone. For example, the *capitulum humeri* is the round prominence at the elbow end of the humerus that articulates with the radius.

capon A castrated male domestic fowl. Capons are rarely found in modern poultry production systems. Surgical caponization, normally at 4–6 weeks of age, was replaced by enemical caponization involving the use of implants, many of which are no longer permitted. The objective was to produce a larger, more tender carcass compared to entire males, and to reduce the incidence of aggression in flocks. Capons were slaughtered at around 14 weeks of age.

capped elbow (capped hock) Chronic inflammation of the bursa overlying the olecranon process (or tuber calcis in the case of the hock), occurring especially in the horse. The lesions usually follow from lying on hard floors or from traumatic irritation caused by the projecting heels of horseshoes. The affected bursae show initial oedema and swelling but after prolonged irritation they develop a firm and fibrous capsule ('cap'). Treatment involves simple anti-inflammatory agents and removal of the cause. In advanced cases the surgical removal of the cap may be indicated, especially when infected or abscessed.

capped hock *See* capped elbow.

caprine arthritis-encephalitis *See* leukoencephalomyelitis-arthritis.

capsid The shell of protein molecules forming the body of a *virus particle or *virion and enclosing the viral nucleic acid.

capsomere The individual protein subunit of the *capsid of an icosahedral *virus. *See also* virion.

capsule 1. A membrane, sheath, or other structure that encloses a tissue or organ. For example, the kidney, lens of the eye, and many glands are enclosed within capsules made largely of fibrous connective tissue. A *joint capsule* is the fibrous tissue, including the *synovial membrane, that surrounds a synovial or freely movable joint. The internal and external capsules are bundles of nerve fibres entering and leaving the cerebral hemispheres of the brain. 2. A soluble case, usually made of gelatin, in which certain drugs are administered. 3. The slimy substance that forms a protective layer around certain bacteria. It is usually made of *polysaccharides.

capsulitis Acute or chronic inflammation of a capsule, especially a joint capsule (*see* arthritis).

captopril A drug used to treat various heart conditions in small animals. It inhibits the action of peptidyl dipeptidase, an *angiotensin-converting enzyme, leading to a decrease in circulating concentrations of angiotensin and aldosterone with consequent arteriolar and venous dilation and increased salt and water excretion at the kidneys. Renal failure has

been reported in some dogs following its long-term use.

carbadox *See* growth promoter.

carbamate poisoning A toxic condition caused by an overdose of a carbamate insecticide. Like *organophosphorus compounds, carbamates inhibit cholinesterase enzymes and can cause salivation, muscular tremors, ataxia, recumbency, and death. Treatment involves the injection of *atropine. Cholinesterase reactivators, such as pralidoxime, are contraindicated.

carbenicillin *See* penicillin.

carbohydrate One of a group of organic compounds based on the general formula $C_x(H_2O)_y$. The simplest carbohydrates are the sugars (*see* monosaccharide, disaccharide), which include glucose and sucrose. *Polysaccharides are carbohydrates of much greater weight and complexity; examples are starch, glycogen, and cellulose. Sugars, notably glucose, and their derivatives are essential intermediates in the conversion of food to energy. Starch and other polysaccharides serve as energy stores in plants, particularly in seeds, tubers, and roots, which provide a major energy source for livestock. Cellulose, lignin, and others form the supporting cell walls and fibrous tissues of plants and are especially important in the diet of grazing animals. Carbohydrates also occur in the surface coat of animal cells, while *mucopolysaccharides are present in many body fluids.

carbohydrate overload (grain overload) A metabolic disorder of ruminants and horses which involves the accumulation of toxic amounts of lactic acid in the rumen and consequent *acidosis following the ingestion of large amounts of barley or other fermentable carbohydrate. *Acute barley poisoning* may ensue when animals gain illicit entry to a feed store or are suddenly introduced to a diet containing a high proportion of barley. Rumen bacteria ferment the carbohydrate to lactic acid so rapidly that the rate of production exceeds the rate of removal and metabolism. The rumen wall undergoes necrosis and the amounts of lactic acid absorbed change the acid/base balance of the blood. Clinical signs rapidly follow, with acute indigestion followed by dullness, staggering gait, coma, and death. *Chronic barley poisoning* involves necrotic lesions of the rumen wall with clumped papillae. Vegetable material or cereal awns become entrapped and induce both local inflammation and liver abscesses. Clinical signs are seen as repeated bouts of indigestion, abdominal pain, and possibly *laminitis. Treatment involves attempts to correct the acidity with oral doses of *sodium bicarbonate – either as a drench for the acute disorder, or as a food additive for chronic poisoning. In severe cases the only option is rumenotomy to remove the rumen contents.

carbolic acid *See* phenol.

carbon dioxide A colourless, almost odourless gas, soluble in water, that is the end-product of aerobic *respiration in living organisms and is required by plants for *photosynthesis. It is present in the atmosphere in small amounts (0.03% by volume). The transport of carbon dioxide in venous blood is enhanced by several mechanisms, principally the presence in erythrocytes of the enzyme carbonic anhydrase; this catalyses the reaction of carbon dioxide (CO_2) with water to form carbonic acid (H_2CO_3), and hence promotes uptake of the gas from tissues. At the lungs, carbon dioxide is given off and discharged during exhalation. An increase in the concentration of this gas in the blood stimulates breathing. The carbonic acid-bicarbonate system is the most important *buffer system in the blood. Carbon dioxide is also produced in the rumen (with *methane) and is discharged by *eructation.

carbon dioxide anaesthesia A method for rendering pigs unconscious before slaughter, in which they are passed through an atmosphere of carbon dioxide and air. When unconscious, the animals are bled. An advantage of this method is that *blood splashing is eliminated.

carbon monoxide poisoning A toxic condition that occurs when animals breathe air containing 0.4% or more carbon monoxide. This may happen when space heaters burning gas, oil, or coal have an inadequate air supply. Absorbed carbon monoxide combines with haemoglobin to form carboxyhaemoglobin, which has a bright-red colour and is unable to combine with oxygen. Affected animals exhibit muscular weakness, stertorous breathing, coma, and rapid death. Treatment must be rapid for success and consists of the inhalation of a mixture of 95% oxygen and 5% carbon dioxide. The latter stimulates the respiratory centre in the brain.

carboxylase An enzyme that catalyses the addition of carbon dioxide to a molecule.

carbuncle A collection of *boils.

carcass *See* meat.

carcin- (carcino-) *Prefix denoting* cancer or carcinoma. Example: *carcinogenesis* (development of).

carcinogen Any agent, particularly a chemical, that causes *carcinogenesis*, i.e. the conversion of a normal cell to a malignant one (*see* cancer). Carci-

carcinoma

nogenic chemicals include polycyclic hydrocarbons, aromatic amines, nitrosamines, asbestos, and chromates. Hormones, such as oestrogen and progesterone, can induce mammary tumours in mice and bitches and renal tumours in experimental animals. A *cocarcinogen* (or *promoter*) is a substance that is not itself a carcinogen but will act with a subthreshold dose of a carcinogen to cause cancer.

carcinoma Any malignant tumour that arises in *epithelium. *Squamous carcinomas* arise from epidermis and squamous mucosae, *adenocarcinomas* from glandular tissue. Carcinomas spread by local invasion of surrounding tissues and by metastasis to form tumour deposits in lymph nodes and internal organs.

cardi- (cardio-) *Prefix denoting* the heart. Examples: *cardiomegaly* (enlargement of); *cardiopathy* (disease of).

cardia 1. The opening at the cranial end of the *stomach that connects with the oesophagus. **2.** The heart.

cardiac 1. Of, relating to, or affecting the heart. **2.** Of or relating to the region of the *stomach adjacent to the cardia. This region varies considerably in extent in different species.

cardiac arrest Cessation of the effective pumping of the heart. It most commonly occurs when the muscle fibres of the ventricles start to beat rapidly without pumping any blood (ventricular *fibrillation) or when the heart stops beating completely (*asystole). Cardiac arrest can have various causes, such as electric shocks, lightning strike, poisoning (e.g. digitalis or molybdenum), or rapid intravenous injection of calcium, magnesium, or potassium salts. Anaesthesia, or even simple restraint of certain animals (e.g. budgerigars) may induce cardiac

arrest. Furthermore, a variety of diseases or tissue changes can lead to heart lesions and culminate in cardiac arrest (*see* cardiomyopathy).

Cardiac arrest causes anoxia of the brain with resultant collapse and loss of consciousness. The animal may gasp for a time but breathing soon stops and death rapidly supervenes. Attempts can be made to restore the heart beat, especially in small animals, by heart massage or direct injection of heart stimulants into the myocardium (*see* artificial respiration; defibrillation). However, such action must be prompt otherwise irreversible brain damage will occur. *Compare* myocardial infarction. *See* heart failure.

cardiac glycosides A group of drugs that stimulate contractions of heart muscle and are used in treating various heart conditions. Digitalis, a preparation obtained from the leaves of foxgloves, contains various cardiac glycosides, including digitoxin, gitalin, gitoxin, and digoxin. These contain a steroid nucleus with a sugar, and are hydrolysed in the body to form aglycones. Purified preparations of digoxin and digitoxin are used therapeutically. Ouabain is a short-acting cardiac glycoside obtained from the seeds of *Strophanthus gratus.*

The potency and duration of action of the cardiac glycosides vary, depending on the sugar residue in the glycoside. Digitoxin is slowly but completely absorbed from the gastrointestinal tract and is highly protein-bound (70–90%) in plasma; it is excreted in bile. Digoxin is rapidly but only partially (60–90%) absorbed from the gastrointestinal tract, and is less protein-bound in plasma (20–30%); it is excreted by the kidneys. These drugs increase myocardial contractility (positive inotropic effect), reduce heart rate, and delay the conduction of impulses through the heart. There is slowing of the heart, which improves cardiac filling, and the increased contractility improves cardiac output, thus raising blood pressure. There is some peripheral vasoconstriction, and diuresis due to the increased renal perfusion.

Cardiac glycosides are used in the treatment of congestive heart failure due to ventricular failure. They are also used to treat atrial fibrillation and atrial or atrioventricular tachycardias. Digoxin is most commonly used in animals because of its high potency and long duration of action. Various methods of *digitalization have been use in animals. Oral dosage is preferred where possible, although slow intravenous injection of crystalline preparations may be used in an emergency. With digoxin or digitoxin, slow digitalization over several days is the safest method. For rapid digitalization, ouabain can be used intravenously but the risk of toxicity is high. Throughout digitalization the patient should be monitored for signs of toxicity, which include anorexia, salivation, vomiting, and diarrhoea. Effects on the heart include atrioventricular block, cardiac arrhythmias, and ventricular tachycardia. If treatment is continued lethargy, weakness, and convulsions can develop. Many factors can increase the animal's sensitivity to cardiac glycosides, such as hypokalaemia, hypomagnesaemia, hypercalcaemia, hypothyroidism, kidney failure, and hepatic disease. Correction of hypokalaemia using oral potassium chloride and the treatment of arrhythmias with lignocaine or beta-adrenergic blockers (e.g. propranolol, timolol) can help mitigate the effects of toxicity.

cardiac muscle The specialized muscle of which the walls of the *heart are composed. It is composed of a network of branching elongated cells (fibres) whose junctions with neighbouring cells are marked by irregular transverse bands known as *intercalated discs*.

cardiography The practice of obtaining a *cardiogram*, i.e. a trace of activity from the heart, using a *cardiograph*. *See also* electrocardiography.

cardio-hepatitis/oedema A condition of turkey poults involving sudden death and characterized by fluid in the body cavity and a swollen liver and heart. It affects poults aged 1–4 weeks, usually the faster growing ones, and males more than females. Affected birds are found dead on their backs. Mortality in outbreaks may be 1–5%, sometimes higher. The cause is unknown but substandard management or stress could be involved.

cardiology The study of the structure, function, and diseases of the heart.

cardiomyopathy Any lesion or disorder of heart muscle. It may be due to a variety of causes, such as deficiency of certain nutrients (e.g. as in mulberry heart disease of pigs) or infection with bacteria, viruses, or protozoa, which can cause inflammation of the heart wall. For example, *parvovirus infection can severely damage the heart wall in young puppies. Chronic myocardial disease is found increasingly in domestic pets, particularly in certain dog breeds. Thickening (hypertrophy) of the heart wall sometimes occurs, reducing the volume of the heart chambers. Alternatively, loss of contractility may occur, with accompanying dilatation. The cause of these lesions is often unknown, though histology reveals *myocarditis and diffuse *fibrosis. *See also* heart failure.

cardiospasm Spasm of the muscle encircling the oesophagus where it opens (via the cardia) into the stom-

cardiovascular system

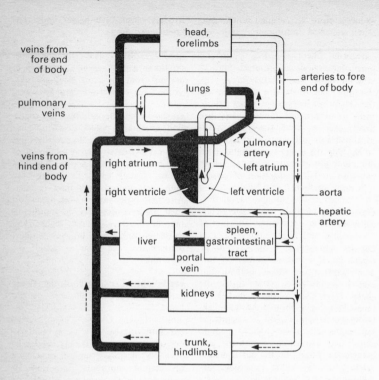

Diagram of the cardiovascular system

ach. Although uncommon in animals it is seen occasionally in horses. Spontaneous spasm may result from drinking ice-cold water or from the sudden introduction of solid food after a long period of debilitation. Also, inflammation of the lower oesophagus, caused, for instance, by the trauma of passing a stomach tube or by the premature rupture of a drug-containing capsule, may cause cardiospasm. Clinical effects resemble those of oesophageal obstruction. The head is extended and the animal makes convulsive attempts at vomiting. Frothy saliva exudes from the mouth. Treatment involves identifying and removing the cause; *spasmolytic agents, such as atropine, may also be administered. *Compare* achalasia.

cardiovascular system (circulatory system) The heart together with the two main networks of blood vessels – the *systemic circulation and *pulmonary circulation (see illustration). The cardiovascular system effects the circulation of blood around the body, which brings about transport of nutrients and oxygen to the tissues and the removal of waste products.

caries *See* dental caries.

carminative A substance that relieves flatulence and colic. It is usually an aromatic oil of vegetable origin, for example from chamomile, cinnamon, or cloves.

carnassial tooth (sectorial tooth) A particularly large shearing tooth present in both jaws of carnivores. In the upper jaw of the dog and cat it is the last *premolar tooth and has three roots. In the lower jaw it is the first molar in the dog and the only molar in the cat and has two roots. In the dog the upper carnassial is frequently a site of root abscesses, which can lead to the development of a *fistula discharging below the eye.

Carolina jessamine *See* yellow jessamine poisoning.

carotenaemia (xanthaemia) Yellow discoloration of blood plasma due to a high intake of *carotenes in the diet. It occurs normally in cattle and sheep grazing on pasture, the carotenes being a natural constituent of herbage. Carotenes serve as precursors for the synthesis of vitamin A, but excess may act as *vitamin D antagonists, exacerbating a tendency to *rickets if vitamin D is marginally deficient in the diet.

carotene One of a class of carotenoid pigments widely distributed in plant and animal tissues. Some, notably α-, β-, and γ-carotenes, are precursors of *vitamin A. Green plants are generally good sources of β-carotene, whereas it is deficient or absent in most concentrates used for livestock feeding, meaning that vitamin A supplementation is required. *See also* carotenaemia.

carotene pigmentation Bright-yellow coloration of the fat. It is found mainly in Jersey and Guernsey cattle, but also occurs in old cows of other breeds, and in sows; the yellow colour of Channel Island milk is due to carotene pigmentation of the butterfat. It is important to distinguish between carotene pigmentation and *jaundice.

carotid artery One of several main arteries in the neck whose branches supply the head region. The right and left common carotid arteries arise from the brachiocephalic trunk (see illustration at artery). They pass forward in the neck between the trachea and oesophagus and end by giving rise to the internal and external carotid arteries and the occipital artery. The *internal carotid* runs inside the skull and supplies the brain. In certain species, notably the ox, the extracranial portion becomes obliterated and converted to a fibrous strand after birth. The intracranial part persists, being fed by branches from the maxillary artery. The *external carotid* mainly supplies structures outside the skull, for example the face, tongue, and jaws.

carotid body A small nodule situated at the furthest division of the common carotid artery. It contains specialized cells surrounded by a dense network of blood capillaries. These cells detect changes in blood pH and oxygen and carbon dioxide levels, and send signals to centres in the brain which control the respiratory and cardiovascular systems.

carotid sinus A slight widening at the terminal division of the common carotid artery. Special nerve endings (*baroreceptors) in the wall detect changes in blood pressure and send signals to centres in the brain that control the heart rate and state of the vascular system.

carp- (carpo-) *Prefix denoting* the carpus.

carpal Relating to the *carpus.

carpitis Inflammation of the *carpus or 'knee' joint. In horses it may occur after strenuous training or as a result of trauma sustained in strenuous exercise, especially in young animals with immature bones. Repeated injury leads to localized overgrowth of bones (*see* exostosis). Similar lesions can occur in cattle that repeatedly lie on hard concrete floors; their knees become grossly thickened. The inflammation and swelling can cause lameness. Rest and the avoidance of further trauma to the knee will aid recovery. However, in more serious cases, fluid may accumulate in the joint, and *corticosteroids may be needed to reduce inflammation.

carpus The region of the forelimb corresponding to the human wrist. In the horse it is often referred to incorrectly as the knee. It comprises several carpal bones, which articulate proximally with the radius and ulna and distally with the *metacarpals. There are typically eight carpal bones arranged in two rows, proximal and distal (see illustration at manus). The first carpal may be absent in the horse, while in ruminants the first is absent and the second and third are fused together. In carnivores the radial and intermediate are fused together forming the *intermedioradial carpal*. Birds have only two separate carpal bones, the radial and ulnar. The distal row is fused with the metacarpals forming the *carpometacarpus*.

carrier 1. An individual that harbours a pathogenic microorganism without exhibiting signs of disease but can transmit the infection to others. **2.** (in genetics) An individual that bears an *allele for an abnormal trait without showing signs of the disorder; the carrier is usually *heterozygous for the gene concerned, and the abnormal allele *recessive. **3.** An animal, usually an insect, that passively transmits infectious organisms from one animal to another. *See also* vector.

car sickness *See* travel sickness.

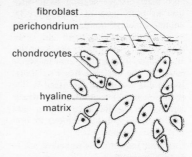

Hyaline cartilage

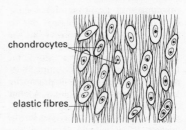

Elastic cartilage

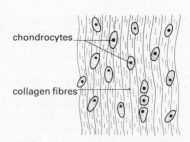

Fibrocartilage

Types of cartilage

cartilage A dense connective tissue composed of a matrix produced by cells called *chrondroblasts*, which become embedded in the matrix as *chondrocytes*. It is a semi-opaque grey or white substance, consisting chiefly of *chondroitin sulphate, that is capable of withstanding considerable pressure. There are three types: hyaline cartilage (*see* hyaline), *elastic cartilage, and *fibrocartilage (see illustration). In the foetus and newborn animal, cartilage occurs in many parts of the body, but most of this cartilage disappears during development. In the adult, hyaline cartilage is found in the costal cartilages, larynx, trachea, bronchi, nose, and at the joints of movable bones. Elastic cartilage occurs in the external ear, and fibrocartilage in the intervertebral discs and tendons.

caruncle A small red fleshy swelling. The *lacrimal caruncle* is the triangular prominence at the inner angle of the eye. It contains glands, may be pigmented, and bears projecting fine hairs. The *sublingual caruncle* is a small paired elevation below the tongue on which opens the submandibular duct and, when present, the major sublingual duct. *Uterine caruncles* are small oval prominences; about a hundred occur in the bovine *endometrium. During pregnancy they greatly enlarge and the numerous crypts on their surfaces receive the villi of the *chorion and contribute to a cotyledonary type of placenta (*see* cotyledon; placentome).

caseation The formation of firm cheeselike matter, rather than pus, as a result of tissue destruction and chronic inflammation. It is characteristic of tuberculosis and certain other chronic diseases. Caseous matter is usually surrounded by a thick fibrous capsule and may eventually calcify.

caseous lymphadenitis (cheesy gland) A chronic infectious disease of sheep and sometimes other ruminants caused by the bacterium *Corynebacterium ovis* (also known as *C. pseudotuberculosis*); it is characterized by the slow development of caseous

(cheesy) swellings in lymph nodes under the skin, in the musculature, and internally. The lesions have a concentrically layered onion-like structure, distinctive at meat inspection; subcutaneous lesions may suppurate. The bacterium survives in discharges and faeces and in contaminated soil; infection commonly occurs through minor skin injuries, such as those sustained during shearing. The disease is generally widespread where sheep are raised, although the UK is free. Severe economic loss occurs in countries exporting sheep meat, such as Australia, since meat from affected carcasses is suitable only for canning. Vaccines give incomplete protection. *See also* ulcerative lymphangitis.

cast 1. A rigid casing for a limb, made of a bandage impregnated with plaster of Paris or a plastic moulding. The cast is moulded around the affected limb, most often to prevent displacement of a fractured bone. This technique is commonly employed in human medicine, but in animals the shape of the limb tends to cause the cast to slip and pressure on the skin can cause ulceration and soft-tissue damage. *Compare* bonepinning. **2.** Describing an animal that has fallen and is unable to rise. This may happen as a result of disease and weakness or may be associated with accidental injury.

castor seed poisoning A toxic condition caused by the ingestion of seeds of the castor oil plant (*Ricinus communis*). The seeds or the residue arising from the pressure extraction of oil from the seeds may be incorporated deliberately or accidentally into animal feedstuffs. Ricin, a phytotoxin contained in the seeds, can be absorbed from the gastrointestinal tract and, after a latent period, cause acute bloody diarrhoea, weakness, and collapse. The toxic dose is variable because previous exposure to sublethal amounts of the toxin can produce a degree of immunity. Treatment ideally involves administration of the specific antiserum but, as this is rarely available, treatment of the clinical signs with sedatives and saline purgatives is recommended.

castration Removal of the testes or ovaries, especially the former. Surgical removal of the testes (*orchidectomy) is routinely performed on males of various species to render them infertile and to reduce undesirable sexual behaviour and aggression in the mature animal by removing the major sources of the male sex hormones (*see* androgen). However, the operation is stressful and causes a growth check, besides carrying a risk of infection or complications. Also, growth rates and food conversion efficiencies of castrated animals (*castrates*) are generally lower than those of noncastrated (*entire*) animals. Hence the increasing popularity of production systems using entire animals, especially *boar pigs and *bull beef. Under current (1988) UK legislation, the castration of cats, dogs, horses, mules, and asses must be performed under anaesthetic by a veterinary surgeon. Castration of other farm animals over 2 months old (or rams over 3 months old) is similarly restricted. Use of the *elastrator (see below) is restricted to animals up to 1 week old. Methods vary according to age and species.

Calves up to 1 week old can be castrated using a rubber ring, which is passed over the testicles using an elastrator and applied to the upper scrotum. This clinches the *spermatic cords causing the testes to wither (atrophy). This method is painful and the risk of infection is high. More popular is the *burdizzo emasculator, a device used with older calves to crush the spermatic cords; the testicles gradually shrink and atrophy. It leaves no open wound and thus carries little risk of infection, but it is

not completely reliable. The third, and totally reliable, option is surgical removal: the scrotal area is cleaned and disinfected, an incision is made in the scrotum, and the testicle is removed, twisting and breaking the cord with its blood vessels or severing and crushing the vessels to minimize bleeding. The procedure is repeated for the other testicle and the wounds are treated with antiseptic powder to counter the risk of infection.

In **sheep** the elastrator can only be used on lambs up to 1 week old, whereas the burdizzo is the best way of castrating older lambs and adult rams. Surgical castration entails cutting off the lower part of the scrotum; each testicle is seized using a pair of forceps and the vessels twisted and broken, or scraped with a scalpel. The wound is then treated with antiseptic and fly repellent before turning the animal out to clean pasture.

In **pigs** the only option is surgical removal of the testis. This should be done as soon after birth as possible, preferably when the animal is 3–5 days old. The scrotal region is cleaned and disinfected. Then each testicle in turn is squeezed against the scrotal wall, an incision is made in the scrotum, and the testicle is pulled out so that the cord can be twisted and severed. Antiseptic is applied to the wound and the piglet is placed in a clean pen.

The castrated male **horse**, known as a *gelding*, is generally less aggressive and thus safer to handle and ride than an entire stallion. The operation can be performed in the first, second, or even third year; delay allows the male temperament and conformation to develop and the potential of the animal to be assessed. A local or general anaesthetic is administered. Each testicle in turn is exposed through an incision made in the scrotum and the vessels of the cord are crushed and severed using forceps and ligatures or an *ecraseur. Castration of colts with a scrotal hernia requires special treatment, as does the castration of *cryptorchids.

In both **cats** and **dogs**, castration entails surgical removal of the testes under general anaesthesia. In cats, castration sometimes prevents the problems of odour and the tendency to roam and fight that are common in entire adult males. The optimum age for the operation is 5 months, although a satisfactory outcome is sometimes achieved in adults. In dogs, castration is performed to prevent promiscuous sexual behaviour and other undesirable traits when adult. The dog should be castrated before attaining sexual maturity; castration of adults can lead to obesity.

Chemical castration involves atrophy of the gonads due to the prolonged influence of sex hormones, either produced in the body or administered as a treatment. It may be used in birds. *Immunological castration* has been proposed as a possible future alternative to surgery. Analogues of sex-hormone releasing hormones, such as luteinizing-hormone-releasing-hormone (LHRH), would be administered to animals in order to stimulate the formation of antibodies able to destroy the animal's own releasing hormones. The resultant decrease in endogenous androgens would lead to gonadal atrophy. *Compare* spaying.

casualty animal An animal affected by injury rather than a pathological condition. In England and Wales under the *Slaughterhouses (Hygiene) Regulations (1977), an injured animal sent for emergency slaughter for human consumption should be accompanied by a veterinary certificate containing: the name and address of the owner of the animal; a description of the animal and its identification marks; the date and time of clinical examination; a signed statement by a veterinarian – "It is my opinion, after making due enqui-

ries and taking and testing any necessary samples, that this animal is not affected with any disease or condition liable to render the whole carcass unfit for human consumption and to the best of my knowledge and belief has not received any medicament, antibiotic, or chemotherapeutic which might do likewise"; the signature and status of the veterinarian; and the date.

cat A carnivorous mammal belonging to the family *Felidae*, which is generally accepted as comprising 38 species grouped into three genera: the large roaring cats (*Panthera*); the nonroaring and generally smaller cats (*Felis*); and the cheetah (*Acinonyx jubatus*), distinguished by having claws that do not retract fully.

The domestic cat, *Felis catus*, shows many of the typical features of the family. Its body is adapted for hunting, and is best suited to short bursts of speed. The sharp retractile claws are used for catching and holding prey, while the long canine teeth are used for killing it. The cats hunt mainly at dawn and dusk, aided by highly developed senses of sight, hearing, and balance. The sense of smell is also well developed, but is used mainly for detecting territorial signals from other cats rather than for tracking prey. The colour and markings of the wild cats have evolved to camouflage them from their prey, although many colour variations have been developed in the modern breeds of domestic cat.

Cat care A proper diet is the first step towards good health, and there is now a variety of reputable brands of prepared foods specifically designed for kittens and for adult cats. Dog foods should not be fed to cats on a regular basis. If fresh food is to be fed, the diet should be balanced and varied and include different meats with some fat, fish, eggs, cheese, and preferably some starchy foods, such as rice or potatoes. A special vitamin and mineral supplement is also needed for cats given fresh food, although an excess can cause as much harm as deficiency. Clean drinking water must be available at all times, especially if dried cat foods are given.

Kittens are normally vaccinated against the viral diseases *cat flu and *feline viral enteritis, and require annual booster doses thereafter. A vaccine against *feline leukaemia is also now available in some countries. These visits to the veterinary surgery provide an ideal opportunity for a regular health check. Other common diseases include ear *mite infestation, *abscesses due to cat fights, and *gastroenteritis, either due to infections or eating contaminated food. Any serious illness requires prompt veterinary attention. Routine care should include grooming of long-haired cats, since swallowing excessive amounts of hair can cause the cat to vomit *hairballs besides leading to a tangled and matted coat, and preventative treatment against *fleas and the common *cat worms. Unless required for breeding, both male and female cats should be surgically neutered (*see* castration; spaying), the former to prevent antisocial behaviour, such as fighting, roaming, and urine spraying, and the latter to prevent pregnancy. Allowing a cat to have a litter has no beneficial effect on its long-term health or life expectancy. Breeding from a queen should only proceed if the kittens are assured of good homes. Cats are generally neutered at 5–6 months of age.

cata- *Prefix denoting* downward or against.

catabolic Describing a metabolic pathway that leads to the breakdown or decrease in complexity of substances in the body, i.e. the processes of catabolism.

catalase An enzyme, present in many cells (including red blood cells and liver cells), that catalyses the breakdown of hydrogen peroxide to water and oxygen.

catalepsy An abnormal nervous state characterized by immobility, loss of voluntary movement, and muscular rigidity but without loss of consciousness. It can be induced by overdosage with *tranquillizers.

catalyst A substance that alters the rate of a chemical reaction but is itself unchanged at the end of the reaction. The catalysts of biochemical reactions are the *enzymes.

cataphoresis The introduction into the tissues of positively charged ionized substances (cations) by the use of a direct electric current.

cataplasia Degeneration of tissues to an earlier developmental form.

cataract Opacity of the lens within the eye causing blurred vision or progressive blindness. Cataracts occur most commonly in dogs and horses, and some individuals have an inherited predisposition. They are also caused by metabolic disease, such as diabetes, or repeated trauma or irritation of the eyeball. In severe cases surgical removal of the lens is indicated, but localized and small cataracts in young animals may scarcely impair vision and can clear up in time.

catarrh Excessive secretion of mucus by mucous membranes, particularly those lining the nasal or air passages. It is often associated with inflammation caused by infection, such as malignant catarrhal fever, atrophic rhinitis, or canine distemper. Inhalation of dust or allergic reactions, for instance to pollen grains, are also common causes. Treatment consists of attending to the primary cause, if appropriate, and the use of a *decongestant or *expectorant to relieve congestion.

catecholamines A group of physiologically important substances, including *adrenaline, *noradrenaline, and dopamine (see dopa), having various different roles (mainly as *neurotransmitters) in the functioning of the sympathetic and central nervous systems. Chemically, all contain a benzene ring with adjacent hydroxyl groups (catechol) and an amine group on a side chain.

cat flu A respiratory infection of cats characterized by fever, nasal and eye discharge, coughing and/or sneezing, and respiratory distress and caused by strains of feline caliciviruses or strains of feline viral rhinotracheitis virus. The incubation period is 2–5 days. Kittens are extremely susceptible and the disease is frequently fatal. Secondary infection may result in *pneumonia or chronic *sinusitis. Cats recovered from flu caused by either calicivirus or rhinotracheitis virus may continue to excrete virus particles for a considerable period or, in the case of rhinotracheitis, for life, particularly at times of stress. Vaccines against these two virus infections are usually given at 9 and 12 weeks of age, together with the *feline viral enteritis vaccine. This has considerably reduced the incidence of the disease, especially since catteries now insist that all boarders are adequately vaccinated.

catgut A fibrous material prepared from the walls of sheep intestines and used to ligate blood vessels and sew up tissues (see suture). It is prepared in a range of diameters and is available either as plain catgut or treated with chromic trioxide to produce chromic catgut. Catgut is gradually broken down by enzymes in the tissues; plain catgut dissolves in about 5–10 days while the chromicized material, which is more resistant, dissolves in approximately 14 days.

cathartic See purgative.

catheter A hollow tube of rigid or flexible material than can be inserted into the body to obtain samples of body fluid or to administer drugs. The length, width, and type of material is dependent upon the site of use. A Foley catheter is one that can be inserted into a body cavity or organ (e.g. bladder or guttural pouch) and kept in place by distension of a balloon around the tip of the catheter. See also catheterization.

catheterization The insertion of a *catheter into a hollow organ, blood vessel, or body cavity. Strict asepsis is required, especially if the catheter is to remain in place. Catheterization requires a knowledge of anatomy and should not be undertaken by untrained personnel. For intravenous catheterization, a blunt catheter is inserted into a vein, through a needle, which is then withdrawn while the catheter is advanced. This minimizes trauma to the vein. Intravenous catheterization is used for administering large volumes of fluid or irritant therapeutic solutions and in cases where repeated intravenous medication is required. The most commonly used vessels are the external jugular, cephalic, recurrent tarsal, and ear veins.

Urinary catheterization, involving the insertion of a catheter via the urethra into the bladder, may be used to obtain a urine sample, to ascertain the presence and location of a urethral blockage, to allow local medication of the bladder, or during contrast radiography of the urethra and bladder. In females a rigid or semirigid catheter is used. Visualization of the urethral orifice by use of a vaginal speculum helps the procedure. In males a long flexible catheter is used, but there are few indications for complete urinary catheterization in male farm animals and the procedure is difficult without general anaesthesia. Sedation (e.g. acepromazine medication) is usually required to achieve sufficient relaxation of the penis in geldings. *Uterine catheterization*, i.e. the insertion of a catheter through the cervix into the uterus, may be used for local medication or drainage and is required for artificial insemination.

cationic detergent Any of a group of surface active agents (surfactants) used as antiseptics and disinfectants. Most are quaternary ammonium compounds. Their bactericidal effect is to alter the surface tension at the bacterial cell membrane and change the cell membrane permeability. Activity is greater against Gram-positive than Gram-negative bacteria; *Pseudomonas* spp., *Mycobacterium* spp., bacterial spores, and viruses are not killed. Their activity is reduced in the presence of soaps and other anionic agents, organic matter, and porous material (e.g. cotton and rubber), but when made up in alcohol as tinctures their activity is enhanced. The principal cationic detergents are benzalkonium chloride and cetrimide. They are nonirritant to tissues but when applied to skin may form a film with fats and are liable to be inactivated by soaps.

cat leprosy A condition in which nodules develop in the skin. It is thought to be caused by the rat leprosy bacterium, *Mycobacterium lepraemurium*. The condition usually remains localized and the nodules are preferably removed surgically.

cat-scratch fever An infectious disease (*zoonosis) transmitted from cats to humans via skin wounds caused by cat scratches, splinters, or thorns. The causal agent remains unknown though most investigators consider it to be a virus. In humans the characteristic signs include local inflammation of lymph vessels and lymph nodes with variable inflammatory lesions at the site of the scratch. In some patients the lymph glands may even accumulate pus and suppurate, while in others a generalized septicaemia with fever occurs. The condition is generally benign with spontaneous recovery.

cattle Ruminant mammals belonging to the genus *Bos* (order Artiodactyla), also called oxen. The two main species are *Bos taurus*, the domesticated cattle of Europe, and *Bos indicus*, the domesticated cattle of India and Africa. Also of agricultural importance is *Bos bubalus*, the domesticated Indian buffalo. In Britain, the major cattle breeds are all *Bos taurus*, although some members of *Bos indicus* have been imported for limited use as sires for beef production. Domesticated cattle have long been bred and reared for their meat, milk, and hides, and as draught animals. Today, they are of great economic and ecological significance worldwide. *See also* cattle husbandry.

cattle husbandry All aspects of the rearing and management of *cattle. In the UK the cattle industry is integrated for the production of milk and meat (*see* beef cattle; dairy cattle). In most other countries milk production and beef production are separate, although dual-purpose breeds are used in some countries for the production of both milk and beef.
Dairy cattle in cool and cold climates are housed through the winter and fed on conserved forages, such as silage or hay, and concentrates. In spring they are turned out to grass, which is supplemented with concentrates, and continue to graze until the autumn. Typically, the calving of herd

members is organized to occur in the same season, usually spring or autumn, although most herds have sporadic calving at other times of the year.

The feeding of a dairy cow is governed largely by its lactation cycle, which determines milk yield, dry matter intake, and changes in live weight and body condition (*see* diet; nutrition). After calving, milk yield rises to a peak at around week 6; but dry matter intake rises more slowly to peak between weeks 12 and 15. Consequently, the cow is usually in negative energy balance for the first few weeks of lactation and loses weight and condition. It is important that a high-energy diet is given at this time to keep weight loss below 0.5 kg per day or 0.5 condition score units per month (*see* condition scoring). Recent evidence has shown that negative energy balance after calving can be virtually eliminated by calving cows in a lower condition (condition score 2) than previously recommended (i.e. condition score 3–3.5), but the success of this approach depends upon a supply of high-energy feed after calving.

Because of their relatively high cost, concentrates are usually allocated to cows individually, either according to current yield or on a flat-rate basis (when the total requirements over the winter period are divided into equal daily allowances). Concentrates are usually fed in the milking parlour during milking, but since no more than 5 kg can be given at one milking it is often desirable to feed concentrates outside the parlour on a group basis. Forages too are usually fed on a group basis, either in troughs or with a self-feed system directly from the silage clamp. On some farms, concentrates and forages are fed together ad lib in controlled proportions as a complete mixed diet. Root crops, such as turnips and kale, are either harvested and fed in troughs or grazed in situ. Grass is either taken to the cows (*see* zero grazing) or grazed in situ according to a particular grazing system (*see* grazing). During the winter, cows are either housed in cowsheds or housed loose in straw-bedded yards or *cubicles (*see* housing). In cowsheds, cows are tied in stalls where they are individually fed and milked. Loose housing means that cows are fed in groups and have to be taken to a milking parlour to be milked (*see* milking).

It is vital that each cow should have some form of identification so that accurate records can be kept of calving, heat, and service dates and also of health, milk yield, and feeding. Cows spend on average four lactations in the dairy herd. The most common reasons for culling are *infertility or other reproductive problems, *mastitis, and lameness.

Beef cattle originate from either dairy herds or *suckler herds. The fattening system employed is determined mainly by the breed and sex of the animal, which govern the rate at which maturity is reached. Intensive systems of beef production are more suited to late-maturing animals; semi-intensive or grass/cereal systems are best for intermediate animals; and extensive or grass-based systems are suited to early-maturing animals. Other things being equal, beef animals reach maturity in the order: heifers; steers; and, finally, bulls. If early-maturing animals are used in an intensive system, they get prematurely fat. Conversely, late-maturing animals used in extensive systems are often difficult to 'finish' for slaughter.

In Britain, beef cattle are commonly reared on one farm and sold as 'stores' for finishing on another farm. This may take place in yards over winter (yard finishing) or at grass over the summer (grass finishing). Intensive fattening systems involve housing animals throughout the fattening period (*see* housing) and are based either on cereals (see barley beef; bull beef) or good quality silage. Animals are slaughtered at 10–15 months of age weighing 380–420 kg. Semi-intensive systems generally employ autumn-born Friesian or Hereford–Friesian cross steers. They are reared over the first winter (see calf husbandry) and turned out to grass in spring at a bodyweight of about 180 kg. They are housed in the autumn to be finished on silage ad lib and 2–5 kg of barley-based concentrate, depending on the quality of the silage and type of animal. They are slaughtered at the end of this second winter, aged 16–20 months and weighing 410–500 kg. Extensive beef systems try to achieve maximum growth from grazed grass using early-maturing animals, such as Hereford–Friesian or Aberdeen Angus–Friesian crosses. Calves are turned out to grass in the spring and stocked at a rate that gives about 0.7 kg per day live-weight gain. In the autumn, the cattle are housed and fed hay or silage plus small amounts of concentrates to give growth rates of 0.5–0.6 kg per day. Because of the lower rate of gain over the winter, these animals should exhibit compensatory growth when turned out to grass in spring. They are slaughtered in late summer, aged 20–24 months and weighing 430–530 kg. See feedlot.

cattle plague See rinderpest.

cauda The tail or a tail-like structure. The *cauda equina* is the bundle of sacral and coccygeal spinal nerve roots that continue beyond the end of the spinal cord to reach their appropriate openings in the vertebral column.

cauda equina neuritis A rare condition of horses involving inflammation (neuritis) of the *cauda equina and resulting in paralysis of the tail, anus, rectum, bladder, and, in males, the penis. There is urinary and faecal retention. Occasionally nonsymmetric cranial nerve paresis may be seen. The neuritis is progressive. Lesions consist of thickening and distortion of extradural sacral and lumbar nerve roots, with discoloration from fresh or older haemorrhages. There may be fibrous replacement of nerve fibres. The aetiology is unknown although suggested factors are an autoimmune phenomenon or an immune reaction associated with previous respiratory disease of herpesvirus origin.

cauda equina syndrome A disorder caused by damage to the nerve roots (cauda equina) that arise at the end of the spinal cord. It is characterized by local dysfunction and pain at the base of the tail; if associated with a spinal fracture or dislocation the result may be *paraplegia with complete loss of sensation in the rear of the hindlimbs and tail. The underlying cause may be a spinal neoplasm or discospondylitis affecting the lumbosacral intervertebral disc; the latter is often associated with bacteraemia and may respond to antibiotic therapy, although frequently it requires surgical drainage. See also cauda equina neuritis.

caudal Relating to the tail end of the body.

caudate nucleus One of the *basal ganglia that forms part of the *corpus striatum in the brain.

caustic soda See sodium hydroxide.

cauterization The application of a heated instrument (a cautery) to cause tissue destruction or to stop bleeding. It is most frequently employed to stop haemorrhage after *dehorning in cattle or to perform *disbudding in calves. A cautery should not be employed to prevent horn growth in goats because of the risk of brain

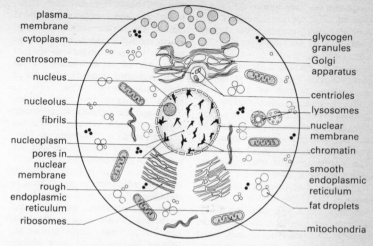

plasma membrane
cytoplasm
centrosome
nucleus
nucleolus
fibrils
nucleoplasm
pores in nuclear membrane
rough endoplasmic reticulum
ribosomes

glycogen granules
Golgi apparatus
centrioles
lysosomes
nuclear membrane
chromatin
smooth endoplasmic reticulum
fat droplets
mitochondria

An animal cell (microscopical structure)

damage through the relatively thin skull. Traditionally, cauteries of different types have been used to treat strained tendons in horses but this practice is now controversial with its adversaries claiming the practice is no better than resting the horse and that unacceptable pain to the animal is involved. *See also* electrocautery.

CCN *See* cerebrocortical necrosis.

celandine *See* blood root poisoning.

-cele (-coele) *Suffix denoting* swelling, hernia, or tumour. Example: *gastrocele* (hernia of the stomach).

celi- (celio-) (*US*) *See* coeli-.

cell The basic unit of all living organisms, which can reproduce itself exactly (*see* mitosis). Each cell is bounded by a *cell membrane* of lipids and protein, which controls the passage of substances into and out of the cell. Cells contain *cytoplasm, in which are suspended a *nucleus and other structures (*organelles) specialized to carry out particular activities in the cell (see illustration).

cell body (perikaryon) The enlarged portion of a *neurone (nerve cell), containing the nucleus. It is concerned more with the nutrition of the cell than with propagation of nerve impulses. A variable number of processes take origin from the cell body. *See* axon; dendrite.

cell count Any method for determining the number or concentration of cells in suspension. Such methods are most often applied to cells in blood, but they can be used on other body fluids, including cerebrospinal fluid, lymph, urine, pathological exudates, and glandular secretions (e.g. milk), as well as artificial suspensions of cells, such as cell cultures.

A *total cell count* measures the total number of all types of cell in a unit volume of fluid. In its most basic form, a cell suspension (or dilution thereof) is introduced into a chamber of known volume. The chamber is then examined under the light micro-

cell culture

scope and the total number of cells is counted. For routine laboratory cell counts, optical counting has largely been replaced by electronic methods. The widely adopted Coulter Counter operates by drawing a known volume of cell suspension through an orifice. The passage of each cell through the orifice is detected electronically and counted. Total cell counts can also be estimated chemically. Addition of anionic detergent to suspensions of cells causes their DNA to aggregate. The viscosity of the resulting aggregate gives an estimate of the original cell count. This principal forms the basis of the *California test* for bovine *mastitis, which is applied to milk.

Differential counts measure the number of given types of cell, either as a proportion of the whole cell population or as an absolute number per unit volume. In some cases, other cell types can be eliminated from the sample by chemical or immunological means (e.g. lysis of red cells using saponin, ammonium chloride, or acetic acid), enabling a differential count using a standard method as above. Alternatively, cell types can often be distinguished by the presence of specific chemical groupings on their membranes. Such groupings can be used to bind very specific antibodies, which in turn may be joined to fluorescent molecules to provide an optical label for the cells of interest (*fluorescent antibody labelling*). The labelled cells fluoresce in ultraviolet light, which allows them to be counted. Alternatively the antibody-binding cells may be lysed by the addition of *complement. Their concentration is then estimated from the difference in total count before and after lysis.

The commonly used *blood leucocyte differential* is estimated from blood smears stained with a *Romanowsky stain, which permits the blood leucocyte types to be differentiated into broad categories: neutrophil; eosino- phil and basophil granulocytes; lymphocytes; and monocytes. Blood smears are systematically screened under the light microscope while the number in each category is counted and recorded as a fraction of the total leucocyte number. Automated methods are also available.

Blood cell counts have major clinical and diagnostic significance, indicating loss, destruction, or underproduction of cells (e.g. in *anaemia or *leucopenia), an unusual demand for cells as in *leucocytosis, or neoplastic proliferation as in leukosis. Particular types of pathogenic organism tend to stimulate production of particular cell types. For instance, pyogenic cocci bacteria stimulate neutrophilia, parasitic worms and hypersensitive responses are associated with eosinophilia, and organisms causing chronic inflammation stimulate monocytosis (*see* leucocytosis).

cell culture (tissue culture) The technique of growing animal cells in culture. Cells can be grown either in suspension or attached to a surface (glass or plastic); in either case a sterile complex growth medium containing vitamins, amino acids, and serum must be supplied. Cells isolated from an organ by limited *proteolysis with trypsin will generally not multiply or do so for only a short time – these are termed *primary cultures*; following a rare event, which is not understood, certain cells can adapt to become established cell lines (e.g. Hela cells). Such cell lines are widely used for fundamental studies in biochemistry, cell biology, genetics, and virology, and for routine drug-testing, clinical virology, and other disciplines.

cell division Reproduction of cells by division first of the chromosomes (karyokinesis) and then of the cytoplasm (cytokinesis). Cell division to produce more body (somatic) cells is by *mitosis; cell division during the formation of gametes is by *meiosis.

cell fusion The process by which the cell *membranes of two animal cells join to form a single cell with two different nuclei (*heterokaryon*). Such fusion is facilitated by the use of inactivated viruses (e.g. Sendai virus) and is an essential stage in the production of *monoclonal antibodies.

cell-mediated immunity Immune responses resulting from cellular activity without the mediation of *antibody (*see* immunity).

cellulitis Inflammation of the soft tissues of the body, particularly soft connective tissues beneath the skin. A common cause is contaminated needles, which introduce infective material to inoculation sites. This is especially a problem during routine mass vaccination where a needle may be reused many times. Similarly, penetrating wounds may lead to spreading infection and inflammation in the surrounding soft tissues. Clinical signs include swelling and pain at the site of infection coupled with fever and toxaemia. Antibiotic therapy may be needed. A specific and fatal form of cellulitis in cattle is *blackleg, caused by the bacterium *Clostridium chauvoei* and characterized by widespread inflammation and destruction of muscles.

cellulose The most abundant plant *polysaccharide, comprising long chains of *glucose residues joined by 1:4β glycosidic bonds. It is digested by the cellulase enzymes secreted by microorganisms present in the gut of most animals, especially herbivores. Cellulose constitutes the bulk of *dietary fibre.

cementum One of the tissues of a *tooth, similar in structure to compact *bone. In brachydont teeth it forms the outer layer of the root and is anchored to the socket by the periodontal membrane. In hypsodont teeth it also covers the outer surface of the enamel in the crown.

-centesis *Suffix denoting* puncture or perforation.

centi- *Prefix denoting* one hundredth or a hundred.

central nervous system (CNS) That part of the nervous system lying in the midline of the body and consisting of the *brain and *spinal cord. The CNS is responsible for integration of nervous activity and for conscious perception of sensations and voluntary control of motor activity. *Compare* peripheral nervous system.

centre (in neurology) A collection of neurones (nerve cells) whose activities control a particular function. The *respiratory* and *cardiovascular centres*, for example, are regions in the *brainstem that control the movements of respiration and the functioning of the circulatory system, respectively.

centri- *Prefix denoting* centre. Example: *centrilobular* (in the centre of a lobule (especially of the liver)).

centric fusion A type of chromosomal *translocation in which two chromosomes, each with their centromere at one end, become fused to give a single chromosome with a centromere towards the middle. *See also* Robertsonian translocation.

centrifugal Moving away from a centre, as from the brain to the peripheral tissues.

centrifuge A device for separating components of different densities in a liquid, using centrifugal force. The liquid is placed in special containers

centriole

that are spun at high speed around a central axis.

centriole A small particle found in the cytoplasm of cells, near the nucleus. Centrioles are involved in the formation of the *spindle during cell division. During interphase there are usually two centrioles in the *centrosome; when cell division occurs these separate and move to opposite sides of the nucleus, and the spindle is formed between them.

centripetal Moving towards a centre, as from the peripheral tissues to the brain.

centromere (kinetochore) The part of a chromosome that joins the two *chromatids to each other and becomes attached to the spindle during *mitosis and *meiosis. When chromosome division takes place the centromeres split longitudinally.

centrosome (centrosphere) An area of clear cytoplasm, found next to the nucleus in nondividing cells, that contains the *centrioles.

centrosphere 1. An area of clear cytoplasm seen in dividing cells around the poles of the spindle. **2.** *See* centrosome.

centrum (*pl.* **centra**) The mid-line primary ossification centre of a *vertebra. It contributes most of the body of the vertebra.

cephal- (cephalo-) *Prefix denoting* the head.

cephalic Of or relating to the head.

cephalosporin Any of a group of beta-lactam antibiotics having a broad spectrum of activity against Gram-positive and Gram-negative bacteria. They were first isolated from *Cephalosporium* moulds, but semisyn-

thetic cephalosporins are now available. Like the penicillins, they inhibit the formation of cross-linkages in the bacterial cell wall, but can also kill penicillin-resistant *Staphylococcus* bacteria that produce the enzyme beta-lactamase.

cercaria (*pl.* **cercariae**) The final larval stage in the life cycle of a *fluke. It develops from the *redia larva in the intermediate host (usually a snail) and resembles the adult, but possesses a tail for locomotion. When mature it leaves the intermediate host and encysts (as a *metacercaria*) on vegetation, developing into an adult when it is swallowed by the primary host. Alternatively it may enter a second intermediate host and encyst until eaten; many types of cercaria penetrate the final host directly through the skin. *See also* miracidium; sporocyst.

cerebellum One of the principal structures of the *brain, situated behind the cerebral hemispheres and above the pons and medulla oblongata (see illustration at brain). It is connected by the rostral, middle, and caudal cerebellar peduncles to the midbrain, pons, and medulla respectively. The cerebellum consists of two lateral hemispheres and a middle region (vermis). The outer layer (cortex) is folded into *folia*, separated by intervening sulci. Within lies white matter, embedded in which are the paired cerebellar nuclei: dentate, interpositus, and fastigial.

The cerebellum maintains muscle tone, balance, and the synchronization of groups of muscles under voluntary control to give smooth coordinated movements. However, initiation of movement is done by the *cerebral cortex.

cerebr- (cerebri-, cerebro-) *Prefix denoting* the cerebrum or brain.

cerebral cortex The outer layer of *grey matter of the *cerebral hemispheres in the brain. Its surface area is greatly increased by being folded into *gyri, demarcated by intervening *sulci (see illustration at brain). Most of the cerebral cortex comprises 6 layers, numbered from the surface inwards. The *pyramidal cells are large cells in layers 3 and 5 and the axons of some of these descend to the spinal cord in the *pyramidal tracts*. Different areas of the cortex are associated with different functions. These areas can be categorized as: *projection areas*, which include the primary motor area responsible for the initiation of muscular activity, the primary somatic sensory area for the perception of the general sensations, and the visual and auditory areas responsible for sight and hearing; *olfactory areas* which receive input from centres in the *rhinencephalon; and *association areas* responsible for collecting and evaluating information, comparing it with previous experience, and selecting a response. The association areas are best developed in the most advanced mammals, notably humans.

cerebral haemorrhage Bleeding from a cerebral artery into the tissue of the brain. It is relatively rare in animals; small haemorrhages are said to occur in cows at parturition but may not produce clinical signs. Brain damage with fatal haemorrhaging may occur in the newborn at birth.

cerebral hemisphere One of the pair of structures in the brain that comprise the *cerebrum. Their size is greatest in the most advanced mammals, notably in humans. Each hemisphere is somewhat C-shaped and contains fluid-filled *ventricles. Anatomically it can be divided into frontal, parietal, temporal, and occipital lobes, which correspond in general to the overlying bones of the skull. The outer layer is the *cerebral cortex of grey matter; within and continous with it is the *white matter. Embedded in this lie the *basal ganglia.

cerebrocortical necrosis (CCN; polioencephalomalacia) A disease of cattle and sheep caused by thiamin (*vitamin B_1) deficiency brought about by microbial breakdown of the vitamin in the rumen. The disease is sporadic and occurs throughout the world. In **cattle** it is most common in calves aged about 6 months. There is sudden onset with blindness, muscle tremor, downward arching of the cervical spine (*opisthotonus), and head pressing. As the disease progresses the animal goes down and displays rapid involuntary movements of the eyes (nystagmus) and convulsions. In **sheep** the disease occurs most commonly in animals aged between 2 and 4 months. The signs are similar to those seen in cattle. The usual treatment is large doses of thiamine given by injection. However, treatment is not particularly effective and mortality rates can be up to 90%.

cerebroside One of a group of compounds occurring in the *myelin sheaths of nerve fibres. They are *glycolipids, containing *sphingosine, a fatty acid, and a sugar (usually galactose or glucose).

cerebrospinal fluid (CSF) The clear watery fluid that surrounds the brain and spinal cord. It is contained in the *subarachnoid space and circulates in the *ventricles of the brain and in the central canal of the spinal cord. The brain floats in the fluid and is cushioned by it from contact with the skull when the head is moved vigorously. The CSF is secreted by the *choroid plexuses in the ventricles, circulates through them to reach the subarachnoid space, and is eventually absorbed into the bloodstream through the *arachnoid villi. Its normal contents are glucose, salts, enzymes, and a few white cells, but no red blood cells.

cerebrum (telencephalon) One of the principal structures of the brain consisting of the paired *cerebral hemispheres and their interconnecting structures, largest of which is the *corpus callosum. The longitudinal cerebral fissure lies between the hemispheres and the transverse cerebral fissure separates them from the cerebellum and the forward part of the brainstem. Some of its more primitive parts constitute the *rhinencephalon.

ceruminous gland tumour A benign or malignant tumour of the ceruminous glands – modified sweat glands that secrete earwax. These tumours occur in the external acoustic meatus of the ear, especially in the cat, where more than half of such lesions are malignant, and in older dogs. They are found in the deeper part of the external canal and are usually less than 1 cm in diameter, pinkish, and dome-shaped. Ulceration with secondary infection is common. The growths are not encapsulated and infiltrate adjacent tissues by forming acinar or papillary structures containing hyaline secretion. Even well-differentiated benign tumours are liable to recur after excision. *Carcinomas are less well-differentiated, locally infiltrative, and inclined to metastasize to local lymph nodes.

cervical 1. Of or relating to the neck. **2.** Of, relating to, or affecting the cervix (neck region) of an organ, especially the cervix of the uterus.

cervicitis Inflammation of the *cervix; it is often accompanied, to a greater or lesser extent, by *metritis (inflammation of the uterus) and *vaginitis (inflammation of the vagina). Cervicitis may impede the entry of spermatozoa to the uterus and so prevent successful insemination. The condition is thus a potential cause of *infertility and therapy, for example using antibiotic pessaries, may be indicated.

cervix The neck or narrow part of an organ, such as the cervix of the *uterus.

cestode *See* tapeworm.

cetrimide *See* cationic detergent.

Chagas disease (American human trypanosomiasis) A disease of humans in South and Central America caused by the protozoan parasite *Trypanosoma cruzi*. This organism infects many wild and domestic mammals but rarely causes disease in these animals, although dogs may occasionally be affected. Its veterinary significance is primarily as a *zoonosis since *T. cruzi* is transmitted from these animals to humans by blood-sucking reduviid bugs. There is no satisfactory treatment and control depends on eradication of the vector bugs. *See also* trypanosomiasis.

chalaza (*pl.* **chalazae**) Any of the twisted strands of albumen in a bird's egg formed during rotation in the oviduct. They lie in the long axis of the egg at either end.

chalazion Swelling of the eyelid due to distension of a sebaceous gland. This is a consequence of inflammation following blockage of the gland's duct. Sometimes it irritates the surface of the eyeball and causes *conjunctivitis, especially if the swelling distorts the eyelid causing an eyelash to turn inwards. Minor surgical intervention with curettage of the gland may be indicated.

Charlier shoe A lightweight shoe fitted to horses that are turned out to grass. The shoe is sunk into the wall of the hoof, the frog is in contact with the ground, and no clips are used. Very skilful fitting is needed.

charlock poisoning *See* brassica poisoning.

chastek paralysis A nutritional disorder occurring in farmed foxes and mink and involving secondary *vitamin B$_1$ (thiamine) deficiency. It arises when animals are fed diets composed largely of raw fish containing the enzyme thiaminase, which destroys the vitamin. Affected animals lose their appetite, show a fall in body weight, and, after paralysis and convulsions, eventually die. The problem resolves if the fish is cooked at 83°C for 5 minutes to destroy the enzyme, or if the raw fish is fed only on alternate days. Subcutaneous injections of 50 mg thiamine hydrochloride promote rapid recovery.

check ligament (accessory ligament) One of three fibrous bands attaching the tendons of the flexor muscles of the digits to parts of the skeleton in the horse. In the forelimb the *superior check ligament* attaches to the superficial digital flexor tendon, and the *inferior check ligament* attaches to the deep digital flexor tendon. In the hindlimb the *check ligament* attaches to the deep digital flexor tendon. They assist in maintaining the extended position of the limbs during standing.

cheil- (cheilo-) *Prefix denoting* the lip(s).

chelating agent A substance that reacts with metal ions to form a ring-shaped molecular complex (*chelate*) in which the metal is held at two or more points. These agents are used in the treatment of heavy-metal poisoning in animals, and include disodium edetate and calcium disodium edetate (*see* EDTA). The calcium or sodium

is displaced by the heavy metal, which is thereby inactivated.

chem- (chemo-) *Prefix denoting* chemical or chemistry.

chemodectoma A tumour arising in chemoreceptor organs, most frequently the aortic and carotid bodies. Older dogs are affected, especially brachycephalic breeds, such as Pekingese. *Aortic body tumour* (or *heart base tumour*) arises at the base of the heart between the aorta and pulmonary artery; *carotid body tumour* occurs at the bifurcation of the common carotid artery in the cranial cervical region. Chemoreceptor tumours are uncommon and are not actively secretory, affecting the animal as a space-occupying lesion or by local infiltration of essential tissue; metastasis to other organs may occur. They are highly vascular tumours and, because of their anatomical situation and intimate connection with blood vessels, are difficult, if not impossible, to remove surgically.

chemoreceptor A cell or group of cells that responds to the presence of specific chemical compounds and initiates nervous impulses. Chemoreceptors include the taste buds of the mouth, the olfactory cells in the nasal mucosa, and the aortic and carotid bodies, which detect changes in the oxygen concentration in the blood.

chemosis Swelling (oedema) of the *conjunctiva. It commonly accompanies *conjunctivitis but is most apparent following insect bites and local allergic reactions. Foreign bodies irritating the eyeball may also be involved. Treatment entails removal of the cause and, if necessary, topical application of *corticosteroids.

chemotherapy The control or treatment of disease by using drugs. The term may refer in a restricted sense to the use of cytotoxic drugs to control various malignant diseases, particularly in cats and dogs. Those used most commonly in dogs include cyclophosphamide, chlorambucil, prednisolone, and vincristine. Most success has been achieved in controlling lymphoid tumours, such as *lymphosarcoma and *leukaemias. However, such treatment is rarely curative and the side-effects may be severe.

cherry laurel poisoning A toxic condition arising from the ingestion of leaves of the cherry laurel, *Prunus laurocerasus*. The leaves contain cyanogenetic glucoside, which is broken down by enzymes in the rumen to produce hydrocyanic acid and cause *cyanide poisoning. The animal staggers and falls, convulsions occur, and death follows rapidly as haemoglobin is converted to cyanohaemoglobin with consequent tissue anoxia. Treatment must be rapid to be successful and consists of the intravenous administration of a solution of sodium nitrite followed by sodium thiosulphate.

Other wild and cultivated trees belonging to the genus *Prunus* include the apricot, peach, Southern mock orange, bitter almond, and various cherries. A clinical condition similar to the above may result from ingestion of the foliage. *See also* Kalmia poisoning.

chestnut The mass of horn on the medial surfaces of the forearm and tarsus in the horse.

Cheyletiella A genus of *mites that are obligate ectoparasites of animals, living on the skin surface and feeding on tissue fluid by means of their biting mouthparts. They are visible to the naked eye (0.8 mm), dorsoventrally flattened, and active. Several species are parasitic on dogs, cats,

and rabbits, producing intense pruritus and exfoliative dermatitis, primarily on dorsal parts of the body. Some animals may not show a marked reaction and act as carriers. Humans may develop a papular urticaria of the arms and trunk when in contact with an infested animal, though the mite does not survive long on humans; repeated scratching may perpetuate pruritus. Diagnosis is by close examination of the pelage, with the examination of brushings and combings under a microscope. Skin 'debris' from infested animals is seen to move, hence the description *walking dandruff*. Treatment is by bathing the infested animal with a suitable *acaricide, which should be repeated 5 days later. All animals in contact with the patient should be dressed and bedding destroyed. Humans in contact with affected animals should change their clothing and bedding. The mites do not survive for more than a few days off their natural hosts.

Cheyne-Stokes respiration Abnormal respiration involving alternating cycles of deep and shallow breathing. It occurs when the sensitivity of the respiratory centres in the brain is impaired, and is common in advanced renal or cardiac disease, or with certain brain tumours. It is usually a terminal event indicating impending death.

chiasma (*pl.* **chiasmata**) 1. (in genetics) The point at which homologous chromosomes remain in contact after they have started to separate in the first division of *meiosis. Chiasmata occur from the end of prophase to anaphase and represent the point at which mutual exchange of genetic material takes place (*see* crossing over). 2. *See* optic chiasma.

chick oedema *See* toxic fat syndrome.

chimera An organism composed of tissues that are genetically different. This may arise as a result of somatic mutation, i.e. mutation of a tissue cell of the developing embryo (*see* mosaicism). More significant, especially in livestock, is a chimera containing cells derived from two different *zygotes. This usually arises because of fusion between placentas during pregnancy and subsequent *anastomosis of the foetal blood circulations. This fusion leads to the chimeric offspring sharing the same cellularly determined characteristics, such as blood types. In many organisms, especially cattle, chimeras between male and female embryos showing external female characteristics are sterile because the production of male determinants by the male cells inhibits development of the *paramesonephric ducts. Such so-called *freemartins occur in cattle, sheep, goats, and pigs. The male, which is also a chimera of male and female cells, is apparently not affected. Chimeras of sheep and goat have been produced experimentally by fusion of zygotes and subsequent implantation in one of the species. These show a mixture of the characteristics of the two species.

Chlamydia A genus of spherical microorganisms that are regarded as Gram-negative *bacteria and that undergo stages of development within host cells. They are widely distributed in nature and can cause disease in animals and humans. The invading rigid-walled infectious form (*elementary body*) is transformed into a larger thin-walled noninfectious form (*initial body*) that divides by binary fission. The large forms then condense to become elementary bodies, which can survive extracellularly and are capable of infecting other cells. Unlike the *rickettsiae the chlamydias do not require arthropod vectors for transmission. *C. trachomatis* is a parasite of humans, causing trachoma, lym-

phogranuloma venereum, and conjunctivitis. *C. psittaci* parasitizes a wide range of hosts, principally birds, in which it causes *psittacosis, a disease that can also affect humans. The organisms are transmitted from host to host by inhalation of fine dust particles. It also causes *enzootic ovine abortion and conjunctivitis, arthritis, and pneumonia in a number of animals. *See also* ornithosis.

chlamydiosis Disease due to infection with microorganisms of the genus *Chlamydia*. *See* ornithosis, psittacosis.

chlor- (chloro-) *Prefix denoting* 1. chlorine or chlorides. 2. green.

chloral hydrate A drug that is occasionally used as an anaesthetic and sedative in farm and laboratory animals. It is dissolved in water for intravenous injection or can be given orally. Within the liver chloral is converted rapidly to trichloroethanol, which is the active compound. Induction of anaesthesia is slow, analgesia is poor, muscle relaxation is good, and there is little respiratory depression. The drug is used for anaesthesia in minor surgical procedures in horses and cattle. A large volume of solution is required, usually administered in a drip set; local anaesthetics may be needed at the surgical site to improve analgesia. Chloral hydrate has been largely superseded by tranquillizers. Chloral is also used to control vermin (*see* alphachloralose).

chloramine A organic compound that liberates chlorine in solution. It is used as a general disinfectant and surgical antiseptic.

chloramphenicol An antibiotic with a broad spectrum of activity against Gram-positive and Gram-negative bacteria and rickettsiae. It was first isolated in 1947 from the bacterium

Streptomyces venezuelae but is now produced synthetically. It is bacteriostatic, inhibiting protein synthesis in bacteria by preventing the binding of messenger-RNA to the ribosome and blocking amino-acid uptake on the growing peptide chain. Although well absorbed from the alimentary tract, it is metabolized to an inactive product by rumen microorganisms. For oral dosing chloramphenicol palmitate is used; for injection it is available as an aqueous suspension or as the more soluble chloramphenicol sodium succinate, which is absorbed better than the suspension when injected intramuscularly and can be injected intravenously.

The use of chloramphenicol in the veterinary field has been limited because of the risk of widespread resistance developing. In food-producing animals chloramphenicol should be used only in life-threatening conditions. It is used to treat *meningitis and various other infections, for example salmonellosis and *Haemophilus* pneumonias, and, being nonirritant, it is used frequently in topical preparations. The aplastic anaemias that occur in humans due to chloramphenicol toxicity are not seen in animals. However, at high doses there may be bone marrow suppression with reduced appetite. Cats and young animals lack the glucuronic acid conjugating mechanism in the liver that inactivates chloramphenicol and bone marrow suppression is more likely to occur in these animals, especially at high doses.

chlorfenvinphos *See* organophosphorus (OP) compounds.

chlorinated hydrocarbons *See* organochlorines.

chloroform (trichloromethane) A colourless volatile liquid formerly widely used as an inhalational anaesthetic. It is still occasionally adminis-

tered to horses by means of a Cox's mask. During induction of anaesthesia chloroform can sensitize the heart to catecholamines, which can lead to ventricular fibrillation and death. Also, it produces respiratory depression and fall in blood pressure. It can also cause necrosis of the liver, kidney, and heart. Chloroform is incorporated in cough mixtures and stomach drenches because of its soothing and antispasmodic properties, and is used extensively as a solvent for fats.

chlorophyll One of a group of green pigments, found in all green plants and some bacteria, that absorb light to provide energy for the synthesis of carbohydrates from carbon dioxide and water (photosynthesis). The two major chlorophylls, a and b, consist of a porphyrin/magnesium complex.

chlorpromazine *See* phenothiazines.

chlortetracycline *See* tetracyclines.

choana (*pl.* **choanae**) One of the paired openings between the *nasal cavity and the *nasopharynx.

choke (oesophageal obstruction) A condition of ruminants and horses caused by blockage of the pharynx or oesophagus with foreign material. In cattle this prevents the normal eructation of gases from the rumen. The consequent accumulation of gas distends the rumen so that it pushes the diaphragm foward, causing compression of the thoracic cavity, progressive respiratory embarrassment, and, if untreated, death. Treatment in uncomplicated cases may simply involve the use of a *probang or *stomach tube to clear the blockage. In cases where the blockage is firmly lodged, muscle relaxant drugs, endoscopy, emergency *tracheotomy, or other surgery may be required. In severe cases temporary relief may be obtained by first releasing gas from the rumen by inserting a *trocar.

choking Excessive restriction of breathing. It can result from constriction or blockage of the airways, or interference with gaseous exchange due to the intake of poisonous gases or other noxious materials. Emergency *tracheotomy may be necessary in extreme cases. *See also* choke.

chol- (chole-, cholo-) *Prefix denoting* bile. Example: *cholemesis* (vomiting of).

cholagogue A drug that increases the flow of bile into the small intestine. The drug has no action on the production of bile but increases the rate of emptying of the gall bladder. Most cholagogues are also *purgatives, for example *calomel and Epsom salts.

cholangiocellular carcinoma A rare tumour arising from the intrahepatic bile duct epithelium. It has been reported in dogs, cats, sheep, and cattle but probably occurs in all species. No breed or sex predisposition is apparent. It usually appears as a solitary primary mass, often with multiple intrahepatic secondary tumours, although multiple primary tumours also occur. Histologically, the cells form bile ducts of varying size that are lined with cuboidal or columnar cells and are often dilated or cystic and filled with mucin. The tumour infiltrates lymph vessels of the portal tracts and, sometimes, the portal vein. Metastases outside the liver frequently occur, with spread to the parietal peritoneum and diaphragm, to the hepatic and other lymph nodes, and to the lungs. Other organs may also be involved. No effective treatment is available.

cholangitis Inflammation of the bile ducts. It is most commonly caused by infestation, such as fascioliasis (liver flukes) in sheep and cattle or *Ascaris lumbricoides* in pigs. In horses cholangitis very rarely results from the spread of inflammation arising from parasitic infestation of the duodenum. The bile-duct lesions and/or the parasites themselves obstruct the bile duct causing jaundice and other signs of liver dysfunction. Treatment is to kill the parasites using appropriate *parasiticides. Cholangitis may also be caused by stones (*see* calculus) blocking the bile duct.

cholecalciferol *See* vitamin D.

cholecystitis Inflammation of the gall-bladder. It is commonly caused by parasitic infestation or irritation of the mucosa by rough-surfaced *gallstones. The lesion causes severe intermittent pain and signs of biliary obstruction, such as jaundice, may become apparent. Surgical removal of the gallstones may be indicated.

cholecystography *Radiography of the gall-bladder. A radio-opaque substance is injected into the circulation to be removed by the liver and concentrated in the bile. The outline of the gall-bladder can then be seen. The technique has been used in small animals as a guide to the position of the liver and to demonstrate biliary stasis.

cholecystokinin A protein hormone secreted by duodenal cells in response to the entrance of peptides, amino acids, fatty acids, hydrochloric acid, and food into the duodenum. It is carried via the blood to the liver where it causes contraction of the gall-bladder. In addition, increased bicarbonate and water are secreted from the pancreas (*see* pancreatic juice).

cholelithiasis 1. The formation of calculi (*see* calculus) or concretions within the gall-bladder and/or the bile duct; they are also known as *gallstones*, *biliary calculi*, or *choleliths*. There may be only one stone present or many small stones. Clinical disease is rare, with up to 75% of cases remaining asymptomatic. Many choleliths are only detected at post-mortem examination. The cause of cholelithiasis is complex and many factors have been suggested. These include infection of the biliary tract, stasis of bile flow, incomplete emptying of the gall-bladder, and saturation of bile with salts. In humans choleliths are of three types: cholesterol choleliths, seen in older patients and associated with obesity and a high-fat low-fibre diet; bilirubin choleliths, which occur in the presence of excessive amounts of unconjugated bilirubin, which is relatively insoluble; and choleliths of mixed origin. Each type has been seen in domestic animals. Clinical signs are due to irritation or obstruction of the biliary tract. They may include vomiting, anterior abdominal pain, jaundice, and passage of pale faeces. Diagnosis is made from a thorough clinical examination together with biochemical and radiographic examination. Treatment usually involves surgical removal of the calculus. Undiagnosed cholelithiasis may lead to rupture of the bile duct and bile *peritonitis. 2. Disease due to the presence of calculi within the gall-bladder and/or bile duct.

cholera 1. Any of several animal diseases. *Fowl cholera is caused by the bacterium *Pasteurella multocida*. Hog cholera is a US synonym for *swine fever. 2. (in human medicine) Asiatic cholera: an enteric disease exclusively of humans, caused by the bacterium *Vibrio cholerae*.

cholesteatoma (cholesterol granuloma) *See* choroid plexus tumour.

cholic acid *See* bile acids.

choline A water-soluble amino alcohol that is usually considered a *vitamin of the B-complex. It is an essential constituent of phosphatidylcholines (or lecithins), which are found in most plant and animal cells. Choline is also an important methyl group donor, is essential in fat metabolism, and is a constituent of the neurotransmitter acetylcholine. Choline can be synthesized in body tissues from the *essential amino acid methionine, and dietary requirements thus depend on the quantity of methionine and fat in the diet. Most foods are good sources of choline.

Choline deficiency is rare because of the compound's wide distribution. Signs of deficiency may be seen in chicks, piglets, and fish, and include poor appetite, slow growth, poor reproduction, stiffness of joints, and fatty infiltration of the liver. Choline has been implicated in the prevention of *perosis (slipped tendon) in chicks and of *splayleg (spraddle) in piglets. Sows given a methionine-deficient diet may have low conception rates and small litters. For diagnosis and treatment *see* vitamin. Other names: **vitamin B$_4$; vitamin B$_7$**.

cholinergic Describing nerve fibres that release *acetylcholine as a neurotransmitter. *Compare* adrenergic.

cholinesterase An enzyme that breaks down a choline ester into its choline and acid components. The term usually refers to *acetylcholinesterase*, which breaks down the neurotransmitter *acetylcholine into choline and acetic acid. It is found in all *cholinergic nerve junctions, where it rapidly destroys the acetylcholine released during the transmission of a nerve impulse so that subsequent impulses may pass. Other cholinesterases are found in the blood and other tissues.

chondr- (chondro-) *Prefix denoting* cartilage. Example: *chondrogenesis* (formation of).

chondroblast A cell that produces the matrix of *cartilage.

chondroclast A cell that is concerned with the absorption of cartilage.

chondrocranium The part of the foetal skull that is formed entirely of cartilage. It is subsequently replaced by bone tissue.

chondrocyte A *cartilage cell, found embedded in the matrix.

chondrodysplasia An inherited condition characterized by defective growth of cartilage in the epiphyses, articular surfaces, and cranial sites, resulting in premature closure of growth plates and therefore shortness of long bones and distorted cranial bones. Affected animals are dwarfs. The condition can be general or restricted to the extremities (*see* achondroplasia). It is seen most commonly in Dexter cattle, where the condition is due to a lethal *recessive allele; homozygous recessive individuals are *bulldog calves, which will normally be miscarried after 4–8 months of gestation. The condition is also seen in Telemark cattle in Norway and in some Hereford and Aberdeen Angus strains in North America and New Zealand. A similar chondrodysplasia of genetic origin is reported in Norwegian elkhounds and the Alaskan malamute dog.

chondrogenesis The formation of *cartilage.

chondroitin sulphate A *proteoglycan that forms an important constituent of cartilage, bone, and other connective tissues. It is composed of glucuronic acid and N-acetyl-D-galactosamine units.

chondroma A rare benign tumour of cartilage, more commonly involving flat bones than long bones. The tumours vary in size and are encapsulated, multilobular, and bluish white to milk white. They grow slowly by expansion, causing deformation of affected bones. Clinical signs are determined by the size and location of the tumour.

chondrosarcoma A relatively rare malignant tumour of cartilage arising within bone or from the periosteum. It has been reported most often in dogs, cats, and sheep; in dogs, it is inclined to affect the larger breeds in middle age, accounting for about 10% of all bone sarcomas. The common sites of occurrence are: in dogs, the ribs, pelvis, and nasal region; in cats, the scapulae, vertebrae, and limbs; and in sheep, the cartilages of the sternocostal region, the scapular cartilage, and the hip. Clinical signs vary with the site of skeletal involvement. Chondrosarcomas form large irregular masses, usually with distinct borders. In the more differentiated tumours, growth can last for months or even longer, with metastases carried in the bloodstream occurring late in the course of the condition. Attempts at local removal usually result in recurrence; however, if the lesion is on a limb, amputation may result in cure.

chord- (chordo-) *Prefix denoting* **1.** a cord. Example: *chordotomy* (surgical incision of the spinal cord). **2.** the notochord.

chorda (*pl.* **chordae**) Any cordlike structure. The *chorda tympani* is a branch of the facial nerve which passes through the tympanic cavity. It supplies the mandibular and sublingual salivary glands and carries taste sensation from the front two-thirds of the tongue. *Chordae tendineae* are fibromuscular cords which pass from the papillary muscles of the ventricles in the heart to the free edges of the cusps of the *atrioventricular valves. They maintain the competence of these valves.

chorea Involuntary jerking or twitching of the muscles due to various degenerative lesions of nerve cells. It is common in dogs with *distemper when the fever has subsided; residual brain damage is revealed as chorea.

chorion The outermost of the *foetal membranes. It is formed from the *trophoblast lined with mesoderm and becomes fused to the *allantois. It thus contributes the foetal part of the *placenta.

chorion epithelioma (choriocarcinoma) A rare tumour arising from the *trophoblast (which forms the wall of the early embryo and contributes to the placenta). It has been reported in dogs, cats, and cattle, and may develop following pregnancy or later from residual placental tissue. Solitary or multiple tumours occur in the uterus, forming large soft masses invading and projecting from the uterine wall. Necrosis and haemorrhage are common and the tumour may rupture the uterine wall to penetrate the peritoneal cavity. The tumour spreads rapidly via the blood, and prognosis is poor.

chorionic gonadotrophin A *gonadotrophin hormone, produced by cells of the placenta, that promotes the maintenance of the *corpus luteum. *Human chorionic gonadotrophin* (or *HCG*), which is produced in the placental villi of humans and some primates and is excreted in the urine, has *luteinizing-hormone-like activity when injected into mammals. It is available as a freeze-dried powder, which is reconstituted in water and

injected intravenously. In male mammals HCG is used as a diagnostic tool to detect the presence of inguinal or abdominal testicles: plasma testosterone is estimated prior to injection of HCG then 1 hour after injection; a rise in plasma testosterone indicates the presence of testicular tissue. However, in some cases abdominal testicles fail to respond. In female mammals HCG can be used to treat cystic ovaries, to induce ovulation prior to service, and to terminate oestrus in species with induced ovulation (e.g. cats and ferrets). In all species ovulation occurs 24–48 hours after treatment with HCG. Tradename: **Chorulon**.

Chorioptes A genus of *mites commonly ectoparasitic on horses, cattle, and sheep, in which it causes *chorioptic mange*. See foot mange.

chorioretinitis Inflammation of the choroid and retina of the eye. This causes blindness in domestic fowls and turkeys, giving the eyes a 'frosted-glass' appearance and a number of physical abnormalities. Young birds show show short-sightedness and wandering behaviour, which becomes quite marked by 6–7 weeks. It has no significant effect on the performance of meat birds, but egg production can be depressed in laying flocks with a relatively high incidence. The cause is thought to be unsuitable regimes of artificial light, particularly duration rather than brightness. In early life, 24-hour lighting should be avoided (*see* light requirements).

choroid The middle, vascular layer of the eyeball between the retina and sclera. It contains many blood vessels, pigment, and in some species has a specialized reflective area termed the *tapetum lucidum. *See* eye.

choroiditis Inflammation of the choroid layer of the eye. It frequently involves the adjacent iris or retina and occurs in many infectious diseases, such as canine distemper and toxoplasmosis. Blindness results if the lesion becomes extensive. Treatment is directed against the primary cause.

choroid plexus A network of blood vessels derived from those in the pia mater which projects into each of the *ventricles of the brain. It actively produces the bulk of the *cerebrospinal fluid.

choroid plexus tumour A tumour arising from the epithelium of the *choroid plexus in the lateral and fourth ventricles of the brain. The commonest types are *papillomas, seen as greyish-white to red cauliflower-like masses growing into a ventricle and compressing adjacent tissue. *Carcinomas also occur; these form a more solid growth with the cells showing anaplasia and frequent division. They tend to spread via the cerebrospinal network. Such tumours are uncommon and are reported mainly in the dog.
Cholesterol granulomas or *cholesteatomas* occur in 15–20% of old horses and are non-neoplastic space-occupying lesions. They consist of accumulations of cholesterol crystals surrounded by granulomatous tissue, which incorporates lipid and haemosiderin-containing macrophages.

Christmas disease See haemophilia.

Christmas Factor (Factor IX; F IX) A blood *coagulation factor, first identified as the missing plasma component in a human family (named Christmas) displaying a sex-linked inherited haemorrhagic disorder. A glycoprotein with a molecular weight of around 56 000 daltons, it is an activator of Factor X and is synthesized in the liver; the final step of its synthesis requires the presence of *vitamin K. In humans, a number of

nonfunctional molecular variants are known, which confer symptoms indistinguishable from the true deficiency. Haemorrhagic conditions associated with Factor IX deficiency or nonfunction are known as Christmas disease or haemophilia B (*see* haemophilia). The disorder has been described in cairn terriers, black-and-tan coonhounds, and St Bernard dogs.

chrom- (chromo-) *Prefix denoting* colour or pigment.

chromaffin Describing cells containing granules that stain brown with chromates. Chromaffin cells occur particularly in the medulla of the *adrenal gland and are of neural crest origin. Adrenaline and noradrenaline are released from the granules when the adrenal gland is stimulated by its sympathetic nerve supply.

-chromasia *Suffix denoting* staining or pigmentation.

chromat- (chromato-) *Prefix denoting* colour or pigmentation.

chromatid One of the two threadlike strands formed by longitudinal division of a chromosome during *mitosis and *meiosis. They remain attached at the *centromere. Chromatids can be seen between early prophase and metaphase in mitosis and between diplotene and the second metaphase of meiosis, after which they divide at the centromere to form daughter chromosomes.

chromatin The material of a cell nucleus that stains with basic dyes and consists of DNA and protein: the substance of which the chromosomes are made. *See* euchromatin; heterochromatin.

chromatography Any of various techniques for separating the components of a mixture by selective adsorption or absorption, for example to separate mixtures of amino acids. In *paper chromatography*, a spot of the mixture to be investigated is placed near one edge of an absorbent paper sheet. The sheet is suspended vertically in a solvent, which rises through the paper by capillary action carrying the components with it. The components move at different rates, partly because they absorb to different extents on the paper. The paper is removed and dried, and the different components form a line of spots along the paper. In *column chromatography* the components are added to a vertical column of adsorbing material (e.g. alumina), in which they are adsorbed to different extents. Solvent is poured through the column, washing out the components at different rates. The components are thereby separated into successive fractions of the solvent, which is collected from the base of the column. *Gel filtration* is a form of column chromatography in which the column contains a gel and through which molecules are separated on the basis of their size. It is used for separating proteins and other polymers.

Gas chromatography is a technique for separating or analysing mixtures of gases or volatile liquids. In *gas-solid chromatography* the components are separated by passing through a tube containing a solid, such as kieselguhr; in *gas-liquid chromatography* the components are separated by a nonvolatile liquid, such as a hydrocarbon oil coated on a solid support. The components are detected as they leave the column, and can be identified by the time they take to pass through the column.

chromatolysis The dispersal or disintegration of the microscopic structures within the nerve cells that normally produce proteins. It is part of the cell's response to injury.

chromatophore A large pigmented cell with many processes occurring in the dermis, uterine caruncles (in sheep), meninges, choroid, and iris.

chromium A metallic element that is probably required in the diet in minute quantities (*see* essential element).

Chromobacterium A genus of motile rod-shaped Gram-negative *bacteria having flagella on the sides and at either end (bipolar). They have a tendency for bipolar staining and usually produce a pigment, *violaceum*. Chromobacteria are widespread in water and soil but only one species is pathogenic – *Chr. violaceum*, which can cause septicaemia or pyaemia in humans and other animals.

Chromosome numbers in various species

Species	Diploid (2n) number
Cat	38
Cattle (*Bos taurus*)	60
Dog	78
Duck	80
Fowl	78
Fox	38
Goat	60
Guinea pig	64
Horse	64
Mink	30
Mouse	40
Pig	38
Rabbit	44
Rat	42
Sheep	54
Turkey	82

chromosome One of the threadlike structures in a cell nucleus that carry the genetic information in the form of *genes. It is composed of a long double filament of *DNA coiled into a helix together with associated proteins, with the genes arranged in a linear manner along its length. It stains deeply with basic dyes during cell division (*see* meiosis; mitosis). The nucleus of each somatic (body) cell in animals contains the full (diploid) number of paired chromosomes, each pair comprising one chromosome of maternal origin and one of paternal origin. Each chromosome can duplicate an exact copy of itself between each cell division (*see* interphase) so that each new cell formed receives a full set of chromosomes. Each sex cell (gamete), formed as a result of meiosis, contains the half (haploid) number of chromosomes. The number of chromosomes present is characteristic of the species (see table).

chronic Describing a long-standing disease or lesion. Chronic disease may follow an initial acute onset, especially where the original cause remains unresolved, or it may develop gradually. *Compare* acute.

chronic obstructive pulmonary disease (COPD) *See* broken wind.

chronic respiratory disease in poultry (CRD) *See* avian mycoplasmosis.

chronotropic Describing the rate and rhythm of heart contractions. A positive chronotropic effect is where the heart rate increases, a negative effect is the opposite.

Chrysops A genus of bloodsucking *flies, commonly known as deer flies or gadflies (*see* gadfly).

chyle The lymph that occurs in the *lacteals following fat absorption from the small intestine. It subsequently flows to larger lymph vessels, then to the cisterna chyli, and then via the thoracic duct to the venous system. The majority (80–90%) of fat absorbed is carried in the chyle as chylomicrons, which are formed within the endoplasmic reticulum of the epithelial cells and are transported out of the cells and pass into the lacteals, which are more permeable to large molecules than the capillaries.

chylomicron A minute fat droplet (approximate diameter 10 μm) and the main form in which absorbed dietary fat occurs in *chyle and blood.

chylothorax A rare condition in which *chyle leaks from a ruptured thoracic lymph duct into the thoracic cavity. If sufficient fluid accumulates the condition may impair breathing by restricting lung capacity. Aspiration of the fluid can give temporary relief.

chyme The semifluid or paste-like contents of the stomach and small intestine, consisting of ingested food well mixed with digestive secretions. It is acidic on leaving the stomach but is neutralized by *bile, *pancreatic juice, and intestinal secretions. It rapidly becomes isosmotic with plasma by the addition or subtraction of water.

chymotrypsin A digestive enzyme that contributes to the degradation of dietary protein in the small intestine. It is derived from the inactive precursor (proenzyme) chymotrypsinogen, which is secreted by the pancreas as a constituent of pancreatic juice. Chymotrypsin hydrolyses peptide bonds on the carboxyl side of aromatic amino acids.

chymotrypsinogen *See* chymotrypsin.

cicatrix A scar: any mark left after the healing of a wound, where the damaged tissues fail to repair themselves completely and are replaced by connective tissue.

-cide

-cide *Suffix denoting* killer or killing. Example: *bactericide* (of bacteria).

ciliary body The part of the middle layer of the *eye that connects the choroid with the iris. It bears an array of *ciliary processes*, which project into the posterior chamber and attach to the zonular fibres of the lens; they also produce *aqueous humour. Smooth muscle fibres in the ciliary body constitute the *ciliary muscle*, which controls the focusing of the lens by altering the tension in the suspensory ligament (*see* accommodation).

ciliary body tumour Any tumour affecting the ciliary body or iris in the eye. They are rare in domestic animals, occurring as *adenomas (benign) or adenocarcinomas (malignant). Ranging from tiny nodules to large masses, they are usually firm in consistency and white to greyish-black in colour, depending on the content of pigmented cells. Adenomas are well differentiated and often resemble the ciliary processes. Adenocarcinomas show greater variation of form, increased cell division, and are locally invasive. Since the tumours rarely metastasize, enucleation involving surgical removal of the eyeball is the treatment of choice for both forms.

ciliate A protozoan of the phylum Ciliophora. They are characterized by having hair-like motile cilia on their cell surface that serve as locomotory organelles. There are two nuclei, a macronucleus and a micronucleus, and a primitive mouth (cytostome). Of the 7200 named species, some 2500 are parasitic, most of which live in the *rumen or large intestine of grazing animals. They are probably harmless commensals and, especially in the rumen, may be beneficial by keeping the rumen bacteria in check and providing a highly digestible form of protein for the host. Never-theless, animals without gut ciliates thrive perfectly well. The only ciliate of pathogenic importance is *Balantidium coli*.

cilium (*pl.* **cilia**) **1.** A hairlike process, large numbers of which are found on certain epithelial cells and on certain (ciliate) protozoa. Cilia are particularly characteristic of an epithelium where movement exists over its surface, for example the upper respiratory tract, where their beating serves to remove particles of dust and other foreign material. **2.** An eyelash or eyelid.

cimetidine An *antihistamine that blocks gastric acid secretion and is used in the treatment of gastric ulcers, uraemic gastritis, duodenal ulcers, and gastro-oesophageal reflux. It acts as a reversible competitive antagonist of histamine at H_2 receptors, with no effect on H_1 receptors. Usually given orally, cimetidine is absorbed rapidly, has a half-life of 2–3 hours, and is eliminated through the kidneys. Side-effects are rare, although cimetidine acts on liver microsomal enzymes, reducing the rate of metabolism of other drugs and reducing hepatic blood flow. Tradename: **Tagamet.**

cingulum (*pl.* **cingula**) A long bundle of nerve fibres concerned with association and lying within the cingulate gyrus of each cerebral hemisphere (*see* cerebral cortex).

circling disease A clinical form of *listeriosis (*Listeria monocytogenes* infection) occurring in cattle and sheep. Usually fatal, it is characterized by circling movements and other nervous signs, including unilateral facial paralysis, swallowing difficulties, blindness, and head pressing, which result from *meningoencephalitis. Penicillin and ampicillin can be effective if treatment is prompt.

circulatory system *See* cardiovascular system.

circum- *Prefix denoting* around; surrounding. Example: *circumanal* (surrounding the anus).

cirrhosis A condition in which fibrous tissue is produced by the liver in response to the injury or death of liver cells. The affected liver is enlarged and may have a 'hobnailed' appearance due to nodules of regenerating liver cells between the fibrous strands. Cirrhosis is a common sequel to *hepatitis, whether caused by infectious agents, parasites (e.g. liver flukes), poisons (e.g. carbon tetrachloride), or poisonous plants (e.g. ragwort). It also occurs as a result of long-standing obstruction of the bile ducts. Complications include *portal hypertension and *ascites. Healing of the lesions and restoration of liver function may occur if the primary cause is removed.

cisterna (*pl.* **cisternae**) An enlarged space. **1.** Cisternae occur in the *subarachnoid space and act as reservoirs for cerebrospinal fluid. The largest is the *cerebellomedullary cisterna* (*cisterna magna*) in the rear of the brain, from where cerebrospinal fluid can be sampled. **2.** The *cisterna chyli* is situated between the crura of the diaphragm. It receives lymph from abdominal viscera and the hindlimbs and gives rise to the thoracic duct.

cistron The section of a DNA or RNA chain that controls the amino-acid sequence of a single polypeptide chain in protein synthesis. A cistron can be regarded as the functional equivalent of a *gene.

citric acid A tricarboxylic acid that is found in many citrus fruits and is an intermediate in the *Krebs cycle (also known as the citric acid cycle) in plant and animal cells.

citric acid cycle *See* Krebs cycle.

citrulline An *amino acid, not found in proteins but a component of the *urea cycle.

clamp A surgical instrument used to stabilize tissue or to prevent passage of material along a tubular structure, for example to prevent bleeding from a cut vessel. *Bone clamps* (e.g. Lowman bone clamps) are used during the surgical repair of fractures to stabilize the bone fragments and to hold a surgical plate in position while it is being screwed to the bone. *Bowel clamps* (e.g. Doyen or Kocher intestinal clamps) are used during surgery involving penetration of the gut. They are designed to close the lumen of the gut and prevent spillage of the gut contents without damaging the underlying gut tissue.

claustrum One of the *basal ganglia in the brain that forms a thin layer of grey matter lying lateral to the external capsule in each cerebral hemisphere.

Claviceps A genus of about 30 fungi that are parasitic upon cereals and grasses. They infect the flowering heads and replace some of the seeds or grains by hard purplish-black elongated *sclerotia (or ergots) of comparable size. Ergots contain a variable mixture of alkaloids that can cause *ergot poisoning in livestock grazing pasture or fed grain or hay containing them. Best known is *C. purpurea*, commonest on rye and wheat but also affecting a number of other cereals and pasture grasses. Other species attack major crops such as sorghum and rice. *C. paspali* includes in its host range watergrass or Dallis grass (*Paspalum dilatum*) – important as a forage crop in many parts of the world. The fungus is responsible for *paspalum staggers.

clavicle A bone that forms part of the *pectoral girdle. It is most highly developed in primates, including humans, in which it is known as the collar bone. In domestic mammals it is much reduced or even absent. In the dog it is represented by a thin bony or cartilaginous plate in the brachiocephalic muscle, and in the cat by a bony bar. In birds the clavicle is frequently a V-shaped bone, otherwise known as the furcula or wishbone, although in some species, for example the budgerigar, it is reduced to a small bony bar.

clavulanic acid A beta-lactam compound used in combination with *penicillins. It is a potent inhibitor of the beta-lactamase enzymes produced by penicillin-resistant bacteria and therefore can protect susceptible penicillins from degradation. For veterinary use clavulanic acid is combined with amoxycillin as Synulox, which has a broad spectrum of activity and resists breakdown by penicillinases.

claw The tough horny structure that covers the third phalange of each digit in birds, certain mammals, and some reptiles. The outer horny layer is a specialization of the epidermis and will continue to grow unless subjected to wear. Underlying this is the highly vascular dermis, termed the *corium*, which nourishes the outer tissue.

cleansing *See* afterbirth; retention of placenta.

clearance (renal clearance) A quantitative measure of the rate at which waste products are removed from the blood by the kidneys. It is expressed in terms of the volume of blood that could be completely cleared of a particular substance in one minute.

cleavage The process of repeated cell division of the *zygote to form a solid ball of cells (*morula). The cells (*blastomeres) do not grow in size between divisions and so progressively decrease in size.

cleft palate (palatoschisis) Incomplete closure of the *palate during embryonic development. It may be associated with *harelip. The resultant palatine fissure creates an opening from the oral to the nasal cavity. This causes suckling difficulties, with most of the milk being lost through the nose. In cattle the condition is found to be associated with *arthrogryposis or *ankylosis, particularly in the Charolais. Links with other skeletal abnormalities have been found in other cattle breeds.

clenbuterol A selective agonist for β_2 *adrenergic receptors that acts on smooth muscle in the bronchi, uterus, and skeletal muscle vasculature, causing muscle relaxation at these sites; it has no significant effects on the heart. Clenbuterol can be given orally or by intravenous or intramuscular injection. It is used in horses to relieve bronchospasm in cases of chronic obstructive pulmonary disease, producing bronchodilation, a reduction in the viscosity of bronchial secretions, reduced airway resistance, and less coughing. These effects last 6–8 hours. Clenbuterol can be used in cattle to cause uterine relaxation in cases of dystocia, or to delay the onset of parturition to allow adequate supervision. When given at the first stage of labour, *parturition is delayed by 6–8 hours; if administered during the second stage of labour, clenbuterol has a much shorter duration of action. Side-effects include sweating, muscle tremors, and weakness. Tradenames: **Planipart**; **Ventipulmin**.

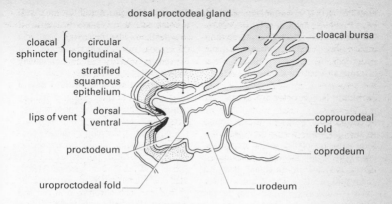

dorsal proctodeal gland

cloacal bursa

cloacal sphincter { circular / longitudinal

stratified squamous epithelium

lips of vent { dorsal / ventral

coprourodeal fold

proctodeum

coprodeum

uroproctodeal fold

urodeum

Median section of the cloaca of a four-month-old hen

clinch (clench) 1. The turned-down end of the horseshoe nail. The nail is twisted to break it, then bent over and hammered down, either straight into the outer wall of the hoof or into a previously rasped clinch bed. **2.** The act of making a clinch.

clips Projections on a horseshoe that prevent it moving on the foot. Toe clips are drawn at the toes opposite the frog to prevent the shoe moving backwards. Side clips can be used as an alternative. Quarter clips are drawn on the hind shoes, half-way between the toe and heel, to prevent sideways movement. Inner quarter clips are sometimes used as well.

clitoris The female counterpart of the *penis. It is composed of erectile tissue which becomes erect following sexual stimulation. It is attached to the ischial arch and its rounded free end or glans lies in a depression in the ventral commissure of the vulva, termed the *fossa clitoridis*. The thin skin lining the glans and fossa constitutes the prepuce of the clitoris.

cloaca 1. The common terminal portion of the digestive and urogenital tracts occurring in most adult vertebrates except placental mammals. The cloaca in developing mammalian embryos subsequently becomes subdivided so that the two tracts have separate outlets. In birds the rectum is continued posteriorly by the first portion of the cloaca, the *coprodeum*, which is partially separated by a mucosal fold from the *urodeum*, into which the ureters and genital ducts (oviduct and ductus deferens) open. The terminal portion (*proctodeum*) is separated by a further mucosal fold. In young birds it has the *cloacal bursa opening in its roof, and in males the *phallus in its floor. It opens to the exterior at the vent (see illustration). **2.** The most caudal part of the embryonic *hindgut.

cloacal bursa (bursa of Fabricius) A diverticulum situated in the roof of the proctodeum in birds (*see* cloaca). It is greatest in size in young birds and shrinks when maturity is reached. It contains much lymphoid tissue in its wall and is the source of the B (bursa) lymphocytes.

cloacitis *See* vent gleet.

clone A group of organisms that are genetically identical and derived asexually from the same *zygote. In animals, cloned individuals are usually produced by embryo splitting. *See also* monoclonal antibody.

clonidine *See* hypotensive agent.

Clonorchis A genus of *flukes found in the Far East, where they are common parasites of fish-eating mammals, especially cats, as well as humans. There are two intermediate hosts, a snail and a fish. The Chinese liver fluke (*C. sinensis*), which lives in the bile duct, pancreatic duct, and duodenum, causes the disease *clonorchiasis*; infestation is caused by eating raw fish.

clonus A short spasmodic contraction of a muscle. Clonic contractions occur in certain types of paralysis and often involve the muscles of an entire limb. For example, spinal lesions may interrupt the central control of reflex movements so that stimulation of a limb triggers a series of involuntary clonic flexions and extensions. Clonic convulsions involve a rhythmic 'paddling' motion in which muscle contraction alternates with relaxation.

clopidol *See* coccidiostat.

cloprostenol *See* prostaglandin.

clostridial enteritis *See* enterotoxaemia.

clostridial haemorrhagic enteritis A necrotizing and usually fatal enteritis typically affecting baby pigs aged less than 1 week; it rarely occurs in piglets older than 4 weeks. The disease is caused by the bacterium *Clostridium perfringens* type C and occurs in the UK, Europe, USA, Canada, and Japan (in the USSR *Cl. perfringens* type B is associated).

There is a high mortality rate, with the peracute form of the disease causing death on the first or second day of life. Affected piglets may have a *dysentery and are usually extremely weak, collapse, and die. The acute form causes death on the third day of life, with a haemorrhagic diarrhoea containing shreds of necrotic mucosa. Persistent, variably haemorrhagic (bloody) or pale-yellow faeces containing necrotic debris characterizes the subacute form; piglets are initially active and alert but become emaciated and dehydrated, succumbing at 5–7 days. The chronic form is less common but affected piglets show intermittent or more persistent mucoid yellow diarrhoea, whilst remaining lively for a week or so. After 10 days growth is retarded and the piglets fail to gain weight normally.

Lesions in affected piglets are found in the small intestine, particularly the jejunum, although the caecum and spiral colon may be involved. Treatment of affected piglets is usually ineffective. Prophylaxis in problem units may be helpful – neonates can be given antitoxin, and appropriate toxoid may be given to actively immunize sows during breeding or gestation.

clostridial myositis *See* gas gangrene (def. 2).

Clostridium A genus of anaerobic or microaerophilic rod-shaped *bacteria, widely distributed in nature. They produce spores, which are usually wider than the bacillus. The position and size of the spores are useful for classifying clostridia, and the spores are very resistant to physical and chemical agents. A number of species produce potent *exotoxins and are of veterinary importance. *Cl. botulinum* causes *botulism in humans and animals. It is a common soil saprophyte worldwide and botulism occurs when animals and humans consume food contaminated with preformed toxins. It also causes *limberneck in fowls and forage poisoning and *lamziekte in cattle.

Cl. perfringens (*Cl. welchi*) are thick rod-shaped capsulated bacteria whose spores are not wide enough to distort the bacillus. They are normally present in the intestinal flora but some factors, including protein-rich diets, enhance their multiplication and production of exotoxins resulting in disease. The species consists of five types – A, B, C, D, and E – depending on the various types of major lethal exotoxins they produce. Type A causes gas gangrene in humans and *yellow lamb disease. Type B is responsible for *lamb dysentery and haemorrhagic *enteritis in sheep and goats. Type C causes necrotic enteritis in lambs, piglets, calves, and chickens and *struck in sheep. Type D causes *pulpy kidney disease in lambs and adult sheep, and type E causes pulpy kidney disease in lambs and calves.

Cl. novyi (*Cl. oedematiens*) is a large anaerobic bacillus that occurs commonly in the soil. It causes necrotic hepatitis or *black disease in sheep and cattle, and a similar condition in pigs, due to toxins produced in association with liver fluke infestation (*see* fascioliasis). *Cl. chauvoei* causes *blackleg in sheep and cattle. The rods appear singly or in short chains, and the oval spores cause the rods to swell in the middle. The organism is commonly found in the soil, particularly in wet pastures. Wounds, especially those associated with docking and shearing, facilitate infection, but cattle with no obvious wounds can develop blackleg.

Cl. septicum causes *braxy in sheep. The bacteria appear as large rods, usually linked to form long chains. The organism is commonly found in the soil, and sheep become infected following wounds to the umbilical cord and the abomasum. In other animals it causes wound infections known as *malignant oedema. *Cl. tetani* is a slender rod-shaped bacterium; spores at the end of the bacillus swell giving it a drumstick appearance. It causes *tetanus in humans and animals due to three types of exotoxins: *tetanospasmin, *tetanolysin (haemolysin), and a nonspasmogenic toxin. The organism is commonly found in the soil and faeces of animals. Humans and animals get infected following deep and penetrating wounds that are quickly closed, creating anaerobic conditions favouring the production of toxins. Umbilical contamination and such practices as *castration, *docking, and shearing are common causes of infection.

clotbur *See* cocklebur poisoning.

clotting (of blood) *See* coagulation.

clotting factors *See* coagulation factors.

cloxacillin *See* penicillin.

Cnemidocoptes A genus of very small round *mites that are widespread ectoparasites of birds. *C. gallinae* is the *depluming mite, which infests the feather shafts of poultry. *C. mutans* burrows under the scales of the legs causing the condition known as *scaly leg in poultry, in which the feet and legs swell and become encrusted. *C. pilae* affects the legs, beak, and feathers of budgerigars.

CNS *See* central nervous system.

coagulation 1. Blood coagulation (blood clotting): the process by which fluid blood is converted to a gel. This takes place as a means of arresting haemorrhage from wounds in which blood vessels are severed. It is also important in other physiological activities, including the repair of wear and

Coagulation factors

Factor	Specific name(s)
Factor I	fibrinogen
Factor II	prothrombin
Factor III	tissue thromboplastin
Factor IV	ionic calcium, essential for cross-linking reactants
Factor V	proaccelerin
Factor VII	proconvertin
Factor VIII	antihaemophilic factor (this exists as at least two subunits: VIIIC, which is the clotting component, and VIIIAg, an inert carrier now known to be identical with von Willebrand's factor)
Factor IX	Christmas factor
Factor X	Stuart Prower factor
Factor XI	plasma thromboplastin antecedent
Factor XII	Hageman factor
Factor XIII	Laki-Lorand or fibrin-stabilizing factor
Factor XIV (provisional)	Fletcher factor or pre-kallikrein
Factor XV (provisional)	Fitzgerald factor, and a high-molecular-weight kininogen

tear in blood vessels, wound healing and inflammation, and the growth of new tissues. The coagulation process consists of a series of reactions involving the sequential activation of inert plasma proteins (*coagulation factors) to active enzymes. The process culminates in the conversion of *fibrinogen to *fibrin, which is cross-linked to form an insoluble matrix in which blood cells are entrapped to form a clot. These reactions also involve *platelets and calcium, and are triggered by injury to blood vessel walls.

There are two alternative initial pathways: a rapid reaction ('extrinsic pathway'), which produces a few molecules of the final enzyme (thrombin) to act upon fibrinogen. This thrombin also feeds back into a slower reaction ('intrinsic pathway') to amplify and accelerate it, so producing much larger amounts of thrombin. At one time these pathways were thought to be initiated separately but it is now recognized that there are common interfaces between the two. At least 14 coagulation factors are involved in the *coagulation cascade*, most of which are synthesized in the liver. Both pathways converge upon Factor X and thereafter the reaction follows a common route. Abnormalities in either pathway or the common phase of the reaction result in a bleeding tendency due to insufficient thrombin generation and hence inadequate conversion of fibrinogen to fibrin.

The terms 'extrinsic pathway' and 'intrinsic pathway' should now be considered obsolete, although they may still be encountered.

2. Any process in which a colloidal liquid changes to a gel.

coagulation factors (clotting factors) A collection of soluble substances (chiefly proteins) that are present in blood plasma and, under certain circumstances, act together in a predetermined sequence to cause blood *coagulation (blood clotting). Although each factor has a name, they are also referred to by Roman numerals, assigned by an international committee (see table). Four of the factors (II, VII, IX, and X) are dependent upon *vitamin K for their full expression in the liver; four (Factors I, V, VIII, and XIII) are *thrombin-dependent; four (Factors XI, XII, XIV, and XV) are known as *contact factors* and are involved with the initiation reactions following injury. Factors III and IV are not proteins but are included because of their crucial roles in the clotting process. Bleeding disorders may be caused by the lack of a particular factor (inherited or acquired), the presence of an inhibitor (e.g. heparin), or the synthesis of an abnormal molecule that is nonfunctional.

cobalt A trace element that is required in the diet, particularly ruminants' diets, for the manufacture of *vitamin B_{12}. The element is employed by gut microorganisms to manufacture the vitamin, which is subsequently absorbed by the animal. Ruminants derive all their vitamin B_{12} from the rumen microorganisms, which thus require an adequate supply of cobalt. Non-ruminants are generally supplied with the vitamin itself. **Cobalt deficiency** This is seen in ruminants grazing on cobalt-deficient pastures. True cobalt deficiency in other species is rare. Sheep are more susceptible than cattle although both species exhibit similar symptoms, namely ill-thrift, loss of appetite, anaemia, and eventual emaciation – collectively known as 'pining'. It may take several months to deplete body reserves of vitamin B_{12} before symptoms appear. The disease can be confirmed by measuring the vitamin B_{12} content of the blood. Prevention involves providing the animals with cobalt-containing *salt licks or dosing them with a slow-release cobalt 'bullet' that remains in the reticulum. Deficient pasture can be top-dressed with cobalt sulphate. Other name: **cobalt pine.**

cocaine An alkaloid derived from the leaves of the coca plant, *Erythroxylon coca*. It can be used as a local anaesthetic, but such use is greatly restricted because of its addictive properties in humans. In animals it was formerly administered topically in the eye or on mucous membranes. Due to its sympathomimetic activity it constricts small blood vessels at the site of application and causes dilation of the pupil. It may also produce clouding of the cornea and is more irritant than agents now in use.

cocarcinogen *See* carcinogen.

coccidia A group of *protozoa within the phylum *Apicomplexa that are parasitic in mammals and birds. They include a number of important pathogens, particularly in the genera *Cryptosporidium*, *Eimeria*, *Isospora*, *Toxoplasma*, and *Sarcocystis*. These are principally parasites of the intestine, in which both asexual and sexual multiplication of the parasite takes place inside host cells. Resistant oocysts are passed in the faeces of the host. One or two hosts may be involved in the life cycle. *See* coccidiosis.

coccidioidomycosis Infection by the *dimorphic fungus *Coccidioides immitis*; it is usually asymptomatic or mild to moderately severe, confined to the upper respiratory tract, and resolves within a few weeks. The infection is not contagious but is acquired by inhaling spores produced by the *mycelium in the soil of hot semi-arid areas of the southwestern USA, Mexico, Guatemala, Honduras, Argentina, Colombia, Paraguay, and

Venezuela. In these enzootic areas the infection is extremely common among humans and animals. Recovery, even from asymptomatic infection, usually confers immunity to reinfection. However, in a small proportion of cases the disease either develops into a benign chronic nodular or cavitary infection of the lung or it eventually progresses to an acute disseminated disease that may involve any tissue of the body.

Bovine coccidioidomycosis is usually reported as a few lesions found in the lungs or lymph nodes during meat inspection. Virtually the only species in which disseminated infection is seen are primates and dogs. Most affected dogs are under 2 years old, show lethargy, weight loss, and fever, with other signs depending upon the site of lesions. Serological tests are valuable in diagnosis and in monitoring the course of the disease. Diagnosis can be confirmed by microscopic observation of the characteristic large ($20-60\ \mu m$) thick-walled spherules containing *endospores ($2-5\ \mu m$) in lesions or their exudate. The organism can be grown in culture from these materials but must be handled with extreme care to avoid liberating the highly infective spores. Coccidioidomycosis is resistant to treatment: *amphotericin B is the drug most often used, but ketoconazole has the advantage of oral administration. In dogs, side-effects and relapses are common. Other names: **California disease; coccidioidal granuloma; desert fever; desert rheumatism; Posadas' disease; San Joaquin Valley disease; Valley bumps; Valley fever.**

coccidiosis An important disease of mammals and birds of worldwide distribution caused by certain protozoa (see coccidia) and characterized by infection of the intestines and diarrhoea. Protozoa of the genus *Eimeria* are by far the most important cause but occasionally other coccidia may

be responsible, e.g. *Isospora*. Coccidiosis is transmitted between animals by the ingestion of *oocysts from the environment and is therefore especially prevalent in intensively kept livestock, notably poultry. Such is the persistence of oocysts in the environment that infection is universal, but disease will only occur in certain situations when nonimmune animals are exposed to very heavy infection, as may occur, for example, in crowded unhygienic conditions. The disease may cause depression, diarrhoea (perhaps with *dysentery), poor growth, and possibly death. Infection produces a good immunity and disease is usually seen only in young animals.

In **domestic fowls** different *Eimeria* species infect different parts of the intestine. *E. tenella* causes severe haemorrhages in the caeca, while *E. necatrix* causes similar lesions in the small intestine. Both these infections can be fatal. *E. maxima* and *E. acervulina* are common infections which are rarely fatal but cause serious impairment of growth and feed conversion efficiency. All *Eimeria* species are extremely host specific – for instance, none of the species infecting fowls infect **turkeys** and vice versa. Infection is thus derived only from environmental contamination by other members of the same host species. There is no vaccine widely available and disease is prevented in broiler chickens by the continuous administration of anticoccidial drugs in feed (see coccidiostat).

Coccidiosis is also an important disease in **sheep**, causing a severe and sometimes fatal diarrhoea in 1–3-month-old lambs. *E. ovinoidalis* is the major pathogenic species. There are several other nonpathogenic species that infect lambs and cause high levels of oocysts in faeces, which may confuse diagnosis. The diarrhoea in lambs rarely contains blood. In **cattle**, the disease can occur in slightly older animals at times of stress, as well as in calves. *E. zuernii* and *E. bovis* are the major pathogenic species and they cause severe dysentery. In **pigs** and **dogs** coccidiosis is associated with *Isospora* spp. infections. In **rabbits**, coccidiosis caused by *E. stiedae* is a severe and possibly fatal condition. This species is unusual in that it infects the walls of the bile ducts in the liver. As well as diarrhoea there may be signs of liver damage, such as jaundice. In all species, outbreaks of disease may be treated with specific drugs given in drinking water or feed.

coccidiostat (anticoccidial) An agent with activity against *coccidia, used to control or prevent *coccidiosis in livestock. The most pathogenic stage in the parasite's life cycle is the second schizont stage, and the parasites must reach this stage to induce immunity in the host. Coccidiostats that kill coccidia at the first schizont stage thus do not permit immunity to be induced. The *sulphonamides were the first effective coccidiostats; the most commonly used compounds are sulphaquinoxaline and sulphadimidine. These drugs kill coccidia at the second schizont stage, thus allowing immunity to develop. The *nitrofurans have anticoccidial as well as antibacterial activity. Amprolium hydrochloride acts as an antagonist to vitamin B_1 (thiamin), which is required in high concentrations by coccidia. However, it can induce thiamin deficiency in the host. Diaveridine is a *folic-folinic acid antagonist used as an anticoccidial, often in combination with sulphonamides to give a synergistic effect – both act on the same metabolic pathway in coccidia. Diaveridine also permits immunity to develop. Ethopabate, a para-aminobenzoic acid antagonist, is used as a coccidiostat, often combined with pyrimethamine or diaveridine. It has no activity against *Eimeria tenella*. The quinolates (e.g. methyl benzoquate, decoquinate, and clopidol) are a group of anticoccidial agents that act against coccidia in epithelial cells. They are poorly absorbed after oral administration. The *ionophore group of antimicrobials, including monensin, lasalocid, and salinomycin, have anticoccidial properties, killing the parasites at an early stage in their development. They are the most commonly used coccidiostats in fattening birds.

Coccidiostats are administered in feed or in water, and various combinations of drugs are used. In fattening poultry they are given continuously until the time of slaughter; the drugs used kill coccidia at an early stage, before the parasites can affect the bird's growth rate. The development of immunity is unimportant. All coccidiostats should be withdrawn immediately before slaughter to prevent contamination of carcasses. In laying poultry and other species the coccidiostats employed should allow some development of the parasites to stimulate immunity. Alternatively, coccidiostats can be used intermittently. Long-term use can be detrimental, producing signs of toxicity, for example, poor egg-laying, tainted eggs, and vitamin deficiencies, depending on the drugs used. Coccidia can become resistant to certain drugs; changing the type of coccidiostat at regular intervals prevents outbreaks of coccidiosis due to parasite resistance. New coccidiostats are being developed constantly to counter parasite resistance.

coccobacillus (*pl.* **coccobacilli**) A bacterium that can appear rod-like (i.e. a bacillus) or spherical (i.e. a coccus), such as *Pasteurella and *Haemophilus.

coccus (*pl.* **cocci**) Any spherical bacterium, such as *Staphylococcus* and *Streptococcus*.

coccy- (coccyg-, coccygo-) *Prefix denoting* the coccyx. Example: *coccygectomy* (excision of).

coccygeal Referring to the coccyx or *tail.

coccyx *See* tail.

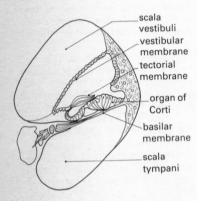

scala vestibuli
vestibular membrane
tectorial membrane
organ of Corti
basilar membrane
scala tympani

Section through a turn of the cochlea

cochlea The organ of the labyrinth of the internal *ear that is concerned with the reception and analysis of sound. It consists essentially of three tubes coiled to form a spiral, with a middle *cochlear duct* (or *scala media*) sandwiched between the *scala tympani* and *scala vestibuli* (see illustration). These latter two are filled with perilymph. The membranous cochlear duct is filled with endolymph and contains, along its length, sensory hair cells of the *spiral organ, which lie on the basilar membrane. The tips of the hairs are embedded in the overhanging *tectorial membrane*. Vibrations transmitted to the internal ear via the fenestra vestibuli are conducted by this fluid-filled system and cause the basilar membrane to vibrate. This distorts the hairs in the sensory cells, which send nerve impulses to the brain via the cochlear

division of the vestibulocochlear nerve. Different parts of the basilar membrane are sensitive to vibrations of different frequencies: the apex of the spiral is most sensitive to low frequencies, while the region nearest the middle ear is sensitive to high frequencies.

cochlear duct (scala media) *See* cochlea.

cochlear nerve *See* vestibulocochlear nerve.

cocklebur poisoning A toxic condition due to the ingestion of various annual herbaceous plants belonging to the genus *Xanthium* (cockleburs), also known as clotburs or sheep burs. They contain the toxic hydroquinone, carboxyatractyloside, which causes gastrointestinal inflammation, haemorrhagic and necrotic hepatitis, and renal tubular degeneration. The clinical signs are anorexia, vomiting, rapid weak pulse, dyspnoea, muscle spasms, convulsions, and death. Treatment is symptomatic.

codeine A *morphine derivative that is much less potent than morphine as an analgesic and as a depressant of the cough centre in the medulla. It is widely used for its antitussive properties in cough syrups, for example codeine phosphate syrup for kennel cough. Because of possible toxic signs (excitement, convulsions) it should not be used in cats.

cod-liver oil A pale-yellow fish oil that is a good source of *vitamins A and D and also unsaturated fatty acids. It was formerly widely used as a vitamin supplement and tonic in young animals, but has been largely superseded by synthetic vitamin preparations.

codominance (in genetics) The condition when both *alleles in a heterozygous organism are fully expressed. *Compare* dominant; recessive.

codon The unit of the *genetic code, consisting of three adjacent nitrogenous bases in the DNA and usually coding for a single specific amino acid.

coefficient of co-ancestry A measure of the degree of relatedness of two animals based on the probability of the transmission of a copy of the same *allele from both. The coefficient of co-ancestry of two animals is the same as the *inbreeding coefficient of their joint offspring.

-coele *Suffix denoting* **1.** a body cavity. Example: *blastocoele* (cavity of blastocyst). **2.** *See* -cele.

coeli- (coelio-) (*US* celi-, celio-) *Prefix denoting* the abdomen. Example: *coeliectasia* (abnormal distension of).

coeliac Of or relating to the abdominal region. The *coeliac artery* is a branch of the abdominal *aorta supplying the stomach, spleen, liver, and gall bladder. The coeliac plexus is the nerve plexus supplying the abdominal organs supplied by the coeliac artery.

coelom The cavity in an embryo between the two layers of mesoderm. It develops into the body cavity, becoming subdivided into pericardial, pleural and peritoneal cavities.

coenurosis Disease caused by infestation with a *coenurus, the larval stage of certain tapeworms. The clinical condition known as gid, or sturdy, in sheep, goats, and other ungulates is caused by the coenurus of *Taenia multiceps*, a tapeworm parasite of the small intestine of dogs and foxes. If sheep ingest eggs from pasture contaminated by dog faeces, these eggs hatch to release an embryo, which penetrates the wall of

the alimentary tract and is conveyed by the blood to the central nervous system, where it develops over a period of about 6 months to a coenurus measuring up to 5 cm in diameter and bearing several hundred scolices. In this form it is often referred to as *Coenurus cerebralis*.

The signs of gid depend on the site and size of the coenurus. Typically, animals with brain coenuri show disorders of gait and stance, often with turning of the head towards the affected side, walking in circles towards the same side, and showing a one-sided blindness on the opposite side. Other signs include excitement, incoordination and prostration (often associated with cerebellar coenurosis), and partial but progressive paralysis with spinal cord involvement. The coenurus may cause a local softening of the skull which, if detectable, is an aid to diagnosis. The only satisfactory treatment is surgical removal of the cyst. Since the life cycle of *T. multiceps* depends on the coenuri being eaten by dogs or foxes, control is best achieved by disposal of all sheep carcasses and remains. Routine treatment of dogs for tapeworms is also advisable. Faeces voided under the influence of anthelmintics may contain tapeworms and should be burned.

Another form of coenurosis occurs under the skin and in other connective tissues of rabbits and hares. This is caused by *T. serialis*, whose life cycle and transmission are similar to *T. multiceps*.

coenurus (*pl.* **coenuri**) The larval stage of the dog tapeworm *Taenia multiceps* (*Multiceps multiceps*). Each coenurus consists of a fluid-filled cyst containing up to 50–60 invaginated tapeworm heads. The cysts develop from eggs eaten by the intermediate host, most commonly sheep, and lodge in the central nervous system, usually the brain, where they cause the disease gid (sturdy) (*see* coenurosis). If the head of a dead infected sheep is eaten by a dog, the coenurus develops into adult tapeworms. Worming dogs regularly, burning their faeces, and disposing properly of the sheeps' heads help prevent gid. *See also* bladderworm.

coenzyme An organic molecule that is required for the action of certain *enzymes. It is an imprecise term since some (e.g. *NAD) are really *substrates while others (e.g. *coenzyme A) act by activating a relatively unreactive substrate. Many are derivatives of the *vitamin B group. *See also* cofactor.

coenzyme A (CoA) A complex organic compound that acts in conjunction with enzymes involved in various biochemical reactions, notably the oxidation of pyruvate via the *Krebs cycle and fatty-acid oxidation and synthesis. It comprises ADP (*see* ATP), the vitamin *pantothenic acid, and β-mercaptoethylamine, the latter of which provides the functionally active sulphydryl group. This activates carboxyl groups by forming a thioester ($-CO-S-$) bond.

cofactor A molecule or ion that is required for the normal catalytic action of certain *enzymes. The term is often applied to metallic ions (e.g. Mg^{2+}), which are essential or stimulatory for many enzymes, especially those using *ATP.

Coggins test *See* agar-gel immunodiffusion test.

coital exanthema *See* equine coital exanthema.

coitus (copulation) The act of sexual intercourse. In higher mammals this comprises *intromission*, i.e. insertion of the erect penis into the vagina of the female, and *ejaculation. Ejac-ulation normally occurs immediately after intromission in rams and bulls, whereas in boars more extensive thrusting movements are required to insert the tip of the penis into the folds of the cervix prior to a lengthy ejaculation of 3–5 minutes. In **birds** the *phallus is the male copulatory organ; this is small and nonprotrusible in most species, including the domestic fowl and turkey, and copulation involves the apposition of male and female vents. However, some birds, for example ducks and geese, have a protrusible penis-like phallus with a seminal groove; this is introduced into the vent of the female during coitus to aid the transfer of semen. *See also* insemination.

col- (coli-, colo-) *Prefix denoting* the colon. Example: *coloptosis* (prolapse of).

colchicine An alkaloid, obtained from the autumn crocus, *Colchicum autumnale*, that has antimitotic properties. It acts as an anti-inflammatory agent in gout arthritis and may occasionally be used in cancer therapy. Colchicine binds to microtubular proteins within cells causing disruption of the mitotic spindle and microtubular structures. Apart from interfering with cell division, this prevents the release of histamine-containing granules from mast cells, inhibits insulin secretion from pancreatic cells, and inhibits the movement of melanin granules in melanophores. Colchicine can be used, albeit rarely, in combination with other drugs (e.g. cyclophosphamide, vincristine, and prednisolone) in cancer therapy. It is absorbed rapidly after oral administration and excreted via the bile into the faeces. Side-effects include disruption of the epithelial lining of the gastrointestinal tract leading to vomiting and diarrhoea, nephrotoxicity, central nervous system depression, and blood dyscrasias.

colchicum poisoning A toxic condition due to the ingestion of the meadow saffron, *Colchicum autumnale*, also known as the autumn crocus. All parts of the plant contain the alkaloid colchicine, a gastrointestinal irritant, which is not destroyed by hay making. Absorption and excretion of colchicine are slow so that the onset of clinical signs is often delayed in animals grazing pastures containing the plant. Treatment is of the clinical signs.

cold cow syndrome An obscure condition of dairy cows, recently observed in southwestern parts of the UK. Outbreaks occur in which the cows become lethargic, lack appetite, suffer diarrhoea, and show a decline in milk yield. Affected animals commonly feel cold to the touch. Clinical signs disappear and milk yield returns to normal in a few days. The cause remains unknown. No consistent metabolic abnormalities have been detected though high concentrations of certain soluble carbohydrates in lush pasture may be important.

colibacillosis Any disease caused by strains of the bacterium *Escherichia coli*. The principal forms of colibacillosis are diarrhoea of newborn or young animals (*enteric colibacillosis of calves, *enteric colibacillosis of piglets, *enteric colibacillosis of lambs), *oedema disease of pigs, *colisepticaemia in calves, lambs, puppies, and poultry, *coliform mastitis in cattle and other species, and *pyometra and urinary tract infections in the dog and cat. Colibacillosis is normally acute, but more chronic forms have been described in poultry (*see* arthritis; Hjarré's disease; omphalitis; osteomyelitis; salpingitis).

colic A condition in which an animal shows signs of severe abdominal pain. The direct cause is usually abnormally vigorous peristalsis in the gastrointestinal tract or distension of the tract. Intestinal obstruction induces colic, whether from *infarction, *intussusception, or impaction with feed or foreign bodies. Distension of the tract results also from the accumulation of gas. However, the pain can be derived from the kidney or ureter (hence *renal colic*), particularly in cases of obstruction with kidney stones. Similar pain may originate in the liver or gall-bladder following obstruction. The affected animal may exhibit such signs as pawing the ground, kicking its abdomen, repeatedly changing its posture, or adopting abnormal postures, such as sitting upright on its hindquarters (dog-sitting). Sweating, rapid pulse, and rapid breathing are additional signs that help in gauging the severity of the colic. Discovery of the cause may be urgent because some forms of colic require prompt surgery. Other forms respond to gentle walking and *analgesics.

coliform bacteria The Gram-negative bacteria in the family Enterobacteriaceae that usually ferment lactose; for example *Escherichia coli*.

coliform mastitis *Mastitis caused by bacteria of the class Enterobacteriaceae, principally *Escherichia coli* and species of *Klebsiella* and *Aerobacter*. E. coli mastitis of **cows** is probably an environmental infection, and occurs frequently in association with the use of sawdust or wood shavings as bedding material. Both severe (acute) and mild forms occur, the former being characterized by its rapid onset, profound toxaemia (often with diarrhoea), and high fatality. Antibiotics are used in treatment. In **sows**, E. coli causes agalactia (cessation of milk secretion) rather than mastitis; it is the commonest udder infection in sows, and causes frequent loss of newborn piglets.

coli granuloma *See* Hjarré's disease.

colisepticaemia Any of a group of septicaemic diseases caused by strains of *Escherichia coli* and occurring mainly in calves, lambs, dogs, and poultry. **Calves** are usually affected in the first week of life. The strains of *E. coli* responsible are often of serogroup O78:K80, some having the ability to extract and utilize iron from infected tissues; they may enter via the umbilicus or nasopharynx. Colostrum deprivation or impairment of gammaglobulin absorption are important predisposing factors. A brief period of fever is followed by the syndrome associated with endotoxin shock (hypothermia, collapse, and rapid death); diarrhoea is not a regular feature (*compare* enteric colibacillosis of calves). Similar septicaemias affect lambs and kids, though not usually piglets. In newborn puppies, fatal colisepticaemia is often due to serogroup O42. Tetracyclines, streptomycin, or other antibiotics are used in treatment.

Colisepticaemia is an important cause of loss in **broiler chickens**, serogroups O2 and O78:K80 being common, and also occurs in **turkey poults** and **ducks**. Broilers aged 6–10 weeks are most susceptible, and, to a lesser extent, those aged 0–2 weeks. Mortality can reach 5%, occasionally more, with morbidity exceeding 20%. Infection is thought not to originate from *E. coli* in the digestive tract but more probably through a respiratory route. Initial signs are often of a respiratory infection, although some cases show only general apathy. There is significant economic loss from unthriftiness and downgrading of carcasses. Predisposing factors may include other respiratory infections (e.g. *avian mycoplasmosis), other diseases (such as *coccidiosis or respiratory virus infections), or poor nutrition. Control depends on good management to reduce the risk of infection, including disinfection of poultry houses and the use of *Mycoplasma*-free chicks. Treatment with nitrofurans and tetracyclines is reasonably successful.

colitis Inflammation of the *colon. It may be caused by bacterial infection (e.g. *Salmonella* or *Campylobacter*) or parasites (e.g. *Trichuris, Coccidia,* or *Toxoplasma*), often with concurrent *enteritis. In young boxer dogs and hounds an ulcerative colitis of unknown cause occurs. Characteristic signs include bloody and possibly mucoid diarrhoea, which may be watery, ill-thrift, and sometimes anaemia. Ulcers may be detected by X-radiography following a barium enema. Severe damage to the colonic mucosa indicates a poor prognosis. Treatment involves a low-residue diet coupled with the administration of antispasmodics (*see* spasmolytic), *kaolin, and appropriate antibiotics or anthelmintics.

Colitis-X occurs sporadically in horses. Although the cause is unknown, the release of bacterial *endotoxins or exhaustive stress may be important factors. Copious watery diarrhoea is the characteristic sign, followed by depression, dehydration, and cardiovascular collapse. Mortality is high. Fluid replacement therapy though logical is commonly unrewarding. *See also* swine dysentery.

collagen A protein that is the principal constituent of the fibres in white fibrous connective tissue (as occurs in tendons). Collagen is also found in skin, bone, cartilage, and ligaments. It is relatively inelastic but has a high tensile strength. *See also* tropocollagen.

collateral 1. Accessory or secondary. 2. A branch (e.g. of a nerve fibre) that is at right angles to the main part.

collateral circulation An alternative route provided for blood by secondary vessels if a primary vessel should become blocked. Collateral circulation is well developed in some tissues and organs, e.g. muscle and gut, but poorly developed in others, e.g. brain, heart, and kidney, where *end arteries occur.

colliculus (*pl.* **colliculi**) A small swelling or projection. For example, the *rostral* and *caudal colliculi* are two pairs of protuberances on the dorsal surface of the midbrain. The rostral colliculi act as relay stations for visual reflexes while the caudal colliculi are centres on the auditory pathways.

collie eye anomaly (CEA) An inherited congenital defect of the canine eye found very commonly in rough collies, smooth collies, and the Shetland sheepdog. The problem involves abnormalities of the retina and the choroid and can be diagnosed with the aid of an ophthalmoscope by around 7 weeks of age, although mild cases will only be detected by an experienced veterinary ophthalmologist. The condition does not usually worsen with age or have any effect on vision; although in severe cases it can cause total blindness. Animals should be checked to ensure they are free from the defect before being permitted to breed.

collodion A mixture of pyroxylin (a nitrocellulose compound), ether, and alcohol. It is painted onto the skin and, as the solvents evaporate, forms a clear flexible protective film, for example for wound closure. Various types of collodion are available incorporating oils, drugs, etc.

colloid A system in which there are two or more phases, with one (the

dispersed or discontinuous phase) distributed in the other (the continuous phase). For example, a *sol* is a colloid in which small solid particles are dispersed in a liquid. In *gels, both dispersed and continuous phases have a three-dimensional network throughout the material and form a jelly-like mass. In *aerosols, the solid or liquid particles are dispersed in a gas.

collyrium A preparation, usually a wash or lotion, for use in the eye.

coloboma A congenital defect of the eye characterized by a gap, notch, or cleft in various parts of one or both eyes. The lids are most frequently affected, although the iris, ciliary body, lens, retina, choroid, or optic nerve may be involved. Impairment of vision depends on the nature and severity of the condition, which is not progressive. An association with incomplete *albinism has been seen in various breeds of cattle, where the disorder is inherited, being controlled by a *dominant autosomal allele. In Charolais cattle the condition is *recessive and associated with *arthrogryposis and *cleft palate.

colon The part of the mammalian large intestine that extends from the caecum to the rectum and which absorbs fluid and electrolytes from the digesta prior to their expulsion as faeces. Its basic form, as seen in carnivores, consists of three parts – the *ascending colon* lying to the right of the abdomen, the *transverse colon* crossing the midline, and the *descending colon* on the left.

In the **horse** the colon is much elongated and is a site for bacterial breakdown of cellulose and absorption of digestion products, such as volatile fatty acids. Its walls have longitudinal bands of smooth muscle (*taeniae) which produce numerous small sacculations (*haustra). The specialized ascending colon and transverse colon together constitute the *large colon*. The ascending colon is greatly developed and forms a long U-shaped loop. The transverse colon leads into a greatly elongated and coiled descending colon, termed the *small colon*.

In **ruminants** and the **pig** the ascending colon is again greatly elongated but twisted to form a spiral loop consisting of centripetal and centrifugal coils. In ruminants this is a flattened structure, compared to a somewhat cone-shaped one in the pig. It leads by a distal loop to the transverse colon. *See* intestine.

colostrum The first secretion produced by the mammary gland in each lactation. Formed shortly before parturition and secreted for a short period thereafter, it is more viscous than true *milk, with a high total protein content, 60% of which is *globulin. The globulin fraction includes many maternal antibodies, which are important in conferring passive immunity on the newborn, provided that the colostrum is consumed within 24 hours of birth while the neonatal alimentary tract is still permeable to proteins. The high proline content and high iron content are both valuable for haemoglobin formation in the young animal.

colour vision The ability to see colours, which is enabled by the activity of the *cones in the retina of the eye. Domestic mammals are believed to perceive colour to a lesser extent than primates or birds.

colp- (colpo-) *Prefix denoting* the vagina.

columella 1. The only auditory *ossicle in birds, extending from the tympanic membrane to the vestibular window. **2.** Any part resembling a small column.

column Any pillar-shaped structure, for example the vertebral column, or any of the main subdivisions of grey or white matter found in the spinal cord.

coma A state of unconsciousness from which an animal cannot be roused, even by painful stimuli. Various diseases may induce coma, including inflammation of the brain (encephalitis), metabolic disorders (e.g. hypoglycaemia, ketosis, and milk fever), heat stroke, and high fever. Brain anoxia and overdoses of anaesthetics have the same result. Comatose animals are often moribund, although specific therapy, for example calcium injection for milk fever, may save them.

comb The fleshy crest surmounting the head in some birds, such as the domestic fowl. There is much variation in form between species and sexes. It is richly supplied with blood vessels. The *snood of turkeys is sometimes termed the nasal comb.

comedo (*pl.* **comedones**) Whitehead or blackhead. A plug of keratin, lipid, and bacteria that occludes the orifice of a hair follicle and protrudes above the skin surface. They may be observed particularly on the ventral abdomen of older dogs that are not groomed regularly, and are also seen in cases of hypothyroidism, hyperadrenocorticism, and hyperoestrogenism. Comedones may be removed by gentle bathing after the application of keratolytic ointments. However, the underlying cause should also be investigated.

commensal An organism that lives in close association with another of a different species without either harming or benefiting it. For example, some microorganisms living in the gut obtain both food and a suitable habitat but neither harm nor benefit their host. *Compare* symbiosis.

commissure 1. A bundle of nerve fibres that crosses the midline of the central nervous system, connecting similar structures on each side. 2. Any other tissue connecting two similar structures, for example the commissure of the eyelids, and commissure of the lips.

common calcaneal tendon (Achilles tendon) A composite tendon attaching to the calcaneal tuberosity on the rear of the hindlimb (*see* tarsus). It comprises the tendons of the *gastrocnemius, superficial *digital flexor, *biceps femoris, *semitendinosus, and *gracilis muscles.

communicans Communicating or connecting. The term is applied particularly to blood vessels or nerve fibres connecting two similar structures.

complement A series of proteins in the blood that plays a major role in the body's immunological defence, by promoting the *phagocytosis of invading cells and other *antigens, and by undertaking the lysis of certain bacteria. Complement is also involved in *inflammation, and may be responsible for some of the damage that occurs in *autoimmune disease and in hypersensitivity.

The series comprises nine distinct protein components, which interact sequentially in a so-called 'cascade' effect: this means that a small triggering event sufficient to activate one of the components generates an amplified effect. In the *classical pathway* of complement activation, the first step is the binding of IgG or IgM *antibodies to specific antigen. The binding action leads to a conformational change in the antibody, which permits the activation of the first complement component, C1. Activated C1 is then able to activate

components C2 and C4, which act jointly as a proteolytic enzyme to cleave component C3 into C3a and C3b. These are thus released in the vicinity of antigen-antibody complexes or at the surface of cells that have bound antibody. C3b stimulates the influx, binding, and phagocytic activities of *macrophages and *neutrophils, and the release of inflammatory substances by *platelets. C3a acts to release *histamine from *mast cells; in this role C3a is known as an *anaphylotoxin*. C3 can also be cleaved by an *alternative pathway*, which bypasses C1, C2, and C4. This pathway is activated by various substances, including bacterial lipopolysaccharide, thrombin and plasmin (*see* coagulation), zymosan from yeast, and various factors in cobra venom and helminth parasites.

Once produced, C3b in conjunction with further proteins – B, D, and P (*properdin) – has the property of stimulating further breakdown of C3. In order to prevent overproduction of C3b, normal serum contains C3b inactivator, the absence of which may result in spontaneous exhaustion of C3. C3b, whether generated by the classical or the alternative pathway, has the additional property of being able to activate C5, which is cleaved to produce C5a, another anaphylotoxin. The remainder of the C5 molecule complexes with C6 and C7 and in this form acquires the power further to attract neutrophils. The activated complex of C567 is finally able to fix components C8 and C9, which thus acquire the power to lyse certain bacteria and other foreign cells.

complement fixation test A test used to establish the presence of, and often also the relative concentration of, particular *antibodies in body fluids (e.g. blood serum), for example in diagnosing certain diseases. If antigen and antibody react they form a complex, which will bind *complement. If such a complex is not formed and complement remains unbound, it is revealed by adding antibody-coated sheep red cells which lyse in the presence of complement. By reacting a standard volume of antigen with a series of dilutions of the antibody in the presence of complement, the relative concentration of the antibody in the initial sample can be quantified. Although still used in diagnosing bovine brucellosis and various virus diseases, the test is now being replaced by simpler and more rapid procedures, such as the *enzyme-linked immunosorbent assay.

compound feed A livestock feed comprising various ingredients that are mixed, ground, and pelleted together. It may be designed as a complete ration or to complement forage intake. Compound feeds can contain a variety of energy and protein sources together with minerals (*see* essential element) and *vitamins. The terms compound feed and *concentrates are often used synonymously by farmers although feed compounders distinguish between them.

conalbumin A *glycoprotein found in egg white that binds ferrous ions (Fe^{2+}).

concave shoe A type of horseshoe used on hunters and other fast-moving horses. The inside edge of the shoe is bevelled off to reduce weight.

concentrate A proprietary feedstuff that constitutes a concentrated source of a particular nutrient (e.g. protein) and is designed for mixing with other feedstuffs (e.g. cereals) to produce a balanced ration. Straights, such as rolled barley, are often misleadingly referred to as concentrates. The term is also used to denote all non-forage feeds. *Compare* compound feed.

conception rate The number of animals pregnant as a proportion of the total number mated or inseminated. In dairy cows it may also be expressed as the reciprocal of the number of inseminations required for successful pregnancy.

conceptus The developing embryo and its surrounding membranes at all stages of development.

concha (*pl.* **conchae**) (in anatomy) Any part resembling a shell. For example, the *concha auriculae* is a depression on the outer surface of the pinna (auricle), which leads to the external auditory meatus of the outer ear. *See also* nasal concha.

concussion A condition involving a limited period of unconsciousness resulting from a blow to the head and consequent injury to the brain. The signs consist mainly of dullness and lack of normal responses, for example diminished pupillary reflexes.

condition scoring A technique for assessing, on a scale of 1 to 5, the body fat reserves of farm livestock. It can be rapidly learned and applied with consistent results although, being a subjective measurement, there is some variation between operators. However, it provides a more reliable assessment of body reserves than liveweight, which is often very variable (*see* weighing methods). **Cattle** are assessed by feeling the amount of fat cover over the transverse processes of the lumbar vertebrae and around the tail head. Beef cattle are assessed on a scale of 1 to 5, where 1 corresponds to an emaciated animal and 5 to a grossly fat animal. Target condition scores for autumn-calving suckler cows are 2.5 at mating, 2 at mid-pregnancy, and 3 at calving. For spring-calving suckler cows, the corresponding targets are 2–2.5, 3, and 2.5. Dairy cows are assessed on a

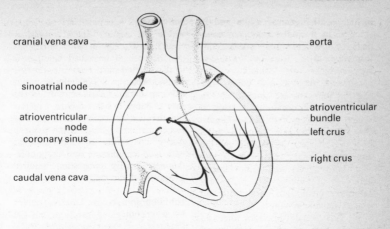

Conducting system of heart

similar basis using a scale of 1 to 4. The target condition score at mating is 2 or above and the target at calving is 2–3.5. If ad lib feeding is not available in early lactation, the target at calving should be 3–3.5.

Breeding **ewes** assessed only over the lumbar vertebrae and scored from 0 to 5. Target condition scores at 3–3.5 at mating, 3 at mid-pregnancy, and 3–3.5 at lambing (housed ewes) or 3.5–4 (out-wintered ewes). **Sows** are also assessed on a 1 to 5 scale and the points of reference are the tail head, loin, ribs, flank, and backbone. There are no set targets for condition score in sows but few sows should be below condition score 2 at weaning and no sow should be condition score 5 at any time.

conducting system (of the heart) The specialized cardiac muscle tissue that stimulates and organizes the contractions of the heart. It consists of the *sinoatrial node, the *atrioventricular node, and the *atrioventricular bundle (see illustration).

condyle A rounded protuberance at the end of certain bones, e.g. femur or humerus, which takes part in the formation of a joint with other bones.

cone One of the two types of light-sensitive cells in the *retina of the eye (*compare* rod). They function best in bright light and are essential for acute vision (receiving a sharp accurate image). The *macula of the retina contains the greatest concentration of cones.

conformation The proportionate shape or contours of a live animal or carcass, usually assessed by comparison with an ideal. *Carcass conformation* usually reflects the value of the carcass to a butcher. In a poor carcass all the profiles are concave with little muscle development; the bones are clearly visible. In an excellent carcass all the profiles are convex with exceptional muscle development; the bones are covered by well-rounded muscle blocks. Conformation is supposed to be assessed independently of fat cover, but in fatter carcasses the rounded appearance can be largely due to fat.

In live animals the conformation of meat-producing animals is a reflection of the desired carcass shape and is assessed in a similar way. However, pedigree breeders often confuse conformation with trueness to breed type, which can contain useless parameters, such as coat colour and whether the ears are pricked up. In dairy cows conformation is assessed rather differently from beef animals. Breed societies rate animals from poor to excellent, depending on the appearance, dairy character, udder shape, legs, feet, size, temperament, and ease of milking. This is a very subjective method of assessment and a more reliable system is *linear assessment*. This method describes where an animal lies between biological extremes for agreed traits, rather than comparing it with an ideal, hence the actual shape of the animal can be deduced. Sixteen traits are currently assessed on a scale from 1 to 9, and a further 32 traits can be reported on if present. The major traits are stature, chest width, body depth, angularity, rump angle, rump width, rear legs (side and rear views), foot angle, fore udder attachment, rear udder width, udder support, udder depth, teat placement (rear and side views), and teat length. In *progeny testing of bulls the average value for all the daughters is compared with the average for the breed.

congenital hypothyroidism (cretinism) A developmental disorder caused by inadequate or absent production of thyroid hormones from birth. Animals born without a thyroid gland often die soon after birth unless supplemented immediately with thyroid hormones. Those producing subnormal quantities of hormone will grow slowly and develop mental retardation. Other clinical signs of hypothyroidism, such as obesity, alopecia, sluggishness, and constipation, may be seen as the animal ages. *See* hypothyroidism.

congestion Accumulation of blood within an organ. *Active congestion* occurs in association with inflammation because of increased blood flow to the affected part. *Passive congestion* occurs because blood fails to drain from an organ, for instance from the liver or lungs in heart failure. Congestion frequently accompanies *oedema (accumulation of fluid in the tissues). Active congestion may be relieved with cold compresses and/or antihistamines. Passive congestion requires treatment of the cause.

conidiobolomycosis Disease caused by a noncontagious infection with the fungus *Conidiobolus coronatus*; a type of *entomophthoromycosis. Occurring in tropical and subtropical areas of Africa, southeast Asia, India, Australia, the USA, and South America, the disease affects humans but is seldom recorded in animals except horses, in which it produces ulcerative granulomas resembling those of *pythiosis and *basidiobolomycosis. These 'equine nasal granulomas' tend to occur around the nostrils and within the nasal passages, often provoking a nasal discharge and causing nasal blockage. The fungus is a pathogen of insects and a soil saprophyte, growing upon moist organic matter, and infection is probably acquired by contact with spores while grazing. The distribution of the lesions tends to distinguish the disease from other types of *equine phycomycosis. Differentiation from these and from cutaneous *habronemiasis can be confirmed by histopathology of tissue containing 'kunkers' (*see* equine phycomycosis) and isolation of the fungus from these bodies. Treatment is by surgical excision where possible, coupled with oral administration of potassium iodide or intravenous sodium iodide.

conjugation The union of two microorganisms in which genetic material

(DNA) passes from one organism to the other. In some bacteria a minute projection on the donor 'male' cell (a *pilus*) forms a bridge with the recipient 'female' cell through which the DNA is transferred. Conjugation is comparable to sexual reproduction in higher organisms.

conjunctiva The delicate mucous membrane that lines the inside of the eyelids (*palpebral conjunctiva*) and covers the front of the *eye (*bulbar conjunctiva*). At the inner angle of the eye it forms a fold termed the *third eyelid. The space between palpebral and bulbar conjunctivae beneath the eyelids is the conjunctival sac, which contains a film of lacrimal fluid.

conjunctivitis Inflammation of the *conjunctiva. Cases include infectious microorganisms, foreign bodies, irritant chemicals, and allergic reactions. For example, in cats infections of mycoplasmas and *Chlamydia* cause conjunctivitis, and herpesviruses produce the condition in most animals. Conjunctivitis may be accompanied by oedema (*chemosis) and the lesion may penetrate causing deep ulceration of the cornea. For instance, in *New Forest disease the ulceration leads to corneal opacity and blindness. Conjunctivitis caused by infection is normally treated by topical application of antibiotics. Otherwise, corticosteroid application may help recovery. *See also* ovine keratoconjunctivitis.

connective tissue The tissue that supports, binds, or separates more specialized tissues and organs or functions as a packing tissue of the body. It consists of an amorphous ground substance of mucopolysaccharides in which may be embedded white (collagenous), yellow (elastic), and reticular fibres, fat cells, *fibroblasts, *mast cells, and *macrophages (see illustration). Variations in chemical composition of the ground substance and in

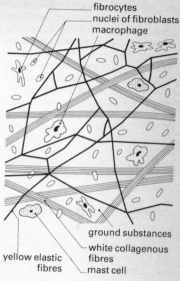

Loose (areolar) connective tissue

the proportions and quantities of cells and fibres give rise to tissues of widely differing characteristics, including bone, cartilage, tendons, and ligaments as well as *adipose, *areolar, and *elastic tissues.

consolidation 1. Solidification of an organ, especially the lung. In pneumonia the normally spongy texture of the lung solidifies as the airways fill with exudate and congestion. **2.** The stage of repair of a broken bone following callus formation, during which the callus is transformed by osteoblasts into mature bone (*see* ossification).

constipation Failure to pass faeces in either the normal quantity or frequency. Typical causes include dehydration, in which there are excessively dry faeces, a low-residue diet, obstruction of the alimentary tract (e.g. with a tumour or foreign body),

contagious abortion

and enlarged prostate. The animal may attempt to defecate but feels pain due to the hard dry material in the rectum. Straightforward constipation may be relieved by means of an *enema of warm water or mineral oil; stubborn cases require manual removal of the faecal material. Laxatives may help during recovery. Constipation in newborns needs urgent attention. Retention of the *meconium (foetal faeces) in foals can be treated by an enema of warm soapy water. In piglets constipation may be due to an imperforate anus, which needs surgical relief.

contagious abortion See brucellosis.

contagious agalactia A contagious disease of sheep and goats characterized by fever, mastitis, conjunctivitis, and arthritis and caused by *Mycoplasma agalactiae*. The disease is enzootic in most of Africa, the Middle East, and India. Infection is by contact but its seasonal incidence suggests that flies may carry pathogens to the udder of susceptible animals; the organisms enter via the teat canal. Following an incubation period of up to 2 months, lactating ewes and goats develop *mastitis and their milk yield is reduced. Flaky yellow clots appear in the milk. The lower joints of the limbs become enlarged and painful, and *conjunctivitis and corneal ulceration may develop. Infected animals lose weight and may succumb to other infections. Chronically infected sheep and goats can excrete M. agalactiae for a considerable time. Vaccines are available to control contagious agalactia, but slaughter of infected animals is recommended in nonenzootic countries.

contagious bovine pleuropneumonia (CBPP) A contagious disease of cattle characterized by fever and cough and caused by *Mycoplasma mycoides mycoides*. The disease is

enzootic in many countries in Africa and possibly also in parts of the Far East. Periodically it spreads into southern Europe. Infection is by inhalation of contaminated moisture droplets and, following an incubation period of between 2 weeks and 6 months, the infected animal develops a fever, loss of appetite, increased breathing rate, and eventually a dry cough. The cough becomes more productive and the animal may adopt a characteristic stance, with both elbows out to relieve pressure on the thorax. Death may occur in 2–3 weeks or the animal may apparently recover. Cattle that have recovered from acute, chronic, or even inapparent disease may become 'lungers'. These animals maintain within their lungs one or more infected foci that have been effectively isolated by the development of a surrounding fibrous capsule. However, this fibrous tissue can break down, when the animal again becomes infectious to susceptible cattle. Blood tests can identify these persistently infected animals, but many veterinary authorities recommend slaughter of all clinically infected cattle and their contacts. Treatment of infected cattle may reduce the mortality rate but produce a larger number of carriers. Clinical diagnosis without laboratory assistance can be difficult because many cattle develop only mild clinical signs. On post mortem the lungs of infected cattle have a characteristic marbled or mosaic appearance. A live attenuated vaccine is used in many of the enzootic areas. CBPP is a *notifiable disease in the UK.

contagious caprine pleuropneumonia (CCPP) A contagious disease of goats characterized by pneumonia and death and caused by *Mycoplasma mycoides capri*. The disease is enzootic in most of Africa, the Middle East, and India although because of the difficulty in diagnosis its true distribution is not known. Infection spreads by inhalation of contaminated moisture droplets and the incubation period is 3–5 weeks, followed by the development of clinical *pneumonia. In the peracute form of the disease death can occur even before the pneumonia is apparent. Mortality rates can reach 100%. Animals that do not die have a long and slow convalescence, becoming thin and emaciated and susceptible to additional lung infections. However, unlike cattle with *contagious bovine pleuropneumonia, affected goats do not persistently excrete the pathogenic organisms. Treatment with tylosine tartrate is effective but in nonenzootic areas a policy of slaughter of all infected animals and their contacts is recommended. Vaccines are employed in enzootic areas. Diagnosis requires the isolation and identification of *M. mycoides capri* in the lung tissue or exudate of an infected goat. CCPP is a *notifiable disease in the UK.

contagious disease Strictly, an infectious disease in which the causative agent(s) are spread by direct animal-to-animal contact. However, it now usually refers to any communicable disease.

contagious ecthyma *See* orf.

contagious epithelioma *See* fowl pox.

contagious equine metritis A contagious disease of mares, caused by the bacterium *Taylorella equigenitalis*, characterized by infertility and abortions. The disease first appeared in Ireland and Great Britain in 1976–77 but was later reported from Europe, USA, and Australia. The causative organism was initially regarded as a member of the genus *Haemophilus* but by 1984 was viewed as sufficiently different to merit a separate genus.

Mares with clinical or subclinical disease harbour the organism in the cervix, urethra, and clitoral fossa. Stallions that serve infected mares transmit infections to other mares, and the organisms can be recovered from the urethra, urethral fossa, penile sheath, and the pre-ejaculatory fluid of stallions.

The disease causes inflammations of the vaginal and uterine mucosa resulting in varying degrees of uterine discharges. The ultimate effect of infection is *endometritis with consequent infertility and early abortions in mares; stallions do not seem to be clinically affected. Diagnosis involves isolation of the organisms, which requires special culture conditions. Treatment of infected animals is with appropriate antibiotics, such as ampicillin, and spread of the disease can be prevented by suitable hygiene measures. It must be remembered that the organisms can persist in the clitoral fossa and urethra of carrier animals.

contagious indigestion *See* avian monocytosis.

contagious porcine pleuropneumonia A disease of pigs caused by infection with the bacterium *Haemophilus pleuropneumonia* and characterized by pneumonia and pleurisy. It may take peracute, acute, or subacute/chronic forms, and affects pigs aged between 6 weeks and 6 months; the more severe form is seen in older, fattening pigs. There is often secondary bacterial invasion, producing abscess formation. Treatment is often ineffective, although broad-spectrum antibiotic coverage of in-contact pigs, with attention to housing and hygiene, may limit the spread of infection.

contagious pustular dermatitis *See* orf.

contamination of lungs A condition occurring during the slaughter of cattle in which blood and ruminal contents are regurgitated and aspirated into the trachea and lungs. A somewhat similar condition is seen in pigs when water enters the lungs during the scalding process.

contemporary comparison A type of *progeny test in which the offspring of one animal (usually a sire) are compared with the offspring of others over the same period and in the same herds. The sire (e.g. a bull) can then be assessed in comparison with all other sires.

contra- *Prefix denoting* against or opposite. Example: *contraversion* (turning away from).

contraception Literally the prevention of conception, although the term also embraces techniques used to prevent *implantation and further development of the early embryo. Contraception is rarely needed in farm species but may be required in pets, for example if a bitch or queen undergoes an unwanted mating during *oestrus. The technique formerly involved the injection of an *oestrogen within 48 hours of the mating, which acted to prolong oestrus. In old bitches, oestrogen injections have been associated with an increased frequency of *pyometra, and in queens oestrogens can be toxic. Current techniques involve an injection of *prostaglandin $F_{2\alpha}$ or *progestogen at an early stage. In mares, if a twin pregnancy is diagnosed at an early stage, it may be possible to destroy one of the embryos by manual compression of the uterus via the rectum, but the technique is not always successful and both embryos may die.

The term contraception may also be extended to include the techniques of *sterilization, such as *vasectomy and *orchidectomy in males. *See also* castration; spaying.

contracted foot (contracted hoof) A musculoskeletal defect, usually congenital, in which the tendons controlling joint flexion are shortened. In the so-called 'contracted' foal many joints are involved producing multiple deformities. An inherited multiple tendon contracture also occurs in calves. Simple contracted flexor tendons occur commonly in calves and foals. Mildly affected animals walk 'on their toes', but in severe cases the animal may be forced to crawl on the front of the fetlocks. *See* contracted tendon.

contracted tendon A condition of horses in which there is excessive pull by the deep flexor tendon on the distal phalanx, and by the superficial flexor tendon on the middle phalanx. This causes changes in the fetlock and pastern of the forefoot of the animal. The condition may be acquired or congenital. *Acquired contracted tendon* can occur in young horses (aged 4 months to 2 years) during periods of rapid growth. One or both forelimbs can be affected. In the early stages the pastern appears upright and the fetlock straight. The coronary band is warm and puffy, and the wall of the foot may flake away at the toe, with possibly some separation between the wall and the sole of the foot at the white line (*see* hoof). The animal rolls the foot from heel to toe when walking. As the condition progresses the weight is taken on the toe and the unused heel grows rapidly, giving the foot a boxy appearance. This progresses to a third stage, in which the animal walks on the front of the foot.

The initial cause of the condition is unknown, but it is always connected with overfeeding and rapid growth. There may be a calcium, phosphorus, or vitamin D imbalance. Treatment in the early stages has a good chance of success, and involves switching the animal to a low plane of nutrition so that growth is reduced; an affected suckling foal must be weaned at once. Animals should be encouraged to exercise. A low-calorie diet should be maintained to guard against recurrence. Surgical section of the inferior check ligament (which reinforces the pull of the deep flexor tendon) is usually beneficial for animals not responding to the starvation diet. Surgery on the deep flexor tendon has serious consequences and is not recommended.

Not uncommonly foals are born with *congenital contracted tendons*. The cause is again unknown. The foal must be helped to stand as normally as possible; straightening and massaging the legs over several days gives good results, and walking also helps to straighten the legs. Protection must be given to areas of the legs likely to be damaged by unnatural posture: splinting or plastering of the limbs may be necessary. Prognosis is good for most cases, although some may be untreatable.

contracture The permanent shortening of a muscle and its fascia resulting in distortion and disability, usually involving an associated limb joint. It is often associated with vascular damage and consequent local ischaemia. Contractures can be associated with the use of casts in fracture fixation, where considerable soft tissue damage may occur, or damage following internal fixation of a fracture.

contraindication Any feature of a patient's condition that indicates against pursuing a certain drug or treatment. For instance, certain opiates are contraindicated in cats because they provoke hyperexcitability. Similarly, some antibiotics are dangerous to guinea pigs because they kill off microbial flora in the large intestine and allow the growth of pathogenic microorganisms.

contralateral On or affecting the opposite side of the body: applied particularly to paralysis (or other symptoms) occurring on the opposite side of the body from the brain lesion that caused them.

contrast medium A substance that is used to improve the visibility of structures during *radiography. Contrast media have the property of absorbing X-rays (i.e. they are *radio-opaque*) and can thus reveal the shape of an organ or structure in which they are present. For example, barium salts can be given orally as contrast media to facilitate radiography of the alimentary tract. Similarly, iodine-containing compounds can be injected intravenously to accumulate in particular organs (e.g. the kidneys) and act as contrast media.

control The part of a study or experiment against which an experimental procedure can be compared and its effects judged. In animal experimentation, control animals are subjected to exactly the same conditions as experimental animals, except for the procedure under investigation. For instance, in vaccine trials the vaccinated (experimental) and unvaccinated (control) animals must be of the same breed, age, and sex distribution and kept under similar conditions if the vaccine's effectiveness is to be conclusively demonstrated.

controlled drugs (UK) Dangerous or otherwise harmful drugs that are scheduled under the Misuse of Drugs Act (1971). Examples are *morphine, *etorphine (Immobilon), and *pethidine. All veterinary surgeons should maintain a register of controlled drugs and keep such drugs in a locked container that can be opened only by the veterinarian or an authorized person.

contusion *See* bruise.

convergence (in neurology) The formation of nerve tracts by fibres coming together into one pathway from different regions of the brain.

convolution A folding or twisting, such as one of the many that cause the sulci and gyri of the cerebral cortex on the surface of the *cerebrum.

convulsion A violent and uncoordinated contraction of muscles, usually with alternating and irregular relaxation. The abnormal muscular activity raises the body temperature. Convulsions or 'fits' are especially common in dogs and may be hereditary in certain breeds. Other causes include organic brain disease (tumours, meningitis, encephalitis), brain swelling, and hyperthermia. In cattle a common convulsive disorder is *cerebrocortical necrosis caused by thiamin (vitamin B_1) deficiency. In foals there is a so-called 'convulsive foal' syndrome.

coonhound paralysis A disease of hunting dogs in the southern USA and other parts of the world, particularly where raccoons are endemic. The disease is associated with bite or scratch wounds received by dogs while hunting raccoons or other wild carnivores. Affected dogs develop hindquarter weakness, which progresses to paralysis and sometimes quadriplegia at 7–14 days postwounding. Facial paralysis and difficulty in swallowing may be seen; spinal reflexes are lost in severe cases. Dogs remain bright, alert, and afebrile, indicating a lack of cerebral involvement. Muscle atrophy is common. The majority of dogs recover in a week to 2 months if given supportive nursing. They are often left with residual weakness and muscle atrophy, and may be sensitive to subsequent exposure. Dogs that develop respiratory paralysis have a poor prognosis; intubation and mechanical ventilation may be attempted.
There is no specific treatment although some beneficial effects are claimed for *corticosteroids. Despite the association of raccoon saliva, no aetiological agent has been identified. A cell-mediated *autoimmune reaction has been suggested. Other name: **idiopathic acute radiculoneuritis**.

copper A metallic element and an essential trace element in the diet of animals. Copper is essential in the body for the production of red blood cells and is a vital component or cofactor in many enzyme systems. It is also involved in the pigmentation of fur, wool, and hair. The copper content of crops, and hence derived animal feeds, is related to copper levels in the soil as well as the species of plant and even drainage conditions. Copper deficiency (*see* hypocuprosis) is an important disease in many parts of the world, principally affecting ruminants. *See also* copper poisoning.

copperbottle A blowfly, *Lucilia cuprina*, which causes blowfly *strike in sheep in Australia and South Africa. *See also* green-bottle fly.

copper poisoning A toxic condition caused by ingestion of copper. Animals vary in their susceptibility to copper poisoning: sheep are highly susceptible, cattle less so, and pigs are relatively resistant. Poisoning may be caused by high levels of copper in herbage, especially where molybdenum levels are low, or by exposure to one of the many copper preparations used in agriculture and horticulture. The oxychloride, chloride, and carbonate of copper are used as fungicidal sprays; copper naphthenate is a wood preservative; and copper sulphate is used as a molluscicide and in footbaths to control footrot of sheep, as well as a fungicide (Bordeaux mixture). Pregnant ewes are injected with copper calcium edetate and other organic preparations of copper to prevent swayback in their lambs.

Acute copper poisoning, due to the ingestion of a single large dose, can occur when thirsty sheep are passed through a footbath of copper sulphate solution. Salivation, purgation, abdominal pain, convulsions, collapse, and death occur. Faeces and intestinal contents are a deep green colour. Another form of acute copper poisoning sometimes follows the injection of a flock of sheep with a standard dose of copper calcium edetate (containing 50 mg copper per dose). Some undersized animals may die suddenly with fluid in the lungs and abdomen, widespread haemorrhages, and focal necrosis of the liver. The condition appears to arise from the rapid absorption of copper from the injection site. Other copper-containing injections which are more slowly absorbed are less harmful.

Chronic copper poisoning is due to the continued absorption of small doses of copper, which accumulate in the liver. It has been reported in sheep grazing sprayed orchards, in housed sheep fed on pig rations (which have a high copper content), and in housed sheep fed on rations containing normally safe levels of copper but inadequate molybdenum. The copper stored in the liver is suddenly released into the bloodstream where it damages the red blood cells and causes *haemolytic anaemia, haemoglobinuria, and jaundice. Further cases can be prevented by ensuring adequate levels of molybdenum in the diet. Although copper poisoning in its various forms mainly affects sheep, the chronic form has been reported in calves fed on milk replacer with a high copper content, and in pigs given rations with a high copper content.

copr- (copro-) *Prefix denoting* faeces.

coprophagy The ingestion of faeces. This is normal in some species, for instance rabbits, which by so doing recycle unabsorbed B-vitamins synthesized by their intestinal flora but evacuated with the faeces. Newborns involuntarily consume maternal faeces when suckling owing to faecal contamination of the teats. Piglets may even supplement their iron intake from this source. However, coprophagy can be an unusual form of depraved appetite or *pica, in which the animal tries to correct a dietary deficiency. Alternatively it may be a vice caused by boredom.

copulation *See* coitus.

coracoid One of the bones of the *shoulder girdle. In mammals it is much reduced and represented by the coracoid process of the *scapula. In birds it is well developed and forms joints with the sternum as well as the other bones of the shoulder girdle, i.e. scapula and clavicle.

corium (*pl.* **coria**) The specialized highly vascular dermis that nourishes the hoof.

'corkscrew' penis A congenital abnormality of the penis occurring in bulls. Very vigorous erection causes spiral deflection because of differences in the elasticity of the dorsal and lateral tunica albuginea. Most bulls overcome this spontaneously by learning to time their insertion before extreme deflection comes on.

corn A localized thickening of the skin or horn of the hoof. Corns commonly occur between the claws of the foot in cattle. They apparently start as a bulge of interdigital fat, which becomes irritated by contact with the ground or the adjacent claws. Overgrowth of the skin produces a protective layer, further enlarging the corn. The result can be pain and lameness; surgical removal of the corn is needed in severe cases.

In **horses** 'corns' are caused by bruising of the sole of the hoof. They are associated with a poorly fitting shoe inflicting undue pressure on the sole. The shape of the hoof may be abnormal or it may be badly trimmed. Bruising leads to inflammation and possibly suppuration, resulting in severe pain and lameness. The 'corn' may need lancing to enable drainage, followed by treatment with foot baths and poultices. Antibiotic therapy helps combat infection.

corncockle poisoning A toxic condition caused by ingestion of the corncockle (*Agrostemma githago*), a plant with reddish-purple flowers that was formerly a common weed of cornfields and may sometimes occur in large numbers. It contains the saponin githagenin, which causes poisoning of pigs and poultry. A single dose of about 5 g/kg of the plant will cause acute signs and continuous feeding of small amounts causes chronic poisoning.

cornea The transparent part of the fibrous layer at the front of the eyeball. It has a smaller radius of curvature than the sclera, which it joins at the corneoscleral junction, or *limbus*. It refracts light rays onto the lens. The cornea contains no blood vessels. *See* eye.

corn lily *See* false hellebore poisoning.

cornu (*pl.* **cornua**) (in anatomy) A horn-shaped structure, such as the processes of the hyoid bone (*see* hyoid apparatus) and *thyroid carti-

lage, the main regions of the *lateral ventricles of the brain, or the two divisions of the *uterus in domestic mammals.

corona (in anatomy) A crown or crownlike structure.

corona radiata 1. The layer of follicular cells surrounding the oocyte after ovulation. **2.** The intermingled mass of fibres connecting the cerebral cortex with the *internal capsule and *corpus callosum in the brain.

coronary arteries The arteries supplying blood to the heart. The *left* and *right coronary arteries* arise from the left and right aortic sinuses respectively, just above the aortic valve.

coronary groove The depression on the inner aspect of the proximal or coronary border of the horse's hoof. It is occupied by the coronary *corium.

coronary sinus The principal vein receiving the veins of the heart. It lies in the coronary groove and drains into the right atrium ventral to the opening of the caudal vena cava.

coronary thrombosis Occlusion of a coronary artery by a blood clot (thrombus). It commonly causes a heart attack in humans but is rare in animals.

coronavirus A family of RNA *viruses having enveloped helical *capsids. They cause respiratory and intestinal diseases in pigs, dogs, and cattle (e.g. neonatal calf diarrhoea).

coronet The part of the *pastern of the horse just above the hoof.

corpora quadrigemina Two pairs of small swellings (colliculi) situated in the midbrain roof in mammals. The anterior (rostral) pair deal with visual reflexes while the posterior (caudal) pair relay auditory stimuli.

corpus (*pl.* **corpora**) Any mass of tissue that can be distinguished from its surroundings.

corpus albicans The residual tissue that remains in the ovary at the point where a *corpus luteum regresses after it ceases its secretory activity. In the bovine ovary the corpus albicans has a white scarlike appearance.

corpus callosum The broad band of nervous tissue that connects the two cerebral hemispheres, forming the largest of the commissures of the brain. Its constituent parts are rostrum, genu, truncus, and splenium. *See* cerebrum.

corpus cavernosum The spongy erectile tissue of the *penis or *clitoris that fills with blood during sexual arousal thereby distending the organ. In the penis it is attached to the ischium by paired crura and surrounded by the ischiocavernosus muscle, and works in conjunction with the *corpus spongiosum. In ruminants and boar much fibrous tissue is present, minimizing the degree of distension during erection, whereas in the stallion and dog much more distension can occur. In carnivores the corpus cavernosum is partly ossified to form the *os penis.

corpuscle Any small particle, cell, or mass of tissue.

corpus luteum (*pl.* **corpora lutea**) The glandular structure in the ovary that forms from a ruptured tertiary follicle after *ovulation. It secretes the hormone *progesterone, which prepares the uterus for implantation of the embryo. If implantation does not occur, the corpus luteum becomes inactive and degenerates. If implanta-

tion does occur, the corpus luteum continues to secrete progesterone until late in pregnancy, when the placenta has taken over this function. *See* ovarian follicle.

corpus spongiosum The spongy erectile tissue that surrounds the urethra within the *penis. Along with the *corpus cavernosum it fills with blood during sexual arousal thereby distending the penis. It enlarges to form the bulb of the penis and the *glans penis.

corpus striatum The region of alternating masses of grey and white matter lying deep within each cerebral hemisphere in the brain. It consists of the caudate nucleus, internal capsule, lentiform nucleus, external capsule, and the claustrum.

corridor disease A type of *East Coast fever caused by the protozoan parasite *Theileria parva lawrencei*, which is contracted by cattle from wild buffalo and is transmitted by the same vector tick as East Coast fever. The disease is clinically similar to East Coast fever but the parasites are scarcer in lymphocytes and red blood cells. The disease is named after the corridor between the Hluhluwe and Umfolozi Game Reserves in Zimbabwe where it was first described, but has been recognized in many areas of East Africa where cattle, buffalo, and the vector tick coexist.

cortex (*pl.* **cortices**) The outer part of an organ, situated immediately beneath its capsule or outer membrane; for example, the *adrenal cortex* (*see* adrenal glands), *renal cortex* (*see* kidney), or *cerebral cortex.

corticosteroid Any steroid hormone synthesized by the cortex of the *adrenal gland, or any related synthetic steroid. There are two main groups of corticosteroids. The *glucocorticoids* are essential for the utilization of carbohydrate, fat, and protein by the body and for a normal response to stress. The *mineralocorticoids* (e.g. *aldosterone) regulate salt and water balance.

The major naturally occurring glucocorticoid hormones are hydrocortisone (cortisol) and corticosterone. Their secretion is controlled by the adenohypophysis via *adrenocorticotrophic hormone, and there is a diurnal pattern of secretion, with a peak in the morning in most species (the peak occurs in the evening in nocturnal animals, e.g. cats). Secretion increases during periods of stress. The corticosteroids are distributed throughout tissues, are metabolized in the liver, and excreted conjugated to glucuronide in the urine (synthetic corticosteroids are metabolized more slowly and can be excreted unchanged in the urine). The effects of glucocorticoids include enhanced *gluconeogenesis (causing increased blood glucose and liver glycogen), muscle catabolism, lipolysis with redistribution of body fat stores, decreased absorption and increased urinary excretion of calcium, reduced levels of growth hormone, decreased bone growth, increased blood haemoglobin, increased numbers of circulating polymorphonuclear cells, decreased circulating lymphoid cells and eosinophils, and suppression of cell-mediated immunity.

The glucocorticoids have marked anti-inflammatory effect, with activity at all stages of *inflammation. They produce a decrease in capillary permeability, reduced exudation and migration of inflammatory cells, stabilization of lysosomal membranes, a reduction in phagocytosis by macrophages, inhibition of the release of arachidonic acid (the precursor of the inflammatory mediators prostaglandins, leukotrienes, and thromboxanes), suppression of granulation tissue formation,

and reductions in collagen formation and fibroblast proliferation thus increasing the time taken for wound healing. Most glucocorticoids have some mineralocorticoid activity, although this is more marked with natural hormones and the early synthetic corticosteroids, such as prednisone and prednisolone. This mineralocorticoid activity mimics the action of aldosterone, causing sodium retention, hypokalaemia, and fluid retention. The more recent synthetic corticosteroids have much less mineralocorticoid and mainly glucocorticoid activity.

Therapeutic uses Hydrocortisone and various synthetic corticosteroids are used therapeutically as anti-inflammatory agents, to treat adrenal insufficiency, and to correct certain metabolic disorders. *Hydrocortisone* has a short duration of action and is used topically, orally, or injected. It penetrates cells rapidly after intravenous injection and is therefore used in the treatment of shock. Long-term systemic use should be avoided because of mineralocorticoid side-effects.

Prednisone and *prednisolone* were the first synthetic corticosteroids. They have increased anti-flammatory activity and less mineralocorticoid activity than the natural steroids. Their duration of action is short and they can be used for alternate-day therapy. *Methylprednisolone* has a longer duration of action. *Flumethasone, betamethasone,* and *dexamethasone* are more potent and have a much longer duration of action, with activity for several days or weeks with some esters. Daily therapy with these drugs causes cumulative effects and possible toxicity. *Betamethasone-17-valerate* and *beclomethasone* are used topically; unlike the other corticosteroids they are poorly absorbed into the circulation. *Triamcinalone* has the least mineralocorticoid effect and has a long duration of action.

The corticosteroids are well absorbed after oral administration or they can be injected intramuscularly; soluble compounds can be given intravenously. The effective dose varies among individuals within a species. Topical preparations are used on skin, eyes, and mucous membranes. Intra-articular injection is used but requires strict asepsis. Corticosteroids are used for their anti-inflammatory properties in, for example, skin conditions, arthritis, allergic respiratory disease, eye inflammation, colitis, autoimmune diseases, and cerebral and spinal oedema. Steroids, especially hydrocortisone, can be given intravenously at high dose rates to maintain tissue perfusion and the microcirculation and thus prevent irreversible shock. Corticosteroids are used to increase blood glucose in the treatment of ketosis and pregnancy toxaemia. They can also be used to suppress immune reactions and hence control autoimmune diseases (e.g. systemic lupus erythematosus, rheumatoid arthritis) and in the chemotherapy of lymphoid tumours. Dexamethasone and betamethasone can be used to induce parturition with a live foetus.

Toxicity is unlikely with a single dose or short-term corticosteroid therapy. Sudden withdrawal of corticosteroids after prolonged use can produce shock, and the animal is unable to respond to stress. The prolonged use of corticosteroids can induce hypokalaemia, alkalosis, oedema, glycosuria, hyperglycaemia, muscle weakness, osteoporosis, increased appetite, increased thirst, hair loss, and increased susceptibility to infection. It is possible to prevent these signs by using alternate-day therapy with short-acting corticosteroids. This allows secretion of natural corticosteroids on the drug-free days. Also the drugs should be given at the peak of natural glucocorticoid secretion.

corticosterone The major glucocorticoid hormone of rodents. See corticosteroid.

corticotrophin See adrenocorticotrophic hormone.

cortisol See corticosteroid.

cortisone A steroid hormone, closely related biochemically to hydrocortisone and corticosterone, found in extracts of adrenal tissue. One of the first adrenal steroids to be isolated and synthesized, it has potent glucocorticoid activity and some mineralocorticoid action; it acts after being converted to hydrocortisone in the body. See corticosteroid.

Corynebacterium A genus of non-motile rod-shaped Gram-positive *bacteria. They do not produce spores but have a tendency for snap division, thus forming clusters resembling 'Chinese letters'. A number of species are commensals, but *C. diphtheriae*, *C. pyogenes*, *C. ovis*, *C. suis*, *C. renale*, and *C. equi* (now renamed *Rhodococcus equi*) are pathogenic (erythromycin/rifampin therapy has reduced mortality to about 10–15%). The term *diphtheroid* is often used to describe corynebacteria other than *C. diphtheriae*, the causative agent of diphtheria in young children. *C. pyogenes* is distributed worldwide and commonly found as a saprophyte on the mucous membranes of healthy animals. However, following abrasion or injury the organism causes localized infections (e.g. umbilical infection), and when the host is weakened due to other infections (usually viral) it is one of the commonest secondary invaders. This species causes widespread pyogenic infections in most domestic animals, *pneumonia, *arthritis, *mastitis, and *abscesses in cattle, and secondary pneumonias after viral infections. *C. pyogenes* and *Streptococcus dysgalactiae* are the main causes of summer mastitis in Europe, for which flies are important vectors. *C. pyogenes* is also associated with pneumonia, arthritis, and other suppurative conditions in pigs and sheep, mastitis in mares, and *pyometra in dogs.

C. equi, a common commensal of the horse, causes pneumonia in young foals with a very high mortality rate (more than 60%). *C. ovis* (also known as *C. pseudotuberculosis*) causes *caseous lymphadenitis in sheep and goats (in North America, subcutaneous abscesses in horses). *C. renale* is responsible for *cystitis and *pyelonephritis in cattle, while *C. suis* causes cystitis and pyelonephritis in sows.

cost- (costo-) *Prefix denoting* the rib. Example: *costectomy* (excision of).

costal Of or relating to the ribs.

cotyledon One of the units of the foetal part of the *placenta in ruminants. It consists of chorionic villi and contributes to a *placentome. *See also* caruncle.

coughing A reflex action causing sudden expulsion of air from the respiratory tract, usually in an attempt to expel foreign particles or exudate. Irritation of almost any part of the respiratory mucosa elicits the coughing reflex. Certain types or patterns of cough may provide specific clinical signs of diagnostic value.

coumarin A lactone derivative of coumarinic acid found in many plants, including the sweet clovers *Melilotus officinalis* and *M. alba*. These are found wild in British pastures but are used as forage crops in North America and Australia. Under certain conditions, for example when sweet clover is weather damaged after cutting and becomes mouldy, the harmless coumarin is converted to *dicoumarol, which is an anticoagulant. Spoiled sweet clover may cause internal or external bleeding in cattle.

cow 1. An adult female ox, generally after its first pregnancy, although the term *heifer may be used until after the second pregnancy. *See* cattle husbandry. **2.** The adult female of various large mammals, such as the elephant, whale, rhinoceros, and seal.

cowbane poisoning *See* hemlock water dropwort poisoning.

Cowdria A genus of *rickettsiae containing a single species, *C. ruminantium*. This causes *heartwater in cattle, sheep, goats, and wild ruminants in many parts of Africa. The disease is transmitted by ticks and the rickettsiae multiply in the white blood cells and blood-vessel endothelium of their host.

cow kennel A form of housing for dairy cows in which *cubicles are provided for individual cows but only the lying-in area of the cubicle is covered. This system combines the advantages of cubicle housing, i.e. reduced bullying and bedding requirements, with low construction costs and better ventilation.

Cowper's glands *See* bulbourethral glands.

cowpox A mild infectious disease of cattle characterized by teat lesions in cows and caused by an orthopoxvirus (*see* poxvirus). The disease is rare and maintained not in cattle but probably in rodents. The virus causes small swellings, particularly on the teats of lactating cows and on the mouths of suckling calves. The swellings become fluid-filled vesicles and then pustules. These rupture and become scabs. However, healing may be delayed by milking procedures, and secondary infection and *mastitis are frequent. The disease spreads quickly through a susceptible herd. Cowpox virus will infect many other mammals, including humans, and may occasionally be seen in zoo and circus animals. In cats, cowpox virus causes pustules on the legs and head and may produce more severe internal lesions. *Compare* bovine herpes mamillitis; pseudocowpox; vaccinia.

cox- (coxo-) *Prefix denoting* the hip. Example: *coxalgia* (pain in).

Coxiella A genus of *rickettsiae in the family Rickettsiaceae consisting of a single species, *C. burnetii*. It is similar to the genus *Rickettsia* in its staining properties and host preferences, but unlike other rickettsiae it is unusually stable outside the host cell. *C. burnetii*, the causative agent of *Q fever, is widely distributed and has been isolated from a variety of ticks and from many animal species, including all the major livestock species. In humans it causes a disease resembling influenza and atypical *pneumonia. It causes abortion in sheep and goats but only mild disease in other animals. *C. burnetii* is very resistant to physical and chemical agents. Meat can remain infected for over a month and the organism can survive for periods exceeding one year in dried tick faeces, the wool of infected sheep, and in skimmed milk. Transmission to humans is by inhalation but other animals are infected by direct animal-to-animal contact or via ticks. Carnivores, such as dogs, may possibly be infected by consuming infected placentas.

Coxsackie virus A subclass of the *enteroviruses, also called echovirus. It includes important pathogens of cattle and pigs.

cracked heel Inflammation of the skin behind the pastern of the horse, characterized by cracks and fissures. Repeated exposure to cold and/or wet conditions underfoot is thought to be the main cause. Pain is usually intense with severe lameness. Treatment entails removing the animal to better conditions, cleaning the affected skin, and dressing with an antiseptic ointment. Recovery usually follows unless the lesions are chronic and well established.

cramp Painful spasmodic contraction of muscles, commonly occurring during and after strenuous exercise. It is common in racing horses and greyhounds and may be related to local accumulation of toxic metabolites in muscles, especially after unaccustomed exertion. 'Crampy' is a hereditary spastic condition of cattle in which the muscle contractions may be so frequent and severe as to require euthanasia. *See also* exercise problems (horses); Scottie cramp.

crani- (cranio-) *Prefix denoting* the skull.

cranial 1. Relating to the cranium. **2.** Relating to the head or front end of the body.

cranial nerves Those nerves that arise directly from the brain. In mammals and birds there are 12 pairs (see illustration), each designated by a Roman numeral and name: I *olfactory; II *optic; III *oculomotor; IV *trochlear; V *trigeminal; VI *abducens; VII *facial; VIII *vestibulocochlear; IX *glossopharyngeal; X *vagus; XI *accessory; and XII *hypoglossal. *Compare* spinal nerves.

craniopharyngioma A rare and benign tumour reported mainly in young dogs and arising from the epithelial remnants of Rathke's pouch in the *pituitary gland. The growths may be located below or above the *sella turcica and consist of alternating solid and cystic areas. They are often large and grow underneath the

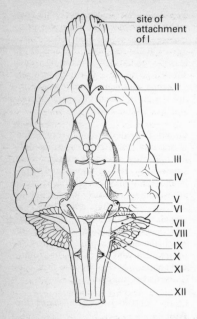

site of
attachment
of I

II

III
IV
V
VI
VII
VIII
IX
X
XI
XII

The cranial nerves attaching to the brain

brain, extending dorsally into the hypothalamus and thalamus. Clinically, they may result in generalized *hypopituitarism or functional abnormality of the brain or cranial nerves.

cranium The part of the *skull that contains the brain, which lies in the cranial cavity.

crazy chick disease See encephalomalacia.

CRD (chronic respiratory disease of poultry) See avian mycoplasmosis.

creatinase An enzyme involved in the conversion of creatine to creatinine.

creatine A molecule found in muscle and derived from arginine, glycine, and methionine. Its phosphate, *creatine phosphate* (*phosphocreatine, phos-*

phagen), acts as a store of high-energy phosphate in muscle and serves to maintain adequate amounts of *ATP (the source of energy for muscular contraction).

creatinine A substance derived from creatine and creatine phosphate in muscle. Creatinine is excreted in the urine. Its concentration in the blood is used as an index of glomerular filtration rate, and hence renal function.

creep feeding The provision of solid food to young mammals prior to *weaning to encourage them to consume non-milk diets. Creep diets are introduced gradually as the digestive enzymes changes to cope with solid food. Such diets should be of good *palatability to promote consumption, be highly digestible, and have a high *nutrient density.

creosote A mixture of *phenols, principally guaiacol and creosol, which are obtained by distillation of wood tar. It is used as an antiseptic, disinfectant, and deodorant, and can be inhaled from a hot solution or given orally in a capsule to treat chronic bronchitis and bronchiectasis. It is a mild expectorant and has an antiseptic action in the airways. Creosote is also used as a wood preservative, and ingestion can cause toxicity (*see* phenol poisoning).

creosote poisoning See phenol poisoning.

crepitation A crackling or cracking sound or feeling. Crepitation may be present on movement of a dislocated or fractured limb. Palpation of subcutaneous emphysema also produces crepitation.

crepitus A grating sound heard when the fractured ends of bones rub together, or when the dry and eroded articular surfaces of a joint rub together in cases of chronic arthritis.

cresol (methylphenol) A *phenol derivative with a characteristic 'pine' smell, that is used as an antiseptic and disinfectant. Cresols act by denaturing protein and are bactericidal but have poor activity against viruses, fungi, and spores. Their effectiveness is reduced by alkaline pH and by the presence of organic debris (e.g. dirt). Cresols are used in 3–5% solutions for routine large-scale disinfection, and can be incorporated in sheep dips as an antibacterial. However, they are irritant to skin and are poisonous if taken internally. Care should be taken when disinfecting premises, especially catteries and kennels. Cresols are also available formulated in soaps.

crest A ridge or linear protuberance, particularly on a bone. Examples include the external sagittal crest (on the skull) and the iliac crest (of the ilium).

cretinism See congenital hypothyroidism.

crib-biting A vice of horses caused by inactivity and boredom. The horse grasps the front of its trough or other fixture between its incisors and, depressing its tongue, swallows air. Eventually this can result in undue wear of the incisors. The horse should be given a more interesting routine or change of environment to prevent the vice becoming established. Woodwork can be removed or treated with repellents in an attempt to combat the habit. A cribbing strap may also be effective. See also wind-sucking.

cricoid cartilage A ring-like cartilage of the *larynx forming joints with the two *arytenoid cartilages and the thyroid cartilage. Caudally it is joined to the trachea.

crista (*pl.* **cristae**) 1. The sensory structure within the ampulla of a *semicircular canal within the inner ear (see illustration). The cristae respond to changes in the rate of movement of the head, being activated by pressure from fluid in the semicircular canals. 2. One of the infoldings of the inner membrane of a *mitochondrion. 3. Any anatomical structure resembling a crest.

crooked toes (deviated toes) Physical deformity of the toes of poultry. It is relatively common, particularly in meat birds and in flocks affected by other leg disorders. The deformity usually starts in young birds but rarely causes walking difficulty, and is not of economic importance. The condition is not thought to be infectious; factors implicated include genetics, brooding under infrared lamps, and faulty hatching.

crop An expansible region of the oesophagus in birds. Situated in the lower part of the neck, its form varies between species, being saclike in the fowl but simply a spindle-shaped enlargement in the duck. It stores food and, in pigeons, produces the nutritive crop milk which is fed to the young. See alimentary tract.

crossbreeding The mating together of animals of different *breeds. The offspring of such a cross will all be identically *heterozygous for any *alleles that distinguish the pure breeds and hence are *homozygous in the parents. Because of this heterozygosity, crossbred animals cannot breed true. The breeds chosen for crossing can be carefully selected to give progeny with particularly useful combinations of parental traits, or in some cases to exploit the phenomenon of *heterosis. Crossbred progeny are widely used for meat production; most beef cattle are crosses between dairy cows and beef breed bulls chosen to produce offspring with optimal carcass qualities. In the sheep industry, meat lambs are often produced by ewes crossbred to be both highly fertile and good mothers, although not necessarily outstanding meat producers themselves. Such ewes are crossed with a ram from a selected meat-producing breed to produce a large crop of high-quality meat lambs. All progeny from crosses between the same two pure breeds are genetically very nearly identical to each other. They therefore have virtually identical husbandry requirements and can be reared successfully in groups, with conditions optimized.

cross-immunity An immune response elicited by one *antigen but directed against another. Such a response may occur in any or all of the possible immune mechanisms, including protection, *hypersensitivity, and *tolerance. Most frequently, cross-reacting antigens are chemically related. *See also* immunity.

crossing over (in genetics) The exchange of sections of chromatids between pairs of homologous chromosomes, which results in the recombination of genetic material. It occurs during *meiosis at a *chiasma.

cross-matching *See* blood typing.

croup The region of the back of a horse behind the saddle.

cruciate ligament One of two powerful ligaments of the stifle joint attaching the tibia to the femur. The *cranial cruciate ligament* runs from the cranial intercondylar area of the tibia to the lateral condyle of the femur. The *caudal cruciate ligament* runs from the caudalmost part of the intercondylar area of the tibia to the medial condyle of the femur. The two form a crosslike arrangement (see illustration). The cranial cruciate liga-

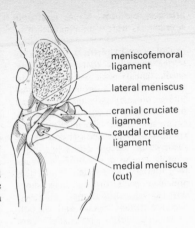

meniscofemoral ligament

lateral meniscus

cranial cruciate ligament

caudal cruciate ligament

medial meniscus (cut)

Cruciate ligaments of left stifle joint, medial aspect

ment is frequently damaged, especially in dogs, causing serious lameness and sometimes necessitating surgical replacement. *See* cruciate ligament rupture.

cruciate ligament rupture Damage to the *cruciate ligaments of the stifle joint. This occurs most often in the dog and usually affects only the cranial (anterior) cruciate ligament, although sometimes there is an associated tear of the medial collateral ligament. The result is instability of the joint; this can be demonstrated by the *anterior drawer sign*, in which the tibia can be displaced forward relative to the distal end of the femur. This injury regularly gives rise to osteoarthritis of the stifle with the development of a marked *synovitis and secondary *exostoses. In the acute stage there is marked disease of the affected leg, and if the ligaments on either side tear at the same time the dog may be temporarily unable to stand. Some cases will make a spontaneous clinical recovery, but many do not and insertion of a cruciate prosthesis or some other stabilizing operation is widely practised.

crude protein (CP) An estimation of the protein content of a feedstuff or diet equal to its percentage nitrogen content multiplied by a factor of 6.25. The value is only approximate since it includes nonprotein nitrogenous compounds, such as amides and amino acids, and does not take into account the varying nitrogen content of different proteins. *Digestible crude protein* (*DCP*) is the amount of crude protein in a diet that can be digested and absorbed by an animal, determined by digestibility trials. Values given are usually apparent not true digestibility. *See also* protein quality.

Cruelty to Animals Act (1876) (England and Wales) An Act of Parliament repealed by the *Animals (Scientific Procedures) Act (1986).

crural 1. Relating to the leg. **2.** Relating to a *crus.

crus (*pl.* **crura**) **1.** An elongated process or part of a structure. The *crura cerebri* are the paired bundles of nerve fibres running from the cerebral hemispheres and forming the ventral part of the midbrain. The right and left crura of the *diaphragm are the parts attaching it to the bodies of lumbar vertebrae. The paired crura of the *penis or *clitoris attach these structures to the ischium. **2.** The leg; i.e. the region of the hindlimb related to the tibia and fibula.

crush A device, usually constructed from tubular steel or wood, for holding or restraining cattle or other animals to enable routine procedures (e.g. worming, trimming feet) to be safely performed. Various designs are available with a range of features. Most restrain the animal by the neck with a moving bar or gate. Removable rear bars and side gates provide greater versatility. *See also* weighing methods.

crutching The shearing of wool from between and behind the legs and the tail of a sheep to reduce the incidence of *strike. It it best done in early to mid spring and again in the autumn.

cry- (cryo-) *Prefix denoting* cold.

cryoglobulin An abnormal plasma protein that gels when cooled. These proteins occur in collagen disorders, lymphoreticular disease, and in multiple *myeloma. In the latter condition in dogs, cryoglobulins have produced circulatory impairment and occlusion of fibrin or platelets to produce peripheral vascular thrombosis and paradoxical bleeding. They may also occur in *systemic lupus erythematosus in dogs.

cryoprecipitate A precipitate produced by freezing and thawing under controlled conditions. For example, a cryoprecipitate of certain plasma proteins is obtained by slowly thawing frozen plasma at around 4°C. It consists mainly of *fibrinogen, *coagulation factors V and VIII, and *plasminogen. The technique is thus a cheap and easy method of concentrating Factor VIII for the successful treatment of haemophilia, especially in dogs. The precipitate has a short storage life and is unstable when thawed, so it must be transfused immediately upon reconstitution.

cryostat 1. A chamber in which frozen tissue is sectioned with a *microtome. **2.** A device for maintaining a specific low temperature.

cryosurgery The use of extremely low temperatures to freeze and destroy unwanted tissues. The target tissues should be subjected to at least two freeze–thaw cycles and the temperatures should be −20°C or below. In veterinary practice either nitrous oxide probes or liquid nitrogen sprays are used. Cryosurgery can be used in areas and tissues not amenable to conventional sharp surgery, such as cutaneous and oral neoplasias and ulcerated areas. There is minimal scar formation. However, care must be taken to ensure that only the required area is frozen, and there is some risk of haemorrhage when the affected tissue sloughs, especially if there are large blood vessels in the area.

crypt A small sac, follicle, or cavity; for example the intestinal crypts (of Lieberkühn), which are intestinal glands. *See* intestine.

crypt- (crypto-) *Prefix denoting* concealed. Example: *cryptogenic* (of unknown origin).

cryptococcosis Disease caused by infection with the capsulated yeast *Cryptococcus neoformans. It affects a wide variety of mammalian species, but is most commonly reported in cats, dogs, cattle, and horses. The disease may be subacute, acute (rarely), or chronic. Granulomatous or mucopurulent lesions may occur in almost any part of the body, most often in the lungs, central nervous system, and nasal, ocular, and oral regions. As in humans, the lung may be the primary site of a sometimes asymptomatic infection, disseminating to other organs by lymphatic or haematogenous spread. In horses ingestion of the organism in swallowed exudate from nasal lesions can apparently lead to the development of granulomatous lesions in the stomach or intestine.

In **cattle**, *cryptococcal mastitis* can be severe, affecting many animals in one herd, but its development is slow and clinical signs are extremely varied. There is evidence of infection by implantation; the disease has been spread among cattle by the use of contaminated milking equipment. Severe swelling and distension of the affected quarter(s) may develop over many days and persist for several weeks, with a progressive reduction and abnormality in the gland secretion but little systemic effect. Other cows may show only a transient or mild swelling of infected quarters, or show no signs. Specific treatment has had little success and the disease is controlled by segregation of infected animals and strict hygiene.

Infection in **cats** and **dogs** usually becomes apparent as subcutaneous swellings, often on the face, or destructive granulomatous lesions involving nasal or oral mucosae. There may be a nasal discharge and signs of central nervous system involvement usually develop. The outcome is usually fatal in spite of treatment.

Diagnosis can be established by the microscopic demonstration in tissue or exudate of the characteristic globose yeast cells having only occasional buds and a wide mucilaginous capsule. Confirmation is by isolation and identification of the fungus in culture.

Cryptococcus A genus of *yeasts that are common inhabitants of the environment. Only *C. neoformans* is pathogenic, causing the disease *cryptococcosis. This organism has a wide capsule and is naturally present in the soil and particularly in accumulations of pigeon droppings.

cryptorchid (rig; ridgling) A male animal in which one or both testes (testicles) are retained in the abdomen or descend incompletely into the scrotum. The condition is hereditary and most frequently occurs in the horse and the pig. *Late cryptorchid* refers to the finding that some piglets may have two testicles at birth, one of which subsequently decreases in size and apparently ascends through the inguinal canal and disappears from the scrotum. A retained testis does not produce sperm but continues normal production of hormones. *Monorchid is often used synonymously with cryptorchid but strictly refers to animals that develop only one testicle.

cryptosporidiosis A disease of mammals (including humans) and birds caused by protozoan parasites of the genus *Cryptosporidium*. Clinical signs depend on the major site of infection. In mammals, the organism primarily parasitizes the intestine and disease is characterized by *enteritis, diarrhoea, and abdominal discomfort. In birds, disease is more usually associated with infection of the respiratory tract or eyes. In farm animals, disease is seen almost exclusively in young stock; older animals develop immunity. It is especially important as a cause of diarrhoea in 1–3-week-old calves, in which cryptosporidia may occur as the only pathogens or in concurrent infection with viruses or bacteria. Diagnosis is confirmed by the detection of cryptosporidial oocysts in stained faecal smears. Normally the disease is nonfatal and resolves within a few days as the host's immunity develops. No drug active against *Cryptosporidium* as yet been found. Bovine infections can infect humans, but most human infections are probably not derived from animals. Cryptosporidiosis appears to be rare in domestic pets.

Cryptosporidium A genus of protozoan parasites that infect a wide variety of mammals, birds, fish, and reptiles and cause the disease *cryptosporidiosis. The genus is probably worldwide in distribution and contains several species, some of which can apparently infect a wide variety of hosts. The parasites inhabit mucous membranes, usually in the

gut but, especially in birds, also in the respiratory tract. After a series of multiplications they produce round cysts, about 5 μm in diameter, which are shed in the faeces 3–5 days after infection. In some situations these cysts may mature inside the host, so beginning the cycle again. This can lead to chronic infections in immunosuppressed hosts. However, most cysts mature outside the host and, being reasonably resistant, will survive for weeks or months, contaminating the environment and providing a source of infection for other animals.

CSF *See* cerebrospinal fluid.

Ctenocephalides A very common genus of *fleas containing the dog flea, *Ctenocephalides canis*, and the cat flea, *C. felis*, both of which are easily transferred from pets to humans. *C. felis* often infests dogs.

cubicle An individual standing for a dairy cow, usually one of many in a cubicle house. The recommended dimensions are 2.2 m long by 1.2 m wide. The sides are generally constructed of tubular steel or wooden rails and cows have free access to and choice of cubicles. Cubicles are normally higher than the dunging passage behind the cow and slope towards the dunging passage. The *bedding, which can be sawdust, sand, peat, or chopped straw, covers a base of concrete or rammed chalk and is retained by a raised lip. *See also* cattle husbandry; cow kennel.

Cuboni test A test for pregnancy in mares involving the detection of high levels of *oestrogens in the urine. It is a laboratory method, requiring one urine sample to be taken between days 120 and 290 of gestation, although the most accurate results are obtained between days 150 and 250. *See also* pregnancy tests.

cud The mixture of fluid and suspended particles that is regurgitated from the reticulorumen of ruminants to be remasticated during *rumination.

Culex A genus of *mosquitoes found worldwide and distinguished by their habit of holding the body parallel to the surface when feeding. Some species transmit the nematode worms, *Wuchereria bancrofti* and *Dirofilaria immitis*, that cause filariasis in humans and *dirofilariasis in dogs.

culmen One of the lobules of the vermis of the *cerebellum in the brain.

culture 1. A population of microorganisms, usually bacteria, grown in a solid or liquid laboratory medium (*culture medium*), which is usually *agar, broth, or *gelatin. A *pure culture* consists of a single bacterial species. A *stab culture* is a bacterial culture growing in a plug of solid medium within a bottle (or tube); the medium is inoculated by 'stabbing' with a bacteria-coated straight wire. A *stock culture* is a permanent bacterial culture, from which subcultures are made. *See also* cell culture. **2.** To grow bacteria or other microorganisms in cultures.

cumulus oophoricus The follicular cells surrounding the oocyte in a mature *ovarian follicle. They are shed with the oocyte at ovulation then regroup around the oocyte to form the corona radiata.

cuneate fasciculus A large paired tract of nerve fibres located in the spinal cord. It transmits impulses from sense organs concerned with touch, pressure, position, and movement in muscles of the forelimb and front part of the trunk. The impulses are received by the *cuneate nuclei in the medulla oblongata of the brain.

cuneate nuclei Discrete masses of nerve cells lying in the medulla oblongata in the brain that receive the fibres of the *cuneate fasciculus from the spinal cord. The *medial cuneate nucleus* relays impulses to the thalamus; the *lateral cuneate nucleus* sends fibres to the cerebellum.

cupola Any of several dome-shaped anatomical structures, e.g. the *cupola pleurae* is the apex of the pleural sac which extends through the thoracic inlet into the root of the neck.

curare An extract obtained from the bark of certain South American vines (*Chondodendron* and *Strychnos* species). It contains D-tubocurarine, which competes for acetylcholine at nerve-muscle junctions and produces flaccid paralysis of skeletal muscles. Hence its local use as an arrow poison. D-tubocurarine was formerly used as a drug to provide muscle relaxation during anaesthesia and in cases of tetanus. In cases of overdosage intermittent positive-pressure ventilation should be used until spontaneous respiration recommences. An *anticholinesterase (e.g. neostigmine or edrophonium together with atropine) will lead to more rapid recovery and has been used as a reversing agent.

curettage The use of a *curette to remove tissue or foreign material from the body. *See also* debridement.

curette A spoon-shaped surgical instrument used for the removal (curettage) of tissue or foreign material from the body. It is useful particularly for firm or calcified tissue, for areas with poor access for other surgical instruments, or for the removal of diseased tissue with an ill-defined border. Veterinary uses include the removal of intervertebral disc material during spinal disc *fenestration, removal of tissue around a sinus tract, and removal of nasal and oral mucosal tumours.

curled toe paralysis An ultimately fatal condition of chicks and poults aged up to 3 weeks, caused by *vitamin B_2 (riboflavin) deficiency in starter diets. It is readily corrected by feeding supplementary riboflavin.

Cushing's disease *See* hyperadrenocorticism.

cusp 1. Any of the cone-shaped prominences on teeth, especially the molars and premolars. **2.** A pocket or fold of the membrane (endocardium) lining the heart or of the layer of the wall of a vein, several of which form a *valve. When the blood flows backwards the cusps fill up and become distended, so closing the valve.

cutaneous Relating to the skin.

cutaneous trunci muscle The sheet of muscle lying immediately below the skin over the lateral wall of the thorax and abdomen. Its contraction results in twitching of the skin.

cutter A meat pig that has reached so-called 'cutting weight', or one that is destined to do so. In Britain the final liveweight is around 80 kg, reached at around 130 days. It is intermediate between the lighter *porker and a *baconer.

cyan- (cyano-) *Prefix denoting* blue.

cyanide Any inorganic salt or complex containing the cyanide ion, CN^-. Cyanides are used in industry, as fertilizers, for sterilization of buildings and soil, and as rodenticides.
Cyanide poisoning In animals this is most likely to occur with hydrocyanic acid (prussic acid), which is formed in the body by the enzymatic hydrolysis of cyanogenetic glycosides (*see* cherry laurel poisoning; linseed

poisoning). These glycosides are inactivated when the plants are dried during hay-making. Ruminants, especially cattle, are more susceptible to poisoning than monogastric animals. Cyanides act rapidly, causing sudden death or, in smaller doses, excitement, salivation, dyspnoea, muscle tremors, convulsions, coma, and death. Cyanide reacts with the enzyme cytochrome oxidase in the mitochondria of cells, inhibiting cell respiration, and the tissues become anoxic. Postmortem examination reveals brightred blood that clots slowly, and a characteristic 'bitter almond' smell of hydrocyanic acid may be detected in stomach contents. Treatment consists in administering 1% sodium nitrite intravenously followed by 25% sodium thiosulphate intravenously, or intravenous sodium thiosulphate alone. The thiosulphate converts cyanide to the nontoxic thiocyanate, which is excreted in the urine. Methaemoglobinuria is a side-effect, although this is less severe when sodium thiosulphate is used alone. Oral administration of sodium thiosulphate can reduce the absorption of cyanide from the gastrointestinal tract.

cyanocobalamin *See* vitamin B_{12}.

cyanosis Bluish discoloration of the skin and mucous membranes due to lack of oxygen in the blood. It occurs in certain conditions affecting the heart and circulatory system, such as *heart failure, and in animals immediately following their birth before proper breathing is established (although discoloration persists if there is congenital heart disease). It also occurs in animals suffering from *pneumonia in which the functioning of the lungs is badly impaired so that the blood is not properly oxygenated. *Methaemoglobinaemia due to nitrate or nitrite poisoning sometimes discolours the blood beneath mucous membranes in a similar way but this must be distinguished from cyanosis.

cyclic AMP (cAMP) *See* AMP.

cyclophosphamide A cytotoxic drug used mainly in small animals in the treatment of various tumours, especially lymphosarcomas and mammary and lung carcinomas. Because of its immunosuppressive properties it is also used in the treatment of rheumatoid arthritis and other immune-mediated diseases. Given orally, it is well absorbed from the gut and is activated by metabolism in the liver. Two toxic metabolites, phosphoramide mustard and acrolein, are also produced. Cyclophosphamide acts as an alkylating agent, binding to DNA and interfering with cell division in rapidly proliferating tissues. Cytotoxicity occurs only in rapidly dividing cells. There is depression of the bone marrow and immunosuppression due to destruction of lymphocytes. Cells can become resistant to the action of cyclophosphamide. Possible side-effects with long-term therapy include lymphopenia, anaemia, occasionally thrombocytopenia, vomiting, and haemorrhagic cystitis. Constant checks on blood cell counts are necessary. The haemorrhagic cystitis is probably caused by the toxic metabolites and its incidence can be reduced by the co-administration of acetylcysteine.

cyclopropane A gaseous anaesthetic, discovered in 1929, that is rarely used nowadays because of its highly inflammable and explosive nature. Insoluble in blood, it gives rapid induction and recovery and therefore can be used to produce anaesthesia quickly during surgery. It is nonirritant with low toxicity to tissues, but causes cessation of breathing (apnoea) and sensitizes the heart to catecholamines producing cardiac arrhythmias.

Cyclops A minute crustacean found worldwide in fresh and brackish waters. It is the intermediate host for the parasitic nematodes *Gnathostoma* (of dogs, cats, pigs, and humans) and the guinea worm (*see* Dracunculus), a parasite of dogs and humans in the tropics.

cypermethrin *See* pyrethroids.

cyst 1. An abnormal sac or closed cavity lined with epithelium and filled with fluid or semisolid matter. Various types of cyst can occur in different parts of the body. *Retention cysts* arise when the outlet of a glandular duct bcomes blocked, as in a sebaceous cyst or a salivary gland cyst. Tumours may become cystic by secreting mucus or other substances, and *ovarian cysts form because of failure of a follicle to rupture. Some cysts are congenital, for example due to the absence of drainage ducts in polycystic kidneys; branchial cysts develop in the neck from remnants of foetal branchial tissue. Surgical removal of cysts may sometimes be necessary. **2.** A dormant stage produced during the life cycle of certain protozoan parasites, such as *Eimeria*, that is capable of infecting a suitable host when ingested. **3.** A structure (hydatid cyst) that forms around larvae of *Echinococcus* tapeworms infesting the tissues of their hosts (*see* hydatidosis).

cyst- (cysto-) *Prefix denoting* **1.** a bladder, especially the urinary bladder. **2.** a cyst.

cysteine *See* amino acid.

cystic 1. Of, relating to, or characterized by cysts. **2.** Of or relating to the gall-bladder or urinary bladder.

cysticercosis Disease due to infestation by cysticerci, the larval forms of tapeworms of the genus *Taenia* (*see* cysticercus) that are found in various vertebrate species acting as intermediate hosts of the tapeworms. Infestation follows the ingestion of eggs deposited in the faeces of a final host, which carries the adult tapeworm in its intestine. The most important veterinary cysticercoses usually cause no signs in the intermediate host but do cause losses by reducing carcass quality. Moreover, there is a risk that humans may become infested with the adults of certain tapeworms by eating cysticerci in undercooked meat, particularly beef and pork.

Infestation of humans by the pork tapeworm (*T. solium*) is more serious than by the beef tapeworm (*T. saginata*) because the former is sometimes associated with a peculiar form of cysticercosis in which a human becomes the intermediate as well as the final host. This condition probably arises from self-infestation with *T. solium* eggs or by eggs being carried by reverse peristalsis from the small intestine to the stomach, where they hatch, penetrate the stomach wall, and grow to cysticerci in various tissues. A severe and possibly fatal form of cysticercosis in the central nervous system may result.

cysticercus (*pl.* **cysticerci**) The larval stage in the life cycle of tapeworms of the genus *Taenia, which parasitize cats, dogs and humans. It consists of a spherical fluid-filled sac in which the head and neck of a single tapeworm are invaginated. The cysticercus develops from the *oncosphere in the intermediate host, usually cattle, sheep, or pigs, where it may cause the disease *cysticercosis, although there may be no symptoms in the intermediate host. In sheep it is known as *Cysticercus ovis* and is the larval stage of *T. ovis*, a parasite of dogs. In cattle it is known as *C. bovis*, an oval structure up to about 1 cm long and the larval stage of *T. saginata*, the

beef tapeworm of humans. *C. cellulosae*, an elongated cyst slightly smaller than *C. bovis*, is the larval stage of *T. solium* of humans and is found in the pig. When the carcass of the intermediate host is eaten by the final host, each cysticercus develops into an adult tapeworm. *See also* bladderworm.

cystine An *amino acid consisting of two molecules of cysteine linked by a disulphide bond. It occurs in extracellular proteins, for example serum proteins, digestive enzymes, and hair.

cystitis Inflammation of the urinary bladder. It is often part of a more widespread infection of the urinary tract. Infection with bacteria, for example *Corynebacterium renale* in cattle, *C. suis* in pigs, or *Escherichia coli* or *Proteus* in dogs, may be responsible. Stones in the bladder may either initiate cystitis, or follow secondarily from the condition (*see* calculus). There are signs of pain and depression, and the animal passes discoloured urine at frequent intervals. Antibiotics effect a temporary cure but relapse is common. *See also* polypoid cystitis.

cystography *Radiography of the urinary bladder. This is undertaken rarely in adult large animals but is commonly used in small animal practice and occasionally in neonates of large animals. Plain radiographs may be helpful but often contrast material is used. A radio-opaque solution can be instilled into the bladder lumen, or air may be used (*pneumocystography*). Alternatively, radio-opaque solution may be instilled then drained, followed by air – i.e. a double-contrast study. This often gives a good outline of the bladder wall. Cystography may be used to aid diagnosis of bladder stones (using air), bladder neoplasia, and bladder rupture.

cystolithiasis 1. The formation of calculi (*see* calculus) or concretions within the urinary bladder. *See* urolithiasis. 2. Disease caused by the presence of such calculi.

cystoscopy The direct visual examination of the interior of the urinary bladder by means of a special optical instrument (*cystoscope*) inserted via the urethra. Diathermy electrodes for removing tumours or biopsy forceps for removing samples of tissue can be used in conjunction with cystoscopes.

cystotomy Surgical incision into the urinary bladder. It is commonly performed for the removal of urinary calculi and for the investigation of bladder lesions.

cyt- (cyto-) *Prefix denoting* 1. cell(s). 2. cytoplasm.

-cyte *Suffix denoting* a cell.

cytidine A molecule containing cytosine and the sugar ribose. *See also* nucleoside.

cytochrome Any of a group of *haem-containing proteins that participate in oxidation-reduction reactions in the cell. Cytochromes form part of the electron-transport chain in *mitochondria; electrons are transferred by reversible changes in the iron of the haem group between the reduced Fe(II) and oxidized Fe(III) states.

Cytoecetes A genus of *rickettsiae that parasitize the white blood cells of sheep and cattle and are transmitted by ticks. *C. phagocytophila* is the causative agent of *tick-borne fever of sheep and cattle and is mainly found in Europe. It can also affect deer and goats. *C. ondiri* causes *petechial fever in East African cattle.

cytogenetics The study of inheritance in relation to cell structure and function, especially the role of the *chromosomes. In veterinary practice this is mostly concerned with the clinical effects of abnormalities of chromosome structure or number that have arisen by *mutation. Such mutations often reduce the fertility of the organism concerned. Chromosomal aberrations are usually diagnosed first from cultured lymphocytes obtained from the peripheral blood circulation, but cultures from other tissues may also be used. In some cases the most useful information comes from studies of meiotic cells obtained by biopsy from the testis.

cytokinesis Division of the cytoplasm of a cell, which occurs at the end of cell division, after division of the nucleus, to form two daughter cells. *Compare* karyokinesis.

cytology The study of cells. *See* anatomy.

cytolysis The breakdown of cells, particularly by destruction of their outer membranes.

cytomegalovirus A group of viruses belonging to the *herpesvirus family and characterized by a relatively slow reproductive cycle and enlargement of the infected cells (cytomegaly). Most members can enter into latent interactions with their host (*see* latency).

cytometer An instrument for determining the number of cells in a given quantity of fluid, such as blood, cerebrospinal fluid, or urine.

cytopenia A deficiency of cells, usually one or more of the various types of blood cell.

cytoplasm The jelly-like substance that surrounds the nucleus of a cell.

cytoplasmic inheritance A form of inheritance in which the genes are carried by a vehicle other than the chromosomes, most usually the *mitochondria (and, in plants, the chloroplasts) in the cytoplasm. The genes do not segregate in the same fashion as chromosomal genes. Since most mitochondria are transmitted in the cytoplasm of the ovum (egg cell), the offspring receive many more cytoplasmic genes from their mother than their father. The young therefore tend to resemble their mother much more than their father in those characters controlled by cytoplasmic genes.

cytosine One of the nitrogen-containing bases (*see* pyrimidine) that occurs in the nucleic acids DNA and RNA.

cytotoxic drug An agent that destroys cells or inhibits their growth. Cytotoxic drugs are used in cancer *chemotherapy and to some extent in the treatment of rheumatoid arthritis. Such drugs exploit the differences in enzyme activity and growth rate exhibited by tumour cells compared to normal cells, and may act at all stages of the cell cycle or only at specific stages of cell division. Combinations of drugs are used to improve the overall kill. All cytotoxic drugs kill normal rapidly dividing cells as well as tumour cells, and toxicity is common, with such side-effects as diarrhoea, vomiting, liver damage, kidney damage, bone marrow depression, anaemia, leucopenia, and increased susceptibility to infection (immunosuppression). Careful monitoring of the patient during therapy is therefore essential. Many tumour cells become resistant to cytotoxic drugs after a period of therapy.

Various groups of cytotoxic drugs are used: alkylating agents, such as *cyclophosphamide and chlorambucil; antimetabolites, for example methotrexate (usually used with folinic acid), cytosine arabinoside, and 5-fluorouracil; antibiotics, for instance *actinomycin D, adriamycin, bleomycin, and mytogillin; plant products, including vinblastine, *vincristine, and podophylotoxin; and other agents, such as procarbazine and nitrosourea compounds. Many of these agents have been used in human cancer chemotherapy and are now being evaluated in animals.

D

dacry- (dacryo-) *Prefix denoting* 1. tears. 2. the lacrimal apparatus.

dactyl- *Prefix denoting* the digits. Example: *dactylomegaly* (abnormal size of).

dairy cattle Cattle bred and maintained specifically for milk production. In the UK the predominant dairy breeds are Friesian, Holstein, Ayrshire, Guernsey, and Jersey. The once popular Dairy Shorthorn has now been superseded. *See* cattle husbandry; milking.

Dallis grass poisoning *See* paspalum staggers.

dangerous dog Any dog that constitutes a danger to the public. In Britain, if a dog is judged by a magistrates' court to be dangerous and not kept under proper control, the court may order the owner to keep the dog under proper control, or order the dog's destruction. *See also* Dogs Act (1906).

dangerous drugs *See* Misuse of Drugs Act (1971).

Dangerous Wild Animals Act (1976) (England and Wales) An Act of Parliament that controls the keeping of dangerous animals. It provides that no person shall keep an animal listed in the Schedule to this Act unless he or she holds a licence granted by a local authority. The Act does not apply to circuses, licensed pet shops, or zoos. The local authority will not grant a licence unless it is satisfied that this would not be contrary to the public interest on the grounds of safety, nuisance, or any other reason. The licensee must be insured against liability for any damage caused by the animal. Each licence lasts until the end of the calendar year. The premises must be inspected by a veterinarian on behalf of the local authority before a licence is granted.

dapsone An antimicrobial sulphone drug used in the treatment of leprosy. It is effective against many spore-forming organisms, including *Bacillus* species and coccidia. It also possesses anti-inflammatory properties. Chemical name: **diaminodiphenylsulphone**.

dark-cutting beef A condition in which the muscles of freshly killed cattle are very much darker than normal. It is much commoner during cold frosty weather and is thought to be due to severe stress.

Darrow's solution A solution of potassium chloride, sodium chloride, and sodium lactate that is used therapeutically for fluid and electrolyte replacement.

dart syringe A piece of equipment for administering tranquillizers to animals too wild or unmanageable to be caught. A special syringe and needle are fired from a gun or crossbow and on striking the animal these inject a precomputed dose of tranquillizer subcutaneously or intramuscularly. Use of this technique has enabled the handling and examination of non-domesticated species.

DDT (dichlorodiphenyltrichloroethane) A chlorinated hydrocarbon compound, that was formerly widely used as an insecticide but is now restricted because of its persistence and toxicity. Insoluble in water but very soluble in fats and oils, DDT is rapidly absorbed when taken orally in solution in vegetable oil and can penetrate intact skin when applied in oil or in an emulsion. After absorption it is stored in body fat and persists there for several months. It is excreted in milk, and high concentrations are found in butter made from contaminated milk. DDT does not have a rapid 'knock-down' effect, and many insects now show resistance. Toxicity in all species is due to damage to the nervous system, with such signs as incoordination, convulsions, paralysis, and death. Other signs include inappetence and, in birds, poor egg hatchability or failure to lay. Toxicity is usually chronic, accompanying a build-up of the compound in adipose tissue. Animals low in body fat and young animals are much more susceptible, as DDT stored in fat is immobilized. However, if the fat reserves are mobilized, for instance during starvation, the DDT is released and acute toxicity can occur.

de- *Prefix denoting* **1.** removal or loss. Examples: *demineralization* (of minerals from bones or teeth); *devascularization* (of blood supply). **2.** reversal.

deadly nightshade poisoning A toxic condition due to ingestion of deadly nightshade (*Atropa belladonna*), not to be confused with woody nightshade (*Solanum dulcamara*). The plant contains the alkaloids atropine, hyoscine, and hyoscyamine, which also occur in henbane (*Hyoscyamus niger*) and thornapple or jimson weed (*Datura stramonium*). Atropine produces dry mouth, rapid pulse, dilated pupils with impaired vision, and constipation. Nervous excitement and delirium are followed by death. Rabbits can eat the plants with impunity as their liver contains an enzyme that inactivates the alkaloids; their muscles have a high alkaloid content, and dogs have died after catching and eating such rabbits. Cattle and sheep are resistant to moderate doses, probably because the alkaloids are diluted and degraded in the rumen. Treatment is by repeated injection of small doses of *physostigmine or *arecoline, until the pupils begin to constrict.

deafness Complete or partial loss of hearing in one or both ears. It may be due to a defect in the conduction of sound from the external to the internal ear, or to a lesion in the cochlea in the inner ear, the auditory nerve, or the auditory centres in the brain. The external ear may become blocked with debris or inflamed; similarly the middle ear may be damaged or destroyed by inflammation and pus (*see* otitis). Excessive noise may damage the auditory nerve and neuroepithelial cells. Also, some drugs (e.g. streptomycin) can impair hearing, and deafness can also be the result of congenital defects or even hereditary tracts. A hearing test coupled with examination may locate the site and nature of the problem. Treatment of simple occlusion of the external ear (e.g. due to mite infestation) can be completely successful. Lesions to the middle and inner ear are much less amenable to treatment.

deamination The replacement of an *amine group of a molecule with oxygen. Enzymatic deamination occurs in the liver and is important in aminoacid metabolism, especially in their degradation and oxidation. The amino group is removed as ammonia and excreted, either unchanged or as urea (in mammals) or uric acid (in birds).

death camas poisoning A toxic condition due to ingestion of perennial herbaceous plants belonging to the genus *Zigadenus* (death camas), which is distributed throughout the USA. They contain steroid alkaloids that cause salivation, vomiting, muscular weakness, convulsions, coma, and death. The treatment is symptomatic.

debeaking The removal of the front portion of the upper beak, and sometimes the point of the lower beak, in birds. It is frequently carried out in poultry to reduce the risk of *cannibalism and *feather pecking. About 30% of the upper beak is removed, using special equipment. If too little is removed, the procedure is largely ineffective; if too much is cut, severe haemorrhage may occur. Debeaking is usually performed at day old and may need to be repeated subsequently. There is some controversy over the degree of pain involved, and objections to the procedure have been raised on humanitarian grounds.

debridement The surgical excision of necrotic or severely damaged nonviable tissue from wounds prior to their closure. Debridement is essential because the presence of necrotic tissue will inevitably lead to wound breakdown if it is incorporated in a wound closure.

debudding *See* disbudding.

dec- (deca-) *Prefix denoting* ten.

decalcification Loss or removal of calcium salts from a bone or tooth.

deci- *Prefix denoting* a tenth.

decidua (*pl.* **deciduae**) The part of the *endometrium that is shed with the *foetal membranes at parturition in carnivores.

declive A lobule in the caudal lobe of the vermis of the *cerebellum, lying just caudal to the primary fissure.

decongestant A substance that reduces or relieves congestion in the upper respiratory tract by reducing local inflammation of the airway. Among the drugs used as decongestants are *adrenergic drugs (e.g. ephedrine), *antihistamines, and nonsteroidal anti-inflammatory drugs (see NSAID). They are often administered by inhalation but some can be given orally. Overuse of inhalational preparations may increase mucosal irritation.

decubitus The recumbent position. It is commonly associated with disease and an inability of the animal to move normally. Because of the prolonged pressure that is applied to the body surface, ischaemic necrosis of the skin is liable to take place resulting in *decubitus ulcers*. Animals affected by various forms of paralysis resulting in recumbency require special nursing to avoid this form of skin damage, which can be very difficult to correct once it has occurred.

decussation A point at which a pair of structures of the body cross to the opposite sides. The term is used particularly for the point at which nerve fibres cross over in the central nervous system.

deep litter A system of keeping laying hens, usually in controlled environment buildings, in which the birds are allowed to roam freely over floors covered with wood shavings or other suitable *litter. Eggs are laid in nesting boxes and thus require manual collection. Although meeting many of the welfare objections to the use of battery cages (see battery systems), deep litter systems may be associated with increased *cannibalism and a high incidence of broken, cracked, or dirty eggs.

defective (in virology) Describing a virus that is incapable of independent growth in a particular host cell. Such viruses may be able to grow in the presence of a helper virus or in a different host cell.

deferent 1. Carrying away from or down from. **2.** Relating to the ductus deferens.

defibrillation The administration of a controlled electric shock to restore normal heart rhythm in cases of cardiac arrest due to *fibrillation. Defibrillation is most often required during surgery. The electrodes of the apparatus (*defibrillator*) may be applied to the chest wall or directly to the heart after the chest has been opened.

defibrination The removal of *fibrin, one of the plasma proteins that causes coagulation, from a sample of blood. It is normally done by whisking the blood with a bundle of fine wires, to which the strands of fibrin that form in the blood adhere.

deficiency disease Any of a wide range of diseases involving deficiency of one or more vital nutrients. Some are simple deficiencies involving only one nutrient while others are complex resulting from multiple deficiencies acting together. The deficiency may follow a shortage or absence of the nutrient in the diet or may arise due to interaction between various components of the diet, for example, excess of one component may restrict the availability of another. Deficiency diseases include several well-known metabolic disorders. For instance, energy deficiency leads to *ketosis, protein deficiency causes *anaemia, deficiencies of *calcium and *phosphorus affect bone development, and magnesium deficiency (*hypomagnesaemia) leads to grass tetany. Trace element deficiencies lead to nonspecific signs of ill-thrift though some specific diseases occur, such as *goitre with iodine deficiency and *muscular dystrophy with selenium deficiency. Deficiencies of the various *vitamins also cause characteristic diseases.

degeneration The deterioration and loss of specialized function of the cells of a tissue or organ. Various causes include defective blood supply, metabolic disorders (e.g. ketosis with fatty change in the liver), nutritional deficiency (e.g. vitamin E/selenium deficiency leading to myopathy), or poisoning. Calcium salts, fat, or fibrous tissue may be deposited in the affected organ or tissue.

degenerative myopathy See Oregon muscle disease.

dehiscence A splitting open, as of a surgical wound.

dehorning The surgical removal of well-established *horns. It is most frequently performed in adult cattle to avoid the risk of accidental injury among the members of a herd. A local anaesthetic is first administered, most commonly by injection in the vicinity of the cornual branch of the zygomatic nerve. In bulls with large horns additional infiltration of anaesthetic around the posterior aspect of the base of the horn is often necessary. The horns can be removed by saw, shears, or embryotomy wire. Bleeding from the cut base of the horn can be partly controlled by haemostatic forceps. *Cauterization of the cut blood vessels can also be employed safely in cattle.

dehydration Excessive loss of water from the body. The common causes are deficient water intake, especially in hot arid countries, disease (e.g. *diarrhoea), or excessive sweating. Animals with an inadequate supply of drinking water normally resorb water from their alimentary tract so that the faeces become unusually dry. In cattle lactation declines and the milk becomes concentrated. Blood changes, which can be used diagnostically, include increased osmolarity and increased concentrations of sodium, protein, and red blood cells. Increasing levels of potassium eventually induce irregularity of heart beat, which may lead to death from *heart block.

In dairy cattle dehydration can be a behavioural problem. Cows tend to drink collectively, so some may remain thirsty if the water trough empties before all receive enough. Very thirsty cattle may suffer from water toxicity when the supply is renewed: a large intake of water causes a sudden decline of osmotic pressure in the gut which in turn induces haemolysis of red blood cells in the intestinal mucosa causing *haemolytic anaemia and *haemoglobinuria.

dehydroepiandrosterone See androgen.

dehydrogenase An *oxidoreductase enzyme that uses a *coenzyme, such as NAD or FAD, as a hydrogen acceptor in the oxidation of a metabolite. An example is lactate dehydrogenase, which catalyses the reaction: lactate + NAD = pyruvate + NADH.

delayed hypersensitivity Type IV *hypersensitivity.

deletion (deficiency) (in genetics) A type of chromosome mutation in which a part of the chromosome, and therefore the genes carried on that part, is lost.

delmadinone acetate A steroid drug that blocks the actions of *androgen hormones. It is available as an aqueous suspension for intramuscular or subcutaneous injection in small animals, and is used in the treatment of testosterone-dependent conditions, for example hypertrophy of the prostate and perianal tumours. Some behavioural problems, including aggression and hypersexuality, may be improved using delmadinone. Tradename: **Tardak**.

deltoid A muscle that runs from the acromion and spine of the *scapula to the humerus. It is an important flexor of the shoulder.

demi- Prefix denoting half.

demodectic mange (follicular mange) A form of *mange caused by parasitic *mites of the genus *Demodex. Unlike other mange mites Demodex live deeply in the skin of their host in the hair follicles. There are many species, each specific to a particular host species. Some hosts, including humans, are affected by two species of Demodex. In many animals Demodex is a harmless parasite, but in dogs, cattle, pigs, goats, hamsters, and to a lesser extent cats, it may be a serious problem. The disease is transferred by an infested female when suckling her young, and does not become apparent for several months, when localized bald patches (alopecia) develop. There may be recovery at this stage; alternatively there may be progression to generalized demodectic mange in which the entire body becomes affected with alopecic thickening of the skin, pustules, and nodule formation (red mange or pustular mange). This may be life-endangering. Demodectic mange is of major importance in cattle in many parts of the world. Mange is diagnosed by the isolation of the parasite in skin combings or in

skin scrapings examined with the microscope. It is treatable with organochloride or organophosphorus preparations with the isolation and disposal of infested fomites. Until recently demodectic mange in dogs was difficult to treat; however, an effective *acaricide is now available.

Demodex A genus of minute ectoparasitic *mites, known as follicle mites because they live in the hair follicles and sebaceous glands of mammals. Follicle mites have a soft elongated body with 8 short legs and piercing mouthparts. The whole life cycle is spent on the host and takes about 2–4 weeks. They are responsible for the condition known as *demodectic mange. D. canis is found on dogs, while D. folliculorum, common on humans in many temperate regions, is also found on cattle, sheep, and dogs.

demulcent A soothing agent used particularly to treat irritated mucous membranes, for instance in cases of inflammation of the throat or alimentary tract. Examples are glycerine, borax, bismuth, olive oil, and arrowroot.

demyelination Breakdown of the *myelin sheaths that surround and support nerve axons in the central and peripheral nervous systems. Copper deficiency leads to *swayback in newborn lambs, in which demyelination of spinal tracts in utero causes the characteristic incoordination and paralysis seen in the lambs.

denaturation Alteration of the three-dimensional structure of a *macromolecule, especially a *protein or nucleic acid. This loss of native structure can be caused by a variety of agents (e.g. heat, extremes of pH, ionic detergents) and usually leads to the irreversible loss of biological activity. Proteins are denatured by cooking, which generally aids their *digestion in the gut.

dendrite One of the shorter branching processes of the cell body of a *neurone, which carries nerve impulses to the cell body. A neurone may have one single or multiple dendrites.

denervation Severance of the nerve supply to a part of the body. This may be caused by injury or disease, or it may occasionally form part of a surgical procedure. Denervated muscles become paralysed and lose their normal tone. The muscle fibres shrink and are replaced by fat. Also, denervation impairs the ability of tissues to heal and renew themselves and exacerbates degenerative changes. However, denervation of a limb or part of a limb removes sensation in that area and is thus potentially useful in preventing pain. It may also be of value in treating certain spastic conditions.

dengue *See* ephemeral fever.

dens A tooth or tooth-shaped structure, particularly the cranially directed process of the *axis otherwise termed the odontoid process.

dent- (denti-, dento-) *Prefix denoting* the teeth. Example: *dentoalveolar* (relating to the teeth and associated jaw).

dental caries Disease of the hard tissue of the tooth, characterized by demineralization and enzymic degradation by bacteria, which are generally derived from pre-existing *dental plaque. It is common in mature horses and sheep, but rare in dogs and cats. Extraction of the affected tooth may be required, followed by attention to accompanying oral conditions, including plaque and *tartar.

dental formula *See* dentition.

dental plaque A dense nonmineralized mass of bacteria (chiefly oral species of *Streptococcus* and *Actinomyces*) and their extracellular polymers that adheres firmly to tooth surfaces, particularly near the gum margins. Plaque formation is accelerated by certain diets, leading to *gingivitis and eventually *dental caries and *periodontal disease. *See also* tartar.

dental pulp The loose connective tissue that fills the pulp cavity of a *tooth. It contains numerous blood vessels and nerves. The peripheral layer of odontoblasts progressively lays down *dentine, so gradually reducing the size of the pulp cavity.

dentate (denticulate) Serrated; having toothlike projections. For example, the dentate nucleus of the *cerebellum or the denticulate ligament of the spinal meninges.

dentigerous cyst A cystic congenital malformation seen mainly in young horses and dogs when active tooth development is taking place. In **horses** dentigerous cysts are found in the temporal region near the base of the ear and, sometimes, in the forehead or in the paranasal sinuses. The lesion is lined by a smooth membrane and usually contains a single tooth, which is either embedded in the petrous part of the *temporal bone or lying free in the lumen. Rupture of the cyst through the skin releases a clear gelatinous fluid and leads to fistula formation with infection frequently occurring. In the **dog** cysts containing one or more teeth are found adjacent to the normal teeth in the mouth.

dentine The layer of tissue that surrounds the pulp cavity of a *tooth. Highly mineralized and resembling

dentition

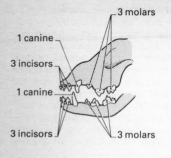

The deciduous teeth of a puppy

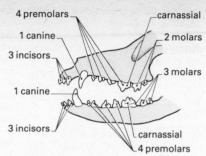

The permanent dentition of an adult dog

Dental formulae of various mammals

Species	Temporary dentition	Permanent dentition
Horse	I 3/3 C 0/0 M 3/3	I 3/3 C 1*/1* Pm 3 or 4/3 M 3/3
Ox	I 0/3 C 0/1 M 3/3	I 0/3 C 0/1 Pm 3/3 M 3/3
Sheep	I 0/3 C 0/1 M 3/3	I 0/3 C 0/1 Pm 3/3 M 3/3
Pig	I 3/3 C 1/1 M 3/3	I 3/3 C 1/1 Pm 4/4 M 3/3
Dog	I 3/3 C 1/1 M 3/3	I 3/3 C 1/1 Pm 4/4 M 2/3
Cat	I 3/3 C 1/1 M 3/2	I 3/3 C 1/1 Pm 3/2 M 1/1

*Usually absent in the mare

modified bone, it is formed throughout life by odontoblasts in the *dental pulp.

dentition The number, type, and arrangement of the teeth (*see* tooth) in the mouth. The *temporary* or *deciduous dentition*, sometimes known as the milk teeth, consists of incisors, canines, and molars and is ultimately replaced by the *permanent dentition*, consisting of incisors (I), canines (C), premolars (P), and molars (M). (See illustration.) The numbers of each type of tooth present in just one side of the mouth is given by the *dental formula*, which varies according to species (see table). Numbers above and below in each fraction refer to the upper and lower jaw respectively.

Each number is doubled to obtain the total present in the mouth as a whole.

deoxycholic acid *See* bile acids.

deoxycorticosterone (11-DOC) A steroid metabolite in the biosynthesis of *corticosterone. Small quantities are secreted by the adrenal gland. Synthetic 11-DOC has potent mineralocorticoid and slight glucocorticoid activity and can be used for the treatment of Addison's disease. *See* corticosteroid.

deoxyribonuclease An *enzyme that catalyses the hydrolysis of *DNA. *See also* endonuclease; exonuclease; restriction endonuclease.

deoxyribose The *pentose sugar found in *DNA.

depilation *See* epilation.

depluming mite A tiny parasitic mite, *Cnemidocoptes gallinae*, that burrows into the feather shafts of poultry causing feather loss. The rump, back, head, and neck of the bird may develop bald patches, and the skin can become red and inflamed. Apart from discomfort, infestation can result in reduced egg output due to the metabolic cost of continual feather regrowth. Individual birds (over 8 weeks old) can be dipped in a solution of a suitable *acaricide. Poultry houses should be thoroughly cleaned and sprayed with an acaricide.

depluming scabies Former name for infestation with the *depluming mite, *Cnemidocoptes gallinae*.

depolarization The sudden surge of charged particles across the membrane of a nerve or muscle cell that accompanies a physicochemical change in the membrane and cancels out, or reverses, its resting potential to produce an *action potential. The passage of a *nerve impulse is a rapid wave of depolarization along the membrane of a nerve fibre.

depraved appetite *See* pica.

depressor A muscle that causes lowering of part of the body. The *depressor labii inferioris* is a muscle that draws down and everts the lower lip.

derm- (derma-, dermo-, dermat(o)-) *Prefix denoting* the skin.

-derm *Suffix denoting* **1.** the skin. **2.** a germ layer.

Dermacentor A cosmopolitan genus of hard *ticks (but restricted to the southwest in the UK) and known as the wood tick or dog tick in the USA. The adults are bloodsucking ectoparasites of humans, dogs, cattle, and horses, while the larvae and nymphs are parasites of smaller mammals. Adults can survive for $1-2\frac{1}{2}$ years without food if a suitable host is not available. They transmit *Rocky Mountain spotted fever to humans and dogs in the USA, the protozoan parasite *Babesia*, which causes fevers in cattle, horses, and dogs in Europe, and in the USA and Canada, their bite can cause *tick paralysis.

dermal Relating to or affecting the skin, especially the *dermis.

Dermanyssus A genus of *mites including the red fowl mite or chicken mite (*D. gallinae*), a bloodsucking ectoparasite of poultry found worldwide. *See* red mite.

dermatitis Inflammation of the skin. It may be caused by pathogens, parasites, sunlight, poor nutrition, allergy, friction, or chemical irritants.

Dermatobia A genus of flies containing the *torsalo fly.

dermatology The medical specialty concerned with the diagnosis and treatment of skin diseases.

dermatome **1.** (in embryology) The part of the *somite in the early embryo that forms the dermis of the skin and associated structures. **2.** (in clinical practice) In the fully developed animal, an area of skin whose sensory nerve supply corresponds to one segment of the spinal cord. These areas form a series of overlapping bands along the trunk and more elongated regions on the limbs. Pinpoint-

dermatomycosis

ing loss of sensation to a particular dermatome can help in diagnosing the level of lesions in the spinal cord. **3.** (in surgery) An instrument used for cutting thin slices of skin for certain skin-grafting operations.

dermatomycosis Infection of the skin by a fungus. This is usually a dermatophyte (the condition is then preferably called *dermatophytosis), but occasionally other fungi invade the skin, such as *Candida albicans* and *Fusarium* spp.

Dermatophagoides A genus of *mites found in house dust and poultry and pig meal in Europe and North America. It may cause allergies, such as *asthma and *dermatitis.

dermatophilosis Disease caused by infection with *Dermatophilus congolensis*, an aerobic actinomycete (filamentous bacterium belonging to the order Actinomycetales). *D. congolensis* causes various skin disorders in a wide range of species. These include *lumpy wool and *strawberry foot rot (both in sheep), *mycotic dermatitis (cattle and sheep), and *rain scald (horses). These conditions may also be referred to as *streptotrichosis. The bacterium has so far been found only in clinical materials from infected animals and humans. It has initially narrow (1–2 μm) branching filaments, which widen and divide transversely into narrow segments, then divide two or three times longitudinally to form a wide band up to eight cells across, each cell forming a coccoid spore. Each spore can, in the presence of free moisture, become a motile biflagellate zoospore, 0.3–0.5 μm in diameter. The zoospores can initiate infection, developing into a new branching system of filaments. However, some skin damage appears necessary for infection to become established, for instance maceration by prolonged exposure to rain or damage by ectoparasites.

dermatophyte Any of various closely related fungi belonging to the genera *Trichophyton*, *Microsporum*, and *Epidermophyton*, distributed worldwide. These organisms can utilize *keratin as a nutrient source and therefore many can parasitize the nonliving cornified integument of animals – feathers, hair, skin, and nails – causing disease (*dermatophytosis), such as *ringworm. Some inhabit the soil, especially where it is rich in shed keratin, occasionally (e.g. *M. gypseum*) or rarely (e.g. *T. ajelloi*) causing infection. Some pathogenic species tend to be confined to humans (e.g. *E. floccosum*); others affecting animals have a wide host range (e.g. *T. mentagrophytes*), some a narrow range (e.g. *M. equinum*). However, most include humans and a few are transmitted to humans frequently (e.g. *M. canis*, *T. verrucosum*). In some animal species, ringworm is caused predominantly by a single dermatophyte (*T. verrucosum* in cattle, *M. canis* in cats). In other host species (e.g. horses) more than one dermatophyte may regularly be involved. Dermatophyte infections are seldom reliably identifiable by the clinical disease they provoke, which may also vary considerably from one host to another.

dermatophytosis Infection by any *dermatophyte fungus. When involving the skin and hair the disease produced may be termed *ringworm or *favus, depending upon its nature; dermatophytosis involving the nail is one form of *onychomycosis. Microsporosis and trichophytosis are more specific terms used when the infecting dermatophyte is known to belong to the genus *Microsporum* or *Trichophyton*, respectively.

dermatosis vegetans An inherited skin disease of pigs, controlled by an autosomal *recessive allele. Skin lesions may be visible at birth but are more likely to develop during the first 3 weeks of life. Areas affected are the belly and the inner surface of the thigh, which develop erythema and subsequently a grey-brown crust. There are also lesions on the coronets of the feet, which become red with the accumulation of blood and fluid (erythema and oedema), and the hoof wall is uneven, brittle, and thickened. The forefeet are more extensively affected than the hindfeet. The performance of affected animals is poor and many die within the first few weeks. Those surviving more than 4 weeks show regression of the lesions. Respiratory dysfunction is also common, with the lungs showing lymphocytic and histiocytic infiltration. Individuals rarely survive beyond 6 months.

dermis (corium) The layer of the skin that lies underneath the *epidermis. It consists of connective tissue and contains blood and lymphatic vessels, sensory nerve endings, hair follicles, and sweat glands and sebaceous glands and their ducts.

dermoid 1. Resembling the skin. **2.** See dermoid cyst.

dermoid cyst A *cyst occurring in the skin and containing hair follicles, sebaceous and apocrine glands, and keratinous material. They are considered to be congenital and/or hereditary in origin, may be single or multiple, and are generally seen in young animals of either sex. There is a predisposition for the condition in Kerry blues and Rhodesian ridgebacks; in the latter breed, it takes the form of single or multiple sinuses along the dorsal midline and is thought to be inherited as a simple recessive trait. Surgical excision is usually curative.

derris An insecticide obtained from the roots of certain leguminous shrubs of the genus *Derris*. The active principle is *rotenone: prepared derris contains about 5% rotenone. Derris is available in dusting powders or combined with soaps and detergents in insecticidal washes. It is relatively nontoxic to mammals, is nonpersistent, and kills insects by contact and ingestion. Fleas and lice are susceptible, but derris is ineffective against mange mites. Treatment should be continued over several days to kill all parasites. Derris is toxic to fish, causing paralysis, convulsions, and death. Toxicity in small animals can result in vomiting and dullness. Local accumulation of the powder in the coat can cause skin irritation in large animals exposed to heavy rain. Lonchocarpus is a similar insecticide obtained from the roots of the related genus *Lonchocarpus*.

desensitization (hyposensitization) A therapeutic process designed to reduce *hypersensitivity in cases of allergy. It involves the administration of antigens in such a way as to alter the balance of the various immune responses. For instance, shifting the balance of *antibody production towards IgG production and away from IgE may produce clinical desensitization. Such a shift can sometimes be induced by administering the antigen parenterally rather than locally.

desmosome See macula adherens.

desnooding The removal of the *snood that lies over the upper beak in turkeys. It should be undertaken as soon as possible after hatching and reduces problems associated with *cannibalism in turkey flocks.

desquamation The process by which the outer layer of the *epidermis is removed by scaling.

detamidine See xylazine.

detergent An agent that is added to water to dissolve fats and oils, thus allowing them to be washed from surfaces. Detergents can be used alone or in combination with antimicrobial compounds to increase their penetration and effectiveness. The *cationic detergents are used as antiseptics and disinfectants. *See also* surfactant.

detoxication (detoxification) The process whereby toxic substances are removed or toxic effects neutralized. It is one of the functions of the liver.

detumescence Subsidence of a swelling.

deut- (deuto-, deuter(o)-) *Prefix denoting* two, second, or secondary.

deviated toes *See* crooked toes.

dew claw The first digit in the paw of the dog. It is regularly present in the forepaw and has a bony connection with the rest of the limb. In the hindpaw, it is frequently absent (although in some cases it can be duplicated) or is attached only by a fold of skin making it particularly liable to accidental damage. Hence, it is frequently removed surgically shortly after birth.

dexamethasone *See* corticosteroid.

dextran A water-soluble polymerized sugar of high molecular weight produced by bacterial action on sucrose. Purified solutions of dextrans with specified average molecular weights are available (e.g. Dextran 40 with an average molecular weight of 40 000) for use as blood volume expanders in the treatment of haemorrhage and shock. The high-molecular-weight polysaccharides remain in the bloodstream thus improving circulation. However, the larger molecules may cause sludging of blood cells in the small capillaries.

dextr- (dextro-) *Prefix denoting* **1.** the right side. Example: *dextroposition* (displacement to the right). **2.** (in chemistry) dextrorotation.

dextrin A *polysaccharide formed by the partial hydrolysis of starch or glycogen. Dextrins are soluble in water and yield maltose and ultimately glucose on further hydrolysis.

di- *Prefix denoting* two or double.

dia- *Prefix denoting* **1.** through. **2.** throughout or completely. **3.** apart.

diabetes insipidus A metabolic disease characterized by excessive thirst (polydipsia) and the production of large volumes of dilute urine. *Primary pituitary diabetes insipidus* is due to a lack of the pituitary hormone *vasopressin. Consequently, water is not properly reabsorbed from the collecting ducts of the kidney. The resultant dehydration causes excessive thirst to compensate for the fluid loss. The disease is treated by replacing the vasopressin using slowly absorbed injectable vasopressin tannate in oil (pitressin) or synthetic arginine vasopressin (DDAVP, desmopressin) as a nasal spray or by drops on the conjunctiva. Transient diabetes insipidus can occur with cranial trauma, although recovery usually follows when swelling subsides and the pituitary stalk becomes revascularized. *Primary nephrogenic diabetes insipidus* (*NDI*), due to lesions or malfunctioning of the kidney tubules, is very rare. More common in animals is *secondary NDI*, which involves severe polyuria and polydipsia. Any factor interfering with the interaction between vasopressin and the renal vasopressin cellular receptors, causing loss of hypertonicity of the renal interstitium, or affecting renal tubular cell function can cause secondary NDI. Examples are *pyometra with resultant coliform endotoxaemia, hypercalcaemia, liver disease, excessive glucocorticoids (*see* corticosteroid), *pyelonephritis, *hyperthyroidism, and *hypokalaemia.

diabetes mellitus A disease involving disordered carbohydrate metabolism caused by inadequate *insulin production by the beta cells of the pancreatic islets. In *Type I diabetes mellitus* (*insulin-dependent diabetes mellitus* or *juvenile diabetes mellitus*) almost no insulin is produced, whereas in *Type II diabetes mellitus* (*non-insulin-dependent diabetes mellitus* or *adult onset diabetes mellitus*) some insulin continues to be secreted. Genetic make-up appears to be a factor in many individuals, and islet cell autoimmune phenomena may be involved in Type I disease. Insulin deficiency causes decreased glucose uptake, a shift to noncarbohydrate forms of energy, acidosis, ketosis, elevated levels of glucose in the blood (*hyperglycaemia), and glucose in the urine (glycosuria). This causes osmotic diuresis, with increased urine production and dehydration, and consequent increased thirst. The condition leads ultimately to coma and death. Type I disease may have a sudden onset, often in young individuals, and the signs are more severe than those of Type II disease, which typically develops gradually in adult animals and has a chronic course.

diakinesis The final stage in the first prophase of *meiosis, in which homologous chromosomes, between which crossing over has occurred, are ready to separate.

dialysis A method of separating particles of different dimensions in a liquid mixture, using a thin semipermeable membrane whose pores are too small to allow the passage of large particles, such as proteins, but large enough to permit the passage of solutes. A solution of the mixture is separated from distilled water by the membrane; the solutes pass through the membrane into the water while the proteins, etc., are retained. The principle of dialysis is used in the artificial kidney.

diamonds Purple or red swollen diamond-shaped areas in the skin of pigs suffering from the mild (urticarial) form of *swine erysipelas. The lesions turn brown and are seen much more clearly after slaughtered pigs have been passed through the hot water in the scalding tank.

diamphenethide A flukicidal drug used to treat acute *fascioliasis in sheep. It is administered orally and is converted to its active form in the liver. The mode of action is unknown but may involve the inhibition of energy metabolism in flukes. This drug has greater activity against the immature parasites in the liver parenchyma than the adults in the bile ducts. Toxicity is low but with overdosage there may be temporary impairment of vision and wool loss. Tradename: **Coriban**.

diapedesis *See* transmigration.

diaphoresis Sweating, especially profuse sweating brought about by the administration of drugs (*see* diaphoretic).

diaphoretic An agent that increases the rate of sweat production (*diaphoresis). Several drugs cause this as a side-effect, including prostaglandins and *pilocarpine.

diaphragm The dome-shaped musculotendinous septum separating the thorax and abdomen. The muscular peripheral part is attached to the lumbar vertebrae by the left and right crura, and to the ribs, costal cartilages, and sternum. The central part is tendinous. The diaphragm plays an important role in breathing, contracting and flattening when air is inspired thereby increasing the capacity of the thoracic cavity. With each expiration it relaxes and returns to its domed shape. The diaphragm is innervated by the phrenic and intercostal nerves, and it has openings through which the aorta, thoracic duct, oesophagus, vagus nerves, and caudal vena cava pass between thorax and abdomen. See illustration.

diaphragmatic rupture/hernia A tear or rupture of the thoracic diaphragm permitting the displacement, or herniation, of abdominal organs into the thorax. It is most commonly the result of injury. Extensive intrusion of abdominal contents into the chest will result in acute respiratory embarrassment. Occasionally only a portion of the liver is displaced through a small hole in the diaphragm and this will cause respiratory embarrassment to develop slowly, as fluid from the congested liver lobe gradually accumulates in the chest. Surgical correction is required in all cases.

diaphysis The shaft (central part) of a long bone, or that part of a long bone which develops from the primary centre of ossification. *Compare* epiphysis.

diaphysitis Inflammation of the diaphysis (shaft) of a bone, through infection or rheumatic disease. It may result in impaired growth of the bone and consequent deformity.

diarrhoea (scouring) Abnormally frequent or copious evacuation of the bowel, usually involving the production of watery faeces. The most important cause is inflammation of the small or large intestines (*see* colitis; enteritis), commonly the result of infection with bacteria (such as *Campylobacter*, *Escherichia coli*, and

Salmonella), *rotaviruses, or protozoa (e.g. *coccidiosis and *cryptosporidiosis). *Johne's disease is a chronic bacterial infection of the intestine in ruminants causing persistent diarrhoea. Heavy infestations of intestinal parasites can also cause diarrhoea, and diarrhoeal movements can be triggered or exacerbated by stress. Absorption of fluid and nutrients is impaired and these are lost in the faeces. Severe or prolonged diarrhoea leads to ill-thrift, wasting, and dehydration of body tissues. The intestinal mucosa may be permanently damaged unless treatment is prompt. The animal may need supportive therapy, such as fluid replacement to counter dehydration.

diarthrosis *See* synovial joint.

diastase An enzyme that hydrolyses starch in barley grain to produce maltose during the malting process. It has been used to aid the digestion of starch in some digestive disorders. *See also* amylase.

diastole The period of the cardiac cycle during which the heart muscle, especially of the ventricles (*ventricular diastole*), is relaxing and the chambers of the heart are refilling. *Compare* systole.

diathermy The production of heat in a part of the body by means of a high-frequency electric current passed between two electrodes. As a form of therapy, diathermy can be used for acute and chronic muscle and joint injuries. The heat produced gives pain relief and promotes healing. In surgery the electrical energy is concentrated in a more limited area: one electrode is in the form of a *diathermy needle* or knife and the other is a moistened pad in contact with the animal's body. This can be used for coagulation of small blood vessels, for transection of tissue where bleeding would otherwise be a problem (such as muscle), and for removal of tissue that would be difficult to remove by other surgical means, for example oral mucosal lesions. It is often used in the surgical treatment of canine anal *furunculosis. Diathermy must be used with care during surgery because it acts by tissue destruction. *See also* electrocautery; electrocoagulation.

diathesis (*pl.* **diatheses**) Predisposition to pathological change or disease. Relatively few syndromes are referred to as diatheses in veterinary medicine, the classic examples being the conditions known collectively as *haemorrhagic diathesis.

diaveridine *See* coccidiostat.

diazepam A tranquillizer and anticonvulsant that is given intravenously to treat status epilepticus (*see* epilepsy) and seizures associated with strychnine poisoning and tetanus. It is also given orally or intramuscularly prior to *myelography to help prevent convulsions, and has been tried in the treatment of aggressive behaviour in dogs. It is thought to act by potentiating the effects of gamma amino butyric acid (GABA), an inhibitory transmitter in the central nervous system, and by reducing the turnover of noradrenaline, dopamine, and C5-hydroxytryptamine.

diazinon *See* organophosphorus (OP) compounds.

diazoxide A drug used in small animals to treat hypertension. It can be administered orally or intravenously, and causes a rapid fall in blood pressure, increased cardiac output, and mild tachycardia. Diazoxide produces dilatation of arterioles but has little effect on large veins; there is marked sodium and water retention and

oedema develops unless diuretics are co-administered.

dichlorophen An anthelmintic drug effective against certain tapeworm infestations (e.g. *Taenia* and *Dipylidium* in dogs and cats and *Monesia* in sheep). Toxicity is low but vomiting and diarrhoea may occur and a large amount of the drug is required for effective dosing. It is now rarely used.

dichlorvos *See* organophosphorus (OP) compounds.

dicoumarol A *coumarin derivative that interferes with the blood clotting mechanism and is used as a rodenticide and an anticoagulant. Dicoumarol and other closely related compounds inhibit *prothrombin production in the liver by competing with vitamin K. Synthesis of coagulation factors VII and X is also affected. Dicoumarol does not affect preformed circulating prothrombin and thus it takes 24–48 hours for the depletion of coagulation factors and clinical signs of poisoning to occur. Toxicity is greater with continuous small doses. The consequences are increased clotting time and greater fragility of blood capillaries with increased likelihood of haemorrhage. Some rats are now resistant to the effects of dicoumarol, probably because they metabolize the drug rapidly. Dicoumarol has been used as an anticoagulant, for example in the treatment of navicular disease in horses.

Dicoumarol poisoning This can occur in dogs, cats, pigs, and other animals that eat the rodenticide (which usually contains bran or oatmeal bait) or contaminated carcasses. Poultry are relatively resistant to dicoumarol poisoning. Clinical signs of poisoning can vary and include haemorrhage subcutaneously, submucosally, and into joints and body cavities, anae-

Dicrocoelium

mia, tachycardia, collapse, shock, and death. Prolonged clotting time is a diagnostic sign. Treatment in severe cases involves transfusion of whole blood (which will contain prothrombin). Otherwise synthetic vitamin K (Konakion) should be given slowly and intravenously, with the dose repeated over several days.

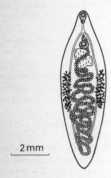

The lancet fluke of sheep,
Dicrocoelium dendriticum

Dicrocoelium A genus of *flukes known as the lesser liver flukes, commonly found as parasites in the bile ducts of herbivorous mammals. *D. dendriticum*, the lancet fluke of sheep, is widespread in Europe, Asia, and North America; in the UK it is restricted to a few parts of northwest England, Wales, and Scotland. It is small and elongated with a complex life cycle involving two intermediate hosts (see illustration). The first is a snail from which the larvae are extruded in balls of mucus. These are eaten by ants of the genus *Formica*, which in turn are ingested by grazing sheep. The effects on the sheep are similar to those of the liver fluke, *Fasciola hepatica*, but sheep can withstand a higher infestation before showing pathological signs. Treatment entails administration of a suitable *anthelmintic. Control of the snail

and removal of ant-hills may assist in prevention.

dicrotic Describing an abnormality in heart rhythm in which a double pulse is felt for each heart contraction.

Dictyocaulus A genus of *lungworms found in the trachea and bronchial system of sheep, horses, and cattle. The life cycle is direct and is exemplified by *D. viviparus*, which causes *husk (or hoose) in cattle. Infestation is also a serious problem in lambs, in which the worms cause a catarrhal bronchitis. This may be followed by secondary infection causing pneumonia, characterized by coughing, mucoid exudate from the nose, and rapid breathing with dyspnoea. Rotational grazing for young stock will help to control infestation. It can be treated with the *benzimidazoles (such as *levamisole or fenbendazole), *ivermectin, or *diethylcarbamazine, which is only effective against the immature larvae. Two vaccines are now available for calves.

dieldrin An *organochlorine compound used as an insecticide. Insoluble in water but soluble in fats, it can penetrate intact skin, even from a dry powder. After absorption it is stored in body fat and residues remain over a prolonged period. In the UK, dieldrin was used in sheep dips until 1965, and as a seed dressing until 1975. It was withdrawn because of problems with environmental contamination and persistence. It is still used to treat timber in buildings. For toxicity *see* chlorinated hydrocarbons.

diencephalon The part of the brain lying between the midbrain and the cerebrum, surrounding the third *ventricle. Its constituent parts are the *epithalamus, *thalamus, *hypothalamus, and *subthalamus.

diesel oil poisoning *See* fuel oil poisoning.

diet The food and water consumed by an individual or group. Animal diets generally consist of a number of individual feedstuffs that, ideally, meet the *nutrient requirements of the animal both qualitatively and quantitatively. This depends upon blending feedstuffs of known nutritive value to achieve a diet that has a nutrient density consistent with the food intake of the animal (*see* voluntary food intake) and will satisfy the animal's requirements. *See also* nutrition.

dietary fibre Broadly, *polysaccharides e.g. cellulose and related substances in food that are resistant to digestive enzymes. In ruminants, fermentation by rumen bacteria allows utilization of a considerable proportion of polysaccharides that are not available to nonruminants. Hence in ruminants dietary fibre is represented largely by the insoluble material of plant cell walls. Dietary fibre is important in all species for maintaining the passage of material through the gut and the removal of toxic substances. In ruminants it is important for rumen fermentation and in lactating dairy cows it affects milk composition (*see* butterfat).

diethylcarbamazine A *piperazine derivative formerly used extensively as an anthelmintic but now largely superseded by modern drugs (e.g. *benzimidazoles and *avermectins). It causes paralysis of the parasites and is administered intramuscularly or orally. The drug is excreted from the body rapidly, usually within 6 hours. Its main use is to treat *lungworm infections in sheep and milking cattle. Immature worms are destroyed better than adult worms, although repeating the treatment daily for 3 days improves the drug's efficacy. It is also used in dogs to kill microfilaria of the heartworm *Dirofilaria immitis* but requires daily oral dosage; it has no activity against the adult heartworms.

diethylstilboestrol A synthetic *oestrogen derived from coal tar. It was formerly used as a growth promoter in beef cattle, but this is now illegal in most countries, including the UK. Diethylstilboestrol is metabolized much more slowly than natural oestrogens and residues in meat and milk have oestrogenic and carcinogenic activity. However, in some countries, it can be given orally as hormone therapy for small animals with, for instance, urinary incontinence, prostatic disease, or hormonal alopecia.

differentiation The process in embryonic development during which unspecialized cells or tissues become specialized for particular functions.

digestibility The proportion of a *diet or individual feedstuff that is not voided in the faeces and is therefore assumed to have been retained by the animal following digestion and absorption. It is usually expressed as a percentage of the dry matter consumed. *True digestibility* (as opposed to *apparent digestibility*) takes into account the faecal output not directly of dietary origin, including digestive enzymes which are not subsequently reabsorbed and cells sloughed off from the mucosal walls during the passage of digesta. Digestibility is influenced by a number of factors, notably the content of *dietary fibre; an increase in this, as is found, for example, in relatively mature crops, is associated with a reduction in digestibility. *See also* D-value.

digestion The physical and chemical processes by which ingested food is broken down in the alimentary tract into a form that can be absorbed and

digit

assimilated by the tissues of the body. Mechanical digestion involves chewing, either before food is swallowed or after regurgitation (see rumination), and churning or grinding by the muscular walls of the gut; this is the chief function of the gizzard (*ventriculus) in birds. Chemical digestion is accomplished by the action of digestive enzymes and other substances (bile, acid, etc.). It begins in the mouth with the action of *saliva, but most takes place in the stomach and small intestine, where food is subjected to *gastric juice, *pancreatic juice, and enzymes of the small intestine.

In herbivores, food is also digested by the enzymes produced by symbiotic microorganisms (bacteria, protozoa, and fungi) that cause *fermentation in various regions of the alimentary tract. This is particularly important in the *rumen of ruminant animals and in the large intestine of other herbivores, such as the horse. Cellulose, the main constituent of plant cell walls, is digested by the microbial cellulases and thus made available to the animal. The digestive and absorptive capabilities of newborn mammals are geared to a milk diet and differ from those of older individuals.

digit One of the distal components of the *manus (forefoot) and *pes (hindfoot), corresponding to the finger or toe in humans. Each digit comprises three bones – the phalanges (see phalanx). Up to five digits (numbered 1 to 5) may be present in each limb, as in the manus of **carnivores**, although in the pes only four are usually present; however, in the canine hindlimb all five digits may be present. In the **pig**, digits 2–5 are present in both the manus and pes; in **ruminants** two principal weight-bearing digits occur in both limbs (numbers 3 and 4), although digits 2 and 5 occur as reduced structures. In the **horse** only number 3 digit is present.

In **birds** three reduced digits occur in the wing, and there are four digits in the foot.

digital cushion A wedge-shaped mass of subcutaneous tissue overlying the frog in the equine *hoof. It is important in absorbing the force of impact of the hoof.

digital extensor muscles The muscles that extend the digits in both limbs. In the forelimb they comprise the *common digital extensor* and *lateral digital extensor muscles*, which also extend the *carpus and the metacarpophalangeal joints (see metacarpus). In the hindlimb they comprise the *long digital extensor* and *lateral digital extensor muscles*, which also flex the *hock and extend the metatarsophalangeal joints (see metatarsus).

digital flexor muscles The muscles that flex the joints of the digits in both limbs. The *superficial digital flexor muscle* inserts to the middle *phalanx and acts only on the proximal interphalangeal joint. The *deep digital flexor muscle* inserts to the distal phalanx and acts on both the proximal and distal interphalangeal joints. In the forelimb both muscles also act to flex the *carpus and the metacarpophalangeal joints (see metacarpus). In the hindlimb they act to extend the *tarsus and flex the metatarsophalangeal joints (see metatarsus).

digitalis An extract prepared from the leaves of foxgloves (*Digitalis* spp.), which contains various *cardiac glycosides. These are used to treat heart diseases.

digitalis poisoning See foxglove poisoning.

digitalization The administration of *digitalis or one of its purified derivatives (*see* cardiac glycosides) to treat heart disease. Digitalization is usually undertaken slowly over several days so that there is a gradual build-up of the drug to therapeutic levels. A rapid build-up may cause toxicity.

digitigrade Describing locomotion in which only the digits are in contact with the ground, as in, for example, dogs, cats, and most fast-running animals. *Compare* plantigrade.

dihydrostreptomycin *See* aminoglycosides.

dihydrotachysterol A synthetic analogue of *vitamin D that, like the vitamin, increases calcium uptake from the gut, causing a rise in plasma calcium, and increases bone mineralization. Given orally and activated by hydroxylation in the liver, it can be used to treat hypocalcaemic tetany (*see* hypocalcaemia) or *hypoparathyroidism. Care should be taken to prevent *hypercalcaemia; chronic hypercalcaemia can lead to calcium deposition in soft tissues, especially the kidney. Dihydrotachysterol is excreted in milk and extraskeletal calcification can occur in the suckling neonate.

dihydroxyanthraquinone A synthetic *anthraquinone drug that acts as a laxative at low doses and causes purgation at higher doses. It is available as a powder combined with a wetting agent (e.g. sodium lauryl sulphate) and is made up in a large volume of water for use in nonruminants to treat impaction and constipation and, occasionally, parasitism. Young animals are susceptible to the drug and lower doses should be used.

diiodotyrosine A precursor of the hormones thyroxine and 3,5,3′-triiodothyronine found in the thyroid gland.

dilatation The enlargement or expansion of a hollow organ (such as a blood vessel) or cavity.

dilator 1. An instrument used to enlarge the internal diameter of a tubular structure or an orifice. The enlargement may be temporary, for example to allow the passage of another instrument, or permanent, for example in the treatment of oesophageal *strictures. *See also* bougie. **2.** A muscle that, by its action, opens an aperture or orifice in the body.

dimercaprol A drug that combines with metals in the body and is used to treat arsenic, antimony, or mercury poisoning. It is a chelating agent given in oil by intramuscular injection. Tradename: **British Anti-Lewisite (BAL)**.

dimethylsulphoxide (DMSO) A solvent used to greatly increase the penetration of substances through the skin. It also acts as a topical *analgesic, and action as an *anti-inflammatory agent has been claimed. A 90% solution is available for local application to treat arthritis, muscle strains, and bone splints. It penetrates intact skin readily and may cause skin irritation and sloughing. The area should not be bandaged after application.

dimetridazole A drug used for the treatment and prevention of *blackhead in turkeys, chickens, and game birds; it should not be used in laying birds. The drug is withdrawn 48 hours prior to slaughter to avoid tissue residues. Dimetridazole also has activity against spirochaetes and thus it is used to prevent and to treat *swine dysentery and post-weaning scours in pigs. It is also used as a growth promoter for pigs and poultry. The drug is available as a premix for incorporation in feed or as a soluble

dimorphic

powder for water medication. Tradename: **Emtryl**.

dimorphic (dimorphous) Having two distinct forms; the term is applied particularly to the small number of pathogenic fungi whose growth in the parasitic phase (i.e. when infecting tissue) is markedly different from their usual saprophytic phase in the environment. In most instances the tissue phase is *yeastlike and the saprophytic phase a *mycelium. The change from one to the other is governed principally by temperature, and is achievable in culture by the use of appropriate conditions. Animal diseases caused by dimorphic fungi include *epizootic lymphangitis, *sporotrichosis, *histoplasmosis, and *coccidioidomycosis.

dinoprost A synthetically manufactured form of *prostaglandin $F_{2\alpha}$, which occurs naturally in the body causing *luteolysis in the ovary. Dinoprost is administered intramuscularly as a luteolytic agent in large animals for the control of oestrus, to induce abortion or parturition, and to treat *pyometra, luteal cysts in cattle, and prolonged *dioestrus in the mare. Side-effects are increased gastrointestinal tract motility, increased respiratory rate, bronchoconstriction, and sweating; these disappear within an hour. Synthetic analogues of prostaglandin $F_{2\alpha}$, such as cloprostenol, fenprostalene, and tiaprost, have reduced side-effects. Dinoprost should not be used in dogs because of toxicity. Also, it is active in humans and care should be taken when handling the drug, especially in the case of asthmatics and pregnant women. The drug can be absorbed from the lungs following inhalation or may penetrate the skin. Tradename: **Lutalyse**.

dioctophymosis Disease due to infestation by parasitic nematodes (roundworms) of the genus *Dioctophyma*, particularly *D. renale*, the largest known nematode, with females sometimes exceeding 1 m in length. The worms inhabit the kidney of the dog and of many wild carnivores in North and South America, the USSR, continental Europe, Africa, and Japan; pigs, horses, cattle, and humans can also become infested. Eggs are passed in the urine of the host and the subsequent life cycle appears to involve species of free-living annelid worms, in which the parasitic larvae develop. They are transferred to the final host by ingestion of the annelid. Infestation often leads to destruction of the affected kidney and death from uraemia may occur; but in the majority of cases the healthy kidney is able to maintain excretory capability and clinical illness is not seen. Treatment is by surgical removal of the worms.

diodone An organic iodide used as an intravenous contrast agent in radiography, mainly for *pyelography. When rapidly injected intravenously it is filtered completely at the glomerulus and secreted by proximal tubules enabling an outline of the kidneys and any defects in renal blood flow and glomerular filtration to be visualized radiographically. Diodone may cause signs of nausea and vomiting in the patient, but it is rapidly excreted.

dioestrus The stage of the *oestrous cycle when a mature corpus luteum is producing progesterone. This results in changes in the *endometrium of the uterus in preparation for *implantation. *See also* oestrus; pro-oestrus.

dioxins Halogenated cyclic hydrocarbons that are highly toxic environmental contaminants, often produced as by-products during the manufacture of herbicides or the incineration of certain chemicals and wastes. Chemically stable and lipid-soluble, dioxins are absorbed orally and through skin and mucous membranes. They are stored in fat tissue and can become concentrated in food chains, with residues remaining in tissues for years after exposure. Young animals are more susceptible to toxicity and signs include weight loss, alopecia, hyperkeratosis, immunosuppression, bone marrow depression, reproductive disorders, and liver enlargement; this produces an overall wasting syndrome. Dioxins have been shown to be both *teratogenic and *carcinogenic. No treatment is available and affected animals should be slaughtered.

dipeptidase An enzyme, found in the lining of the small intestine, that splits *dipeptides into their constituent *amino acids.

dipeptide A molecule consisting of two amino acids joined together by a *peptide bond (e.g. glycylalanine, a combination of the amino acids glycine and alanine). See dipeptidase.

diphenhydramine An *antihistamine that acts on H_1 receptors. It can be administered orally, parenterally, or topically, and has a long duration of action (up to 24 hours). The drug reduces the initial inflammation in various allergy-linked conditions, such as laminitis or chronic obstructive pulmonary disease. It is also used to treat insect stings and pruritus, and is useful in preventing travel sickness. Overdosage may lead to hyperexcitability and possibly convulsions. Intravenous injection may cause myocardial depression.

diphtheresis The formation of a 'false membrane' (i.e. *diphtheroid membrane*) similar to that characteristically formed in diphtheria. This occurs most commonly in cases of *calf diphtheria, where large areas of necrosis in the mouth and larynx develop membranous coverings. These may interfere with breathing. Similar diphtheretic lesions may be found in the uterine tracts of cows and sheep where *Fusobacterium necrophorum* infection is established. Dogs with uraemia due to chronic renal failure may suffer necrotic lesions of the endocardium, which are sometimes described as diphtheretic. The cause is unknown.

diphtheria See calf diphtheria; fowl pox.

Diphyllobothrium A genus of *tapeworms, also known as *Dibothriocephalus*, found worldwide although now probably absent from Britain. There are several species, the commonest being *D. latum*, the broad or fish tapeworm, a parasite in the intestine of humans and fish-eating mammals, including dogs and cats. It is a large tapeworm, up to 12 m long and comprising as many as 4000 proglottids. There are two intermediate hosts: a crustacean, such as *Cyclops*, and a freshwater fish. When fish waste is eaten by dogs or cats, or raw fish is eaten by humans, the second stage larvae develop into adults. Infestation with the adult tapeworms can cause severe anaemia, while the larva or sparganum may cause the disease *sparganosis.

dipl- (diplo-) *Prefix denoting* double.

diplegia Paralysis of both sides of the body. *Compare* hemiplegia; paraplegia.

diplococcus (*pl.* **diplococci**) Any of a group of spherical bacteria that occur in pairs, such as *Neisseria* and *pneumococci.

diploid Describing a nucleus, cell, or organism in which each chromosome is represented twice. The diploid number is designated as $2n$. This is the case in all cells in mammals except for the gametes (spermatozoon and ovum), which are *haploid.

diprenorphine A drug used to antagonize the actions of the potent morphine-like drugs (e.g. *etorphine). It can be injected intravenously, intramuscularly, or subcutaneously. Tradename: **Revivon**.

Diptera See fly.

Dipylidium

Dipylidium A genus of *tapeworms occurring as parasites in the small intestine of dogs, cats, and occasionally humans. It includes *D. caninum*, distributed worldwide and the commonest tapeworm of dogs in towns. Its intermediate host is a flea, such as *Ctenocephalides canis*, *C. felis*, or *Pulex irritans*, or the biting louse, *Trichodectes canis*. The dog or cat relieves the irritation caused by the bites of these insects by eating them and thus the adult tapeworm develops in the primary host. Hooks on the tapeworm's head damage the intestinal mucosa and may cause inflammation. The mobile proglottids passing out with the faeces may cause itching around the anus. Treatment entails dosing with an *anthelmintic effective against the larvae and adults. Worming should be augmented by bathing the animal with a suitable insecticidal shampoo to destroy any fleas or lice, and insecticidal treatment of the bedding etc. of the dog or cat.

dipyrone See NSAID.

diquat poisoning See paraquat poisoning.

Dirofilaria A genus of parasitic *nematodes, also known as heartworms, found mainly in dogs in the tropics and subtropics and causing the disease *dirofilariasis. *D. immitis*, the most common species in dogs, is found in the right ventricle of the heart or pulmonary artery, and the female worm may grow to 30 cm in length. The life cycle is indirect, with mosquitoes as the intermediate hosts. *Microfilariae are taken up in the mosquito's blood meal and migrate to the Malpighian tubules (excretory organs), where they develop. They move to the insect's mouthparts for final development into the infective stage, which is injected into the final host when the mosquito

feeds. The cycle within the mosquito takes 8–17 days. Initially the injected microfilariae stay near the bite but within 3–4 months the young adults are found in the heart, and after a further 2 months they have matured and produce microfilariae. Other species include *D. repens*, found in subcutaneous connective tissue of dogs in Italy, India, Sri Lanka, Indo-China, and Kenya, *D. scapiceps*, found in rabbits, and *D. tenuis*, found in raccoons.

dirofilariasis Disease due to infestation by parasitic nematodes of the genus *Dirofilaria*. It normally affects dogs, and occasionally cats, caused by *D. immitis*, the canine heartworm. A heavy worm burden may impede the blood circulation causing congestion and cirrhosis of the liver. Hydrothorax and oedema of dependent parts follows. Affected dogs cough, are listless, breathe rapidly, and have a noticeable heart murmur; any sudden exertion results in collapse. The disease is ultimately fatal. The microfilariae can be controlled with *diethylcarbamazine, which may also be given prophylactically in mosquito-infested areas. Arsenical compounds are more effective against adult worms, but if too many adult worms are killed suddenly it can cause the dog's death. Thiacetarsamide is normally given intravenously, but dogs should receive a vitamin supplement two weeks before each treatment. The trivalent antimony compound Fouadin has been used for many years; it is best administered by slow intravenous injection, but can also be given intraperitoneally or intramuscularly.

dis- Prefix denoting separation.

disaccharide A molecule consisting of two linked *monosaccharide units. The most common disaccharides are *maltose, *lactose, and *sucrose.

disarticulation Complete separation of the bones and supportive structures (joint capsule, ligaments, etc.) forming a joint. The term tends to be used in connection with the cadaver rather than the live animal, in which total disarticulation is rare. It may occasionally happen following a severe injury or be performed surgically during amputation.

disbudding **(debudding)** The removal of the horn buds in calves to prevent the growth of horns. This is best done by applying a caustic compound during the first week of life. Alternatively, a *disbudding iron* can be used at 4–6 weeks. This is similar to a soldering iron and is heated either by gas or electricity. Firstly, a local anaesthetic is injected over the ridge of bone halfway between the eye socket and the horn. After a short interval the hot iron is applied for about 10 seconds to the horn bud to kill the horn-forming tissues. The area is then sprayed with *antibiotic.

disc (in anatomy) A rounded flattened structure, such as an *intervertebral disc or the *optic disc.

Disciplinary Committee A committee of the Council of the Royal College of Veterinary Surgeons, charged with the statutory duty of considering and determining any disciplinary case against a veterinarian referred to them by the *Preliminary Investigation Committee, and applications for the restoration of a name to the *Register of Veterinary Surgeons or *Supplementary Veterinary Register.

discospondylitis Inflammation of one or more intervertebral discs with an *osteomyelitis of the contiguous vertebrae. The condition is most common in pigs (in the UK), occurs less commonly in large male dogs and sheep, and is uncommon in cats, cattle, and horses. Although usually the result of a primary *bacteraemia or *septicaemia, discospondylitis may also occur secondarily to a chronic localized infection from a wound.

In **pigs** bacteria, such as *Erysipelothrix rhusiopathiae* or *Brucella suis*, are usually isolated as the causal organisms, although streptococci and *Staphylococcus aureus* are not uncommon. Most porcine cases seem to be associated with tail-bite lesions, infected wounds or bites, and castration or injection sites. Affected animals show an initial stiffness and reluctance to move with an ataxia or weakness culminating in spasticity. There is often tail paralysis, with or without faecal and urinary incontinence. The vertebral osteomyelitis frequently results in pathological fracture and this in turn causes sudden onset of spinal cord compression with acute paralysis. Cervical, thoracic, and lumbar regions may be affected although in the pig the lumbar discs are more often involved.

In **sheep** docking wounds or navel infections are often thought to be the origin of the initial infection by *Corynebacterium pseudotuberculosis*. *Salmonella* organisms have been isolated from lesions in **foals** and *Brucella* spp. from adult **horses**. In **dogs** the affected animals (usually male) are initially feverish but then become depressed and anorexic. Initial spinal pain is replaced by stiffness and then neurological signs and ataxia, caused by spinal cord compression. Radiographic examination shows sclerosis and irregularity of intervertebral disc spaces with bone lysis of vertebral bodies. *Staphylococcus aureus* is frequently isolated from blood and/or urine. Domestic **cats** may be affected as a result of infected bite wounds at the base of the tail. This results in coccygeal discospondylitis with stiffness and pain in the lower vertebral column.

Diagnosis is usually made on clinical evidence, with radiographic examina-

Diseases of Animals Act (1950)

tion in small animals, and appropriate bacteriological examinations. Screening of cerebrospinal fluid may be helpful also. Treatment of cases diagnosed early may be accomplished with long courses (4–6 weeks) of broad-spectrum antibiotics. Where neurological signs are present then surgery to relieve cord pressure or nerve compression may be attempted, but this is often unsuccessful, particularly in large animals. The situation is complicated, with a poorer prognosis, if associated vertebrae are fractured or affected by osteomyelitis. Other name: **vertebral osteoarthritis.**

Diseases of Animals Act (1950) (England and Wales) An Act of Parliament repealed by the *Animal Health Act (1981).

Diseases of Animals (Waste Food) Order (1973) (England and Wales) A Parliamentary Order that requires the processing of waste food by an authorized method before being fed to animals. The Order also lays down requirements for the holding, storage, and transportation of waste food intended for animal consumption.

disinfectant An agent that destroys microorganisms and is used to sterilize inanimate objects and surfaces. Strong acids, strong alkalis, oxidizing agents, and reducing agents can all be used as disinfectants. *Phenols and substituted phenols are used as disinfectants but have poor efficacy against viruses and spores. However, they are comparatively cheap and are widely used as general disinfectants for buildings. Other disinfectants include iodine compounds and *cationic detergents. Strong solutions of chlorine compounds or *formalin are used to disinfect buildings after disease outbreaks, and in the UK, a list of approved products is produced by the Ministry of Agriculture, Fisheries, and Food.

disjunction The separation of pairs of homologous chromosomes during meiosis or of the chromatids of a chromosome during *anaphase of mitosis or meiosis.

dislocation (luxation) Displacement of the bones forming a joint. The surrounding soft tissues are stretched and the ligaments of the joint may be torn. In young animals the growth plate of the immature bone may give way rather than the joint dislocate, resulting in an *epiphyseal fracture. The anatomical arrangements of a joint largely determine the clinical features of its dislocation. The most common dislocation affects the hip joint of the dog, often due to a road traffic accident. The femoral head typically moves upwards and forwards over the rim of the acetabulum, causing the affected leg to be shortened compared with its neighbour and the foot and stifle turned inwards. Treatment requires replacement of the femoral head into the acetabulum under general anaesthesia, by employing a combination of traction on the foot, to overcome the action of the muscles of the hip area, and rotation of the limb to cause the femoral head to pass over the rim of the acetabulum and back into the cup of the joint. When reduction is effected the joint will move (extend and flex) smoothly. The leg must be strapped up in a flexed position, with hock out and stifle in for at least four days to ensure that dislocation does not recur.

Dislocation of the *elbow* in dogs involves the anconeal process of the ulna moving laterally in relation to the humerus, and requires the joint to be fully flexed during reduction. If either colateral ligament is torn, this must be sutured or the joint will remain unstable. Dislocation at the *hock* joint involves fracture of the lateral malleolus; frequently there is marked lateral angulation of the foot with a wound in the skin medial to the joint and exposure of the articular surface of the tibia. Reduction requires operative correction of the malleolar fracture to provide stability. Dislocation of the *jaw* causes inability to close the mouth because the teeth cannot occlude properly. Correction involves forcing the articular condyles of the mandible downwards by employing a fulcrum between the teeth and forcing the incisors together. Dislocations of *vertebrae* most often occur with fracture of the intervertebral articular facets. The clinical consequences depend principally upon the degree of damage to the spinal cord. In many cases the affected animal will show paralysis of the hindlimbs, often with sensory loss. If the lesion is sufficiently high, respiratory embarrassment may be associated with intercostal paralysis, and may result in death. Low spinal dislocations produce less nervous damage if they occur behind the end of the spinal cord. Fixation of spinal dislocations involves plating or fusing the vertebrae to prevent further nervous tissue damage, and is most useful where only nerve roots are present in the vertebral canal. *See also* luxating patella.

displaced abomasum (slipped stomach) A condition in which the *abomasum (fourth stomach), which normally lies to the right of the rumen, is displaced below and to the left of the rumen. It principally affects dairy cows, although it can occur in bulls and in other species, such as goats, and results in abnormal digestion leading to poor appetite, diarrhoea, and *ketosis. Cows are most commonly affected in the 6 weeks after calving. Clinical examination of affected animals reveals a characteristic 'pinging' sound on *auscultation of the left abdomen. Casting and rolling affected animals can replace the abomasum in its proper

position. However, relapses often occur. Permanent cure can be effected by a simple surgical operation which anchors the organ in position. A more severe form is occasionally encountered where the abomasum is displaced but remains in the right-hand side of the abdomen. In these circumstances twisting (*torsion) and dilatation may occur. High levels of concentrates or the presence of other active disease, such as mastitis or metritis, are thought to predispose an animal to the disease.

dissection The cutting apart and separation of body tissues along the natural divisions of the organs and different tissues in the course of a surgical operation. Dissection of dead bodies is carried out in anatomy.

disseminated Widely distributed throughout an organ or body. The term can refer to pathogenic organisms or to pathological changes. For instance, a malignant tumour spreading with metastases throughout the body may be described as disseminated.

disseminated intravascular coagulation (DIC) An acquired haemorrhagic disorder that arises due to abnormal activation of the *coagulation (blood clotting) mechanism by various factors, including tissue breakdown products, inflamed blood vessels, exposed collagen, or tumour cells. This leads to the formation of blood clots in the blood capillaries (microcirculation), the initiation of *fibrinolysis, depletion of *platelets and *coagulation factors, and the production of fibrin degradation products (FDPs), which are anticoagulant and potentiate bleeding. Laboratory findings include low platelet counts, prolongation of coagulation tests, elevated FDPs, and fragmented plasma cells. DIC may be associated with infectious diseases, septicaemia, peritonitis, shock, severe trauma, heat stroke, and various neoplastic conditions. The underlying condition must be treated aggressively and the microcirculation restored. Shock and electrolyte imbalances should be corrected, and if bleeding persists plasma transfusion and heparinization (*see* heparin) may be indicated.

distal (in anatomy) Situated away from the origin or point of attachment or from the median line of the body. For example, the term is applied to a part of a limb that is furthest from the body; to a blood vessel that is far from the heart; and to a nerve fibre that is far from the central nervous system. *Compare* proximal.

distemper A serious contagious disease of dogs, foxes, ferrets, and mink caused by a *morbillivirus and characterized by fever, *gastroenteritis, bronchopneumonia (*see* pneumonia), and nervous signs. Infection is usually by the inhalation of virus-contaminated breath from an infected animal and, following an incubation period of 4–5 days, a fever develops. Diarrhoea, vomiting, pneumonia, and, in pregnant bitches, abortion, together with incoordination and loss of appetite, are the typical clinical signs. Some strains of virus also cause thickening of the skin of the nose and pads causing the condition known as *hardpad*. About half of affected dogs may die and those that recover frequently show persistent involuntary limb jerks or nervous tics. Puppies may be protected by maternal antibody up to 12 weeks of age, and this can be supplemented with vaccination with a live attenuated vaccine. However, because maternal antibody can interfere with the effectiveness of vaccination, puppies vaccinated against distemper before 12 weeks of age must be given a second injection at 12 weeks. Distemper vaccines are usually combined with vaccines against parvovirus, leptospirosis, and canine hepatitis. Puppies born to infected bitches may also develop distemper, although occasionally they appear clinically normal but persistently excrete distemper virus.

distillers' grains (distillers' draff) A by-product of whisky production used in the feeding of cattle and sheep. It consists of the residue of fermented grains after alcohol production, which is filtered and sold wet or dried. The composition varies within the ranges of 200–280 g/kg crude protein and 9.5–10.8 MJ/kg metabolizable energy. *See also* brewers' grains.

distomiasis Disease due to infestation by distome *flukes, i.e. flukes characterized by the possession of two suckers near their anterior end for attachment to the host.

diuresis Increased formation of urine by the kidneys. This normally follows the drinking of more fluid than the body requires, but it can be stimulated by the administration of a *diuretic.

diuretic An agent that increases the rate of *urine formation and hence water loss from the body. They are used to treat *oedema. There are various types of diuretics, differing in their mode of action. Substances that are freely filtered at the glomerulus but not reabsorbed (e.g. mannitol, glucose) raise the osmotic pressure in the renal tubule and cause osmotic diuresis. *Xanthines cause increased blood flow to the kidneys, leading to an increased glomerular filtration rate and mild diuresis. Other diuretics (e.g. aldosterone antagonists, carbonic anhydrase inhibitors, *frusemide, and *thiazides) act by inhibiting sodium reabsorption from the kidney tubules with a resultant loss of water by osmosis. Very rapid removal of oedema fluid can lead to fluid and electrolyte imbalances and *shock. Diuresis may also cause *hypokalaemia due to loss of potassium in the urine. This can be treated using potassium chloride administered orally.

diverticulum A pouch formed by the wall of an organ. For example, the *diverticulum ventriculi* is a flattened conical blind pouch of the left extremity of the stomach in the pig. The *preputial diverticulum* is an ovoid pouch in the dorsal wall of the prepuce of the pig. It contains urine and decomposing epithelium producing a foul odour. The diverticulum of the *auditory tube (guttural pouch) is a large saclike ventral pouch of the auditory tube in the horse, lying between the base of the skull and the pharynx.

DNA (deoxyribonucleic acid) The genetic material of all cells and many *viruses; it is a major constituent of *chromosomes and carries the *genetic code for determining hereditary characteristics. DNA is a double-stranded *polynucleotide containing *deoxyribose, *phosphate, and the bases *adenine, *guanine, *cytosine, and *thymine. The two strands of nucleotides are wound round each other and linked by hydrogen bonds between specific complementary bases – adenine with thymine, and guanine with cytosine. This forms a spiral ladder-shaped molecule – the *double helix* (see illustration). Its molecular weight ranges from about two million (for the smallest DNA viruses) to 10^{12} for the largest animal chromosomes. The sequence of the bases in DNA carries the genetic code for the synthesis of *proteins and is functionally divided into *genes; each gene encodes for a single protein or protein subunit. Although a small amount of DNA is found in the *mitochondria and, in plants, in the

chloroplasts, the vast bulk of the DNA of higher organisms resides in the chromosomes of the nucleus.

Prior to cell division, the hydrogen bonds between the two strands of the parent DNA are cleaved and the strands unwind. Each strand then acts as a template for the assembly of a new complementary strand, resulting in two identical double-stranded DNA molecules, one of which passes to each daughter cell. Errors in DNA replication may lead to a *mutation.

DNOC (dinitro-ortho-cresol) poisoning A toxic condition due to the ingestion of DNOC or related compounds, which are used as herbicides and form yellow or orange solutions. They cause persistent staining of wool and hair. Ingestion of the undiluted or partially diluted concentrate by animals, usually from open containers or contaminated streams, uncouples oxidative phosphorylation and prevents the synthesis of ATP by the tissues. Animals become listless

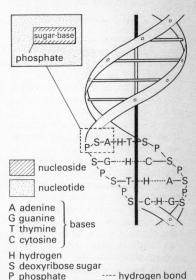

A adenine
G guanine
T thymine } bases
C cytosine

H hydrogen
S deoxyribose sugar
P phosphate   ---- hydrogen bond

nucleoside
nucleotide
sugar-base
phosphate

Structure of DNA

and inactive, develop a very high temperature, become prostrate, and die rapidly. There is no antidote; intravenous fluids may give relief but ataractic drugs should be avoided.

docking The removal of the tail or part of the tail. Docking of sheep is performed to help prevent the accumulation of faeces around the hindquarters and thus reduce the risk of ,*strike. Hill sheep may be left undocked to afford protection against the weather. A tight-fitting rubber ring is applied to the tail, causing the lower part of the tail to wither and die. Sufficient tail should remain to cover the vulva (female) or anus (male). Current UK legislation restricts use of the rubber ring without anaesthetic to the first 7 days of life. Docking of lambs may also be performed surgically (with local anaesthesia), usually in the first month. Docking of horses (except for veterinary reasons) is illegal in the UK, while docking of dogs for cosmetic reasons is now generally frowned on.

Surgical amputation of the tail or part of the tail may be needed in any species following, for example, damage to the tail. This requires the administration of a local anaesthetic to the base of the tail, and suturing of the wound afterwards.

Docking and Nicking of Horses Act (1949) (England and Wales) An Act of Parliament that prohibits the docking or nicking of horses except where a veterinary surgeon, after examining the animal, has certified in writing that the operation is necessary for the health of the horse – because of disease or injury to the tail. The Act also restricts the import of docked horses to those animals that HM Customs are satisfied will be exported from Great Britain as soon as possible. 'Docking' is defined as

the deliberate removal of any bone or part of a bone from the tail of a horse; 'nicking' is defined as the deliberate severing of any tendon or muscle in the tail of a horse.

dock poisoning *See* oxalate poisoning.

dog A carnivorous mammal belonging to the family *Canidae*, which contains 37 species, including wolves, jackals, and foxes. The domestic dog, *Canis familiaris*, is thought to have evolved as a species in the Middle East 10 000–12 000 years ago from the wolf and possibly other species of wild dog. It has developed a close relationship with man due to its value as a guard dog, for herding animals, as a draught animal, for hunting, and as a companion. Although the latter use has become predominant in recent times, dogs are also trained for many more functions, such as rescue work, guidance for the blind, and scent detection.

The British *Kennel Club divides pedigree dogs into six groups, broadly based on their function: working dogs; gundogs; terriers; hounds; toy dogs; and utility breeds; each group contains numerous breeds. Dogs are basically carnivorous although they can readily adapt to an omnivorous diet when meat is in short supply. They retain many of the attributes of their wild ancestors, who hunted in packs and used their keen senses of smell and hearing, and to a lesser extent sight, to identify and track prey.

Dog care Dogs need regular exercise, grooming, and human companionship. It is best to feed either one of the reputable prepared dog foods, which are available canned, dry, or in a semimoist form, or fresh meat together with dog biscuit and a balanced vitamin and mineral supplement. There is normally no need to supplement prepared dog foods, since vitamins and minerals are added and an excess of these can be harmful. Feeding household scraps may not provide a balanced diet and can also lead to chronic digestive problems or obesity. Clean drinking water must be provided at all times.

Puppies should receive a veterinary examination soon after purchase to check for any signs of congenital disease or infection, when advice on vaccinations, worming, etc., can also be sought. Dogs are normally vaccinated against *distemper (hardpad), *canine viral hepatitis, *leptospirosis, and *canine parvovirus infection, as well as *rabies in areas where the disease is enzootic. It is also possible to vaccinate dogs against the agents that cause *kennel cough, although this is often only carried out when a dog is due to enter a boarding kennel. Dogs also need to be checked regularly by the owner for signs of ear infections, skin disease, and dental disease, which are all very common. Adult dogs require annual booster vaccinations, which also allow regular veterinary examination. As the dog becomes older, these examinations may need to become more frequent in order to check for the common diseases of old age, including chronic *nephritis, heart disease, and *cancer. Surgical neutering of female dogs (see spaying) prevents womb infections, *false pregnancies, and *mammary tumours, as well as alleviating the behavioural problems when a bitch is in season and the risk of accidental mismating.

It is vital that puppies commence gentle obedience and toilet training as early as possible, since behavioural problems are very common in dogs. Most of the dog's behaviour in a family relates to its natural behaviour patterns in a pack, and it is essential that a dog learns its place and is not allowed to dominate the family. Dogs should always be under control when off the lead, and never allowed to wander alone. They should also wear a collar and identifying name tag at all times.

dogbane See Apocynum poisoning.

Dogs Act (1906) (England and Wales) An Act of Parliament that gives a police officer power to seize any dog, found in a highway or public place, that he has reason to believe is a stray dog and to detain it until its owner has claimed it and paid all expenses incurred in its detention. After seven days, and if the owner has not claimed the dog and paid all expenses, the dog may be sold or destroyed humanely, but not given or sold for the purposes of vivisection.

Dogs (Protection of Livestock) Act (1953) (England and Wales) An Act of Parliament that provides for the punishment of persons whose dogs worry livestock on agricultural land. 'Worrying' is defined as attacking livestock or chasing them in such a way as may reasonably be expected to cause injury, suffering, or, in female animals, abortion or loss of or diminution of produce.

dog's mercury poisoning A toxic condition in grazing animals caused by the ingestion of dog's mercury (*Mercurialis perennis*). Poisoning usually occurs in the winter months when grazing is sparse or hidden by snow and foraging animals find patches of the plant in the shelter of walls and hedgerows. The plant has two main effects: one is an acute *gastroenteritis due to an unidentified irritant substance; the other is a *haemolytic anaemia also due to an unidentified agent. Affected animals develop diarrhoea and pass dark-coloured urine. They should be denied access to the plant and given *demulcent preparations orally and *haematinics.

dog tick A hard *tick that is an ectoparasite of dogs. These include *Ixodes canisuga* and *I. hexagonus*, common on suburban dogs and cats in the UK, the sheep tick, *I. ricinus*, which is also found on dogs in farming areas, the American dog ticks, *Dermacentor variabilis* and *D. reticulatus*, the European dog tick, *Rhipicephalus sanguineus*, and the African/Australasian dog tick, *Haemaphysalis leachi*.

dolich- (dolicho-) *Prefix denoting* long.

dolichocephalic Describing a long narrow skull, as in wolfhound dogs. *Compare* brachycephalic.

dominant 1. (in genetics) Describing the activity of an *allele that, in the *heterozygous state, conceals the presence of the other, *recessive, allele. *Compare* recessive. **2.** (in animal behaviour) Describing an animal that has priority over other members of its group (e.g. in access to food, mates, etc.) because of its success in previous aggressive encounters. *See* bunt order; peck order.

dopa (3,4-dihydroxyphenylalanine) A derivative of the *amino acid tyrosine that acts as a *neurotransmitter. It can be decarboxylated to dopamine, which is an intermediate in the synthesis of adrenaline, noradrenaline, and melanin.

dopamine *See* dopa.

dors- (dorsi-, dorso-) *Prefix denoting* **1.** the back. **2.** dorsal.

dorsal Relating to or situated at or close to the back of the body.

dose A carefully measured quantity of a drug given to a patient at any one time. This is calculated with reference to the weight of the animal, the amount of drug needed to give a desired effect, and the duration of action of the drug. Recommended dose rates are given on data sheets compiled by the drug manufacturer.

dosimeter A device to record the amount of radiation received by workers with X-rays or other radiation, usually consisting of a small piece of photographic film in a holder attached to the clothing. At regular intervals the film is examined to discover the amount of radiation it (and therefore the wearer) have received.

double muscling (muscular hypertrophy) A condition occurring occasionally in cattle and sheep in which there is a marked increase in the size of the muscles due to a greater number of muscle cells (i.e. not literally double muscles). The muscles most often affected are those of the neck, shoulder, and hindlimbs, and there is a decrease in the subcutaneous muscle and fat. Therefore in carcasses the condition shows up very clearly as each muscle is clearly delineated.

double scalp A mineral deficiency disease of sheep associated with thinning of the bones of the skull. Eventually the degeneration of bone progresses to the point where affected animals cannot eat properly and they fail to thrive. The primary cause is probably phosphorus deficiency, though phosphorus supplementation of the diet does not always reverse the clinical signs – probably because established lesions fail to resolve completely.

douche A stream of hot or cold water, possibly containing a dissolved antiseptic or antimicrobial agent, that is directed onto parts of the body or into a body cavity. It may be employed in the treatment of infected wounds, uterine infections, and bladder infections or for rectal or colonic irrigation in cases of constipation or for emptying the rectum prior to X-ray examination or before surgery involving the rectum and anus.

dourine A venereally transmitted disease of horses and asses caused by the protozoan parasite *Trypanosoma equiperdum*, which is morphologically indistinguishable from *Trypanosoma brucei*. Confined to localized regions of Asia and Africa, the disease runs a chronic course, commencing with swelling of the genitalia, slight fever, and genital discharges. Later, transient circumscribed weals appear on the flanks and then muscular paralysis appears, which is progressive and usually fatal unless treated. The parasites can be found in smears made from genital membranes, the skin swellings, or blood. Several drugs are effective as treatment and the disease has been eradicated from many areas by the detection of carriers using blood tests, and by the control of mating. Dourine is a *notifiable disease in the UK.

downer cow syndrome A condition of dairy cows, usually occurring after an attack of *milk fever, in which the animal apparently recovers from the effects of calcium insufficiency (*hypocalcaemia) but cannot rise. It appears alert, but seems to suffer paralysis of the hindlimbs. One cause is trauma inflicted when the cow originally collapses; this may involve severe lesions or even fractures of the pelvis or femur. More common, however, is pressure damage to the sciatic nerve or muscles of the hindlimbs following prolonged recumbency; the recumbency may be due to obturator paralysis following parturition (*see* obturator nerve). Also, continued lying on hard concrete floors restricts blood supply and causes widespread ischaemic *necrosis of muscles.

The treatment and outcome depend on the underlying problems. The first requirement is to ensure that blood concentrations of calcium, phosphorus, and magnesium have returned to normal after the milk fever. If not, further medication may be necessary. Secondly, high levels of such enzymes as glutamyl oxalotransaminase and creatine phosphokinase in the blood may indicate muscle damage, in which case good nursing and regular turning from side to side may aid recovery. Damage to the sciatic nerve may be gauged by the animal's ability to flex its hocks or fetlocks. Evidence of paralysis indicates that recovery will be prolonged or unlikely. Most cows recover within 1 week, but if 2 weeks pass without improvement the animal should be sent for slaughter. Various mechanical slings and lifting devices are available but their use requires care.

doxapram A drug that is used as a respiratory stimulant, most commonly to treat *apnoea with anaesthetic overdose or in neonates to initiate respiration. The effect is transient, lasting for about 5–10 minutes. It can be administered intravenously, intramuscularly, subcutaneously, or sublingually. With high doses there may be convulsions due to stimulation of the central nervous system.

Dracunculus A genus of parasitic *nematodes, also known as guinea worms. *D. insignis* is found in raccoons in North America and occasionally in mink and dogs. The female attains an enormous length (60–120 cm) compared to the minute male and lives deep beneath the skin, rising to the surface to expel larvae. The larvae are only released on contact with water, where they invade the intermediate host. *D. medinensis* (100–400 cm) causes the disease dracontiasis in humans, which results from drinking water contaminated

drain

with infected water fleas (*Cyclops*) – the intermediate hosts.

drain A device used to draw off fluid or gas from a part of the body by means of capillary action, gravity, and/or suction. They are particularly useful following thoracic or abdominal surgery to prevent the accumulation of fluid that may become infected or cause a build-up in pressure. The drain should be brought out through a stab incision in the skin away from the primary wound repair, otherwise healing of the wound is delayed. There is a possibility of infection tracking up the drain and it must be removed as soon as possible, and certainly within 5–7 days. The end of a tubular drain may be incorporated into an automatic suction device to provide continuous removal of fluid in a controlled and relatively clean fashion.

drainage The removal of fluid from a body cavity or tissue. This may occur as a natural bodily response through an open wound, sinus, or fistula, and can be facilitated, for example following surgery, by the insertion of a *drain.

drenching The oral administration of a liquid medication. The neck of the drenching bottle should be placed on top of and towards the back of the tongue, to prevent spillage and to stimulate swallowing. Large volumes of liquid should be delivered in several stages so the animal can swallow each mouthful, otherwise there is a risk that liquid may be aspirated into the lungs. The bottle should be shatterproof (e.g. tough plastic), not glass. Routine drenching with anthelmintics is often performed with a *drenching gun*. This delivers a preset dose of the drug with each squeeze of the trigger, enabling rapid dosing of large numbers of animals. However, care must be taken to ensure that the barrel or nozzle does not damage the animal's throat when inserted. Hence the animal must be properly restrained, particularly its head.

dressing Material used to cover and protect wounds or operation sites. Dressings may be self-adhesive or held in place by bandages, and can serve to apply pressure to the site if required. Special dressings may incorporate antiseptics or antibiotics. The dressing may be prevented from sticking to the wound by using paraffin gauze on the wound or proprietary nonadhesive film, which will allow the wound exudate to be absorbed by a pad.

dried grass Grass or lucerne (alfalfa) that is conserved by rapid artificial drying (at temperatures of 100–1000°C) to a dry matter of 900 g/kg. Available as wafers, cobs, or pellets, it has a nutritive value similar to the *grass from which it is made. Variations in quality are usually denoted by a star rating (1–5 stars) according to *D-value and crude protein content. *Compare* hay; haylage; silage.

drip (meat inspection) The watery blood-stained fluid that exudes from frozen meat as it thaws out. The loss in weight may be up to 3%.

drom- (dromo-) *Prefix denoting* movement or speed.

dropped sole A condition affecting horses' hooves following repeated attacks of *laminitis. This disease damages the sensitive laminae that produce the horn of the hoof wall. The weakened horn allows the wall to spread outwards so that the sole is no longer supported and seems to drop towards the ground.

dropsy *See* oedema.

Drosophila A genus comprising the fruit or vinegar *flies, so called because the adults lay their eggs in decaying and fermenting fruit and vegetables, on which the developing larvae feed. Adults of the species *D. repleta* sometimes feed on faeces and therefore may transmit diseases. *D. melanogaster* is used in genetic studies.

drug A substance administered for the prevention, diagnosis, or treatment of disease or to restrain animals. In the UK drugs are classified according to their availability to the public. The legal categories are: *GSL* (*general sales list*), which are available for purchase without restriction; *P* (*pharmacy* medicine), which can be sold by retail pharmacists; *PML* (*product on the merchants' list*), which can be sold by retail pharmacists and agricultural merchants to commercial keepers of animals; *POM* (*prescription only medicines*), which are available for animal use under the supervision of a veterinary surgeon; and *CD* (*see* controlled drugs), which require special prescriptions.

Drug Enforcement Agency (DEA) (USA) An agency in the US Department of Justice that is responsible for the enforcement of the laws concerning controlled substances. It regulates the legal trade in narcotics and dangerous drugs, and initiates programmes for suppressing the illegal use of such substances.

drug resistance Lack of susceptibility or response to a drug, particularly as exhibited by microorganisms and parasites. Drug resistance is usually genetically determined; some organisms are naturally resistant to certain drugs, or resistance may develop due to mutation, transduction, transformation, or conjugation. There are various mechanisms of drug resistance, including increased ability of the organism to metabolize the drug, the production of drug antagonists, alteration in drug receptors, reduced drug uptake, and increased excretion of the drug. The speed of development of resistance in populations depends on the type of drug. Resistance to one drug may confer resistance to other drugs with a similar structure and mode of action (*side-resistance*), or to chemically unrelated drugs with differing actions (*cross-resistance*). *Multiple-resistance* involves resistance to a wide variety of compounds. The use of certain antimicrobial agents in veterinary medicine has been restricted to reduce the risk of resistant populations of pathogens evolving and becoming widespread in the environment, with the consequent potential threat to human health. Hence, the antimicrobial growth promoters used in livestock farming are not ones that are used routinely in treating human diseases.

drumstick (in cytogenetics) A lobe protruding from the nucleus of polymorphonuclear *leucocytes (white blood cells) and shaped like a drumstick. They are found in some nuclei in some female mammals and are probably related to the number of inactive X chromosomes. Drumsticks can be used to determine the number of X chromosomes present in species where *Barr bodies are difficult to see. The number of X chromosomes equals the number of drumsticks plus one.

drunken lamb syndrome Alcohol intoxication of lambs (or calves) fed milk replacer diets containing fat-free milk but with added glucose. This mixture is fermented to alcohol in the stomach by the yeast *Torulopsis glaborata* and concentrations of up to 5 g of ethanol per litre may result. The alcohol may be sufficiently absorbed into the bloodstream to induce clinical signs of drunkenness or even death. Newborn animals are especially susceptible because their livers possess very little alcohol dehydrogenase, the enzyme capable of metabolizing the alcohol. Prevention depends on particular care when lambs are weaned early (*see* weaning).

drying off (cows) The procedure for terminating the lactation in a dairy cow. Milking is stopped either when the milk yield is uneconomically low, or at about 8 weeks before calving to give the optimum length of dry period. If milk production is still high, it can be lowered by reducing the concentrate allocation to the cow. At drying off, antibiotics are usually administered (dry cow therapy) to reduce the risk of *summer mastitis.

duck A member of the large family Anatidae. Wild ducks are distributed worldwide and are hunted as game in many countries. Domestic ducks are also reared commercially for their meat and for egg production; common breeds include the Campbell, Orpington, Aylesbury, and Pekin.
Ducks in general do not compare favourably with domestic fowls in terms of productivity and carcass composition, and duck meat is considered a luxury in most European countries. The demand for duck eggs is insignificant. *See* duck husbandry.

duck husbandry All aspects of the production of *ducks. Ducks are frequently reared for meat production in *intensive husbandry systems. In Great Britain, the Pekin duck is preferred; this is slaughtered at approximately 8 weeks of age at a liveweight of about 2.5 kg. However, the proportion of lean meat is small and fat levels are excessive. The Barbary duck is more popular in France because of its relative leanness. Time of slaughter is critical as *food conversion ratios deteriorate rapidly after approximately 11 weeks of age in males.

Conditions during rearing are similar to those for *broiler chickens except that the duck is hardier and can tolerate lower environmental temperatures. In addition, no litter is provided as ducks produce copious amounts of liquid excreta and prefer to splash in water. Consequently they are raised on mesh floors and the slurry produced is channelled away. In addition to duck meat, duck down is a valuable by-product, used for quilts and cushions.

duck plague *See* duck virus enteritis.

duck septicaemia *See* anatipestifer infection.

duck virus enteritis (duck plague) A highly infectious disease of ducks, caused by a herpesvirus, that can cause mortality of up to 90%. The chief clinical sign is a disinclination to walk. Both ducklings and adults are affected. Vaccines can be used for prevention, but are normally employed to prevent the spread of an outbreak.

duck virus hepatitis (DVH) An acute and highly infectious viral disease of ducks, causing mortality of up to 90%. Birds aged up to 3 weeks are most susceptible, but older birds can be affected, while adults are generally resistant. Death usually follows within an hour of the onset of signs, which are seen as sluggishness in movement. In the terminal stages, the birds fall over onto their sides, and may perform paddling motions with their feet before dying. The virus survives fairly well outside the body, and contaminated footwear, vehicles, and equipment can transmit the disease from site to site, as can wild birds. A live vaccine is available.

duct (ductus) A tubelike structure or channel, especially one for carrying glandular secretions.

ductless gland *See* endocrine gland.

ductule A small duct or channel.

ductus (*pl.* **ducti**) *See* duct.

ductus arteriosus A blood vessel in the foetus connecting the left pulmonary artery at its origin with the aortic arch, so bypassing the pulmonary circulation. It normally closes after birth, becoming converted to the *ligamentum arteriosum*. Failure of the ductus to close (*patent ductus arteriosus) produces a continuous *murmur.

ductus deferens (vas deferens) (*pl.* **ducti deferentes**) One of a pair of ducts that convey spermatozoa from the *epididymides of the testes to the *urethra. It is one component of the spermatic cord and has a thick muscular wall, which aids in ejaculation. Its terminal part enlarges to form an ampulla in the horse, bull, ram, and dog and opens along with the duct of the *seminal vesicles (when present) on the lateral side of the colliculus seminalis. In birds it opens into the cloaca.

duo- *Prefix denoting* two.

duodenal juice A viscous mucus-rich alkaline secretion produced by compound tubular glands (Brunner's glands) in the wall of the first part of the duodenum. Rich in hydrogencarbonate (bicarbonate), its function is to protect the duodenum from attack by acidic *chyme. The secretion of duodenal juice is stimulated by direct mechanical and chemical influences, by impulses from the *vagus nerve, and by hormones, especially *secretin. Failure of its secretion, for instance due to excessive sympathetic nervous activity, will lead to ulceration of the duodenal mucosa.

duodenoscope An *endoscope designed for visualization of the duodenum. It is passed down the oesophagus, through the stomach to the duodenum, and is used to locate abnormalities, such as ulceration, neoplasia, or strictures, and to assist the taking of biopsies.

duodenostomy An operation to create a permanent opening into the duodenum. This may be from the surface of the body, for example to study gut functions experimentally, or to join the duodenum to another section of the alimentary tract to bypass a diseased part of the gut.

duodenum The first part of the small *intestine, leading from the stomach. In **mammals** it forms a U-shaped loop consisting of cranial, descending, transverse, and ascending parts, and leads into the *jejunum at the *duodenojejunal flexure*. Its structure is generally similar to the remainder of the small intestine, with the additional presence of submucosal glands. Two papillae may occur near the junction of the cranial and descending parts: the *major duodenal papilla* is the site of the opening of the *bile duct and, when present, the *pancreatic duct; the *minor duodenal papilla* is where the accessory pancreatic duct discharges. In **birds** the duodenum succeeds the *ventriculus and is a much elongated loop consisting of descending and ascending parts. Bile and pancreatic ducts open into the terminal region of the ascending part. *See* alimentary tract.

dura mater The outermost layer of the *meninges, composed of thick tough fibrous connective tissue. It surrounds the brain and spinal cord and is separated from the underlying *arachnoid mater by the *subdural space, which contains a film of fluid. The spinal part is surrounded by the *epidural space, but in the cranium the dura mater is fused to the internal surface of the cranial bones and has projecting folds extending between various parts of the brain: the *falx cerebri lies between the two cerebral hemispheres; the *tentorium cerebri is between the cerebral hemispheres and the cerebellum; and the diaphragma sellae between the diencephalon and the pituitary gland.

D-value The percentage of digestible organic matter in the dry matter of ruminant feedstuffs. It can be calculated by summing the digestible nutrients or by laboratory analysis. The *metabolizable energy content of feedstuffs can be calculated by multiplying the D-value by a factor of 0.14 for straw, 0.155 for hay and dried grass, or 0.16 for silage, roots, grasses, legumes, other green feeds, cereals, and by-products. The D-value is sometimes inaccurately used to refer to the *digestibility of dry matter or organic matter.

dwarfism A growth defect in which animals fail to achieve normal stature. It may or may not be accompanied by anatomical deformities. There are several causes. Dwarfism due to a malfunctioning pituitary gland and consequent lack of growth hormone occurs in German shepherd dogs, in which it seems heritable. It may be related to pituitary cysts or tumours. The newborn pups appear normal but their growth is retarded. Eventually there is loss of hair and bald patches (alopecia) appear. Blood levels of growth hormone are low. Treatment is by administration of canine growth hormone. Pedigrees should be assessed in an attempt to breed out the defect. In cattle, the form of dwarfism known as an 'acorn' calf seems to be due to a nutritional deficiency of the mother in mid-pregnancy. Although the hungry cow may be seen to eat acorns (hence 'acorn'

calf) these do not cause the defect. *Achondroplasia is a form of inherited dwarfism in which the animal has shortened and deformed head and legs. Again, carriers of the defect need to be detected and excluded from breeding. See also bulldog calf.

dwarf tapeworm See Hymenolepis.

-dynia Suffix denoting pain.

dys- Prefix denoting difficult, abnormal, or impaired.

dysautonomia Dysfunction of the *autonomic nervous system. It occurs in cats affected by the *Key-Gaskell syndrome and in horses with *grass sickness. The cause is unknown. Histologically there is degeneration of the autonomic ganglia; both sympathetic and parasympathetic divisions of the autonomic nervous system are affected. The degree of dysfunction is variable, but often severe, with animals showing anorexia, difficulty or inability to swallow, absence of salivation and tear secretion, cessation of defecation, and, in horses, considerable amounts of mucus in the rectum. Dehydration occurs rapidly and the animal appears very dull and depressed; collapse follows. In horses, patchy sweating occurs and muscular tremors are a frequent feature. In many cases death comes rapidly, although it can be delayed by the administration of intravenous fluids sufficient to maintain circulation and renal function. The small proportion of cases that survive show marked weight loss; recovery is slow and often incomplete. Other name: **autonomic polyganglionopathy.**

dyscrasia Abnormal composition of the blood, particularly where the aetiology or pathogenesis of the condition is uncertain. The term is seldom used in modern veterinary medicine.

dysentery Disease of the intestinal tract causing severe diarrhoea with blood and mucus. It may be a feature of various conditions in which there is haemorrhage and inflammation of the intestines and is particularly associated with certain bacterial and parasitic infections, such as *salmonellosis and *coccidiosis. In veterinary medicine the principal forms are *lamb dysentery, *swine dysentery, and *winter dysentery. Humans are affected by *bacillary dysentery*, due to the bacterium *Shigella dysenteriae* and related forms, and *amoebic dysentery, caused by the protozoan *Entamoeba histolytica*, which can also affect dogs.

dysgenesis Faulty development of an organ or part of the body.

dysgerminoma A rare *ovarian tumour occurring in most species. It is generally confined to one ovary, and is large and soft with areas of haemorrhage and necrosis. Metastasis may occur, producing secondary lesions in the regional lymph nodes, liver, and kidney. In the dog such tumours have been associated with hormonal disturbance.

dyspepsia Gastric indigestion. Causes include excessive intake (gorging) of food, foreign bodies, excess stomach acidity, *gastritis, or peptic ulceration. *Antacids are usually prescribed although severe or long-standing cases need careful diagnosis and possibly surgical intervention.

dysphagia Difficulty in swallowing. Obstruction or severe inflammation of the throat are among the causes. Spasm of the throat muscles causes the characteristic dysphagia seen in rabies cases.

dysplasia A disorder of cellular organization and development. In animals the most important type is disordered development of joints, the best known being canine *hip dysplasia, in which the head of the femur fails to fit exactly into the acetabulum. *Physeal dysplasia* of horses occurs in fast-growing foals exercising on dry hard ground. The growth plates of the long limb bones become damaged and inflamed. Prevention and treatment require an adequate and balanced mineral intake; overweight animals are more prone to the condition.

dyspnoea Laboured or difficult breathing. It usually implies that oxygen supply is inadequate to match metabolic demands. Obstruction or blockage of the air passages is a common cause, whether due to a foreign object or to disease, such as pneumonia or emphysema. Environmental factors may increase the likelihood of dyspnoea: for example, high altitude alone can provoke dyspnoea, even in resting animals. Other diseases decrease oxygen supply or oxygen-carrying capacity and thus cause dyspnoea, for example anaemia or heart failure.

dystocia Difficult birth: i.e. one in which the young cannot be delivered by maternal effort alone. The overall incidence depends on species and breed, but in the domestic species dystocia is most common in cattle. Dystocia can be classified as either maternal (where the essential cause involves the mother) or foetal (where some aspect of the foetus is responsible). *Maternal dystocia* may result from the absence or weakness of uterine contractions (uterine inertia), which in turn may be caused by a deficiency of hormones, such as *oestrogens, *oxytocin, or *prostaglandin $F_{2\alpha}$, or minerals, such as calcium. Overstretching of the *myometrium, myometrial degeneration due to ageing, or even psychological inhibition of labour due to environmental dis-

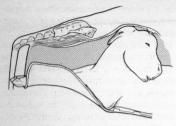

Anterior presentation with head and neck retained (calf)

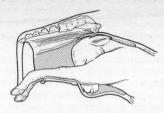

Anterior presentation with downward displacement of the head (calf)

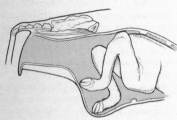

Posterior presentation with downward displacement of hind legs (calf)

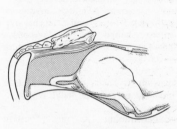

Breech presentation (calf)

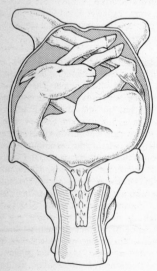

Dorsotransverse presentation (foal)

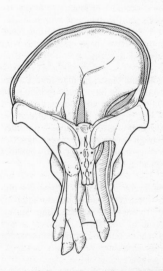

Ventrotransverse presentation (foal)

turbance can also lead to inertia. Likewise, any factor affecting the abdominal musculature can also tend to prevent expulsion of the foetus, as will uterine *torsion. In addition, any maternal anatomical abnormality that obstructs the birth canal will result in dystocia; examples include failure of the cervix to dilate fully (*see* ringwomb), congenital defects of the vagina or vulva, or inadequacy of the pelvis (due to breed, immaturity, or injury). *Foetal dystocia* is more common. Causes include disproportion of foetal size compared with the maternal birth canal; this may be due to foetal oversize resulting from a prolonged gestation or to conditions such as *hydrocephalus. In addition, many cases of dystocia involve an abnormal *presentation of the foetus in the birth canal.

In **cattle**, dairy breeds are most affected and dystocia usually results from foetal factors, frequently when a heifer is carrying a crossbred foetus sired by a bull of a large beef breed. Ringwomb, abnormal presentations, and twin births when there is simultaneous presentation of parts of both foetuses can also cause problems. Likewise, in **sheep**, the causative factors are usually foetal in origin and especially relate to abnormal presentation and twinning. Dystocia is not very common in **horses** and is usually due to foetal factors. In **pigs** maternal dystocia is the most frequent although the general incidence is low; likewise in **cats**. In **dogs** dystocia is generally maternal in origin, the incidence varying with breed; it is high in certain terriers and miniature breeds where selective breeding has exaggerated various features of conformation.

dystrophy Failure to maintain the normal function and mature size of an organ. It is usually caused by impaired supply of nutrients or other materials. For example, *muscular dystrophy may be due to deficiency of selenium and vitamin E, which leads to the accumulation of toxic peroxides on the muscle cell membrane. Muscle fibres so affected degenerate and die. Osteodystrophy in the adult is usually due to mineral deficiency or imbalance so that the bone is demineralized and structurally weakened. Fibrous material is deposited in the weakened bone. Lameness results with the likelihood of spontaneous fractures.

dysuria Difficulty in passing urine, often associated with pain. Causes include weakness of the bladder wall or obstruction of the urethra by calculi (*see* calculus). Inflammation of the bladder (*cystitis) or urethra (*urethritis) may have a similar effect. Catheterization may be indicated to give temporary relief followed by surgery to remove any obstruction. Antibiotic treatment should be given for an infected bladder.

E

ear The sense organ concerned with hearing and balance. The *external ear* consists of the *auricle, or pinna, which receives sound waves and directs them into the external acoustic meatus. At the far end of the meatus is the tympanic window (eardrum), which vibrates in response to sound waves and divides the external ear from the *middle ear*. This consists of the tympanic cavity – an air-filled slitlike chamber that connects to the nasopharynx via the *auditory tube (Eustachian tube). Vibrations are transmitted across this cavity by the auditory *ossicles – malleus, incus, and stapes – which stretch from the tympanic membrane to the vestibular window (fenestra vestibuli).

ear ballooning of pigs

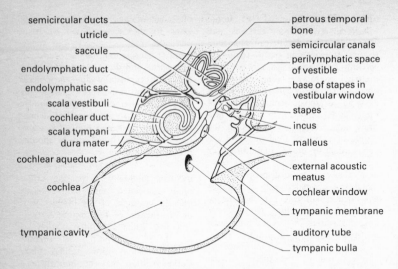

semicircular ducts — petrous temporal bone
utricle —
saccule — semicircular canals
endolymphatic duct — perilymphatic space of vestibule
endolymphatic sac —
scala vestibuli — base of stapes in vestibular window
cochlear duct — stapes
scala tympani —
dura mater — incus
cochlear aqueduct — malleus
cochlea — external acoustic meatus
— cochlear window
— tympanic membrane
tympanic cavity — auditory tube
— tympanic bulla

Middle ear and inner ear of the dog

The *internal ear* consists of a *bony labyrinth* within the temporal bone of the skull. This accommodates the membranous structures of the *membranous labyrinth*: the cochlear duct, which is part of the spiral *cochlea and is concerned with the reception and analysis of sound; the three *semicircular canals, which are concerned with balance; and two structures concerned with sensing the position of the head – the *saccule and *utricle – which lie within the vestibule. The bony labyrinth is filled with a fluid (perilymph), and this fluid surrounds the membranous structures, which are themselves filled with endolymph. Vibrations of the vestibular window are transmitted through this fluid-filled system and converted to nerve impulses in the cochlea. The impulses are then transmitted to the brain and interpreted as sound (see illustration).

Inflammation of the ear (*otitis) commonly affects the external ear and may spread to the middle ear. Dis-

eases of the internal ear can affect hearing and balance.

ear ballooning of pigs Swelling of the ear flap (auricle) in pigs due to *haematoma formation following injury, generally as a result of fighting.

ear mange *See* otodectic mange.

ear tipping The practice of removing, under anaesthetic, the tip of the left ear of feral cats when they are neutered as a distinguishing mark in order to prevent them being recaptured later.

easing the heel (opening the heel) 1. A procedure for treating corns and bruised heels in horses, in which the lower edge and bar of the heel is rasped away so it does not press on the shoe. 2. The removal of the connection between the wall and bars of the heel – a malpractice that leads to contracted heels.

East Coast fever (ECF; bovine theileriosis) An acute and frequently fatal form of *theileriosis affecting cattle. It is caused by the protozoan parasite *Theileria parva and transmitted by the brown ear tick, *Rhipicephalus appendiculatus*. The tick, and hence the disease, are confined to East and Central Africa, where ECF is a major constraint on cattle production. In exotic susceptible animals the disease is characterized by fever and enlarged lymph nodes, which become apparent some 10–15 days after infected ticks feed on the host. The first node to become enlarged is the parotid lymph node below the ear, the feeding site of the tick. As the disease progresses the animal becomes severely depressed and ceases to eat and ruminate. There may be diarrhoea and discharges from the nose and eyes. Breathing becomes laboured due to oedema of the lungs, from which death may occur 1–2 weeks after the onset of illness. Among native cattle in enzootic areas, many animals recover and become carriers of the infection. Moreover, cattle exposed to ticks under range conditions may be simultaneously infected with several *Theileria* species and strains, producing a more complex syndrome, which may include anaemia due to *T. mutans* infection (*see* tzaneen disease). Diagnosis is based on clinical signs, together with the demonstration of parasites in stained smears of lymph-node biopsies or blood. A good immunity develops in recovered animals. However, strain differences in the parasite have presented problems in vaccine development, although prototype multistrain live vaccines are now in advanced experimental use. Control relies on strict and frequent treatment of cattle with *acaricides to combat the tick vector. A specific and effective drug, parvaquone, is now available to treat cases should control

measures fail. *See also* corridor disease.

ec- *Prefix denoting* out of or outside.

ecbolic An agent that causes uterine contraction; it may be used to produce abortion or accelerate parturition. Various hormones are used, including *prostaglandins, *oestrogen, and *oxytocin. The ergot alkaloids were the earliest ecbolic drugs, and *ergot poisoning can cause abortion in livestock.

ecchymosis (*pl.* **ecchymoses**) A purple discoloration of the skin similar to a bruise and caused by bleeding from underlying vessels into the skin beneath the dermis. Damage to the blood-vessel walls which results in ecchymoses is found in *septicaemia, *purpura haemorrhagica, and *warfarin poisoning. *See also* petechia.

eccrine *See* merocrine.

ecdysis The act of shedding skin; *desquamation.

ECG *See* electrocardiography.

echinococcosis *See* hydatidosis.

Echinococcus A genus of *tapeworms found worldwide (in Britain commonly in central and South Wales). The adults are parasites in the small intestine of carnivores, dogs, wolves, and jackals. They are small, up to 8 mm long, with usually three proglottids. They cause little or no damage in dogs, but the eggs pass out with the faeces and when eaten by an intermediate host, chiefly sheep, cattle, horses, pigs, or humans, each egg develops into a spherical fluid-filled cyst, the *hydatid cyst, usually in the lungs or liver (see illustration). This cyst can reach 150 mm in diameter, contains numerous secondary cysts, and is responsible for hydatid

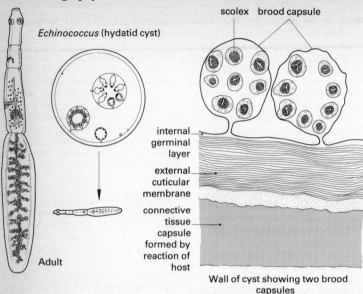

Echinococcus (hydatid cyst)

scolex brood capsule

internal germinal layer

external cuticular membrane

connective tissue capsule formed by reaction of host

Adult

Wall of cyst showing two brood capsules

The tapeworm *Echinococccus granulosus*

disease (*hydatidosis). Routine worming of dogs helps to prevent the spread of the tapeworm.

echocardiography   The use of ultrasonic waves directed through the chest wall to obtain an *echocardiogram*, i.e. a recording of the movement and structures of the heart. This is useful in the diagnosis of pericardial and valvular disorders and of congenital lesions of the heart.

echography   The use of ultrasonic waves directed through the body to differentiate between tissues of different density. The waves are reflected to different degrees by different tissues and converted into a visual image, the *echogram*.

echovirus   *See* Coxsackie virus; enterovirus.

eclampsia   A convulsive condition which occurs in late pregnancy, immediately after parturition, or in early lactation. The cause is unknown although *hypocalcaemia may contribute and administration of calcium borogluconate may alleviate the symptoms. Clinical signs include restlessness, increased respiratory rate, convulsions, pyrexia (fever) (up to 42.7°C), mastitis, and sometimes purulent vulval discharge. Bitches and queens are most commonly affected. Mares can exhibit similar signs in early lactation or associated with stress, but are not usually pyrexic (*see* lactation tetany). They should be treated with calcium and magnesium salts. Severely affected animals often die, but response to treatment is good in mild cases. Other name: **puerperal tetany**.

E. coli   *See* Escherichia.

econazole *See* imidazoles.

ecraseur A surgical instrument, consisting of a chain on a ratchet, that may be used in the *castration of the larger domestic animals. The scrotum is incised to expose the testis and the ecraseur applied to the spermatic cord, thereby crushing the blood vessels inside the spermatic cord and destroying the blood supply to the testis. The process is then repeated with the other testis.

ect- (ecto-) *Prefix denoting* outer or external.

ectasia (ectasis) The dilatation of a tube, duct, or hollow organ.

ecthyma *See* orf.

ectoderm The outer of the three *germ layers of the early embryo. It gives rise to the nervous system and sense organs, the teeth and lining of the mouth, and the *epidermis and its associated structures (hair, claws, etc.).

-ectomy *Suffix denoting* surgical removal of a segment or all of an organ or part.

ectoparasite *See* parasite.

ectoparasiticide An agent used to kill ectoparasites, particularly arthropod parasites that live or feed on the skin, either permanently or for short periods. Compounds used as ectoparasiticides include *organochlorines, *organophosphorus compounds, carbamates, *pyrethroids, *derris, sulphur compounds, and *ivermectin. They can be applied variously in, for example, sprays, washes, dips, powders, pour-ons, spot-ons, or impregnated collars, or injected parenterally. Many (e.g. *dieldrin) have a persistent effect, both on the host and

in the environment, hence their use is restricted.

ectopia 1. The misplacement, due either to a congenital defect or injury, of a bodily part. *Ectopia cordis* is congenital displacement of the heart into the neck, completely outside the thoracic cavity; it is most commonly seen in calves, and affected animals can survive for several years. 2. The occurrence of something in an unnatural location.

ectopic 1. Describing a tissue or organ that is displaced from its normal position due to a congenital defect or injury. For example, an ectopic tooth is one in which the embryonic tooth-forming tissue persists within the jaw to subsequently grow into a *dentigerous cyst or *odontoma. Ectopic ureters in the bitch may drain into the vagina instead of the bladder and thus cause incontinence; surgical correction is indicated. 2. Describing the occurrence of something in an unnatural location. For example, an ectopic heart beat (extrasystole) is one due to a nerve impulse generated somewhere outside the sinoatrial node. *See also* ectopic pregnancy.

ectopic pregnancy A pregnancy in which the embryo or foetus develops outside the uterus, most commonly in the uterine tube. Such pregnancies are usually unsuccessful.

ectro- *Prefix denoting* congenital absence.

ectromelia A contagious disease of mice characterized by skin eruptions and ulcers and caused by orthopoxvirus (*see* poxvirus). Infection is by inhalation or entry of the virus through a skin abrasion. Seven days after experimental inoculation of ectromelia virus a skin lesion develops at the site of inoculation; this is followed 2 days later by a generalized rash. Some mice die before the appearance of these secondary skin eruptions. On post mortem small white areas may be seen on the liver and spleen. Animals that recover may carry the virus for a considerable time, while some mice may completely fail to show clinical signs of disease but remain carriers of the virus.

The appearance of ectromelia varies with strains of mice, strains of virus, and infecting dose of virus. Ectromelia virus is closely related to *vaccinia virus, and its absence from wild mice has led to the suggestion that ectromelia may not have originated in mice. Vaccinia has been used to control ectromelia in mouse colonies, but the only effective method of control is complete destruction of the colony and disinfection. Mice entering a colony should be quarantined and blood-tested for the virus. The presence of ectromelia in a colony of mice being used for experimental work can affect the validity of experimental results, and its presence in colonies being used for the production of vaccines or reagents can result in the ectromelia virus being unintentionally included in these products.

eczema An obsolete term in veterinary medicine, literally meaning 'boiling over', formerly used to describe severely itchy skin conditions. More appropriate terms are atopic dermatitis (*see* atopy), *allergic dermatitis, and *allergic contact dermatitis. In human medicine it refers to various noncontagious inflammations of the skin characterized by papules and vesicles, which rupture to give a moist surface to the lesion.

ED₅₀ Effective dose 50 or median effective dose: the dose of a drug found to be effective in 50% of animals tested.

edrophonium A reversible *anticholinesterase that can be used to reverse competitive neuromuscular blocking agents. It is also used in the diagnosis of *myasthenia gravis in dogs prior to the use of longer-acting compounds in treatment (e.g. neostigmine, pyridostigmine, and ambenonium). It is injected intramuscularly, intravenously, or subcutaneously and has a short duration of action (3–10 minutes).

EDS *See* egg-drop syndrome.

EDTA (ethylenediamine tetraacetic acid) A compound used (in the form of its calcium salt) as a *chelating agent to treat heavy metal poisoning, especially *lead poisoning. Being poorly absorbed from the gut, it is injected slowly intravenously. When used in lead poisoning, the lead accumulated in bone tissue is chelated, displacing calcium from the EDTA, and subsequently excreted. The lead in soft tissues is redistributed to the skeleton, so reducing signs of toxicity. Several treatments with calcium EDTA are needed to remove large quantities of lead. EDTA has a toxic effect on the kidneys, causing *nephrosis. This may be due to the rapid removal of chelated metals at the renal tubules; these effects usually disappear when treatment is halted. EDTA (as the acid or sodium salt) is also used as an anticoagulant in blood samples taken for certain tests.

EEG (electroencephalogram) *See* electroencephalography.

effective population size The number of individuals that, if bred in the manner of an idealized population, would give rise to the same rate of inbreeding as the population under consideration. It allows for, e.g., different numbers of males and females to be taken into account in calculat-

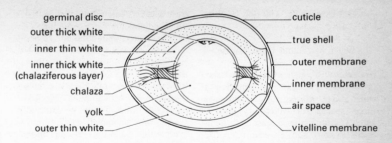

germinal disc — cuticle
outer thick white — true shell
inner thin white — outer membrane
inner thick white (chalaziferous layer) — inner membrane
chalaza — air space
yolk — vitelline membrane
outer thin white —

Structure of the egg

ing the average *inbreeding coefficient for the population.

effector An organ, such as a muscle or gland, that carries out an activity, especially under the control of the nervous system.

efferent 1. Designating nerves or neurones that convey impulses from the brain or spinal cord to muscles, glands, and other effectors; i.e. any motor nerve or neurone. 2. Designating vessels or ducts that drain fluid (such as lymph) from an organ or part. *Compare* afferent.

egg 1. *See* ovum. 2. The shelled egg in birds and other egg-laying vertebrates. In **birds** it has the following components: the *germinal disc*, which is a small white spot on the surface of the yolk consisting of cytoplasm and the remains of the nucleus; the *yolk*, consisting of *white yolk* – very rich in protein and including the *latebra*, which extends from the centre to a disc below the germinal disc – and *yellow yolk* – very rich in fat, which may consist of various strata differing in composition. The yolk is surrounded by: several *yolk membranes*; the *albumen*, including the twisted strands (*chalazae) that suspend the yolk; the *inner* and *outer shell membranes*, which sep-

arate at the blunt end of the egg to enclose the *air space*; the *shell*, composed of smooth hard calcareous material; and the *cuticle*, which is a thin transparent permeable coating. See illustration.

egg-bound *See* impacted.

egg-drop syndrome (EDS) A condition of laying hens involving depression in laying performance. It is due to an adenovirus infection and was of major economic importance in the late 1970s and is still seen today. Egg production fails to hit peak target or is depressed subsequently, and shell quality is seriously affected, often with loss of pigment. Birds in deep-litter or barn systems show a high incidence of floor-laying. Other signs may include poor appetite or diarrhoea. There is no treatment but effective vaccines are in general use.

egg-eating A vice in laying hens where the shell is broken open and the contents consumed. The initial egg breakage may be accidental, but subsequent incidents are deliberate, as the hen appears to develop a taste for the egg contents. It is observed in both extensive and intensive systems (*see* poultry husbandry) although less so in battery units as eggs are rapidly removed from cages. The only remedy is to cull persistent offenders.

egg heart *See* round heart disease.

Ehrlichia A genus of *rickettsiae transmitted by ticks and affecting a wide range of animals. There are three species of veterinary importance, causing the disease *ehrlichiosis. *E. canis* and *E. equi* parasitize circulating white blood cells of dogs and horses respectively, causing fever and anaemia. The organism multiplies mainly in the lymphocytes and monocytes but can also affect the neutrophils. *E. riscistici* causes a severe enteritis in horses. *See also* equine ehrlichiosis.

ehrlichiosis Any disease due to infection with rickettsiae of the genus *Ehrlichia*, which are transmitted by ticks. Ehrlichiosis of **dogs** is characterized by fever, nasal and eye discharges, and emaciation and caused by *E. canis*. The disease is widespread in the tropics and subtropics in areas where the dog tick *Rhipicephalus sanguineus* is distributed. Following an incubation period of 1–3 weeks affected dogs develop a fluctuating fever and a nasal and eye discharge, which becomes mucopurulent. Dogs avoid the light and haemorrhages may sometimes be seen on the skin. Nervous signs may also develop. Dogs that survive the first week become anaemic and very thin with sunken eyes and a foul breath. Treatment with *tetracyclines is recommended although recovered dogs become carriers and may relapse. Wild dogs, coyotes, foxes, and jackals may show only mild clinical signs. Weeks or months after apparent recovery, dogs may develop a severe and sometimes fatal nosebleed. The fever returns, appetite is lost, and respiratory distress develops. The nosebleeds continue and the dog usually dies within a week. This sequel to ehrlichiosis is known as canine tropical pancytopenia: it is immunologically mediated and does not respond to treatment. Control of ehrlichiosis entails strict control of *tick infestation.

Various species of *Ehrlichia* infect **ruminants** in Africa. Such infections, known as 'mild disease' of cattle and sheep, are characterized by intracytoplasmic inclusions in the *monocytes and the presence of excess fluid in the pericardial sac (*compare* heartwater). The agents are tentatively named *E. bovis* and *E. ovina* and are transmitted respectively by ticks of the genus *Hyalomma*, and *Rhipicephalus bursa. See also* equine ehrlichiosis.

Eimeria A genus of coccidian protozoa (*see* coccidia) that are intracellular parasites of mammals and birds. Most *Eimeria* species parasitize the intestinal tract but some are found in other organs, such as the liver or kidney. Many are important pathogens, causing the disease *coccidiosis. *Eimeria* are highly host specific, and there may be several species in each host. Consequently hundreds of species have been described.

Animals become infected by ingesting infective *oocysts. In the gut, *sporozoites liberated from the oocysts invade host cells and begin to grow and divide (see illustration). A series of asexual multiplicative cycles (*merogony) occurs in which large *meronts may form, causing tissue destruction. This is followed by a sexual process resulting in the formation of oocysts, which are shed into the gut and excreted in faeces. This cycle may take as little as 4 days in birds, but longer (18–21 days) in sheep or cattle. In this time one ingested oocyst can give rise to hundreds of thousands of daughter oocysts. Oocysts are not immediately infective but must mature and divide (sporulate or undergo *sporogony) outside the host. This normally takes 1–2

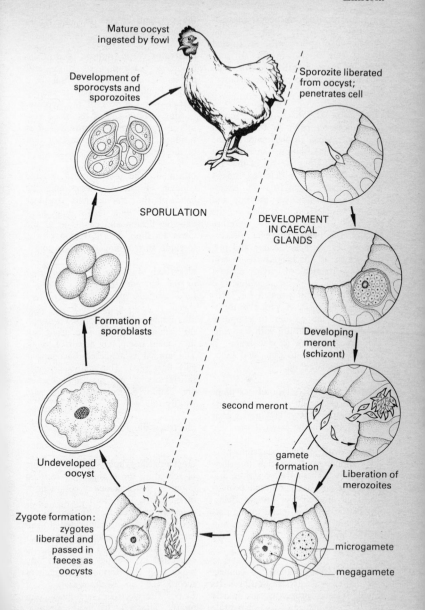

Mature oocyst
ingested by fowl

Development of
sporocysts and
sporozoites

Sporozite liberated
from oocyst;
penetrates cell

SPORULATION

DEVELOPMENT
IN CAECAL
GLANDS

Formation of
sporoblasts

Developing
meront
(schizont)

second meront

gamete
formation

Liberation of
merozoites

Undeveloped
oocyst

Zygote formation:
zygotes
liberated and
passed in
faeces as
oocysts

microgamete

megagamete

Life cycle of the coccidian protozoan, *Eimeria tenella*

days and results in an oocyst containing four sporocysts, each of which contains two sporozoites. Sporulated oocysts can survive in the environment for many months and are resistant to most commonly used disinfectants.

ejaculation The discharge of *semen from the erect penis at the moment of sexual climax in the male. At the instant of ejaculation, spermatozoa are propelled from the tail of the epididymis and ductus deferens, mixed with seminal plasma from the accessory genital glands (e.g. prostate and seminal vesicles), and expelled via the powerfully contracting urethra through the penis. However, in certain species, such as the dog and pig, the semen is discharged as several successive fractions of varying content and consistency. *Electroejaculation* is a method of collecting semen for *artificial insemination. A probe is introduced into the rectum to stimulate the genital musculature with low-voltage pulses, leading to ejaculation. It is most successful in rams and bulls. *See also* insemination.

elastic cartilage A type of *cartilage in which elastic fibres are distributed in the matrix. It is yellowish in colour and is found in the external ear.

elastic tissue Strong extensible flexible *connective tissue rich in yellow *elastic fibres*. These are long, thin, and branching and are composed primarily of an albumin-like protein, *elastin. Elastic tissue is found in the dermis of the skin, in arterial walls, and in the walls of the alveoli of the lungs.

elastin A *protein found in connective tissue, especially elastic fibres. Its unique elastic properties are partly due to cross-linkage of its polypeptide chains by desmosine, an amino acid only found in elastin and formed by the covalent linkage of four lysine residues.

elastrator An instrument, used in the bloodless *castration of lambs and calves, that enables the stretching of a strong rubber ring so that it can be placed over the neck of the scrotum, causing compression of the blood vessels in the spermatic cords and thus resulting in the ultimate degeneration of the testicles.

elbow 1. The joint formed by the condyle of the *humerus and the head of the *radius and trochlear notch of the *ulna. It is a hinge joint allowing flexion and extension of the lower forelimb. **2.** The region of the forelimb surrounding the elbow joint.

electrical stunning A method used in the humane slaughter of certain food animals, particularly pigs and sheep. A low-voltage (70 V for pigs) alternating current is passed through the brain of the animal using an instrument resembling a pair of tongs. The animal is rendered unconscious and then bled. The method is only satisfactory if experienced operators are employed and instructions are strictly followed.

electrocardiogram *See* electrocardiography.

electrocardiography The technique of recording the changes in electrical potential that accompany contractions of the heart. This electrical activity is detected by electrodes applied to the body surface and connected to an amplifier and recording apparatus (*electrocardiograph*). The signals are converted to tracings on a moving paper strip, thus forming a permanent record (i.e. an *electrocardiogram* or *ECG*). The electrodes are most commonly attached to both pectoral limbs, one pelvic limb, and the thoracic wall. By selective switching between the electrodes it is possible to obtain different ECG patterns, with varying diagnostic applications. The technique can be used to detect alterations in cardiac rhythm, abnormalities of electrical conductivity in the heart muscle, dissociation of the normal sequence of muscle contraction, or the occurrence of abnormal muscle contractions.

electrocautery 1. The destruction of diseased or unwanted tissue by means of an electrically heated wire or needle. **2.** The instrument used for this operation. *Compare* diathermy.

electrocoagulation The destructive coagulation of tissues by means of a high-frequency electric current concentrated at one point as it passes through them. The technique prevents or reduces haemorrhage and can be used as an alternative to crushing bleeding vessels with artery forceps or to ligating such vessels. It is a rapid and convenient method of haemostasis but must be used with care. *See also* diathermy.

electroencephalography The technique of recording the electrical activity of the brain. Electrodes are applied at points on each side of the midline of the skull and connected to an apparatus (*electroencephalograph*) that amplifies the signals and converts them to a tracing on a paper strip, called an *electroencephalogram* or *EEG*. The recording of EEGs in animals is often more difficult than in humans because of the electrical activity of muscles overlying the skull. Electroencephalography can detect loss of electrical activity from areas where brain damage has occurred, and abnormal electrical patterns from areas of the brain with electrical instability, as in sites associated with fits, for instance.

electrolyte A liquid that conducts electricity due to the presence of positive or negative ions. In biochemical usage, the term often refers to the ions themselves. The major ions in biological systems are Na^+, K^+, Cl^-, Ca^{2+}, Mg^{2+}, HCO^-_3, and *phosphate, which occur in aqueous solution. Clinically, the electrolytes in blood *plasma are of great importance. Their concentrations are maintained within close limits by homeostatic mechanisms (*see* homeostasis) in order to provide the optimum ionic environment for the proper structure and function of tissues and organs in the animal. Concentrations of various electrolytes are altered by many diseases, in which electrolytes are lost from the body (as in vomiting or diarrhoea) or are not excreted and accumulate (as in renal failure). Severe depletion of electrolytes requires therapeutic replacement of the appropriate substance, either by mouth or intravenously.

electromyography The continuous recording of the electrical activity of a muscle by means of electrodes inserted into the muscle fibres. The trace (*electromyogram*) is displayed on an oscilloscope. The technique can be used experimentally, for example to study the actions of muscles, the effects of drugs, or to aid in the diagnosis of muscular disorders.

electron microscope A microscope that uses a beam of electrons for viewing the specimen. The resolving power (ability to register fine detail) is a thousand times greater than that of an ordinary light microscope. The specimen must be examined in a vacuum, which necessitates special techniques for preparing it, and the electrons are usually focused onto a fluorescent screen (for direct viewing) or onto a photographic plate (for a photograph, or *electron micrograph*). A *transmission electron microscope* is

electron transport chain

used to examine thin sections at high magnification. A *scanning electron microscope* is used to examine the surface of objects at various magnifications; its great depth of focus and contoured view is advantageous.

electron transport chain *See* respiratory chain.

electrophoresis A method of separating charged molecules or ions in solution by subjecting them to an electric field. Molecules migrate at different rates depending on their net charge and size and so separate into distinct bands on the electrophoretic medium – usually a gel or paper. The technique is commonly applied to the analysis of serum proteins in clinical diagnosis. *See also* immunoelectrophoresis.

electrotherapy The use of electricity in the treatment of disease. *See also* diathermy.

elf fire *See* alveld.

ELISA *See* enzyme-linked immunosorbent assay.

elixir A preparation, containing glycerine or alcohol, that is used as a vehicle for administering unpleasant-tasting drugs. Flavourings, such as oil of aniseed, fennel, orange, lemon, or coriander, may be incorporated. Elixirs are occasionally made up for the oral administration of drugs to dogs and horses.

Elizabethan collar A device, resembling an upturned lampshade and made out of heavy-duty plastic or thick cardboard, that is fitted over the neck of an animal, usually a dog, to prevent self-mutilation, particularly following surgery.

Elokomin fluke fever A fluke-borne rickettsial disease of dogs, occurring in the same regions as *salmon poisoning and transmitted by the same fluke. Although the agent is a *Neorickettsia*, recovered animals show no immunity to salmon poisoning.

elongated soft palate A condition, commonly found in *brachycephalic dogs, in which the relative shortening of the nose makes the mobile soft *palate too long, so that it cannot be properly withdrawn from the airway when the dog breathes. In mild cases this simply results in noisy breathing, but in severe cases the dog may collapse when stressed due to lack of oxygen. In the latter instance, surgical correction may be needed. Other name: **hyperplasia of the soft palate**.

Elsoheel *See* spastic paresis.

em- *Prefix. See* en-.

emaciation Wasting of the body caused by malnutrition or chronic debilitating disease (e.g. Johne's disease, tuberculosis, parasitic diseases). In meat inspection, emaciated carcasses are characterized by wasting of the muscles and reduction in the amount of fat, which is soft, wet, and gelatinous in advanced cases. The flesh is soft, wet, and flabby and does not set. The condition should not be confused with *poorness.

embedding (in microscopy) The fixing of a specimen within a mass of firm material in order to facilitate the cutting of thin sections for microscopical study. The embedding medium, e.g. paraffin wax for light microscopy or Araldite for electron microscopy, helps to keep the specimen intact.

embolism The condition in which an *embolus becomes lodged in an artery and obstructs the blood flow. If the embolus is a blood clot (thrombus), it forms in the heart or within a

embryo transplantation

vein. When released the clot follows the blood flow until it obstructs an artery, thus impeding or stopping the local blood supply and causing the death of tissue supplied by the artery (*infarction). Thus an embolus coming from a vein may pass through the heart and lodge in the narrowing pulmonary arteries producing *pulmonary embolism* and an infarct within the lung. Cardiac thrombi, which form on the heart valves, are common in endocarditis; if dislodged they can produce kidney infarcts. In horses a verminous *aneurysm of the anterior mesenteric artery may give rise to an embolus that is liable to break loose and occlude the iliac arteries with consequent collapse of the hindlimbs.

embolus (*pl.* **emboli**) Material, such as a blood clot, fat droplet, or a foreign body, that is carried by the blood from one point in the circulation to lodge at another, especially where the arterial system narrows to obstruct its passage (*see* embolism). An embolus of fat droplets commonly originates from a fractured bone when fat in the bone marrow accidentally enters the circulation. *See also* thrombosis.

embrocation A preparation that is rubbed locally into intact skin. It may contain a *rubefacient drug, which causes local vasodilatation, and the friction during application increases this effect. Most embrocations are oily emulsions containing methyl salicylate, ammonia, capsicum, or aconite as the rubefacient. They are used as counterirritants and to provide heat to areas of muscle strain and arthritis.

embryo An organism in the course of its development. In **mammals** the term refers to the early stages of prenatal development during which the main organ systems develop (*compare* foetus). In **birds** the term includes all stages up to hatching.

embryology The study of the embryo, otherwise known as developmental anatomy. *See* anatomy.

embryonic disc The early stages of development of the embryo when it is a flat sheet of tissue, initially continuous at its margins with the *trophoblast. Later it is bounded dorsally by the amniotic cavity (*see* amnion) and ventrally by the *yolk sac. The formation of the *primitive streak in the embryonic disc determines the orientation of the embryo, which then becomes progressively transformed into a three-dimensional structure.

embryo transplantation The process by which an *embryo is recovered from a donor animal and transferred into the uterus or oviduct of a recipient of the same species to complete its development. Embryo transplantation is successful because of the immunological *tolerance shown by the oviducts and uterus towards embryos containing foreign *antigens – 50% of embryonic antigens are of paternal (and hence foreign) origin normally. In addition, the mammalian embryo undergoes a free-floating period before implantation, and in domestic species this period is quite long so that embryos can be transplanted at quite late stages. This allows assessment of recovered embryos so that unsuitable embryos can be rejected. The major commercial use of the technique is in the multiplication of superior genotypes; embryo transplantation gives an increased rate of genetic improvement since, not having to accommodate the foetus in utero, the most valuable dams are able to produce many offspring in their lifetime. The technique also has advantages in the import and export of stock, since transportation of embryos is considerably cheaper than that of breeding animals. It can also be used to produce twinning in

263

emesis

beef cows, which increases biological efficiency.

The same basic procedures of embryo transplantation have been used in all the agriculturally important species. The dam is *superovulated by injection of pregnant mare's serum gonadotrophin (*PMSG) so that many oocytes develop. *Artificial insemination (AI) is performed using semen from a selected sire, then the embryos are collected, usually at the late *blastocyst stage. Collection may be surgical, in which case *laparotomy is used to locate the oviducts and facilitate the introduction of a flushing medium to dislodge any embryos present. In nonsurgical collection the embryos are flushed out of the conscious animal by means of a three-way catheter introduced into the vagina and cervix. Surgical collection gives higher success rates at present, but has all the disadvantages of general anaesthesia and may only be repeated a few times due to the formation of uterine and ovarian *adhesions. Nonsurgical collection is much easier to carry out on the farm, besides being cheaper and repeatable. After collection, the embryos are assessed microscopically on the basis of their morphology; only viable embryos are transplanted. It is vital that embryos are transferred into a recipient uterus that is at exactly the same stage of the oestrous cycle as the donor; this may be achieved through the use of synchronizing agents, such as *progestogens or *prostaglandin $F_{2\alpha}$. Alternatively, embryos may be stored for short periods in culture media; for long-term storage they may be frozen in liquid nitrogen at $-196°C$. Success rates for transferring thawed frozen embryos are lower than for fresh embryos.

Transplantation may be performed surgically, involving general anaesthesia, or nonsurgically through the cervix using a version of the AI *catheter. Either technique is suitable for cows and mares, but in sows and ewes the tortuous cervix is not easily penetrated so surgery is necessary. Future commercial applications of the technique may involve embryo splitting (to produce identical twins or quadruplets), sexing of embryos (e.g. to ensure heifer calves for milk production), and cloning (see clone) to produce large groups of identical individuals. See also ovum transplantation.

emesis See vomiting.

emetic An agent that causes *vomiting (emesis). Many substances, including sodium chloride, sodium carbonate (washing soda), copper sulphate, zinc sulphate, and mustard, can act as emetics by causing local irritation of the gastric mucosa, thereby initiating the vomiting reflex. Others, e.g. digitalis and apomorphine, act centrally. Antimony tartrate and potassium tartrate (tartar emetic) are no longer used as emetics because of toxicity. In small animals, solutions of sodium chloride, sodium carbonate, or mustard can be administered orally, for example following the ingestion of toxic substances. Vomiting occurs within 15 minutes of administration but the effect can be variable. These substances are non-toxic, even if vomiting does not occur. However, if no vomiting is induced after administering zinc or copper sulphate (1% solutions), gastric lavage may be necessary to prevent toxicity due to absorption of copper or zinc. *Apomorphine is a reliable emetic in small animals but it is now a *controlled drug. *Xylazine produces emesis in cats and frequently in dogs, and can be used in some cases of poisoning. Vomiting is not possible in ruminants, horses, and rodents, but regurgitation of stomach contents may occur, with expulsion through the nose in horses.

-emia (*US*) *See* -aemia.

eminence A projection, often rounded, on an organ or tissue, particularly on a bone. An example is the *intercondylar eminence* on the tibia.

emollient A substance used to soften skin, remove desquamating (flaking) skin, and reduce skin irritation. Various oils, paraffin-based ointments or creams, fat emulsions, and oily emulsions are used. Dusting powders containing, for example, French chalk, are also used but are less effective. Emollients are nonirritant and are not absorbed through the skin.

emphysema An abnormal accumulation of air within the body tissues. *Pulmonary emphysema* involves distension of the alveoli in the lungs, leading to destruction of alveolar tissue. This may rarely result from overdistension during assisted ventilation under general anaesthesia, especially in small animals, but is more likely to occur as part of a disease process, such as *broken wind or chronic *bronchiolitis in horses. In *subcutaneous emphysema* air accumulates in subcutaneous tissues. This may be due to injury of the respiratory tract allowing air to escape, surgery, or the presence of gas-producing organisms, such as *Clostridium* bacteria. Gradual resorption of the air into the blood will occur if there is no ongoing leakage or infection.

empirical Describing a system of treatment based on experience or observation, rather than on logic or reason.

empyema Accumulation of pus in a body cavity. Empyema of the pleural cavity surrounding the lungs can arise due to a purulent infection of the lungs or pleura (e.g. pneumonia or pleurisy). Empyema may also develop in the guttural pouch of the horse as a result of streptococcal infection spreading from the upper respiratory tract during an attack of *strangles.

emulsion A *colloid in which small droplets of one liquid are dispersed in another liquid. Emulsions of oils or fats in water are often stabilized by using *detergents as *emulsifiers*. These ensure that the small globules of fat or oil remain in suspension. Some drugs can be prepared as emulsions and used topically or orally.

en- (em-) *Prefix denoting* in; inside.

enamel The insensitive outer covering of the crown of a *tooth. It is the hardest tissue in the body and is composed of long hexagonal prism-like rods of *hydroxyapatite.

enarthrosis *See* ball-and-socket joint.

encapsulated (of an organ, tumour, etc.) Enclosed in a capsule.

encephal- (encephalo-) *Prefix denoting* the brain.

encephalin (enkephalin) *See* endorphin.

encephalitis (*pl.* **encephalitides**) Inflammation of the substance of the brain. If the inflammation also involves the membranes enclosing the brain, the condition is termed *meningoencephalitis* (*see* meningitis). Many encephalitides extend to involve the spinal cord (i.e. *encephalomyelitis*); inflammation of the cord only (*myelitis) is less common. Infection is almost invariably the cause. *Viral encephalitis* may be caused by the viruses of rabies, Aujeszky's disease, *Japanese encephalitis, malignant catarrhal fever, spontaneous bovine encephalomyelitis, louping ill, scrapie, swine fever, African swine fever, swine vesicular dis-

encephalomalacia

ease, Teschen disease of pigs, infectious *equine encephalomyelitis, canine distemper, and *infectious avian encephalomyelitis. Other viral encephalitides include Murray Valley, St Louis, California (La Crosse), Powassan, Russian spring-summer, Central European, and Kyasanur Forest. All are potentially transmissible to humans, although humans are not part of the natural cycle of the viruses, which usually involves a tick or insect and bird. Other domestic mammals may be accidentally affected when they are introduced into a new habitat. The diseases are usually of restricted distribution but are characterized by periodic epizootics in areas previously clear of disease. *Bacterial encephalitis* may be caused by *Listeria monocytogenes* and *Haemophilus somnus*. In all cases the signs are mainly nervous, including excitability, mania or depression, circling, head-pressing, tremors, ataxia, paresis, and coma. When the cause is bacterial, antibiotics can be used; there is no specific treatment for the viral forms.

encephalomalacia Degeneration (literally 'softening') of the brain. It is due to a variety of causes. Among them are plant or other toxins. For example, horses eating large amounts of the yellow star thistle (*Centaurea solstitalis*), found in the USA, may suffer localized softening of the globus pallidus and substantia nigra in the brain, i.e. *nigropallidal encephalomalacia. Crazy chick disease* is a form of encephalomalacia, usually seen in chicks and poults, caused by a dietary deficiency of *vitamin E or by interference with the vitamin's metabolism. Affected birds show uncoordinated behaviour followed by paralysis and death. *Cerebrocortical necrosis, which affects cattle and sheep, is a form of encephalomalacia due to thiamin (*vitamin B_1) deficiency.

encephalomyelitis Inflammation of the brain and spinal cord, often caused by viral or bacterial infections (*see* encephalitis). *See also* infectious avian encephalomyelitis.

encephalomyocarditis (EMC) virus A *picornavirus of mice that has been extensively used as an experimental virus for laboratory investigation.

encysted Enclosed in a cyst.

end- (endo-) *Prefix denoting* within or inner. Example: *endonasal* (within the nose).

Endangered Species Act (USA) A federal law giving the Secretary of the Interior the power to list a species as protected, to determine its critical habitat, and to protect it from being taken.

endarteritis Inflammation of the inner lining of an artery. In animals it is most commonly caused by parasites. For example, the migrating larvae of *Strongylus vulgaris* commonly cause inflammation in the anterior mesenteric artery in the horse. This can lead to a weakening of the arterial wall (*aneurysm) which may rupture and cause a fatal haemorrhage. Arteritis also occurs in *malignant catarrhal fever in cattle and *equine viral arteritis. Such lesions induce local clotting of the blood (thrombosis) and the risk of arterial obstruction (embolism) as the clots dislodge.

end artery The terminal branch of an artery, which does not communicate with other branches. The tissue it supplies is therefore probably completely dependent on it for its blood supply.

endemic Describing diseases that occur in certain localities or populations. Strictly, it is a term used in human medicine, *enzootic being the equivalent term for diseases of animals.

endocardiosis Chronic thickening of the heart valves leading to their distortion and impaired function. It commonly results in progressive *heart failure, particularly in older dogs, which gradually develop pulmonary congestion, a persistent cough, and reduced ability for exercise.

endocarditis Inflammation of the endothelial lining of the heart (endocardium). It is usually caused by bacterial infection, especially *Streptococcus* spp., *Erysipelothrix rhusiopathiae*, and *Corynebacterium pyogenes*. It commonly affects the heart valves leading to valvular insufficiency as they become distorted and fibrosed. In addition large clots (thrombi) may build up on the valvular surface (*vegetative endocarditis*); if portions of these break off they may cause *embolism and consequent tissue death (*infarction) elsewhere in the body. Prolonged *antibiotic therapy may control the infection giving remission of the clinical signs.

endocardium The internal layer of the wall of the heart. It is lined by a layer of endothelial cells, under which lies connective tissue. Flaps of the endocardium form the *cusps of the heart valves.

endocrine gland (ductless gland) A gland that manufactures *hormones and secretes them directly into the blood, in which they are carried to some distant target tissue to exert a specific action. Endocrine glands include the pituitary, thyroid, parathyroid, and adrenal glands, the ovary and testis, the placenta, and parts of the pancreas. *Compare* exocrine gland.

endocrinology The study of the *endocrine glands and the substances they secrete (*hormones).

endoderm The inner of the three *germ layers of the early embryo that gives rise to the lining of most of the alimentary tract and its associated glands – the liver, gall-bladder, and pancreas. It also forms the lining of the bronchi and alveoli of the lung and most of the urinary tract.

endogenous Arising within or derived from the body. *Compare* exogenous.

endolymph The fluid contained within the membranous labyrinth of the inner ear.

endometriosis Abnormal location and growth of the cells that normally form the membranous lining of the uterus (endometrium). Such unusual growth, seen only in primates, often occurs within the muscle coat of the uterine wall or in the ovary, frequently without clinical signs. However, they may become cystic, cause pain, and need surgical removal.

endometritis Inflammation of the membranous lining of the uterus (*endometrium). It is commonly caused by bacterial infection at parturition or abortion, or occurs as a sequel to a retained placenta. *Brucella abortus*, *Escherichia coli*, streptococci, or staphylococci are the usual pathogens. Affected animals develop fever, become depressed, and show a vaginal discharge. Therapy involves the administration of *antibiotics to combat infection; *prostaglandins or *oxytocin may help to evacuate the infected contents of the uterus. Endometritis often occurs as part of a more generalized inflammation of the uterus (*metritis) with the muscular components of the uterine wall also affected (*see* myometritis). It is a common cause of infertility.

endometrium The mucous membrane lining the uterus. It contains connective tissue, blood vessels, and endometrial glands. During the *oestrous cycle the endometrium becomes thickened, with an increased blood supply, in preparation for implantation of the embryo(s). If pregnancy is not established it returns to its previous state; in some primates, including humans, the endometrium breaks down and is discharged at menstruation. Inflammation of the endometrium (*endometritis) can cause infertility. *See also* involution.

endomyocarditis Inflammation of both the lining (endocardium) and the muscular wall (myocardium) of the heart. The lesion is an extension of *endocarditis into the deeper tissues of the heart wall.

endomysium The fine connective tissue sheath that surrounds a single *muscle fibre.

endoneurium The fine connective tissue sheath that surrounds individual fibres within a *nerve.

endonuclease An *enzyme that catalyses the hydrolysis of a *nucleic acid at an internal position on the *polynucleotide chain. Endonucleases may hydrolyse both *DNA and *RNA, but are more commonly specific (i.e. *endo DNase* or *endo RNase*). Hydrolysis leads to the generation of 3'- or 5'-phosphate termini, depending on the enzyme, and to the production of shorter oligonucleotides of varying lengths. *Compare* exonuclease. *See also* restriction endonuclease.

endoparasite *See* parasite.

endopeptidase *See* peptidase.

endoplasmic reticulum (ER) A system of membranes present in the cytoplasm of cells. ER is described as *rough* when it has *ribosomes attached to its surface and *smooth* when ribosomes are absent. It is the site of manufacture of proteins and lipids and is concerned with the transport of these products within the cell (*see also* Golgi apparatus).

end organ A specialized structure at the end of a peripheral nerve fibre, acting as a receptor for a particular sensation. Taste buds, in the tongue, are end organs subserving the sense of taste.

endorphin One of a group of polypeptides, similar to encephalins, that have analgesic activity and are released in the body in response to injury or other stimuli. They act at the same receptors as the opiate drugs, causing depression of the central nervous system with analgesia and narcosis. The injection of endorphins has effects similar to *morphine, with problems of dependence and withdrawal. The actions of endorphins are reversed by opiate antagonists (e.g. naloxone, nalorphine, and diprenorphine). It is thought that the release of endorphins is stimulated during acupuncture producing analgesia.

endoscope A rigid or flexible instrument used to visualize internal body structures. Most consist of a tube with a light at the end and an optical system for transmitting an image to the user's eye. Endoscopy can be performed in the conscious or anaesthetized animal. The various types of endoscope are designed for examining specific parts of the body (*see* duodenoscope; gastroscope; laparoscope; laryngoscope; proctoscope). *See also* fibrescope.

endospore The spore formed within a cell or microorganism, either singly or in large numbers, by cleavage of the cell contents. Examples are the resting nonvegetative stage of certain bacteria. Some fungi also produce endospores.

endosteum The membrane that lines the marrow cavity of a bone.

endothelium (*pl.* **endothelia**) The single squamous layer of cells that lines the heart, blood vessels, and lymphatic vessels. *Compare* epithelium.

endothermic Describing a chemical reaction associated with the absorption of energy in the form of heat. *Compare* exothermic.

endotoxaemia A form of *toxaemia resulting from the dissemination of endotoxins of Gram-negative bacteria through the bloodstream. The endotoxins are lipopolysaccharides present on the bacterial surface, and are liberated when the cells lyse. Endotoxaemia usually results from a septicaemia, such as *colisepticaemia, but may also arise from local infection, as in the profound toxaemia of *coliform mastitis. Signs are not specific for the infecting bacterium, and any of those described for toxaemia may be present. Shock may be more marked than in other toxaemias: pooling of blood in the splanchnic circulation rapidly leads to hypotension, hypothermia, collapse, and death, with little evidence of illness. Otherwise, pyrexia (fever) is the most regular feature, arising both from the direct action of endotoxin on the hypothalamus and the liberation of *pyrogenic substances from damaged leucocytes. Treatment is as given for toxaemia.

endotoxin A toxic substance produced by certain bacteria that is released when the organisms die and disintegrate.

endotracheal anaesthesia A technique for administering volatile or gaseous anaesthetics (*inhalational anaesthetics) through a tube inserted, via the mouth and larynx, into the trachea of the patient. The tube is usually inserted after general *anaesthesia has been induced by an intravenously injected agent, and the gaseous mixture is delivered through the tube by an anaesthetic machine. Various types of anaesthetic circuit may be used, providing nonrebreathing of expired gases, partial rebreathing with a leak of gases (with or without carbon dioxide absorption), or total rebreathing (closed circuit) with full carbon dioxide absorption. All circuits are designed to enable the anaesthetist to control the concentrations of anaesthetic, oxygen, and carbon dioxide in the gaseous mixture, thereby regulating the depth of anaesthesia. The endotracheal tube is commonly fitted with an inflatable cuff to provide an airtight seal in the tracheal lumen. On completion, anaesthetic administration is stopped and the animal is allowed to breathe air through the tube until signs of the swallowing reflex return, when the tube is removed.

end-plate The area of striated muscle cell membrane immediately beneath the motor nerve ending at a *neuromuscular junction. Special receptors in this area trigger muscular contraction when the nerve ending releases its *neurotransmitter.

enema (*pl.* **enemas** or **enemata**) A solution administered through the anus into the rectum. A special enema *syringe (*Higginson's syringe*) may be used, and the procedure must be done slowly, gently and with lubrication to minimize trauma and pain due to rectal and colonic distension.

To treat constipation, a laxative enema, such as warm soapy water or a mixture of glycerine and water, can be effective. An enema can also be given for retained *meconium in the foal. In radiography, a laxative enema prior to radiography of the caudal, abdominal, and pelvic regions is useful to encourage defecation. A barium enema (*see* barium sulphate) may be given during radiographic examination of the terminal alimentary tract. This can aid the diagnosis of abnormalities, such as diverticuli, strictures, or neoplasms. *See also* suppository.

energy The capacity to do work. The chemical energy supplied to an animal in a particular diet or feedstuff can be expressed in several ways. The *gross energy* (*GE*), measured in MJ/kg, is the amount of energy released during complete combustion of the material in a calorimeter, although this is not an accurate estimate of the energy available to the animal after ingestion, since some of the gross energy is lost during digestion, absorption, and metabolism. Thus *digestible energy* (*DE*) is the gross energy of the ingested food less the gross energy of the corresponding faecal output. The determination of further losses associated with gaseous products (principally methane in ruminants) and urine gives the *metabolizable energy (ME). Further deduction of the *heat increment* gives the *net energy* (*NE*). (Heat increment is essentially the energy spent in the digestion, absorption, and metabolism of the food.)

Net energy is the most accurate expression of the amount of ingested energy available to the animal, but it is complex to estimate and difficult to apply in practice. Digestible energy is used widely in Great Britain when considering pigs, since most variable losses of ingested gross energy are associated with the faeces. Metabolizable energy is preferred for poultry

and ruminants. The above terms are used to describe both the dietary energy requirements of animals and the energy values of diets or feedstuffs for particular species.

enflurane A halogenated ether used as an inhalational anaesthetic. It was introduced in 1973 as a possible alternative to *halothane and has a low blood solubility, giving rapid induction and recovery from anaesthesia. Muscle relaxation is better than with halothane and increases with depth of anaesthesia. However, respiratory depression is greater than with halothane, and during induction abnormal motor activity and seizures can occur. Also, it is a poor analgesic and it is comparatively expensive.

enilconazole *See* imidazoles.

enkephalin *See* endorphin.

enlarged hock syndrome A condition of 2–6-week-old turkey poults characterized by swollen hocks and bowed legs. Nutritional deficiencies are thought to be involved, particularly *vitamin E, and also *choline and *nicotinic acid.

enophthalmos Retraction of the eye into the eye socket (orbit). In animals the commonest cause is malnutrition or starvation, which leads to resorption of the periorbital fat allowing the eye to sink back into its socket.

ensilage *See* silage.

Entamoeba A genus of amoeban protozoa that are parasitic in the digestive tract; most of them are nonpathogenic. The normal feeding stage is nucleated and varies in shape as the organism moves by extending pseudopodia. *Entamoeba* also form nucleated rigid-walled cysts that are passed in faeces. The only species causing disease in mammals is *Enta-*

moeba histolytica, which causes *amoebic dysentery in humans and occasionally in other primates and dogs but rarely in other species. It may be distinguished from other nonpathogenic species by the number of nuclei in the cyst, and by its habit of engulfing red blood cells.

enteque seco The Spanish name for a toxic condition affecting grazing animals in South America, the West Indies, and other tropical and subtropical parts of the world. It is due to the ingestion of *Solanum malacoxylon* or related plants, which contain 1,25-dihydrocholecalciferol, a metabolite of *vitamin D$_3$ that promotes calcium absorption from the diet and causes calcification of the large arteries and bone abnormalities. Affected animals become thin, develop an abnormal gait, and when exercised or herded may die suddenly due to rupture of the damaged arteries. Other name: **Manchester wasting disease.**

enter- (entero-) *Prefix denoting* the intestine. Example: *enterolith* (calculus in).

enteral (enteric) Of or relating to the intestinal tract.

enteralgia Abdominal pain or *colic.

enterectomy Surgical removal of part of the intestine. This is necessary if a part has been irreversibly damaged by the loss of its blood supply or by the presence of a foreign body, or if some other abnormality is present, such as a stricture or neoplasm. An *anastomosis must then be performed to restore continuity of the gut. *See also* enterostomy; enterotomy.

enteric colibacillosis of calves (white scours) A common condition of calves under 1 week of age, characterized by enteritis with diarrhoea

and caused by enterotoxigenic strains of *Escherichia coli*. A limited number of OK *E. coli* serogroups are responsible: many, though not all, possess K99 colonization pili and produce enterotoxin STa. Mixed infections with rotaviruses or other agents sometimes enable these strains to cause disease in older calves. Predisposing factors include poor hygiene, stress (e.g. transportation), and deprivation of colostrum, which contains *E. coli* antibodies, though not usually K99 antibody. The faeces are loose or, when the disease is due to K99 strains, very watery, whitish or yellowish, with a rancid odour. If untreated, death usually occurs after a varying period of debility. Tetracyclines, streptomycin, and other antibiotics given orally are effective, and rehydration therapy is desirable.

enteric colibacillosis of lambs A condition of lambs in the first few days of life, characterized by acute enteritis and caused by strains of *Escherichia coli*, some of which produce K99 pili and enterotoxin STa. The faeces of affected animals are yellow and watery, and death follows rapidly, generally associated with a septicaemia (*see* colisepticaemia).

enteric colibacillosis of piglets An enteritis and diarrhoea of pigs up to 12 weeks of age caused by enterotoxigenic strains of *Escherichia coli*, often O149, although strains of other O groups occur. The enterotoxins may be LT or STa or both, sometimes with STb as well, and most strains have colonization pili of types K88, K99, 987P, or F41. The common forms are a rapidly fatal neonatal diarrhoea (occurring in the first 4 days of life), and a severe but generally nonfatal post-weaning diarrhoea; in the latter, *rotaviruses may also be implicated. Tetracyclines or other antibiotics can be given to the piglets, or to the sow before farrowing to protect piglets from the neonatal form of the disease. Vaccines containing *E. coli* strains selected from appropriate serological groups are available. For the neonatal condition, sows are vaccinated with a preparation containing LT, which confers passive protection on the piglets up to weaning. Natural exposure to intercurrent strains during this period induces resistance to the post-weaning form of the disease as well. Other names: **piglet diarrhoea**; **piglet scours**.

enteritis Acute or chronic inflammation of the mucosa of any part of the intestines. The typical signs are diarrhoea or dysentery, abdominal pain, malabsorption, dehydration, electrolyte loss, and acid-base imbalances. Enteritis may be classified according to the pathological changes occurring the the mucosa; the principal ones are: catarrhal, haemorrhagic, diphtheritic, necrotic, or ulcerative. It is often accompanied by *gastritis (gastroenteritis) leading, in dogs, cats, and pigs, to vomiting.

The causes are very numerous and include: various microbial infections, either largely confined to the intestinal tract or part of a more extensive clinical picture; parasitic infestations; poisoning; prolonged oral medication with antibiotics; dietary deficiencies or imbalances; digestive (enzymic) malfunctions; anaemia; allergies; and certain congestive circulatory conditions involving cardiac or renal damage. Enteritic diarrhoea in young stock may cause a growth check, rapid loss of condition, or even death. The major infections and infective conditions associated with enteritis are shown in the table. For effective treatment, the cause of the enteritis must be identified so that appropriate drugs (e.g. antibiotics, sulphonamides, antiprotozoals, anthelmintics) can be administered. Fluid and electrolyte replacement, and dietary adjustment or supportive measures may also be needed. Oral mixtures for diarrhoeas frequently contain *kaolin and other absorbent or protective substances.

Enterobius *See* pinworm.

enterocentesis Puncture of the intestine. This may be performed intentionally to collect a sample of intestinal contents or to relieve intestinal distension, or it may occur inadvertently during surgical puncture of other parts.

enterogenous Borne by or carried in the intestine.

enteroglucagon *See* glucagon.

enterolith An intestinal stone (*calculus). They are typically made up of alternate layers of insoluble fatty acid esters and precipitated phytates or ammonium magnesium phosphate. Clinical signs are not always apparent, but intestinal obstruction and colic may result. In severe cases surgical removal of the stone is required. *See also* hair ball.

enteropathy Disease of the intestine, particularly the small intestine. *See* colic; enteritis; haemorrhagic bowel syndrome.

enterostomy The surgical creation of an artificial opening from the intestine either through the abdominal wall to the skin surface or to another part of the intestine. The former is rarely required due to disease in animals although a temporary enterostomy of the colon (*colostomy*) is used in horses that have sustained a tear of the rectum; it is used more often in experimental animals to study gut functions. The latter may be used following the surgical removal of part of the gut or to bypass diseased gut; for example a *gastrojejunostomy* to join the stomach and jejunum (*see* gastrostomy), or a *jejunocaecostomy* to join the jejunum to the caecum. *Compare* enterectomy; enterotomy.

enterotomy Surgical incision into the lumen of the intestine. This is a common procedure in small animals to remove foreign bodies that have been swallowed. It is required more rarely in farm animals but is used in horses for removing solid concretions known as *enteroliths or faecoliths. The operation may also be used to decompress distended intestine or to assess intestinal viability as indicated by the colour of the gut mucosa. *Compare* enterectomy; enterostomy.

enterotoxaemia 1. Any of a group of acute often fatal diseases resulting from the absorption of *exotoxins produced in the intestine by various types of the bacterium *Clostridium perfringens* (types B, C, D, and E) or in the liver by *Cl. novyi* (types B and C). (It should be noted that these exotoxins have no similarity to the *enterotoxins of some Gram-negative enteric bacteria.) The bacteria occur harmlessly in the intestinal tract; *Cl. novyi* may additionally occur in normal liver. An accessory factor (e.g. dietary or tissue damage) initiates disproportionate multiplication of the clostridia; in the *Cl. perfringens* enterotoxaemias, an additional, unknown, factor increases intestinal permeability. Definite diagnosis requires serological toxin-neutralization tests in laboratory mice to identify the toxin in intestinal contents or liver specimens from dead animals. Highly effective vaccines can be prepared from the toxins of each bacterial agent. *See* bacillary haemoglobinuria; black disease; lamb dysentery; pulpy kidney disease; struck.
2. An alternative name for *oedema disease of pigs; it should be avoided because of possible ambiguity.

enterotoxin A toxic substance produced in the intestine by the rapid multiplication of bacteria, mainly *Clostridium welchii* type C or D.

enterovirus A genus of the *picornavirus family. Several infect bovine and porcine hosts.

entomophthoromycosis Chronic granulomatous, ulcerative, or inflammatory subcutaneous disease caused by infection with the fungi *Conidiobolus coronatus* (*conidiobolomycosis), *Basidiobolus haptosporus* (*basidiobolomycosis), or other fungi of the order Entomophthorales; a type of *zygomycosis. *See also* equine phycomycosis.

entropion Malformation of the eyelid and eyelashes, which turn onto the eyeball inflicting pain, inflammation, and ulceration. Although sometimes caused accidentally, the condition is hereditary in many breeds of dog. The malformation can be surgically corrected but the animal should not be used for breeding.

enuresis The involuntary passing of urine. It is a type of *incontinence and is most often caused by stress, but may also be a sign of disease, such as degenerative lesions in the spinal cord.

envelope A membranous structure enclosing the protein shell (*capsid) of certain groups of *viruses. It is acquired by new *virions from membranes of the infected host cell and contains lipid and viral proteins (often *glycolipids and *glycoproteins). It apparently serves to enhance the *infectivity of the virus. The envelopes of some viruses are rather amorphous, while those of others have a characteristic shape under the electron microscope, for example the 'bullet' shape of *rabies virus.

environment Any or all aspects of the surroundings of an organism (external environment) or of its individual cells (internal environment), which influence its growth, development, and behaviour.

enzootic 1. Describing a disease of animals that is restricted to a locality or population. It is synonymous with the term 'endemic' in human medicine. 2. An enzootic disease. *Compare* epizootic.

enzootic ataxia *See* swayback.

enzootic bovine leukosis A persistent infection of cattle characterized by the development of tumours and caused by bovine leukosis virus. The disease was introduced into the UK with the importation of infected cattle from Canada in 1972 and 1973. Following an incubation period of 4–7 years, there is enlargement of superficial or internal *lymph nodes with consequent disease in other essential organs associated with pressure or obstruction by the tumours. However, because the majority of cattle in the UK are slaughtered before 6 years of age, very few cases of clinical enzootic bovine leukosis have been seen. In other countries where the virus is enzootic, some herds have reported a high incidence of clinical disease. Transmission is probably by biting insects, but iatrogenic transmission by contaminated needles or vaccines has occurred. Enzootic bovine leukosis is a *notifiable disease in the UK, although following the identification of the infected imported cattle and their contacts, the prevalence of the virus there is now very low.

enzootic ovine abortion A disease of sheep characterized by abortion and caused by the bacterium *Chlamydia psittaci*. The disease is distributed worldwide and is a cause of serious economic loss. Infection is usually by ingestion following contact with infected foetal membranes, but the organism is also passed in the faeces of infected ewes. Abortion usually occurs in the final month of pregnancy, but can occur earlier; stillborn or weak lambs may be produced at term. The aborting ewe may retain the foetal membranes and develop uterine infection (*metritis), otherwise infection in the ewe is without clinical signs. The *placenta is the main organ affected. The cotyledons are dark-red or grey and the area between is thickened and appears yellow or grey in colour. Ewes that have aborted rarely do so again, but there are a number of different strains of *C. psittaci* and these do not give cross immunity. This has hampered the development of an effective vaccine.
Following confirmation of the disease, all aborting ewes should be segregated and the foetal membranes, dead lambs, and contaminated bedding destroyed or buried. Thorough disinfection is essential. It is recommended that aborting ewes and suspect ewes, which are potential sources of future infection, be culled and sold for slaughter. If enzootic abortion is anticipated in a synchronously lambing flock, treatment with long-acting *tetracyclines at 6 and 3 weeks before lambing may be helpful. Replacement ewes should be bought from enzootic abortion-free flocks and if possible segregated from the main flock during the last month of pregnancy. *C. psittaci* also infects many other species of mammals and birds and has been associated with abortion in humans.

enzootic pneumonia of pigs A common, economically important, and highly contagious *pneumonia of young pigs caused by *Mycoplasma hyopneumoniae* (*M. suipneumoniae*), usually with other microorganisms, including *M. hyorhinis* and *M. flocculare*. Affected animals show coughing and retarded growth; at slaughter, reddish or grey consolidated areas are found in the lungs. Concomitant infection with the bacteria *Pasteurella multocida* or *Bordetella bronchiseptica* frequently exacerbates the condition. Individual animals may be treated with *tetracyclines, but eradication of the disease from a herd using antibiotics alone is not feasible. Some control can be achieved by reducing stocking density and improving housing. Eradication is possible by removing all pigs and, after 30 days, restocking completely with pregnant gilts from *specific pathogen free herds. However, vigilance is necessary to prevent reinfection.

enzootic pneumonia of sheep An infectious disease of sheep, caused by the bacterium *Pasteurella haemolytica*, that is characterized by acute pneumonia and septicaemia. Biotypes A of this organism cause enzootic pneumonia and septicaemia in young lambs, while biotypes T cause systemic infections in older or adult sheep. The organisms are distributed worldwide and commonly found in the nasopharynx of healthy ruminants. It is thought that such factors as inclement weather, transportation, castration, docking, or other stressful events may help to precipitate disease. The disease has usually a sudden onset, with sudden deaths in young lambs due to acute pneumonias and septicaemias. In older lambs and adult sheep there is acute or subacute pneumonia with coughing and nasal discharge. The incidence of disease may be reduced by eliminating stress and improving housing. Vaccines are commercially available but they are of doubtful efficacy.

enzootic posthitis A serious condition of castrated male sheep (wethers), particularly of the Merino breed, and to a lesser degree rams, occurring in Australia and less commonly in Britain and North America. The lesions consist of necrotic foci extending over large areas of the *prepuce and adjacent glans penis and urethral process, with ulceration. Sloughing of the prepuce often follows an accumulation of urine and ammonia production. The causal agent is the bacterium *Corynebacterium renale*, but there are important associated factors, such as high alkalinity of urine, high oestrogen content of pasture, high protein or legume content of pasture, high-calcium and low-phosphorus content of diet, and wetness of the pasture. In bad outbreaks the flock should be removed to drier pastures and their nutritional plane temporarily reduced. For badly affected wethers, irrigation of the preputial lesions with 5–10% copper sulphate solution or cetrimide disinfectant with antibiotic coverage is recommended. Where the prepuce is obstructed or there is extensive preputial necrosis, cutting open the prepuce to release the accumulated urine and necrotic debris is advocated. Control measures in affected areas include dietary management to reduce urea content and lower pH of the urine, and the use of antiseptic creams in wethers and ewes to reduce *C. renale* infection. The use of subcutaneous *testosterone implants in wethers is helpful.

enzyme A protein that acts as a catalyst in biochemical reactions. Each enzyme is specific to a particular reaction or group of similar reactions. Many require the association of *cofactors in order to function. The molecule(s) undergoing reaction (the *substrate*) binds to a specific *active site on the enzyme to form a short-lived intermediate; this greatly increases the reaction rate. Enzyme activity is influenced by substrate concentration and by temperature and pH, which must lie within a certain range. Other molecules may compete for the active site, causing inhibition of the enzyme or even irreversible destruction of its catalytic properties.

enzyme-linked immunosorbent assay

Enzyme production is governed by a cell's *genes. Enzyme activity is further controlled by pH changes, alterations in the concentrations of cofactors, feedback inhibition by the products of the reaction, and activation by another enzyme, either from a less active form or an inactive precursor. Such changes may themselves be under hormonal or nervous control.

The names of most enzymes end in -*ase*. There are six classes, namely the *oxidoreductases*, which catalyse oxidation-reduction reactions (*see* dehydrogenase; oxidase); *transferases*, which catalyse group transfer reactions; *hydrolases*, which catalyse bond cleavage by *hydrolysis; *lyases*, which catalyse removal of a group, leaving a double bond, or the reverse; *isomerases*, which catalyse the formation of isomers; and *ligases*, or *synthetases*, which catalyse the combination of two molecules with the concomitant hydrolysis of a high-energy bond (e.g. in *ATP).

enzyme-linked immunosorbent assay (ELISA) A test in which specific antibodies or antigens are indicated by an enzyme-catalysed colour change. The technique enables rapid analysis of multiple samples and is now used for the diagnosis of many animal diseases. Firstly, antibody or antigen is adsorbed onto a solid substrate, such as a plastic multiwell plate. A solution of test material (e.g. infected tissue or serum) is then allowed to interact with the adsorbed reagent. Any matching antigens and antibodies will form complexes, which adhere to the substrate; any uncomplexed material is washed away. An indicator is then put on the plate; this is either a second antibody to the antigen in the test material, or an antispecies antibody prepared against the antibody in the test material. The indicator has previously been conjugated to an enzyme; this causes a colour change in a fourth reagent, which

is placed on the plate. The colour change is assessed either by eye or spectrophotometer, and its intensity indicates the presence and even concentration of antibody or antigen in the test material. The test has many advantages over previous test procedures, which required the use of animals or tissue culture facilities, and has now been adopted for a large number of diagnostic procedures.

eosin A red acidic dye, produced by the reaction of bromine and fluorescein, used to stain biological specimens for microscopical examination. Eosin may be used in conjunction with haematoxylin, a contrasting blue alkaline dye taken up by different parts of the same specimen.

eosinophil A white blood cell (*leucocyte) of the granulocytic series whose granules have affinity for the dye eosin. Eosinophils are produced in the bone marrow (*see* haemopoiesis), which also has a large storage capacity for these cells. On release from the marrow eosinophils enter the tissues after a few hours in the circulation. The mature eosinophil is incapable of replication and dies in the tissues after a few days.

Eosinophils have surface receptors for IgG and IgE *antibodies, *complement components, glucocorticoids (*see* corticosteroid), and *histamine and these substances can exert a chemotactic effect on eosinophils, attracting the cells into areas of inflammation. This is especially true when the inflammation is complement- or histamine-mediated or when helminth parasites are involved. Eosinophils destroy bacteria by *phagocytosis and by producing hydrogen peroxide (*see* neutrophil). They can also exert parasiticidal effects, by producing both hydrogen peroxide and a major basic protein, which is released from the eosinophil granule. Eosinophils also regulate hypersensitive inflammatory reactions (*see* hypersensitivity), probably by phagocytosing antigen-antibody complexes and by inactivating histamine and other inflammatory substances.

eosinophilia *See* leucocytosis.

eosinophilic granuloma complex A group of related conditions affecting the skin and oral cavity of cats, causing raised plaques of inflammatory tissue to develop, either on the lips, within the mouth, or on the skin. These usually cause intense irritation, and if they are in accessible areas rapidly become ulcerated due to continual licking. Care must be taken with the diagnosis to avoid confusion with squamous cell *carcinomas. The precise cause of the condition is unknown, but it is often thought to be triggered by an allergic reaction. Treatment may involve the exclusion of possible allergens, long-term medical therapy, or *cryosurgery of the lesions. Other names: **eosinophilic plaque**; **indolent ulcer**; **rodent ulcer**.

eosinophilic myositis A condition of cattle and dogs in which foci of dead tissue infiltrated with *eosinophils are seen in the muscles. The cause is unknown, but *Sarcocystis* infestation is one possibility. A similar disease, also of unknown cause, occurs in the muscles of German shepherd dogs. The jaw muscles are affected and become swollen. Repeated attacks give rise to gradually increasing atrophy and loss of muscle function so that the dog cannot eat. There is no treatment.

eparterial Situated on or above an artery.

ependyma The extremely thin membrane, composed of cells (*ependymal cells*), that lines the ventricles of the brain and the choroid plexuses. It is responsible for helping to form cerebrospinal fluid.

ependymoma A tumour of the *ependyma membrane in the brain. Ependymomas have been reported in horses, cattle, dogs, and cats but are rare in any species. They may arise at any point in the ventricular system, most commonly in the lateral ventricles. Such tumours form large ill-defined bulging masses that are highly cellular and vascular. Malignant forms show *anaplasia and frequent cell divisions; metastasis via the cerebrospinal network leads to invasion of other sites in the ventricular system and of the meninges.

Eperythrozoon A genus of *rickettsiae that are obligate blood parasites of various domestic and wild animals. Transmission is by arthropod vectors, such as ticks and lice, or by injection of blood. A few species are of veterinary importance. These include *E. suis*, which is transmitted by lice and causes a disease characterized by *anaemia and *jaundice in pigs. *E. ovis* causes anaemia in sheep, with high mortality in lambs, and *E. felis* has been associated with anaemia in cats (*see also* Haemobartonella).

ephedrine A naturally occurring alkaloid drug that has been used to treat asthma. It has *sympathomimetic properties and causes bronchodilatation, peripheral vasoconstriction, cardiac stimulation, and mydriasis, but has been superseded by more specific β_2 adrenergic agonists.

ephemeral fever An acute but transient disease of cattle caused by a *rhabdovirus and characterized by fever, lameness, and sometimes collapse. It is enzootic in Africa, the Middle East, Asia, and north Australia. Transmission is by tropical and subtropical species of midge, and distribution of the disease is therefore determined by that of the vector, although ephemeral fever can be introduced into previously disease-free areas by infected midges carried by strong winds or even in aircraft. Infected cattle develop a high fever, nasal and eye discharge, swollen lymph nodes, and muscular pain. Milk production is dramatically reduced in lactating cows. The animal may become unable to stand and can injure itself. Recovery is usually complete within a week, although milk yields remain low for the remaining lactation. Fatality is rare. Dead and attenuated vaccines have been used to control the disease. Other names: **dengue; three-day sickness**.

epi- *Prefix denoting* above or upon.

epiblepharon An inflammatory lesion in which the edge of the eyelid adheres to the conjunctival surface of the eyeball. If long continued the adhesion fibroses and becomes permanent. Surgery is indicated.

epicardium The external layer of the wall of the heart. It is a *serous membrane and effectively forms the visceral or inner layer of the *pericardium.

epicondyle The protuberance above a *condyle at the end of a bone, especially the humerus and femur.

epidemic 1. A term used in human medicine to describe a disease affecting many people in the same locality at the same time. The term *epizootic is used to describe similar diseases in veterinary medicine. **2.** An epidemic disease. *Compare* endemic.

epidemic diarrhoea A highly infectious disease of pigs characterized by diarrhoea and caused by a *coronavirus. The disease is similar to *transmissible gastroenteritis but less severe. It appears as two distinct syndromes, one affecting pigs under 10 weeks of age and causing diarrhoea and vomiting, the other affecting pigs of all ages. The disease is not usually fatal unless complicated by additional disease problems, and recovery is generally complete after a week.

epidemic tremors *See* infectious avian encephalomyelitis.

epidemiology The study of *epidemic disease. Although strictly relating to human disease the term is in common usage for animal diseases. Epidemiology embraces many aspects, including the way a disease spreads and the factors involved in the animal's susceptibility, such as housing, overcrowding, and nutrition.

epidermal inclusion cyst A nodule-like *cyst occurring in the skin and filled with keratin and fragments of hair shafts. They may be single or multiple, are often compressible, and are lined with a simple squamous epithelium. They sometimes rupture to discharge a cheesy material. The cysts are common in the dog but rare in the cat, and are mainly situated on the head, neck, trunk, and upper limbs. They may originate from blocked hair follicles or from the traumatic implantation of epidermal fragments into the dermis or lower epidermis. Simple surgical excision gives complete cure.

epidermis The outermost layer of the *skin comprising successive layers of squamous keratinized *epithelium. It is highly variable in thickness, being much thicker at sites of abrasion, for example foot pads. The deepest proliferative layer is the *stratum basale*, succeeded by the *stratum spinosum*, *stratum granulosum*, *stratum lucidum* (only recognizable in non-hairy skin), and the keratinized *stra-*

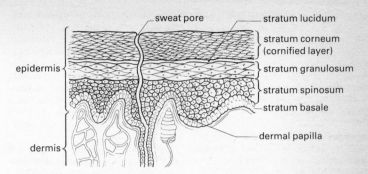

A section of epidermis

tum corneum on the surface (see illustration).

epidermoid Having the appearance of epidermis (the outer layer of the skin): used to describe certain tumours of tissues other than the skin.

epididymis (*pl.* **epididymides**) The highly coiled duct conveying spermatozoa from the *testis to the *ductus deferens. The head of the epididymis receives the efferent ductules of the testis and is succeeded by the body and tail of the epididymis. Sperm take 10–15 days to pass through the epididymis, undergoing maturation during this time, and collect in the tail of the epididymis and ductus deferens ready for *ejaculation.

epididymitis Inflammation of the epididymis. It commonly involves the associated testis as well (*see* orchitis). Causes include injury and bacterial infections, and the resulting pain is usually severe. There may be sterility, either temporary or permanent. Surgical castration may be necessary, although broad-spectrum antibiotics often resolve the infection. *See also* ram epididymitis.

epidural (extradural) On or over the dura mater (the outermost of the three membranes covering the brain and spinal cord). The *epidural space* is the space between the dura mater of the spinal cord and the vertebral canal. *See also* spinal anaesthesia.

epidural anaesthesia *See* spinal anaesthesia.

epigastric Referring to or relating to the abdominal wall. For example, the epigastric arteries are the main blood vessels supplying the abdominal wall.

epigastrium The central part of the forward (cranial) abdominal region.

epiglottis (*pl.* **epiglottises** or **epiglottides**) One of the several cartilages of the *larynx. It lies to the rear of the tongue and helps seal off the larynx during swallowing.

epilation (depilation) The removal of hair by its roots. It is usually performed in situations where the hair is causing a clinical problem. Plucking or clipping produce only very temporary results and are unsatisfactory where permanent epilation is required. This is achieved by *electrolysis* (*catholysis*) in which a fine electrode is inserted into the skin alongside the hair follicle; the passage of a direct current of low amplitude produces permanent damage to the hair follicle and gives permanent epilation. Epilation is most often employed for the removal of extra hairs from the margins of the eyelids in cases of canine distichiasis.

epilepsy A brain disorder characterized by sudden loss of consciousness and convulsions. It is seen most often in dogs, although rare heritable forms of epilepsy are known in cattle. A typical epileptic seizure lasts for only a few minutes, the animal falling onto its side and performing running movements with its legs. Often it involuntarily defecates and urinates. After the convulsions the dog recovers spontaneously and returns to normal very quickly. Although the cause is frequently unknown, epilepsy may be associated with vitamin deficiency, especially B vitamins, intestinal worms, or fever. Susceptibility is high in certain breeds, where there appears to be a genetic predisposition. Various drugs, such as *primidone or phenobarbitone (see barbiturate) control the seizures. *Status epilepticus* is the occurrence of repeated epileptic fits without any recovery of consciousness between them. If prolonged it causes serious imbalance of the salts (electrolytes) in the body and is life-threatening.

epimysium (*pl.* **epimysia**) The fibrous connective tissue that surrounds a *muscle.

epinephrine *See* adrenaline.

epineurium The outer sheath of connective tissue that surrounds a *nerve.

epiphenomenon An atypical clinical sign that appears during a disease process but is not necessarily directly related to it. It may lead to a wrong diagnosis or suggest an unusual complication.

epiphora A condition in which tears run down the cheeks, usually due to blocked tear ducts, which normally drain into the nose (*see* lacrimal apparatus). Some breeds of dog, such as King Charles spaniels, normally overspill their tears.

epiphyseal cartilage (epiphyseal disc) The plate of cartilage that separates the *epiphysis and the *diaphysis in a growing long bone. It is an important site of cell division and hence growth in a bone's length. Progressive conversion of its diaphyseal surface forms a layer of new bone tissue called the *metaphysis.

epiphyseal fracture A fracture involving the *epiphysis of an immature long bone. It can involve disruption of the epiphyseal plate and displacement or separation of the epiphysis, or a fracture of the epiphysis itself. Epiphyseal separation is possible in any of the long bones, but occurs most commonly at the distal end of the femur in the **dog** and **cat**.

epiphysis (*pl.* **epiphyses**) **1.** The rounded extremity of a long bone. In mammals, though not in birds, it develops as one or more secondary centres of ossification, which are separated by the *epiphyseal cartilage* from the primary centre in the *diaphysis. It eventually fuses with the diaphysis when growth is complete to form a complete bone. **2.** Epiphysis cerebri: *see* pineal gland.

epiphysitis Inflammation of the end (*epiphysis) of a long bone. It is especially common in intensively reared animals in which the immature bones must bear the weight of a rapidly grown and prematurely heavy body, and is often exacerbated by the trauma inflicted by certain flooring materials, such as slats. Vitamin D deficiency or mineral imbalances that weaken bone development may also be present. Clinical signs include swelling of the ends of the long bones, pain, and lameness. In very advanced cases the head of the femur may separate from the shaft. Prevention depends on good husbandry, with special attention to flooring and optimum nutrition.

epiplo- *Prefix denoting* the omentum. Example: *epiplocele* (hernia containing omentum).

episio- *Prefix denoting* the vulva.

episome A length of *DNA (usually circular) found in certain bacterial cells in addition to the bacterial chromosome. A single cell may have 10–20 molecules of the episomal DNA, which carries a small number of genes and replicates either with the bacterial chromosome or autonomously (*see* plasmid). The presence of an episome usually confers certain properties (e.g. antibiotic resistance) upon its host bacterium. Some have been widely used in gene cloning (*see* clone) and *genetic engineering. Certain episomes are bacterial *viruses, and the term has been applied to similar states occurring when animal viruses establish a latent infection (*see* latency) in animal cells (e.g. certain *herpesviruses, such as Epstein-Barr virus).

epistasis The phenomenon where an *allele of one gene suppresses the action of the alleles of another gene. The most obvious case is where the expression of the alleles of the second gene is dependent on the product of one of the alleles of the first. Where the first gene is represented by alleles that do not produce the required product, the second gene cannot show its effect. The term is sometimes used for any interaction between genes. *Compare* hypostasis.

epistaxis *See* nosebleed.

epithalamus The uppermost part of the *diencephalon in the brain, surrounding the roof of the third ventricle and including the *pineal gland.

epithelium (*pl.* **epithelia**) The tissue that covers the external surface of the body and lines hollow structures (except blood and lymphatic vessels). Epithelial cells may be flat and scale-like (*squamous*), *cuboidal*, or *columnar*. The latter may bear cilia or brush borders or secrete mucus or other substances (*see* goblet cell). The cells rest on a common *basement membrane*, which separates epithelium from underlying *connective tissue. Epithelium may be either *simple*, consisting of a single layer of cells; *stratified*, consisting of several layers; or *pseudostratified*, in which the cells appear to be arranged in layers but in fact share a common basement membrane (see illustration). *See also* endothelium; mesothelium.

epizootic 1. Describing a disease that affects many animals of a particular species or type at the same time. Epizootic diseases characteristically spread rapidly through a population and are followed by a return to a disease-free state. It is synonymous with the term 'epidemic' in human medicine. **2.** An epizootic disease. *Compare* enzootic.

epizootic lymphangitis (pseudo-farcy) A chronic infectious disease of horses, mules, and donkeys that is caused by the fungus *Histoplasma farciminosum*. It is enzootic in some areas bordering the Mediterranean and northern parts of Africa, notably Iraq, Egypt, and Sudan, and also occurs in China, the USSR, and elsewhere. The disease mainly affects the

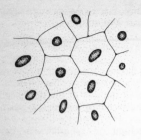

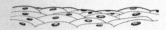

Stratified squamous epithelium, surface view above and sectional view below

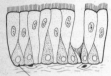

basement membrane
Simple cuboidal epithelium

goblet cell

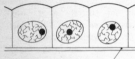

Ciliated columnar epithelium

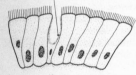

basement membrane
Pseudostratified ciliated epithelium

Types of epithelium

limbs, with chronic indurative ulceration of the skin, thickening of superficial lymph nodes, and enlargement of regional lymph nodes. When the lymph nodes become abscessed they rupture, discharging a thick purulent exudate. Lymphatic channels connecting the involved lymph nodes develop a cordlike appearance beneath the skin (*compare* farcy).

Mucous membranes and internal organs are rarely involved, although conjunctival, nasal, and primary pulmonary infections are said to occur in Sudan. A presumptive diagnosis can be made by demonstrating cells of the parasitic yeast phase of this *dimorphic fungus in pus or tissue from granulomatous lesions consistent with the disease. The round to oval cells, no larger than $2-5 \mu m$ in diameter, occur mostly within macrophages or giant cells and are indistinguishable from those found in *histoplasmosis. Diagnosis is established by isolation of the causative organism from infected tissues, although this may require culture on enriched media for periods of $1-3$ weeks. Intravenous administration of sodium iodide has been reported as beneficial in some cases, and spontaneous recovery has also been reported. However, most cases persist as chronic infections. Epizootic lymphangitis is a notifiable disease in the UK.

epoophoron *See* mesonephros.

epulis (*pl.* **epulides**) A benign tumour of the mouth occurring mainly in dogs. Epulides consist of firm grey-pink masses that often project from between the teeth or from the hard palate near to the teeth. They occur commonly in the region of the carnassial and canine teeth of the *brachycephalic breeds of dog. Because of their location, they are subject to trauma and are often ulcerated and infected. *Metaplasia of the underlying stromal tissue produces bone matrix and bone in many cases. Complete surgical excision is curative, but the anatomical situation often makes this impossible and regrowth takes place. Epulides may be an example of *hyperplasia rather than neoplasia.

equi- *Prefix denoting* equality.

equine autoimmune haemolytic anaemia (haemolytic disease of the newborn foal) An *autoimmune disease of foals in which an acute *anaemia is induced as a result of destruction of red blood cells by antibodies in the foal's blood. The antibody is acquired in the colostrum and can be absorbed into the foal's circulation during the first 12–24 hours of life. The blood group of a foal is determined partly by the sire, and a proportion of mares will therefore carry foals whose blood group is incompatible with their own. Injury to the placenta can expose the mare to incompatible foetal red cells leading to the production of specific antibody by the mare. The chance of such an immunization occurring increases with the number of pregnancies. The signs of the anaemia may be acute or subacute, beginning from a few hours to 5 days after the foal's first suckling. There is prostration and lethargy, breathlessness, fast heart rate, and sometimes staining of the urine with haemoglobin. The membranes of the mouth and eyes show progressive jaundice.

Diagnosis is supported by the presence of antibody on the foal's red cells – demonstrated by the *Coombs test – and made virtually certain by the presence of antibody to the foal's red cells in maternal serum or colostrum. If investigation is made prior to the birth, the latter finding also allows the problem to be anticipated and avoided. Foals whose dams possess potentially haemolytic antibody should be allowed to suckle a 'safe' foster mare for the first 48 hours or be bottle-fed safe colostrum, which can be kept deep-frozen for the purpose. The condition can also be avoided by mating mares only to stallions who do not have the offending incompatible blood groups. It is also possible to monitor mares during pregnancy for the appearance of any antibody to the sire's red cells, this being a good indication that immunization of the mare has taken place.

Treatment is by conservative nursing in mild cases and by replacement blood transfusion in severe ones. Replacement assists in the removal from the circulation of some of the bilirubin that accumulates owing to haemoglobin release during haemolysis. The preferred material for transfusion consists of saline-washed red cells of the dam herself, since these are certain to be insusceptible to haemolysis by maternal antibody.

A type of spontaneous autoimmune haemolytic anaemia that is analogous to *canine autoimmune haemolytic anaemia may occur in the horse, but this has not been reported frequently.

equine babesiosis A disease of horses caused by the protozoan parasites *Babesia caballi* or *B. equi*. *B. caballi* is pear-shaped, 2–5 μm long, and resembles *B. bigemina* of cattle. *B. equi* is smaller (2–3 μm long) and occasionally forms linked groups of four organisms in a Maltese cross shape. Both are widely distributed throughout the world, generally in tropical and subtropical areas. They are transmitted by ticks of the genera *Dermacentor*, *Hyalomma*, and others. The parasites multiply in their host's red blood cells causing fever, anaemia, jaundice, and sometimes also *haemoglobinuria. Other clinical signs also occur and the disease can be fatal. Diagnosis is confirmed by the finding of parasites in stained blood smears during the early stages of disease. In recovered animals parasites persist, but cannot easily be detected. Serological tests may be used to detect carrier animals and prevent their importation into areas free of disease. The disease can be treated with drugs and tick control measures may be used to prevent infection. There is recent evidence that *B. equi* also parasitizes lymphocytes and is probably more closely related to *Theileria* than to *Babesia*. See also babesiosis. Other names: **equine biliary fever**; **equine piroplasmosis**.

equine biliary fever See equine babesiosis.

equine coital exanthema A mild genital infection of mares and stallions transmitted venereally and characterized by pustular lesions on the external genitalia. It is caused by a *herpesvirus. The disease is rare in the UK.

equine contagious metritis See contagious equine metritis.

equine ehrlichiosis 1. A febrile disease of horses caused by the rickettsia *Ehrlichia equi, reported from certain regions of the USA (Sacramento Valley). It is characterized by anaemia, oedema of the limbs, lymphadenopathy, and thrombocytopenia. **2.** A severe enteritis of horses caused by *Ehrlichia riscistici*, occurring in parts of North America. Other name: **Potomac horse fever**.

equine encephalomyelitis A mosquito-transmitted infection of horses, mules, and donkeys characterized by fever and neurological signs and caused by *alphaviruses. The viruses are classified into three antigenically related groups: western (WEE); eastern (EEE); and Venezuelan (VEE). EEE is distributed in eastern North America from Canada to the Caribbean and Central and South America. WEE is distributed throughout North and South America but is apparently absent from Central America. VEE is restricted to northern South America and Central America. Within each of the three groups there are a number of distinct subtypes of virus. The viruses circulate in cycles involving mosquitoes, wild birds, rodents, rep-

tiles, and amphibians. However, enzootics of disease occur when infected mosquitoes start to feed on horses, and these are usually associated with climatic conditions that favour insect activity. Except for some strains of VEE horses do not become part of the virus cycle, and have been termed 'dead-end hosts'.

The development of clinical disease in horses is dependent on the strain of virus, the infecting dose, and the individual susceptibility of the horse, and can range from mild or inapparent to severe and fatal. WEE is usually less severe than EEE or VEE. Following an incubation period of 2 days a fever develops which subsides and then returns 3–4 days later. The affected animal at first loses its appetite and becomes depressed, hanging its head almost to the ground. Weight loss is dramatic. Some animals may become hyperexcitable and show other evidence of neurological disturbance, and horses infected with EEE frequently develop severe skin irritation and may mutilate themselves. Death occurs up to 10 days after infection and although the majority of animals that recover subsequently appear normal, some animals may show persistent evidence of central nervous system damage. Pheasants may become fatally infected with equine encephalitis virus, which can also cause severe disease and death in humans. Control is by vaccination of susceptible horses and measures to reduce *mosquito numbers.

equine filariasis A disease of horses caused by small parasitic filarial *nematodes, *Setaria equina*, which are found in the peritoneal cavity. The larvae are transmitted by mosquitoes and biting flies. The disease, which occurs in South and Central Europe, Asia, and America, is debilitating rather than serious, causing anaemia and general malaise. However, movement of the nematodes to other sites can cause conjunctivitis and oedematous swellings. Affected animals are normally treated with *diethylcarbamazine.

equine glandular dermatitis *See* equine phycomycosis.

equine infectious anaemia A persistent infection of horses, mules, and donkeys caused by a *retrovirus and characterized by intermittent fever, anaemia, and wasting. It is enzootic in South and Central America, Africa, Asia, Australia, and parts of Europe and North America. It is seen particularly in low-lying, swampy regions. Transmission is by contact with infected horses, including infected semen, and the disease may be spread by biting insects. Foals born to infected mares are also infected. The incubation period is 1–3 weeks, followed by a fever, discharge from the eyes and nose, and swelling of the legs. Small haemorrhages may be seen under the tongue. Death may occur during this initial stage, but more usually the horse recovers and suffers intermittent relapses. The work capacity of chronically infected horses is progressively reduced. Mortality may reach 70% but, commonly, infected horses are destroyed because of recurring ill health.

Infected animals develop high levels of specific antibodies against the virus but these are unable to inactivate and eliminate the infection. The antibodies and viral antigens form complexes, which concentrate in the kidneys and interfere with renal function. Chronically infected animals die from kidney failure. The antibodies can be detected in the serum of infected animals using an *agar-gel immunodiffusion test (*Coggins test*). The virus is resistant to many commonly used disinfectants and can persist in dried blood for many months. The disease is usually introduced into

new areas by the movement of carrier animals. There is no treatment or vaccine, and infected animals and contacts should be destroyed. Equine infectious anaemia is a *notifiable disease in the UK and in most of North America. Other name: **swamp fever.**

equine infectious bronchitis *See* equine influenza.

equine influenza An infectious disease of horses characterized by fever, cough, and loss of appetite and caused by equine *influenzavirus A type 1 or type 2. Virus particles are carried on moisture droplets in the air and breathed in by the animal, which develops a fever after 1–3 days. The horse is depressed and has a persistent dry cough, exacerbated by dusty stable conditions. Recovery may be complete in a week, but frequently secondary bacterial infection prolongs the course of the disease, and if the horse is not completely rested permanent lung damage may result. Control is by vaccination against both virus types, but this may not be totally effective due to the development of new strains, particularly within the type 2 equine influenza group. The Jockey Club in the UK will not allow horses to race unless they have been adequately vaccinated against this disease. This involves two vaccinations 3–12 weeks apart, followed by annual boosters. Other names: **equine infectious bronchitis; Newmarket cough; stable cough.**

equine leukoencephalomalacia *See* fusariotoxicosis.

equine papilloma One of a rash of wartlike growths typically found on the lips and muzzle of horses and caused by a *papovavirus. The virus particles can be transmitted by direct contact between infected and susceptible horses, and possibly also by bit-

equine papular dermatitis

ing flies and contaminated brushes and tack. Horses are usually infected when yearlings or 2-year-olds and recovery is usually spontaneous without any treatment, although autogenous vaccines have been used in stubborn cases. Immunity is lifelong following recovery.

equine papular dermatitis *See* equine papilloma.

equine phycomycosis Any disease of horses caused by infection with fungi traditionally placed in the class Phycomycetes. The commonest clinical form is known variously as cutaneous or subcutaneous phycomycosis, hyphomycosis destruens equi, bursattee, granular dermatitis, equine granuloma, leeches, Florida horse leech, or swamp cancer. Frequently these terms have been applied indiscriminately to any of several clinically very similar diseases: cutaneous *habronemiasis, *pythiosis, *basidiobolomycosis, and *conidiobolomycosis. All produce roughly circular ulcerating cutaneous granulomatous lesions containing yellowish granular bodies known as 'kunkers' or, due to frequent mistaken identification as such, 'leeches'. The diseases differ in details of the nature and distribution of their lesions and can be differentiated definitively by microscopic and cultural examination of the kunkers. Individually these conditions may also differ in their geographical distribution throughout the areas where 'equine phycomycosis' is common – tropical and semitropical areas of India, Indonesia, Papua New Guinea, Australia, and South America, and Gulf regions of the USA.

equine piroplasmosis *See* equine babesiosis.

equine protozoal myeloencephalitis A disease of the central nervous system of horses caused by an untyped protozoan, possibly of the genus *Sarcocystis. It is most frequently recognized in the eastern states of North America, but occurs throughout the continent in all breeds of mature horses. Clinical signs are very variable and include ataxia and signs of cranial nerve damage. Specific antiprotozoal therapy may help some horses.

equine rhinopneumonitis An infectious disease of horses, mules, and donkeys characterized by fever, coughing, and abortion in pregnant mares and caused by equine *herpesvirus 1. Two subtypes of the virus are recognized: subtype 1 causes respiratory disease, abortion, and (rarely) neurological disorders; subtype 2 causes predominantly respiratory disease. Both subtypes are enzootic worldwide. Pregnant mares may abort up to 4 months after infection. Foals born from infected mares may be weak, show respiratory distress, and fail to thrive. Some horses become persistently infected and continue to shed virus, particularly when subjected to stress, such as training or additional disease. Dead and live attenuated vaccines are available but are not considered particularly effective.

equine sarcoid A common benign skin tumour of horses, similar to the *fibropapillomas seen in cattle. They most frequently affect the legs, ventral trunk, ears, and mouth. Multiple occurrence is common and the tumours appear as raised pedunculated or sessile lesions; superficial ulceration is common. Sarcoids are locally infiltrative but do not metastasize. They are liable to recur after surgical excision. However, a large percentage of such lesions will regress spontaneously, although this may take years. Bovine papilloma virus genome can be detected in some sarcoids and the lesion has been reproduced experimentally following intradermal inoculation of the virus.

equine serum hepatitis A form of hepatitis of viral origin that usually occurs in horses following injection with equine serum tissue preparations or toxins (e.g. *Clostridium perfringens*), 40–60 days after inoculation. The disease resembles human type B viral hepatitis. Death occurs in 6–24 hours, with jaundice, ataxia, and neurological disturbance. At autopsy affected livers are usually of normal size but may be shrunken or enlarged. Gross sections of liver show mottling, and histologically there is severe fatty degeneration.

equine verminous arteritis A condition of horses involving thickening and fibrosis of arterial walls caused by irritation from *Strongylus vulgaris* larvae. It normally affects the cranial mesenteric artery. The inflammation and damage weakens the arterial wall allowing the formation of an *aneurysm, which may burst causing a fatal haemorrhage. Also, the inflammation may lead to the development of a thrombus, portions of which can break away to cause multiple gangrenous infarctions in the intestines, with consequent severe pain; treatment at this stage is of no avail because many parts of the intestines may be affected at once. However, anthelmintics are effective in the early stages of the infestation.

equine viral arteritis An infectious disease of horses caused by a *pestivirus and characterized by fever, subcutaneous haemorrhages, and respiratory and intestinal signs. The disease is present in Europe and North America but not in the UK. The virus causes necrosis of the walls of the smaller arteries with consequent escape of blood into the surrounding tissues. When this occurs superficially haemorrhages may be seen, classically under the tongue, and soft swellings may be apparent, such as swelling of the eyelids. Pregnant mares may abort. Some animals remain persistently infected, particularly when infected in utero, and can be responsible for the introduction of disease into a stable. A live attenuated vaccine is available.

equisetum poisoning *See* bracken poisoning.

erectile Capable of causing erection or becoming erect. The penis is composed largely of erectile tissue.

erection The state of increased rigidity and size of the *penis during sexual excitement that enables coitus to take place. In some species, for instance the dog and horse, the spongy tissue of the penis becomes engorged with blood causing the penis to increase in both length and diameter. In other animals, such as ruminants and pigs, the penis is fibroelastic and changes little in actual size during erection; it is extended by relaxation of the muscle controlling the sigmoid flexure along its shaft. Deflection of the penis to one side during erection is a defect that can cause mating difficulties and render a male unfit for service. However, the semen can be collected by artificial procedures and used for artificial insemination.

erector spinae muscle The main muscle mass lying on the dorsal surface of the vertebral column (spine) throughout its length. It acts to extend the vertebral column.

erg- (ergo-) *Prefix denoting* work or activity.

ergocalciferol *See* vitamin D.

ergometrine An ergot alkaloid used to induce abortion and for the treatment of uterine inertia and postpartum uterine haemorrhage. It acts as a direct stimulant of uterine smooth muscle. At low doses the force and frequency of uterine contractions are increased; with higher doses contractions are more prolonged and uterine spasm occurs. It can be given orally but is generally used intravenously, and is effective at all stages of gestation, especially on the gravid uterus. Toxicity can occur with large doses (see ergot poisoning). *Prostaglandins, *corticosteroids, or *oxytocin are now preferred to ergometrine for controlling parturition.

ergosterol A *sterol found in yeast which can be converted to vitamin D by the action of ultraviolet light.

ergot (anatomy) A small mass of horn overlying the back of the fore and hind fetlocks in the horse.

ergot poisoning (ergotism) A toxic condition caused by the ingestion of *sclerotia (ergots) of fungi belonging to the genus *Claviceps, notably C. purpurea, which infects the flowering heads of cereals (especially rye and wheat) and certain pasture grasses. The ergots usually contain alkaloids, some of which are poisonous, particularly ergotamine, ergotoxine, and ergometrine. These stimulate the contraction of smooth muscle thereby restricting the flow or arterial blood. Cattle are most often affected; sheep and pigs appear less susceptible. The main effect in pigs is agalactia. In cattle, the disease can take either of two forms – nervous or gangrenous. The former is rarely caused by C. purpurea. However, it has been reported in the USA, producing in cattle a prancing gait, staggers, and vertigo as its main signs. *Paspalum staggers is a nervous form of ergotism caused by C. paspali.

The most prominent effects of gangrenous ergotism in cattle are lameness and dry *gangrene of the extremities. Signs of pain or an abnormal gait, often affecting first the hindlimbs, are followed by swelling extending upwards from the coronary band, subsequently developing into an area of cracking and gangrenous skin clearly demarcated from normal tissue. Sloughing of that skin and separation of the hoof may follow, and other extremities (e.g. ears and tail) may be affected. Cold weather accentuates these effects. There is no useful treatment apart from the control of local bacterial infection and withdrawal from the source of ergots. Evidence of the ingestion of large amounts of ergot is necessary to confirm a diagnosis. A similar syndrome of unknown aetiology but apparently unconnected with ergot has been seen on several occasions. Ergotism must also be differentiated from *fescue toxicosis. Bovine abortion has been attributed to ergotism on several occasions, but the link remains unsupported by experimental studies and remains controversial.

Ergots in pastures can be avoided by preventing the grass from flowering. Grazing alone may be insufficient and periodic cutting necessary, especially in late summer. Grain should be inspected for ergots, but in small numbers or in milled grain they are best detected by laboratory examination.

erogenous Describing certain parts of the body, the physical stimulation of which leads to sexual arousal.

eructation The expulsion of gas from the stomach. In ruminants eructation is essential for removing the gas produced by fermentative *digestion in the reticulorumen. Tension receptors in the wall of the reticulorumen detect raised pressure, and a forward moving contraction of the dorsal sac of the *rumen pushes the gas cap towards the cardia, which relaxes (*see* reticulum). Gas enters the oesophagus and passed very rapidly to the buccal cavity, from where much of it may be inhaled with the next inspiration; the remainder is voided from the mouth. The whole process is coordinated by neural reflexes. Eructation is inhibited if the region of the cardia is surrounded by fluid, as in frothy bloat, or because of lateral recumbency of the animal. It is also inhibited by factors that interfere with stomach motility, such as pain, hypocalcaemia (e.g. in *milk fever), and drugs (e.g. atropine and general anaesthetics). Failure of eructation causes death due to *bloat.

eruption 1. Any lesion that appears at the surface of the skin and is characterized by its prominence and redness. It can apply to a wide range of lesions, from simple transient reddening to widespread development of pustules. **2.** The emergence of a growing tooth from the gum into the mouth.

erysipelas A disease of poultry, caused by infection with the bacterium *Erysipelothrix insidiosa* (*rhusiopathiae*) characterized by sudden death. It principally affects turkeys over 3–4 months old, but can occur in younger birds, and in fowls, ducks, game birds, and some mammals. Usually there are no warning signs, although sometimes there is cyanosis (blueness) of the head, diarrhoea, and a high temperature. Mortality ranges from 1 to 50% of infected birds. Acute cases take the form of a general septicaemia, while chronic infections cause arthritis. The most effective treatment is intramuscular injection of the whole flock with a suitable antibiotic, although food or water medication can be tried in an emergency. Prevention consists in routine vaccination with a killed vaccine; this can also be given during outbreaks. Turkeys reared for breeding purposes should be vaccinated between 10 and 20 weeks, followed by a second dose just before laying. Some vaccines are combined with a *Pasteurella* vaccine. Infected carcasses can transmit *erysipeloid infections to humans through wounds. *See also* swine erysipelas.

erysipeloid (erythema serpens) An infection of the skin and underlying tissues with the bacterium *Erysipelothrix rhusiopathiae*. It usually affects people handling poultry, fish, or meat. Infection enters through scratches or cuts on the hands, and is normally confined to a finger or hand, which becomes reddened; sometimes systemic illness or valvular heart lesions develop. Treatment is with antibiotics.

Erysipelothrix A genus of rod-shaped aerobic pleomorphic Gram-positive *bacteria comprising a single species, *E. rhusiopathiae*. It is widely distributed in the soil and is also present in healthy pigs and other species. It is responsible for *swine erysipelas, *erysipelas in poultry, the skin infection erysipeloid in humans and other animals, and arthritis in sheep. Infections are spread by direct or indirect contact. The organism is very resistant to chemical agents (e.g. phenol) and physical agents (e.g. drying) but is readily killed by moist heat (15 minutes at 55°C). Farms can remain infected for a long time.

erythema Reddening of the skin due to congestion of the superficial blood vessels. It may be patchy or diffuse and can be caused by various factors; it is often a sign of inflammation and infection.

erythr- (erythro-) *Prefix denoting* **1.** redness. Example: *erythuria* (excretion of red urine). **2.** erythrocytes.

erythroblast Any of the precursor cells whose division leads to the production of *erythrocytes.

erythroblastosis The presence of the nucleated precursors of red cells (*erythroblasts) in the blood.

erythrocyte (red cell; red blood corpuscle) A mature blood cell that contains *haemoglobin, the pigment responsible for transporting oxygen. Erythrocytes comprise most of the cells in blood, being present normally at a concentration of about 5–10 million per microlitre of blood, depending on species. They account for about half the volume of circulating blood, the remainder being occupied largely by the *plasma, with a small contribution from white cells and platelets. Mammalian erythrocytes are disc-shaped and lack a nucleus, which is extruded during the later stages of their formation in the bone marrow (*see* haemopoiesis). In other vertebrates, the erythrocytes are oval and nucleated. Erythrocytes have a limited lifespan in the circulation, typically 50–150 days, depending on species. During this period the cells produce substantial amounts of reduced NADP (*see* NAD), which assists in the maintenance of reduced *glutathione; this is probably important in maintaining the reducing conditions within the cell necessary to preserve the cell's major constituent, haemoglobin.

Oxygen is carried by the iron-containing haem subunit of the haemoglobin molecule. The affinity of haemoglobin for oxygen is reduced by the presence of carbon dioxide, so that the transported oxygen is easily released from the erythrocytes in the tissues. Erythrocytes also contain the enzyme carbonic anhydrase, which catalyses the formation of bicarbonate ions from carbon dioxide and water. The erythrocytes thus readily take up carbon dioxide from tissues, in the form of bicarbonate ions, and transport it to the lungs.

erythrocyte mosaicism A mixture of blood types caused by prenatal joining of the placental blood vessels in nonidentical twins.

erythrocyte sedimentation rate *See* ESR.

erythromycin *See* macrolide antibiotics.

erythropenia *See* anaemia.

erythropoiesis *See* haemopoiesis.

erythropoietin A protein hormone, produced by the kidney, that stimulates the production of additional red blood cells (*see* haemopoiesis) in response to low oxygen tension in the blood. *Androgens will also stimulate erythropoietin production.

eschar A scab or covering of dead skin at the site of a burn or cauterization. The lesion, which penetrates all the layers of the epidermis and dermis, heals to form a fibrous scar (cicatrix).

Escherichia A genus of motile rod-shaped lactose-fermenting Gram-negative bacteria, widely distributed in nature. *E. coli* is the only known pathogenic species, commonly subdivided into many biotypes and serotypes. It is the most common aerobic commensal in the gastrointestinal tract, but certain serotypes, the *enteropathogenic strains*, are pathogenic due to the enterotoxins they produce and/or their invasiveness. Most of these serotypes seem to be host specific but some can affect more than one species.

Strains possessing one or more *virulence factors* are capable of causing disease, particularly in the weakened, stressed, or young animal. These virulence factors have been extensively studied; they include: two classes of gut-active *enterotoxins – one heat-labile (LT), the other heat-stable (STa; STb); external structures (fimbriae; often termed 'colonization pili') of several types (K88, K99, 987P, and F41) mediating attachment to the gut wall; O antigens of the pyrogenic cell-wall lipopolysaccharide (LPS), important in strains causing colisepticaemia; certain K antigens (present either in the LPS or, in certain groups, forming a capsule); a high-affinity iron-uptake system allowing multiplication in host tissues; and the oedema disease principle (EDP), produced by some porcine isolates.

Most outbreaks of disease due to *E. coli* (colibacillosis) occur in young animals and involve diarrhoea and/or bacteraemia (*see* colisepticaemia). In **cattle** a number of *E. coli* strains cause an acute and fatal disease in young calves, known as *enteric colibacillosis of calves, or white scours, characterized by severe diarrhoea and whitish faeces. These strains usually produce enterotoxins and are identified by the adhesive antigen K99. Other strains cause septicaemia in newborn calves, often associated with lack of sufficient colostrum. These strains are highly invasive and multiply in the blood and tissues other than the gastrointestinal tract. *E. coli* commonly causes *mastitis in dairy cattle, associated with environmental contamination.

In **pigs** *E. coli* causes neonatal *diarrhoea during the first week of life in piglets kept under intensive conditions. This disease is caused by enterotoxin-producing serotypes, usually associated with K88 colonization pili (which correspond to K88 'adhesive antigens'). In older piglets, the bacterium may cause post-weaning diarrhoea, which is aggravated by the change of diet. The mortality rates are higher in newborns, being as high as 90% (*see* enteric colibacillosis of piglets). *Oedema disease is associated with enterotoxin-producing serotypes; it also occurs commonly during the post-weaning period but can affect other age groups. In **sheep** serotypes of *E. coli* similar to those that cause colibacillosis in calves (K99) also cause enteric disease in lambs less than 1 week old (*see* enteric colibacillosis of lambs). Other serotypes cause septicaemia and sudden death. In **horses** *E. coli* strains may cause abortions in mares and diarrhoeas and septicaemias in newborn foals.

esophag- (esophago-) (*US*) *See* oesophag-.

ESR (erythrocyte sedimentation rate) The rate at which red cells (erythrocytes) settle out of suspension in blood plasma, measured in vitro under standardized conditions. Changes in the rate can indicate abnormalities of plasma proteins associated with disease. When blood, to which an *anticoagulant has been added, is allowed to stand undisturbed, the red cells form characteristic aggregations (rouleaux). *Rouleau formation is promoted by changes in plasma *globulin and *fibrinogen concentrations, and because rouleaux sediment faster than individual red cells, the degree of change in these protein concentrations correlates with the ESR. The test is therefore a useful but nonspecific indicator of diseases involving globulin and fibrinogen changes. Compared to other domestic animals, normal horses have a very high ESR, and normal ruminants a low ESR, hence ESR is not usually measured in these species.

Plasma viscosity also correlates with plasma protein concentration, and viscosity estimations can therefore be used to some extent as a substitute for ESR measurement.

essential amino acid

essential amino acid An *amino acid that an organism cannot synthesize itself in sufficient quantities and that must be supplied in its diet or culture medium. Animals generally require the following ten essential amino acids: arginine; histidine; isoleucine; leucine; lysine; methionine; phenylalanine; threonine; tryptophan; and valine. Deficiency of one or more of these in the diet can lead to retarded growth and other clinical signs. However, ruminants and other herbivores normally obtain sufficient amounts by the digestion of their gut microorganisms, which can synthesize the essential amino acids.

For monogastric animals, the dietary value of proteins (*see* protein quality) is determined by their content of essential amino acids. Proteins from animal sources, such as meat, eggs, and milk, usually contain all the essential amino acids and are of high nutritional quality; plant proteins, particularly cereal proteins, tend to be deficient in one or more essential amino acids and must be balanced by another complementary protein when devising a ration (*see* diet).

essential element Any of a number of elements required by living organisms to ensure normal growth and maintenance. Apart from the elements found in organic compounds (i.e. carbon, hydrogen, oxygen, and nitrogen), animals, plants and microorganisms all require a range of elements in inorganic form, depending on the type of organism. The *major elements*, present in tissues in relatively large amounts (greater than 0.005%), are *calcium, *phosphorus, *potassium, *sodium, chlorine, *sulphur, and *magnesium. They fulfil a variety of metabolic roles in the body. The *trace elements* occur in tissues at much lower levels and the amounts required in the diet are of the order of several milligrams per day or less, compared to requirements measured in grams

per day for major elements. The principal trace elements are: *chromium, *cobalt, *copper, *iodine, *iron, *manganese, *molybdenum, *selenium, and *zinc. Other elements may be required in even smaller amounts. If given in large amounts, many are toxic, especially copper, selenium, and molybdenum. The trace elements may serve as *cofactors or as constituents of complex molecules, for example iron in *haem and cobalt in *vitamin B_{12}.

essential fatty acid One of a group of long-chain *fatty acids that must be supplied in the diet of all domestic animals. They are polyunsaturated, i.e. contain two or more double bonds, and each double bond is separated by a single methylene group, i.e. the double bonds are not conjugated. This confers important fluid properties on the membranes of animal cells. The major types are linoleic (C18:2), linolenic (C18:3), and arachidonic (C20:4) acids. Arachidonic acid is also the precursor of the *prostaglandins. The oilseeds used in pig and poultry feeds are good sources, while grazing animals obtain adequate supplies from herbage. Hence deficiency, characterized by skin lesions and poor growth, is rare under normal conditions.

essential oil A volatile oil, consisting largely of terpenes, derived from various aromatic plants. They are used in various pharmaceutical preparations.

ester A molecule formed by the condensation reaction between an *acid and an *alcohol with the elimination of water. The acid involved may be organic, for example acetic acid as in *acetylcholine, but many esters of biological importance are derivatives of inorganic phosphoric acid, for example *AMP, glucose-6-phosphate, *phospholipids, and *nucleic acids. *Triesters*, molecules containing three ester groups, are major constituents of oils and fats (*see* triglyceride).

estradiol *See* oestradiol.

estro- (est-) (*US*) For words beginning with this prefix, see words beginning **oestro-** or **oestr-**.

estrogens *See* oestrogen.

estrone *See* oestrone.

etamiphylline *See* xanthine.

ethanol (ethyl alcohol) *See* alcohol.

ether (diethyl ether) A volatile and highly-inflammable liquid that is still used as an inhalational anaesthetic for small animals. It has a high blood solubility leading to slow induction of anaesthesia and slow recovery. Although nontoxic to organs such as the liver it is an irritant and animals should be given *atropine to reduce the production of respiratory and salivary secretions. Ether gives good muscle relaxation, and it has a synergistic action with *curare-type muscle relaxants. Analgesia is very good and effects on the cardiovascular system are minimal since direct depression of the heart is offset by increased sympathetic drive.

ethidium bromide *See* homidium bromide.

ethmoid A bone in the skull that contributes to the boundaries of the cranial cavity, nasal cavity, and orbits. Its perpendicular plate contributes to the bony part of the nasal septum, while its *cribriform plate* forms the roof of the nasal cavity and is perforated to allow passage of the *olfactory nerve filaments from the nasal cavity to the brain. The complex *ethmoidal labyrinth* on either side consists of scroll-like *ethmoturbinates*.

ethmoid haematoma (ethmoidal giant cell tumour; progressive haematoma) A lesion found in horses, usually as an ulcerated haemorrhagic mass in the posterior nasal cavity. It tends to enlarge progressively resulting in a haemorrhagic or mucopurulent nasal discharge. It is possibly not a true tumour but the product of chronic infection or repeated haemorrhages. Excision is possible but recurrence is likely.

ethopabate *See* coccidiostat.

ethyl chloride (chloroethane) A highly inflammable gas, formerly used as an *inhalational anaesthetic but superseded by safer compounds. It has also been used in a spray as a local anaesthetic; it evaporates rapidly from the surface producing an area of frozen insensitive tissue. However, this can cause tissue necrosis if freezing is prolonged.

ethylene glycol poisoning (antifreeze poisoning) A toxic condition most commonly occurring in cats and dogs that have drunk water containing ethylene glycol, which is used in engine cooling systems as an antifreeze. Pigs and poultry are also affected. Ethylene glycol is metabolized to oxalic acid, and calcium oxalate crystals are deposited in the kidney tubules. Affected animals vomit and develop ataxia and convulsions, followed by death. Intraperitoneal injections of 20% ethanol and 5% sodium bicarbonate are recommended as treatment.

ethylene oxide (epoxyethane) A colourless flammable gas used for sterilization. It is toxic and should be used in an enclosed chamber. Its sterilizing activity is optimal at 33% humidity and 20–56°C. The gas kills microorganisms, including spores, and is used to sterilize plastics and heat-sensitive material. Tissues also can be sterilized in ethylene oxide without their structure being damaged. After sterilization, items should be left in a well-ventilated area for 24–48 hours. The toxic ethylene oxide is removed by passing it through water, producing ethylene glycol.

etiology *See* aetiology.

etorphine A narcotic *analgesic that is used in combination with a tranquillizer to produce neuroleptanalgesia (*see* Immobilon) for the control of wild and aggressive animals. It is also used in domestic species such as the horse and dog. It can be administered by projectile syringe fired from a dart gun or blowpipe. Etorphine has properties similar to *morphine but is about 1000 times more potent. There are species differences in the response to etorphine: humans are very susceptible, and very small doses injected or penetrating through skin wounds are fatal. The effects of etorphine can be reversed by specific narcotic antagonists (e.g. *diprenorphine or naloxone).

eu- *Prefix denoting* **1.** good, well, or easy. **2.** normal.

eubacteria An obsolete term used to describe all the chemosynthesizing and photosynthesizing *bacteria.

euchromatin Chromosome material (*see* chromatin) that stains most deeply during mitosis and represents the major genes. *Compare* heterochromatin.

Euphorbia *See* spurge poisoning.

euploidy The condition of cells, tissues, or organisms in which there is one complete set of chromosomes or a whole multiple of this set in each cell. *Compare* aneuploidy.

Eustachian tube *See* auditory tube.

euthanasia Humane destruction; the killing of an animal without causing fear or suffering. In small animals (dogs, cats, etc.) the most commonly employed technique is the rapid intravenous injection of a concentrated *barbiturate. Occasionally it may prove necessary to administer the drug intracardially (into the heart) or intrathoracically (into the thorax). Very small mammals or birds are usually placed in a small airtight container with some volatile anaesthetic – usually *halothane – and not removed until dead. Horses are most commonly shot, employing a free bullet; this is satisfactory only in skilled hands. Horses injured on a racetrack and unable to rise may be exsanguinated (bled) by cutting the caudal vena cava through the rectum. This causes the horse to die without struggling. The blood will be contained by the anal sphincter, thus minimizing distress to spectators. In North America all horses are given intravenous drugs to kill them.
The humane slaughter of food animals usually involves stunning, either by a captive-bolt gun, *electrical stunning apparatus, or carbon dioxide anaesthesia, followed by exsanguination to prepare the carcass for hanging.

evagination The protrusion of a part or organ from a sheathlike covering or by eversion of its inner surface.

evening trumpet flower *See* yellow jessamine poisoning.

eventration Protrusion of the omentum or intestine through the abdominal wall. Small protrusions of this kind commonly occur through the umbilicus of piglets and puppies. When the protrusion is large, surgery is indicated; small protrusions heal spontaneously. The term is rarely used in veterinary surgery. *See* hernia.

eversion The turning outwards of a structure. Eversion of the uterus may occur soon after parturition, especially in cattle and sheep (*see* prolapsed uterus). *Compare* inversion.

ex- (exo-) *Prefix denoting* outside or outer.

exanthema (*pl.* **exanthemas** or **exanthemata**) **1.** A skin rash. **2.** Any disease characterized by such a rash.

exchange transfusion *See* transfusion.

excise To cut out tissue, an organ, or a tumour from the body.

excision arthroplasty Surgical removal of the head of the femur. It is usually carried out as a last resort to salvage an irreparably damaged hip joint, allowing it to form a fibrous false joint. Cats and small dogs usually regain surprisingly good use of the limb after this operation, but a return to normal use may be a problem in the larger breeds of dog.

excitation (in neurophysiology) The triggering of a conducted impulse in the membrane of a muscle cell or nerve fibre. During excitation a polarized membrane becomes momentarily depolarized and an *action potential is set up.

excoriation The destruction and removal of the surface of the skin or the covering of an organ by scraping, the application of a chemical, or other means, for instance as a result of chafing.

excrescence Any abnormal outgrowth from the body surface, such as a *papilloma.

excreta Any waste material discharged from the body, especially faeces.

excretion The removal of the waste products of metabolism from the body, principally through the action of the *kidneys (*see* urine) but also by the liver and the sweat glands of the skin. In prenatal life the main organ of excretion is the *placenta. The term is also used to include the egestion of *faeces.

exercise problems Various conditions noticed in working or competition animals, particularly horses and dogs, characterized by poor performance and possibly distress during strenuous activity. Such problems may be related to any body system, but the cardiovascular, respiratory, and musculoskeletal systems are especially important, and any disease process can result in an unwillingness or inability to exercise well. *Exhaustion* is characterized by dehydration, increased body temperature, heart, and respiratory rates, cardiac arrhythmias, generalized muscle twitching, and disorientation. It may occur, for example, in horses during long-distance endurance rides. Treatment involves hydration, correction of acid/base and electrolyte imbalances, cooling, rest, and anti-inflammatory drugs. Horses in similar situations may also suffer a form of cramp known as *synchronous diaphragmatic flutter*. This is thought to be provoked by temporary metabolic derangements, such as hypocalcaemia, hyperkalaemia, or alkalosis. Other causes of exercise problems in horses are *azoturia (tying-up syndrome) and *aortoiliac thrombosis. In dogs, *myasthenia gravis causes rapid fatigue of the animal on exercise. *See also* cramp.

exhalation (expiration) The act of breathing air from the lungs out through the mouth and nose. *See* breathing.

exo- *Prefix. See* ex-.

exocrine gland

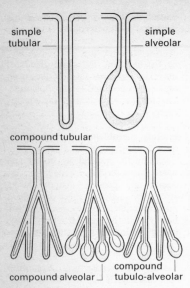

simple tubular

simple alveolar

compound tubular

compound alveolar — compound tubulo-alveolar

Types of exocrine gland

exocrine gland A gland that discharges its secretion by means of a duct, which opens onto an epithelial surface. An exocrine gland may be *simple*, with a single unbranched duct, or *compound*, with branched ducts and multiple secretory sacs. The illustration shows some different types of these glands. Examples of exocrine glands are the sebaceous and sweat glands. *See also* secretion.

exogenous Originating outside the body or part of the body: applied particularly to substances in the body that are derived from the diet rather than built up by the body's own processes of metabolism. *Compare* endogenous.

exonuclease An *enzyme that catalyses the hydrolysis of a *nucleic acid at a terminus of the *polynucleotide chain. Exonucleases may hydrolyse both *DNA and *RNA, but are more commonly specific (i.e. *exo DNase* or

exo RNase). They usually lead to the production of single nucleotides and are described as $3' \rightarrow 5'$ or $5' \rightarrow 3'$ (*see* phosphodiester) depending on the direction of hydrolysis. *Compare* endonuclease.

exopeptidase *See* peptidase.

exophthalmos An inherited eye disorder, controlled by a *recessive allele. It is not apparent at birth and can only be diagnosed later in life. Defective vision is the first sign, followed by progressive protrusion and sideways deviation of the eyeballs. In Jersey cattle the condition has been reported from 6 months of age, but in American shorthorns (where the condition is widespread) it does not appear until lactation has started.

exostosis (*pl.* **exostoses**) An outgrowth of bone. It is commonly caused by chronic irritation or trauma to ligaments and tendons at the point of their attachment to the bone. An inherited form of the disease known as *multiple inherited exostosis* occurs in thoroughbreds and Quarter horses. It may cause little harm but the outgrowths are visible or can be felt on limb and rib bones. *See also* osteophyte.

exothermic Describing a chemical reaction in which energy is released in the form of heat. *Compare* endothermic.

exotic Describing an animal or disease occurring in a region or country far from its normal distribution range.

exotoxin A toxic substance produced by certain bacteria and released by the living organisms.

expectorant An agent that increases the rate of removal of secretions from the airways. Expectorants may be *mucolytics, which act by decreasing the viscosity of secretions and therefore facilitate their removal from the bronchi and bronchioles, or the *parasympathomimetic drugs (e.g. pilocarpine), which act directly to increase bronchial secretions. Plant-derived preparations of volatile oils (e.g. Friars' balsam, balsam of Tolu) have also been used; these can be inhaled and cause local irritation, thus increasing the fluidity of bronchial secretions.

explant 1. Live tissue transferred from any organism to a suitable artificial medium for culture. The tissue grows in the artificial medium and can be studied for diagnostic or experimental purposes. Tumour growths are sometimes examined in this way. **2.** To transfer live tissue for culture outside the body.

extension veterinarian (USA) A veterinarian, employed in part by the federal government but usually based on a state facility, such as a university, who provides information and advice to livestock producers and their veterinarians.

extensor Any muscle that causes the straightening of a limb or other part.

external capsule The band of nerve fibres within each cerebral hemisphere in the brain lying between the lentiform nucleus and the claustrum. *See* corpus striatum.

exteroceptor A sensory nerve ending in the skin or in a mucous membrane that is responsive to stimuli from outside the body. *See also* chemoreceptor; receptor.

extirpation The complete surgical removal of tissue, an organ, or a growth.

extra- *Prefix denoting* outside or beyond.

extracellular Situated or occurring outside cells; for example, *extracellular fluid* is the fluid surrounding cells.

extraembryonic coelom (exocoelom) The cavity, lined with mesoderm, that surrounds the embryo in the earliest stages of its development. It communicates temporarily with the *intraembryonic coelom. With further development it becomes obliterated by the growth of the *amnion and *allantois, which fuse with the *chorion.

extraembryonic membranes *See* foetal membranes.

extrapyramidal system A group of nerve tracts and pathways connecting parts of the cerebral cortex, basal ganglia, thalamus, cerebellum, and reticular formation with motor neurones in the spinal cord not contained in the *pyramidal tract. The extrapyramidal system is mainly concerned with the regulation of stereotyped muscular activity without direct voluntary control.

extrasystole *See* ectopic (def. 2).

extrauterine Outside the uterus.

extravasation The escape of blood or fluid from vessels into the surrounding tissues, usually over considerable areas. Very large haemorrhages cause tumour-like swellings (*see* haematoma). Injury is the usual cause, although deformations (*aneurysms) of arterial walls may burst and allow the escape of blood. *Compare* ecchymosis; petechia.

extrinsic muscle A muscle, such as any of those controlling movements of the eyeball, that has its origin

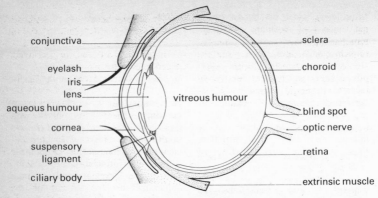

conjunctiva

eyelash

iris

lens

aqueous humour

cornea

suspensory ligament

ciliary body

vitreous humour

sclera

choroid

blind spot

optic nerve

retina

extrinsic muscle

The eye (sagittal section)

some distance from the part it acts on. *See also* eye.

exudation The formation of *exudate*, an abnormal tissue fluid with a high protein and *leucocyte (white cell) content produced characteristically in injury or *inflammation.

exudative diathesis A condition of young domestic fowls and turkeys involving breakdown of the blood capillary walls due to nutritional deficiency. There is slight haemorrhage through small lesions in the capillaries, and also leakage of plasma due to increased capillary permeability. A gelatinous yellow fluid accumulates beneath the skin, particularly on the breast and under the wings, and within the muscles. Also, a severe anaemia develops, characterized by excessively large red cells (i.e. *macrocytosis). The condition responds rapidly to dietary supplementation with vitamin E or selenium. *See also* muscular dystrophy.

eye The organ of sight, specialized for receiving light and converting light stimuli to nerve impulses, which are transmitted to the brain. It is a roughly spherical three-layered structure: the outer fibrous coat consists

of the *sclera and the transparent *cornea; the middle vascular layer comprises the *choroid, *ciliary body, and *iris; and the inner sensory layer is the *retina (see illustration). Light enters the eye through the cornea, which refracts it through the *aqueous humour onto the lens. By adjustment of the shape of the lens (*see* accommodation) light is focused through the *vitreous humour onto the retina. The arrangement of the eyes varies in different species; they are directed more to the front to provide *binocular vision in predators, whereas in herbivores they are more

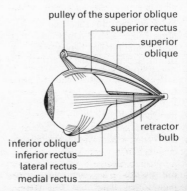

pulley of the superior oblique

superior rectus

superior oblique

retractor bulb

inferior oblique

inferior rectus

lateral rectus

medial rectus

Extrinsic muscles of the eye

to the side to give a wider visual field. Each eye is contained within an *orbit in the skull, and its movement is controlled by three pairs of extrinsic eye muscles – dorsal and ventral rectus, lateral and medial rectus, and dorsal and ventral oblique – and by the retractor bulbi (see illustration).

eyelash See cilium.

eyelid (palpebra) The protective covering of the *eye. The upper and lower eyelids each consist of skin, muscle, a thickened plate of connective tissue (*tarsus*), and glands. Their inner surface is lined by palpebral *conjunctiva. The upper and lower lids close in blinking to protect the eye and spread lacrimal fluid over the front of the eye. The third eyelid (nictitating membrane) is a fold of the conjunctiva at the inner (medial) angle of the eye, containing a plate of cartilage and glands. It is highly mobile and when the eye is drawn back into the orbit, for example during blinking, the third eyelid sweeps across the surface of the cornea.

eyeworm Any of various parasitic *nematodes that occur on or in the eye. Worms of the genus *Thelazia* infect dogs, ruminants, and occasionally humans. They normally remain in the inner corner of the eye, preferring the conjunctival sac and nasolacrimal duct, but can sometimes be seen creeping over the eyeball surface. The worm's rough cuticle abrades the surface of the eyeball and the irritation stimulates tear flow and dilatation of the blood vessels. Scar tissue may develop leading to blindness in severe cases. Secondary infections may arise, with consequent keratitis, conjunctivitis, ophthalmia, and a purulent discharge, which may cause the eyelids to gum together. The intermediate hosts are flies (*Musca* spp.), which often collect around the eye. Treatment involves local application of diethylcarbamazine or dosing with levamisole or tetramisole. This should be followed by application of an antibiotic eye ointment.

In monkeys and humans the filarial worm *Loa loa* wanders beneath the skin causing an itching sensation. It can also migrate to the eye. The motile embryos are present in the blood and the intermediate hosts are certain biting flies (mango flies).

F

F_1 (first filial generation) The first generation of offspring resulting from a cross between selected parents, especially between parents from different inbred lines, in which case the offspring (F_1 hybrids) may show *heterosis.

face fly See autumn house fly.

facet A small flat surface on a bone or tooth, especially a surface of articulation.

facial eczema A type of hepatogenous *photosensitization that occurs in sheep and cattle in New Zealand and in cattle in Australia. It affects animals grazing rapidly growing ryegrass pastures when conditions of temperature and moisture facilitate the rapid multiplication of the fungus *Pithomyces chartarum*. The spores of this fungus contain the mycotoxin *sporidesmin, which causes necrosis of liver cells. The necrotic areas are infiltrated by new cells and there is fibrosis and proliferation of disorganized bile ducts. The excretion of bilirubin and phylloerythrin is impeded and because the latter is a *photodynamic agent the animals become sensitive to sunlight. Their face and ears swell and become scabby and necrotic, resembling eczema. Some affected animals die; others recover partially but liver damage persists and growth is poor.

facial nerve The seventh *cranial nerve (VII). It runs through the facial canal in the temporal bone of the cranium, close to the middle ear, before leaving the skull at the *stylomastoid foramen*. Within the facial canal it gives off branches that supply the salivary glands, lacrimal gland, glands in the nasal cavity and palate, and the taste buds in the front two-thirds of the tongue. Outside the skull it enters the parotid gland and divides into a number of branches that supply the facial muscles. Damage to the facial nerve within the parotid gland or in the face leads to paralysis of the face, but does not impair sensation in the skin (*see* nervus intermedius).

facial paralysis Dysfunction of the *facial nerve, which principally supplies motor nerve fibres to the muscles of facial expression. Loss of muscle action produces relaxation of the face, with loose lips and cheek and absence of blinking. If only one side is affected, there is displacement of the face towards the normal side; this is most noticeable in animals with a mobile muzzle, such as the horse and sheep, and is much less apparent in animals with a firmly fixed muzzle, like cattle and dogs. The commissures of the lips cannot be retracted and there may be a tendency for food to drop from the mouth or collected between the cheek and teeth. In horses the nostril movements are under facial nerve control, consequently marked respiratory obstruction can occur on exercise and this must be controlled, especially with bilateral facial paralysis. Facial paralysis can be caused by injury to the nerve branches within the face by a wound

or by pressure from a buckle, etc. or by damage to the nerve as it courses through the parotid gland due, for example, to sepsis. Many cases recover spontaneously but all patients should have a detailed neurological examination.

-facient *Suffix denoting* causing or making. Example: *abortifacient* (causing abortion).

facilitation (in neurology) The phenomenon that occurs when a neurone receives, either through a number of different synapses (spatial summation) or repeatedly from the same synapse (temporal summation), impulses that are not powerful enough individually to start an *action potential but whose combined activity brings about some *depolarization of the membrane. In this facilitated state a small additional depolarization will suffice to trigger off an impulse in the cell.

factitious Describing experimental results or clinical signs produced artificially, either by design or accident. They may confuse the interpretation of experimental data or prevent an accurate diagnosis.

facultative Describing an organism that is not restricted to one way of life. A *facultative parasite* can live either as a parasite or, in different conditions, as a nonparasite able to survive without a host. *Compare* obligate.

FAD (flavin adenine dinucleotide) A *coenzyme, derived from riboflavin (vitamin B$_2$), that takes part in many important oxidation-reduction reactions. It consists of riboflavin, ribitol, adenine, ribose, and two phosphate groups.

fading puppy syndrome A condition in which the puppies in a litter gradually fail to thrive and stop sucking, usually resulting in the death of the whole litter within 3 weeks of birth. Many agents have been incriminated, but it is now thought that infection with *canine herpesvirus is the most likely cause. Since the virus grows at low body temperatures, keeping the puppies at a slightly higher temperature than normal may be beneficial. Bitches suspected to be carriers of the virus should not be bred.

faeces The waste material that is voided via the anus. It consists of food residues plus cellular debris, secretions from the alimentary tract, and bacteria. The quantity and composition vary with species and diet. For example, the fibre content is high in horses, whereas the water content is high in cattle but much lower in sheep and goats. Colouring depends mainly on the content of derivatives of bilirubin, a *bile pigment. See also meconium.

fainting See syncope.

falciform ligament The sickle-shaped midline fold of peritoneum that extends from the liver to the diaphragm and ventral abdominal wall as far as the umbilicus. It is a remnant of the ventral *mesentery and carries the obliterated *umbilical vein. It may acquire considerable quantities of fat.

Fallopian tube See uterine tube.

false hellebore poisoning A toxic condition due to the ingestion of various perennial herbaceous plants belonging to the genus *Veratrum* (false hellebores), particularly *V. californicum* and *V. viride*, also known as corn lily and Indian poke respectively. They occur throughout the USA and contain steroid alkaloids that cause salivation, diarrhoea, frequent urination, general muscular weakness, slow irregular heartbeat,

laboured respiration, prostration, convulsions, and death. Congenital deformities occur in the lambs of sheep fed *V. californicum* between the 12th and 14th days of gestation. Treatment is symptomatic.

false pregnancy A physical and behavioural syndrome that quite commonly occurs in the bitch 2–3 months after oestrus (heat). There is mammary gland development, lactation, and maternal behaviour, such as nesting and mothering an inanimate object. Other less frequently noted signs include vomiting, diarrhoea, excessive urination (polyuria), increased drinking (polydipsia), and anorexia. The cause is unknown. Treatment entails simply normal care and observation unless the animal is in extreme discomfort, in which case *megestrol acetate may be administered. The only preventive measure hitherto has been removal of the ovaries and uterus (ovariohysterectomy). However, elevated levels of circulating *prolactin have recently been demonstrated in the bitch with false pregnancy, and treatment with drugs that suppress prolactin secretion has given encouraging results.

False pregnancy occurs frequently in the **goat**. After what is considered a normal gestation (146–151 days) the doe voids a large volume of cloudy fluid (referred to as a 'cloudburst'), the abdomen returns to normal size, and lactation begins. The cause is obscure and common theories include early foetal death with continued fluid production and hydrometra.

If ovulation is induced in **cats** and no pregnancy results, the corpora lutea produce progesterone for about 20 days and cease to produce it at 40 days. Signs of pseudopregnancy are therefore confined to uterine endometrial hyperplasia, rather than the mammary development or behavioural changes seen in the bitch.

False pregnancy is rare in the sow and not reported in the ewe or cow. Other names: **phantom pregnancy; pseudocyesis; pseudopregnancy.**

falx A sickle-shaped structure. The *falx cerebri* is the fold of *dura mater that projects from the surface of the cranium between the cerebral hemispheres of the brain. It helps to stabilize the brain during movements of the head.

farcy An early name for any clinical condition in which the principal signs are nodular swellings of the superficial lymph nodes ('farcy buds') and thickening of the associated lymph vessels ('farcy pipes'). The term derives from the 'stuffed' appearance of these enlargements, and is still used for cutaneous *glanders and *bovine farcy, and sometimes for *epizootic lymphangitis of horses (Japanese farcy).

farmer's lung *See* allergic alveolitis.

Farriers (Registration) Act (1975) (England and Wales) An Act of Parliament that permits only persons registered under the Act to perform farriery. It thus seeks to prevent unnecessary suffering to horses in the hands of unskilled people and to ensure that farriers and shoeing smiths are properly trained. The Act defines farriery as "any work in connection with the preparation or treatment of the foot of a horse for the immediate reception of a shoe thereon, the fitting by nailing or otherwise of a shoe to the foot or finishing off of such work to the foot." Veterinarians are granted the right to carry out farriery.

farrowing The act of *parturition in pigs. Farrowing usually occurs 115 days after insemination, although this may vary from 112 to 117 days. The mammary gland (udder) undergoes considerable growth in the last 2 weeks of gestation, and in the 3–4 days prior to farrowing the individual glands become clearly demarcated and *colostrum may be expressed. The vulva swells and reddens, and in the 24–48 hours prior to farrowing the behaviour of the sow or gilt often changes dramatically, with an increase in restlessness becoming evident as well as frequent attempts at nest-building (even in conditions where no bedding is provided). With the imminent delivery of the first piglet, abdominal straining may be apparent in addition to vigorous twitching of the tail and the discharge of foetal fluids from the vulva. Due to the small foetal size compared with the dam, *dystocia resulting from foetal malpresentation is very uncommon. Piglets are delivered randomly from both horns of the uterus, and the mean interval between successive births is approximately 15 minutes. About half the foetuses show an anterior *presentation and the remainder posterior. Many piglets have intact umbilical cords; the length and elasticity of these is considerable and may even allow piglets to suckle before rupture occurs. Approximately 5% of piglets are stillborn, the majority having died from *anoxia during birth. The duration of farrowing is exceedingly variable, ranging from under 1 hour to more than 24 hours, but most are completed in 2–4 hours. Individual placentae may be passed at any stage but they frequently fuse together and are passed en masse a few hours after the last piglet. *Retention of the placenta is very uncommon.

Under intensive husbandry conditions, farrowing occurs in a special *farrowing crate, and the sow/gilt is moved into this some days prior, usually having been wormed and treated against ectoparasites. Many sows and gilts show intense stereotyped behaviour (such as bar biting) before farrowing, and the incidence of this can be reduced by the provision of bedding for nest-building. Newborn piglets are very susceptible to crushing and *hypothermia, and require a specially heated creep area where they can rest safely. Common veterinary problems in the sow include the metritis-mastitis-agalactia syndrome (see MMA), which normally occurs within 24 hours of farrowing. In gilts, instances of hysteria during farrowing leading to savaging of piglets are not uncommon. The main infectious cause of mortality in newborn piglets is neonatal diarrhoea, frequently caused by *Escherichia coli* bacteria (see enteric colibacillosis of piglets).

farrowing crate A structure into which a sow or gilt is placed immediately prior to *farrowing. It is usually constructed of metal struts embedded in a concrete floor within a larger pen and is designed to contain the sow so that she is able to stand but not turn around. Rolling over on one side to expose her teats during suckling can only be achieved slowly: thus the risk of crushing her piglets is reduced considerably.

fascia (*pl.* **fasciae**) Connective tissue forming membranous layers of variable thickness in all regions of the body. Fascia surrounds the softer or more delicate organs. The *superficial fascia* is found immediately beneath the skin and contains a variable quantity of fat. The *deep fascia* forms sheaths for muscles and is composed of dense fibrous tissue.

fasciculation 1. (in pathology) Jerky spontaneous visible contractions of groups of muscle fibres supplied by a single motor nerve fibre. The condition is an involuntary reaction to an abnormal discharge of a single or several spinal motor neurones, resulting usually in ripple-like contractions under the skin. The cause of fasciculation is unknown but is thought to involve abnormality of acetylcholine levels, since *neostigmine (an inhibitor of cholinesterase) can induce fasciculation experimentally. In humans, fasciculation is usually associated with motor neurone disease, which is accompanied by neurogenic atrophy of groups of muscles. 2. (in anatomy) The formation of a *fasciculus.

fasciculus (fascicle) (*pl.* **fasciculi**) A bundle, e.g. of nerve or muscle fibres.

fasciitis Inflammation of the *fascia – the bands of connective tissue surrounding certain structures, such as bundles of muscle fibres. The term is not commonly used in veterinary medicine.

Fasciola A genus of parasitic flukes including the liver *fluke, *Fasciola hepatica*, found worldwide in the bile ducts of most herbivores (see illustration). It is of most importance in cattle and sheep, causing *fascioliasis; a heavy infestation in sheep can lead to the appearance of *black disease. *F. gigantica* is a larger species found in sheep and cattle in tropical Africa and Asia.

fascioliasis Disease due to infestation by flukes of the genus *Fasciola*. The most widespread species is the liver fluke *F. hepatica*, which infests principally sheep, goats, and cattle, although many other mammalian species, including humans, are susceptible. Part of the life cycle is spent in an intermediate host, a snail of the genus *Lymnaea*, from which cercariae emerge to form cysts (metacercariae) attached to vegetation. When a final host ingests metacercariae, the young parasites emerge from the cysts in the intestine, penetrate the peritoneal cavity, and enter the liver, where they cause tissue destruction by feeding on the liver parenchyma. This phase of parasitism lasts 6–7 weeks, after which the flukes enter the bile ducts,

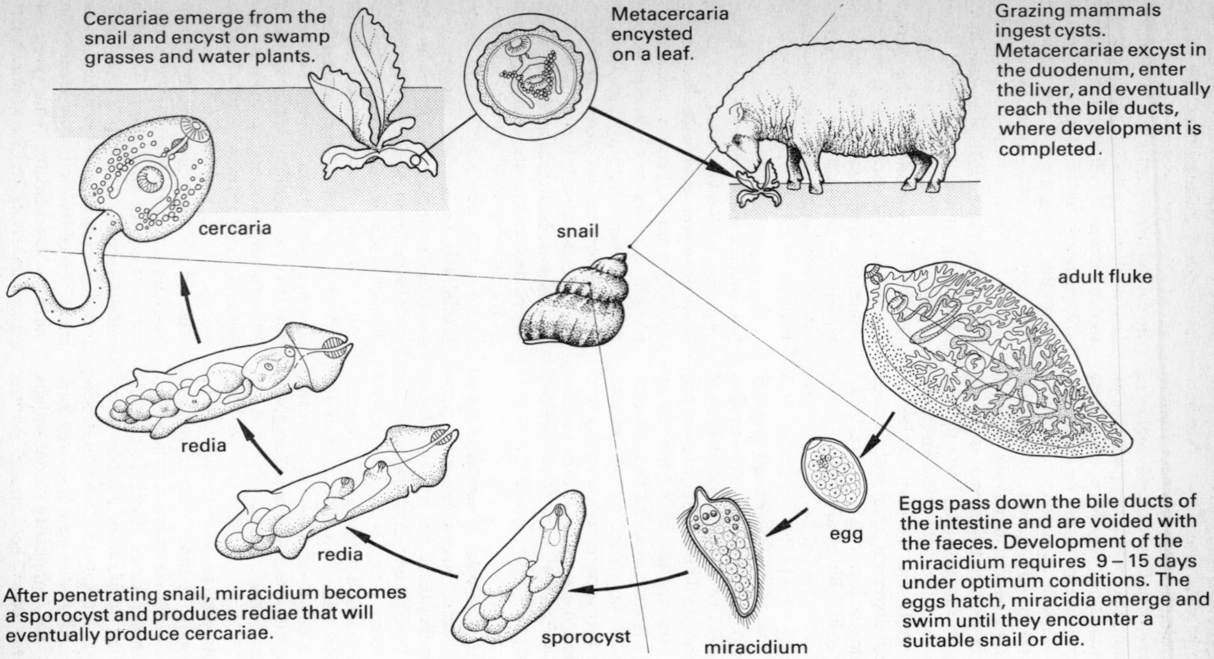

Grazing mammals ingest cysts. Metacercariae excyst in the duodenum, enter the liver, and eventually reach the bile ducts, where development is completed.

adult fluke

Metacercaria encysted on a leaf.

Cercariae emerge from the snail and encyst on swamp grasses and water plants.

Eggs pass down the bile ducts of the intestine and are voided with the faeces. Development of the miracidium requires 9 – 15 days under optimum conditions. The eggs hatch, miracidia emerge and swim until they encounter a suitable snail or die.

egg

miracidium

sporocyst

snail

redia

redia

cercaria

After penetrating snail, miracidium becomes a sporocyst and produces rediae that will eventually produce cercariae.

Life cycle of the liver fluke, *Fasciola hepatica*

reach maturity, and lay eggs, which appear in the faeces.

The ecology of the parasite is much influenced by weather conditions, hence the degree of liver fluke infestation tends, especially in temperate zones, to vary from year to year. *Acute fascioliasis* is the rarer form of the disease and is largely restricted to sheep. It results from simultaneous liver infestation by large numbers of young flukes following the release of many cercariae from well-developed snails that were infested at the time of their maximum abundance, usually mid- to late summer. Acute fascioliasis tends to follow warm wet summers in which both snail numbers and rates of snail infestation are high. Owing to the time required for the parasite to develop in the snail, acute fascioliasis is usually evident in sheep late in the year, causing sudden death. Blood may be present at the mouth and anus of the carcass. The condition is sometimes complicated by the toxaemia due to bacterial infection known as *black disease. Liver destruction and the presence of the young parasites are evident at post mortem.

Chronic fascioliasis occurs as a result of the gradual acquisition of parasites over a period. It is the commoner form, particularly in mammals other than sheep. The primary lesion is a chronic usually progressive fibrosis of the liver. The bile ducts frequently show hyperplasia and, later, loss of their epithelium; their walls are thickened and may eventually become calcified. Affected animals also tend to show progressive anaemia, low plasma albumin, submandibular oedema ('bottle jaw'), depression, and weight loss. These changes are less common in cattle than sheep. In adult dairy cows, reduction in milk yield may occur. Clinical signs appear only when sufficient parasites have been acquired, hence the chronic form is much less clearly seasonal than the

acute form. Diagnosis of fascioliasis is confirmed by demonstrating *F. hepatica* eggs in the faeces.

In principle, prevention can be achieved by draining land or applying molluscicides to remove snails. Study of meteorological records enables forecasting of heavy cercarial release so that in bad years the worst affected pastures can be avoided. *Anthelmintics give clinical benefit and also reduce egg output so restricting snail infestation.

In Africa and India *F. gigantica* is the predominant liver fluke. The life cycle and pathogenicity are generally similar to *F. hepatica*, with various species of *Lymnaea* serving as intermediate host.

fat A mixture of lipids, chiefly *triglycerides, that is solid at normal body temperatures. Fats occur widely in plants and animals as a means of storing food energy. In vertebrates, fat is deposited in a layer beneath the skin (subcutaneous fat) and deep within the body as specialized *adipose tissue (*see also* brown fat). The insulating properties of fat are also important, especially in animals lacking fur (e.g. pigs) or inhabiting cold climates.

Fats derived from plants and fish generally have a greater proportion of unsaturated *fatty acids than those derived from mammals. Their melting points thus tend to be lower, causing a softer consistency at room temperatures. Highly unsaturated fats are liquid at room temperatures and are therefore more properly called *oils.

fatty acid An organic acid with an aliphatic hydrocarbon chain and a terminal carboxyl group, general formula $C_nH_{(2n+1)}COOH$, in which n varies from zero (formic acid, HCOOH) to 20 or more. Most naturally occurring fatty acids have an even number of carbon atoms. Short-chain fatty acids such as acetic (ethanoic), propionic (propanoic), and butyric (butanoic) acids are important in metabolism, especially in ruminants (see volatile fatty acids), and in milk. However, the most abundant in the animal body are the long-chain fatty acids (C14–C18), which may be saturated or unsaturated. They most commonly occur as constituents of certain lipids, notably *glycerides, *phospholipids, sterols, and waxes, in which they are esterified with alcohols. Polyunsaturated fatty acids contain two or more double bonds; some, comprising the *essential fatty acids, are required in the diet.

The physical properties of fatty acids are determined by chain length, degree of unsaturation, and chain branching. Short-chain acids are pungent liquids, soluble in water. As chain length increases, melting points are raised and water-solubility decreases. Unsaturation and chain branching tend to lower melting points.

fatty degeneration A pathological change in a tissue involving the deposition of abnormally large amounts of fat in its cells. Such deterioration is commonly seen in the liver, kidney, and heart. Factors such as poor blood supply or poisoning injure the cells, resulting in defective metabolism and the accumulation of fat droplets. Fatty degeneration of the liver may lead eventually to the death of affected cells and thence to complete liver failure. However, some degree of fatty degeneration of the liver occurs normally in recently calved cows (see fatty liver). Furthermore, in the cat the kidney is normally fatty and the accumulation of fat in the tubule cells is no evidence of fatty degeneration.

fatty liver (of cattle) A metabolic condition affecting cows that calve when excessively fat. They suffer from a reduced appetite which leads to rapid use of fat from the body stores and its accumulation in the liver. Affected animals are more prone to *ketosis, *infertility, and *mastitis. Laboratory tests on blood samples can reveal characteristic changes and are a useful aid to diagnosis. To prevent the condition, cows should not be overfed in late lactation or during the dry period and should be condition score 3 (see condition scoring) at calving.

fatty liver and kidney syndrome (FLKS) A fatal nutritional disorder of chicks. It is strongly associated with a shortage of *biotin, and also with rations low in fat and protein, particularly wheat-based diets. Clinical signs appear suddenly in apparently healthy birds between 1 and 4 weeks of age. The chicks collapse and seem paralysed, often resting on their breasts with heads lying in front; death tends to follow within hours. Post-mortem examination shows excessive fat in the liver and kidneys, which are also enlarged; the liver and heart are abnormally pale. The condition usually affects just a few birds in a flock but in exceptional outbreaks the mortality can approach 20%. Feeding supplementary biotin has proved beneficial as a preventive measure in both experimental and field conditions. Outbreaks of FLKS can be triggered by sudden environmental stress. Compare fatty liver haemorrhagic syndrome of hens.

fatty liver haemorrhagic syndrome of hens A condition of laying hens in which excessive amounts of fat accumulate in the liver. It typically appears in flocks sporadically or as a spate of sudden deaths, caused by haemorrhage from the ruptured liver. However, productivity can also be affected, with reductions in egg output of up to 30%. The synthesis of excess fat in the liver seems to be linked to high feed consumption, and affected birds are usually overweight.

Contributory factors apparently include hot weather, high rates of lay, lack of exercise (as in caged birds), a genetic component, and possibly an unsuitable carbohydrate source in the diet. There is no clearly effective treatment, but dietary vitamin supplementation can be tried. *Compare* fatty liver and kidney syndrome.

fauces (oropharynx) The part of the *pharynx that lies behind the mouth and oral cavity, with which it communicates through the isthmus of the fauces. The palatine tonsil is situated in its lateral wall.

favus A severe skin disease caused by infection with certain *dermatophyte fungi, which produce characteristic dense masses of *mycelium, spores, and epithelial debris in the form of cup-shaped crusts called *scutula*. Masses of these structures may resemble a honeycomb (*favus* is Latin for a honeycomb). In humans favus is most often caused by *Trichophyton schoenleinii*, in gallinaceous birds (e.g. domestic fowls) by *Microsporum gallinae* ('fowl favus'), and in mice by *T. mentagrophytes* var. *quinckeanum*.
Fowl favus is reported in domestic **poultry** worldwide but is generally sporadic or rare. Infection typically produces dull-white patches or crusts on the comb and wattles ('white comb'), and the disease sometimes spreads to other parts of the body and involves the feathers. The infection is contagious and may be transmitted to other animals or to humans.

feather One of the outgrowths of the epidermis of birds that form the body covering. They are composed of the protein *keratin. The *contour feathers* are arranged in regular rows on the body, giving the body its streamlined shape. Each has a central shaft with a flattened vane on each side. Each vane is composed of two rows of fila-

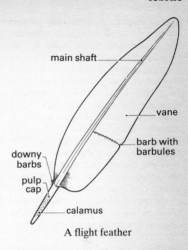

A flight feather

ment-like barbs, which are connected to each other by means of hooked barbules to form a smooth surface (see illustration). The flight feathers of the wing (*remiges*) are divided into *primaries*, carried on the manus, and *secondaries*, carried on the antebrachium. The *rectrices* are the flight feathers of the tail. The small fluffy *down feathers* (*plumes*) cover and insulate the whole body. In newly-hatched chicks they are the only feathers; in adults they lie between and beneath the contour feathers.

feather pecking A vice occasionally found in housed poultry flocks, in which birds acquire the habit of pecking the feathers of other individuals. Lack of stimuli and boredom may be predisposing factors. In its mild form it results in feather loss, which besides being unsightly may give rise to follicle infections, thus downgrading carcasses. More seriously, exposed areas of skin are liable to attract further pecking (*see* cannibalism).

febrile Relating to or affected with *fever.

feed additive A substance that is added to animal rations in relatively low concentrations. It may be an antimicrobial agent (e.g. *antibiotic) to prevent or treat disease, a nutrient supplement (e.g. *essential element or *vitamin), or a *growth promoter. One of the main problems when using feed additives to treat disease is ensuring uniform intake of the drug throughout a group of animals. The additive must be thoroughly mixed with the ration, and each animal in the group must obtain a sufficient quantity of the ration. The addition of antimicrobials to commercially prepared rations (e.g. for pigs or poultry) requires a veterinary written directive.

feedback The coupling of the output of a process to the input. Feedback mechanisms are important in regulating many physiological processes; for example, hormone output and enzyme-mediated reactions. In *negative feedback*, a rise in the output of a substance (e.g. a hormone) will inhibit a further increase in its production, either directly or indirectly. In *positive feedback*, a rise in the output of a substance is associated with an increase in the output of another substance, either directly or indirectly.

feed block A hard block of concentrated dietary supplements, such as minerals and vitamins, to which animals usually have free access. Intake is controlled by the hardness or saltiness of the block; nevertheless, wide variations in intake occur. *See also* salt lick.

feeding *See* diet; nutrient; nutrition.

feedlot A mainly North American system of housing *beef or *dairy cattle in a large pen, or group of pens. Land around the feedlot is used not for grazing but for growing high-energy crops, such as forage maize, that are transported to the feedlot and given to the cattle along with cereals or agricultural by-products. Some US feedlots are extremely large, with a capacity of up to 32 000 cattle.

feed refusal and emetic syndromes *See* fusariotoxicosis.

Feline Advisory Bureau A UK charity, founded in 1958, that is dedicated to promoting research and giving advice on all aspects of feline care and health. The organization publishes a members' bulletin, holds regular meetings throughout the country, and funds a specialist feline veterinary scholarship at Bristol Veterinary School. It also publishes a wide range of leaflets giving advice on specific disorders and other topics relating to cats. Address: 350 Upper Richmond Road, Putney, London, SW15 6TL.

feline calicivirus infection *See* cat flu.

feline infectious anaemia A disease of cats characterized by *anaemia and caused by the rickettsia species *Haemobartonella felis*. During this characteristically chronic illness parasite numbers fluctuate in the blood and the parasites may be very difficult to detect. The parasite is probably transmitted by fleas or lice. The disease is treatable with tetracycline antibiotics.

feline infectious enteritis *See* feline viral enteritis.

feline infectious peritonitis A disease of cats caused by a *coronavirus and occurring in two distinct forms: the 'wet' form is by far the most common and causes an accumulation of fluid in the abdomen and/or in the chest; the 'dry' form causes inflammation in any of various places in the body, and neurological disorders are frequent when the disease affects the nervous system. Cats are very commonly found to be carrying the virus, but only a small proportion of infected animals develop the disease, which then usually takes a slow and insidious course. There is no effective treatment, and the disease is invariably fatal once clinical signs develop. Control of the disease in a cattery or breeding colony is by the removal of infected animals. *See also* peritonitis.

feline influenza *See* cat flu.

feline juvenile osteodystrophy *See* feline nutritional secondary hyperparathyroidism.

feline leukaemia A cancer of cats frequently associated with feline leukaemia virus infection. Virus-induced leukaemia is characterized by *anaemia and foetal death in the pregnant queen. Infection with feline leukaemia virus may also be manifested by the development of tumours in the *thymus, intestinal tract, or *lymph nodes. Cats infected as kittens usually become persistently infected and may develop disease as 1- or 2-year-olds, whereas infection in older cats is usually overcome by an effective immune response. The virus is transmitted by close contact with a persistently infected cat that is excreting virus. These persistently infected animals also have a reduced ability to resist other diseases and may die without the involvement of feline leukaemia virus being suspected. The presence of the virus may be confirmed by a blood test. Removal of infected cats from breeding colonies is considered essential. A vaccine is available in North America.

feline miliary dermatitis An intensely itchy chronic skin disease of adult cats characterized by numerous small papules arranged in groups over the body. Most cases are the result of a *hypersensitivity reaction to flea bites. The animal may scratch or rub affected areas of skin, breaking the hairs of the coat or creating bald patches. Fleas should be excluded from the cat's environment and *anti-inflammatories prescribed to control the itching (pruritus) and inflammation. If untreated, intestinal hair balls may result from the persistent licking of the itchy papules. Other names: **miliary eczema**.

feline nutritional secondary hyperparathyroidism A disease, characterized by reduced mineralization of the skeleton, normally seen in young kittens, particularly Siamese kittens, fed a meat-rich diet that is low in calcium. Signs include lameness, bending of the long bones, and a tendency for the bones to fracture very easily. Correcting the diet will rapidly prevent further development of the condition, but cannot reverse the existing pathological changes. Other names: **feline juvenile osteodystrophy**; **nutritional osteopenia**; **juvenile osteopenia**.

feline panleukopenia *See* feline enteritis.

feline pneumonitis An infection of the upper respiratory tract in cats, caused by the microorganism *Chlamydia psittaci*. The clinical signs may be similar to those of *cat flu, with discharge from the nose and eyes, although in some cases there may be only a chronic *conjunctivitis without any other signs. Treatment may involve a long course of tetracycline antibiotics. Prevention by vaccination is available in some countries. Other name: **chlamydiosis**.

feline progressive arthritis A noninfectious form of *polyarthritis, usually affecting male cats aged 18 months to 5 years. It may occur in an acute erosive form or as a more chronic proliferative disease. The acute disease is less common and resembles *rheumatoid arthritis, with pain and stiffness. It occurs in older cats in carpal and metaphalangeal joints, producing joint instability and deformities. The more common chronic disease is characterized by *osteoporosis with periosteal new bone and ankylosis of joints over a period of 2–8 weeks. Periarticular erosions and fibrous ankylosis may occur but deformity of joints is not a feature. The exact aetiology is unknown but feline syncytia-forming virus (FeSFV) and feline leukaemia virus (FeLV) have been isolated from affected cats. It has been suggested that the condition is an unusual manifestation of FeSFV infection, potentiated by FeLV presence. Treatment with *corticosteroid or immunosuppressive drugs (such as cyclophosphamide) is said to be beneficial. The latter agents, however, may suppress bone marrow function.

feline pyothorax A condition of cats involving an accumulation of pus due to infection within the pleural cavity surrounding the lungs. The infection may be introduced by a penetrating injury of the pleural cavity or be spread in the bloodstream from another source. The major presenting sign is usually laboured breathing, accompanied generally by high temperature, dullness, and inappetence. Radiography and *pleurocentesis may assist with the diagnosis. Some cases may respond to systemic antibiotic therapy alone; more severe cases can require surgical insertion of a chest *drain so that the pus can be repeatedly drawn off and antibiotics injected directly into the chest cavity.

feline urological syndrome (FUS) A disorder of the urinary system of cats caused by the deposition of mineral crystals within the tract. It is most common in overweight neutered male cats with a sedentary lifestyle, and a major factor in its cause is the consumption of foods with a high magnesium content, particularly some of the dried cat foods. In female cats the crystals usually cause a chronic irritation of the urinary bladder, resulting in recurrent bouts of *cystitis. However, the narrower *urethra of the male cat means that obstruction to urine outflow can rapidly occur due to a plug of crystals. Cystitis can be treated with antibiotics, together with permanent changes to the diet to try to dissolve any crystals and prevent recurrence. Urinary obstruction is an acute emergency that must be corrected immediately to avoid permanent damage to the kidneys and bladder. Owners that notice a male cat straining must take care to differentiate this condition from constipation, which is less serious.

feline viral enteritis An acute disease of domestic and wild cats caused by a *parvovirus and characterized by diarrhoea, dehydration, prostration, and death. The disease is highly contagious with an incubation period of about 1 week. However, death may occur in young animals before the development of clinical signs. *Pancytopenia develops rapidly and early so that within 10 days of infection the total leucocyte count in the blood may be reduced to 1000 cells/ μl or less. The leucopenia is evidently caused by direct viral destruction of the white cell-producing stem cells in the bone marrow and lymphoid organs. Red cell- and platelet-producing stem cells are also affected. Recovery is marked by a gradual return to normal of the leucocyte count, with the appearance of juvenile white cells in the blood, often with bizarre cellular morphology.

Treatment is by fluid and electrolyte replacement, with antibiotics to combat secondary bacterial infection. The virus is very resistant and may persist in the environment. Kittens may be protected up to 12 weeks of age by maternal antibody. Subsequent protection can be provided using dead or live attenuated vaccine. Annual vaccination is recommended. Other names: **feline infectious enteritis; feline pancytopenia; feline panleucopenia.**

feline viral rhinotracheitis *See* cat flu.

feminization A condition in which a male individual develops female secondary sexual characteristics. It is due to persistently elevated levels of *oestrogens, which typically result in decreased muscle mass, pendulous prepuce, mammary development, and some hair loss. This is common in *Sertoli cell tumours in dogs and can be seen with other testicular and adrenal tumours. Lack of libido and infertility are common clinical signs. Therapy usually involves surgical removal of the causal lesion. *See also* hyperoestrogenism.

femoral Of or relating to the thigh or to the femur.

femoral artery The principal artery of the thigh region, where it is the continuation of the external iliac artery. It runs superficially on the inner (medial) side of the thigh in the femoral triangle, where it is the routine site for feeling the pulse in the dog and cat.

femoral nerve A nerve arising from the lumbar plexus to supply the iliopsoas and quadriceps femoris muscles and giving rise to the *saphenous nerve.

femoral paralysis Dysfunction of the *femoral nerve, which supplies motor fibres to the quadriceps femoris muscles of the hindlimb. It results in inability to extend the stifle and consequent difficulty in weight bearing and in advancing the leg. There is also loss of sensation in a small area

of the medial side of the hindlimb, and, in dogs, in the medial toe.

femur The long bone in the thigh region of the hindlimb. The head of

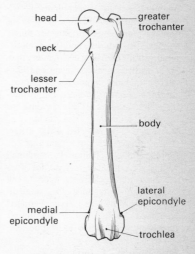

Left femur of dog, cranial aspect

the femur articulates with the acetabulum of the os coxae at the hip joint. At the base, the medial and lateral condyles articulate with the tibia, and the trochlea articulates with the patella at the stifle joint (see illustration).

fenbendazole *See* benzimidazoles.

fenestra (in anatomy) An opening resembling a window. The *fenestra vestibuli* is the opening between the middle *ear and the vestibule of the internal ear. It is closed by a membrane to which the stapes is attached. The *fenestra cochleae* is the opening between the scala tympani of the cochlea and the middle ear. Sound vibrations leave the cochlea through the fenestra cochleae which, like the fenestra vestibuli, is closed by a membrane.

fentanyl A synthetic narcotic *analgesic with properties similar to *morphine but about 80 times more potent. It is used in combination with a tranquillizer to produce a state of *neuroleptanalgesia suitable for minor surgical procedures, and is administered intramuscularly; excitement may occur with intravenous injection. Side-effects include hypotension, bradycardia, respiratory depression, twitching, and movement in response to external stimuli. The action of fentanyl can be reversed using a narcotic antagonist (e.g. naloxone or diprenorphine). Fentanyl combined with a tranquillizer is used for Caesarean section because the neonate can be given the antagonist drug immediately following delivery. Fentanyl combined with the tranquillizer fluanisone is marketed as Hypnorm.

fermentation A form of anaerobic *respiration carried out by certain microorganisms. The end-product varies widely between organisms; examples include ethanol (see alcohol), *lactic acid, and *propionic acid. Each of the different mechanisms allows the organism to generate some energy (in the form of *ATP) from its food molecules (e.g. *glucose) without the complete oxidation possible under *aerobic conditions. Fermentation is particularly important in the nutrition of ruminants and other herbivores because of the anaerobic conditions prevailing in the rumen, caecum, and large intestine.

ferri- (ferro-) Prefix denoting iron.

ferritin The main storage form of *iron in the animal body, comprising a complex of the protein apoferritin and ferrous iron. It is most abundant in the liver. See also transferrin.

fertilization The fusion of a *spermatozoon and an *ovum. The penetration of a secondary *oocyte by a spermatozoon is followed by rapid changes in the oocyte membrane that prevent other spermatozoa from penetrating. Penetration stimulates the completion of *meiosis and the formation of the ovum and second polar body. The male and female *pronuclei now fuse thus forming a *zygote with the diploid number of chromosomes.

fescue toxicosis Any of several disorders, probably involving fungal toxins (mycotoxins), occurring in cattle grazing tall fescue, Festuca arundinacea, an important pasture and fodder grass, especially in North and South America. One syndrome, fescue foot, progresses from early signs of a roughened coat, reduced weight gain, a slightly arched back, and evident soreness in the hindlimbs, to a dry *gangrene of the extremities not readily distinguishable from that found in *ergot poisoning. However, it occurs where there is no infection of grass with the ergot fungus – Claviceps, although fungi closely related to Claviceps are widespread in tall fescue and many perennial weed grasses. These fungi grow within the stems and leaves of apparently healthy grasses, and are thought to produce ergot alkaloids.
Summer syndrome, a widespread disorder in cattle grazing fescue in hot weather, has been firmly linked to a high level of infection in the grass by the fungus Acremonium coenophialum. Affected animals lose the ability to tolerate heat, their body temperature and respiratory rate rise, and they seek shade or wade into water. Reduced weight gain and milk yield lead to substantial economic losses.

fetlock 1. The joint formed either between the *metacarpus and the phalanges (in the forelimb) or between the *metatarsus and the phalanges (in the hindlimb), especially in the horse. **2.** The region of the limb surrounding these joints in the horse.

feto- *Prefix denoting* a foetus.

fetoscopy The process by which an *endoscope is inserted through the abdominal and uterine walls in order to visualize the foetus.

fetus *See* foetus.

Feulgen reaction A method of demonstrating the presence of DNA in cell nuclei. The tissue section under investigation, after hydrolysis with dilute hydrochloric acid, is treated with *Schiff's reagent. A purple coloration develops in the presence of DNA.

fevered flesh A condition of the carcass of an animal that has been slaughtered while fevered. The flesh is a darker red than normal, with small scattered haemorrhages, giving the whole carcass a dull-red appearance.

fever (pyrexia) A clinical state in which the *body temperature rises above normal. Fever develops as a prominent clinical sign in several infectious diseases, due partly to toxins produced by the infecting microorganisms and partly to pyrogens (*see* pyrogenic) released by *neutrophils in the blood. The rise in body temperature plays a vital role in combating infection, but also affects bodily functions. The febrile animal is typically dull and depressed and fails to eat. It shivers and seems apparently cold. Pulse rate and breathing rate increase. Prolonged fever gives rise to dehydration and disturbances in salt metabolism due to loss of water and sodium chloride in sweat. Severe fever leads to convulsions, and death usually occurs if the temperature rises more than 5°C above normal. Treatment depends on the primary cause, but the fever can be reduced by administering *antipyretic drugs. The provision of shade or the application of cold water or ice will help if the environmental temperature is high. Convulsions induced by fever may be controlled by sedation with *barbiturates.

fever root A North American plant, belonging to the genus *Cicuta*, that contains the toxic alkaloid cicutoxin (*see* hemlock water dropwort poisoning).

fibr- (fibro-) *Prefix denoting* fibres or fibrous tissue.

fibre 1. (in anatomy) A threadlike structure, such as a muscle cell, a nerve fibre, or a collagen fibre. **2.** (in dietetics) *See* dietary fibre.

fibre optics The use of bundles of parallel fibres (*optical fibres*) having special properties for transmitting light waves, and therefore visual images, by internal reflections within the fibre bundles. Fibre-optic systems are employed in instruments (*fibrescopes) to examine internal body cavities.

fibrescope An *endoscope that uses fibre optics for imaging. Its great advantage over older endoscopes is its flexibility, which enables thorough examination of passages or cavities, especially the upper respiratory and upper alimentary tracts, thoracic and abdominal cavities, urethra, and urinary bladder.

fibril A very small fibre or a constituent thread of a fibre (for example, a *myofibril of a muscle fibre).

fibrillation Rapid and uncoordinated contractions of individual muscle fibres. It may occur in any muscle but is of especial importance in heart muscle, where it may result in death. Fibrillation of the heart ventricles (*ventricular fibrillation*) occurs in the terminal stages of most fatal diseases and toxic conditions. Fibrillation of the atria (*atrial fibrillation*) is not necessarily fatal. It commonly follows from lesions in the heart wall. Affected racehorses may start a race well but rapidly fade thereafter. A similar condition occurs in draught horses and also in cows with metabolic disease. Success in the treatment of atrial fibrillation depends on the degree of damage to the atrial musculature. *Digitalis and *quinidine sulphate have been used. *See also* arrhythmia.

fibrin The final product of the blood *coagulation (clotting) mechanism, produced by the action of the enzyme *thrombin upon the protein precursor, *fibrinogen. The fibrin polymerizes to form an unstable network, which, by the further action of activated Factor XIII, is strengthened into an insoluble clot by the introduction of covalent calcium crosslinks between the fibrin molecules. Once a fibrin plug has served its purpose in wound healing it is digested by the fibrinolytic enzyme *plasmin.

fibrinogen The protein precursor from which the insoluble component of blood clots (*fibrin) is formed in the final stage of *coagulation. Fibrinogen is a very large molecule whose plasma concentration exceeds that of any other individual protein. It consists of three dissimilar pairs of polypeptide chains (alpha, beta, and gamma) linked together by disulphide bonds. It is converted into fibrin by the action of *thrombin, with the evolution of two short-chain peptides (fibrino-peptides A and B).

fibrinolysis The process by which the insoluble *fibrin of blood clots is broken down into soluble *fibrin degrada-tion products* (*FDPs*), which involves the fibrinolytic enzyme *plasmin. Although the exact mechanism remains controversial it is generally regarded that physiological and pathological fibrinolysis are identical processes regulated by endogenous inhibitors and dependent upon a number of activators for initiation. These activators are present in all body tissues, including plasma, but not in the liver. High concentrations are found in vascular endothelium, which is the principal source of the plasma activator activity. Activators are also secreted by *granulocytes in the blood and by some types of malignant neoplasm, which produce abnormally large amounts. This gives rise to pathological bleeding states induced by nonspecific lysis of clotting proteins other than fibrin. Examples of this have been described in *prostatic carcinoma and in mast cell *leukaemia in dogs.

fibroblast The basic cell of *connective tissue that is responsible for the production of extracellular *fibres and *ground substance. Typical protein-producing cells, fibroblasts contain much rough *endoplasmic reticulum and a prominent *Golgi apparatus.

fibrocartilage A tough kind of *cartilage in which there are dense bundles of fibres in the matrix. It is found in the intervertebral discs.

fibrocyte An inactive cell present in fully differentiated *connective tissue. It is derived from a *fibroblast.

fibroelastosis Excessive proliferation of elastic fibres in connective tissue. The relatively rare disease *congenital fibroelastosis* occurs in cats, calves, and piglets. The lining of the heart wall and heart valves becomes covered in a thick layer of elastic·fibres. The heart muscle enlarges (hypertrophies) to compensate but *heart failure results. Less severe cases show no clinical signs.

fibroid A tumour of smooth muscle with a high fibrous tissue content. They arise in the wall of the uterus, cervix, vagina, or vulva, and are found in dogs and cats. The growths may be multiple and large, and are often pedunculated so that they protrude from the vulva. Histologically they comprise a mixture of smooth muscle cells, fibroblasts, and collagen fibres. It has been suggested that the lesions are related to hormonal malfunction. Fibroids must be excised completely to avoid recurrence.

fibroma A benign tumour consisting of varying proportions of fibroblasts and collagen fibres. The main sites affected are the skin, uterus, and vagina; in the latter organs the tumour is often combined with muscle tissue to form *fibroleiomyomas*. The dog, cat, and horse are most commonly affected and, as these tumours are generally discrete and encapsulated, surgical excision is curative.

fibropapilloma A form of *papilloma in which the proliferation of fibrous tissue equals or is greater than that of the epithelial tissue. Such lesions are seen especially in young cattle, although other ruminants may also suffer. In **cattle** fibropapillomas affect the epithelium of the penis and vulva, the interdigital skin of the feet, and the teats. They appear as solitary flat or raised masses with a crusty or horny surface; occasionally they are pedunculated, and they are frequently ulcerated and infected, especially on the external genitalia. Regression is normal over a period of months although recurrence often follows attempts at surgical removal. In bulls the tumours may haemorrhage during copulation or erection, and because of

the pain animals may refuse to serve. Larger tumours on the penile sheath may prevent retraction of the penis causing contamination with urine and possible infection. In cows the tumours may interfere with calving. *See also* equine sarcoid.

fibroplastic nephritis (white spotted kidney of calves) A condition found in the kidneys of young calves, characterized by numerous white nodules (up to 8 mm in diameter) in the cortex of the kidney. The cause is unknown, and the condition regresses with age; it is not found in older animals.

fibrosarcoma A malignant tumour arising from *fibroblasts in connective tissue. They occur in all species but are more frequent in the dog and cat. In the dog the skin, subcutaneous tissue, and oral and nasal cavities are the common sites, while in the cat the subcutaneous tissue is mainly affected. The tumours are nonencapsulated and poorly demarcated from the surrounding tissue, are firm or fleshy in consistency, and vary in size and shape. Microscopically they consist of interwoven bundles of fibroblasts with associated collagen fibres. Rapid infiltrative growth is common with a high risk of local recurrence and metastasis in the most poorly differentiated tumours. A retrovirus has been incriminated in the causation of fibrosarcomas in cats.

fibrosis Thickening and scarring of connective tissue. Fibrosis is most often a response to inflammation or injury. *See also* cirrhosis.

fibrositis Inflammation of fibrous connective tissue, especially in relation to joints, as in rheumatic diseases.

fibrous tissue *See* connective tissue.

fibula The more slender of the paired lower long bones of the hindlimb. With the tibia it extends between the stifle (knee) and tarsal joint (ankle). Typically, as in the dog, the fibula forms joints with the *tibia at either end, and at the lower end a lateral projection, the *lateral malleolus*, takes part in the formation of the tarsal joint. In the **horse** the fibula is incompletely ossified and the lateral malleolus is present as a part of the tibia. In **ruminants** the upper end is fused to the tibia forming a short bony spur, while the lateral malleolus is present as a separate bone (see illustration at tibia).

fièvre boutonneuse (Marseilles fever; Kenya tick typhus; Indian tick typhus) *See* spotted fever.

filament A very fine threadlike structure or constituent of a fibril (for example, a myofilament of a myofibril).

filaria (*pl.* **filariae**) Any of various long threadlike nematodes that, as adults, are parasites in the blood or lymphatic systems, connective tissue, body cavities, eye sockets, or nasal cavities. They include members of the genera *Brugia*, *Dirofilaria*, and *Onchocerca*. Their larvae (*microfilariae*) occur in the host's blood or lymph, and the intermediate hosts are normally blood-sucking arthropods.

filariasis Disease caused by infestation with filarial nematodes, for example *dirofilariasis*, *stephanofilariasis*.

filiform Shaped like a thread; for example, the threadlike *filiform papillae* of the *tongue.

filum (*pl.* **fila**) A threadlike structure. The *filum terminale* is the slender tapering terminal section of the spinal cord.

fimbria (*pl.* **fimbriae**) A fringe or fringelike process, such as any of the fingerlike projections that surround the opening of the ovarian end of the *uterine tube. The fimbria of the hippocampus in the brain is formed by the fibres leaving the hippocampus and is continued by the *fornix.

fishmeal A by-product of the fish processing industry based on offal or whole fish and used as an animal feedstuff. It is of variable nutritional value, depending on the original material, but is an excellent source of protein, essential amino acids, energy, minerals, and vitamins. Excessive heating during drying may reduce protein availability for nonruminants (*see* protein quality).

fish oil A by-product of fish processing which, after refining and purification, may be incorporated in animal diets. It is a good source of energy and essential fatty acids but is too high in free fatty acids to be used without prior blending with other fats and oils. Moreover, dietary levels of fish oil above approximately 10 g/kg are associated with fishy taints in the carcass.

fish solubles A by-product of the fish processing industry used as an animal feedstuff. High in protein and vitamins, it is the dried residue remaining after the extraction of *fish oil.

fission A method of asexual reproduction in which the body of a protozoan or bacterium splits into two equal parts (*binary fission*), as in the amoebae, or more than two equal parts (*multiple fission*), for example sporozoite formation in the malarial parasite (*see* Plasmodium). The resulting products of fission eventually grow into complete organisms.

fissure 1. (in anatomy) A groove or cleft; e.g. the longitudinal *fissure* is the groove that separates the two cerebral hemispheres in the brain. **2.** (in pathology) A cleftlike defect in the skin or mucous membrane caused by some disease process; e.g. an *anal fissure* is a break in the skin lining the anal canal.

fistula (*pl.* **fistulae**) An abnormal opening or channel connecting a cavity or lumen of an organ with the skin surface or with another cavity or lumen. Fistulae may be congenital or acquired as a result of, for example, injury, surgery, infection, or neoplasia. A *rectovaginal fistula*, joining the rectum and vagina, may occur during parturition due to penetration of the tissue by the foot of the foetus, especially in mares. Faeces then enter the vagina and ascending infection of the reproductive tract causes infertility. Surgical repair is required and this can be a difficult procedure. *See also* fistulous withers; poll evil.

fistulous withers A condition of the horse involving inflammation of the bursa overlying the 1st to 5th thoracic vertebrae, leading to formation of *fistulae between the bursa and the skin in the region of the withers (the base of the neck, just in front of the position of the saddle). Infection with *Brucella* bacteria is generally assumed to be the cause, from either direct penetration or haematogenous spread. The condition has decreased in prevalence as the problem of bovine *brucellosis has lessened. Isolation of the organism is difficult, especially if secondary infection occurs. Serum antibody levels may be helpful in confirming the diagnosis. Treatment is problematical: antibiotics are not likely to be curative, vaccination may help, and radical surgical interference is often required. This is a major procedure and not always successful. Brucellosis can be trans-

mitted to humans, especially with an open discharging lesion, and owners must be aware of this hazard. *Compare* 'poll evil'.

fit A convulsive seizure (*see* convulsion) in which the animal loses consciousness, falls onto its side, and makes running movements with its legs. Treatment involves correction of any obvious cause or control of the convulsions by a *sedative drug.

fitweed *See* blood root poisoning.

fixation A procedure for the hardening and preservation of tissues or microorganisms. Fixation kills the tissues and ensures that their original shape and structure are retained as closely as possible. It also prepares them for sectioning and staining for microscopy. The specimens can be fixed by *perfusion or immersed in a chemical *fixative or subjected to freeze-drying, which allows the making of frozen sections of tissues, for example for studying tissue enzymes.

fixative (fixing agent) A chemical agent, e.g. alcohol or osmium tetroxide, used for the preservation and hardening of tissues. *See* fixation.

flaccid 1. Flabby and lacking in firmness. **2.** Characterized by a decrease in muscle tone (e.g. flaccid *paralysis).

flagellate A *protozoan that bears one or more *flagella. Members of the four genera *Trypanosoma*, *Trichomonas*, *Giardia*, and *Histomonas* are flagellates.

flagellum (*pl.* **flagella**) A fine long whiplike thread attached to certain types of cell (e.g. spermatozoa and some unicellular organisms). Flagella are responsible for the movement of the organisms to which they are attached.

flatworm *See* Platyhelminthes.

flav- (flavo-) *Prefix denoting* yellow.

flavin adenine dinucleotide *See* FAD.

flavin mononucleotide *See* FMN.

flavivirus A genus of the *togavirus family, formerly called *arbovirus B group.

flavomycin *See* growth promoter.

flavoprotein A protein containing *FAD or *FMN (called *flavins*). Flavoproteins are constituents of several oxidoreductase enzyme systems involved in metabolism.

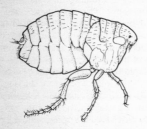

Ctenocephalides felis, the cat flea (female)

flea A small wingless insect belonging to the order Siphonaptera. Fleas are ectoparasites of mammals and birds, living in the coat or (rarely) just beneath the skin and feeding on the blood of their host. Their mouthparts are specialized for biting and sucking; the body is laterally compressed to facilitate movement over the host's body, and the limbs are adapted for clinging and for jumping from host to host (see illustration). The eggs hatch into whitish wormlike larvae, which feed on organic matter, for example in the host's nest or bedding. After two moults the larva spins a cocoon and undergoes metamorphosis into the adult.

Many species infest more than one host. The dog flea, *Ctenocephalides canis*, can also occur on cats and humans. It causes severe irritation and, if infestation is severe, anaemia in young animals. The host's immune system may become sensitized to flea bites resulting in a form of *eczema. Similar conditions are caused in their respective hosts by the cat flea, *C. felis*, and the human flea, *Pulex irritans*, and all three species may transmit the tapeworm, *Dipylidium caninum*, initially ingesting tapeworm eggs in the larval flea stage. The rat fleas, *Nosopsyllus fasciatus* and *Xenopsylla cheopis*, may transmit plague to humans, and the European rabbit flea, *Spilopsyllus cuniculi*, transmits *myxomatosis to rabbits. The chicken flea or 'stick-tight', *Echidnophaga gallinacea*, is common in poultry, especially in tropical regions, and can cause skin ulcers. *Jiggers, or chigoes, are fleas of the tropical genus *Tunga*, found in America and Africa. They can infest humans and all domestic livestock.

In all cases, treatment entails dressing the animal's coat with flea powder or aerosol spray containing a suitable *insecticide. Precautions should be taken to prevent inhalation or contact with the eyes. Pets can also be treated with an insecticidal shampoo or fitted with a *flea collar. To prevent reinfestation, housing and/or bedding should be thoroughly cleaned and treated with insecticide. Ideally, old bedding materials should be burnt.

flea collar An insecticide-impregnated collar that is used on dogs and cats to prevent flea infestations. The material in the collar spreads through the sebum layer in the skin to give some protection against the parasites. Flea collars have a limited lifespan and should be replaced at frequent intervals, according to the manufacturer's instructions. Toxicity can occur, especially in cats. An area of hair loss and skin irritation may develop underneath the collar, requiring its removal.

fleece rot (wool rot) A superficial mild dermatitis of sheep caused by proliferation of bacteria at the skin surface. It follows prolonged wetting and results in a seropurulent exudation that produces a layer of matted fleece adjacent to the skin. Sometimes there is staining of the fleece, usually in shades of green, yellow, or brown, due to the involvement of chromogenic bacteria. The condition is distinguished from *mycotic dermatitis, in which the causal organism invades the epidermis and follicles. The two diseases may coexist in a single animal or flock. Fleece rot reduces the quality of the fleece and predisposes towards fly strike.

flexor Any muscle that causes bending of a limb or other part.

flexure A bend in an organ or part, such as the *sternal*, *pelvic*, and *diaphragmatic flexures* of the large *colon of the horse.

flip-over syndrome See acute death syndrome.

flocculation Aggregation of insoluble material into a *flocculate*, or light fluffy precipitate; for example the flocculation of *glycoprotein, etc., sometimes occurs when urine is left to stand.

flocculonodular lobe In evolutionary terms, the most ancient part of the *cerebellum in the brain, consisting of the paired *flocculus of the hemisphere and the midline nodulus of the vermis. It receives input from the semicircular canals of the internal *ear and the *vestibular nuclei and is concerned with the maintenance of balance.

flocculus (*pl.* **flocculi**) A small ovoid lobule of the hemisphere of the cerebellum. *See* flocculonodular lobe.

floor space The amount of floor area allocated to each individual animal, particularly when housed in a group. Space allocation in practice is a compromise between biological requirements and overall output per house. *Welfare codes for farm animals recommend minimum floor space allocations according to species and size of animal. *See* stocking rate.

Florida horse leech See equine phycomycosis.

flour mite infestation Infestation of flour or other cereal-derived meals with any of various species of flour *mite or forage mite. Heavy infestation affects the value of the feedstuff and can also be of medical and veterinary significance – people and stock in contact with contaminated meal may suffer irritation and dermatitis.

fluanisone (haloanisone) A tranquillizer of the *butyrophenone group. It is used in combination with the analgesic drug *fentanyl to produce neuroleptanalgesia in animals.

fluid replacement therapy The administration of fluids to replace body fluids lost due to disease or other circumstances. The composition of the fluid administered is determined by the nature of the fluid loss, but is either isotonic saline solution or some physiological variant, such as Ringer's lactate (*see* Ringer's solution). The volume of fluid required is determined by the accrued fluid loss: calculation of this must account for any shortfall in fluid intake as well as urinary, faecal, and respiratory losses, the period of time over which the loss has occurred, and the bodyweight of the animal. Acute losses must be replaced rapidly, usually by intravenous administration. Fluids can be given by other routes, such as subcutaneously or intraperitoneally, where the requirement is less pressing.

fluke (trematode) A parasitic flatworm (*see* Platyhelminthes) belonging to the class Trematoda. They have short unsegmented flattened bodies, covered by a protective cuticle, and bear hooks or suckers for attachment to their host. There are two main groups: the Monogenea, which are mostly parasites of the skin and gills of fish, and the Digenea. These parasitize the intestine, biliary system, vascular system, and urogenital tract of vertebrates, and include several important pathogens of domestic animals and humans, such as the liver fluke, *Fasciola hepatica* (*see* fascioliasis), and the schistosomes (*see* schistosomiasis).

Typically, digenetic flukes are hermaphrodite. Their eggs develop and hatch after leaving the host to produce a ciliated larva, the *miracidium. This finds and penetrates an intermediate host, usually a gastropod mollusc, before developing further to form a *sporocyst. In turn this gives rise to a further larval stage, the *redia. The final larval stage, the *cercaria, leaves the mollusc to infect, via various routes, the final host, where it grows into the mature fluke.

flumethazone See corticosteroid.

flunixin See NSAID.

fluoracetate poisoning A toxic condition arising from the ingestion of sodium fluoracetate or fluoracetamide. Both compounds are used as rodenticides, but they are not selective and their accidental ingestion by other species produces toxic effects by

lethal synthesis. Fluoracetate is converted by tissues to fluorcitrate, which blocks the enzyme aconitase by replacing its substrate citrate. This interference with the *citric acid cycle, mainly in the heart and brain, produces cardiac irregularities and convulsions. Theoretically, the administration of acetate should be able to compete with fluoracetate and relieve the citric acid cycle block, but its value is doubtful. Treatment of the clinical signs, including the injection of barbiturates to control convulsions, may be helpful.

fluorescein An orange dye used (as fluorescein sodium) in ophthalmology to detect ulceration of the cornea. When the dye is placed on the cornea, areas of damage show intense green fluorescence and foreign bodies can be identified. It is also used to test for patency of the nasolacrimal ducts. After use it should be washed from the eyes using sterile water to prevent irritation. Fresh sterile fluorescein should be used because some microorganisms (e.g. *Pseudomonas*) can grow in the dye.

fluorescence The emission of light by a molecule following absorption of visible or invisible radiation (e.g. ultraviolet rays or X-rays). *See* fluoroscope.

fluorescent antibody labelling See cell count.

fluorine A halogen element, found in nature mainly in the form of fluoride ion. Fluoride can replace hydroxide in hydroxyapatite, a constituent of teeth, making teeth more resistant to decay. Molecular fluorine (F_2) is a highly toxic gas. Gaseous industrial effluent containing fluorine can contaminate pasture to levels that have toxic effects on livestock (*see* fluorosis).

fluoroscope A piece of equipment on which X-ray images can be viewed directly without taking and developing X-ray photographs. The area of the body being examined appears on a screen, where the image is the reverse of that usually seen on radiographs – i.e. bone appears dark and gas appears white. The movement of body organs and their contents can be seen. However, the fluoroscope is less useful in large animal practice due to the greater tissue densities encountered and high levels of radiation involved.

fluorosis A toxic condition due to the long-term ingestion of fluorine. Fluorosis mainly affects grazing animals whose pasture is contaminated by effluent from the chimneys of factories producing aluminium, bricks, cement, steel, glass, or fertilizers from materials that contain fluorine. Fluorosis can also arise from the ingestion of mineral supplements containing rock phosphate contaminated with fluorine. Ingested fluorine accumulates in bones and teeth. Teeth become pigmented and pitted; bones become weakened and exostoses develop near to joints. Spontaneous bone fractures, especially of the os pedis, cause sudden lameness. When fractured ribs heal, the resultant callus causes their shape to be distorted. Cattle and sheep are mainly affected, horses less so, and pigs and poultry rarely because they are usually kept intensively. The source of fluorine should be detected and its ingestion prevented, possibly by a change of husbandry and by the continual use of an alleviator, such as aluminium sulphate, which reduces the absorption of fluorine and its deposition in bones.

fluprostenol *See* prostaglandin.

flux An abnormally copious flow of fluid from an organ or cavity. It can be applied, for example, to the flow of purulent material from an infected uterus or of watery diarrhoea from a calf with enteritis.

fly An insect (*see* Insecta) belonging to the order Diptera. They are relatively small and possess two pairs of wings, although only the forewings are used for flight; the hindwings have evolved to function as small, club-shaped balancing organs (halteres). Adults may have piercing and sucking mouthparts for feeding on plant fluids, decaying organic matter, or blood. The eggs hatch into grub-like larvae (*maggots); eventually a pupa forms in a barrel-like puparium, in which metamorphosis to the adult takes place. Many flies are pests, disease vectors, or parasites of animals and humans, either as adults or in their larval stages. Even non-biting flies, such as the *autumn house fly and *headfly, are an irritation to grazing livestock, interfering with their resting and feeding and causing loss of condition. Flies with blood-sucking adult stages, for example, the *buffalo gnat, *gadfly, *keds, *midges, *stable flies, and *horn flies, inflict a painful bite causing distress and interrupting feeding. Cattle may be provoked into gadding, with the risk of exhaustion or injury and consequent reduction in milk yield. Sheep may rub their fleece to alleviate the irritation, thus damaging the wool. The fly-inflicted wounds attract other flies and may become secondarily infected; allergies may develop.
Flies are also important vectors of disease. The non-biting house fly (*Musca domestica*) and the bluebottle (*Calliphora* spp.) visit faeces and human food, and the latter lays its eggs on meat, spreading such diseases as bacterial dysenteries and gastroenteritis. The house fly and headfly play an important role in the spread of *mastitis in cattle: the bacteria are picked up in fly excreta and saliva on

an infected udder and carried to uninfected cows. Other bacterial and virus diseases transmitted by flies include *bluetongue in sheep (carried by midges and mosquitoes), *equine encephalomyelitis (mosquitoes), and *anthrax (house flies, gadflies, and stable flies). Parasites too are transmitted by flies. For example, some act as intermediate hosts for parasitic nematode worms, which cause diseases such as filariasis in humans, *dirofilaria in dogs (mosquito), and *onchocerciasis (buffalo gnat or blackfly). Others transmit protozoan blood parasites that cause diseases, including *surra in domestic animals (gadflies and stable flies), sleeping sickness in humans and *nagana in cattle (tsetse flies), malaria (mosquito), and *leishmaniasis (sandfly). The larval stages of certain flies are themselves parasites. For instance, green-bottle fly larvae cause blowfly *strike of sheep and warble fly larvae damage the hides and meat of cattle. Fly control measures are thus of great economic and veterinary importance. Nets give some protection but many flies are small enough to pass through. Insect repellents can be used either on screens in animal houses or sprayed directly onto the animals themselves or used in special repellent ear tags. They have a limited residual effect and must be renewed regularly. Suitable *insecticides can be used for spraying animal houses, or used in dips or sprays for the animals themselves, or applied as dressings to wounds. Effective control may entail the clearance, drainage, and selective spraying with residual insecticides of local fly breeding-grounds. Biological methods of control, such as the introduction of fly parasites or of sterile males, may also be used.

FMN (flavin monucleotide) A derivative of riboflavin (vitamin B_2) that is the immediate precursor of *FAD and functions as a *coenzyme in various oxidation-reduction reactions.

foal heat diarrhoea A mild diarrhoea occurring in foals between 6 and 14 days of age. It is not clinically important: foals remain bright and alert and continue to nurse. The condition occurs at the same time as the mare's first oestrous cycle after the birth but is not caused by changes in the mare's milk. It probably reflects a change in gut function, particularly absorption of water, as the foal matures.

foal husbandry Essential aspects of caring for the foal and its mare. The newborn foal should stand and suckle fairly soon after delivery, normally within 30 minutes to two hours. If this does not happen, take 100–175 g milk from the mare, transfer the milk to a baby's bottle fitted with a lamb's teat, and feed it to the foal. The milk must be at blood temperature. After one or two such feeds the foal should stand up and suckle from the mare. The mare may not stand long enough for a newborn foal to feed; if she is restless hold her head, and if irritable hold a foreleg up as well. Avoid holding the foal's head because this unbalances it. Put a small amount of milk on the foal's muzzle to encourage sucking. Weak foals can be supported when feeding by a sack held under the abdomen. An infrared lamp can be placed in a corner of the stable to provide warmth for a weak foal. A very young foal normally suckles every 5–8 minutes. After a few days this interval is extended to 1½ hours or so, and by 3 weeks suckling is every 3 hours. A newborn foal usually voids the *meconium within about 24 hours of delivery. If this has not occurred, liquid paraffin may be administered orally as a lubricant.

In summer, foals can live outdoors with the mare from an early age. This may be from birth for native ponies, but will vary according to the weather for other types. Watch for signs of chilling in the first month. If possible, stabled mares and foals must be turned out for part of every day. This opportunity for exercise is important for the foal's growth. Foals born either early or late in the year, when the weather is colder, will grow thick coats and can be turned out for a short time on milder days. A covered or sheltered yard is adequate for exercise.

Catch the foal (in the company of its mare) and stroke it frequently in the first few days of life so it forms a good bond with humans. After a few days lead the foal around the box by means of a soft cloth placed around the neck and a hand around its quarters. Similarly, lead the foal behind the mare when they are turned out. Gradually accustom the foal to wearing a headcollar but do not lead on the headcollar until the foal is about a month old.

Feeding The mare should be fed from a tough on the ground to allow the foal to nibble some solid feed from 1–2 weeks of age. Either damp the feed or mix it with soaked sugar-beet shreds to reduce dust. Rolled barley and oats, flaked maize (corn), soaked sugar-beet shreds, soya-bean meal, linseed meal, and dried grass are all suitable for both mare and foal. Feed twice a day unless good grass is plentiful. The quantity of concentrate feed required by the mare depends on the time of the year and hence the quality and quantity of grass available. Most mares and foals can graze outside with no extra feed during late spring and early summer. For highly bred animals, extra feeding is needed from late summer onwards when the feed value of the grass declines. Ponies and hardy types will continue thriving on this poorer grass. From the age of 2 months, the foal is given its own concentrate ration, for example starting with a handful each of rolled oats and crushed linseed cake. For stabled animals, fresh water and clean soft hay should always be available within reach of the foal. *See also* horse husbandry; weaning.

foaling *Parturition in the mare. Foaling occurs after a gestation period of 335–345 days, although wide variations (up to 14 days or more) are common between expected and actual foaling dates. About 1 month before foaling the mare's udder begins to increase in size. If the mare is stabled, the amount of bulky feed in the diet should be progressively reduced to avoid an overloaded abdomen, and succulent food (e.g. carrots, swedes, apples) can be given. Regular exercise should be continued, whatever the weather. 12–24 hours before foaling, 'waxing' occurs: this is the release of a honey-like secretion from the teats, forming blobs or strings. 12–18 hours before foaling there is a noticeable increase in udder size, the teats balloon, the quarters collapse either side of the root of the tail, and the mare may be restless. Imminent foaling is recognized by pawing the ground, frequent lying down and rising, and slight sweating on the shoulders. Foaling takes place very quickly. The mare should be left lying quietly as long as possible, after moving the foal so the mare can lick it.

The mare can foal outdoors in warm weather, being put to graze with a quiet companion in a small easily watched paddock. Keep a headcollar on the mare to facilitate catching her. When she starts to foal, her companion should be quietly removed. Newborn foals can easily roll under fences or into ditches, so the paddock must be secure and free of potential hazards. In warm dry weather hardy types of newborn foal can be left out overnight; otherwise move the mare and foal into a stable. Very young or weak foals can be carried in a blanket, with the mare following. Stronger foals can be coaxed to follow the mare as she is led. The foal should be pushed into the stable ahead of the mare.

In cold or wet weather, or to observe the mare more easily, foaling should take place indoors, either in a special foaling box or the mare's own loosebox. Immunity to the pathogens present in the mare's box will be passed onto her foal. Immunity to pathogens present in foaling boxes may not be acquired by the foal. The foaling box or loosebox should be thoroughly cleaned and disinfected prior to use. Spread fresh sawdust or shavings on the floor and cover this with an even layer of straw, carefully banking it up the walls. Fill dead space (e.g. under wall-mounted mangers) with straw bales and place bales against any projections on which a stumbling foal could injure itself. Keep the stable clean, and spread a thin layer of clean straw after mucking out. Remake the whole bed if the mare has not foaled within a day or two. *See also* foal husbandry.

focal distance (of the eye) The distance between the lens and the point behind the lens at which light from a distant object is focused.

focal osteodystrophy *See* tibial dyschondroplasia.

focus (*pl.* **foci**) **1.** The starting point or principal site of a disease process. **2.** A localized area of disease. For example, focal necrosis in the liver involves the death of several small areas of liver cells scattered throughout the organ. **3.** The point at which rays of light converge after passing through a lens. **4.** To cause light rays to converge at a point (the focus). This is done by the lens in the eye, which focuses light onto the retina (*see* accommodation).

fodder beet poisoning A toxic condition that arises when fodder beet, a useful winter feed, is introduced too rapidly into the diet of cattle. Although the oxalate content and resultant hypocalcaemia is responsible for many cases (*see* oxalate poisoning), it is believed that other constituents of the beet may have toxic effects.

foetal membranes (extraembryonic membranes) The membranous structures that surround and protect the foetus and contribute to the *placenta and *umbilical cord. They consist of the *amnion, *chorion, *allantois, and *yolk sac. See illustration.

foetus (fetus) A mammal in the later stages of prenatal development when its recognizable characteristics have been formed. *Compare* embryo.

fog fever An acute and commonly fatal respiratory disease of cattle caused by ingestion of the amino acid L-tryptophan. This is metabolized in the rumen to 3-methyl indole, which is absorbed. Typically it occurs in the autumn on 'foggage' or aftermath pasture. Some cattle recover spontaneously after a brief period of overbreathing. Others show acute distress with characteristic extrusion of the tongue and drooling of saliva. At post-mortem examination the lungs are consolidated and there is extensive *oedema and *emphysema. A characteristic change is *hyperplasia of the alveolar cells lining the alveoli. Affected animals should be handled and driven carefully to avoid undue stress. There is no cure, but removal of animals from the offending pasture helps. Other names: **bovine atypical interstitial pneumonia**; **acute bovine pulmonary emphysema and oedema**.

folic acid (folacin) A *vitamin of the B-complex that, with *vitamin B_{12}, is required as a cofactor in the

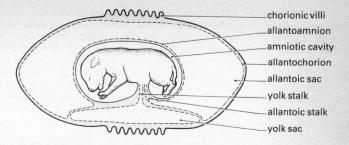

- chorionic villi
- allantoamnion
- amniotic cavity
- allantochorion
- allantoic sac
- yolk stalk
- allantoic stalk
- yolk sac

Foetal membranes of the dog (longitudinal section)

enzymatic transfer of one-carbon groups in the metabolism of proteins and nucleic acids. Rapidly growing tissues (e.g. intestinal mucosae, haemopoietic system, embryos) have the greatest requirements. Dietary requirements are affected by intakes of vitamin B_{12}, iron and methyl group donors (choline, methionine), and fat. Folic acid is synthesized by some plants and by microorganisms in the reticulorumen and large intestines, although the latter require adequate supplies of para-aminobenzoic acid (PABA). Good sources of folic acid are meat meals, yeast, wheat middlings, soya-bean meal, spinach, and legumes; however, its bioavailability is decreased by organic binding. It is moderately stable to air and heat but is degraded by light, alkalis, and acids.

Folic acid deficiency This is rare except in chicks and turkey poults, for which maternal supplies of folic acid are important. Deficiencies may occur in animals given prolonged courses of antimicrobial agents, especially *sulphonamides, which interfere with microbial metabolism of PABA. Deficiency signs are principally poor growth, anaemia, and, in some cases, diarrhoea. Chicks may also show increased mortality, poor feathering, leg and hock disorders, and decreased hatchability of eggs with increased

abnormalities of embryos. Turkey poults may show cervical paralysis. For diagnosis and treatment *see* vitamin. Other names: **vitamin B_9; vitamin M; pteroylmonoglutamic acid**.

folium (*pl.* **folia**) A thin leaflike structure, such as any of the folds of the cortex on the surface of the cerebellum.

follicle A small secretory cavity, sac, or gland. A *hair follicle* is a sheath of epidermal cells and connective tissue that surrounds the root of a *hair. *See also* ovarian follicle.

follicle-stimulating hormone (FSH) A hormone (*see* gonadotrophin) produced by the adenohypophysis of the pituitary gland and responsible for the stimulation of follicular growth in the ovaries and the initiation of *spermatogenesis in the testes.

follicular mange *See* demodectic mange.

folliculitis Inflammation of hair follicles in the skin.

fomentation *See* poultice.

fomes (*pl.* **fomites**) Any object that has been in contact with an animal suffering from an infectious disease and may therefore be contaminated with the infective microorganisms and thus be capable of transmitting the disease to other animals or man. Bedding, feed troughs, and harness are common fomites.

food *See* diet; nutrient.

Food Act (1984) (England and Wales) An Act of Parliament that provides for the making of Orders and Regulations on food hygiene. The Act has seven Parts: (1) general food provisions; (2) milk and dairies; (3) markets; (4) hawkers; (5) cold stores; (6) administration; (7) general matters.

Food and Drug Administration (FDA) (USA) A unit within the Department of Health and Human Services of the federal government. The FDA is divided into six bureaux: biologics, drugs, foods, radiologic health, veterinary medicine, and medical devices. The Bureau of Veterinary Medicine evaluates, for safety and efficacy, preparations and devices proposed for use in veterinary medicine. Animal drugs and animal-feed additives must be approved by the FDA before being used in the USA or exported. Veterinarians in private practice may, however, use any legally obtainable drug in accordance with their best professional judgment.

Food and Drugs Act *See* Food Act (1984).

food conversion ratio The amount of food consumed per unit liveweight gain. Thus a food conversion ration (FCR) of 2.5:1 indicates that 2.5 kg of food produced a 1 kg gain in liveweight. To promote optimum ratios the *diet must be of high *digestibility and supply all the necessary *nutrients for high growth rates. Generally, the highest FCRs are achieved with good-quality diets fed

*ad lib to rapidly growing nonruminants. Ruminants are fed traditionally on poorer quality diets, which are associated with lower FCRs. There is usually a reduction in FCR with age. Furthermore, FCR is heritable and varies between animals of the same species. Consequently it figures in breeding programmes in the selection of improved genotypes.

Food Safety and Inspection Service (USA) *See* United States Department of Agriculture.

foot The lower part of a limb that makes contact with the ground. In quadrupeds the terms 'forefoot' and 'hindfoot' are frequently employed, although in anatomy the term 'foot' or *pes refers exclusively to the hindlimb. In the forelimb the corresponding region is termed the *manus.

foot abscess of sheep A suppurative condition of the foot of lambs and adult sheep caused by *Fusobacterium necrophorum* in association with *Corynebacterium pyogenes* and sometimes *Escherichia coli*. It is most frequent in wet seasons. Lameness occurs due to the development of an abscess, which may be either at the toe or the heel of one foot. Surgical dressing, together with the intravenous administration of a soluble sulphonamide preparation, is effective. *Compare* foot rot.

forage poisoning A toxic condition of horses and cattle caused by the ingestion of contaminated fodder; *botulism can be incriminated in some cases.

foot-and-mouth disease A highly infectious disease of cloven-footed animals, including cattle, sheep, pigs, and goats, characterized by fever and the development of vesicles in the mouth and on the feet and teats, and caused by *aphthoviruses. In young animals lesions also occur in the muscles, particularly of the heart. Coypus, moles, and hedgehogs may also be affected. The disease is enzootic in Africa, South America, the Middle East, and Asia, and occurs sporadically in eastern and southern Europe. Transmission is by the respiratory or oral route. Large amounts of virus are excreted in the milk of infected cattle and in the breath of infected animals, particularly pigs. Typical sources of infection are: in cattle, a virus-containing aerosol produced by exhalation; in pigs, uncooked infected swill (kitchen waste food); and in calves, infected milk. The incubation period is 2–14 days followed, in cattle, by a fever and the appearance of vesicles on the gums, palate, tongue, feet, and teats. These quickly rupture, particularly in the mouth, and large areas of epithelium may be lost from the surface of the tongue. Lactating animals show a dramatic drop in milk yield, and secondary bacterial infection may cause *mastitis. Recovery is prolonged, with consequent loss of condition in both dairy and beef cattle. There may be high mortality in young animals. Pigs, sheep, and goats usually develop only mild clinical signs, although there may be severe losses in young stock. Deer occasionally suffer severe clinical foot-and-mouth disease with death occurring even in adult animals.

There are seven types of foot-and-mouth disease virus, each producing similar clinical disease. However, animals recovering from infection with one type are still fully susceptible to infection with one of the others. Within each type (designated A, O, C, Asia 1, SAT 1, SAT 2, and SAT 3) are a number of subtypes, which are constantly evolving, often enabling them to overcome the immunity of previously infected or vaccinated animals. Consequently, there is a constant need to identify and monitor current strains of the virus to ensure that existing vaccines are still effective. This task is performed by the World Reference Centre for Foot-and-Mouth Disease at the Animal Virus Research Institute, Pirbright, England, which advises on the current worldwide distribution of the seven viral types and on suitable vaccines.

Control of the disease is by slaughter of infected animals and those animals in contact with them. Where this is not practised, animals are given twice-yearly vaccinations with a dead polyvalent vaccine incorporating the subtypes of virus prevalent in the area or those most likely to be introduced. Foot-and-mouth disease is a *notifiable disease in the UK, USA, and Canada (among other countries). Other name: **aphthous fever.**

foot bath A shallow bath or trough through which livestock can walk for routine disinfection of the feet. A bath 2–3 m long and 1.5 m wide is used for cattle, usually dairy cows, to reduce the incidence of foot troubles, e.g. *foul-in-the-foot. The disinfectant is normally a 5% solution of formalin or a 2.5% solution of copper sulphate. For best results the bath should be used twice a week during the winter housing period, the ideal site being at the exit to the milking parlour. For sheep, a foot bath is placed at the exit of a pen or fold and filled with similar disinfectant to prevent *foot rot.

foot mange (itchy leg) A form of *mange affecting the lower limbs of the horse and due to the *mite *Chorioptes equi*. Formerly very common it is now seldom seen, possibly due to better husbandry and a reduction in the number of horses with excessive feathering of the lower limbs. The resulting irritation causes shuffling, stamping, and biting of the feet and may be sufficiently severe to interfere with the animal's rest. Other members of the genus *Chorioptes* cause lesions on the rump and hindquarters of cattle and the ventral body and limbs of sheep.

foot rot An infectious disease of sheep and goats that affects the horny structures and associated soft parts of the foot. It is caused by the bacterium *Bacteroides nodosus*, sometimes accompanied by the spirochaete *Treponema penortha*. Infection is often associated with warm wet conditions and the bacteria commonly enter the foot via a cut or other injury. Signs are lameness in the affected foot with swelling between the clays in the interdigital space; the soles and walls of the hoof tend to separate from the rest of the foot, which contains a foul-smelling greyish discharge. Mobility can be badly impaired and the animal loses condition. Treatment involves paring away the affected horn and cleaning the foot in an antiseptic solution. An antibiotic spray or ointment is applied to the foot and the animal may be given an antibiotic injection. Vaccination of the flock coupled with the use of disinfectant footbaths (e.g. containing 3% formalin or 5% copper sulphate) and removal to clean pasture can effectively control the disease. Sheep brought in to a flock should also be treated in the footbath.

The term is also applied colloquially to a variety of erosive and degenerative foot infections in other species. Various nonspecific erosions can affect the feet in pigs, and *B. nodosus* infection, environmental factors, and the composition of the hoof horn all play a part; nutrition is an important factor. Topical chemotherapy or antibiotic sprays may be useful in treating affected feet, but prevention is paramount – ensuring that flooring is clean, dry, and nonabrasive. Other name: **progressive foot rot**. *See also* foot abscess of sheep; foul-in-the-

foot; ovine interdigital dermatitis; strawberry foot rot.

forage mite A *mite that normally lives in forage but is sometimes an ectoparasite of horses, damaging the skin. Examples: *Tyroglyphus* and *Glyciphagus*.

foramen (*pl.* **foramina**) An opening or hole, particularly in a bone. The *foramen magnum* is a large hole in the occipital bone through which the spinal cord passes. The *foramen ovale* is the opening between the two atria of the foetal heart that allows blood to flow from the right to the left side of the heart by displacing a membranous valve.

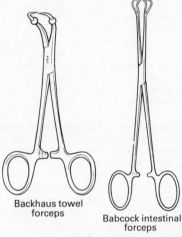

Backhaus towel forceps

Babcock intestinal forceps

Examples of forceps

forceps A surgical instrument with two opposing blades or jaws designed to hold or compress tissue. Many different types are used in veterinary surgery, falling into four major categories (see illustration). *Towel forceps* (or *towel clamps*), such as the Backhaus or Lane types, are used to hold sterile drapes in place around the surgical site. They have a device to keep the jaws closed. *Tissue forceps*, for example the Allis or Babcock types, are used to grasp tissue without causing irreversible damage, and to move unwanted tissue away from the plane of surgery. They also are self-retaining with a ratchet device.

Dissecting forceps, for instance the Ramsey or Waugh types, are used to stabilize tissue during dissection. Their jaws may be toothed (*rat-tooth forceps*) or non-toothed (*smooth* or *dressing forceps*), and the jaws may or may not be serrated. The type used depends on the delicacy of the tissue, and also the preference of the surgeon. *Artery forceps* (*haemostats*), such as the Halsted mosquito or Spencer Wells types, are used to grasp and compress blood vessels to prevent or stop haemorrhage. Large vessels must be ligated (*see* ligature) prior to removal of the forceps, but the crushing action of the forceps is sufficient to stop bleeding from smaller vessels.

forebrain 1. (in embryology) The most rostral (i.e. nearest the snout) part of the embryonic brain, which eventually develops into the *cerebrum and *diencephalon. 2. (in anatomy) A collective term for the parts of the brain that have developed from the embryonic forebrain, i.e. the cerebrum and diencephalon.

foregut The upper part of the embryonic gut. During development of the embryo the most cranial part forms the pharynx, thyroid gland, parathyroid glands, thymus, and the lower respiratory tract. The remaining lower part forms the oesophagus, stomach, part of the duodenum, liver, and pancreas. *Compare* midgut; hindgut.

Forest fly *See* New Forest fly.

forging An abnormality of gait, seen in some horses, in which the toe of the hindfoot strikes the underside of the forefoot when trotting. This is often due to youth or to tiredness. It can be prevented by bevelling the inside of the fore shoe and the toe of the hind shoe. The hind shoe can also be set further back. *Compare* overreaching.

formalin A solution containing about 40% formaldehyde (methanal) in water, with some added methanol to prevent the formation of paraformaldehyde. It is used as a disinfectant and is active against bacteria, fungi, and viruses. With potassium permanganate it produces formaldehyde gas, which is used to fumigate buildings. Premises are disinfected with formalin after disease outbreaks (e.g. foot-and-mouth disease). Formalin is also used as a fixative to preserve organic tissues prior to sectioning for microscopy. Formerly it was used in foot baths for cattle and sheep and as an *antizymotic, but it is carcinogenic and damaging to tissues. Protective clothing should be worn when using formalin.

fornix (*pl.* **fornices**) An arched or vaultlike structure. In the brain the fornix is a large fibre bundle leading from the *hippocampus to the hypothalamus. The *fornix of the vagina* is the ringlike recess at the cranial end of the vagina, around the cervix of the uterus. The conjunctival fornix is the point of reflection of the conjunctiva from the inner surface of the eyelid to the anterior surface of the eyeball.

fossa (*pl.* **fossae**) A depression or hollow. The *acetabular fossa* is the nonarticular depression in the *acetabulum. The *fossa glandis* is the deep depression surrounding the urethral process in the horse. The *ischiorectal* *fossa* is the deep wedge-shaped depression on either side of the terminal parts of the digestive and urogenital tracts.

foul-in-the-foot (fouls) A contagious disease of cattle, known as infectious foot rot in the USA and interdigital phlegmon in the Netherlands, characterized by severe lameness and caused by a bacterium, *Fusobacterium necrophorum*. This organism infects the skin between the claws of the foot resulting in severe foot lameness, which appears suddenly and is accompanied sometimes by a slight fever (39–40°C). Swelling of the leg just above the hoof is also common. The skin between the claws typically has a fissure with foul-smelling dead tissue covering a raw area. The infective organisms can be transmitted via contaminated bedding or muck, and the disease is more common during wet humid weather or when there are wet conditions underfoot. Cattle of all ages can be affected although the disease is more common in adults. Treatment involves cleaning and disinfecting the foot, making sure that there are no thorns or stones trapped in the foot. The wound should receive topical application of bactericidal or antibiotic spray, and penicillin can be injected intramuscularly to combat systemic infection. The response is usually rapid. The use of a footbath containing 2.5% *formalin can help prevent the disease. Other name: **interdigital necrobacillosis.** *See also* foot rot.

fovea (*pl.* **foveae**) (in anatomy) A small depression or pit. The *fovea capitis* is a small circular pit on the middle of the head of the femur to which a ligament attaches. In the vertebrate eye the fovea is a small depression in the back of the retina directly opposite the pupil and lens. It contains densely packed *cones and is the area of greatest acuity of vision in daylight. Two retinal foveae are present in some birds, for sharp forward and lateral vision.

fowl cholera (haemorrhagic septicaemia) A highly infectious and often virulent disease of poultry and other birds, characterized by septicaemia and internal haemorrhages. It is caused by the bacterium *Pasteurella multocida* and is of worldwide importance. Waterfowl are particularly susceptible. Among poultry, older birds are more usually affected, typically turkeys aged over 2 months and domestic fowls over 3 months. The severity of outbreaks varies a great deal and depends largely on the strain of *P. multocida* involved. Three forms of the disease are recognized: peracute, chronic, and a localized wattle infection (*wattle cholera*) or a joint infection. In the *peracute form*, mortality may reach 95%, with birds found dead without warning. In other outbreaks there may be signs over a period lasting from a few hours to a few days; these include darkening of the head (*cyanosis), swollen discoloured wattles, fever, diarrhoea with green foul-smelling faeces, a discharge from the beak, nose, and eyes, lethargy and depression, ruffled feathers, and a refusal to eat. There is severe septicaemia and post-mortem examination reveals multiple tiny internal haemorrhages. The *chronic form* tends to cause much lower mortality but morbidity remains high and significant economic loss still results. Signs include respiratory distress, tracheitis, and conjunctivitis; the infection can also invade the joints and middle ear, leading to lameness and wry-neck (torticollis).

The disease can be spread by wild birds and rodents, and in the UK is a major problem for the turkey industry where birds are kept in pole barns. There is typically no opportunity to treat peracute fowl cholera, but more chronic forms respond to antibiotics, albeit variably. Birds can act as carriers of the infection after recovery, and there is a risk of further flare-ups. Vaccines are available.

fowl coryza (infectious coryza of chickens) A catarrhal condition of the upper respiratory tract of domestic fowls and other poultry caused by the bacterium *Haemophilus paragallinarum (H. gallinarum)*, sometimes developing concurrently with *avian infectious laryngotracheitis or *infectious bronchitis. There is discharge from the beak, and purulent exudate distends the infraorbital sinuses. Treatment and prevention are by antibiotic medication in the drinking water.

fowl paralysis *See* Marek's disease.

fowl pest *See* Newcastle disease.

fowl plague *See* avian influenza.

fowl pox An infectious viral disease of poultry and other birds causing lowered performance and variable mortality. It is caused by the avian poxviruses and is most commonly seen in domestic fowls, turkeys, pigeons, canaries, and game birds. The various strains of the virus that have been isolated are primarily host specific, although there is a degree of cross-infectivity; for example, pigeon-pox virus can be used in vaccines for poultry as well as fowl-pox virus. There are two principal forms of the disease: a diphtheretic form (*avian diphtheria*), which causes whitish caseous (cheesy) membranes in the mouth and trachea; and a more common skin form (*avian contagious epithelioma*), which starts with grey spots on the comb, wattles, eyelids, and beak that enlarge into brownish wartlike lesions and spread over the face. A third form is relatively rare but very severe, with cutaneous pox over the entire body. Both major forms result in economic loss from reduced weight gain and egg output, but the diphtheretic form can cause greater mortality due to obstructed breathing. Older birds aged up to about 12 months are most commonly affected. Infection can occur through skin abrasions, and spread of the disease in a flock is comparatively slow. Biting and blood-sucking insects are important vectors. The incubation period is 3–14 days, and an outbreak may run for up to 3 months in a flock. During an outbreak there is no treatment for infected birds, which should be culled. The rest of the flock can be vaccinated. Routine vaccination is only necessary in areas where fowl pox is enzootic or on infected premises. The virus survives for years outside the body, so rigorous hygiene is essential after an outbreak. Vaccination can take place after 6 weeks of age but is most usual at 3–5 months, just prior to lay.

fowl typhoid A form of *salmonellosis occurring in fowls, mainly growing and adult birds, caused by *Salmonella gallinarum*. The severity and mortality vary, but outbreaks among the more susceptible breeds give rise to acute enteritis and many deaths. Recovered birds remain carriers and infection may pass via the egg to chicks, producing a condition resembling *pullorum disease; eradication methods are similar.

foxglove poisoning A toxic condition caused by ingestion of the foxglove (*Digitalis purpurea*). The plant, characterized by tall flower spikes in summer, is a biennial, and seedlings persisting through the winter provide a convenient source of green food for grazing animals. Clearance of woodlands stimulates dormant seeds leading to a copious growth of seedlings. The plant contains digitonin and other cardiac glycosides, which cause vomiting, diarrhoea, and slowing of the heart rate. The strength of heart contractions is increased in the initial stages causing increased blood pressure and an increase in urinary output. Later, the pulse weakens and anuria develops followed by collapse, coma, and death in 24–48 hours. Ingestion of 100 g of the plant is toxic to a horse and about 15 g causes signs in a pig. Treatment includes the use of emetics and purgatives and *atropine to control the heart rate. Other plants with similar toxic effects include the lily of the valley (*Convallaria majalis*) and the hellebores, such as the stinking hellebore (*Helleborus foetidus*), the green hellebore (*H. viridis*), and the Christmas rose (*H. niger*).

fracture Breakage of a bone, most commonly resulting from trauma. Fractures are classified according to various features (see illustration). A *simple fracture* is one with no associated disruption of the overlying skin, and therefore it is not subject to contamination. (A fracture in which the affected bone is broken into two parts may also be referred to as a 'simple fracture'.) A *compound fracture* (or *open fracture*) is one in which the overlying skin has been broken; the fractured ends of the bone may be exposed, or may have retracted into the soft tissues. In all compound fractures, contamination of the fracture site, to a greater or lesser extent, must be assumed. *Comminuted fractures* are characterized by multiple fracture lines and the presence of multiple bone fragments. A fracture may be *complete*, where the bone is broken right through, or *incomplete*, where it is broken only partway across, as in a *greenstick fracture. *Complicated fractures* are those in which some other structure, such as a nerve or blood vessel, has been damaged. *Impacted fractures* occur when one end of a fractured bone is forced inside the other, not uncommonly

resulting in longitudinal splits in that fragment. *Depressed fractures* occur when an area of bone is pushed below the surface of the surrounding bone; it most often refers to a skull fracture. *Distracted fractures* are those in which the fractured ends are pulled apart, most often by muscular contraction. *Epiphyseal fractures involve the growth plate of a developing long bone.

The most common cause of fractures is trauma due to road traffic accidents. Falls, kicks, and, occasionally, violent muscular activity by the animal itself can also result in fractures. A *dislocation may occur in conjunction with a fracture (i.e. *fracture-dislocation*). Pathological processes, such as neoplastic destruction of bone or malformation of bone due to nutritional deficiency, can result in *pathological fracture*. The major sign in most cases is loss of use of the affected area, commonly with associated distortion. If the fractured ends of the bone rub against each other a grating sound (*crepitus) can be heard. The area of fracture usually has local soft-tissue swelling as a result of haemorrhage, and almost invariably pressure on the site will produce pain. Examination of a fracture site should be conducted as gently as possible, and no attempt should be made to induce crepitus. Radiography of the suspected fracture will assist in determining the type of fracture and form of treatment.

In most instances reduction and realignment of the fracture is necessary, along with some means of immobilization to hold the fractured bone in position to allow it to heal. External fixation by plaster *cast or *splints is not always successful in animals because the shape of the limb tends to cause the cast to slip downward. Internal fixation, employing either *bone pinning or bone plating, has become widely employed, especially in dogs and cats. However, care

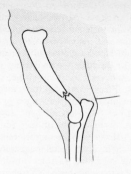

Simple transverse fracture

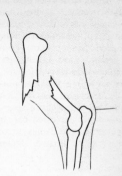

Compound fracture

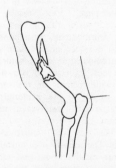

Comminuted fracture

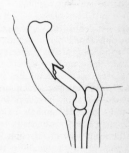

Impacted fracture

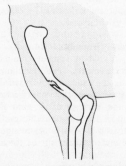

Greenstick fracture

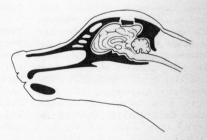

Depressed fracture of skull

Various types of fracture

is required, with strict *asepsis to avoid possible infection of the fracture site, which can cause serious complications. The mechanics of bone realignment and fixation have been extensively studied, and highly specialized techniques developed for specific fracture sites. In a small proportion of cases fractures may be left untreated and will heal well. In severe cases, excision of the fractured part is indicated because of the likelihood of degeneration due to loss of blood supply.

fraenum (frenum) (*pl.* **fraena**) *See* frenulum.

framycetin *See* aminoglycosides.

Francisella A genus of very small nonmotile rod-shaped Gram-negative *bacteria comprising a single species, *F. tularensis*, the causative agent of *tularaemia. It occurs naturally in rabbits and wild rodents, which are the main reservoirs of infection for humans and domestic animals. The bacterium may be transmitted by ticks but the usual way of infection is by the consumption or handling of infected carcasses.

freemartin A female calf (*heifer) that is born infertile due to incomplete development of the reproductive tract. Such calves are usually born twin to a normal bull calf, although the condition can occasionally occur in single heifers when the original twin male foetus dies in early pregnancy. Normally, a common blood supply to the twin foetuses is established early in pregnancy. The male foetus starts to produce hormones before the female, so influencing the female's early sexual differentiation. Later, the female foetus produces its own hormones, so at birth its external reproductive organs appear almost normal. However, internally the ovaries, uterus, and cervix may be abnormal or missing, and the vagina is often only a third of the normal length. About 85% of heifer calves born twin to a bull calf are freemartins; the rest are normal because the common blood supply was not established or the male foetus did not produce sufficient levels of male hormones. Freemartins can be detected by measurement of the length of the vagina, by the larger than normal clitoris, or by a tuft of hair on the vulva. However, the most reliable detection involves rectal palpation or analysis of blood samples to detect the presence of male XY chromosomes.
The condition also occurs in sheep, goats, and pigs.

freezer burn (meat inspection) A condition that occurs in frozen meat, offal (particularly kidneys), and poultry carcasses. It occurs as brown, yellow, or whitish areas on the surfaces and is due to over-prolonged or excessive freezing, resulting in surface desiccation.

fremitus The sensation of turbulence in a part of the body that can be detected by feeling with the fingers (*palpation). Fremitus can be detected on palpating the uterine arteries in early pregnancy in cattle, or in thoracic palpation in cases of cardiac valvular disease.

frenulum (fraenum, frenum) (*pl.* **frenula**) A fold of mucous membrane between structures. The frenulum of the lip is the mucosal fold extending from the centre of the upper or lower lip to the corresponding gum. The frenulum of the tongue is the midline fold between the floor of the mouth and the under surface of the tongue.

freshening *See* calving.

Fresh Meat Export (Hygiene and Inspection) Regulations (1981)

(UK) A statute implementing EEC directives and laying down the requirements that must be met by slaughterhouses approved by the Ministry of Agriculture for the export of fresh red meat to other member states of the EEC.

frog (anatomy) The wedge-shaped mass lying between the *bars in the equine *hoof. It is composed of relatively soft elastic horn.

frog pad *See* bar pad.

frontal 1. Of or relating to the forehead. The frontal bone of the *skull forms the forehead, and the frontal lobe of each cerebral hemisphere in the brain underlies this frontal bone. **2.** Relating to the frontal *plane, which is a horizontal plane through the body in the anatomical (standing) position.

frostbite Tissue destruction, usually in the extremities or exposed parts of the body, resulting from prolonged exposure to severe cold. The body reacts to cold by constricting the blood vessels that supply the skin in order to conserve heat. Although exposed extremities may actually freeze, more often prolonged ischaemia (lack of blood supply) suffices to cause tissue death. *Gangrene may follow and the affected parts eventually slough away. The condition is relatively common in young animals born outdoors and exposed to extreme cold. The skin becomes pale and bloodless and eventually swollen and painful. In severe cases a sharp demarcation line between normal and affected areas appears and the destroyed tissue eventually sloughs off leaving a raw and bleeding surface. Treatment depends on the stage and severity of the lesions. Early frostbite is treated by warming the affected part. In more advanced cases the necrotic areas may have to be

removed surgically followed by the application of *antiseptic to the open wound. Sometimes extensive lesions to the hooves may entail surgical amputation of the foot, or even euthanasia.

frost stud (frost nail; frost peg) A shoeing feature giving improved grip. The nail head is not driven into the horseshoe to be flush but is left proud and partially flattened. Anti-slip frost studs, either tapered or threaded, can be fitted into a prepared socket in the heel of the shoe. Blanks keep the socket clear when a stud is not in use.

fructose A *hexose sugar, occurring in green plants, fruits, and honey, and sweeter-tasting than *sucrose, of which it is a constituent. Fructose is the main sugar in semen and is used as an energy source by the spermatozoa. Phosphate esters of fructose are important intermediates in *glycolysis.

frusemide (furosemide) A potent *diuretic that is used to treat oedema in, for example, congestive heart failure, liver failure, blocking of lymphatic drainage, cerebral oedema, allergic reactions, salt poisoning, postoperative oedema, and mammary oedema. It has a sulphonamide structure and is thought to act in the kidney at the ascending limb of the loop of Henle, inhibiting active chloride reabsorption thus reducing both sodium and water reabsorption and causing intense diuresis. Frusemide can be administered orally or as an intravenous injection for more rapid effect. In the kidneys it is secreted into tubular fluid at the proximal tubules. Diuresis is about 8–10 times greater than with *thiazide diuretics, occurs rapidly after drug administration, and lasts for 3–4 hours. Very rapid removal of oedema fluid can cause large fluid and electrolyte losses leading to shock. Frusemide causes slightly increased potassium loss and hypokalaemia can develop; this may be a problem especially if frusemide is used with *cardiac glycosides because low plasma potassium sensitizes the heart to the effects of these drugs. Hypokalaemia can be corrected by oral administration of potassium chloride. *Bumetanide* is a diuretic similar to frusemide but about 4 times more potent.

FSH *See* follicle-stimulating hormone.

fuel oil poisoning A toxic condition due to the ingestion of kerosene (paraffin oil) or diesel oil (gas oil), both of which consist of mixtures of hydrocarbons. Cattle and goats have been poisoned by drinking from fuel-oil containers. They become weak, perhaps bloated, and die mainly from aspiration of the oil into the lungs. Treatment of the clinical signs is rarely successful. Use of kerosene as a skin dressing for pigs has caused dermatitis and haematuria. Sea birds are often unable to fly when their feathers become matted following immersion in crude oil. They should be cleansed by careful application of oil solvents, such as butter, margarine, soap, or detergent solution.

-fuge *Suffix denoting* an agent that drives away, repels, or eliminates.

fuller The groove in the lower (ground) surface of a horseshoe that accommodates the heads of the nails and assists grip on the ground.

fullering The formation of a groove in the lower (ground) surface of a horseshoe to accommodate the heads of the nails, thus reducing wear on the nail heads and also providing additional grip.

fulminating Describing a clinical sign or disease with a very severe and sudden onset. A typical example is *anthrax of cattle, in which the affected animal undergoes a brief episode of fever and dies within a few hours.

fundus (*pl.* **fundi**) **1.** The base of a hollow organ: the part farthest from the opening; e.g. the fundus of the stomach, reticulum, or uterus. **2.** Part of the interior of the eye that is situated opposite the pupil as seen with the *ophthalmoscope.

fungicide An agent used to inhibit the growth of fungi. Chemical fungicides are used, for example, on stored potatoes, as seed dressings, to protect stored grain, and as timber preservatives. Toxicity to livestock can occur when treated grain is fed inadvertently to animals. Among the compounds used are organomercury compounds, copper compounds, sulphur-containing compounds, thiram, chlorophenols, dodine, zineb, and maneb. *See* antimycotic; organomercury poisoning.

fungoid 1. Resembling a fungus. **2.** A fungus-like growth.

fungus (*pl.* **fungi**) Any of a major group of eukaryotic organisms constituting the taxon Mycota (Fungi). They lack chlorophyll and may consist of single cells (e.g. most yeasts) or a multicellular *mycelium, which consists of filamentous branching *hyphae of microscopic dimensions but sometimes aggregated into a visible mat (*mould) or a large reproductive structure (e.g. toadstool; *sclerotium). Most fungal cells are multinucleate and have rigid cell walls composed chiefly of chitin. Originally (and sometimes still) classified with green plants, fungi are now placed by many authorities in a separate taxonomic kingdom. A few groups of fungi that produce motile water-borne spores are transferred by some to the kingdom Protista, which contains the protozoa and most algae.

Most fungi live as *saprophytes, of which a number are also able to infect animals. Fungi are also a major cause of plant disease, and many plant pathogens can survive only as parasites. Several fungal diseases are of considerable veterinary importance, such as *ringworm, *phycomycosis, *blastomycosis, and *mycotic abortion. Moreover, fungi of different groups produce various toxic substances, some of which are released into the material on which the fungus is growing. These substances include *antibiotics, which are exploited therapeutically, and *mycotoxins, which cause diseases known as *mycotoxicoses. Mycelial fungi characteristically produce large numbers of microscopic, often air-borne, spores by which means they spread and colonize new sites or infect new hosts. This means that many fungi can be recovered in culture from places in which they are not growing but are merely present as contaminant spores. This has important implications in the diagnosis of animal diseases in which fungi may be involved.

funiculus (*pl.* **funiculi**) A cordlike structure. The dorsal, lateral, and ventral funiculi are the three main subdivisions of the white matter in each half of the *spinal cord.

furaltadone *See* nitrofurans.

furazolidone *See* nitrofurans.

furcula (*pl.* **furculae**) The fused right and left *clavicles in birds.

furfuraceous Describing a dry *eczema with scaling of the skin in which the scales resemble bran or dandruff. The term is uncommon in veterinary medicine.

furuncle *See* boil.

furunculosis 1. An inflammatory skin condition involving multiple or recurrent *boils (furuncles). The presence of a carbuncle (i.e. group of boils) causes sloughing of the overlying skin. Local furunculosis may result from trauma, for example from a tick or insect bite, which introduces infecting bacteria (usually *Staphylococcus aureus*); if extensive it may indicate generalized ectoparasitism causing self-excoriation (e.g. demodectic mange), or an animal in which the resistance to infection is lowered as a result of poor nutrition, systemic disease (e.g. hypothyroidism, diabetes mellitus), or immune incompetence. Antibiotics are used to treat the bacterial infection.
2. A specific disease of adult trout and, sometimes, salmon, caused by the bacterium *Aeromonas salmonicida*. Ulcers develop on the skin and fins, and abscesses in the kidneys; a generalized infection then leads to death. Sulphamerazine has been used in controlling the disease.

FUS *See* feline urological syndrome.

fusariotoxicosis Any of several widely differing diseases caused by ingesting feed containing *mycotoxins (*fusariotoxins*) produced by fungi belonging to the genus *Fusarium*. Many different fusariotoxins are known (some species produce more than one) and several are the cause of animal disease.

Oestrogenic syndrome (*oestrogenic mycotoxicosis*) is produced by the mycotoxin zearalenone (sometimes called F-2 toxin) to which pigs are the most sensitive farm animal. The disease has been reported from many European countries, North America, USSR, Australia, and elsewhere. The toxin is a product of *F. graminearum* (= *F. roseum*; the asexual state of *Gibberella zeae*), which is a common and worldwide cause of cob rot in maize (corn) and of scab in cereal grains. Other species, notably *F. culmorum*, can also produce zearalenone. Maize cobs infected in the field develop a red rot spreading from the tip; the toxin is commonest in cobs harvested and stored when wet, though it can occur in grain or compound feed allowed to become damp and moulded by fusaria in storage.

Affected gilts and sows may appear to be in oestrus but not receptive to the boar. Vulval and mammary enlargement often occurs; in severe cases there may be vaginal and rectal prolapse. Young males show swollen mammary glands and atrophy of the testes. Treatment is limited to withdrawal of contaminated or suspect feed; regression of clinical signs should follow within 2–3 weeks.

Feed refusal and emetic syndromes in pigs are usually associated with the same *Fusarium* species affecting maize or other cereals but are caused by different fusariotoxins, of which deoxynivalenol ('vomitoxin') is probably the most important. Feed refusal is reflected in decreased weight gain; ingestion of small quantities of the feed may cause vomiting. The syndromes have been reported mostly from North America and Europe.

Equine leukoencephalomalacia is an often fatal disease of horses, donkeys, and mules caused by an unknown mycotoxin, most often associated with an infection of maize and other cereals by *F. moniliforme*. Sometimes called 'mouldy corn disease', it occurs in North and South America, Egypt, and South Africa. Producing first apathy, somnolence, and often an abnormal gait, the disease may have a sudden onset and run a rapid course over just a few days. Affected animals soon behave as if blind, colliding with any obstruction, and may become frenzied before recumbency and death ensue. The most characteristic lesions are focal areas of necrosis and liquefaction in the white matter of the cerebral hemispheres of the brain.

Fusarium A genus of fungi abundant worldwide in cultivated soil and as saprophytes. Some species are responsible for important plant diseases, a number produce toxins that cause *fusariotoxicoses in animals, and a few cause *opportunistic disease in humans and, very rarely, in other animals. Mycotic keratitis and skin infections account for nearly all reported animal infections, mostly in reptiles.

fusiform Spindle-shaped; tapering at both ends.

Fusobacterium A genus of rod-shaped strictly anaerobic Gram-negative *bacteria. They vary from small *coccobacilli, with tapered or pointed ends, to filamentous forms, and are obligate parasites of the mouth and intestine of humans and animals, causing various necrotic infections. Of the many species only *F. necrophorum* is of veterinary importance. It is a common inhabitant of the gastrointestinal tract, multiplying in damaged tissues following trauma or other infections (*see* necrobacillosis).

G

GABA *See* gamma-aminobutyric acid.

gadfly A large heavily built *fly, also known as the horse fly, deer fly, cleg (in Britain), and march fly (in Australia). Gadflies have powerful wings and are strong fliers. The females are ectoparasites of humans and domestic animals, particularly horses and cattle, feeding on their blood with biting dagger-like mouthparts. The eggs are laid near water and hatch into semi-aquatic caterpillar-like larvae, which develop into pupae in nearby soil or mud. Gadflies, belonging to such genera as *Chrysops*, *Tabanus*, and *Haematopota*, are found worldwide. They are active during daylight, especially on hot sultry days, and can inflict a painful bite, which may cause animals to stampede, or gad. This can cause a reduction in milk yield in cattle. They also transmit a number of serious diseases, such as *surra, *equine infectious anaemia, *anthrax, and *tularaemia. Control is difficult. Breeding sites can be drained, sprayed with oil or paraffin so that the larvae cannot breathe, or sprayed with a suitable *insecticide. Nets can be used to protect animals from the adults.

galact- (galacto-) *Prefix denoting* **1.** milk. Example: *galactosis* (formation of). **2.** galactose.

galactose A *hexose sugar that is a constituent of *lactose (milk sugar) and of *glycoproteins. It is derived from the enzymatic breakdown of dietary lactose by *lactase, absorbed from the gut, and converted to *glucose in the tissues, particularly the liver.

gallamine triethiodide A drug that, like *curare, competes with acetylcholine at nerve-muscle junctions, so preventing the transmission of nerve impulses from nerve to muscle. This produces muscle weakness then flaccid paralysis. The muscles controlling fine movement are affected first, followed by those of the limbs, and ultimately the intercostal muscles and diaphragm. The drug can be used in anaesthesia to prevent movement of the patient, but facilities for artificial ventilation of the animal are needed because of respiratory paralysis. Many of the volatile anaesthetics, especially ether, potentiate the neuromuscular blocking effects. Overdosage can be treated by artificial respiration coupled with the administration of

*neostigmine, preceded by atropine, which antagonizes the blocking action in skeletal muscles.

gall-bladder A pear-shaped sac, lying in contact with the liver, in which *bile is stored and concentrated. Bile enters and leaves the gall-bladder via the cystic duct; in addition some may enter from the liver via small hepatocystic ducts. The gall-bladder is absent in the horse. *See also* bile duct.

gallsickness *See* anaplasmosis.

gallstone A stone or concretion within the biliary tract or gall-bladder. *See* cholelithiasis.

GALT (gut-associated lymphoid tissue) *See* lymph nodule.

game bird A wild bird that is hunted. Examples include pheasants, partridges, and ducks. Game birds can make a significant contribution to the overall profitability of a farming enterprise, especially if their hatching, rearing, and subsequent distribution are carefully managed. The production of young chicks, particularly pheasants, is frequently a sophisticated and high-cost enterprise. If they are to provide good sport, following the hatching and rearing stages contact with humans should be kept to a minimum. Careful management of farm or estate is extremely important if adequate numbers of wild game birds, whether artificially reared or not, are to be maintained. This may include the provision and care of hedgerows, trees, and shrubs as cover, all of which enhance the value of farmland for other wildlife. There is frequently a conflict between arable land management and game bird management and such activities as cultivations, spraying, and straw-burning should be arranged to minimize harm to wildlife.

gamete A mature sex cell: the
*ovum of the female or the *sperma-
tozoon of the male. Gametes are haploid, containing half the normal
number of chromosomes.

gametocyte Any of the cells that are
in the process of developing into
gametes by undergoing *gametogenesis. *See also* oocyte; spermatocyte.

gametogenesis The process by which
spermatozoa and ova are formed. In
both sexes the precursor cells undergo
*meiosis, which halves the number of
chromosomes. However, the timing of
events and the size and number of
gametes produced are very different
in the male and female. *See* oogenesis; spermatogenesis.

gamma-aminobutyric acid (GABA)
A *neurotransmitter, formula NH_2-
$(CH_2)_3COOH$, that is derived from
glutamic acid (*see* amino acid) and
concentrated in the synaptic vesicles
of the *synapses of nerve cells.

gamma globulin Any of a group of
proteins present in serum and separable and identifiable by *electrophoresis: gamma (γ) globulins take up a
characteristic position near the cath-
ode of the electrophoretic field. They
contain most, but not all, of the
*antibody activity of serum.

gangli- (ganglio-) *Prefix denoting* a
ganglion.

ganglion (*pl.* **ganglia**) Any structure
in the *peripheral nervous system
containing a collection of nerve cell
bodies and often also *synapses for
relaying impulses between nerve cells.
A spinal ganglion occurs on the dorsal (sensory) root of each *spinal
nerve and is composed of cell bodies
of sensory neurones but not synapses.
The *sympathetic nervous sytem has
a paired chain of interconnected ganglia situated ventral to the vertebral

column throughout its length. Each
ganglion contains both cell bodies
and synapses and is connected to its
corresponding spinal nerve by a
*ramus communicans. In the cervical
region, however, they are reduced in
number to form three *stellate ganglia*
– the cranial cervical, the middle cervical, and the cervicothoracic. In the
*parasympathetic nervous system, the
synaptic relays are located mainly in
nerve plexuses in or close to the
organ concerned. However, a number
of parasympathetic ganglia occur in
the head, such as the ciliary, pter-
ygopalatine, otic, mandibular, and
sublingual, and in the pelvic region.

ganglion blocker A drug that blocks
the transmission of nerve impulses
through ganglia of the *autonomic
nervous system. Such drugs act by
blocking *nicotinic acetylcholine
receptors, and include the alkaloids
nicotine (which causes initial ganglion
stimulation then blockade), hex-
amethonium, and pentamethonium.
These drugs were formerly used in
man as hypotensive agents, since they
block sympathetic stimulation and
cause a reduction in blood pressure.
They are no longer used therapeutically, having been superseded by
adrenergic blocking drugs. *Halothane
causes ganglion blockade as a side-
effect during anaesthesia.

ganglioneuroma A benign slow-
growing tumour associated with the
sympathetic nervous system and consisting of a mixture of ganglion cells,
Schwann cells, and nerve fibres. Of
embryonic origin, it is rare in domestic animals but has been reported in
the dog – frequently in the brain or
in cranial nerve ganglia – and in cattle, associated with the abdominal
sympathetic nerve plexuses.

ganglioside One of a group of
*glycolipids found in the *plasma
membrane of animal cells and in

*neurones. Each consists of a branched oligosaccharide (comprising up to seven sugar residues) attached to a sphingolipid.

gangrene Death and decay of part of the body due to deficiency or cessation of blood supply. *Dry gangrene* is caused by circulatory loss or blockage, which results in withering and mummification of the dependent part. In *moist gangrene*, death of tissue is followed by its putrefactive decay due to bacterial infection. Gangrene may be caused by injury (e.g. due to extreme heat or cold, trauma, chemicals, pressure), arterial obstruction or closure (e.g. due to senile change, Raynaud's disease, ergot poisoning, arteriosclerosis, neurological disorders), obstruction in the venous return, thrombi, or emboli. *Gas gangrene* is the result of *Clostridium* bacteria (e.g. *Cl. oedematiens*, *Cl. welchii*, *Cl. septicum*, *Cl. chauvoei*) invading the tissues via surgical wounds or injuries; these bacteria are common in the environment.

The initial clinical signs are usually those of inflammation (redness, heat, swelling), followed by black/green discoloration of the tissue, a foul smell, tissue breakdown, and systemic illness. With gas gangrene there is in addition various amounts of gas, crepitus, and emphysema. Treatment is by surgical removal of the necrotic tissues, antibiotic therapy, and supportive treatment for shock. Preventive measures include thorough cleansing of wounds (both surgical and traumatic), the use of antiseptics and antibiotics, and, in some cases, immunization using clostridial vaccines.

gangrenous dermatitis A local bacterial infection of the skin of poultry, causing necrosis and gangrene. Both *Staphylococcus aureus* and *Clostridium* spp. can be involved. Birds of all ages are susceptible but there can be significant mortality in chicks aged 3–7 weeks. The causes are not understood and there are no known preventive measures or treatment. It is sometimes associated with *avian malignant oedema.

gangrenous mastitis One form of very acute *mastitis in milking cows, sheep, and goats due to infection with the bacterium *Staphylococcus aureus*. In the cow, the disease usually occurs shortly after calving: the inflamed udder rapidly becomes swollen, reddish-purple, and later greenish-black and cold, and the secretion from the udder is bloody or purulent. The condition is even more rapid and severe in the ewe, being known as *black garget*. In all species death from toxaemia generally results, although ewes sometimes recover when the gangrenous quarter sloughs off. Systemic treatment with an antibiotic must be commenced early to be effective, bearing in mind that many strains of S. aureus are penicillin-resistant. *See also* summer mastitis.

gapes A parasitic disease of domestic fowls, turkeys, and other birds involving infestation of the trachea and bronchial tubes with gapeworms. Affected birds may gasp, cough, and straighten the head upwards with opened beak in a characteristic 'gaping' action in an effort to assist breathing. It is usually caused by the nematode worm *Syngamus trachea*, although other species may be encountered. The life cycle is maintained through earthworms and other worms, such as brandling worms, which are eaten by birds, hence the condition is largely confined to traditional production systems, such as free-range. It is thus rare in modern commercial units, but it may occur in turkeys kept on straw in pole barns. Treatment is with suitable anthelmintic drugs.

gap junction *See* nexus.

garden nightshade (black nightshade) poisoning *See* solanine poisoning.

garget A term for *mastitis in ruminants, now rarely used except in reference to sheep. *Black garget* is *gangrenous mastitis; *stone garget* is chronic mastitis with induration of one or both quarters.

gas gangrene 1. A fulminating primary *gangrene of muscle and subcutaneous tissue arising from contamination of wounds and other injuries with bacteria of the genus *Clostridium* and sometimes other bacteria of intestinal origin, often several together. It is characterized by rapid necrosis, the development of a haemoglobin-stained oedema containing gas bubbles, local greenish discoloration or blackening of tissue, and profound toxaemia resulting in death. In animals, *Cl. perfringens* type A, *Cl. novyi* type A, *Cl. sordellii*, and other *Clostridium* species occur. In humans, *Cl. perfringens* type A usually predominates. Antibiotic treatment is effective if given sufficiently promptly. **2.** A general name for clostridial infections characterized by acute necrosis of muscle (myositis) or *cellulitis, with accompanying toxaemia (*compare* enterotoxaemia). It includes both miscellaneous infections with *Clostridium septicum*, *Cl. chauvoei*, *Cl. perfringens* type A, or *Cl. sordellii*, and the specific conditions *blackleg, *braxy, and *big head. *See also* malignant oedema; avian malignant oedema.

gas oil poisoning *See* fuel oil poisoning.

Gasterophilus *See* horse bot.

gastr- (gastro-) *Prefix denoting* the stomach.

gastralgia Stomach pain. It usually occurs as a result of indigestion (*dyspepsia), the presence of gas, parasitic infestation, or inflammatory disease (*gastritis).

gastrectasia (gastrectasis) Dilation of the stomach. This occurs if gas is produced in excessive amounts or is unable to escape via the pylorus or cardia. Gastric torsion or twisting can occur in dogs, especially in deep-chested breeds, such as the boxer, Irish wolfhound, and Afghan hound. This can lead to gastrectasia and consequent shock, collapse, and death if the dog is untreated. If the passage of a *stomach tube does not release the gas, surgical correction is indicated. *See also* bloat.

gastrectomy Surgical removal of the stomach. In veterinary surgery, a partial gastrectomy is occasionally performed in small animals and very rarely in foals, particularly when there are irreversible changes in the gastric tissue, most commonly due to neoplasia. The procedure is difficult as access is limited. *Compare* gastrostomy; gastrotomy.

gastric Relating to or affecting the stomach.

gastric glands Glands located in the mucosa of the *stomach wall that secrete some or all of the constituents of *gastric juice. There are three types: the cardiac glands secrete mainly mucus; the gastric glands proper secrete all the elements of gastric juice; and the pyloric glands are similar but do not secrete hydrochloric acid.

gastric juice The exocrine secretion of the *gastric glands in the stomach. In the adult it contains hydrochloric acid, pepsinogens, *intrinsic factor, and mucus; *rennin is an additional component in the calf, lamb, and pig before weaning. *Hydrochloric acid provides the low pH required for optimum activity of the pepsin enzymes. Pepsinogens are inactive precursors of the *pepsins, and are converted to active pepsins when the pH falls below 5, and also by autocatalysis, i.e. pepsin activates further conversion of pepsinogen. Pepsins catalyse the hydrolysis of peptide bonds of food proteins, and, in young animals, cause the coagulation of milk. They are inactivated by the alkaline contents of the small intestine.

Gastric juice is secreted in response to both unconditional and conditional reflexes. In the *cephalic phase* of secretion, the *vagus nerve acts directly on the gastric glands and also causes liberation of the hormone *gastrin, which in turn stimulates acid secretion. In the *gastric phase* of secretion the presence of food in the stomach causes central and local neural reflexes, initiated by distension of the stomach wall. Further hormonal stimulation may occur when *chyme enters the duodenum. *Histamine is a powerful stimulant of gastric acid secretion and may be involved in the response to vagal stimulation and gastrin. As antral (*see* antrum) pH falls below 2.0 gastrin release is inhibited and gastric secretion reduced, until the pH rises again. Hormonal and neural inhibitory influences also arise from the duodenum and small intestine.

gastric ulcer (peptic ulcer; stomach ulcer) A small necrotic focus involving both mucosal and submucosal layers of the stomach wall. Occasionally severe ulceration can result in perforation and rupture of the wall. Gastric ulcers may be present without causing signs of disease, and they are quite often found incidentally at autopsy. Hypersecretion of stomach acid and/or deficient resistance of the stomach mucosa is

thought to predispose to ulceration. Pyloric obstruction or incompetence with gastric reflux, neoplasms, ingestion of toxic chemicals or foodstuffs, drugs, parasites, and stress have all been implicated. Reduced local blood flow (ischaemia) may be an important factor in stress-related ulceration. Clinical signs include pain, melaena (black faeces), vomiting, anorexia, and anaemia.

Pigs are particularly susceptible to gastric ulceration and often die as a result of massive haemorrhage subsequent to ulceration and perforation. There are two types: the first affects the glandular mucosa of young piglets and is caused by a fungal infection (*mucormycosis). The second occurs in all age groups and affects the pars oesophageus, which is covered by highly susceptible squamous epithelium. This second type is usually severe, results in gastric haemorrhage and death, and is thought to be of dietary aetiology.

Various systemic diseases (e.g. *swine fever, *mucosal disease) cause widespread ulceration of epithelium, both in the gastrointestinal tract and at other sites. High-copper rations, whey feed, and finely ground rations have been suspected of causing gastric ulcers in swine. There is a comparatively higher incidence of gastric ulceration in feedlot cattle, which are fed a highly concentrated diet and are relatively stressed. Gastric ulcers are a cause of sudden death in foals.

Treatment is often supportive, maintaining body fluid balance and preventing dehydration by intravenous *fluid replacement therapy. The diet should be bland, soft, and easily digested. *Antacids and histamine blockers may prevent the ulcers from becoming larger. Large perforating ulcers may require *gastrectomy, and euthanasia is indicated in severe cases.

In **dogs**, gastric ulcers occur infrequently as painful chronic lesions that cause persistent vomiting, often with blood present. The lesions have thickened margins of mucosal tissue with deep craterlike centres, and they often perforate leading to haemorrhage and/or peritonitis. The causes are uncertain, but hypersecretion of acid together with raised glucocorticoid (*see* corticosteroid) levels and associated liver disease appear to be important. Treatment, if feasible, should aim at reducing inflammation and infection by demulcent antibiotic therapy. Partial *gastrectomy is usually necessary.

In **cattle**, gastric ulceration is usually seen in the abomasum of young calves as a result of stress. In older animals ulcers and scars from healed ulcers are associated with high levels of grain in the diet, and local fermentation together with abomasal stasis are thought to be important. Perforation with ensuing peritonitis or haemorrhage is common.

gastrin A hormone produced by the duodenum in response to gastric dilatation or the ingestion of peptides and amino acids. Gastrin promotes gastric acid and pepsinogen secretion, motility of the pyloric *antrum, and gastric mucosal growth.

gastritis Inflammation of the lining (mucosa) of the stomach. It commonly occurs together with inflammation of the intestine (*enteritis) as gastroenteritis. *Acute gastritis* is usually defined where there are microscopic acute inflammatory cellular infiltrates in the stomach wall. These are associated with superficial erosion, *gastric ulcers, infarction of gastric veins, clostridial bacteria, fungi, and some acute systemic viral infections, for example canine parvovirus or canine distemper virus. *Chronic gastritis* as described in humans is rarely recognized in domestic species. Uncommonly the stomach is involved in *canine eosinophilic gastroenteritis,

and canine amyloidosis rarely causes a form of histiocytic gastritis. Also in dogs, especially the basenji, chronic hypertrophic gastritis (Menetrier's disease of humans) causes characteristic hypertrophy of the folds of mucous membrane lining the stomach (i.e. rugal hypertrophy). In any species, chronic irritation by reflux of gastric secretion may cause hypertrophy of the antral region of the stomach.

In **ruminants**, inflammation of the lining of the abomasum (fourth stomach), i.e. *abomasitis*, is often associated with systemic viral diseases that affect the gastrointestinal tract. Also, abomasitis is one of the consequences of clostridial disease in sheep.

In all cases, gastritis may cause vomiting, pain, anorexia, and depression, besides the clinical signs of any underlying disease. Treatment is often to relieve the signs, and can involve resting the gastrointestinal tract for 24 hours from solid food while maintaining fluid intake, either orally or intravenously. Pain-killers (*analgesics) may also be administered. *See also* rumenitis.

gastrocnemius A fleshy muscle, divided into lateral and medial heads, located in the back of the leg. Its origin is from the distal end of the femur and it inserts to the *calcaneus via the common calcaneal tendon (Achilles tendon). On contraction it flexes the stifle joint and extends the hock joint.

Gastrodiscus A genus of *flukes widespread in the tropics and subtropics. *G. aegyptiacus* is a common parasite in the large intestine of horses and other equids, and also of pigs. It is large and pear- or disc-shaped with a ventral sucker at the rear of its body. The eggs are larger than those of other flukes and the intermediate host is a water snail. The presence of large numbers in the intestine of young stock may cause inflammation leading to loss of condition, poor growth, and persistent diarrhoea, which may be fatal.

gastroenteritis Inflammation of both the stomach and intestines (*see* gastritis; enteritis). *See also* haemorrhagic gastroenteritis; parasitic gastroenteritis; transmissible gastroenteritis.

gastrolith A stomach stone (*calculus). It usually consists of a central core, which may be a small irritant foreign body, and an outer shell, often of tightly packed vegetable matter. Gastroliths are more common in herbivores and omnivores than in carnivores.

gastrorrhoea An excessive secretion of gastric juice (*gastrosuccorrhoea*) or of mucus (*gastromyxorrhoea*) by the glandular lining of the stomach.

gastroscope An *endoscope designed for visualization of the interior of the stomach. It is passed down the oesophagus to allow inspection of the stomach lining and facilitate the taking of biopsies. Gastroscopy is useful for the diagnosis of ulceration, neoplasia, and stricture formation. The technique is feasible in all species but the length of scope required in adult large animals may exceed that of standard medical endoscopes.

gastrostomy The surgical creation of a permanent opening into the stomach. This may be done to connect the stomach to the surface of the body (performed to study gut functions) or to another section of the alimentary tract to bypass diseased gut; for example in a *gastrojejunostomy* the opening in the stomach is brought through the wall of the jejunum so bypassing the pylorus and duodenum. In this latter case, care must be taken to allow bile from the liver and pancreatic secretions to reach the jejunum. *Compare* gastrectomy; gastrotomy; rumenotomy.

gastrotomy Surgical incision into the lumen of the stomach. The most common indication in small animals is for the removal of ingested foreign material or to inspect or facilitate biopsy of the lining of the stomach. *See also* rumenotomy. *Compare* gastrectomy; gastrostomy.

gastrula (*pl.* **gastrulas** or **gastrulae**) The stage of vertebrate embryonic development succeeding the *blastocyst, during which the embryo develops into a bilaminar then a trilaminar germ disc and the primitive gut (*archenteron) is formed.

gel A colloidal suspension that has coagulated to a rigid or jelly-like solid. Agarose or polyacrylamide gels are frequently used as media for *electrophoresis and for immunological techniques.

gelatin A jelly-like substance formed when tendons, ligaments, etc. containing *collagen (a protein) are boiled in water.

gelatin sponge A haemostatic *dressing used in operation sites to control oozing blood. It is prepared as foamed *gelatin and supplied presterilized in glass or paper packs. The sponge remains in situ but is subsequently completely absorbed and produces little tissue reaction. Its use is particularly indicated where many small vessels are bleeding and cannot be controlled by other means.

gel filtration *See* chromatography.

gemmule One of the minute spines or surface extensions of a *dendrite, through which contact is made with another neurone at a *synapse.

gene

gene A portion of *DNA, corresponding to a particular sequence of the *genetic code, that carries the information to govern the change at some point in a biochemical pathway. *Structural genes* direct the synthesis of specific polypeptide chains that make up proteins. These genes may be associated with a controlling *operator gene*, forming an *operon* unit, which in turn is regulated by a *regulator gene*. Most genes are carried on the *chromosomes; higher animals possess two sets of chromosomes, and hence two sets of genes (except for some on the sex chromosomes). Genes can be represented by different forms called *alleles; different alleles of the same gene affect the same point in a biochemical pathway but in different ways.

-genesis *Suffix denoting* origin or development. Example: *spermatogenesis* (development of spermatozoa).

genetic code The means by which genetic information in *DNA controls the manufacture of specific *polypeptides by the cell. The code takes the form of a series of triplets (*codons*) of bases in DNA, from which is transcribed a complementary sequence of codons in messenger *RNA (*see* transcription). The sequence of these codons determines the sequence of *amino acids during *protein synthesis. There are 64 possible triplet combinations of the four bases present in DNA and RNA and only 20 amino acids present in body proteins: some amino acids are coded by more than one codon, and some codons have other functions.

genetic drift The phenomenon, most important in populations of limited size, in which there are random changes in the frequency of particular *alleles due to the sampling nature of their inheritance. Thus, over successive generations, alleles can 'drift'

toward higher or lower frequencies, particularly alleles that are not being actively selected. Animals carry a random selection of these nonselected alleles, and if, for instance in a breeding programme, only a few animals are chosen to breed then a high proportion may, by chance, carry copies of nondesired recessive alleles. Since each allele has a 50% chance of being transmitted to any offspring these alleles can become common in the next generation. In subsequent generations they may commonly appear in the *homozygous state, thus allowing their undesired effect to be expressed. Therefore, genetic drift can be accelerated by selective breeding programmes, and is an especial problem in breeds where a single male is used to mate many females. *See also* inbreeding.

genetic engineering The techniques of altering the genetic make-up of a cell or individual by inserting into its DNA genes from other sources (e.g. from another organism or species). The resultant altered DNA, known as *recombinant DNA*, is usually produced with the aid of a *plasmid. Once inserted, the foreign gene may, for example, use the cell's machinery to synthesize a particular desired protein. These techniques are now widely used to obtain drugs from microorganisms, allowing the construction of super-productive strains containing multiple copies of genes whose products are desired. Similar techniques have been used in some mammals, notably sheep, to produce animals that secrete large quantities of useful drugs in milk. *See also* restriction endonuclease.

genetics The study of inheritance in all its aspects. *See also* cytogenetics.

-genic *Suffix denoting* 1. producing. 2. produced by.

geniculate body Either of two projections that constitute the *metathalamus*, part of each *thalamus in the brain. The *lateral geniculate body* is associated with visual pathways and the *medial geniculate body* with auditory pathways.

genital Relating to the reproductive organs or to reproduction.

genitalia The reproductive organs of either the male or the female. The term external genitalia is usually used in reference to the external parts of the reproductive system.

genito- *Prefix denoting* the reproductive organs. Example: *genitourinary* (relating to the reproductive and excretory systems).

genome The total of all the *genes carried by an organism, breed, or species.

genotype 1. The genetic constitution of an individual or group as determined by the particular set of genes it possesses. **2.** The genetic information carried by a pair of alleles that determines a particular characteristic. *Compare* phenotype.

gentamicin *See* aminoglycoside.

gentian violet A purple dye with some antibacterial and antifungal activity that is used topically either as a marker or for the treatment of some skin conditions, such as wounds and foot rot. It retains its activity in the presence of organic debris.

geo- *Prefix denoting* the earth or soil.

ger- (gero-, geront(o)-) *Prefix denoting* old age.

germ cell (gonocyte) Any of the embryonic cells that have the potential to develop into spermatozoa or ova. The term is also applied to any of the cells undergoing gametogenesis and to the gametes themselves.

germinal 1. Relating to the early developmental stages of an embryo or tissue. **2.** Relating to a germ.

germinal epithelium The epithelial covering of the ovary, which was formerly thought to be the site of origin of *oogonia. These are now known to originate from the yolk sac endoderm in the young embryo.

germ layer Any of the three distinct layers of tissue present in the very early stages of embryonic development (*see* ectoderm; mesoderm; endoderm). These layers subsequently differentiate to form the tissues of the body.

gestation The period from *fertilization up to the time of birth (*parturition), during which, in mammals, development occurs within the uterus (*see* pregnancy). The length of gestation varies with species (see table).

Getah virus An *alphavirus.

giant cell Any large cell. They may contain one or more nuclei, and occur in various situations, for example in chronic inflammation.

Giardia A genus of *flagellate protozoa distributed worldwide and infecting the upper small intestine of mammals, occasionally causing the disease *giardiasis. A number of species of *Giardia* have been named from different hosts, such as humans, dogs, and cattle, but it is unresolved whether these are distinct species and to what extent cross-infection occurs between hosts of different species. The organism is shaped like a pear cut longitudinally in half, about 10–20 μm long, and carries eight flagella. They lie in the intestinal lumen with their flat face apposed to the gut lining. They also form oval cysts, which are excreted in the faeces.

giardiasis A disease of mammals (including humans) caused by protozoa of the genus *Giardia* and characterized by diarrhoea. Of worldwide distribution, this is one of the commonest parasitic infections of humans in temperate regions. In animals the disease is uncommon but probably occurs most often in dogs. It is uncertain to what extent infections are transmitted from animals to humans or vice versa. Human infections are often related to poor hygiene in food preparation or infected water supplies. Diagnosis is confirmed by the detection of the organisms in faeces. The disease can be treated with specific drugs.

gid *See* coenurosis.

gilt A young female pig between weaning age and the time of its first litter. The term is also applied to female pigs kept for meat production.

gingiv- (gingivo-) *Prefix denoting* the gums.

gingiva (*pl.* **gingivae**) The gum: the dense fibrous tissue covered with smooth mucous membrane overlying the alveolar processes and margins of the jaw bones.

gingivitis Inflammation of the gums. This may be acute or chronic, and caused by local irritation and infection or systemic disease. Dental plaque, infection from elsewhere in the mouth, trauma, foreign bodies, caries, and broken teeth may all cause gingivitis. Systemic diseases that predispose to gingivitis or in which gingivitis is a sign include diabetes, vitamin B deficiency, uraemia, leptospirosis, and, in cats, *feline leukaemia and certain respiratory virus infec-

tions. Clinical signs may include salivation, reddening and swelling of the gums, pain and difficulty in chewing, dropping food, anorexia, and halitosis (bad breath). In severe cases there may be a purulent discharge from the gum margin. Treatment involves removing the cause of local irritation where applicable (e.g. removal of plaque or extraction or repair of carious teeth). Systemic diseases must be treated accordingly. Supportive therapy may often be required to overcome the pain associated with eating. *See also* periodontal disease.

gizzard *See* ventriculus.

gland An organ or group of cells that is specialized for synthesizing and secreting certain fluids, either for use in the body or for excretion. There are two main groups of glands: the *exocrine glands, which discharge their secretions by means of ducts, and the *endocrine glands, which secrete their products – hormones – directly into the bloodstream. *See also* secretion.

glanders A contagious disease of horses, donkeys, and mules that can be transmitted to humans. It is characterized by ulceration of the respiratory mucosa or skin and is caused by the Gram-negative bacterium *Pseudomonas mallei*. Glanders is enzootic in the Middle and Far East. Infection is by ingestion of contaminated food or water or by inhalation. Horses are the most susceptible, and following an incubation period of up to several months they develop a fever, nasal discharge (sometimes bloodstained), and a cough, with enlarged and painful submaxillary lymph glands. Nodules develop on the nasal mucosa, which rupture to leave ulcers; the nasal discharge becomes mucopurulent. Nodules may also develop in the lungs and lymph nodes and in the superficial lymph vessels of the hindlimbs – *cutaneous glanders* or 'farcy'. The nodules on the hindlimbs rupture to form ulcers and discharge thick pus.

Horses may be affected without showing clinical signs, or develop only mild disease from which they recover, or develop chronic glanders. Mules and donkeys usually develop the acute form of the disease and death can occur in 2–3 weeks. Carnivores may be infected by eating 'glandered' meat. Treatment of livestock is not recommended, even in countries where the disease is enzootic. The preferred policy is slaughter and eradication where feasible. Although humans are quite resistant to the disease, the acute form may lead to death in 2–20 days unless treated. In the more common chronic form, patients survive without treatment. Administration of sulphonamides or streptomycin is usually effective. Both glanders and farcy are *notifiable diseases in the UK.

gland of the third eyelid The glandular tissue surrounding the cartilage of the third *eyelid. The *superficial* (*nictitans*) *gland* occurs in all domestic species and produces a secretion similar to that of the *lacrimal gland. The *deep* (*Harderian*) *gland* occurs only in the pig and produces a fatty secretion.

glans penis The terminal expanded portion of the *corpus spongiosum surrounding the corpus cavernosum in the penis. Its form varies among species, being mostly vascular in carnivores and in the stallion, mostly fibrous in ruminants, and practically absent in the boar.

Glasser's disease An infectious polyserositis and arthritis of pigs, caused by the bacterium *Haemophilus parasuis*. *Mycoplasma hyorhinis* and *Escherichia coli* may produce a clinically similar syndrome. *See* polyserositis.

glaucoma A disease of the eye in which there is abnormally high pressure inside the eyeball, usually due to increased production and/or restricted drainage of *aqueous humour. This fluid is produced by the ciliary body and drained by a specialized venous system in the filtration angle of the eye (between the ciliary apparatus and the sclera in the anterior chamber of the eye). Increased pressure makes the eyeball bulge and protrude from the lids. Other signs include conjunctival congestion, scleral congestion, corneal oedema, and dilated fixed pupil. Ophthalmic examination often reveals a dislocated lens, cupped optic disc, retinal atrophy, or some combination of these signs. Most cases are secondary to some inflammation and obstruction of the filtration angle.

Certain dog breeds have a predisposition to glaucoma. These include wirehaired terriers, basset hounds, beagles, cocker spaniels, poodles, and Norwegian elkhounds. Treatment aims to decrease aqueous humour production, increase outflow, and decrease intraocular volume and pressure. *Mydriatic and *miotic drugs are given in turn to treat blockage of the filtration angle by debris. Surgery is required if the lens is dislocated and lying in the anterior chamber. Late detection of the condition often makes it impossible to treat, and in these cases complete surgical removal of the eye is indicated.

glenohumeral Relating to the glenoid cavity and the humerus: the region of the shoulder joint. The glenohumeral ligaments are thickened parts of the shoulder joint capsule.

glenoid cavity The socket of the shoulder joint: the oval shallow depression of the *scapula into which the head of the humerus fits.

gli- (glio-) *Prefix denoting* **1.** neuroglia. **2.** a glutinous substance.

glia *See* neuroglia.

gliadin One of the two main components of gluten, the mixture of proteins present in the endosperm of wheat. Its presence in the diet can cause coeliac disease in susceptible individuals. *See also* glutelin.

glioma Any tumour of non-nervous cells (*neuroglia) in the nervous system. They may be composed of mature cells resembling astrocytes (*astrocytomas), oligodendrocytes (*oligodendrogliomas), or ependymal cells (*ependymomas), or anaplastic variants of such cells. The more primitive or undifferentiated the cells are, the more rapid is their growth. Gliomas do not metastasize but may be disseminated by the cerebrospinal fluid to other parts of the nervous system.

globin One of a group of proteins, found in the body, that can combine with iron-containing porphyrin to form the *haemoglobins (found in red blood cells) or *myoglobin (found in muscle).

globulin Any of a wide variety of proteins that can be precipitated from serum by ammonium sulphate. The globulins can be partially separated by *electrophoresis into alpha (α), beta (β), and gamma (γ) fractions: alpha globulins take up a position nearest to, and gamma globulins furthest from, the anode in the electrophoretic field. Alpha and beta globulins contain many of the lipoproteins, glycoproteins (e.g. *haptoglobin), and metal-transporting proteins (e.g. *transferrin and caeruloplasmin). *Antibody activity is found predominantly in the gamma fraction, and *complement in the beta fraction.

globulinuria The presence of globulins in the urine. This is usually an indication of abnormal kidney function.

globus A spherical or globe-shaped structure; for example the *globus pallidus*, part of the *lentiform nucleus in the brain (*see* basal ganglia).

glomerulitis Inflammation associated with the glomeruli of the kidney (*see* glomerulus). *See* glomerulonephritis.

glomerulonephritis A condition of the kidney, usually due to the deposition of immune complexes in the basement membrane of the glomeruli (*see* glomerulus). It is common in dogs and cats but rarely diagnosed in farm animals. Fixation of complement by these complexes damages the basement membrane, leading to increased permeability of the glomerular capillary. The clinical signs are of acute renal failure, such as uraemia, oliguria (reduced volume of urine), and proteinuria. The condition may resolve or progress into chronic renal failure, with subcutaneous oedema, ascites, hypoalbuminaemia, albuminuria, and anaemia. Treatment is usually supportive, maintaining body fluids by intravenous *fluid replacement therapy and performing *dialysis, via either the peritoneum or intravenously.

glomerulus (*pl.* **glomeruli**) **1.** The network of blood capillaries contained within the cuplike end (glomerular capsule or Bowman's capsule) of a *nephron in the kidney. It is the site of primary filtration of waste products from the blood into the nephron. The glomerulus and glomerular capsule together constitute a *renal corpuscle*. **2.** Any other small rounded mass.

glomus (*pl.* **glomera**) An encapsulated group of *arteriovenous anastomoses. The arterial vessels have a thick wall with numerous epithelioid muscle cells, which are richly innervated.

gloss- (glosso-) *Prefix denoting* the tongue. Example:

glossectomy Surgical removal of the tongue. Partial glossectomy is occasionally required in animals, usually following a severe traumatic injury. *glossopharyngeal* (relating to the tongue and pharynx).

Glossina *See* tsetse fly.

glossitis Inflammation of the tongue.

glossopharyngeal nerve The ninth *cranial nerve (IX), which supplies the stylopharyngeus muscle of the pharynx, parasympathetic fibres to the parotid gland, and sensory fibres to the posterior third of the tongue and the pharynx.

glossopharyngeal paralysis Dysfunction of the *glossopharyngeal nerve. It results in difficulty in swallowing due to loss of local sensation and muscular activity, and also loss of taste from the caudal part of the tongue.

glottis (*pl.* **glottises** or **glottides**) The part of the *larynx formed by the vocal processes of the arytenoid cartilages and the vocal folds. These structures surround a narrow opening, the *rima glottidis*, which can be closed during swallowing or to increase the pressure in the airway caudally, for example in coughing.

gluc- (gluco-) *Prefix denoting* glucose. Example: *glucosuria* (urinary excretion of).

glucagon A protein hormone produced by the alpha cells of the pancreas in response to *hypoglycaemia, and by cells of the upper intestine (*enteroglucagon*) in response to the ingestion of glucose or fat. Glucagon stimulates the breakdown of stored glycogen in the liver, thus causing an increase in blood sugar levels, and also directly stimulates the release of *insulin.

glucocorticoid *See* corticosteroid.

gluconeogenesis The metabolic process by which *glucose can be manufactured in body tisues from certain other metabolites, including some non-carbohydrate sources. Most gluconeogenesis occurs in the liver, where it is important in helping to maintain the supply of glucose to the blood by converting other metabolites, such as lactate produced by skeletal muscles, to glucose. When carbohydrates are in short supply, for example during starvation, certain amino acids can also give rise to glucose via gluconeogenesis. The process is very important in ruminants, where propionic acid is one of the principal energy sources (*see* volatile fatty acid) absorbed from the rumen. However, it can only be fully utilized after first undergoing conversion to glucose in the liver via gluconeogenesis.

glucosamine An amino sugar derived from *glucose. It is an important constituent of *glycoproteins and some *polysaccharides.

glucose (dextrose) A *hexose sugar, which, with its phosphate esters (glucose-1-phosphate and glucose-6-phosphate), plays a central role in the metabolism of all living organisms, particularly as a source of energy. The concentration of glucose in the blood is under close hormonal control (*see* glucagon; insulin) and the brain is very sensitive to changes in its level. Excess glucose is stored as *glycogen, principally in the liver and

glucoside

skeletal muscle. Liver glycogen acts as a hormonally regulated reservoir of blood glucose, being mobilized by *phosphorylase to replace depleted glucose or being synthesized when blood glucose is in excess. Defects in this mechanism lead to *diabetes mellitus. Abnormally low blood glucose (*hypoglycaemia) or excessively high blood glucose (*hyperglycaemia) can both cause pathological effects.

glucoside *See* glycoside.

glucuronic acid A derivative of glucose which, in the liver, can be added (from UDP-glucuronic acid) to other molecules to detoxify them and make them more water soluble, for example bilirubin diglucuronide (*see* bile pigments).

glutamate oxaloacetate transaminase *See* AST.

glutamate pyruvate transaminase *See* ALT.

glutamic acid (glutamate) *See* amino acid.

glutaminase The enzyme that deaminates the *amino acid glutamine by catalysing the reaction: glutamine + water = glutamate + ammonia. It is important in the transport of amino groups around the body.

glutamine *See* amino acid.

glutathione A tripeptide (*see* peptide) (gamma glutamyl-cysteinyl-glycine or GSH) that occurs in all animal cells. The sulphydryl (-SH) group of the cysteinyl residue is important in maintaining the correct reducing condition within the cell by oxidizing disulphide bonds, for example:
R-S-S-R + 2GSH = 2RSH + G-S-S-G (oxidized glutathione). More than 90% of cellular glutathione is in the reduced form. It is particularly important in the protection of red blood cells against the harmful action of peroxides, as the selenium-containing enzyme glutathione peroxidase.

glutelin (glutenin) One of the two major proteins of wheat gluten (*see also* gliadin). Maize glutelin is one of the two main proteins of the maize (corn) kernel, along with *zein.

gluteus (*pl.* **glutei**) One of three paired muscles in the hip region – the superficial, middle, and deep gluteal muscles. They extend and abduct the *hip joint.

glyc- (glyco-) *Prefix denoting* sugar.

glyceride (acylglycerol) A fatty-acid ester of glycerol. Esterification can occur at one, two, or all three hydroxyl groups of the glycerol molecule producing mono-, di-, and triglycerides respectively. *Triglycerides are the major constituents of fats and oils found in living organisms. Alternatively, one of the hydroxyl groups may be esterified with a phosphate group forming a phosphoglyceride (*see* phospholipid) or to a sugar forming a *glycolipid.

glycerine *See* glycerol.

glycerol (glycerine; propane-1,2,3,-triol) A trihydric alcohol that is a colourless sweet-tasting viscous liquid. It is a constituent of the *triglycerides and *phospholipids found in living organisms. Glycerol is used in the treatment of hypoglycaemia, encountered in *ketosis in cattle and *pregnancy toxaemia in ewes. It is given orally and provides a source of readily available energy. Repeated dosing is usually necessary because of its short duration of action. It is also used as a carrier and solvent for drugs.

glycerophosphate An intermediate in triglyceride synthesis in the body. It is also administered orally to stimulate fat metabolism, most commonly as calcium glycerophosphate, which can be incorporated in tonics and feed supplements.

glyceryl guaiacolate (guaiphenesin) A centrally acting muscle relaxant used in horses. It probably acts at interneurones in the spinal cord and brain stem, causing skeletal muscle relaxation and flaccid paralysis. The cardiovascular and respiratory systems are not greatly affected unless there is overdosage. Analgesia is poor and surgical operations should not be carried out with this drug alone. Glyceryl guaiacolate is infused intravenously as a 5% solution in dextrose. More concentrated solutions are irritant and high concentrations cause haemolysis. After administration it is conjugated to glucuronide by the liver and excreted in the urine. Recovery takes 20–60 minutes. Overdosage is indicated by rigidity of extensor muscles, and this can be followed by muscle relaxation and cardiac arrest unless infusion is halted. The drug has also been used successfully to induce muscle relaxation in cases of *strychnine poisoning in dogs. In the horse it has been used as a casting agent, but it is preferable to use lower doses and induce anaesthesia with a reduced dose of a thiobarbiturate.

glycine *See* amino acid.

glycocholic acid *See* bile acids.

glycogen A polysaccharide consisting of a branched polymer of glucose found principally in liver and skeletal muscle and to a lesser extent in the kidney. It acts as a readily available store of glucose, and its synthesis (*glycogenesis) and degradation (*glycogenolysis) are controlled by the opposing actions of the hormones *insulin, which promotes glycogenesis, and *adrenaline and *glucagon, which promote glycogenolysis. The glucose derived from muscle glycogen has to be used within the muscle, but that from liver glycogen can be released from the liver by the action of the enzyme glucose-6-phosphatase in order to maintain the level of blood glucose.

glycogenesis The process by which *glycogen is synthesized in the animal body from an activated form of glucose (UDP-glucose). *See also* glycogenolysis.

glycogenolysis The process by which *glycogen is broken down in the animal body by the enzyme glycogen *phosphorylase to yield glucose-1-phosphate. *See also* glycogenesis.

glycolipid A *lipid with one or more sugar residues attached. They are commonly found among cell-membrane lipids, with the sugar orientated on the outside of the cell.

glycolysis (Embden-Meyerhof pathway) The series of biochemical reactions by which a molecule of *glucose is converted into two molecules of pyruvate (or lactate) with the production of usable energy in the form of two molecules of *ATP. It is central to the generation of energy in the cell and can operate under either anaerobic conditions (e.g. leading to the excretion of lactate by strenuously exercising muscle) or aerobically in conjunction with the *Krebs cycle to produce CO_2 along with 38 molecules of ATP.

glycoprotein A protein with a number of sugar residues attached. Many membrane proteins and most plasma proteins (except albumin) are glycoproteins. The proportion of carbohydrate in the molecule ranges from a few percent to well over half in different glycoproteins.

glycoside A compound formed by replacing the hydroxyl (-OH) group of a sugar by another group. If the sugar is glucose, the derivative is termed a *glucoside*; similarly, *galactosides* are derivatives of galactose, and *fructosides* of fructose. Some glycosides have important pharmacological properties, for example digoxin, which is a heart stimulant (*see* digitalis). *Cyanogenetic glycosides*, which occur in various plants, can liberate hydrogen cyanide when hydrolysed and are thus potentially toxic to animals (*see* linseed poisoning).

glycosuria The presence of glucose in the urine. This is often used as a preliminary test for *diabetes mellitus, but care must be taken in interpretation as shocked animals and cats under stress may be glycosuric. A series of blood glucose levels taken during a 24-hour period, with documentation of feed times, is needed to confirm any diagnosis of diabetes mellitus. Dipstick tests (e.g. Urostix) are available to detect glucose in urine.

gnath- (gnatho-) *Prefix denoting* the jaw.

Gnathostoma A genus of parasitic *nematodes occurring in the stomach of wild and domestic cats, fish-eating carnivores, pigs, and occasionally humans. The adult worms are short and thick and are found in tumours in the liver, stomach, and oesophagus. Extensive destruction of tissue follows; in the liver this results in yellow mosaic streaks on the surface. The tumours can rupture into the body cavity and the resulting peritonitis may be fatal. Infestation occurs mainly in Asia and North America. The two intermediate hosts are water

fleas (*Cyclops*), and then fish, frogs, or reptiles. There is no recognized treatment and diagnosis may be hampered due to the difficulty in finding eggs.

gnotobiotic 1. Describing an environment that contains only one or a few types of known microorganisms or no microorganisms whatsoever. **2.** Describing an animal that has been delivered and reared so that it is free of pathogenic organisms. The young are delivered by Caesarean section and maintained without any contact with their dams; all their food is sterilized. Such animals are produced for experimental purposes, especially to investigate disease processes.

goad A device for encouraging animals to move. Excessive use of sticks can cause bruising so battery-powered electric goads are preferable. They have spring-loaded contacts that give the animal a mild electric shock. Excessive use of the electric goad should be avoided since this may induce panic.

goat pox An infectious disease of goats characterized by fever and generalized pocks, caused by capripoxvirus (*see* poxvirus). The distribution, epidemiology, and clinical signs are the same as described for *sheep pox. Although most strains of capripoxvirus show a preference for a particular host species, whether sheep, goats, or cattle, the viral strains that cause goat pox will also infect sheep; indeed, some strains are equally virulent in goats and sheep. European breeds of goat are highly susceptible to goat pox and many strains of capripoxvirus will cause 100% mortality in British goats. Control is by vaccination using a live attenuated vaccine. Single vaccines are available that control both sheep and goat pox. Goat pox is a *notifiable disease in the UK. *See also* orf.

goblet cell A flask-shaped secretory cell found in the *epithelium of the respiratory and intestinal tracts. Goblet cells secrete the principal constituents of mucus.

going light *See* avian tuberculosis.

goitre Enlargement of the thyroid gland, usually due to *iodine deficiency. There are two types of goitre. The first is due to iodine deficiency in the soil and occurs in young animals. Therefore, distribution is often localized. Newborn animals show enlarged thyroids and in severe cases may be stillborn or partially hairless, and too weak to suckle. The second type is caused by the presence of *goitrogens* in the diet. These are substances, found in such plants as kale, cabbage, and raw soya beans, that are capable of inducing thyroid enlargement in animals of any age. Iodized salt (sodium chloride) prevents both types of goitre but may be of little value for treating established lesions.

goitrogen A substance that when ingested gives rise to *goitre. An example is 1,5-vinyl-2-thio-oxazolidine, found in some plants of the genus *Brassica* (*see* brassica poisoning).

golden corydalis *See* blood root poisoning.

golden eardrops *See* blood root poisoning.

golden slippers The golden-yellow feet (hooves) of foetal calves.

Golgi apparatus A collection of vesicles and folded membranes in a cell, usually connected to the *endoplasmic reticulum. It stores and later transports the proteins manufactured in the endoplasmic reticulum. The Golgi apparatus is well developed in cells that produce secretions, e.g. pancreatic cells producing digestive enzymes.

gonad The male or female gamete-producing organ, namely the ovary in the female and the testis in the male.

gonadorelin A synthetic analogue of *gonadotrophin releasing hormone (GnRH) that acts on the anterior pituitary causing the release of endogenous gonadotrophins (FSH and LH). It is injected intramuscularly. In cattle it is used to treat ovarian cysts, stimulate ovulation in the postpartum period, and induce ovulation (usually given on the day of artificial insemination). Gonadorelin is not effective in the mare, but the related synthetic analogue *buserelin*, which has greater potency and a longer half-life, is effective in stimulating ovulation of a mature follicle in the mare. Tradenames: **Fertagyl** (gonadorelin); **Receptal** (buserelin).

gonadotrophin Any of several hormones that act on the ovaries or testes (gonads) to promote the production of sex hormones and either ova or spermatozoa. They include *follicle-stimulating hormone, *luteinizing hormone, *chorionic gonadotrophin, and *prolactin. *See also* PMSG.

gonadotrophin-releasing hormone (GnRH) A hormone that causes the release of both *luteinizing hormone and *follicle-stimulating hormone from the adenohypophysis of the pituitary gland; it is often referred to as luteinizing hormone-releasing hormone (LHRH).

Gongylonema A genus of parasitic *nematodes found in the oesophageal wall or stomach (rumen) of ruminants and other grazing animals. *G. pulchrum* occurs in cattle, sheep, goats, buffaloes, horses, and camels; *G. verrucosum* is found in ruminants in tropical regions. The adult worms inhabit tumours on the gut wall. Eggs are passed in the faeces and are ingested by dung beetles, in which the larvae develop. The larvae are then passed or the beetles may be eaten directly by the host. Infestation does not cause disease. Humans may be infested by accidental ingestion of the beetles. The larvae do not develop properly but may cause creeping eruption in the cheeks and lips.

goni- (gonio-) *Prefix denoting* an anatomical angle or corner.

gossypol poisoning A toxic condition occurring in nonruminant animals fed on rations containing cotton seeds. These contain the aromatic aldehyde gossypol, which can cause inappetence and loss of weight. Continuous feeding may cause dyspnoea, emaciation, and death. Ferrous sulphate added to the ration has a protective effect. Cottonseed meal should not constitute more than 5– 10% of pig and poultry rations.

GOT (glutamate oxaloacetate transaminase) *See* AST.

gout A metabolic disease, particularly of humans but also other animals, such as poultry and reptiles, caused by a defect in uric acid metabolism and consequent deposition of urate crystals in the body resulting in pain and swelling. In *articular gout*, white semisolid urate deposits accumulate around joints, particularly the feet. In *visceral gout*, the white urate deposits are found under the serosal surfaces of the abdominal organs and within the kidney, leading to blockage of the ureters. Shortage of drinking water may be a precipitating cause. The disease commonly occurs in intensively housed poultry but other cage and fancy birds may be similarly affected. Treatment involves the encouragement of drinking – especially water made alkaline by the addition of small quantities of sodium bicarbonate. Gout also occurs in reptiles due to dehydration, excessive protein intake, or kidney disease. Obstruction of the ureters is a common sequel.

Governing Council of the Cat Fancy The premier organization governing the registration of pedigree cats in the UK. It is also responsible for licensing shows for pedigree cats throughout the country, and organizes its own annual show, the Supreme Show. Address: 4– 6 Penel Orlieu, Bridgwater, Somerset.

GPT (glutamate pyruvate transaminase) *See* ALT.

Graafian follicle A mature 'tertiary' *ovarian follicle prior to ovulation. It consists of a ball of cells with a fluid-filled central cavity in which the *oocyte develops. The follicle grows under the influence of *follicle-stimulating hormone and gradually migrates to the surface of the ovary. Here it distends the ovary surface and eventually bursts, releasing the oocyte to the oviduct. The follicle then becomes a *corpus luteum.

gracile fasciculus A large tract of nerve fibres in the dorsal *funiculus of the *spinal cord which transmits sensory impulses concerned with touch, pressure, and *kinaesthesia from the hindmost part of the body, including the hindlimb.

gracile nucleus A nucleus in the medulla oblongata in the brain that receives the sensory nerve fibres of the *gracile fasciculus in the spinal cord. Fibres from the gracile nucleus cross over (decussate) to join the medial *lemniscus on either side.

gracilis muscle A broad sheet of muscle lying superficially on the medial side of the thigh. It acts to adduct the hip joint.

graft 1. Any organ, tissue, or other material that is implanted into the body to replace an existing body part. An *autograft* is derived from the same individual; examples are *skin grafts and bone grafts. A *homograft* is derived from another individual of the same species, for example a kidney or cornea. A *heterograft is taken from an individual of another species; for example denatured cartilage or specially prepared and sterilized compact bone. Tissue matching and/or immunosuppressive therapy may be required to prevent the recipient's immune system rejecting homografts. Heterografts may be used as temporary implants, or they can be specially treated before insertion to avoid rejection. **2.** To surgically implant such a graft.

-gram *Suffix denoting* a record; tracing. Example: *electrocardiogram* (record of an electrocardiograph).

Gram's stain A method of staining bacterial cells, used as a primary means of identification. A film of bacteria on a glass slide is stained with a violet dye, treated with decolorizer (e.g. alcohol), and then counterstained with red dye. *Gram-negative* bacteria lose the initial stain but take up the counterstain, so that they appear red microscopically. *Gram-positive* bacteria retain the initial stain, appearing violet microscopically. These staining differences are based on variations in the structure of the cell wall in the two groups.

granulation The growth of small rounded outgrowths, made up of small blood vessels and connective tissue, on the healing surface of a wound or ulcer. Granulation tissue forms as a normal part of the healing process. *See also* proud flesh.

granulocyte A white blood cell (leucocyte) that has granular cytoplasm. *Neutrophils, *eosinophils, and *basophils are all granulocytes.

granuloma A chronic inflammatory lesion produced in response to a variety of stimuli, such as bacterial or protozoan invasion, or a foreign body. It is composed chiefly of macrophages and lymphocytes in a well-vascularized stroma, the macrophages usually containing intact microbial cells or other ingested particles. This produces a hard usually flesh-coloured mass in the skin, often with a verrucose surface; they may be multiple. Discrete lesions tend to undergo concentric zonation, with necrosis or caseation in the centre and an outer zone of fibrosis; suppuration, when present, is most often due to *secondary infection, although some organisms provoke pyogranulomatous inflammation and can be considered the primary cause of the response.

'Infective granulomas' are a category of microbial diseases characterized by progressive granuloma formation. They include *tuberculosis, *Johne's disease, *actinomycosis, *actinobacillosis, *glanders, some forms of *brucellosis, *botriomycosis, coligranuloma (*see* colibacillosis), and most internal (systemic) fungal diseases. In a minority of the infective granulomas (actinomycosis, actinobacillosis, and botriomycosis) are seen distinctive structures, or 'granules', centred around small colonies of the microorganism; these must be distinguished from granulomas. *Compare* granulation.

granulomatous Having the characteristics of a *granuloma.

granulopoiesis The production and development of *granulocytes. *See* haemopoiesis.

granulosa cells The epithelial cells of an *ovarian follicle.

granulosa (theca) cell tumour The commonest of the *ovarian tumours, recorded in all domesticated species. Generally confined to one ovary, the tumours are solid or cystic spherical often large masses that are white to yellow, depending on the amount of lipid present in the cells. Although benign the tumours often produce excessive amounts of steroid hormones, leading to *anoestrus or persistent oestrus in bitches, cows, and mares; mares exhibit stallion-like behaviour, while bitches undergo cystic hyperplasia of the endometrium. Surgical removal of the tumour is successful and cures the hormonal conditions.

-graph *Suffix denoting* an instrument that records. Example: *electrocardiograph* (instrument recording heart activity).

grass A monocotyledonous herb of the family Gramineae. Grasses comprise the staple food of most ruminants and many nonruminant herbivores; they are also used in some pig and poultry production systems. The major grass species in British pastures are perennial ryegrass (*Lolium perenne*), Italian ryegrass (*Lolium multiflorum*), timothy (*Phleum pratense*), cocksfoot (*Dactylis glomerata*), and the fescues (*Festuca* spp.). The nutritive value of grasses varies with species and also with stage of growth – the younger the grass the higher the proportion of leaf and the higher the content of energy and protein. The supply of grass is influenced by species of grass, application of fertilizer, climate, and frequency of grazing or cutting.

In spring, when grass growth is rapid, care must be taken to avoid *bloat and *hypomagnesaemia, especially in cattle. Hence, grazing animals should be introduced to lush pasture gradually, with supplementary feeding of roughage for the first few weeks. The burden of gastrointestinal worms and other parasites can be minimized by rotating the area grazed and by regular dosing with *anthelmintics.

Grass crops are conserved as livestock feedstuffs in various forms, principally *silage, *hay, *haylage, and *dried grass. *See also* grazing.

grass sickness A usually fatal disease of horses, occurring in the UK and parts of Europe, typically seen in animals at pasture and characterized by obstruction of the large intestine and decreased gastrointestinal motility. The acute form of the disease can result in death within 12–72 hours. There is also a chronic form, which may extend over weeks or months. A neurotoxic factor has been isolated from affected animals, but this may be a product rather than a cause of the disease. However, the disease characteristically involves degeneration of the autonomic ganglia, which supports some form of neurotoxicity. The clinical signs include depression, restlessness, increased heart rate (tachycardia), sweating, muscular *fasciculations over the shoulder, drooling of saliva, difficulty and pain associated with swallowing, and discharge of stomach contents through the nostrils. There is also gastric tympany and/or excess fluid contents, an impacted large colon, and scanty hard faeces. Additional findings at necropsy include linear ulceration of the oesophageal mucosa and a massive accumulation of fluid in the stomach and small intestine. There is no satisfactory treatment. *See also* dysautonomia.

grass staggers *See* hypomagnesaemia.

gravel 1. Sediment or small stones in the urinary tract, which may be passed in the urine. It is usually composed of calcium phosphate, calcium oxalate, or uric acid, and follows the excretion by the kidneys of abnormally high amounts of the corresponding substance. **2.** Infection of a horse's foot extending from the white line to the coronary band (*see* hoof).

grazing The selection and cropping of vegetation by herbivorous animals. The principal domesticated herbivores graze chiefly on *grass, although legumes and other forage crops are also important. The amount of time spent grazing will vary with sward conditions, weather, and the individual animal; both cattle and sheep spend approximately equal periods grazing, ruminating, and resting in each day. Cattle in temperate climates tend to have two peaks of grazing activity, in the early morning and early evening, with little or no grazing during darkness. In hotter climates this pattern may be changed, with up to two-thirds of grazing taking place during darkness. Sheep tend to have shorter and more frequent grazing periods than cattle. The amount of available herbage influences the time spent grazing, but cattle will not spend more than about 9 hours per day grazing so supplementary feeding is necessary for high-producing animals when herbage is short.

Sheep are more selective grazers than cattle and tend to nibble the more succulent leafy parts of the grass plant. Cattle tend to pull at grass with their tongue (if the grass is long enough) and consume a higher proportion of stem material. Sheep are able to graze closer to the ground than cattle and it is sound practice to let sheep follow grazing cattle to utilize the grass remaining.

greasewood poisoning A toxic condition resulting from the ingestion of foliage of the large deciduous shrub, *Sarcobatus vermiculatus* (greasewood),

which occurs in the western USA. It contains soluble oxalates, which interfere with calcium metabolism and cause the clinical signs of listlessness leading to incoordination, prostration, coma, and death. Calcium oxalate crystals are deposited in the kidney tubules and nephrosis occurs. Treatment is by oral and intravenous administration of calcium, along with symptomatic therapy. *See* oxalate poisoning.

greasy pig disease A contagious skin disease of suckling piglets caused by the bacterium *Staphylococcus hyicus* and characterized by exudative or seborrhoeic *dermatitis. The peracute form is fatal; less severe cases respond to penicillin.

green-bottle fly A large metallic-green blowfly of the genus *Lucilia*, also known as the sheep maggot fly and responsible for blowfly *strike of sheep in most temperate countries as well as in southern Africa and Australia. The eggs are laid on any decomposing animal substance, in wounds, or on wool soiled with urine, faeces, or blood, most commonly in the soiled area below the root of the tail and especially when the faeces are loose due to grazing on lush pasture. The larvae attack the skin causing inflammation and consequent local discharge of body fluids, on which they feed. When mature, they leave the host and pupate on the ground. Prevention entails immersing the sheep in a dip containing one of the many suitable *insecticides, some of which may be used in dressings for the wounds resulting from blowfly strike.

green leg *See* ruptured gastrocnemius tendon.

greenstick fracture A type of *fracture occurring in young animals in which the fracture line extends only partly across the bone, which then splits lengthways, rather like a partly sawn green branch.

green wool A form of *lumpy wool in which secondary infection with the bacterium *Pseudomonas aeruginosa gives a green pigmentation to the soiled wool.

grey matter The darker coloured tissue of the central nervous system, composed principally of the cell bodies of neurones, branching dendrites, and neuroglia (compare white matter). In the brain grey matter forms the *cerebral cortex and the outer layer of the *cerebellum as well as other nuclei; in the spinal cord the grey matter lies centrally, surrounded by the white matter.

griseofulvin An antifungal antibiotic produced by certain fungi of the genus *Penicillium and used clinically in the treatment and prevention of *ringworm. It is fungistatic, possibly by disrupting the mitotic spindle during cell division. Griseofulvin is given orally, usually incorporated in feed. It is only sparingly soluble in water, and its absorption from the alimentary tract is aided by providing the drug in fine particles and feeding in combination with fatty material. Subsequent metabolism in the liver causes its inactivation.

Griseofulvin from the bloodstream is incorporated into keratin as it is formed. Consequently all new growth of the hair shafts, nails, and cornified layer of the skin produced during the period of treatment is resistant to further invasion by the infecting fungus. However, fungi in existing keratin remain unaffected by the drug and are a potential source of reinfection or cross infection. Reinfection is uncommon provided treatment is maintained for a sufficient period, which may be several weeks or months. Presumably an immune response to the original lesions is by then protective, but animals given the drug prophylactically are again susceptible soon after treatment is stopped. Toxicity is uncommon but the drug should not be used in pregnant animals because of its possible teratogenic effects.

grit Mineral particles, either soluble (e.g. limestone) or more usually insoluble (e.g. granite), that are provided for housed poultry being fed coarsely ground or whole-cereal feeds. After ingestion, the grit particles are retained in the gizzard where they aid digestion by producing a grinding action. Grit is seldom required with mashes, meals, and pellets.

grootlamsiekte The condition, occurring in southern Africa, in which sheep experience a prolonged gestation after ingesting the shrub *Salsola tuberculata* during the last 50 days of pregnancy.

ground hemlock A North American plant, *Taxus canadensis*, that contains the same toxic alkaloid as yew (see yew poisoning).

groundnut meal A feedstuff consisting of the residue following the extraction of oil from groundnuts (peanuts). It has a high fibre and relatively low protein content and is usually considered only for inclusion in ruminant diets. Contamination with *Aspergillus* fungi may lead to *aflatoxicosis.

groundsel See ragwort poisoning.

ground substance The matrix of *connective tissue, in which various cells and fibres are embedded.

growth hormone See somatotrophin.

growth plate See epiphyseal cartilage.

growth promoter An agent used to improve the growth rate and/or the feed conversion efficiency of livestock. Several classes of compounds are used, but the two major groups are antibacterials and anabolic hormones. Growth-promoting antibacterials are used in pigs, poultry, sheep, and cattle, being added to the rations over prolonged periods. Their use is controlled to minimize any possible impact on the development of bacterial resistance to therapeutic antibacterials in both animals and humans. Any resistance associated with growth promoters must be very slowly developing and not transferable to other organisms. Also, there should be no cross-resistance with drugs used therapeutically. Tissue residues of the antibacterials should be negligible, hence the use of compounds that are poorly absorbed from the gastrointestinal tract. Many drugs are withheld prior to slaughter to avoid residues in the carcass.

The main groups of antibacterial growth promoters have activity against Gram-positive organisms, but their mode of action has not been fully defined. One possible mechanism is by controlling subclinical disease, for example decreasing toxins produced by the gastrointestinal flora thereby reducing the depth of the gut mucosa and improving absorption. Another is by changing the gastrointestinal flora and removing organisms that metabolize dietary nutrients to waste products, for example reducing methane production in ruminants or organic acid production in pigs. Growth-promoting antibacterials used in animals include arsenicals, copper, *avoparcin, *macrolide antibiotics, *bacitracin, bambermycin, flavomycin, *dimetridazole, *ionophores, olaquindox, carbadox, noxythiolin, and halquinol. The incorporation of antibacterials into animal feedstuffs requires a veterinary written directive.

Hormonal growth promoters were formerly used extensively but have now been banned in EEC countries because of concern over possible residues in meat. In castrated animals, androgens such as *trenbolone acetate – given either alone or in combination with *oestrogens, e.g. oestradiol or *zeranol – produce marked improvements in growth rates. Androgens have also been used to improve growth rates and carcass quality in beef heifers and cull cows.

Other growth-promoting agents being investigated are the β_2 adrenergic agonist drugs (e.g. *clenbuterol), which have been found to improve growth rates and carcass quality, and growth hormone.

guanine One of the nitrogen-containing bases (*see* purine) that occurs in the nucleic acids DNA and RNA.

guanosine A compound containing guanine and the sugar ribose. *See also* nucleoside.

Guard Dogs Act (1975) (England and Wales) An Act of Parliament that makes it an offence to use a guard dog at any premises unless a person (the 'handler'), who is capable of controlling the dog, is present on the premises and the dog is under the control of the handler at all times, except while the dog is secured. A notice warning of the guard dog's presence must be clearly shown at each entrance to the premises.

gubernaculum (*pl.* **gubernacula**) The paired fibrous strands of tissue that connect the gonads to the inguinal region in the foetus. In the male they guide and possibly draw the testes through the inguinal canal into the scrotum before birth. In the female the ovaries descend only slightly within the abdominal cavity and the gubernacula persist as the round ligaments of the uterus, connecting the ovaries and uterus to the inguinal region.

Guide to Professional Conduct A code of ethics and guide to the conduct of veterinary practice in the UK published by the *Royal College of Veterinary Surgeons. The Guide deals with relations between practitioners and clients and with interprofessional relations and provides information on veterinary obligations in particular situations.

guinea worm *See* Dracunculus.

gum (in anatomy) *See* gingiva.

Gumboro disease *See* infectious bursal disease.

gustation The sense of taste or the act of tasting.

gustatory Relating to the sense of taste or to the organs of taste.

gut 1. *See* intestine. **2.** *See* catgut.

guttate Describing lesions in the skin that are shaped like drops.

guttural pouch A large saclike ventral pouch (diverticulum) of the *auditory tube in the horse, lying between the base of the skull and the pharynx.

guttural pouch diphtheria (guttural pouch mycosis) A condition of horses and other equines in which infection causes *diphtheresis of the mucous membranes lining the *guttural pouch. Bacteria (usually *Streptococcus* or, rarely, *Pasteurella*) or fungi (*Aspergillus*) are commonly isolated from cases. Clinical signs include a mucopurulent nasal discharge (which may be unilateral or bilateral), fever, nosebleed, difficulty in swallowing, respiratory upsets, and facial paralysis. Diagnosis entails

endoscopy and radiographic examination. Treatment is by catheterization and irrigation of the pouches and parenteral administration of antibiotics. Early treatment may be successful. Severe cases may require surgical drainage of the pouches or ligation of bleeding vessels. If the condition damages the cranial nerves and carotid arteries, the prognosis is poor. Since fungal spores occur in healthy guttural pouches, suspected mycotic infection should be confirmed by direct microscopic examination of fragments of material from the lesions for evidence of mycelial growth.

guttural pouch emphysema (guttural pouch tympany) Distension of the *guttural pouch in the horse, due to obstruction of the pharyngeal opening of the auditory tube. It results in a painless swelling behind the angle of the jaw, which is resonant on percussion. The condition is relieved by creating an alternative opening to the guttural pouch.

gyr- (gyro-) *Prefix denoting* **1.** a gyrus. **2.** a ring or circle.

gyrus (*pl.* gyri) A raised convolution of the *cerebral cortex, between two sulci (clefts).

H

Habronema A genus of parasitic *nematodes that infest horses and cause the disease *habronemiasis. There are three main species: *H. microstoma*, *H. macrostoma*, and *H. muscae*. The adults are found in the gut, while the larval stages may be found in open wounds. The eggs are passed in the faeces and ingested by the larvae of stable flies and house flies, in which they themselves develop into larvae; they remain with the fly larva until it becomes an adult fly. The horse becomes infested either by swallowing the adult fly or by migration of the nematode larvae from the fly's mouthparts to open wounds on the horse.

habronemiasis A disease of horses caused by parasitic nematodes of the genus *Habronema*. The adult worms are found in nodules on the stomach wall or embedded in the gastric mucosa, depending on the species of parasite involved. The result is chronic inflammation of the stomach, which interferes with gastric function. The larvae are spread by flies and may infest open wounds, causing a condition known as *summer sores*. The horse may bite the affected part until the skin is quite raw, and larvae may be transferred to the horse's mouth and be swallowed to resume normal development to the adult. In Australia a granular conjunctivitis known as *swamp cancer* is believed to be caused by *Habronema* larvae. There may be also be a growth on the inner corner of the eye. Treatment is with *ivermectin.

haem An iron-containing compound (a *porphyrin) that combines with *globins to form *haemoglobin, or *myoglobin. It is also found in the *cytochromes.

haem- (haema-, haemo-, haemato-) (*US* hem-, *etc.*) *Prefix denoting* blood. Example: *haematogenesis* (formation of).

Haemaccel Tradename for a blood plasma-volume expanding solution. It is formed from degraded bovine gelatin and contains polypeptides (with molecular weights in the range 5000–50 000) and salts. It is infused intravenously in cases of shock and hypovolaemia. Blood losses of up to 25% of the total blood volume can be replaced by Haemaccel. The polypeptides are nonallergenic and those of low molecular weight are filtered at the kidneys, ensuring that urine flow is maintained to prevent renal failure. *See also* dextran.

haemagglutinating encephalomyelitis of piglets *See* vomiting/wasting disease.

haemal lymph nodes Small dark-red nodes, up to 20 mm in diameter, found in ruminants in close association with lymph nodes. They consist of lymphatic tissue with sinuses containing blood, and are most easily seen in sheep carcasses, associated with the lymph nodes in the lumbar and pelvic areas.

haemangioma *See* angioma.

haemangiopericytoma A common tumour found only in the dog and nearly always in the subcutaneous tissues of the limbs of middle-aged to old animals. Occasionally, it may be seen on the trunk or at other sites. They are slow-growing nonencapsulated lesions, often large and forming multinodular firm swellings in the dermis and subcutaneous layers of the skin. Histologically, the tumour consists of spindle-shaped (fusiform) cells arranged in bundles or in tight whorls forming a characteristic 'fingerprint' pattern. The tumour cells may infiltrate between muscle bundles, tendons, and nerves, making complete surgical excision extremely difficult. Where there is recurrence of the tumour following excision, amputation may be considered as metastasis from the limb to other parts of the body is rare.

haemangiosarcoma *See* angiosarcoma.

haemarthrosis **(intra-articular haemorrhage)** Bleeding into the joints. It is most common in cases of injury and *haemorrhagic diathesis; haemophiliacs are prone to repeated episodes (*see* haemophilia).

haematemesis The act of vomiting blood. This may be a result of injury, rupture, gastritis, parasitic infestation, neoplasia, or poisoning (e.g. warfarin).

haematidrosis A rare condition in which blood or blood pigment is secreted in sweat.

haematin A chemical derivative of *haemoglobin formed by removal of the protein part of the molecule and oxidation of the iron atom from the ferrous to the ferric form.

haematinic A substance that promotes the formation of red blood cells. They are used to treat anaemia. Ferrous or ferric salts are given orally as haematinics in many species. Neonatal piglets are routinely given an intramuscular injection of iron-dextran to prevent *piglet anaemia.

haematocele (haematocoele) A blood-filled swelling outside the normal circulatory system. A common example is swelling of the testis secondary to haemorrhage into the tunica vaginalis.

haematocolpos A build-up of menstrual blood in the vagina anterior to an imperforate hymen. Strictly this applies only to primates in which menstruation occurs (e.g. humans). A persistent hymen may cause a similar problem in the bitch after the pro-oestral bleeding just prior to oestrus.

haematocrit *See* packed cell volume.

haematocyst A cyst containing blood. *See also* haematocele.

haematogenous 1. Derived from or carried by the blood. 2. Relating to

the production of blood or its components: haemopoietic (*see* haemopoiesis).

haematoma An accumulation of blood within the tissues that clots to form a solid swelling. This occurs when the bleeding is confined to a space, for example within the capsule of such organs as the kidney, liver, or spleen, or beneath the skin, as in the aural haematoma, found in the dog and cat. Almost always, haematomas arise following traumatic injury and/or some blood coagulation problem (e.g. haemophilia or warfarin poisoning), or occasionally neoplasms.

haematometria An accumulation of blood in the uterine cavity. This is a rare condition and may occur as a result of embryonic or foetal death, trauma, poisoning (e.g. warfarin), infection, a bleeding disorder, or a neoplasm.

haematomyelia Bleeding into the tissues of the spinal cord. This usually occurs following trauma but it can be a result of *telangiectasis.

haematopoiesis *See* haemopoiesis.

haematoporphyrin A type of *porphyrin produced during the metabolism of haemoglobin.

haematosalpinx *See* haemosalpinx.

haematothorax *See* haemothorax.

haematuria The presence of blood or red blood cells in the urine. It may be the result of injury, infection, a neoplasm in the urinary tract, or a generalized blood coagulation disorder.

haemo- *Prefix. See* haem-.

Haemobartonella A genus of *rickettsiae found in association with the red blood cells of animals. They are transmitted by arthropods. Unlike the *anaplasmas, these usually coccoid organisms are found on the surfaces of red blood cells or invaginated within their membrane. In some animals they cause anaemia and jaundice. Species affecting domestic animals include *H. felis*, which causes severe anaemia in cats, *H. bovis*, found in cattle in association with *anaplasmosis, and *H. canis*, found in dogs but without any known clinical effect.

haemobartonellosis (bartonellosis) Any of various infectious diseases caused by arthropod-borne rickettsiae of the genus *Haemobartonella*. They are usually mild or inapparent, with the one exception of feline haemobartonellosis, caused by *H. felis*, which is characterized by high fever, anaemia, and rapid loss of weight. Diagnosis is established by staining blood smears with Giemsa or acridine orange. Treatment with tetracyclines and chloramphenicol is effective.

haemoconcentration A decrease in plasma volume, which causes a concomitant increase in the proportion of red blood cells relative to the plasma. Haemoconcentration may occur in any condition in which there is a severe loss of water from the body.

haemodilution An increase in plasma volume, which causes a concomitant decrease in the proportion of red blood cells relative to the plasma.

haemoglobin One of a group of *proteins that occur widely in animals and function as oxygen carriers in the blood. Vertebrate haemoglobin is contained within the red blood cells or *erythrocytes and is responsible for their colour. The haemoglobin molecule consists of the protein globin,

which comprises four polypeptide chains; each chain carries an iron-containing *haem group. The iron in haemoglobin is in the reduced Fe(II) state and remains so after oxygen has bound reversibly to the iron atom (i.e. the reaction is an oxygenation not an oxidation). Oxidation of the iron to Fe(III) produces methaemoglobin (*see* methaemoglobinaemia), which is subsequently unable to bind oxygen. At the lungs, haemoglobin takes up oxygen to form *oxyhaemoglobin*. In the capillaries, dissociation takes place and oxyen is made available to the oxygen-depleted tissues.

Haemoglobin also has a buffering effect on the large amounts of hydrogen ion released by the formation of bicarbonate from carbon dioxide in the tissues, a reaction catalysed by the enzyme carbonic anhydrase, which is present in erythrocytes.

When erythrocytes die their haemoglobin is degraded by an elaborate pathway designed to conserve their iron content. This degradation is largely dependent on fixed cells of the *macrophage system present in liver, bone marrow, and spleen. Free haemoglobin released into the plasma is first bound to *haptoglobin for transport, a device which prevents loss of haemoglobin via the kidneys. After removal of the haem complexes from globin, the iron is conveyed to the bone marrow with the help of the transport protein *transferrin, and the remaining pigment is converted to the yellow compound, bilirubin, taken by the blood to the liver hepatocytes and excreted in the *bile. Iron may also be stored as *ferritin or *haemosiderin in macrophages.

haemoglobinometer An instrument for estimating the concentration of *haemoglobin in solution. All of the various types use either colorimetric or spectrophotometric principles to compare the light absorption of blood haemoglobin with a standard. Usually the haemoglobin is first converted to a more suitable form, such as acid haematin, oxyhaemoglobin, or cyanmethaemoglobin.

haemoglobin reactive protein *See* haptoglobin.

haemoglobinuria The presence of haemoglobin in the urine. This is usually indicative of increased breakdown of the red blood cells (*haemolysis), so that the released haemoglobin cannot be taken up rapidly enough by blood proteins. It can occur following strenuous exercise (e.g. in racing or working horses) or the ingestion of certain poisons (e.g. *brassica poisoning), and in some infectious diseases, notably *babesiosis. *Postparturient haemoglobinuria affects newly calved dairy cows. *Compare* azoturia. *See also* bacillary haemoglobinuria.

haemolysin A substance capable of destroying red blood cells (erythrocytes), i.e. causing haemolysis.

haemolysis The destruction of red blood cells (*erythrocytes). *See* haemolytic anaemia; haemolytic disease.

haemolytic Causing, connected with, or resulting from the destruction of red cells (i.e. haemolysis).

haemolytic anaemia *Anaemia caused by destruction of the red blood cells. There are many causes. Certain poisons are able to induce haemolysis, including copper, to which sheep are particularly susceptible, lead, phenyl hydrazine, many organic compounds related to benzene and phenol, phenothiazine, ricin, and many snake and spider venoms. Some toxins of the bacteria *Clostridium oedematiens* type B and C. *haemolyticum* and of some staphylococci and streptococci are haemolytic (although haemolysis is not a major sign in infections by these organisms). Even some foodstuffs contain haemolytic factors; thus, high levels of kale feeding have been associated with haemolysis in cattle.

*Autoimmune diseases produce haemolysis usually by the action of autoantibodies. *Transfusion of mismatched blood is liable to result in haemolysis due to the action of the recipient's immune system. The danger of haemolysis increases with second and subsequent transfusions. Deficiency of enzymes involved in sugar metabolism, and of certain other enzymes, is known to make haemoglobin vulnerable to oxidation and irreversible damage, with the formation in the cell of visible haemoglobin precipitates known as *Heinz bodies. Affected red cells have a reduced life span. The inability to synthesize certain enzymes is inherited, and is responsible for a number of human haemolytic anaemias. A type of hereditary anaemia has also been described in Basenji dogs, attributed to deficiency of the enzyme pyruvate kinase.

Bacterial infections causing haemolysis are chiefly *leptospirosis and bacillary *haemoglobinuria caused by *Clostridium haemolyticum*. Haemolytic viral conditions include *equine infectious anaemia and *ehrlichiosis in dogs and horses. Protozoal haemolytic infections, in which destruction of the red cells is caused by the reproducing organisms within, chiefly involve several species of *Eperythrozoon*, *Haemobartonella*, and *Plasmodium*, and *anaplasmosis and *theileriosis. Physiological imbalance, for instance in *postparturient haemoglobinuria, can cause haemolysis. Haemolysis due to water intoxication has been reported in animals, usually calves, that have accidentally been deprived of water and then allowed to drink to excess.

Treatment of haemolytic anaemia always depends primarily on identification and removal of the cause. Supportive therapy in the form of blood transfusion or oxygen is sometimes indicated.

haemolytic disease Any disease involving destruction of the red blood cells (*haemolysis). *See* bovine autoimmune haemolytic anaemia; canine autoimmune haemolytic anaemia; equine autoimmune haemolytic anaemia; haemolytic anaemia.

Haemonchus A genus of parasitic *nematodes containing members that cause *parasitic gastroenteritis in livestock. For example, *H. placei* affects cattle in warmer regions, and *H. contortus* is important in sheep. The adults are found in the mucosa of the abomasum, and pass eggs in the host's faeces. When the larvae have hatched and developed they migrate up the leaves of wet herbage, from where they are ingested by the host to settle in the abomasum. In **ewes** immunity to the worms may decrease before parturition causing an increase in egg production, which places lambs at an increased risk of infestation. Lambs may also be infested by larvae from a previous year, and can suffer severe anaemia in the summer months before natural immunity has time to develop. Affected animals may be constipated and suffer oedematous swelling at the throat ('bottle jaw'). Treatment is by thiabendazole, fenbendazole, etc.; ivermectin is an excellent newer drug (*see* benzimidazole).

haemopericardium The presence of blood within the pericardial cavity surrounding the heart (*see* pericardium). This may be the result of trauma, a blood coagulation disorder, poisoning (e.g. warfarin), or a neoplasm. In ruminants it may also occur when sharp objects penetrate deeply through the wall of the reticulum (*see* traumatic reticulitis).

haemoperitoneum The presence of blood in the abdominal cavity (*see* peritoneum). This may be the result of trauma, a blood coagulation disorder, poisoning (e.g. warfarin), or a neoplasm. Any condition affecting the friability of the spleen, liver, or kidneys is particularly likely to lead to haemoperitoneum. Also, it may be due to postsurgical haemorrhage, for example in the frequently performed spaying and castration operations.

haemophilia A sex-linked inherited bleeding disorder in which the blood clots very slowly due to a deficiency or structural defect of one of the *coagulation factors. *Haemophilia A* is characterized by deficiency of coagulation Factor VIII (F VIII) and occurs in many breeds of dogs, in cats, and horses. The tendency to bleed is usually severe, associated with F VIII levels below 1% of normal, but moderate (F VIII 2–5%) and mild forms (F VIII above 5%) are encountered. The F VIII gene lies on the *X-chromosome, and affected animals are generally male. Female carriers usually have F VIII levels that are 40–60% of normal and they are asymptomatic. However, female progeny of a mating between an affected male and a carrier female may show the disease. Severely affected animals suffer from major spontaneous haemorrhage into muscles, joints, and body cavities and often die before reaching adulthood. Management of the bleeding requires infusion of the deficient coagulation factor in the form of plasma or plasma concentrates; whole blood is rarely effective. Other names: **'classical' haemophilia**; **Factor VIII deficiency**.
Haemophilia B is characterized by a deficiency of Factor IX (F IX) and has been reported in several breeds of

Haemophilus

dogs and British shorthaired cats. The clinical expression and severity are similar to haemophilia A, but this condition is much less common. The pattern of inheritance, clinical picture, and management of the condition are identical to haemophilia A. Other names: **Christmas disease**; **Factor IX deficiency**.

Haemophilus A genus of pleomorphic aerobic Gram-negative *bacteria. They can grow only in the presence of certain factors (factors X and V) found in blood or other animal or plant tissue and are hence strict parasites, infecting mucous membranes. Pathogenic species include *H. suis*, which causes pneumonias in pigs in association with *swine influenza virus; *H. parasuis*, which has been associated with *Glasser's disease in pigs; *H. pleuropneumoniae*, which causes *contagious porcine pleuropneumonia; *H. gallinarum*, which causes acute or chronic respiratory disease and air-sac infections in the fowl, often in conjunction with viral infections; and *H. agni* and *H. somnus*, which are associated with *septicaemia in lambs, bronchopneumonia in adult sheep, and *Haemophilus septicaemia of cattle.

Haemophilus septicaemia of cattle
A septicaemic condition of young cattle caused by the bacterium *Haemophilus somnus* (*H. agni*), accompanied by meningoencephalitis, synovitis, pleuritis, and pneumonia. It has been recognized in Britain, the USA, Germany, and Switzerland. Death often occurs 8–12 hours after the first appearance of clinical signs. *Tetracycline antibiotics are used in treatment. In-contact animals are closely observed for the first signs so that they may be treated promptly. Other names: **Haemophilus somnus meningitis**; **sleeper syndrome**.

haemopneumopericardium The presence of blood and air in the pericardial cavity surrounding the heart (*see* pericardium). This may occur following traumatic injury (e.g. *traumatic reticulitis) or other disease.

haemopneumothorax The presence of blood and air in the pleural cavity. This may occur following trauma or surgery.

haemopoiesis (haematopoiesis) The production and development of blood cells. Haemopoiesis begins in embryonic life in the tissues of the yolk sac, and is later continued in the liver and spleen. By the time of birth, the *bone marrow has become the main site of haemopoiesis, where it is restricted to the red marrow, which is packed with haemopoietic cells. Yellow bone marrow, by contrast, contains fat but no haemopoietic cells. The cell from which all classes of blood cell are derived is the *haemopoietic stem cell* (*haemocytoblast*), which maintains its numbers by continuous mitosis. Some of these cells differentiate into stem cells that give rise to the various blood cell types.
In *granulocyte production (*granulopoiesis*), the stem cell is called a *myeloblast*, which matures into the *promyelocyte* – the earliest stage to show cytoplasmic granulation. Further development enables the three types of granulocyte – *basophil, *neutrophil, and *eosinophil – to be differentiated according to the staining properties of their granules. Maturation involves alteration of the nucleus from a spherical to a kidney shape, then to a band, and finally to the polymorphonuclear or lobed form. The mature nucleus cannot divide, hence the granulocyte is incapable of any further multiplication.
*Monocytes, which have become mononuclear phagocytes of the *macrophage system, are produced by the division of *monoblasts*. Monocytes are

capable of replication throughout life in any of the many tissues where they take up residence.

*Lymphocytes are produced in several organs in addition to the bone marrow. These include the *thymus, *lymph nodes, *spleen, *cloacal bursa, *tonsils, and *Peyer's patches. Lymphocytes develop from the large ancestral *lymphoblast* with a large nucleus, becoming small mature cells with a compact nucleus and very reduced cytoplasm. The process of differentiation is reversible; small lymphocytes reassume the lymphoblastic appearance prior to beginning a new cycle of division. The principal stimulus for this is foreign *antigen (*see* immunity). Adequate production and differentiation of lymphocytes depends on the presence of an intact thymus and, in birds, a cloacal bursa. A final stage of lymphocyte differentiation is the plasma cell, a form committed to *antibody production (*see* lymphocyte).

*Erythrocyte production (*erythropoiesis*) begins with the *proerythroblast*, which matures into an *early normoblast*, a smaller but otherwise similar cell. Thereafter, the successive types become progressively smaller and stain a pink-tan colour due to their *haemoglobin content. There is also progressive loss of the nucleus which, in mammals, is eventually extruded; in other vertebrates the nucleus is retained. Immature erythrocytes (*reticulocytes*) are released from the bone marrow to the circulation, where they may be distinguished by relatively *basophilic staining and large size. Red-cell production is controlled by the hormone *erythropoietin, which is released by the kidney in amounts determined by the tissues' need for oxygen.

*Platelets develop from a *megakaryoblast*, which undergoes nuclear division without division of the cytoplasm to form a multinucleate *megakaryocyte*. Platelets are then formed by fragmentation of the megakaryocyte cytoplasm.

Haemopoiesis is finely regulated according to the body's need. A raised level of erythropoiesis is usually evidence of blood loss or destruction. Moreover, abnormally high rates of division in a particular cell type may be an indication of a cancerous disorder. Depressed rates of production result from the action of a number of poisons, including that of an agent in bracken, which is able to depress platelet production (*see* bracken poisoning). Haemopoiesis is also markedly depressed by ionizing radiation.

haemoptysis The spitting or coughing up of blood from the lungs or airways. This follows pulmonary or bronchial haemorrhage, which may result from injury, infectious disease, neoplasm, or poisoning (e.g warfarin).

haemorrhage (bleeding) The escape of blood from a ruptured blood vessel, externally or internally. Rupture of a major vessel can lead to rapid loss of blood and consequent *shock, collapse, and death, if untreated. Signs of internal bleeding include vomiting or coughing up of blood (*haematemesis, *haemoptysis), blood in the faeces (*melaena), and blood in the urine (*haematuria). *See also* haemostasis; haemostatic.

haemorrhagic Causing, associated with, or resulting from blood loss (haemorrhage).

haemorrhagic bowel syndrome A peracute or acute haemorrhagic enteritis affecting weaned pigs aged 4–9 months (less commonly at 1–2 months), usually in high health status herds or groups. The condition has been reported in the UK, Europe, the USA, Asia, and Australia. Affected young gilts and boars previously in good condition show dysentery with copious fresh blood in diarrhoeic faeces and they rapidly become anaemic if not found dead. At autopsy there is haemorrhagic enteritis of the ileum with the colon frequently involved. Free blood and fibrin casts with thickening of the mucosa are seen macroscopically. Microscopic examination of the ileum shows extensive necrosis of the mucosa with haemorrhage, fibrin thrombosis, and an eosinophil cellular reaction. The reaction resembles acute bacterial enteritis with a Type I hypersensitivity reaction. The thickened mucosa resembles lesions associated with porcine intestinal adenomatosis (PIA) seen in younger pigs (*see* adenomatosis). There is a strong relationship between PIA, necrotic enteritis and regional enteritis, and the presence of *Campylobacter sputorum mucosalis* bacteria. Unlike PIA there are few or no *Campylobacter* organisms present in lesions of haemorrhagic enteritis, and transmission experiments have failed to establish a causative role for the bacterium. Some authorities have suggested that haemorrhagic bowel syndrome is an acute manifestation of PIA, whilst others have postulated that the haemorrhages result from an unidentified bowel insult that predisposes to invasion and proliferation of *Campylobacter* organisms. Treatment with antihistamines, corticosteroids, and broad-spectrum antibiotics (tylosin and chlortetracycline) is said to be effective although pigs with the peracute syndrome usually die. Control in other pigs in the unit is effected by use of antibiotics. Other name: **proliferative haemorrhagic enteropathy.**

haemorrhagic diathesis A condition in which there is a tendency for abnormal bleeding. It is due to a defect or deficiency in one or more of the components of *haemostasis: vessel wall contractility (rarely); platelets; or coagulation proteins. It may be caused by substances that interfere with the blood-clotting mechanism (e.g. as occurs in *warfarin poisoning), the result of immune-mediated *thrombocytopenia or *disseminated intravascular coagulation, or caused by an inherited disorder, such as *haemophilia or *von Willebrand's disease.

haemorrhagic enteritis An *adenovirus infection of turkeys causing inflammation and haemorrhage of the intestine. It occurs worldwide. Birds are frequently infected but rarely show clinical disease. The infection also occurs in fowls and pheasants.

haemorrhagic gastroenteritis of pigs Any of various diseases of pigs that can cause haemorrhagic *gastritis and/or haemorrhagic *enteritis. The most significant such conditions are *clostridial haemorrhagic enteritis, which usually affects newborn piglets (under 1 week); *swine dysentery, found chiefly in weaned pigs; and *haemorrhagic bowel syndrome, again affecting weaned pigs (4–9 months). Similar lesions may also be associated with *gastric ulcers, and with intestinal *torsion. The latter condition may occur in weaned and fattening animals, especially in whey-fed and overcrowded pigs. The cause is not known, but overfeeding and genetic factors have been proposed.

haemorrhagic septicaemia A fatal acute septicaemia of cattle and buffaloes caused by certain serotypes of the bacterium *Pasteurella multocida. In contrast to other forms of *pasteurellosis, haemorrhagic septicaemia is a primary infection specific to these serotypes. The disease is common in south and southeast Asia, the Middle East, and in Africa, occurring usually during wet and humid weather. Buffaloes and cattle are mainly affected, although sheep and goats are also susceptible. The disease is characterized by very high fever, diarrhoea, and oedema, with animals showing difficulty in breathing. At necropsy extensive haemorrhages are seen in the serous cavities, with blood-stained fluid in the thorax and abdomen; enteritis and oedema of the subcutaneous tissue are also common. Control measures include programmes of vaccination. *See also* fowl cholera.

haemorrhagic syndrome (of poultry) A condition of young domestic fowls and turkeys characterized by numerous usually small haemorrhages in the skin, muscles, and internal organs and causing poor performance and mortality. The causes are unclear, but *vitamin K deficiency appears to be involved. It was once a significant cause of economic loss on broiler growing units, with mortality up to 40–50%, but it is now relatively uncommon. The signs are ruffled feathers and general debility followed by death, although birds may die without showing signs. In less severe cases there can be downgrading of carcasses, unthriftiness, and reduced egg output in laying birds. When the syndrome was common there was an apparent link to the sulphonamide coccidiostats, now far less widely used; these are known to increase vitamin K requirements. *Compare* fatty liver haemorrhagic syndrome of hens.

haemosalpinx (haematosalpinx) An accumulation of blood in the oviduct. This can be associated with a tubal pregnancy.

haemosiderin An iron-containing storage complex found in animals that are receiving excessive amounts of dietary iron. It occurs principally in the liver, spleen, and bone marrow and has no fixed composition, containing variable amounts of iron along with protein and polysaccharides.

haemosiderosis The excessive accumulation in the tissues of the pigment *haemosiderin. This is caused by an abnormally high rate of destruction of red blood corpuscles in the region, with consequent release of haemoglobin. The iron component of the haemoglobin is then incorporated into haemosiderin. These biochemical reactions take place inside tissue *macrophages, in which the haemosiderin is subsequently stored. Several different disease processes may lead to haemosiderosis, including local haemorrhage and congestion, in which case the haemosiderosis is similarly local, and haemolytic diseases, where pigment accumulation is largely in the spleen (*see* haemolytic anaemia). A particular instance of haemosiderosis is seen in heart failure, where the lungs are affected as a result of passive congestion and have the gross appearance described as *brown induration*. Here the pigment-loaded macrophages (often visible under the microscope as *heart-failure cells*) give the lung tissue a golden-brown appearance. A similar congestive haemosiderotic process may operate in the liver during heart failure.

haemostasis The arrest of bleeding (haemorrhage). This includes the natural physiological processes of *blood coagulation and the contraction of damaged blood vessels. The term is also applied to various first-aid and surgical procedures used to stop bleeding. These include the application of pressure pads and *tourniquets to temporarily seal vessels near the body surface; the use of *cauterization or *diathermy to cut and seal vessels by heating; and *ligatures for tying vessels. *See also* haemostatic.

haemostatic (coagulant) An agent that stimulates blood coagulation (clotting), thereby stopping or preventing haemorrhage. Preparations of natural coagulants can be applied locally to aid blood coagulation at wounds and during surgery. Thromboplastin, extracted from bovine brain, is used to reduce capillary oozing. Bovine thrombin can be used alone to reduce capillary haemorrhage, or with fibrinogen (obtained from human blood) or fibrin foam strips, which are used to establish a framework for further blood coagulation (thrombin converts fibrinogen to fibrin). These agents cannot be injected intravenously. Oxidized cellulose is a white gauze material that is applied dry to an area of haemorrhage; it then swells forming a gelatinous mass. It can be used to pack dead spaces or bleeding cavities and is absorbed over 7–10 days. Oxidized cellulose inactivates penicillin. Calcium alginate or combined sodium and calcium alginates are available as a powder or as a presoaked dressing. The salts are soluble in sodium citrate solution and can be used on wounds or internally during surgery. *Gelatin sponge can be used to stimulate coagulation or to fill dead spaces after surgery. Absorption takes about 6 weeks.

Malonic and oxalic acids act as coagulants in vivo and can be injected intramuscularly or intravenously to reduce haemorrhage, for example in nosebleed, postpartum, or after surgery. Adrenaline can be used locally as a haemostatic or used prophylatically to cause local vasoconstriction prior to surgery. Ferric chloride, aluminium ferrous sulphate, silver nitrate, and tannic acid have been used as astringents to block the ends of blood vessels and enhance coagulation, but they tend to be irritant. *See also* haemostasis.

haemothorax (haematothorax) The presence of blood in the pleural cavity. The possible causes include trauma, a blood coagulation problem, poisoning (e.g. warfarin), or a neoplasm.

hair One of numerous threadlike keratinized outgrowths of the epidermis of the mammalian *skin that help to protect and insulate the skin and provide colours and patterns for camouflage, warning and display. Each hair develops inside a tubular *hair follicle*. The part above the skin consists of three layers: an outer *cuticle*; a *cortex*, forming the bulk of the hair and containing the pigment that gives the hair its colour; and a central core (*medulla*), which may be hollow. The *root* of the hair, beneath the surface of the skin, is expanded at its base to form the *bulb*, which contains a matrix of dividing cells. As new cells are formed the older ones are pushed upwards and become keratinized to form the root and shaft. A hair may be raised by a small erector muscle in the dermis, attached to the hair follicle.

The wool fibres forming the fleece in sheep are fine hairs of small diameter that lack a medulla. Coarse kemp and hairy fibres also occur. The characteristics of the fleece vary greatly in different breeds of sheep and determine its use for different purposes.

hair ball (trichobezoar) An accumulation of hair, usually ball-shaped and firm, found in the stomach or other part of the gastrointestinal tract. Hair balls form as a result of persistent licking and swallowing of hair, and may cause indigestion or even impaction (*see* impacted). They are common in cats, which often vomit them instead of passing them in the faeces. Long-haired or Persian-type breeds are particularly prone. Calves may also suffer from hair balls, especially if denied adequate roughage, when they may compulsively lick their own coat or that of other calves. Hair balls can also affect rabbits, especially long-haired breeds. In caged animals, excessive grooming can be a sign of stress. The best treatment is dosing with *liquid paraffin, which helps lubricate expulsion of the hair ball with the faeces.

hair loss *See* alopecia.

hairy shaker disease *See* Border disease.

half-life (of a drug) The time taken for the concentration (usually the plasma concentration) of a drug to fall by 50%. The half-life is used to estimate the frequency of dosage needed to maintain an adequate concentration of the drug over a given period but prevent accumulation of the drug in the body. It can vary with species and age of animals. For example, drug metabolism is slow in neonates, therefore the half-life is extended.

halogeton poisoning A toxic condition due to the ingestion of the annual herbaceous plant *Halogeton glomeratus* (halogeton), which occurs in the western USA. It contains soluble oxalates and oxalic acid, which cause a haemorrhagic and oedematous rumen, pale swollen kidneys, and the deposition of calcium oxalate crystals in the kidney tubules. The clinical signs are depression, weakness, respiratory difficulty, salivation, coma, and death. Treatment is by oral and intravenous administration of calcium and fluids. *See also* oxalate poisoning.

halothane **(trifluorochlorobromo-ethane)** An extremely widely used inhalational anaesthetic. It is a noninflammable volatile liquid that forms nonexplosive mixtures with air and oxygen, is nonirritant to tissues, and has an intermediate blood solubility, allowing rapid induction of and recovery from anaesthesia. There is respiratory depression and hypotension due to myocardial depression, ganglion blockade, and vasodilatation in relation to dose. Halothane gives only fair analgesia and muscle relaxa-

tion, although nitrous oxide used in conjunction improves the analgesia. Halothane is metabolized in the liver and some of the reduction metabolites are hepatotoxic.

halothane challenge test A test used in pigs to screen breeding stock and detect animals susceptible to the inherited condition of *malignant hyperthermia (porcine stress syndrome). Animals are exposed to the anaesthetic *halothane for 5 minutes and blood levels of creatinine phosphokinase are measured. A rise of 20–100-fold in creatinine phosphokinase between samples taken prior to and after anaesthesia indicates susceptibility to malignant hyperthermia. Using succinylcholine with halothane may increase the sensitivity of the test.

halquinol *See* growth promoter.

hamartoma A non-neoplastic tumour-like malformation that arises because of localized disorder in the relationship of normal tissues and consequent overproduction of one or more tissue elements. They appear before or soon after birth, grow with the individual, and cease to grow when body growth finishes. They may be composed of a single type of cell, such as melanocytes in pigmented lesions, a particular type of tissue, or a mixture of tissues.

haploid **(monoploid)** Describing a nucleus, cell, or organism in which each chromosome is present only once. The gametes (i.e. spermatozoon and ovum) are haploid.

hapten A substance that binds specifically to *antibody but is unable to elicit the formation of the antibody when injected into an animal (*compare* antigen). Haptens usually have molecular weights of less than 5000. Alone, they cannot activate helper T-cells (see lymphocyte) and so trigger antibody production. However, if a hapten is conjugated to a protein antigen prior to administration, the conjugate can elicit both T- and B-cell activity with the resultant production of antibody specific for the hapten.

haptoglobin A serum protein, in the alpha *globulin class, that binds free *haemoglobin in the plasma and prevents its loss via the kidneys. Instead, the bound haemoglobin is transported to the liver, bone marrow, and spleen for degradation. In the event of *haemolysis, circulating haptoglobin is depleted; estimates of plasma haptoglobin concentrations are therefore used to detect recent haemolytic events.

Harderian gland The deep *gland of the third eyelid.

hardpad See distemper.

harelip A congenital deformity in which there is failure of fusion between the maxillary and medial nasal processes during embryonic development, resulting in a cleft in the upper lip. It is often associated with *cleft palate.

harvest mite See Trombicula.

haustrum (pl. **haustra**) One of the small pouches (sacculations) that occur in rows in the wall of the caecum and colon in the horse and pig.

Haversian canal The central canal of an *osteone.

Haversian system See osteone.

hay *Grass and other herbage dried to a moisture content of 150–200 g/kg for use as conserved fodder for livestock. The herbage is cut and dried in the field, drying time depending on the weather and initial moisture content. When the moisture content is low enough to inhibit degradation by plant and microbial enzymes, the crop is baled and stored. Alternatively, for barn-dried hay, the hay is baled soon after cutting, stacked in a barn, and air blown through the stack to reduce the moisture content. Traditionally the crop is cut when mature to reduce its moisture content and therefore the drying time, although this drastically reduces the nutritive value of the hay. To avoid dependence on weather conditions or the need for expensive drying equipment, *silage has increased in popularity as an alternative method of conserving grass. Compare dried grass.

hay fever An allergic inflammation of the nasal passages caused by *hypersensitivity to pollen.

haylage A form of *silage with a moisture content intermediate between *hay and normal silage. Grass is wilted before being chopped and ensiled. Haylage often suffers by combining the higher nutrient losses in the field associated with haymaking with the higher losses of nutrients after harvest associated with ensiling.

headfly A small non-biting *fly, Hydrotaea irritans. Headflies greatly irritate cattle and sheep, settling on an animal often in very large numbers and feeding on secretions from the eyes, nose, or small wounds. They often accumulate on cows' teats, transmitting bacteria such as those that cause *summer mastitis. In the UK, damage to sheep is largely confined to those breeds with relatively little wool on their heads, although quite severe head wounds can result. Headflies can be controlled by the use of suitable *insecticides, and insect repellents. Sheep can be pro-

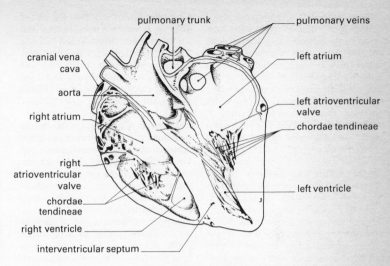

Section of heart of horse

tected by head caps although these are inconvenient to use.

health mark (EEC) A mark, in a prescribed form, applied to carcasses and portions of red meat and poultry meat and to containers of meat products indicating that they have been produced and inspected in accordance with the appropriate EEC Directive and may be used in trade between member states of the Community.

heart A hollow muscular cone-shaped organ, situated in the thorax between the lungs with the pointed end (apex) directed downwards and tailwards. Its wall consists largely of cardiac muscle (*myocardium), with an inner lining (*endocardium) and an outer protective *pericardium. It is divided by a septum into separate right and left halves, each of which is divided into a dorsal atrium and ventral *ventricle (see illustration). Deoxygenated blood from the *venae cavae and *coronary sinus passes through the right atrium to the right ventricle. This contracts

and pumps blood to the lungs via the *pulmonary trunk. The newly oxygenated blood returns to the left atrium via the *pulmonary veins and passes to the left ventricle. This forcefully contracts, pumping blood out to the body via the *aorta. The direction of blood flow within the heart is controlled by *valves, and the muscle contractions are organized by the heart's specialized *conducting system.

heart attack An acute form of *heart failure, causing some degree of collapse and often death of the patient. The term is not commonly used in veterinary medicine. See cardiac arrest; myocardial infarction.

heart base tumour See chemodectoma.

heart block A condition in which the pumping action of the heart is impaired due to an abnormality of the *conducting system of the heart. Damage to the specialized conducting

heart failure

fibres, either of a physiological or pathological nature, will affect the synchrony between the contractions of the atria and ventricles. Heart block may be only partial, in which case the impulses are delayed or not all of them are conducted, or complete, in which case the ventricles beat at their own intrinsic rate. It may be further subdivided into *right-sided* and *left-sided* block. *See also* heart failure.

heart failure An inability of the heart to provide sufficient output to maintain the blood circulation. It may be caused by any of various congenital defects or diseases that reduce the efficiency of contraction of the heart muscle, affect nervous control of heart muscle, or overload or damage the heart muscle. The most common are *endocarditis, *myocarditis, *pericarditis, and *valvular disease. *Acute heart failure* causes rapid collapse and coma or sudden death (*see* cardiac arrest). *Subacute heart failure* has less rapid onset and is associated with coughing, faster breathing rate, a fast weak pulse, abnormal heart sounds (*murmurs), and irregularities in the heart rhythm (*see* arrhythmia). The oral and ocular mucous membranes are often pale or blue. In *chronic heart failure*, any of the above signs may develop over a period. The condition may affect a particular side of the heart: *left-sided failure* is associated with coughing and increased breathing rate; *right-sided failure* leads to fluid accumulation and hence swelling in the abdomen and limbs (ascites and oedema).

Four main drug groups are used to treat heart failure in domestic animals. Cardiac *glycosides (e.g. *digitalis) have a positive *inotropic effect on the heart muscles causing increased strength of contraction. *Vasodilators widen the blood vessels and increase the vascular space, thereby encouraging fluid to move

from the tissues. *Diuretics act on the kidneys to increase urine output and so relieve the oedema and ascites. Finally, xanthines act on the heart muscle to strengthen contractions and encourage a normal rhythm and beat. *See also* cardiomyopathy; heart block; myocardial infarction.

heartwater A tick-transmitted disease of domestic and wild ruminants characterized by fever, convulsions, collapse, and death and caused by the rickettsia *Cowdria ruminantium*. The disease is enzootic in Africa south of the Sahara, its distribution being determined by that of the tick vector, namely *Amblyomma* spp. Following an incubation period of 1–4 weeks, cattle develop a high fever with a gradual onset of nervous signs, such as circling, abnormal gait, drowsiness, and then hyperexcitability with eventual collapse, convulsions, and death. Feeding and rumination continue well into the course of the disease. Nonindigenous cattle are particularly susceptible to the acute form of the disease and may collapse and die before the onset of nervous signs, whereas indigenous animals may develop only a transient fever or show no clinical signs. Very young animals have a high natural resistance to the disease. Control is by elimination of the *tick vector or by inducing immunity with deliberate infection followed by treatment with *tetracyclines. Other name: **veld sickness.**

heartworm *See* Dirofilaria.

heat exhaustion (heat stroke; hyperthermia) Distress due to an excessive rise in *body temperature, resulting from either an unduly hot environment or abnormally high production of body heat. The signs are extreme weakness, trembling, and collapse. Rapid pulse and breathing commonly occur and body temperature is greatly elevated, possibly as high as 43°C. Urgent treatment is required otherwise convulsions and death rapidly ensue. Options include immersion in cold water and moving the animal into shade. Improved ventilation helps prevent the problem. However, it is vital to distinguish the effects of *fever from those of heat exhaustion.

Various factors affect susceptibility to heat exhaustion. Not only temperature of the environment but also the relative humidity and ventilation are important. For example, dogs left in cars on sunny days without adequate ventilation are particularly vulnerable. Species differ in their methods of cooling. Horses sweat profusely when dissipating heat generated by galloping, whereas ruminants sweat very little but increase their breathing rate to promote heat loss from the lining of the nostrils and respiratory passages. Dogs pant actively with a protruded tongue to give additional surface for cooling. Birds too rely principally on heat loss from respiratory surfaces. In all species, cooling via the skin depends on the dilation of subcutaneous blood vessels and demands an increased blood volume and hence water intake. Water is also used for dissipating body heat by evaporation from the skin surface (sweating) and mucosa. Therefore lack of body water is a crucial factor in susceptibility to heat exhaustion. Another factor is loss of salt (sodium chloride) in sweat, which may lead to imbalance of tissue electrolytes and heat cramps. *See also* malignant hyperthermia; porcine stress syndrome.

heat stroke *See* heat exhaustion.

heaves *See* broken wind.

heavy hog A large meat pig that is too heavy to be sold as a *baconer. It is used mainly for the manufacture of meat products and is also referred to as a manufacturing pig.

hecto- *Prefix denoting* a hundred.

heifer A young female ox from birth until slaughter or until its first, or sometimes second, pregnancy, after which it becomes a *cow. *See* cattle.

Heinz body An abnormal microscopic inclusion within the cytoplasm of certain red blood cells (erythrocytes). It is probably caused by the precipitation of denatured *haemoglobin, the cause of which is supposedly some oxidative disturbance. The phenomenon is frequent in poisoning by haemolytic substances, such as phenothiazine and phenyl hydrazine. A structure indistinguishable from a Heinz body occurs in a proportion of the red cells of some normal domestic cats and of other members of the cat family.

helc- (helco-) *Prefix denoting* an ulcer.

Helenium poisoning A toxic condition due to the ingestion of any of various perennial or annual herbaceous plants of the genus *Helenium*, distributed throughout the USA and including the bitterweeds, staggerweed, and sneezeweeds (*H. tenuifolium*, *H. autumnale*, *H. nudiflorum*, *H. microcephalum*, and *H. hoopesii*). The toxic principles are a glycoside (dugaldin) and the sesquiterpene lactones, helenalin and hymenoxin. These cause depression, weakness, salivation, pronounced vomiting, emaciation, and death. Treatment is of the clinical signs.

helicopter chicks *See* runting and stunting syndrome.

helio- *Prefix denoting* the sun.

helminth A general name for any parasitic worm, i.e. one of the *flukes (trematodes), *tapeworms (cestodes), or *roundworms (nematodes).

hem- (hema-, hemo-, hemat(o)-) (*US*) *See* haem-.

hemeralopia (day blindness) The condition in which vision is comparatively good in dim light but poor in bright light. It is difficult to assess in animals.

hemi- *Prefix denoting* the right or left half of the body.

hemiplegia Paralysis or weakness affecting one side of the body. In animals it commonly results from predominantly unilateral damage to the spinal cord associated with intervertebral disc protrusions or explosions, spinal neoplasia, or occasionally vertebral canal stenosis (narrowing) associated with vertebral malformation and instability. In humans the most common cause is damage to the motor areas of the cerebral cortex, for instance due to impaired blood supply as in a 'stroke'.

hemisphere *See* cerebral hemisphere; cerebellum.

hemizygous Describing genes that are carried on unpaired chromosomes, for example the genes on the unpaired *sex chromosomes in male mammals or female birds. Thus, only one *allele of each hemizygous gene is present. *Compare* heterozygous; homozygous.

hemlock poisoning A toxic condition arising from the ingestion of hemlock (*Conium maculatum*), also known as California fern in the USA. All parts of the plant contain coniine, an alkaloid with a nicotine-like action (*see* nicotine poisoning). For example, 2 kg of the plant is fatal for a horse. It causes dilated pupils, staggering gait, rapid pulse, and laboured breathing, which fails rapidly. On post-mortem examination, the characteristic mousy smell of the plant is noticeable. Treatment includes the use of purgatives and also atropine to assist cardiac function. The ingestion of hemlock by pregnant sows has produced abnormalities in their offspring.

hemlock water dropwort poisoning A toxic condition caused by ingestion of hemlock water dropwort (*Oenanthe crocata*). The plant is found on the banks of streams and in other marshy places, such as ponds and ditches. All parts of the plant, but particularly the tubers, are attractive to grazing animals, and access is facilitated by ditching and draining operations, which leave the stems and tubers lying in adjacent fields. Ingestion by cattle of 0.5 kg or more is followed by the rapid onset of clinical signs, which are due to an alkaloid, oenanthotoxin, with a strychnine-like action. The pupils become dilated, there is salivation and abdominal pain, and muscular spasms lead to violent convulsions and death from asphyxia. Ingestion of a sublethal dose will produce clinical signs followed by recovery. Convulsions may be controlled by the injection of *diazepam or by intravenous barbiturates. Pigs can survive a potentially lethal dose by vomiting. Cowbane or water hemlock (*Cicuta virosa*) is found in the same habitats and contains the alkaloid cicutoxin, which causes similar toxic effects. *See also* strychnine poisoning.

henbane poisoning *See* deadly nightshade poisoning.

hepadnavirus A family of DNA *viruses characterized by having DNA that is partly double stranded and partly single stranded. The best understood member is the human hepatitis B virus.

heparin A mucopolysaccharide *anticoagulant found in the granules of *mast cells. It acts by antagonizing the action of thrombin on fibrinogen (*see* coagulation). An extracted purified form of heparin is used to prevent and treat blood coagulation disorders, and to prevent coagulation in blood samples taken for laboratory investigation.

hepat- (hepato-) *Prefix denoting* the liver. Example: *hepatorenal* (relating to the liver and kidney).

hepatic Relating to the liver.

hepatitis Strictly any inflammatory condition of the liver, including the biliary system. The term may properly be used to describe liver lesions that are known to be caused by or associated with infectious or parasitic agents, or lesions exhibiting a true inflammatory response irrespective of cause. Hepatitis thus encompasses some degenerative conditions of unknown aetiology that invoke a coexisting inflammatory response. The inflammatory changes may be focal or diffuse; acute, subacute, or chronic. Although many such conditions specifically affect the liver, some primarily nonhepatic diseases produce secondary hepatitis. Nonspecific hepatitis with no overt clinical disease is a relatively common autopsy finding in many species.

Hepatitis may sometimes be precipitated or preceded by *cholangitis, although inflammation of the intrahepatic bile ducts and canaliculi alone (*cholangiolitis*) is rare. More commonly seen is *cholangiohepatitis*, involving portal tracts and surrounding periportal hepatic parenchyma, particularly in farm animals (e.g. sheep, cattle). This is usually associated with parasitic infestation in the biliary system, which predisposes to secondary bacterial infection. Cholangitis resulting from bacterial infection alone follows bile stasis in the major or common bile ducts. Such situations

may arise with occluding neoplasia of the pancreas (e.g. in dogs and cats), scarring of the pancreatic and hepatic major ducts following acute or chronic *pancreatitis (e.g. in dogs, cats, and horses), or *lymphadenitis of hepatic hilar nodes (e.g. in ruminants and pigs). Cholangiohepatitis due to biliary calculi is rare but does occur in the ox.

The many causes of hepatitis fall into several categories (see table). Among viral diseases, hepatitis is a feature of, most notably, *canine viral hepatitis, *Wesselbron disease, *Rift Valley fever, and *equine serum hepatitis. Hepatitis may also occur in *canine parvovirus infection and in feline parvovirus infection (*see* feline viral enteritis). Herpesvirus infection can cause hepatitis in foals, calves, lambs, and puppies; liver lesions may be seen especially in aborted foetuses from infected mares and cows.

Hepatitis due to bacterial infection is common in farm animals and horses, but uncommon in dogs and cats. In ruminants and pigs contiguous spread of inflammation/infection from adjacent peritoneal lesions to involve the liver is common, and in cattle direct implantation of bacteria may occur (as occurs in *traumatic reticulitis). Haematogenous spread of bacterial infection via the hepatic artery or hepatic portal vein is common in large animals, and spread of infection via umbilical veins is seen in calves, piglets, lambs, and foals (*see* navel ill; omphalophlebitis). In the dog and cat bacterial hepatitis is associated with ascending infections of the bile ducts. A wide spectrum of bacterial pathogens cause focal hepatitis in different species (see table).

Nonspecific liver abscesses in beef cattle may be associated with ruminal ulceration caused by feeding high-cereal rations (*see* rumenitis). *Black disease (infectious necrotic hepatitis), caused by the bacterium *Clostridium noyvi*, is most common in sheep and

hepatitis

Types of hepatitis and their principal causes

Type	Principal causes	Particular species affected
VIRAL HEPATITIS	Herpesviruses	Foals, calves, lambs, puppies
	Canine viral hepatitis (adenovirus)	Domestic and wild canids
	Parvovirus infections	Felids and dogs
	Feline infectious peritonitis (coronavirus)	Domestic cats
	Rift Valley fever	Lambs, calves (adult ruminants)
	Wesselbron disease	Lambs (calves) and birds
	Equine serum hepatitis	Horses
BACTERIAL HEPATITIS	*Listeria monocytogenes*	Foetal/neonatal lambs, calves, piglets
	Shigella equinilis	Foals
	Pasteurella pseudotuberculosis	Lambs (dogs/cats)
	Pasteurella haemolytica	Lambs
	Haemophilus agni	Lambs
	Salmonella spp.	All species
	Mycobacterium tuberculosis	All species
	Nocardia asteroides	Dogs
	Clostridium noyvi	Cattle
	Clostridium haemolyticum	Cattle
	Bacillus piliformis	Foals, cats, mice
FUNGAL HEPATITIS (rare)	Possibly secondary infection or associated with blastomycosis, histoplasmosis, coccidioidomycosis	
PARASITIC HEPATITIS	*Fasciola*	Sheep, cattle
	Dicrocoelium	Sheep, cattle
	Opisthorchis	Dogs, cats, other carnivores
	Ascaris (milkspot liver)	Pigs
	Taenia (cysticercosis)	Sheep, cattle
	Echinococcus (hydatidosis)	Horses, sheep
TOXIC/DRUG-RELATED HEPATITIS	Inorganics (e.g. copper, iron, arsenic, phosphorus, mercury, tannic acid) Organic compounds (e.g. carbon tetrachloride, chloroform, dieldrin, tetrachlorethane, dimethylnitrosamine, cresols, pitch, gossypol)	

Type	Principal causes	Particular species affected
	Poisonous plants (e.g. ragwort, heliotrope) Fungal toxins (e.g. aflatoxins) Drugs (e.g. tetracyclines, rifampicin, steroid contraceptives, novobiocin, isoniazid, arsenicals, mebendazole, acetaminophen)	
NUTRITIONAL/ METABOLIC HEPATITIS	Methionine, cystine deficiencies	Rats
	?Vitamin E/selenium imbalance	Pigs
	?Cobalt deficiency (white liver disease)	Sheep
	?High-clover pastures	Sheep
	Disordered copper metabolism (inherited)	Certain dog breeds
CHRONIC ACTIVE HEPATITIS	Autoimmune-mediated?	Dogs

is strongly associated with liver damage due to fluke infestation (e.g. *Fasciola hepatica* in the UK and *Dicrocoelium dendriticum* in France). Bovine *haemoglobinuria caused by *Clostridium haemolyticum* involves liver lesions similar to those of black disease. *Bacillus piliformis* infection causes *Tyzzers disease in foals, cats, and laboratory mammals, such as mice and Rhesus monkeys. At autopsy the liver is very enlarged with multiple necrotic foci.

Hepatitis caused by fungal agents alone is rare; secondary fungal growth may occur following an initial necrotizing insult. In dogs in North America, however, hepatitis associated with *blastomycosis, *histoplasmosis, and *coccidioidomycosis has been reported.

Parasites, principally helminths, are probably the most important cause of hepatitis in farm animals worldwide. Many helminths inhabit the bile ducts and cause liver damage incidentally or as a result of their excretory or metabolic activities. Alternatively, the adult forms may be gut parasites that travel through hepatic parenchyma as part of their normal life cycle or accidentally. Damage may take the form of trauma (necrosis and haemorrhage) with eventual healing and scarring, or parasite larvae may encyst in liver tissue resulting in chronic, often calcifying, lesions.

Nematode parasites cause relatively little hepatitis, although the larval forms of *Ascaris suum* are responsible for chronic focal hepatitis, known as *milkspot liver in pigs. Tapeworm larvae may cause focal hepatitis of varying degrees of severity, for example the larval forms of *Taenia* in sheep and cattle (*see* cysticercus). Generally, however, aberrant cysts of these tapeworms become abortive and eventually form small foci with no apparent clinical signs. *Echinococcus* spp. may produce large cysts in the liver of horses and sheep (*see* hydatidosis).

The most important parasites causing hepatitis are the flukes, notably liver flukes of the genus *Fasciola*, which affect sheep and cattle worldwide (*see* fascioliasis). *Dicrocoelium dendriticum*, the lancet fluke, is normally found in the bile ducts of sheep and cattle. It causes a less severe cholangiohepatitis than *Fasciola hepatica*, with fibrous thickening and marked mucous gland hyperplasia of the larger bile ducts. *Platynosomum concinnum*, a parasite of cats in southern Asia and South America, is similar to *D. dendriticum*. Heavy infestations of *Opisthorchis* flukes can cause hepatitis in dogs, cats, and other carnivores. The protozoan parasite *Toxoplasma gondii*, of cats, dogs, and sheep, may occur in the liver and provoke foci of necrosis.

Hepatitis due to toxic agents or drugs occurs sporadically and can be dramatic. Duration of exposure to the agent is crucial. The hepatitis may be mild with cloudy swelling only, or more severe with widespread necrosis, depending on the dose of toxic agent and its affinity for liver tissue. Female animals are said to be more susceptible, and deficiencies of carbohydrate and protein enhance the effects of toxicity. A wide range of agents have been implicated (see table). Poisonous plants are frequently hepatotoxic (e.g. ragwort, heliotrope), while fungal toxins, notably aflatoxins (*see* aflatoxicosis), can cause lipidosis or chronic hepatitis with fibrosis.

Drug-induced hepatitis may be manifested as cytotoxic or cholestatic hepatitis, or a combination of the two. The cytotoxic types have a more severe prognosis, with chronic active hepatitis (CAH; *see* canine chronic active hepatitis), fatty change, fibrosis, and hepatic vein thromboses as sequelae. Drugs may damage the structural integrity of hepatocytes (e.g. chloroform, carbon tetrachloride), or they may block metabolic pathways of hepatocytes leading to secondary structural change (e.g. ethanol, tetracyclines). Others cause allergy-like sensitization with repeat dosing, or are metabolized to hepatotoxic products resulting in necrosis and jaundice (e.g. mebendazole, acetaminophen in cats). Nutritional/metabolic hepatitis is sporadic. Methionine and cystine deficiencies cause cirrhosis and hepatic necrosis respectively in rats. There is some evidence that vitamin E and selenium imbalance in the diets of pigs may result in hepatic necrosis, although this may be part of a nutritional myopathy syndrome (*see* porcine stress syndrome). Cobalt deficiency has been associated with a 'white liver disease' in young sheep in New Zealand, and hepatic necrosis is reported in lambs in California grazing high levels of trefoil clover pastures. Bedlington terriers and some other breeds of dog (e.g. West Highland white terriers) have a genetic predisposition (autosomal recessive) to the accumulation of copper in hepatocytes. The condition manifests itself either as an acute usually fatal disease in young adults associated with stress, or as a more chronic progressive condition. A third group may be asymptomatic clinically. Canine chronic active hepatitis, thought possibly to be an autoimmune disease, may also have a genetic predisposition.

hepatization The pathological alteration of a normally spongy tissue into firm liver-like tissue. It may be used to describe consolidated lung tissue in cases of severe pneumonia.

hepatocellular carcinoma A malignant liver tumour seen especially in cattle, sheep, and dogs but also reported in other species. The lesion is generally a large multilobulated mass that is sharply demarcated from adjacent normal liver tissue, which it progressively replaces. The colour is variegated, with grey, yellow, red, brown, and green areas representing tumour tissue, necrosis or fatty change, haemorrhage, surviving hepatocytes, and bile-staining respectively. Prognosis is poor because of the replacement of normal with nonfunctional tissue, possible rupture of the liver with fatal intra-abdominal haemorrhage, or metastases to regional lymph nodes, peritoneum and omentum, and the lungs.

hepatocyte One of the principal cells of the liver. They are arranged in cords, forming the liver *parenchyma. The surface of the hepatocytes facing into the perisinusoidal space (*see* sinusoid) has numerous microvilli to facilitate the exchange of various substances with the blood. The hepatocytes produce bile, which is secreted into the tiny bile canaliculi interposed between the hepatocytes.

hepatoid Describing cells that resemble or are arranged in a similar pattern to liver cells. For example, a hepatoid *adenoma occurs in the para-anal region in the dog.

hept- (hepta-) *Prefix denoting* seven.

herbicide poisoning *See* paraquat poisoning; sodium chlorate poisoning.

heredity *See* genetics.

heritability A measure of the amount of variation due to genetic causes present in a given population in a speci-

fied environment. Estimates of heritability are important in devising selective breeding programmes. It is desirable that any trait to be improved has a high heritability, with its variation controlled by the alleles of a large number of genes. Characters such as final adult weight, carcass traits, and morphological features tend to have greater heritability than characters associated with reproduction and survival of the young. The heritability of a trait can be measured (and expressed numerically from 0 to 1) by statistical comparison of sibs, of mothers with offspring or of fathers with offspring, or by half-sib relationships. As a selection programme proceeds so the heritability of the selected trait falls as the undesired alleles at the various genes are removed, so causing the genetic variability to drop. When a population breeds true for any trait, the heritability of that trait is nil.

hermaphrodite An animal with both male and female reproductive organs including both ovarian and testicular tissue. This condition is very rare. *Pseudohermaphrodites* possess gonadal tissue of only one type, and are either male or female. The condition is more common and usually affects goats and pigs. *See* intersex.

hernia The protrusion of a tissue or organ outside the cavity in which it normally lies. In domestic animals hernias may be congenital or acquired, internal or external. *Internal hernias* affect internal organs, principally the intestines, without the formation of a hernial sac. Internal hernias through natural orifices are uncommon, but loops of small intestine may pass through the foramen of Winslow (epiploic foramen) in the equine omentum. Omental and mesenteric hernias occur when bowel loops pass through acquired tears in the greater or lesser omentum and mesentery respectively; they are uncommon.

An *external hernia* consists of a hernial sac, usually formed from an out-pouching of the peritoneum, covered by subcutaneous or connective tissue with an outer skin layer. A hernial ring is sometimes present as a potential constricting structure; it can be a natural orifice or an acquired pathological aperture.

The more common types of hernia seen in veterinary species are as follows:

Umbilical hernia Probably the commonest type, these are often congenital and may be an inherited defect. The hernial sac is formed by abdominal peritoneum and skin and its contents vary from omental or peritoneal fat to loops of small or large intestine, largely depending on the size of the hernial ring. Complications arise when bowel loops or omentum become trapped (*incarcerated*) in the hernial sac with resulting necrosis or degeneration and ensuing peritonitis. Umbilical hernia is common in pigs, calves, puppies, and foals. Repair is usually effected by reduction of the contents and sac by appropriate surgical techniques; large hernial rings may require the use of synthetic inserts to close the defect.

Inguinal/scrotal hernia These occur when portions of omentum, peritoneal fat, or loops of bowel pass down the inguinal canal and, in the male, occupy the cavity of the tunica vaginalis alongside the testis or its vascular supply. The degree of herniation depends on the diameter of the patent internal inguinal ring. In males this orifice normally remains open but its size and therefore the tendency to herniation is inherited. Scrotal hernias of some duration usually result in testicular degeneration or atrophy as a result of hypoxia following vascular congestion or ischaemia. These types of hernia are not uncommon in cattle, sheep, and horses, and are common in pigs presented for open castration, where eventration of bowel loops may occur. Such hernias can be opened and the hernial sac reduced and obliterated by suturing appropriately. Females are not usually affected by inguinal hernias although the bitch does have a normally patent inguinal ring which, if large enough, may allow herniation of the vaginal process and possibly a uterine horn. The latter event is particularly serious if the bitch is pregnant or develops pyometra since the enlarged horn may become incarcerated in the inguinal region.

Perineal hernia This is usually seen in adult male dogs, often ones with enlarged prostates. There is possibly an inherited predisposition but a hormonal influence in the weakening of perineal fascia and the coccygeal muscle/anal sphincter region has also been implicated. Abdominal straining produces herniation of retroperitoneal pelvic fat initially, with progression to involve the rectum, prostate, and more rarely the bladder. Inclusion of the bladder usually precipitates an acute urethral obstruction. The herniation is usually unilateral but may affect both sides. Surgical repair aims to repair the pelvic diaphragm by the use of coccygeal or similar muscle transfixation. More recently attempts at repair using heterograft implants of collagen (e.g. pig skin preparations) have had limited success. Recurrence of the herniation following continued tenesmus is often a problem and any investigation and therapy should seek to remove predisposing causes, such as prostatic hypertrophy.

Ventral hernia These affect the ventral abdominal peritoneum. Although uncommon, they may occur in horses, sheep, and cattle, typically appearing during pregnancy as a result of the combined weight of alimentary organs and gravid uterus; previous trauma or weakening is a predisposing factor. The degree of tearing of peritoneum is usually so great that surgical repair is not entirely successful, if attempted.

Femoral hernia These are rare, developing from peritoneal outpouching through the triangular space between the abdominal wall and course of the femoral artery supplying the hindlimb. Such hernias are associated with congenital conditions or with exercise trauma and may be rarely seen in animals engaged in strenuous exercise, such as showjumping or steeplechase horses. *See also* diaphragmatic rupture/hernia.

hernio- *Prefix denoting* a hernia.

herpes mamillitis *See* bovine herpes mamillitis.

herpesvirus A family of DNA *viruses, members of which infect most domestic animals. They have enveloped icosahedral *capsids containing a large DNA molecule (MW = 10^8). Herpesviruses can interact with their host cells to give a lytic infection or enter a latent state (*see* latency), which can cause recurrent infections. Diseases caused by herpesviruses include *Aujeszky's disease, *infectious bovine rhinotracheitis, and equine abortion, plus a number of generally mild skin diseases. The family includes the *cytomegaloviruses, but these are substantially different in their physical and biological properties from other herpesviruses.

Hertztod disease *See* porcine stress syndrome.

heter- (hetero-) *Prefix denoting* difference; dissimilarity.

heterochromatin Chromosome material (*see* chromatin) that stains most deeply when the cell is not dividing. It is thought not to represent major genes but may be involved in controlling these genes, and also in controlling mitosis and development. *Compare* euchromatin.

heterogametic Producing two kinds of *gametes – one carrying male determinants, the other lacking such determinants or carrying female determinants. Male mammals and female birds are heterogametic (*see* sex chromosome).

heterograft An old term for *xenograft.

heterograft (xenograft) A living tissue graft that is made from one animal species to another. For example, attempts have been made to graft animal tissues into humans.

heterokaryon A cell containing nuclei of two different genetic constitutions. This forms part of the normal life cycle in some fungi. Some mammalian cells, even of different species, can be fused in the laboratory; there is frequently preferential loss of the chromosomes of one species, and analysis of gene function in such cells allows genes to be assigned to specific chromosomes.

heteroplasty The grafting of tissue from an animal of one species to another.

heterosis (hybrid vigour) The superiority of a crossbreed over either of its parents (in fitness, performance, etc.). The degree of heterosis shown by an animal is related to the proportion of its genes that are *heterozygous. Animals showing marked heterosis are thus highly heterozygous and cannot breed true. Each *F_1 generation must be produced anew by crossing parents from two unrelated inbred lines that are *homozygous for all or most genes. Only crosses between particular inbred lines show heterosis, and many different such lines need to be tested to find the

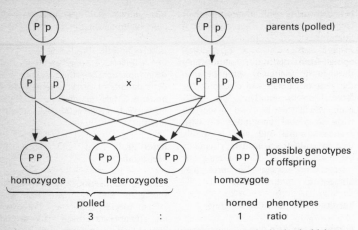

Diagram illustrating the results of a cross between two cattle, both of which are heterozygous for the polled gene [P (polled) is the dominant allele; p (horned) is recessive]

optimum parental pairing. Although highly heterozygous, all the members of a cross between two inbred lines are genetically identical, since they all receive identical sets of alleles from each parent. This genetic homogeneity allows optimum husbandry conditions for the F_1 generation to be precisely defined, enabling maximum production efficiency of the particular genotype.

Heterosis is a property of the entire *genome rather than of individual genes, and there is now some evidence that its origins relate more to optimal interactions between gene products than to direct superiority of the heterozygote. *See also* inbreeding.

heterotrophic (organotrophic) Describing those organisms (known as heterotrophs) that use complex organic compounds to synthesize their own organic materials. This group includes the majority of bacteria and all animals and fungi.

heterozygous Describing an organism having two different *alleles for

any pair of its genes. If there is no dominance between the alleles or if they show *codominance, the characteristics of the heterozygote will be intermediate between the two homozygotes for either allele (*see* homozygous). If there is complete dominance (*see* dominant) between the alleles the heterozygote will be indistinguishable phenotypically (*see* phenotype) from an organism having two copies of the dominant allele (the homozygous dominant). Hence, if a heterozygote is mated to a homozygous recessive, 50% of the offspring can be expected to carry the dominant allele from the heterozygote and thus show the dominant trait. If a heterozygote is mated to a dominant homozygote, all the offspring will carry at least one dominant allele and will be phenotypically identical. The cross between two heterozygotes will, if dominance exists between the alleles, produce a 3:1 ratio of young showing the dominant trait to those showing the recessive (see illustration). Heterozygotes will not therefore breed true since crosses between them will always produce some homozygotes.

Some breeds are characterized by the heterozygous states, e.g. Manx cats and dexter cattle, and the breeder of these must accept the continual production of some unsuitable types. There is some evidence that many genes are at their most efficient in an organism when they are in the heterozygous state. Animals that are highly heterozygous (i.e. heterozygous at a very large number of genes) can be produced by crossing specific inbred lines. These animals may show much enhanced performance over their parents and over the general population and are said to exhibit *heterosis or hybrid vigour. *See also* carrier.

hex- (hexa-) *Prefix denoting* six.

hexacanth *See* oncosphere.

hexachlorophane A chlorinated diphenol antiseptic with bactericidal properties but poor activity against viruses, fungi, and spores. Also its activity is reduced in alkaline pH and in the presence of organic matter. It is used as a skin antiseptic prior to surgery, but is highly lipid-soluble and can penetrate intact skin. Its use as an antiseptic has declined because of reports of toxicity in babies and puppies. The central nervous system is affected causing blindness and convulsions.

hexamine A urinary antiseptic and diuretic which is now rarely used. It is given orally and is excreted at the kidneys, where it is active in acidic urine (pH below 5.5), releasing ammonia and formaldehyde. These have antibacterial actions in the bladder and lower urinary tract, the diuretic effect resulting from irritation of tubular cells. High doses may cause gastrointestinal or urinary tract irritation, with vomiting, albuminuria, and haematuria. Hexamine is used in

combination with urinary acidifiers (e.g. sodium acid phosphate, ascorbic acid).

hexamitiasis A parasitic disease of turkeys, game birds, and occasionally chicks caused by the flagellate protozoan *Hexamita meleagridis*. Clinical signs are diarrhoea, lethargy, weight loss, and occasionally death. Drugs used for control are the same as for *blackhead.

hexoestrol A synthetic *oestrogen that was formerly used as a growth promoter for livestock. Its use in food-producing animals is now illegal in the UK and many other countries due to the occurrence of oestrogenic and carcinogenic tissue residues in carcasses.

hexokinase An enzyme that catalyses the conversion of glucose to glucose-6-phosphate. This is the first stage of *glycolysis.

hexosamine The amino derivative of a *hexose sugar. The two most important hexosamines are *glucosamine and galactosamine.

hexose A *monosaccharide with six carbon atoms. Hexose sugars are the sugars most frequently found in food. The most important hexose is *glucose.

hiatus An opening or aperture. For example, the diaphragm contains hiatuses for the oesophagus and aorta.

Hibitane Tradename for chlorhexidine hydrochloride, an antiseptic and disinfectant with a broad spectrum of activity against Gram-positive and Gram-negative bacteria. It is used in teat dips for dairy cattle, for preoperative skin preparations, in eye ointments, and in antiseptic pessaries for the treatment of metritis. Toxicity is low with a low incidence of local skin irritation, and it remains active in the presence of tissue debris and pus. It can be used in alcoholic or aqueous solution or in combination with quaternary ammonium compounds.

hidr- (hidro-) *Prefix denoting* sweat. Example: *hidropoiesis* (formation of).

hilus (*pl.* **hila**) A hollow situated on the surface of an organ, such as the kidney or spleen, at which structures such as blood vessels, nerve fibres, and ducts enter or leave it.

hindbrain 1. (in embryology) The most caudal part of the embryonic brain, which eventually develops into the *cerebellum, *pons, and *medulla oblongata. 2. (in anatomy) Those parts of the brain that have developed from the embryonic hindbrain, i.e. the cerebellum, pons, and medulla oblongata.

hindgut The caudal part of the embryonic gut, which gives rise to the descending colon, rectum, urinary bladder, and much of the urethra. *See also* cloaca (def. 2.).

hip 1. The joint formed by the *acetabulum of the *os coxae and the head of the femur. It is a ball-and-socket type of joint and allows flexion, extension, abduction, adduction, and rotation of the hindlimb. 2. The region of the body surrounding the hip joint.

hip dysplasia Abnormal development of the hip joint causing a tendency for the head of the femur to slip out of the acetabulum. The condition is common in most large breeds of dog, with the notable exception of the greyhound. It most commonly causes problems while the dog is rapidly growing (at 4–8 months old) or later in life when secondary arthritic changes have occurred in the hip. Clinical signs include pain on rising,

reluctance to exercise or climb, and a rolling gait. It is best diagnosed by radiography under general anaesthesia. Mild cases may be treated with rest and possibly painkilling drugs, whereas more severe cases may need corrective surgery or even replacement of the joint with an artificial hip. The disease is caused by a combination of heredity and environmental factors, such as feeding and exercise. The *British Veterinary Association runs a screening programme in conjunction with the *Kennel Club: a panel of experts gives each hip a score of between 0 and 53; the lower the score, the lesser the degree of hip dysplasia. In North America a similar programme is run by the Orthopedic Foundation for Animals. Breeders can then select their breeding stock from dogs and bitches with the best hips possible.

hippocampus (*pl.* **hippocampi**) A long curved portion of the cerebral cortex in the brain that projects into the temporal horn of the lateral ventricle. Fibres leaving the hippocampus form a thin layer of white matter on its ventricular surface (the *alveus of the hippocampus) and converge to form the *fimbria of the hippocampus, which is continuous with the *fornix. The hippocampus and its connections form parts of the *limbic system.

hist- (histio-, histo-) *Prefix denoting* tissue.

histaminase An *enzyme that degrades *histamine.

histamine An *amine derived from the amino acid histidine. It is produced in many diferent tissues, especially by *mast cells, and is involved in the inflammatory response. It has pronounced pharmacological effects, including the dilation of blood capillaries and contraction of smooth muscle. Histamine is responsible for some of the clinical signs occurring in *anaphylaxis and allergic reaction (*see* hypersensitivity), and its effects can be countered by the administration of *antihistamine and *anti-inflammatory drugs.

histidine *See* amino acid; histamine.

histiocyte A connective tissue *macrophage.

histiocytoma A skin tumour comprising masses of histiocytic cells and occurring in dogs. It mainly affects young animals, particularly on the pinna of the ear and the distal extremities. It grows rapidly, reaching a diameter of 1–2 cm in a few weeks and producing a well-circumscribed dome-shaped lesion that is freely movable over the underlying tissues. Hair is lost from the affected region and epidermal ulceration is common. Spontaneous regression normally takes place over a period of months. Surgical excision is generally curative although a few lesions recur locally.

histiocytosis A condition in which there is an abnormal accumulation and/or proliferation of connective tissue macrophages, otherwise known as reticuloendothelial cells or *histiocytes. The condition occurs in association with a large number of enzyme deficiencies, which are well described in humans and occasionally reported in other animals. These deficiencies lead to the accumulation in the histiocytes of glycogen, lipids, or mucopolysaccharides. Histiocytosis also occurs in the canine cutaneous *histiocytoma, a lesion with a frequently benign clinical course.

histochemistry The study of the identification and distribution of chemical compounds within and between cells, by means of stains, indicators, and light and electron microscopy.

histocompatibility The degree to which the immune system of an animal will tolerate the presence of foreign tissue. Histocompatibility is the principal factor in determining the acceptance or rejection of grafts, and it is partly governed by the genetic relationship between the donor and recipient of the graft. Thus grafts transferred between sites on the same body (*autografts*) normally elicit no immune response. Grafts between genetically identical individuals, such as identical twins (*isografts*), are similarly compatible. However grafts between unrelated members of a species (*allografts*) or members of different species (*xenografts*) are targets for strong immunological rejection. This is so even when the recipient is not immunologically presensitized to the grafted *antigens. Second or subsequent grafts from the same donor are rejected at an accelerated rate.

The cause of graft rejection is the presence in nearly all tissues of potent histocompatibility *antigens. There are three known classes of histocompatibility antigen, which, in the small number of species so far studied, are found to be encoded by genes close together on the DNA comprising a region known as the *major histocompatibility complex* (*MHC*). *Class I antigens* are present on most nucleated cells; they stimulate both graft rejection and specific antibody production when administered to incompatible individuals. Because of the latter property, Class I antigens are said to be *serologically defined.* One major biological purpose of the Class I group is to serve as markers for cytotoxic *lymphocytes. These attack and destroy body cells that are virus-infected or whose surfaces bear foreign antigens, but only if the cell also bears self Class I antigens. Apparently, the lymphocyte must simultaneously recognize Class I and foreign antigen before it will undertake further action.

histogenesis

Class II antigens are normally present only on cells of the immune system, i.e. lymphocytes and certain accessory cells, including *macrophages. Most immune responses are the result of cooperation between macrophages and lymphocytes and between lymphocytes of different categories (*see* immunity). This cooperation will not take place if one group of cells has foreign Class II antigens. When confronted with incompatible Class II antigens, lymphocytes undergo transformation into lymphoblasts (*see* haemopoiesis) and divide. Most strikingly, this response occurs in a large proportion (up to 5%) of normal unprimed lymphocytes. Owing to this effect on lymphocytes, Class II antigens are described as *lymphocyte defined*. Additionally, Class II antigens may play a part in graft rejection, and they, or some closely associated molecular structures, also elicit specific antibody formation. Since Class II antigens have a pronounced role in governing intercellular cooperation, they are sometimes found to influence the overall reactivity of individuals to certain antigens. In humans, susceptibility to particular diseases is found in association with certain histocompatibility antigens. This may prove increasingly to be true of animals as data becomes available.

Both Class I and II antigens are proteins with some resemblance to antibody immunoglobulin. However, the genes encoding antibodies are known to be separate from the MHC. Class I and II are also notable for *polymorphism, with, in vertebrates, up to 25 alternative alleles for each locus within the MHC. Furthermore, the genes are codominant, i.e. both paired alleles at each of several loci are expressed. The potential number of antigenic combinations is therefore very great, making the matching of tissues for grafting correspondingly difficult.

Class III genes also form part of the MHC. They encode for some of the components of *complement and also regulate complement production.

histogenesis The formation of tissues.

histoid 1. Resembling normal tissue. **2.** Composed of one type of tissue.

histology The study of the structure of tissues by means of special staining techniques combined with light and electron microscopy. *See* anatomy.

Histomonas A genus of protozoan parasites containing a single species, *H. meleagridis*. The organism is amoeba-like with one or more flagella. It varies in size (from $4-30\,\mu m$ diameter) and shape depending on the stage in its life cycle and the site of parasitism. *H. meleagridis* is an extremely common and normally benign parasite of the large intestine of domestic fowls and turkeys, but it may occasionally invade the intestine wall and liver provoking severe disease in turkeys (*see* blackhead).

Cysts are shed in the faeces of infected birds but usually do not survive direct transmission to other birds by the oral route. Instead, the parasite has evolved a remarkable symbiotic relationship with the parasitic roundworm *Heterakis gallinarum*. This common nematode inhabits the caecum with *Histomonas*, which it ingests. The protozoan invades the ovaries of female roundworms and passes from the host within the worm eggs, which are excreted in faeces. Within the thick-shelled egg *Histomonas* can remain viable in the soil for many months or even years. When the eggs are ingested by other birds the worm larvae hatch and the histomonads are liberated and able to parasitize their new host. As a further refinement to this life cycle, earthworms can ingest the *Heterakis* eggs, which in turn contain *Histomonas*. In this way the spread and survival of the histomonads may be further enhanced. Many outbreaks of histomoniasis in free-range turkeys were historically associated with heavy rain, which brought large numbers of earthworms to the soil surface.

histomoniasis *See* blackhead.

histone A basic protein that combines with a *nucleic acid to form a *nucleoprotein.

histoplasmosis 1. A noncontagious infection of humans and other animals caused by the fungus *Histoplasma capsulatum*, an organism found worldwide inhabiting soil, especially where this is enriched by the excreta of bats or birds. Where infection is enzootic, notably in southeastern states of the USA, it is very common in both wild and domestic animals but clinically evident in only a few, mostly dogs. The initial infection is pulmonary, due to inhalation of spores. This usually resolves spontaneously but sometimes becomes chronic and progressive, or disseminates to almost any organ of the body, with a predilection for those of the *reticuloendothelial system.

Clinical manifestations of the disease vary widely. Common signs in **dogs**, and in the occasional infected cat, are a chronic cough, diarrhoea, weight loss, and fever. Diagnosis tends to rely upon the microscopic demonstration of the yeast phase of the organism within macrophages, to be found in stained preparations of biopsy material, exudates, or body fluids. The yeast forms are not easily differentiated from those of several other infections and confirmation by isolation of the organism in culture is desirable. Serological tests used in human medicine have not been fully evaluated for veterinary use. Treatment with *amphotericin B and

ketoconazole has had limited success but relapse is common. Other names: **cave disease**; **Darling's disease**; **Ohio Valley disease**; **reticuloendothelial cytomycosis**; **Tingo Maria fever**.
2. Any infection by a fungus belonging to the genus *Histoplasma*, such as *epizootic lymphangitis of horses, caused by *H. farciminosum*, and African histoplasmosis, which is caused by *H. duboisii* and affects primates in Africa.

Hjarré's disease (coli granuloma) A disease of domestic fowls due to infection with various strains of the bacterium *Escherichia coli*. It occurs only sporadically and involves the development of granulomatous lesions in the caecum, liver, and intestines, which can ultimately cause death. Older laying hens are most susceptible, and the condition may be initiated by the activities of internal parasites.

hock The tarsal or ankle region (*see* tarsus) or the region surrounding the joints formed by the tarsal bones (tarsal or hock joint).

Hodgkin's disease A malignant disease of lymphatic tissues in humans, characterized by painless enlargement of lymph nodes. It is questionable whether Hodgkin's disease as described for humans actually occurs in other animals. However, a Hodgkin's-like *lymphoma has been described in the dog, with firm often fibrous enlarged lymph nodes; multiple greyish-white nodules are found in the liver, spleen, and lungs where dissemination has taken place.

hog Specifically a castrated male pig but, more generally and particularly in North America, any pig. It formerly meant a wild boar in its second year.

hog cholera *See* swine fever.

hogg An infrequently used term for an uncastrated male pig.

holo- *Prefix denoting* complete or entire.

holocrine Describing a gland or type of secretion in which the entire cell disintegrates when the product is released.

homatropine *See* atropine.

homeo- (homoeo-) *Prefix denoting* similar; like.

homeopathy A system of medicine based on the theory that 'like cures like'. The patient is treated with minute quantities of remedies that would themselves produce clinical signs similar to the patient's condition if they were given in a toxic dose. Modern homeopathy was established by Samuel Hahnemann (1755–1843) for treating human patients. It has been adapted for use in animal patients and is employed by certain practitioners, sometimes as an adjunct to conventional therapy. There is a British Association of Homeopathic Veterinary Surgeons.

homeostasis The physiological process by which the internal systems of the body (e.g. blood pressure, body temperature, acid-base balance) are maintained at equilibrium despite variation in external environmental conditions.

homidium bromide (ethidium bromide) A trypanocidal drug active against *Trypanosoma congolense, T. vivax,* and *T. brucei* but inactive against *T. evansi.* It is thought to act by binding to trypanosome DNA, preventing protein synthesis and cell division. It is given by deep intramuscular injection to reduce local reaction to the drug, although there may be localized swelling and stiffness after injection. Homodium can be used in the treatment of trypanosomiasis and is prophylactic for about a month. When the drug is combined with *suramin the prophylactic effect is increased. Homidium bromide is carcinogenic and teratogenic.

homo- *Prefix denoting* the same or common.

homogametic Describing the sex whose gametes all carry the same kind of *sex chromosome. In mammals this is the female, whose gametes carry only the X chromosome; in birds the male is the homogametic sex, carrying only Z chromosomes in its gametes. *Compare* heterogametic.

homogenize To reduce material to a uniform consistency, e.g. by crushing and mixing. Organs and tissues are homogenized to determine their overall content of a particular enzyme or other substance.

homograft An old term for *allograft.

homoiothermic Warm-blooded: able to maintain a constant body temperature independently of, and despite variations in, the temperature of the surroundings. Mammals (including humans) and birds are homoiothermic. *Compare* poikilothermic.

homologous 1. (in anatomy) Describing organs or parts that have the same basic structure and evolutionary origin, but not necessarily the same function or superficial structure. 2. (in genetics) Describing a pair of chromosomes of similar shape and size and having identical gene loci. One member of the pair is derived from the dam; the other from the sire. The members of each homologous pair become closely associated during *meiosis.

homozygous Describing an organism that carries identical *alleles for any particular pair of its genes. Homozygotes thus produce only gametes carrying that particular allele, and breed true if crossed with organisms that are similarly homozygous. The degree of homozygosity in a population or group is increased by *inbreeding. *Compare* heterozygous.

hoof (ungula) The horny covering of the distal end of the digit in the limb of ungulate mammals, which include horses, pigs, and ruminants. The **horse's** hoof is composed of the wall, sole, and frog. The *wall* is the part of the hoof that is visible when the animal is standing; it can be divided into the *toe*, the *quarters*, and the *heels*, which reflect inwards as the *bars. The *sole* constitutes the greater

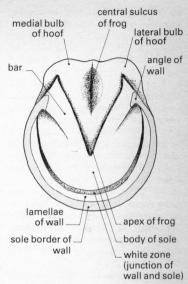

Right fore hoof of horse, ground surface

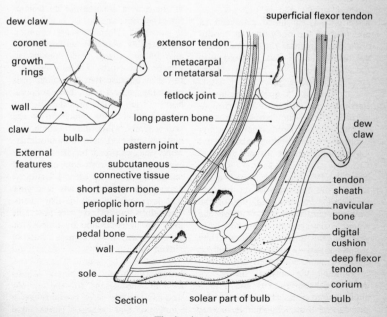

The bovine hoof

393

part of the hoof surface in contact with the ground. The *frog is the wedge-shaped mass lying between the bars. The hoof is avascular and derives its nutrition from the underlying *corium. See illustrations.

hookworm The common name for *nematodes belonging to the family Ancylostomidae. They are intestinal parasites characterized by having a mouth capsule with ventral teeth or plates inside the opening. They normally have a direct life cycle and can infect their host by direct penetration of the body surface or by ingestion. Hookworms cause a chronic debilitating condition and are particularly important in humans in tropical areas. See also Ancylostoma; bunostomiasis.

hoose See husk.

hordeolum See stye.

hormone A substance produced in one part of the body (by an *endocrine gland, such as the thyroid, adrenal, or pituitary) and released into the bloodstream to be carried to another specific target organ or tissue, where it elicits a specific response. Examples of hormones are *corticosteroids (from the adrenal cortex), *somatotrophin (from the adenohypophysis of the pituitary gland), and *thyroxine (from the thyroid gland).

horn 1. The hard keratinized tissue forming the epidermis of the hoof of the horse, ruminants, and pig, or the claw of carnivores. **2.** One of the paired structures that project from the head in ruminant species. They are composed of a hard keratinized epidermis and an underlying dermis surrounding the cornual process of the frontal bone. The size and form is highly variable and characteristic of a species and breed. Ruminants lacking horns are described as polled.

Removal of the horns (see dehorning; disbudding) is performed routinely in cattle to reduce the risk of injury to other cattle and stockpersons. **3.** A crescent-shaped organ or part, such as the horns of grey matter of the *spinal cord or the horns of the lateral *ventricle in the brain. See cornu.

Horner's syndrome A combination of clinical signs that indicate damage to the cervical or thoracic sympathetic nerves, due, for example, to direct pressure from a tumour or from swelling of an infected guttural pouch. There is sweating and excessive heat on one side of the head and neck; the corresponding eyelid droops and the pupil of the same eye constricts. Cure depends on removing the cause of pressure on the affected nerve.

horn fly A small bloodsucking *fly of the genera Haematobia or Lyperosia. They are known as buffalo flies in Australia. Horn flies are common ectoparasites of cattle and occasionally horses, sheep, and humans in Europe and North America and are so-called because they are often seen swarming round the base of the horns. The adults persistently bite their hosts causing much irritation, skin wounds, which may become secondarily infected, and even anaemia. Milk yield can also be affected. The eggs are laid in fresh cow dung, and moisture is essential for the larvae to develop. Hence, any means of drying the dung quickly will destroy them. The adults rarely leave the host and they can be controlled by dipping or spraying the host with a suitable *insecticide.

horse A hoofed mammal, Equus caballus, belonging to the family Equidae, which also contains asses (donkeys) and zebras. Horses are believed to have evolved from small browsing forest dwellers, such as eohippus. Later ancestors were progressively larger, becoming fast-moving grazing animals with well-developed senses. The outer toes of the foot were reduced as the central toe gradually enlarged to form the hoof. Modern breeds can be traced back to various Asian and European ancestors, such as Przewalski's horse and the tarpan.

Horses have long been domesticated for riding and as draught animals. They are also used for recreation and a range of equestrian sports and activities, such as steeplechasing, showjumping, eventing, and dressage. The breed, age, and sex of a horse are all important in determining its suitability for a particular activity and the way it is cared for. Horses mature at 3½–5 years of age, depending on breed, and can live for 20–35 years. They are measured in hands (1 hand = 4 in = 10.16 cm) to the top of the shoulders (withers). A pony is a horse that does not exceed 14½ hands (1.47 m). *See also* horse husbandry; foal husbandry.

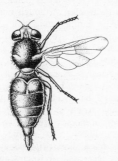

Gasterophilus haemophilus, the commonest UK horse bot

horse bot One of several large hairy flies whose larvae are parasites of horses, elephants, and, occasionally, dogs, pigs, and humans (see illustration). The adults are short-lived with only rudimentary mouthparts and do not feed. The eggs are cemented to hairs on the horse's body, the precise site depending on the species of horse bot. The most common, *Gasterophilus intestinalis*, lays its eggs on the forelimbs. The eggs hatch when licked by the horse and the larvae burrow into the tissues of the mouth, eventually passing down the alimentary tract to various sites in the digestive system, where they attach themselves by mouth hooks causing inflammation and ulcers. Rarely, the normal passage of digesta through the tract can be affected; some horses develop a hypersensitive reaction (*see* hypersensitivity) to the excretory products of the larvae. Eventually the larvae leave with the faeces and develop into pupae in the soil. Treatment entails dosing the horse with either trichlorphon or ivermectin or adding dichlorvos to the feed. Regular grooming procedures will free the horse of eggs.

horse husbandry Essential aspects of keeping a horse. The care and management of horses varies considerably, depending on the type of horse and what it is used for (see below). For instance, the amount of time horses are stabled as opposed to grazing outdoors depends on their breed or type (and therefore ability to withstand adverse weather) and the amount of work they are doing. Feeding also depends on breed and type and the amount of work done. Racehorses are fed mainly on energy-rich cereals (e.g. oats), while native ponies doing little work will thrive on rough grass, hay, and other bulky feeds.

Feeds suitable for most horses include whole or rolled oats, rolled barley, flaked maize (corn), broad bran, and well-soaked sugar beet shreds. High-protein feeds can include linseed, soya-bean meal, dried alfalfa, dried grass, and milk powder. All young horses benefit from succulent feeds, such as carrots, and from bonemeal in their diet. Horses have comparatively small stomachs so concentrates must be fed in small quantities and frequently: horses in fast work are usually fed concentrates four times per day; hacks and brood mares two or three times per day; and ponies once or twice per day. Since a horse at grass grazes up to 22 hours per day, stabled horses should ideally always have hay available (except in special cases, i.e. the racehorse).

Clean straw makes excellent bedding for stables but dusty or mouldy straw can lead to respiratory troubles for horses in poorly ventilated stables. A dust-free environment is particularly important for competition horses, which are often bedded on shredded paper or wood shavings; this also avoids the problem of horses eating straw and increasing their roughage intake. For roughage, *haylage, or similar moist products avoid possible problems associated with dusty or mouldy hay. An air vent should be fitted to the highest part of the stable roof, and the top half of the stable door should remain open in all but the most severe weather to provide adequate ventilation.

Grooming Horses and ponies at grass simply need any mud on the coat brushing off before riding. The natural oil in the coat waterproofs it. Stabled horses and ponies need thorough regular grooming to remove the oil and clean the coat. In the autumn as the winter coat grows, and at intervals throughout the winter, horses in hard work are clipped or partially clipped. This reduces sweating and, as the sweat evaporates, chilling. Most horses and ponies at grass grow thick winter coats and do not need rugs. Fine-coated horses or clipped horses at grass require a New Zealand rug, which is windproof and waterproof.

Competitive horses

Racehorses, including flat racehorses, steeplechasers, hurdlers, and point-to-point horses, are all thoroughbreds. Their highly specialized training and feeding bring them to peak fitness for certain days. Their diet consists mainly of best-quality oats, with limited amounts of high-quality hay. They are usually stabled throughout the year.

Eventers and showjumpers are thoroughbreds and crossbreds. A more sustained level of fitness is required compared to racehorses, and feeding and exercise are balanced to give a very fit horse carrying no excess weight. The diet again comprises a high proportion of oats, but more hay or haylage than allowed for racehorses. They are stabled throughout the time they are working.

Hunters may be thoroughbreds or thoroughbred-crosses, or they may be of unknown breeding. All horses with a suitable temperament and the ability to jump can be hunted. Traditionally hunters are turned out to grass for the summer then brought indoors at the end of the summer to be made fit by weeks of slow work. However, it is possible for a horse to be both ridden during the summer and hunted in the winter. Although normally stabled during the hunting season hunters can live out if provided with a New Zealand rug and given additional feed.

Dressage horses are often thoroughbreds, warm-blood horses, or crossbreds, but Welsh cobs, Arabs, and Anglo-Arabs are also suitable. These very fit horses are fed an oat-based diet. Ideally they should be turned out for a short period daily for some free exercise, fresh air, and a little grass.

Endurance horses can be any horses with the qualities needed for long-distance riding. Arabs or part-Arabs are particularly suitable. A diet high in carbohydrates is required, and oats, rolled barley, flaked maize, and good-quality hay are suitable.

Show horses (all classes) are well-muscled animals covered by a layer of fat to enhance their appearance. All are usually stabled throughout the show season and their cereal intake (oats, barley, or maize) balanced according to behaviour and appearance. Soaked sugar beet is often used for show horses.

Noncompetitive horses

Working horses include hacks, riding-school horses, and children's ponies (see below). In summer it may be possible to work these horses off grass if enough good-quality pasture is available. If stabled and given a cereal-based diet, they benefit from being turned out to grass for part of every day: the grass is nutritionally beneficial, the exercise keeps their temperament calm and sensible, and the fresh air helps avoid respiratory troubles. Significant quantities of oats are not required by this group and may be harmful, causing excitability and difficulty in controlling the horse. This is particularly a problem associated with feeding oats to children's ponies. A typical diet may include rolled barley, bran, soaked sugar beet shreds, flaked maize, and hay. The quantity is adjusted to balance the quality and quantity of grass available, and the amount of work being done. Bran and soaked sugar beet are not fed together at the same feed as both are bulky feeds.

Children's ponies (excluding show ponies) Both crossbred and native-type ponies can live out at grass all year round. A thick hedge, wall, or field shelter is needed to give protection against strong winds and driving rain, and hay should be fed in winter; concentrate feeds are also given if the animal is working hard. Ponies of thoroughbred type can live out at grass in summer but must be stabled in winter or rugged with a New Zealand rug. Moreover, in winter they require a small amount of concentrate feed daily, with extra if they are working. Care must be taken to limit the grazing of ponies, especially when there is a sudden growth of grass in spring or autumn. This high-protein grass, or very plentiful summer grass, can cause *laminitis in overfed ponies.

Heavy horses (e.g. Shire, Clydesdale, Suffolk punch, Percheron) are traditionally used as draught animals, pulling implements on farms or drays in towns. On farms, heavy horses are kept at grass and given extra feed according to the work done. In towns they are stabled with perhaps a two-week 'holiday' at grass each year. Feed for heavy horses is bulky – often chopped hay or straw with a third in volume of broad bran. Low-protein mixes based on rolled barley can also be used. Feeding is often up to seven times a day. Few commercial farms now use horses, but they are used by companies for promotion and advertising, and are shown competitively. *See also* foaling; foal husbandry.

horse nasal bot fly (Russian gadfly) A small *fly, *Rhinoestrus purpureus*, also called the horse nostril fly, found in central Europe, the USSR, and North Africa. The larvae are parasites of the horse, the adult female fly depositing them into and around the nostrils where they feed on mucous secretions; they later migrate to the pharynx or larynx of their host.

horse nettle A North American plant, *Solanum carolinense*, that contains the toxic alkaloid solanine (*see* solanine poisoning).

horsepox A contagious disease of horses characterized by skin eruptions on the lower legs or in the mouth and caused by orthopoxviruses (*see* poxvirus). It is sometimes colloquially referred to as 'grease'. The disease is present in Europe, but is now probably extinct in the UK. The 'leg form' is characterized by the appearance of nodules, vesicles, pustules, and scabs on the back of the pasterns. In the 'buccal form' lesions first appear on the inside of the lip and may affect the whole mouth. Recovery is usual in 3 weeks.

Horse Protection Act (USA) A federal Act, administered by the *United States Department of Agriculture, prohibiting the use on horses of methods and devices that cause pain or inflammation. Such procedures were formerly used in an effort to make horses perform better, particularly those showing Tennessee walking horses.

horseradish poisoning A toxic condition arising from the ingestion of herbaceous plants of the genus *Armoracia* (*A. rusticana* or *A. lapathifolia*). They contain an irritant volatile oil, similar to that of the mustards and with similar clinical effects (*see* brassica poisoning).

horsetail poisoning *See* bracken poisoning.

host An animal or plant in or upon which a parasite lives. An *intermediate host* is one in which the parasite passes its larval or asexual stages; a *definitive* or *final* host is one in which the parasite develops to its sexual stage. A *transport host* is one in which the parasite does not undergo developmental changes but is merely distributed in the environment.

host range (virology) Those cells or animals that can serve as host for a particular virus. The host range varies between virus types and is of obvious significance in determining the potential spread of a viral disease between host species.

housing Structures designed for shelter, control, or protection. Under cold environmental conditions mammals and birds use food energy to generate body heat, hence less food energy is available for productive purposes. For rapidly growing meat animals and laying hens the result is a significant reduction in liveweight gain, a worsening *food conversion ratio, and, for laying hens, a fall in egg output. For newborn animals cold stress can quickly prove fatal (*see* hypothermia). In all cases the effects of cold are exacerbated by wind and precipitation. There is consequently a need to provide shelter, insulation, and possibly heat, depending on the type of livestock.

Ventilation must be adequate otherwise the resulting build-up of gases (e.g. ammonia) may present health risks to both stock and personnel. Increased humidity predisposes towards respiratory problems, particularly in ruminants. Additional heat is provided for young stock, especially chicks; these are maintained at approximately 35°C at hatching, falling gradually to 21°C by around 3 weeks of age. Similarly, newborn piglets require warmth at birth. For older livestock in temperate climates, effective insulation of walls and roofs coupled with good ventilation is usually adequate. *Bedding or *litter may be provided, except in *intensive husbandry systems with automatic waste transport and disposal. For cattle, *cubicles make better use of available space and are cleaner. Lighting intensity (*see* light requirements) and photoperiod are critical for pullets and laying hens, to manipulate the onset of egg production, and for *broilers, to promote feed intake (*see* light requirements). *See also* bull husbandry; floor space.

Humane Slaughter Act (USA) A federal Act requiring that livestock are slaughtered only by humane methods. Cattle, calves, horses, mules, sheep, swine, and other livestock must be rendered insensible to pain by a single blow to the head, gunshot, or electrical, chemical, or other means that is rapid and effective, before being shackled, hoisted, thrown, cast, or cut. However, the Act also makes provisions for slaughter in accordance with the ritual requirements of the Jewish or other religious faiths whereby the animal suffers loss of consciousness by simultaneous and instantaneous severance of the carotid arteries.

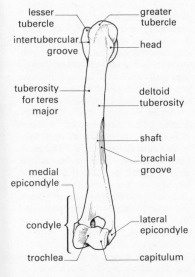

lesser tubercle
greater tubercle
intertubercular groove
head
tuberosity for teres major
deltoid tuberosity
shaft
brachial groove
medial epicondyle
condyle
lateral epicondyle
trochlea
capitulum

Left humerus of dog, cranial lateral aspect

humerus (*pl.* **humeri**) The single long bone of the upper forelimb. The head of the humerus articulates with the scapula forming the shoulder joint, while distally the capitulum and trochlea articulate with the radius and ulna to form the elbow joint (see illustration).

humoral immunity *Immunity mediated by soluble agents, such as antibody and complement, and not involving direct intervention by cells.

humour A body fluid. *See* aqueous humour; vitreous humour.

husk (hoose) A disease of cattle caused by invasion of the lungs with the parasitic nematode (lungworm) *Dictyocaulus viviparus*. It occurs in many temperate and cold areas of the world, particularly the UK, where it affects principally calves aged between 4 and 6 months. The mature lungworms live in the bronchi and air passages, where they lay their eggs. These hatch to form larvae, which are coughed up, swallowed, and passed out with the faeces onto the pasture. After two further developmental stages these larvae become capable of infecting another animal. Ingestion of grass contaminated with larvae results in migration via the bloodstream to the lungs where they develop to adults, thus completing the life cycle. The disease is therefore usually confined to grazing animals.

The adult worms in the airways cause irritation (*parasitic tracheobronchitis*) and the migrating larvae bring about *pneumonia. Therefore, signs include increased rate and depth of breathing, a harsh 'husky' cough, and raised body temperature. The disease may last as long as 3–4 weeks and there is often considerable loss of bodyweight. Cases may be complicated by a secondary bacterial pneumonia. An oral vaccine (Dictol) is available for immunizing calves prior to their first grazing season. Treatment involves administration of *anthelmintics, such as *levamisole or fenbendazole (*see* benzimidazole). Other names: **parasitic bronchitis; verminous pneumonia.**

hyal- (hyalo-) *Prefix denoting* **1.** glassy; transparent. **2.** hyaline. **3.** the vitreous humour of the eye.

hyaline (hyalin) Any translucent glasslike material that is deposited in or on tissues or surface epithelia; it is usually associated with degenerative changes or disease. Membrane-like deposits of hyaline (*hyaline membranes*) are often described in pulmonary alveoli in the early stages of viral pneumonias in sheep and calves. Their composition may be of *fibrinlike material, glycosaminoglycan, or coagulated surfactant. Similar membranous deposits line the alveoli and airways in *acute respiratory distress syndrome, being known as the *asphyxiation membranes*. Multifocal accumulations of macrophages and giant cells containing hyaline deposits are seen beneath the pleura of old dogs as an incidental finding at autopsy. Hyaline deposits in the kidney are often associated with canine and feline *glomerulonephritis or other diseases (e.g. diabetes mellitus, amyloidosis).
Hyaline cartilage is the most common type of *cartilage. It is bluish-white flexible material with a matrix of chondroitin sulphate in which fine collagen fibres are embedded.

hyaline membrane 1. The membrane separating the outer root sheath and inner fibrous layer of a hair follicle. **2.** A membrane-like deposit of *hyaline.

hyaloid Referring to the *vitreous humour of the eye. The *hyaloid canal* runs through the vitreous humour and contains the *hyaloid artery*, which is a foetal artery supplying the lens of the eye.

hyaluronic acid An acid *mucopolysaccharide that acts as the binding and protective agent of the ground substance of connective tissue.

It is also present in the synovial fluid around joints and in the vitreous and aqueous humours of the eye. It is injected intra-articularly to treat some types of arthritis in the horse.

hyaluronidase An enzyme that hydrolyses *hyaluronic acid. It is found in the testis and seminal plasma and is involved in the penetration of the ovum by the sperm. The enzyme decreases the viscosity of intracellular tissue, allowing increased diffusion of substances. It can be administered to improve the spread of drugs from an injection site and to reduce oedema.

H-Y antigen An antigen present in mammals on the cells of males only. It is believed to be encoded on the Y chromosome and can elicit a wide variety of immune responses, including graft rejection. It may thus be regarded as a *minor histocompatibility antigen* (*see* histocompatibility).

hybrid The offspring of a cross between two genetically distinct lines, strains, breeds, or species. The progeny of crosses between species are usually sterile, as is the mule (a cross between a horse and a donkey). Hybrids produced within a species are typically highly *heterozygous and thus incapable of breeding true. *See also* heterosis.

hybridoma A type of cell formed by the fusion of two or more cells, at least one of which is cancerous. The most usual type involves the fusion between a B-lymphocyte and a plasma tumour cell. *See also* monoclonal antibody.

hybrid vigour *See* heterosis.

hydatid cyst The larval stage in the life cycle of tapeworms of the genus *Echinococcus, such as *E. granulosus* and *E. multilocularis*. It consists of a large spherical fluid-filled cyst containing hundreds of secondary cysts, or brood capsules, in each of which grow a number of tapeworm heads. The hydatid cyst develops in the liver, lungs, or brain of the intermediate host, usually in sheep, pigs, or horses but also in humans. It may grow to the size of an orange, 150 mm in diameter, and causes *hydatidosis (hydatid disease). *See also* bladderworm.

hydatidosis (hydatid disease) Disease due to infestation by *hydatid cysts of the tapeworms *Echinococcus granulosus* or *E. multilocularis*. Hydatidosis can affect many mammalian species, including humans. These species function as intermediate hosts for the parasite. Infestation occurs following ingestion of the tapeworm eggs, which are present in the faeces of a final host. In the case of *E. granulosus*, dogs or related species are the final hosts; with *E. multilocularis*, foxes are additional sources of infection. Although hydatidosis shows no host specificity, most strains of *Echinococcus* hydatid, especially *E. granulosus*, seem to have a predilection for certain mammalian species. *E. granulosus* hydatids are found worldwide; *E. multilocularis* is found in Central Europe, the USSR, parts of North America, and the Middle and Far East.

The growth rate of hydatids is variable and almost any tissue can be infested. The signs are therefore indefinite. Domestic animals do not usually show any signs of infestation, but heavy infestations in horses, which are common hosts in Great Britain, occasionally result in respiratory difficulty and anaphylaxis (*see* hypersensitivity). Sheep, goats, pigs, cattle, and camels usually exhibit no signs, even though the liver and/or lungs may show heavy parasitism. In humans, hydatid disease is potentially serious, owing to the large size that

hydatid cysts may attain and the tendency for the cysts to rupture and release daughter cysts, which can spread to distant organs (i.e. undergo metastasis) and form new hydatids. *E. multilocularis* hydatids are multiple cysts and show continuous proliferation, invasion, and metastasis, so that their growth is very similar to that of a malignant tumour; infestation carries a grave prognosis. *E. granulosus* hydatids are single cysts, and clinical course and prognosis depend on the site, size, and operability of the cyst.

Diagnosis is by radiography in humans and other species of comparable size. A large number of immunological tests have been designed but none has been universally adopted, possibly due to the unpredictable nature of immunity to hydatids, particularly by antibody-producing cells and local defensive mechanisms. Surgical removal is the usual treatment but it carries two main dangers: induced metastasis and anaphylactic reaction (*see* hypersensitivity). Experimentally, the use of anthelmintics, such as albendazole and mebendazole (*see* benzimidazole), against hydatids has shown promise.

hydr- (hydro-) *Prefix denoting* water or a watery fluid.

hydraemia A condition in which the blood plasma contains an excess of water.

hydralazine *See* hypotensive agent.

hydrallantois A condition is which there is excess allantoic fluid in the *allantois during development of the embryo. Such an excess results from inadequate placental drainage and, in a cow, the quantity of fluid can increase from a normal 15–20 l to 170 l. Most cases abort and those which do not often result in a dead foetus. It is most common in the cow and occurs rarely in the mare. *Compare* hydramnios.

hydramnios (hydrops amnii; hydrops amnion) A condition in which there is an excess of *amniotic fluid in the amniotic cavity and oedema of the amnion. This is often associated with inherited or acquired malformation of the foetus, which normally controls the amount of amniotic fluid by foetal swallowing. Many cases are resolved by abortion, and in those which reach term the foetus is often dead. *Compare* hydrallantois.

hydrocele The accumulation of fluid in a body cavity or sac from which there is no free drainage. It may occur in the scrotum or within the fibrous connective tissue surrounding a testis.

hydrocephalus An abnormal increase in the amount of cerebrospinal fluid in the ventricles of the brain. It is most common in the newborn, in which it causes the skull to swell or appear dome-shaped. Affected animals show a variety of nervous signs, which soon prove fatal. The condition may be hereditary and affected family lines should not be bred; *bulldog calves of Dexter cattle are typical examples. Other species may be affected. Adults also can be affected, but the rigidity of the skull means that swelling does not occur.

In the horse the growth of a cholesteatoma (*see* choroid plexus tumour) in the brain may obstruct the outflow of cerebrospinal fluid and induce hydrocephalus. The condition is commonly fatal and not usually worth treating in domestic animals. However, in cases of hydrocephalus due to *vitamin A deficiency, either directly in the diet of young animals or indirectly in animals born to vitamin A-deficient mothers, vitamin A supple-

ments may be effective for prevention or even cure.

hydrochloric acid An acid secreted by the oxyntic cells of the *gastric glands into the stomach, where its concentration can be as high as 0.1 mol (pH 1). It is important in the denaturation of dietary protein and the activation of pepsinogens to *pepsins. After the gut contents leave the stomach their pH is raised in the intestine by the secretion of bicarbonate in the bile and pancreatic juice.

hydrochlorothiazide *See* thiazide diuretics.

hydrocolpos An unusual accumulation of fluid or mucus in the vagina. The condition is rare but has been described in cattle in association with an *imperforate hymen.

hydrocortisone (cortisol) *See* corticosteroid.

hydrogenase An enzyme that catalyses the addition of hydrogen to a compound in reduction reactions.

hydrogen bond An electrostatic interaction between a hydrogen atom bound to an electronegative atom (e.g. O, N, F) and another electronegative atom. Along with other weak (i.e. noncovalent) forces, such as hydrophobic interactions, hydrogen bonds are very important in maintaining the three-dimensional native structure of proteins and nucleic acids. The unique properties of water, which are so central to the function and behaviour of all living things, are mainly due to the extensive hydrogen bonding between water molecules.

hydrogen peroxide An oxidizing agent used as an *antiseptic and deodorant. It is available as an aqueous solution, which is stable in acidic conditions but decomposes in the presence of alkali, organic material, and metals. The concentration of the solution is expressed in volumes of oxygen released by it; the standard solution is 20 volumes. Contact with organic tissue causes hydrogen peroxide to release oxygen, catalysed by the tissue enzyme catalase. This produces a cleansing action, which persists while oxygen is being liberated. The effect is rapid and transient in the presence of organic debris, and many microorganisms (e.g. bacterial spores) are not killed. Hydrogen peroxide is used as an antiseptic and cleaning agent in the treatment of abscesses.

hydrolase An enzyme that catalyses the *hydrolysis of a molecule.

hydrolysis The chemical reaction by which a bond in a molecule is broken by the addition of the elements of water across the bond.

hydroma See hygroma.

hydronephrosis Cystic dilatation of the pelvis of the kidney. This is due to obstruction of the free flow of urine from the kidney. Clinical signs may be absent because the blockage affects only one kidney and the opposite kidney adequately compensates for the loss. Ureteral obstruction is commonly due to a *calculus (stone), but congenital maldevelopment or other ureteral anomaly may induce the lesion, especially in pigs. Hydronephrosis of both kidneys leads inevitably to *uraemia and death.

hydropericardium The accumulation of excess fluid in the *pericardium. It is common in cases of *heart failure in conjunction with *oedema elsewhere in the body, and also occurs in debilitating diseases, such as protein deficiency, anaemia, parasitic infestation (e.g. liver fluke), or chronic liver

disease. Obstruction to lymphatic drainage may also be a factor. Clinical signs of panting and fatigue become apparent if heart function is severely impeded. Treatment involves withdrawal of the fluid by *paracentesis and attendance to the primary cause.

hydropneumopericardium Gas and fluid in the *pericardium. The cause is commonly an infection of the pericardium.

hydropneumothorax Air and fluid in the pleural cavity. Air may enter from the lung or from the outside via a penetrating wound; the fluid may be an effusion due to debilitating disease, or an inflammatory exudate due, for example, to pneumonia.

hydrosalpinx The accumulation of serous fluid in an oviduct. It is commonly the end result of an infection (see salpingitis), which may leave fibrous scars obstructing the oviduct. Reduced fertility or infertility may result if sperm cannot reach and fertilize ova in the oviduct.

hydrothorax The accumulation of serous fluid in the pleural cavity. This may result from congestive heart failure or from a debilitating disease, such as protein deficiency, anaemia, parasitism, or liver cirrhosis. Lung volume may be restricted causing respiratory distress. Furthermore the large veins draining into the base of the heart may be constricted. Drainage of the fluid (see pleurocentesis) gives temporary relief but cure depends on alleviating the primary cause.

hydroureter Localized distension of a ureter with urine due to blockage with a calculus (stone) or some other obstruction. Complete obstruction causes *hydronephrosis.

hydrovarium The accumulation of serous fluid in the ovary. This is frequently a sequel to infection, which may leave fibrous adhesions that obstruct the outflow of fluid from the ovaries down the oviducts. Infertility follows if both ovaries are affected.

hydroxyapatite The inorganic material that impregnates the fibrous matrix of *bone. It comprises variable amounts of calcium phosphate and calcium hydroxide.

hydroxyproline One of two *amino acids found especially in the connective-tissue protein *collagen (the other is hydroxylysine). It is formed by the hydroxylation of the amino acid proline in procollagen, in a reaction involving vitamin C.

hygr- (hygro-) *Prefix denoting* moisture.

hygroma (hydroma) A cyst-like swelling of the knee (stifle) joint containing serous fluid. In cattle this is a common lesion in *Brucella abortus* infection. However, hygromas can occur as a result of repeated trauma, for example inflicted by the concrete edges of cow standings.

hymen The membrane that covers the entrance to the vagina in the young.

Hymenolepis A genus of small *tapeworms found worldwide (see illustration). Most are parasites in the intestines of birds, such as ducks and geese, in which case the intermediate hosts are aquatic crustaceans. Two species that parasitize rodents and occasionally humans are the dwarf tapeworm, *H. nana*, which is only 25 –40 mm long and is a common tapeworm in the USA, and *H. diminuta*. The larva of the dwarf tapeworm lives in mealworm beetles or fleas but can also develop in the intestine of the primary host. The intermediate hosts for *H. diminuta* are various species of moths and beetles. Heavy infestations of these tapeworms may produce diarrhoea, loss of weight and appetite, and nervous disorders. Treatment entails a course of *anthelmintics.

Hymenoxus poisoning A toxic condition due to the ingestion of various perennial or annual herbaceous plants belonging to the genus *Hymenoxus*, which is distributed throughout the western USA and northern Mexico and includes the bitterweeds and rubberweeds. These contain an unknown toxic principle, which appears to be cumulative and causes inflammation of the gastrointestinal tract, with depression, incoordination, muscle tremors, salivation, vomiting, and diarrhoea. Treatment is symptomatic. *See also* Helenium poisoning.

hyo- *Prefix denoting* the hyoid apparatus. Example: *hyoglossal* (relating to the hyoid bones and tongue).

hyoid apparatus An arrangement of rods of bone and cartilage that attaches to the temporal bone on the base of the skull and extends around the pharynx to provide attachment for various muscles and for the cartilages of the larynx. The number and form of the bones varies between species.

hyoscine (scopolamine) *See* atropine.

Hyostrongylus A genus containing the parasitic *nematode *H. rubidus*, which is found in the stomach wall of pigs and occurs worldwide. Eggs are passed in the faeces and the larvae are swallowed by the host with vegetation. They pass to the stomach and attach to the gastric mucosa for final development. Adult worms begin to lay eggs three weeks after ingestion.

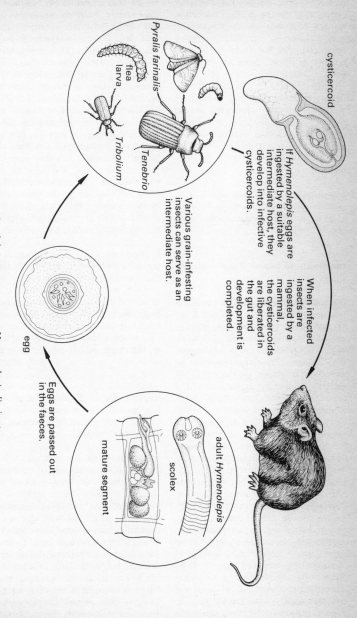

cysticercoid

Pyralis farinalis

flea
larva

Tribolium

Tenebrio

If *Hymenolepis* eggs are
ingested by a suitable
intermediate host, they
develop into infective
cysticercoids.

Various grain-infesting
insects can serve as an
intermediate host.

When infected
insects are
ingested by a
mammal,
the cysticercoids
are liberated in
the gut and
development is
completed.

adult *Hymenolepis*

scolex

mature segment

Eggs are passed out
in the faeces.

egg

Life cycle of the rat tapeworm, *Hymenolepis diminuta*

A rise in egg production normally occurs after farrowing, thus increasing the risk of infestation for piglets. The worms cause a gastritis condition associated with nodule formation and sucking of blood from the stomach wall. Anaemia, diarrhoea, and unthriftiness are the general clinical signs. The larvae are very susceptible to desiccation and cleanliness in the piggery is paramount in preventing infestation. Affected animals can be treated by giving parbendazole in the feed (*see* benzimidazole) or ivermectin.

hyp- (hypo-) *Prefix denoting* **1.** deficiency, lack, or small size. **2.** (in anatomy) below; beneath. Example: *hypoglossal* (under the tongue).

hyper- *Prefix denoting* **1.** excessive; abnormally increased. **2.** (in anatomy) above.

hyperadrenocorticism The condition resulting from excess production of glucocorticoid hormones (*see* corticosteroid) by the adrenal cortex or excess exogenous steroid administration. *Primary hyperadrenocorticism* or *Cushing's syndrome* is the result of glucocorticoid-secreting tumours of the cortex or adrenal hyperplasia. *Pituitary-dependent hyperadrenocorticism* or *Cushing's disease* is due to tumours of the hypothalamus or anterior pituitary gland, which can cause excess production of *adrenocorticotrophic hormone (ACTH), thereby stimulating adrenal hypertrophy and hyperplasia and excess glucocorticoid secretion. Pituitary-dependent and primary lesions can be differentiated by using an ACTH assay, a dexamethasone suppression test, or a metyrapone suppression procedure. *Iatrogenic Cushing's disease* can result from chronic overmedication with exogenous steroids. An ACTH response test may assist in confirming this. In dogs, excess glucocorticoids can cause

weight gain, polyuria, polydipsia, skin and muscle atrophy, weakness, hair loss, decreased immune response, and liver disease. Horses show an excess hair coat, often noticed in the spring when the animal fails to shed. Therapy for pituitary-dependent hyperadrenocorticism is often chemically accomplished by using o,p-DDD (dichlorodiphenyldichloroethane). Surgical excision of the adrenal glands (adrenalectomy) and pituitary (hypophysectomy) have also been successful. Adrenal tumours can be removed surgically, but adrenal adenocarcinomas (*see* carcinoma) have often metastasized by the time a diagnosis is made. Iatrogenic Cushing's disease is best treated by weaning the animal from the exogenous steroid.

hyperaemia Congestion of tissues or organs with blood. It may result from excessive inflow of blood (*active congestion*), as occurs in inflammation, or from obstruction to the veins (*passive congestion*). Much of the hyperaemia occurring in inflammation is induced by various mediating substances, such as histamine, which dilate the arterioles and capillaries of the affected area.

hyperaesthesia Excessive sensibility. For example, hyperaesthesia results in intense itching and scratching in sheep with *scrapie.

hypercalcaemia An abnormally high concentration of calcium in the blood. This rarely occurs because blood calcium is normally strictly regulated by two hormones (*parathyroid hormone and *calcitonin) and any tendency to hypercalcaemia is soon corrected. For instance, the very high calcium levels that follow intravenous infusion of calcium in *milk fever therapy can fall to normal in only an hour or so. However, massive doses of vitamin D given to prevent milk fever can produce more sustained hypercalcaemia lasting 5–10 days and with calcium levels rising from a normal of 2.4 mmol/l to 3.25–3.75 mmol/l. Also, excessive dietary calcium will induce variable mild and transient hypercalcaemia followed by *hypocalcaemia. Furthermore, in dogs, horses, and cats, hypercalcaemia may be induced by various tumours. These may secrete substances that act like parathyroid hormone. As a result serum calcium may rise to over 4 mmol/l with correspondingly low levels of inorganic phosphorus. In all cases, hypercalcaemia causes cardiac irregularity, constipation, and muscular weakness. Long-term effects include the deposition of excess calcium beneath the endothelium of arteries and of the heart.

hypercalcinuria An excessively high calcium concentration in the urine, usually occurring as a result of *hypercalcaemia. The urine of ruminants is alkaline and normally contains very little calcium (or phosphorus) otherwise these minerals would precipitate forming renal and bladder calculi (*see* calculus). However, high intakes of phosphorus can stimulate bone resorption, raise the level of blood calcium, and at the same time render the urine acidic so that hypercalcinuria occurs. Massive doses of vitamin D_3, given to prevent milk fever, also provoke both hypercalcaemia and hypercalcinuria with the possibility of renal calculi. Horses normally have very high amounts of calcium in the urine, which is precipitated as calcium carbonate and accounts for the cloudy appearance of equine urine.

hypercapnia The presence in the blood of an abnormally high concentration of carbon dioxide. This commonly results from disease, such as pneumonia, which causes respiratory insufficiency and prevents adequate gaseous exchange in the lungs. The build-up of carbon dioxide in the blood stimulates the respiratory centre in the brain to increase the breathing rate in an attempt to compensate. Hypercapnia can also occur in livestock housed with inadequate ventilation and hence excessive carbon dioxide in the atmosphere.

hyperchloraemia An abnormally high concentration of chloride anions in the blood. It is comparatively rare because excess chloride is readily excreted in the urine under normal circumstances. However, shortage of drinking water and consequent dehydration cause the concentration of blood chloride (and sodium – *see* hypernatraemia) to increase. In contrast, dehydration due to water loss from the body, as during excessive sweating or in diarrhoea, involves the loss of chloride in the secretions thus counteracting any tendency towards hyperchloraemia. *Compare* hypochloraemia.

hypercholesterolaemia An abnormally high concentration of cholesterol in the blood. In humans it is associated with atherosclerosis and cardiovascular disease, whereas in animals its significance is as an indicator of liver and thyroid disorders.

hyperemesis Excessive and persistent vomiting (*see* vomiting).

hypergammaglobulinaemia An excess of *gamma globulin in the blood. Gamma globulins are a class of proteins, separable by *electrophoresis, that contain much of the serum antibody, or immunoglobulin. Elevation of gamma globulin occurs in neoplasias and chronic inflammation and infection. It is particularly characteristic of malignant *myeloma, a cancerous condition of the antibody-producing lymphocytes or plasma cells in which these cells produce a single homogeneous type of

hyperglycaemia

immunoglobulin. This is seen as a pronounced 'spike' in the electrophoretic protein profile.

hyperglycaemia An abnormally high concentration of glucose in the blood. In dogs and (very rarely) cats, it is usually caused by *diabetes mellitus, in which production of the hormone insulin is impaired. Insulin normally corrects hyperglycaemia by removing glucose from the blood for metabolism in the tissue cells. In the absence of insulin blood plasma glucose accumulates, rising from the normal value of 4.13–5.5 mmol/l to as high as 27.5 mmol/l. Values above 6.6 mmol/l are diagnostic of diabetes. Excess glucose enters the urine giving it high osmolarity, thus inducing the excretion of excess urine (polyuria).

In horses, the causes of hyperglycaemia are excitement, pituitary tumours, previous treatment with xylazine, and – very rarely – phaeochromocytomas. *Compare* hypoglycaemia.

hyperidrosis (hyperhydrosis) Excessive sweating. Horses commonly sweat profusely during and after arduous exercise, and in extreme cases this may lead to dehydration and depletion of electrolytes so that fluid replacement therapy may be necessary. Fevers may also induce excessive sweating.

hyperimmune serum The serum of an individual that has been repeatedly immunized with a given *antigen so as to produce high *titres of specific *antibody.

hyperinsulinism The condition resulting from excess levels of the hormone *insulin. This may arise due to excessive insulin administration in therapy for diabetes mellitus, or be due to the presence of an insulin-secreting tumour (*insulinoma). Excess insulin results in low blood sugar (*hypoglycaemia) and can lead to coma and death. Varied neurological signs are present, such as lethargy, muscle tremors, stumbling gait, and seizures. These signs most commonly occur following insulin therapy, with the animal refusing to eat a meal. Therapy for low blood sugar consists in intravenous administration of glucose followed by oral glucose and carbohydrate when the acute crisis is over. An insulin assay contrasting the insulin and glucose concentrations in the blood is highly diagnostic for insulinomas. Surgical removal of the tumour should be attempted, although many will have metastasized by the time diagnosis is made.

hyperkalaemia (hyperpotassaemia) An abnormally high concentration of *potassium in the blood. Most potassium is intracellular, and its concentration in blood, which is controlled indirectly by the hormones *angiotensin II and *aldosterone, is not necessarily indicative of tissue concentrations. Hyperkalaemia is common, occurring in all species. The causes include oliguric or anuric renal failure, *acidosis (especially when associated with dehydration), tissue damage, tissue catabolism (especially when associated with dehydration), adrenal insufficiency (*see* Addison's disease), excessive oral or parenteral intakes of potassium, and excessive doses of some diuretics. In ruminants it has been associated with *hypomagnesaemia. Clinical signs of hyperkalaemia include increased thirst, diminished reflexes, muscular weakness (aesthenia), bradycardia, cardiac failure, and death. Treatment is directed to overcoming any cardiac irregularities, as well as correcting the underlying causes. *Compare* hypokalaemia.

hyperkeratosis An increase in thickness of the stratum corneum, the outermost layer of the *skin. It may occur naturally as a protective response to pressure, or indicate the presence of disease.

hyperlipaemia (lipaemia) An abnormally high concentration of lipids, mainly triglycerides, in the blood. The suspended lipid makes the blood appear opalescent or milky. It is normal in animals that have recently ingested a meal with a high fat content, for example carnivores, such as dogs and cats, and milk-fed ruminants. In sick and anorexic horses hyperlipaemia occurs to a mild degree and without clinical signs. It is of greatest clinical significance in small fat ponies, especially those in late gestation or early lactation, and those in negative energy balance due to starvation, pregnancy, lactation, parasitism, or transportation. In these ponies there may be massive release of lipid into the plasma causing metabolic dysfunction and clinical signs. These include, in progression, dullness, lethargy, poor appetite, rapid loss of body condition, trembling, staggering gait, ventral oedema, fever, diarrhoea, and high mortality rates after about 10 days of illness. There is hepatic and renal dysfunction and marked fatty infiltration of many tissues, including liver, kidneys, and heart. Treatments include improving feed intake and administration of glucose and insulin. Hyperlipaemia may also occur in hepatic lipidosis in cats, and in some severe cases of diabetes mellitus, hypothyroidism, hepatitis, and pancreatitis in dogs.

hypernatraemia An abnormally high concentration of *sodium in the blood. The blood concentration of sodium ions is controlled by the hormones *angiotensin II and *aldosterone, and sodium is excreted via the kidneys and intestines. Hypernatraemia is uncommon but can occur in all species, causing decreases in intracellular volume with marked changes in cellular function. The causes include dehydration (especially when secondary to *renal disease, hyperthermia, and deficient intakes of sodium); *diabetes insipidus; hyperaldosteronism (*see* hyperadrenocorticism); and excessive intakes of sodium (e.g. in *salt poisoning) and/or restricted intakes of fresh drinking water. In diabetes insipidus and water deprivation it may occur with *hypovolaemia, whereas in hyperaldosteronism it may occur with *hypervolaemia. Signs and treatment of hypernatraemia depend on the cause, but circulatory collapse and correction of dehydration are features of most cases. *Compare* hyponatraemia.

hypernephroma (renal carcinoma) A malignant tumour of kidney cells occurring in most species in middle-aged and older animals. In **dogs**, males are more often affected than bitches, and presenting clinical signs are blood in the urine and a palpable abdominal mass. The tumour arises in the renal cortex from one pole of the kidney and may grow to replace a large part of the organ, with occasional extension into adjacent tissues. On post-mortem examination the lesion is usually well demarcated from normal renal tissue, which is atrophied and compressed. Invasion of the renal pelvis, ureter, renal veins, and hilar lymphatics occurs, with metastases especially in the lungs and liver. Removal of the affected kidney is curative providing the tumour has not spread to other organs.

hyperoestrogenism A syndrome involving abnormally high levels of circulating oestrogens. It is well defined in males, and is seen most commonly in dogs with a Sertoli cell tumour (*see* feminization). The condition may also occur in females with cystic ovarian disease, but this condition is less well defined. *Iatrogenic*

hyperparathyroidism

hyperoestrogenism has been reported in bitches that have been treated for mismating with synthetic oestrogens. Blood dyscrasias and clotting deficiencies have been reported and some animals have died as a result.

hyperparathyroidism A condition resulting from excess production of *parathyroid hormone (PTH) by the parathyroid gland, which can result in high blood calcium (*hypercalcaemia) and, if untreated, consequent mineralization of soft tissues, kidney failure, and heart failure. *Primary hyperparathyroidism* is usually caused by tumours of the parathyroid; the tumours are usually *adenomas, which are benign and can be surgically removed. More common is *pseudohyperparathyroidism* –due to tumours elsewhere in the body (e.g. *lymphomas and anal adenomas) that have the ability to produce PTH-like substances that also mobilize calcium and result in identical syndromes. Radioimmunoassay for PTH and blood calcium quantitation can differentiate between these conditions. *Secondary hyperparathyroidism* is also common; it can be nutritional or renal in origin. When the kidney fails to resorb calcium properly, the parathyroid secretes PTH to compensate for the low blood calcium. A vicious cycle results since calcium continues to be lost into the urine and the high concentration of PTH continues calcium mobilization from bone. Eventually demineralization can occur and *rubber jaw syndrome develop. Chronic malnutrition can also cause high PTH – in an attempt to compensate for low blood calcium. Dietary lack of vitamin D, low calcium, or excessive phosphorus are common causes.

hyperplasia The increased production and growth of normal cells in a tissue or organ. The affected part becomes larger but retains its normal form. For example, the mammary gland undergoes hyperplasia in late pregnancy as a result of hormonal stimuli. The skin or other epithelial surface may show hyperplastic thickening in response to chronic irritation. Lymph nodes show reactive hyperplasia in response to persistent infection. *Compare* hypertrophy; metaplasia; neoplasm.

hyperpnoea An increase in the rate of breathing that is proportional to an increase in metabolism; for example, on exercise. *See also* hyperventilation.

hyperpyrexia A state of high *fever (pyrexia) in which body temperature is markedly elevated above normal. *See also* heat exhaustion.

hypersensitivity A condition in which an allergic process leads to tissue damage and/or to clinical illness (*see* allergy). Four types of hypersensitivity reactions are recognized. *Type I reactions* are brought about by an *antigen reacting with tissue *mast cells bearing specific *antibodies on their membranes. The result is the release by the mast cells of substances which cause inflammation. Antibodies mediating Type I reactions are also known as *reagins or homocytotropic antibodies and are of the IgE class. Genetic predisposition to manufacture reagins is known as *atopy. The signs of Type I hypersensitivity may be generalized (*anaphylaxis) and can vary with the species; they typically include respiratory distress (caused by bronchial constriction), diarrhoea, vomiting, salivation, abdominal pain, and *cyanosis. Dogs tend to exhibit vascular shock owing to pooling of blood in the portal system. The reaction may also be localized, most typically seen as inflammation of the skin or nasal mucosa. *Type II reactions* are a form of cell damage induced by antibody; *complement or cytotoxic cells may also be involved. Such reactions may injure any tissue but blood cells are particularly susceptible. The result is most strikingly seen in haemolytic responses to incompatible blood transfusions where foreign red cells are destroyed by acquired specific antibody. In other cases, however, the damage is mediated by an *autoantibody (see autoimmune disease; serum sickness).

Type III reactions are caused by antigen-antibody complexes, which are formed in or carried to the walls of small blood vessels, where they activate complement. In *Type IV reactions* antibody is not involved; instead the hypersensitivity is mediated by *lymphocytes whose membranes bear receptors capable of binding with *antigen. Tissue damage is brought about either directly by the lymphocyte itself or indirectly by lymphocyte secretions that activate other leucocytes in the area. The classical instance of a Type IV reaction is the dermal response to tuberculin shown by specifically presensitized cattle. Although Type IV responses may be considered essentially protective rather than damaging, a number of diseases seem to occur as a result of uncontrolled Type IV processes. These include contact hypersensitivity, autoimmune *thyroiditis, and a number of granulomatous conditions associated with chronic infections.

hypersplenism Excessive destruction of blood cells by the spleen. There is associated enlargement of the spleen and deficiency of red cells and sometimes of other cells. In true hypersplenism the changes in blood cells are halted by removal of the spleen. This is not the case if, as is more common, the spleen's overactivity is a consequence of damage to the red cells (see haemolytic anaemia).

hypertension Abnormally high *blood pressure. This is rarely diagnosed in animals due to difficulty in taking measurements.

hyperthermia See heat exhaustion; malignant hyperthermia.

hyperthyroidism A condition resulting from increased secretion of thyroid hormones from the *thyroid gland. It has recently become common in older cats, which have a very rapid heart rate, excessive appetite, diarrhoea, polyuria, polydipsia, and weight loss. There is often a palpable lesion in the neck. The disease can be confirmed by finding elevated serum thyroid hormone concentrations. Therapy is directed toward decreasing thyroid hormone output with propylthiouracil or methimazole. Surgical removal of the thyroids is quite successful; alternatively the thyroid can be destroyed in situ by administering radioactive iodine. Presently, the cause of the disease and its recent increase in prevalence are unknown. The disease is less common in other veterinary species, but does occur occasionally in dogs.

hypertonic 1. Describing a solution that has a greater osmotic pressure than another solution. See osmosis. **2.** Describing muscles that demonstrate an abnormally high degree of *tonicity.

hypertrophy Increase in the size of a tissue or organ due to enlargement of its cells rather than cell multiplication (as occurs during normal growth or tumour formation). Muscles undergo hypertrophy in response to exercise. Also, similar changes occur in the musculature of the uterine wall in response to pregnancy. However, the increased load may be due to disease. For example, heart muscle undergoes hypertrophy in response to cardiovascular disease. Compensatory hypertrophy occurs in paired organs, such as the kidneys: when the function of one is impaired the other grows to compensate. *Compare* hyperplasia.

hyperuricaemia The presence of an abnormally high concentration of *uric acid in the blood. Although uncommon in mammals it is liable to occur in poultry and other birds, in which uric acid is the end-product of nitrogen metabolism. Thus birds normally have relatively high levels of uric acid in the blood. Dalmatian dogs lack the liver enzyme uricase, which converts uric acid to allantoin. Hence blood uric acid tends to be elevated in this breed. The detection of hyperuricaemia has been recommended as a sensitive indicator of liver failure.

hyperuricuria The presence of an abnormally high concentration of *uric acid in the urine. It occurs in Dalmatian dogs, which cannot convert uric acid to allantoin in the liver. This makes them susceptible to the formation of urate calculi (stones) in the bladder (*see* lithiasis). Other dogs may suffer similarly if liver function is impaired. In cases of liver failure ammonia is excreted as well, and calculi of ammonium urate tend to form.

hyperventilation Breathing at an abnormally rapid rate. It occurs if the carbon dioxide level in the blood is abnormally high as a result of impaired gaseous exchange in the lungs, which can occur, for example, in pneumonia.

hypervitaminosis Disease caused by excessive intake of a *vitamin. It tends to occur more readily with the fat-soluble vitamins, which are stored in the liver, but is less common with water-soluble vitamins, which can be excreted in the urine. For example, cats fed mainly on liver, which is rich

in vitamin A, can suffer hypervitaminosis. Also cats or dogs fed too much fish-liver oil may suffer vitamin D toxicity, signs of which include vomiting and diarrhoea, the production of large volumes of urine (polyuria), and bone disease with calcification of the soft tissues. A similar problem occurs in cattle given massive doses of vitamin D_3 to prevent milk fever, and has also been reported in horses.

hypervolaemia An abnormal increase in the volume of circulating blood. Excessive intakes of salt cause temporary hypervolaemia due to the higher osmolarity of the blood; the blood volume later falls as the salt is excreted. A pathological cause is *heart failure, in which vascular congestion is accompanied by failure to excrete excess water. Blood volume rises as oedema of the body tissues develops. Hypervolaemia can also result from excessive transfusion of plasma or blood.

hypha (*pl.* **hyphae**) A threadlike tubular filament with a refractile rigid wall, usually forming part of a branching system known as a *mycelium – the main growth form of most *fungi. Hyphae may or may not develop cross-walls (septate or aseptate hyphae, respectively) and they grow by extension from the tip, invading organic material aided by the secretion of enzymes. Fungal hyphae tend to retain their form and refractility even when the cytoplasm within them has died or migrated to another part of the mycelium; they can thus still be detected or examined microscopically in such a state.

Hyphomyces destruens The former name for the nonsporulating fungal mycelium found in the lesions of many cases of *equine phycomycosis. The organism has since been identified as a species of *Pythium* and this form of the disease is now termed *pythiosis.

hypn- (hypno-) *Prefix denoting* **1.** sleep. **2.** hypnosis.

Hypnorm *See* fentanyl.

hypnotic A drug that induces drowsiness or, at higher doses, sleep or a light plane of anaesthesia. Hypnotics are used in veterinary medicine as premedicants prior to anaesthesia, to facilitate animal handling, and in the treatment and prevention of epileptiform seizures. Examples are the benzodiazepines (e.g. *diazepam), *barbiturates, *chloral hydrate, and *metomidate. Most produce central nervous system depression as well as sleep, and high doses produce a state of general anaesthesia (except the benzodiazepines). *Compare* sedative.

hypo- *Prefix. See* hyp-.

hypoadrenocorticism (Addison's disease) A syndrome resulting from atrophy of the adrenal cortex, which results in inadequate mineralocorticoid and glucocorticoid (*see* corticosteroid) production and severe sodium and potassium imbalance. Most dogs with classical Addison's disease have atrophy of both the mineralocorticoid and glucocorticoid portions of the adrenal glands, probably from autoimmune phenomena. Glucocorticoids, such as cortisol and corticosterone, have slight mineralocorticoid activity, but their concentrations are so great compared to aldosterone (about 1000 times more) that they provide a significant mineralocorticoid effect as well. Therefore, for the syndrome to occur the entire adrenal cortex must be atrophied. Dehydration occurs, resulting in very poor organ perfusion. Clinical signs include vomiting, diarrhoea, anorexia, lethargy, and collapse. Specific electrical changes due to elevated serum potas-

sium (hyperkalaemia) can be detected by electrocardiography, and the heartbeat is often slow. Tentative diagnosis can be made based on the low serum sodium and high potassium. Aldosterone and cortisol assays can confirm the adrenal atrophy. Therapy is accomplished by hormone replacement using synthetic mineralocorticoids, such as 11-DOC or florinef, and by adding sodium to the diet.

hypoaesthesia Diminished sensitivity to pain and other stimuli. *Compare* anaesthesia; hyperaesthesia.

hypocalcaemia An abnormally low concentration of *calcium in the blood. Transient hypocalcaemia may occur in animals given diets low in calcium and/or high in phosphate, but this is usually corrected by mobilization of calcium reserves in the bones. A more acute and severe hypocalcaemia usually occurs because of failure of the homeostatic mechanisms controlling blood calcium concentrations. This happens especially at the end of pregnancy and at the beginning of lactation, when there are sudden demands for calcium and the skeletal reserves have not hitherto been mobilized. In dairy cattle this form of hypocalcaemia is generally termed *milk fever, and may be accompanied by *hypomagnesaemia, *hypophosphataemia, and *ketosis. Sheep may suffer a similar condition preceded by deprivation of food (*see* lambing sickness). Hypocalcaemia also occurs in beef cattle, horses, dogs, and, rarely, cats, mink, poultry, goats, and pigs. It causes excitability, spastic paralysis, incoordination, muscle tremors, increased respiratory rates, convulsions, coma, and death. In these species it is associated with either pregnancy and lactation (*see* eclampsia; lactation tetany) or, in both sexes of horses and ruminants, transportation for long periods of time (*see* transit tetany). Hypocalcaemia may also occur in laying poultry given diets deficient in calcium and phosphate, and in dogs with acute *pancreatitis. In all species, treatment with parenteral solutions of calcium (e.g. calcium borogluconate) in the early stages of the condition is usually successful. Special preventive measures can be taken for dairy cattle (see milk fever). Compare hypercalcaemia.

hypocapnia See acapnia.

hypochloraemia An abnormally low concentration of chloride in the blood. Chloride concentration normally follows that of sodium, hence hypochloraemia and *hyponatraemia occur together in salt (sodium chloride) deficiency. Exceptions apply in certain diseases. For example, in persistent vomiting the loss of chloride anions by way of the acid secretion of the stomach leads to hypochloraemia, and the resulting relative excess of sodium induces metabolic *alkalosis. Although this is a common sequel to persistent vomiting in single-stomached animals it also occurs in ruminants with abomasal disorders or gut obstruction. Therapy consists of isotonic saline solution containing excess chloride administered orally or intravenously, depending on circumstances. Compare hyperchloraemia.

hypochlorite An *antiseptic that slowly releases chlorine when exposed to air or organic material. The released chlorine is an oxidizing agent and destroys microorganisms; it also acts as a deodorizing agent. The chlorine is inactivated by reacting with organic material to form chloramines, which release chlorine only very slowly. Sodium hypochlorite is used in teat dips and as a general antiseptic and disinfectant. It acts as a bleach and may cause temporary skin irritation; care should be taken when handling concentrated solutions. Other names: **chlorinated soda; Dakin's solution.**

hypocupraemia An abnormally low concentration of copper in the blood. It usually indicates copper deficiency (*hypocuprosis), although caution is needed in interpreting the results of blood tests – not all hypocupraemic animals show signs of copper deficiency or respond beneficially to supplementation. Also, genuinely copper-deficient animals can maintain their blood copper concentration for long periods using reserves stored in the liver. In hypocupraemia, blood copper can fall from the normal of about 100 $\mu mol/l$ to 16–60 $\mu mol/l$.

hypocuprosis Disease caused by copper deficiency. Low concentrations of blood copper (*hypocupraemia), ceruloplasmin, or liver copper, found in diagnostic tests, confirm the condition. The disease is not always due to a simple deficiency of copper but can be caused by the interaction of excess molybdenum, which restricts copper absorption. High intakes of protein can exert a similar effect because sulphur in certain amino acids precipitates the copper as unavailable sulphide. Cattle usually suffer copper deficiency on pasture where the soil is copper-deficient or has high molybdenum levels (see teart soils). Clinical signs include diarrhoea coupled with bone disorders (*osteoporosis), anaemia, and a characteristic failure of hair pigmentation, especially around the eyes. The wool of affected sheep lacks its usual crimp and is termed 'stringy' or 'steely'. Production is affected, with ill-thrift, poor growth rates, and infertility. Copper deficiency in pregnant ewes induces *swayback (enzootic ataxia) in their lambs, which have lesions of the brain stem and spinal cord. Copper deficiency also occurs in goats, deer, and pigs. Dietary supplementation relieves the problems although excess copper can cause *copper poisoning, especially in sheep.

Hypoderma A genus containing many of the *warble flies, whose larvae are internal parasites of cattle.

hypodermic Beneath the skin: usually applied to subcutaneous *injections. The term is also applied to the syringe used for such injections.

hypoglossal nerve The twelfth *cranial nerve (XII). It supplies the muscles of the tongue.

hypoglycaemia An abnormally low concentration of glucose in the blood. It is especially common in ruminants, which absorb little or no glucose from their alimentary tracts and rely on the liver to synthesize essential supplies, e.g. for lactation. Hypoglycaemia commonly occurs in early lactation in high-yielding dairy cows and may indicate the onset of *ketosis. Similarly in sheep, hypoglycaemia in late pregnancy may be an early warning sign of *pregnancy toxaemia. Hypoglycaemia is of special significance in newborn animals, such as piglets. These have little body fat and rely on their glycogen reserves to provide energy during their first few hours. Failure to suckle or cold weather during this critical period can induce hypoglycaemia, followed by a fall in body temperature (*see* hypothermia), incoordination, and death. An injection of 5% glucose, given intraperitoneally, often gives a rapid response. Hypoglycaemia also occurs in severe liver disease, after excess administration of insulin, or with insulin-secreting tumours. *Compare* hyperglycaemia.

hypoglycaemic agent A substance that reduces the concentration of glucose in the circulation. The hormone *insulin regulates blood glucose in

normal animals, and in cases of *diabetes mellitus daily injections of insulin together with dietary management can control the hyperglycaemia. Oral hypoglycaemic agents, such as the sulphonylureas (tolbutamine and chlorpropamide) and the biguanides, cause hypoglycaemia in normal animals following oral administration. They have little effect in dogs with diabetes mellitus, possibly because the disease is too far advanced when treatment is initiated.

hypogonadism Decreased function of the gonads, which may be due to gonadal lesions or lesions in the hypothalamus or pituitary gland. It results in decreased trophic hormone production and consequent impaired reproductive activity or absence or impairment of secondary sexual characteristics. Determining the location of the specific lesion is difficult since few species-specific trophic hormone assays are presently available for diagnostic use. Therapy is often based upon the findings during a thorough clinical examination and history.

hypoidrosis Diminished ability to sweat. This rarely occurs in animals. *Compare* anidrosis.

hypokalaemia An abnormally low concentration of potassium in the blood. It most commonly occurs as part of a complex metabolic disturbance known as metabolic *alkalosis. This follows persistent vomiting, abomasal disorders, or obstructions of the alimentary tract in which excessive amounts of chloride anions are lost in the digestive secretions. Potassium cations are then excreted in the urine to restore the acid-base balance. Hypokalaemia occurs rarely as a result of decreased dietary intake, for example, in intensively reared beef cattle fed diets containing almost no roughage (roughage normally contributes ample potassium in ruminant diets). Horses undertaking endurance rides may also suffer hypokalaemia due to loss of electrolytes in sweat. In all cases, hypokalaemia causes severe muscular weakness and exhaustion, sometimes with muscular tremors and irregular heart beat. Therapy may involve the administration of a solution of potassium salts, although care must be taken to avoid giving excess potassium (*see* hyperkalaemia).

hypomagnesaemia An abnormally low concentration of *magnesium in the blood. This is usually related to a dietary deficiency of magnesium, and can lead to depletion of magnesium reserves in the bones, convulsions, tetany, and death. *Hypomagnesaemic tetany* (*grass staggers*) is a condition of adult ruminants with an acute or chronic onset. The acute form most often occurs when animals are turned out to young succulent pasture in the spring. Dairy cows are usually affected after turnout, whereas beef cows may also suffer from the disease in autumn and winter. The signs are incoordination, muscle tremors, and excitability with animals often having a 'wild' look. The disease progresses to convulsions and death if not treated. Measurement of blood magnesium levels by laboratory tests confirms the diagnosis. Treatment entails careful slow intravenous or subcutaneous injection with magnesium sulphate. The disease can be prevented by ensuring animals receive supplementation with *calcined magnesite (magnesium oxide) in the feed during the period of risk. Cows should receive about 50 g/head/day, calves 7–15 g, and lactating ewes about 7 g.

hypomyelinogenesis The former term for a group of congenital viral infections causing nervous signs and abnormal gait in newborns. These include *Border disease in lambs, progressive ataxia in cattle, and con-

genital tremor syndrome in piglets. The *pestiviruses responsible cross the placenta of the dam to infect the foetuses, and cause deficient development of *myelin in nervous tissue, hence the clinical signs.

hyponatraemia An abnormally low concentration of sodium in the blood. It can occur as a result of sodium deficiency or excessive loss of sodium in body secretions. Sodium levels are under strict hormonal regulation and any tendency towards hyponatraemia is rapidly corrected by preventing loss of sodium via the digestive secretions or urine. However, ruminants grazing pastures in areas with sodium-deficient soils often become hyponatraemic, although this may take up to 1–2 months to develop. This process is accelerated if the animals suffer subclinical or clinical *mastitis, which entails losses of sodium in the milk. The sodium deficiency can be easily corrected by providing *salt licks, although care must be taken to avoid overindulgence and *salt poisoning. Hyponatraemia also occurs with *diarrhoea because of the loss of sodium ions through the inflamed intestinal mucosa. In severe cases this causes decreased blood volume, low blood pressure, and reduced osmolarity leading eventually to circulatory failure. Hyponatraemia can also affect certain marine mammals kept in fresh water, for example, seals kept in zoo parks. *Compare* hypernatraemia.

hypoparathyroidism The condition resulting from atrophy of the parathyroid glands or accidental removal of the glands during thyroidectomy. This causes reduced levels or complete absence of *parathyroid hormone (PTH); the disease can be confirmed using a PTH assay. Without PTH blood calcium falls precipitously (*see* hypocalcaemia), which can result in hypocalcaemic tetany and death. Therapy for the acute condition entails intravenous administration of calcium. Long-term therapy is accomplished with dietary calcium supplements and the administration of active metabolites of *vitamin D.

hypophosphataemia An abnormally low concentration of *phosphate in the blood. Blood phosphate is not under direct hormonal control, hence concentrations vary widely and in phosphate deficiency they may fall quickly. Hypophosphataemia is commonly accepted as evidence of a nutritional deficiency of *phosphate. However deficient animals may maintain blood levels for a time by calling on mineral reserves. Phosphate deficiency in young animals gives stunted growth and *rickets. In older cattle reduced milk yield and infertility occur. Hypophosphataemic animals may show *pica (depraved appetite) and will chew bones.

Dietary phosphate deficiency is common in livestock grazing phosphate-deficient pastures, which occur extensively worldwide. Livestock in these areas require supplementation of the diet with ground rock phosphate; this is usually an ingredient of mineral licks and premixes. Phosphate deficiency is rare in meat-eating species, such as dogs and cats; poultry too are seldom affected because of their predominantly grain-based diets.

hypophysis See pituitary gland.

hypopituitarism (panhypopituitarism) A syndrome caused by subnormal activity of the *pituitary gland and involving multiple endocrine disorders, including *hypogonadism, *hypothyroidism, *hypoadrenocorticism, and dwarfism. This complete syndrome is rare, but there is the possibility for selective cellular loss from the pituitary gland, which can result in more narrowly defined syndromes.

hypoplasia Underdevelopment or incomplete development of an organ or tissue. There may be a disproportionate reduction of particular cellular components. For example, hypoplasia of the bone marrow leads to anaemia or leucopenia, depending on which cell lines are hypoplastic.

hypoproteinaemia An abnormally low concentration of protein in the blood. The term usually applies to serum *albumin and *globulins, which constitute the major osmotic components of blood.

Hypoproteinaemia has various causes, including persistent blood loss due to heavy infestation with blood-sucking parasites, kidney disease (which allows blood protein to leak into the urine), certain enteric diseases (which interfere with protein digestion and absorption), dietary deficiency of protein, and liver disease (which interrupts albumin synthesis by the liver). The osmotic pressure of the blood falls and fluid accumulates throughout the body, especially subcutaneously and in the various body cavities. Treatment consists of correcting the primary cause.

hyposensitive Less than normally sensitive to a given *antigen.

hyposensitization See desensitization.

hypostasis 1. (hypostatic congestion) The accumulation of fluid or blood in a part of the body owing to poor circulation. Affected organs and tissues become deprived of oxygen; muscles fail to function and the skin succumbs to pressure sores. In *generalized hypostasis* the return of blood to the heart slows allowing congestion in part or the whole of the venous circulation. The primary cause is commonly some kind of *heart failure, such as valvular incompetence. Blood accumulates in the major organs,

hypotension

which appear swollen, discoloured, and congested. If congestion persists the lung and liver undergo 'brown induration' due to the accumulation of *haemosiderin, a pigment derived from the destruction of red blood cells. *Local hypostasis* may be caused by cirrhosis of the liver, which obstructs blood flow from the abdominal viscera. It may also follow the restriction of venous blood flow by pressure from tumours or the occlusion of a vein with a thrombus. Hypostasis also occurs in animals that are recumbent for long periods, for example *downer cows. **2.** (in genetics) The phenomenon where the action of a gene is dependent on the previous action of another gene. *Compare* epistasis.

hypotension A condition in which the arterial *blood pressure is abnormally low. It is rarely diagnosed in animals because no simple and effective technique for measurement exists. Acute hypotension occurs in cases of shock, *anaphylaxis, and certain other hypersensitive reactions. Treatment involves the prompt administration of adrenaline. Chronic hypotension occurs in various diseases, especially *heart failure.

hypotensive agent Any of a group of drugs used to reduce blood pressure. These drugs are used in the treatment of heart conditions (e.g. congestive heart failure), mainly in small animals. Blood pressure is maintained by the smooth muscles of the blood vasculature, which are under the control of the *sympathetic nervous system via adrenergic receptors (adrenoceptors). Hypotensive agents act by reducing vascular resistance, which reduces the workload on the heart and improves cardiac efficiency. This in turn reduces valvular incompetence, cardiac dilatation, and myocardial tension.

There are various types of hypotensive agent. Prazosine acts by blocking the α_1 adrenoceptors, thus reducing the peripheral resistance without any tachycardia or blocking of noradrenaline action on α_2 receptors (*see* alpha blocker). *Beta blockers act by reducing heart rate and also causing a fall in peripheral resistance and circulating blood volume. The *phenothiazines act as sedatives and also have an alpha-blocking effect. Clonidine acts as an agonist at α_2 adrenergic receptors in the central nervous system and periphery, reducing cardiac output and peripheral resistance. *Halothane acts as a ganglion-blocking drug, causing a fall in blood pressure as a side-effect during anaesthesia. *Reserpine acts locally and centrally to deplete noradrenaline stores in sympathetic neurones, thereby causing a fall in blood pressure.

Other drugs used to induce hypotension can act directly on the smooth muscle of blood vessels. Hydralazine is administered orally or parenterally, producing arterial vasodilatation with a reflex tachycardia. Sodium nitroprusside can be used to induce hypotension by reducing peripheral resistance and causing venodilatation with a reflex tachycardia. Nicotinic acid is used orally to cause vasodilatation in superficial blood vessels. Nitrites (e.g. amyl nitrite, *sodium nitrite) and nitrates that are converted to nitrites in the body are used to cause smooth muscle relaxation in blood vessels with vasodilatation, especially of veins. Verapamil and nifedipine act as arteriolar vasodilators by interfering with calcium uptake into smooth muscle. *Captopril acts as an *angiotensin-converting enzyme inhibitor, causing vasodilatation and inhibiting the secretion of *aldosterone. There is general vasodilatation and a reduction in fluid retention.

Many of these drugs may have side-effects, such as tachycardia, heart arrhythmias, and reduced myocardial activity. They are often also expensive.

hypothalamus The region of the *diencephalon in the brain lying below the thalamus and around the floor of the third ventricle. It is connected to the *pituitary gland by the infundibulum. The hypothalamus contains several important centres controlling body temperature, thirst, hunger, water balance, and sexual drive. It is also closely involved with emotional activity and sleep through its connection with the *limbic system, and functions as a centre for the integration of hormonal and autonomic nervous activity through its control of pituitary secretion.

hypothermia Abnormally low body temperature, usually following exposure to cold. *Body temperature is maintained at about 38.5°C in mammalian livestock species and about 41.5°C in birds. In hypothermia it may fall to 25°C or lower. The condition commonly occurs in the newborn, especially when born in cold environments or when the mother's milk fails. Piglets are especially at risk because they have relatively little body fat to provide reserve energy or heat insulation. Lambs are more cold-resistant but can easily succumb to hypothermia if cold and wet. Animals born prematurely with a low birthweight are more susceptible. Treatment entails the intraperitoneal administration of warm glucose solution and providing shelter and an infrared lamp for warmth. Hypothermia as a sequel to fever is a bad sign that often indicates imminent death. Prolonged anaesthesia, especially in neonates or very small animals, tends to result in hypothermia unless preventive measures are taken.

hypothyroidism A syndrome resulting from a lack of thyroid hormone production. Thyroid hormones are necessary for normal growth and development in the young and for normal metabolism in young and adults. Low hormone concentrations result in cretinous dwarfism during development. Adults show weight gain, sluggishness, decreased mental activity, hair loss, infertility, decreased body temperature, and in some instances, *myxoedema. Many hypothyroid animals have autoimmune *thyroiditis (Hashimoto's disease), which results in thyroid atrophy. Farm animals often demonstrate *goitre with hypothyroidism due to inadequate dietary iodine. Decreased hormone production can be assayed with *radioimmunoassay. However, a number of nonthyroidal illnesses can cause decreased thyroid hormone concentrations and a false indication of hypothyroidism. Dietary iodine deficiency can be avoided by feeding iodized salt. In small animals, hypothyroidism can be corrected by administering synthetic thyroid hormone orally on a daily basis. Both *thyroxine and *triiodothyronine (T3) are commercially available. See also congenital hypothyroidism.

hypotonic 1. Describing a solution that has a lower osmotic pressure than another solution. See osmosis. **2.** Describing muscles that demonstrate diminished *tonicity.

hypovolaemia (oligaemia) A decrease in the volume of circulating blood. See shock.

hypoxaemia The presence in the blood of an abnormally low concentration of oxygen, usually as a result of inadequate uptake of oxygen in the lungs because of lung disease. See also anoxia.

hypoxia A deficiency of oxygen in the tissues. *See also* anoxia; hypoxaemia.

hyster- (hystero-) *Prefix denoting* the uterus.

hysterectomy Surgical removal of the *uterus (womb). This forms part of the routine *spaying (neutering) operation in female dogs and cats (*see also* ovariohysterectomy). It is performed extremely rarely in large animals but may be necessary in any species where uterine disease is unresponsive to medical therapy, for example neoplasia or haemorrhagic ulceration.

hysterocoele Hernia of the uterus. This is a rare condition in animals.

hysteroscope (uteroscope) An *endoscope designed to aid visualization of the uterus. It is inserted via the vagina and cervix, and may be useful in diagnosing uterine disease or facilitating the taking of biopsies from specific areas of uterine tissue or in swabbing uterine contents or mucosa.

hysterotomy Surgical incision into the lumen of the uterus. This is generally undertaken as part of a *Caesarean section.

I

-iasis *Suffix denoting* a diseased condition.

iatrogenic Describing a condition induced by treatment, as either an unforeseen or inevitable side-effect.

IB *See* infectious bronchitis.

IBD *See* infectious bursal disease.

IBR *See* infectious bovine rhinotracheitis.

ibuprofen *See* NSAID.

ichthyosis A rare congenital condition of cattle, dogs, and humans in which the skin is thickened, fissured, and scaly due to a defect in *keratinization. It varies in severity.

ICSH (interstitial-cell-stimulating hormone) *See* luteinizing hormone.

icterus *See* jaundice.

identical twins *See* twins.

idiopathic Describing a disease of unknown cause.

idiosyncrasy An unusual and unexpected reaction by an individual to a certain drug or food. This may be due to an individual having a sensitivity outside the 'normal' range or to hitherto unsuspected factors, such as disease.

ile- (ileo-) *Prefix denoting* the ileum. Examples: *ileocaecal* (relating to the ileum and caecum); *ileocolic* (relating to the ileum and colon).

ileitis Inflammation of the ileum (lower small intestine). The ileum is involved in most forms of *enteritis, the commonest being neonatal diarrhoea, which is caused by a variety of infectious agents; outbreaks and even individual cases are frequently associated with mixed infections. Treatment is generally with antibiotic therapy. Prevention is aided by ensuring that newborns receive adequate colostrum and are not overcrowded. A specific form of ileitis is *Johne's disease, which causes clinical signs in cattle over 2 years old. The bacterium multiplies in the intestinal mucosa, eventually causing a severe and persistent diarrhoea. Pigs can be affected by a specific ileitis that resembles Crohn's disease in humans. The intestinal mucosa thickens, ulcerates, and may perforate leading to acute and fatal peritonitis. The cause is unknown. Terminal ileitis of lambs can resemble Johne's disease, but some cases are caused by intestinal parasites.

ileocolitis Inflammation of the ileum and colon. It usually involves a simple extension of *ileitis.

ileostomy The surgical creation of a permanent opening into the lumen of the ileum. This may be done to connect the ileum to the surface of the body (e.g. to study gut functions), or to another section of the gut to bypass diseased gut. For example an *ileocolostomy* involves connecting the ileum to the colon to bypass the ileocaecal junction. *See also* enterostomy.

ileum (*pl.* **ilea**) The short terminal part of the small intestine leading from the jejunum and to which the ileocaecal fold is attached. *See* alimentary tract.

ileus Obstruction of the gastrointestinal tract, preventing the normal passage of food, fluid, and gas through the gut. *Mechanical ileus* is due to physical obstruction, such as an impaction (*see* impacted), *intussusception, *strangulation, or *torsion. *Physiological* (*adynamic*) *ileus* results from an inability of the gut to propel material along the lumen. *Postoperative ileus* occurs after surgery, usually following an abdominal operation, and is a form of physiological ileus. The causes include altered nervous control of the gut musculature, electrolyte imbalances, distension and hypoxia, severe *peritonitis, or *endotoxaemia. Treatment depends on the cause. Impaction of the gastrointestinal tract is due to the accumu-

lation of ingested material; the material is not propelled along the gut and therefore obstructs the passage of food and secretions. It may occur in any part of the gut but particularly in the stomach of the dog and horse; the omasum of cattle; and the ileum and pelvic flexure of the horse. It can be due to overeating, poor dentition, lack of fluid intake, or gut motility disorders. Treatment may involve the administration of lubricants, or surgical removal of the obstruction. *See also* choke; colic.

ili- (ilio-) *Prefix denoting* the ilium.

iliac Relating to or part of the *ilium. The paired *external* and *internal iliac arteries* arise from the caudal end of the aorta. The external iliac artery becomes the *femoral artery and supplies most of the hindlimb. The internal iliac artery supplies organs of the pelvic cavity, the perineum, and the hip region. *External* and *internal iliac veins* drain fields similar to the arteries and join to form the *common iliac vein*, which drains into the caudal vena cava.

ilium One of the bones that fuse to form the *os coxae in the adult hip.

ILT *See* avian infectious laryngotracheitis.

imidazoles A group of antifungal agents having similar structures and properties. They include clotrimazole, econazole, enilconazole, ketoconazole, miconazole, and also thiabendazole; thiabendazole (*see* benzimidazole) has anthelmintic as well as antifungal properties. They have a broad spectrum of activity against dermatophytes, yeasts, actinomycetes, and also some Gram-positive bacteria and anaerobes. The drugs interfere with fungal membrane permeability, prevent the synthesis of ergosterol (the primary cellular sterol of fungi), and inhibit fatty acid synthesis.

Ketoconazole is the only imidazole used systemically to treat mycoses. Given orally, it is absorbed best from an acidic environment. However, it is highly protein-bound and penetrates poorly into cerebrospinal fluid. It is metabolized in the liver and excreted in the bile and urine. Toxicity can occur, with vomiting, hepatotoxicity, and reproductive disorders. The other imidazoles are mainly used topically to treat ringworm and other infections. The drugs penetrate into the stratum corneum of the skin and can have a persistent effect. Miconazole is available as Conoderm cream for use in small animals, and enilconazole as Imaverol for large animals.

imidocarb An antiprotozoal drug, with the properties of a reversible cholinesterase inhibitor, used in the treatment and prevention of babesiosis and anaplasmosis. It is well absorbed when used subcutaneously or intramuscularly and distributes throughout the tissues, where it becomes bound to proteins. It is excreted unchanged in the urine and faeces. High doses in cattle can protect against babesiosis for up to one month, but toxicity can occur – the drug has a low *therapeutic index. Animals should not be slaughtered for at least 28 days after treatment. Tradename: **Imizol.**

Immobilon Tradename for a neuroleptanalgesic (*see* neuroleptanalgesia) containing both a tranquillizer and also the narcotic analgesic *etorphine. It is marketed as small-animal and large-animal preparations, but is not available in the USA. *Small Animal Immobilon* contains methotrimeprazine and etorphine, and is used in dogs to produce neuroleptanalgesia of about one-hour duration – suitable for minor surgical operations. It can be used

intravenously or intramuscularly. Side-effects include tachycardia or bradycardia, hypotension, respiratory depression, twitching, and sudden reaction to noise. The effects of etorphine can be reversed using *diprenorphine (Revivon). When used as an anaesthetic for Caesarean operations, respiratory depression in the neonate(s) can be counteracted by using diprenorphine. Immobilon should not be used in cats.

Large Animal Immobilon contains acepromazine (*see* phenothiazines) and etorphine, and is marketed for use in horses, donkeys, cattle, sheep, and pigs. It can be used intravenously or intramuscularly. Horses and cattle can be immobilized for up to 45 minutes, sheep and pigs for 25 minutes. Side-effects in horses are tachycardia, hypertension, muscle spasms, rigidity, and tremors. The drug should not be used in animals with signs of cardiovascular disease. Again, the effects of etorphine can be reversed with diprenorphine, but animals should be supervised in case of remission several hours later.

Immobilon is potentially very dangerous to humans, with relatively small doses proving fatal. Signs of toxicity in humans include dizziness, nausea, pupillary constriction, respiratory depression, hypotension, cyanosis, and cardiac arrest. When using Immobilon the reversing agent, naloxone, should be available at all times.

immunity The body's ability to resist infection or invasion by other ('foreign') agents or organisms and to counter any harmful effects they may cause. A great variety of mechanisms are involved in immunity. Innate mechanisms, such as the production of mucus in the alimentary and respiratory tracts, are part of the animal's normal physiological constitution. Some innate mechanisms are inherited. Vertebrates have a unique additional mechanism, that of *acquired immunity*, which may be of two types. *Active acquired immunity* is the process whereby exposure to disease organisms or to foreign *antigens confers resistance to subsequent infections. It is also specific in that the mechanism of resistance is directed only against the *antigen that elicited the original response. The immune response involves the production of *antibodies which have the power to physically bind the specific antigen, to activate *complement, and to assist *phagocytosis by *leucocytes. Other acquired immune mechanisms are mediated directly by cells of the lymphoid-macrophage system (*see* lymphocyte; macrophage). Artificial active immunity can be produced by the injection of antigens or organisms; this is the basis of *vaccination. *Passive acquired immunity* is produced by the transfer of antibodies from an immune to an unprotected animal. This occurs when antibodies are transferred from mother to foetus via the placenta, or from mother to the newborn via the *colostrum. It provides an important means of natural protection for young mammals. In birds, passive transfer of antibodies occurs via the yolk. Passive immunity may also be conferred by administering *antiserum. In all cases, passive immunity is short-lived.

immunization The production of *immunity. This occurs as part of the normal immune mechanism of the body, or it may be produced by artificial means. *Active immunization* involves the administration of specially treated *antigens (e.g. bacteria, viruses, or their toxins) to stimulate the body to produce *antibodies; this is the procedure of *vaccination. *Passive immunization* involves the administration of preformed antibodies (*see* antiserum); it provides only short-lived immunity.

immuno- *Prefix denoting* immunity or immunological response.

immunodeficiency A state in which one or more of the mechanisms of the immune system (*see* immunity) is deficient. Immunodeficiency may be inherited as a genetically determined defect, or acquired, for example when the lymphoid system is affected by virus infection or neoplasia.

immunoelectrophoresis A technique for identifying antigenic fractions in blood serum or other body fluids according to their electrophoretic and immunological properties. The molecules, usually proteins, are first separated by *electrophoresis. Antiserum containing a particular antibody is then poured into a slot cut in the gel support. The antibody and antigens diffuse through the gel and form a precipitate where they interact. The presence of particular antigens can thereby be detected and the amount present is indicated by the intensity of the precipitin line.

immunoglobulin *See* antibody.

immunological tolerance *See* tolerance.

immunology The science and study of *immunity, and of related phenomena, including *tolerance, *hypersensitivity, and *allergy.

immunophoresis *See* immunoelectrophoresis.

immunostimulation Stimulation of an immune response (*see* immunity).

immunosuppression Suppression of the immune response, whether specifically in relation to a particular *antigen, or nonspecifically in relation to immune responses in general (*see* immunity). It may occur naturally as the result of the activity of suppressor cells, or artificially as a result of drugs that inhibit lymphocyte activity (*see* lymphocyte).

impacted Firmly wedged. An *impacted tooth* is one that cannot erupt into a normal position because it is obstructed by other tissues, such as a tooth of a previous set. *Impacted fractures* of long bones occur when the splintered end of one shaft wedges into the open end of the marrow cavity of the other. *See also* impaction of the oviduct.

impaction of the oviduct (egg binding) A build-up of eggs in the oviduct of laying poultry, due to inability to lay the eggs. It can be caused by an oversized egg, or weakness or exhaustion of the hen. The affected bird shows signs of distress and makes repeated attempts to lay. After smearing the vent with a lubricant (e.g. Vaseline), the egg can be gently eased towards the vent with the fingers. Prolonged impaction may cause inflammation of the oviduct, while breakage of impacted eggs is likely to damage the oviduct leading to infection (e.g. peritonitis) and death.

imperfect bleeding Impaired bleeding of a carcass following slaughter. It occurs because the live animal was weak (e.g. due to disease) or was very stressed. The flesh of the carcass is dark red and the organs (e.g. lungs and kidneys) contain a lot of blood. The carcass sets badly and is unfit for human consumption.

imperforate Lacking an opening. *Imperforate anus* is the failure of the anal membrane to break down. It is most common in cattle and pigs. *See also* atresia.

imperforate hymen A condition in which a fibrous membrane stretches across the vagina. This is not uncommon in maiden fillies, and if complete may lead to the accumulation of uterine, cervical, and vaginal secretions, sometimes even causing distension of the vagina. Signs may vary from apparently mild discomfort during urination to marked straining and even vaginal prolapse in severe cases. If left untreated it will cause reduced fertility. Surgical penetration of the membrane is readily achieved. A similar condition is occasionally seen in cattle, where it is usually associated with *white heifer disease.

impetigo A contagious pustular disease of the skin caused by streptococci or staphylococci invading the epidermis and producing a number of small focal lesions, usually yellowish green. They are frequently seen on the ventral abdomen of young puppies, but also occur in horses on the saddle area or other regions in contact with tack. The condition usually follows breaks in the epidermis due to insect bites, scratches, or friction from tack. Improved husbandry, such as adjustment to ill-fitting tack, can often reduce the incidence of the disease. Swabs may be taken to determine the bacteria present so that the appropriate antibiotic may be prescribed, if necessary in addition to local antisepsis.

implant A substance (such as a drug) or a tissue graft that is inserted into the subcutaneous tissues of the body (e.g. beneath the skin). Drug implants are typically formulated as a pellet so that the drug is released slowly from the site of administration over a period of several weeks or months. This allows blood concentrations of a drug to be maintained over long periods without the need for frequent handling of animals. Implants have been used to administer growth-promoting hormones.

implantation 1. The attachment of the conceptus to the tissues of the uterus, which commences at the *blastocyst stage of development. In domestic mammals the conceptus remains within the uterine cavity (*central implantation*). In primates, including humans, the conceptus invades maternal tissue and becomes entirely surrounded by it (*interstitial implantation*), whereas in rodents the conceptus settles within a uterine crypt (*eccentric implantation*). **2.** The placing of a substance (e.g. a drug or nutrient) within a tissue or an organ.

impotence The inability to copulate. The term is most often applied to the male and in domestic animals physical and hormonal causes are most likely. Physical causes may include hereditary or acquired abnormalities of the external genitalia, such as *phimosis, traumatic lesions, tumours, etc. Hormonal causes may include imbalance of thyroid, pituitary, adrenal, or gonadal hormones. Other diseases causing more general muscular or nervous weakness may also be responsible.

impulse (in neurology) *See* nerve impulse.

in- (im-) *Prefix denoting* **1.** not. **2.** in; within; into.

inappetence Lack of desire for food.

inbreeding The mating of individuals that are more closely related than the average degree of relatedness of all individuals in the population. Inbreeding increases the likelihood that offspring inherit the same *alleles from both parents, and leads to a build up of homozygosity in the population (*see* homozygous). Homozygosity for particular alleles means that animals will breed true for the characteristics determined by those alleles. However, inbreeding carried

out to establish homozygosity for selected desired alleles (and hence characteristics) will also establish homozygosity for other alleles, causing a considerable random loss of genetic variation. With successive generations, this eventually leads to a loss of performance in the individuals, a phenomenon known as *inbreeding depression. However, by demonstrating the presence of recessive deleterious alleles, inbreeding can allow the elimination of such alleles from the group. The most severe inbreeding regime is the mating of parent and offspring or full brother and sister, both of which will produce homozygosity at 25% of the genes. Mating of half sibs gives 12.5% homozygosity, as does aunt/uncle × nephew/niece. Full-cousin matings give 6.25% homozygosity. *Line breeding, which is another form of inbreeding, will also slowly build up homozygosity. *See also* inbreeding coefficient.

inbreeding coefficient The probability that the two alleles at any gene pair in an individual are alike by descent from some ancestor common to both parents. This can be calculated in various ways and can apply to the population as a whole or to a specific individual. The greater the value of the inbreeding coefficient, the greater the degree of homozygosity in the genome (*see* inbreeding). *See also* effective population size. *Compare* coefficient of co-ancestry.

inbreeding depression The loss of performance of an inbred population associated with loss of genetic variability (i.e. increasing homozygosity) over successive generations. It is believed to arise because many genes work best in the heterozygous state. Also, recessive deleterious but hitherto concealed characters may be brought to light by homozygosity;

some of these can have lethal consequences. *See also* inbreeding.

incidence The number of animals affected by a disease as a proportion of the population at risk. It may be expressed as a fraction or percentage.

incision **1.** The surgical cutting of soft tissues, such as skin or muscle, with a knife or scalpel. **2.** The cut so made.

incisor One of the front teeth, usually conical or chisel-shaped for cropping or cutting. In ruminants, only the lower jaw bears incisors, which work against a horny pad on the upper jaw. *See* dentition.

incisure (in anatomy) A notch, small hollow, or depression.

inclusion body A discrete area within a cell that preferentially takes up a specific histological stain. Inclusion bodies are usually *acidophilic, and may occur in the nucleus (*intranuclear inclusion bodies*) or in the cytoplasm (*intracytoplasmic inclusion bodies*); some are surrounded by a clear area or halo, which remains completely unstained. Inclusion bodies appear in certain cell types that are infected with adenoviruses, poxviruses, herpesviruses, or rabies virus, and are of considerable diagnostic importance.
Negri bodies are intracytoplasmic inclusion bodies seen in certain nerve cells of the central nervous system following infection with rabies virus, and represent accumulations of virus-induced protein. Poxviruses also cause the development of intracytoplasmic inclusion bodies, these are either areas of viral morphogenesis (*type B inclusions*, *Guarnieri bodies* of smallpox) or areas of virus-induced protein matrix containing mature virus particles (*type A inclusions*, *Bollinger bodies* of cowpox, *Marchal bodies* of

ectromelia, *Downie bodies* of fowl pox, *Borrel bodies* of sheep pox). Herpesvirus infections produce acidophilic intranuclear inclusions (*Cowdry type A inclusions*), and adenoviruses, such as *canine hepatitis virus, cause basophilic intranuclear inclusions (*Cowdry type B inclusions*).

inclusion body hepatitis A disease of domestic fowls and other birds possibly due to adenovirus infection, causing poor performance and increased mortality. It chiefly affects growing broilers aged 4–7 weeks and produces a sudden rise in mortality. In a broiler flock the disease normally takes 1–2 weeks to run its course and may result in up to 10% mortality. Birds show reduced growth rate and suboptimal feed conversion. Internally the liver and kidneys become enlarged and subject to haemorrhages, while the bursa of Fabricius is shrunken. Under the microscope, *inclusion bodies can be seen in the nuclei of liver cells. No treatment or vaccine is available, and the mode of transmission is not understood.

incompetence Impaired function, particularly of the valves of the heart, which sometimes fail to seal on closure thus allowing the backflow of blood. *See* valvular disease.

incontinence The tendency of an organ to void its fluid contents inappropriately. Incontinence can apply to the urinary bladder, bowel, and mammary gland. However, urinary and faecal incontinence is difficult to determine in animals other than housetrained pets. It usually follows from a lesion in the central nervous system, especially in aged animals. Mammary incontinence commonly follows from lesions of the teat sphincter, although some dribbling of milk is normal in high-yielding dairy cows, especially in early lactation.

incoordination (in neurology) Inability to perform harmonious body movements, often with irregular and uncontrolled muscular activity. It can be caused by disorder in any part of the nervous system.

incubation The period from the laying of a fertile egg until hatching, during which the embryo develops. In commercial poultry production it is almost exclusively carried out under artificial and precisely controlled conditions following the collection of fertile eggs from the breeder flock. To ensure maximum hatchability, such factors as temperature and relative humidity need to be carefully controlled; mechanical ventilation is crucial in removing gaseous waste products and providing fresh air. To minimize disease, precautions include the sterilization of equipment between batches, the fumigation of all incoming eggs to reduce the risk of transfer of disease from parent to offspring, and the avoidance of cross infection. Average incubation periods are: fowl 21 days, duck 28 days, turkey 28 days, goose 30 days, pheasant 24 days, canary 14 days, budgerigar 18 days.

incubation period 1. The interval between exposure to infection and the onset of clinical signs. **2.** (in bacteriology) The period of development of a bacterial culture. *See also* incubation.

incus A small anvil-shaped bone in the middle *ear that articulates with the other auditory ossicles – the malleus and stapes.

Indian hemp *See* Apocynum poisoning.

Indian poke *See* false hellebore poisoning.

Indian tobacco *See* Lobelia poisoning.

indicator A compound that changes colour to allow visualization of chemical reactions or to indicate completion of a reaction. Many indicators are used to determine the acidity or alkalinity of solutions, or to detect redox reactions. A *universal indicator* is a mixture of indicators that gives various colour changes to determine pH over a wide range of values. In veterinary medicine indicators impregnated in strips of paper are used to test for various constituents in blood and urine.

indigestion Failed or disordered digestion, usually accompanied by abdominal pain. In **ruminants** irregular food intake disturbs fermentation in the rumen and predisposes to indigestion, while excessive intake of rapidly fermentable carbohydrate induces ruminal *acidosis with damage to the rumen wall. Large and rapid intake of lush grass can cause *bloat, with distension of the rumen by gas or foam.
In **horses** indigestion can arise due to irregular feeding or unsuitable food and may involve accumulations of gas or impacted ingesta in the colon, leading to *colic. Indigestion is also common in **dogs** and **cats**, which may feed on unsuitable bones or decayed meat and consequently suffer abdominal pain with bouts of vomiting. Also, grooming may lead to *hair balls in the stomach followed by persistent episodes of retching. *See also* dyspepsia.

indole A derivative of the amino acid *tryptophan produced by bacteria in the large intestine. It is the substance mainly responsible for the odour of faeces.

indomethacin *See* NSAID.

induction 1. (in anaesthesia) Initiation of *anaesthesia. The most frequently employed technique is the intravenous administration of a soluble agent, commonly a barbiturate. **2.** (in obstetrics) The artificial initiation of *parturition. It may involve dilatation of the uterine cervix or the administration of drugs, such as *prostaglandins, to trigger muscle contractions. **3.** (in embryology) The phenomenon by which the development of one structure leads to the development of another. For example, the presence of the notochord causes induction of the neural plate from the overlying ectoderm.

induration Abnormal hardening of a tissue or organ. For example, the udder may become indurated and fibrosed due to chronic *mastitis. Lungs may undergo *brown induration*, in which the lung tissue not only hardens but also accumulates brown pigment haemosiderin from the breakdown of red blood cells.

infarction The death of part or all of an organ due to obstruction of its arterial blood supply by a blood clot or embolus. Hence, infarction of the heart wall results from obstruction of the coronary arteries; infarctions of the kidney in pigs commonly result from emboli shed from the heart valves as a consequence of *swine erysipelas infection.

Infected Area (England and Wales) An area, declared by the Minister by special Order under the *Animal Health Act (1981), surrounding an *Infected Place. The movement of animals and the conduct of markets within the Area may be restricted.

Infected Place (England and Wales) Premises on whose occupier Notice has been served by a local authority of Ministry of Agriculture Inspector, where the Inspector has been told or suspects a *notifiable disease exists. Movement and activity of persons and animals on and off the premises

may be restricted or prohibited. *See also* Infected Area.

infection Invasion of the body by harmful organisms (pathogens), such as bacteria, fungi, protozoa, rickettsiae, or viruses. The infective agent may be transmitted by direct contact with another infected animal (*carrier), or by the inhalation of moisture droplets or dust particles contaminated with the pathogen, or by ingestion of contaminated food or drink. Pathogens may also be transmitted venereally during *coitus, or passed from an infected dam to her foetus (es) during pregnancy or birth. Some infectious organisms are carried and introduced by animal vectors, notably flies and ticks. The pathogens enter via a wound or bite or through mucous membranes. After an incubation period, clinical signs appear in the host. Different host species may be susceptible to infection with a given pathogen, and show varying signs of disease or no disease at all. Also, individuals that have developed immunity to a particular organism may still be carriers. *See also* secondary infection.

infectious avian encephalomyelitis (epidemic tremors) An infectious disease of domestic fowls, turkeys, and other birds due to a picornavirus. It causes nervous signs and heavy mortality in chicks and poults, and a brief dip in egg production in older birds. The virus is transmitted both through the egg from breeding flocks and orally from bird to bird. The nervous signs are seen only in birds up to 6 weeks old; they comprise tremors and ataxia, which usually progresses from slight incoordination to eventual paralysis and death. In the early stages birds typically sit on their hocks. The tremors are not seen in all outbreaks or in all birds; they chiefly affect the head and neck but can spread to the rest of the body.

Although some birds may recover, all affected birds should be culled since subsequent performance is likely to be impaired. Incubation periods are 1–7 days for infected eggs, and 11 days or longer for oral infections. This can result in a two-stage outbreak in a flock of newly hatched chicks, with egg-infected chicks showing clinical signs during the first week, and cross-infected chicks showing signs after 2 weeks.

An outbreak in laying birds is less significant, involving a drop in egg production (usually 5–10% over a period of 5–14 days) and a loss of hatchability of 5% in breeder flocks. There is no treatment and control depends upon vaccination. Pullets should be vaccinated at 9–14 weeks old; this prevents a fall in egg production and blocks egg transmission to chicks. Proper cleaning out and disinfection between flocks is also recommended.

infectious bovine keratoconjunctivitis *See* New Forest disease.

infectious bovine pustulovaginitis (IPV) A disease of cattle and buffalo characterized by fever and a vulval or preputial discharge and caused by a *herpesvirus. A closely related virus causes *infectious bovine rhinotracheitis (IBR). The fever associated with IPV is lower than seen in IBR. Erosions develop on the vulva or prepuce and the infected animal exhibits signs of severe irritation. Transmission is usually by the venereal route and lesions develop within 3 days of mating. Bulls may develop adhesions and subsequently be unable to serve a cow. Recovery usually occurs after a few weeks but animals remain persistently infected. Other name: **coital vesicular exanthema.**

infectious bovine rhinotracheitis (IBR) A disease of cattle and buffalo caused by a *herpesvirus and charac-

terized by fever and nasal and eye discharge. Infection with a closely related virus can cause *infectious pustular vulvovaginitis in cattle. IBR occurs worldwide. Transmission is by contact with infected animals, and occurs by the respiratory route. The virus will also cross the placenta of pregnant animals causing abortion. Following an incubation period of up to 7 days, the infected animal develops a fever and lactating cattle suffer a dramatic drop in milk yield. Eye and nasal discharges, at first clear, start to contain pus, and a cough associated with a bronchopneumonia develops. Recovered animals remain persistently infected. IBR can be controlled with a live vaccine which prevents or reduces the severity of clinical disease but does not prevent infection with the virus.

infectious bronchitis (IB) A highly infectious disease of domestic fowls, caused by a *coronavirus and characterized by respiratory signs and substantially lowered production. Of major economic significance worldwide, it can cause high mortality in very young chicks but is more typically a problem in older birds. In laying hens IB causes reduced output and lowered egg quality, while in broilers, growth rate and feed conversion are depressed.

Infection is by the respiratory route, with transmission occurring between birds or wind-borne between flocks. The virus multiplies in three main sites – the lungs, oviduct, and kidneys – giving rise to the three main groups of clinical signs, although these can vary widely in severity. Classical IB in a laying flock begins with respiratory signs about 2 days after infection. There is coughing, sneezing, gasping, swelling of the face, nasal discharge, watery eyes, and general weakness and depression with greenish wet droppings. After a few days, egg output drops sharply (by up to 50%) and may remain depressed for many weeks. About 3–4 weeks after the appearance of clinical signs egg quality deteriorates; eggshells can be thin, weak, misshapen, or soft, show roughness, scoring, and pale coloration, or be absent altogether. Internal laying can occur. The albumen can be thin and watery, the yolk may become detached, and there may be blood spots. Post-mortem examination of affected birds reveals lesions in the trachea and lungs. In the renal form the kidneys may be pale and swollen, the ureters dilated, and urate deposits occur throughout the body (*compare* gout).

An outbreak spreads in days and normally runs its course in 1–2 weeks. Virtually all birds are affected but few die, although an outbreak in very young birds can cause mortality of up to 30%. The severity and nature of outbreaks varies greatly with the virulence and strain of the virus, as well as flock age, the weather (outbreaks tend to be more severe in winter), and the presence of other infections (e.g. *avian mycoplasmosis). Secondary infections, such as *colisepticaemia and mycoplasmosis, may develop. Many mild outbreaks in layers or broilers manifest themselves only as reduced egg production.

There is no treatment; control depends on vaccination. Various serological types of virus have been recognized, including the Massachusetts, which is used for vaccines in the UK. Despite widespread vaccination, unexplained problems with egg quality and falls in egg production are regularly encountered in the egg industry throughout the world. These are thought to be due to new or variant mild IB strains. Various vaccination programmes can be used. If an early challenge is likely, spray vaccination with the most attenuated live vaccines at day old is recommended. Subsequent or later initial vaccination takes place at 3–5 weeks, usually adminis-

tered in the drinking water. Mild respiratory signs may follow for up to 2 weeks. For protection during lay a stronger vaccine is used at 12–16 weeks. Some IB vaccines are combined with *Newcastle disease vaccine. The disease should be distinguished from Newcastle disease, *avian infectious laryngotracheitis, avian mycoplasmosis, and *egg-drop syndrome.

infectious bursal disease (IBD; Gumboro disease) A highly contagious viral disease of domestic fowls, causing variable mortality and immunosuppression, and affecting birds from 1 to 16 weeks of age, most often from 3 to 6 weeks. The course of the disease is rapid. Soon after the appearance of white watery diarrhoea, the birds stop eating and become depressed and lethargic with ruffled feathers; the first deaths may occur within 2 days. Some birds exhibit trembling. The mortality, which typically peaks and subsides within a week, is usually less than 10% but can reach 30% or more. Most of the flock tend to show clinical signs to some extent, and although surviving birds recover quickly and seem normal, the flock's weight gain and feed conversion is likely to suffer permanently. Post-mortem examination shows the *cloacal bursa (bursa of Fabricius) to be enlarged and inflamed, with widespread loss of the B-lymphocytes. This severely disables the bird's immune system and can reduce the response to routine vaccination for other diseases, such as infectious bronchitis and Newcastle disease. The kidneys may be pale and swollen, which led to the early name of 'infectious avian nephrosis', now discarded. The liver may also be affected, and there may be dehydration and haemorrhages in the muscles.

The virus is resistant to a wide range of temperatures (subzero to over

infectious pancreatic necrosis

60°C), pH values, and cleaning agents, although compounds based on formalin and iodine are the most useful. Hence, eradication of the virus from infected units is difficult and it will tend to recur. Control of the disease is achieved through vaccination. Commercial broilers are normally protected by maternally derived antibodies from vaccinated breeder hens, although they can be given a live vaccine at day old in spray or by injection. Breeder hens are given a live vaccine when they are being reared, followed by an oil adjuvant at point of lay. There is no treatment. The disease was first identified in the town of Gumboro, Delaware, in the USA. Other name: **infectious bursitis**.

infectious bursitis See infectious bursal disease.

infectious canine laryngotracheitis See kennel cough.

infectious haematopoietic necrosis An infectious disease of salmon and trout characterized by lethargy, prominent eyes (exophthalmia), distended abdomen, and death. It is caused by a *rhabdovirus and is found in North America, Japan, Australia, and northern Europe. Mortality may reach 90% in fish under 2 months old but rarely exceeds 10% in fish over 2 years old. The severity of the disease is increased by water temperatures below 15°C. Affected fish accumulate fluid in the abdomen and develop exophthalmia, dark skin, and haemorrhages at the base of the fins. Fish that survive infection persistently excrete virus so that slaughter of all stock and disinfection of premises are the only effective means of control. It is a *notifiable disease in the UK. *Compare* viral haemorrhagic septicaemia.

infectious nasal granuloma A chronic inflammation of the nasal mucosa of cattle, goats, and horses caused by infestation with the parasitic fluke *Schistosoma nasalis*. The disease occurs in the Indian subcontinent. The mechanism of inflammation is similar to that in other schistosome infestations (*see* schistosomiasis). Similar pathological changes may be caused by the fungus *Rhinosporidium*.

infectious necrotic hepatitis See black disease.

infectious nucleic acid The nucleic acid (*DNA or *RNA) extracted from a *virus and purified in such a way that it is able to initiate an infective cycle leading to the production of complete *virions. However, some viruses (such as *poxvirus, the *retroviruses, and *negative-strand RNA viruses) carry essential enzymes in their virion, so it is not possible to initiate an infection with the pure viral nucleic acid. *See also* reverse transcriptase.

infectious pancreatic necrosis (IPN) An infectious disease of young salmon and trout caused by an unclassified RNA virus and characterized by lethargy, distended abdomen, abnormal swimming motion, and death. The virus is found in North America, Europe, and Japan. Disease is rare in fish over 6 months old. In young fish susceptibility is increased in overcrowded conditions and at temperatures between 9 and 11°C. Susceptibility also varies with species and even with strains of fish. Mortality ranges from very low to over 90%, and is influenced, moreover, by the strain of virus involved. Affected fish develop a distended abdomen, dark skin, and a circular swimming motion. Recovered fish persistently excrete virus, and control of the disease is by slaughter of all stock. IPN is a *notifiable disease in the UK.

infectious pustular vulvovaginitis (IPV) *See* infectious bovine pustulovaginitis.

infectious serositis *See* anatipestifer infection.

infectious sinusitis of turkeys *See* avian mycoplasmosis.

infectious synovitis of poultry A condition of young domestic fowls, turkey poults, and guinea fowl caused by infection with *Mycoplasma synoviae* or a reovirus. It is characterized by inflammation of joints, bursae, and tendon sheaths, leading to lameness and arthritis. Loss of condition occurs but the mortality rate is low. The infection can spread by contact or by egg transmission. Medication with chlortetracycline (*see* tetracyclines) and other antimicrobials temporarily insuppresses the disease but does not eliminate it from a flock. *Compare* infectious bursal disease (Gumboro disease).

infectivity A measure of the potency of a preparation of a virus, commonly measured by a *plaque assay.

inferior (in anatomy) Lower in the body in relation to another structure or surface. In quadrupeds the use of the term is limited to certain structures in the head, for example lips and eyelids.

infertility Reduced fertility (*compare* sterility); as applied to most domestic species it means the inability to mate, conceive, or carry a viable *foetus to term (*see also* abortion). Infertility may be *anatomical*, *functional*, or *infectious*. The causes of infertility are numerous but affect the female more often than the male. Infertility tends to be of most economic importance in cattle, horses, and pigs but is increasing in importance in sheep. In cattle and pig enterprises, profitability is largely dependent upon the *calving index and farrowing index.

In the **cow**, anatomical causes of infertility include ovarian hypoplasia (inadequate development of the *ovaries), intersexuality (*see* freemartin), and acquired abnormalities, such as scar tissue *adhesions on the ovaries and tumours of the reproductive tract. Functional causes include *anoestrus, *ovarian cysts, and *suboestrus. Infectious causes are also important and include *endometritis, *metritis, *campylobacteriosis (of cattle), *brucellosis, and *trichomoniasis.

In **ewes**, structural and functional abnormalities are much less common than in cows; many of the problems with sheep infertility lie with the male (see below) and failure to carry a viable foetus to term. *Enzootic ovine abortion, *toxoplasmosis, *campylobacteriosis (of sheep), *salmonellosis, and *listeriosis are particularly important.

In **mares**, infertility is commonly associated with the inappropriate timing of mating, which should take place on the second day before the end of *oestrus. Anoestrus, suboestrus, and irregular heats are also common causes. Endometritis may be associated with delayed uterine *involution and also with vaginal defects. Foetal loss is often associated with twinning. The most important infectious causes of abortion are virus infections, such as *equine rhinopneumonitis and *equine viral arteritis.

In **sows**, anatomical problems can be quite common, usually involving lack of development of uterine structures. Anoestrus and inappropriate mating times may also be responsible for infertility, while *porcine parvovirus infection is an important infectious cause. Endometritis and metritis may also be common causes (*see also* MMA). In very intensive pig units, environmental stress (e.g. close confinement) may be a predisposing factor.

In **bitches** the most common causes are anoestrus (due to lack of development of the ovaries), *pyometra, and endometritis.

In male animals infertility may be caused by failure to copulate or failure to fertilize the female. Among the causes of copulation failure are lack of libido, anatomical defects, disease or injury to the penis (e.g. fracture of the penis), and locomotor problems, such as severe lameness. Failure of fertilization is due to inadequate levels of viable spermatozoa in the *semen. This may be related to inadequate development of the testis (testicular hypoplasia), *cryptorchidism, or *orchitis (see also brucellosis). The treatment of infertility largely depends upon determining the underlying cause.

infiltration 1. The abnormal entry of a substance (*infiltrate*) into a tissue or organ. For example, inflamed tissue becomes infiltrated with leucocytes and oedemal fluid. Infiltration with cancerous cells is an important feature in the spread of malignant tumours; whereas fatty infiltration commonly occurs in the liver or kidney as a degenerative change. **2.** The injection of a local anaesthetic solution into the tissues to cause local *anaesthesia.

inflammation A reaction of tissues to injury (physical or chemical) or infection; it may also arise as part of certain hypersensitive responses (see hypersensitivity). *Acute inflammation* involves local dilatation and increased permeability of blood vessels and the migration of white blood cells (*leucocytes) to the affected site. Inflamed tissues develop the cardinal signs of heat, swelling, redness, and pain. The leucocytes form part of an exudate from the local arterioles, capillaries, and venules. This exudate

has a diluting effect on local toxins, and contains proteins, notably *fibrin and *antibody, which can limit the spread of bacteria. Many of the leucocytes can phagocytose invading organisms (see neutrophil); the activity of leucocytes may lead to the formation of *pus.

Inflammation is mediated by a number of soluble agents. *Histamine, a product of *mast cells, is particularly important in hypersensitive inflammation and acts by dilating blood vessels and increasing their permeability, especially in the earlier phase of inflammation. *Kinins, which are produced in inflamed tissues from precursor molecules called kininogens, are chiefly represented by bradykinin and kallidin; these are responsible for promoting the later stages of inflammation. *Complement is important in mediating histamine release and the accelerated migration of leucocytes. *Prostaglandins exert a wide variety of physiological effects: prostaglandin E causes vasodilatation and increased capillary permeability, particularly in late prolonged phases of inflammation. This effect is often antagonized by aspirin (see NSAID), which prevents the conversion of arachidonic acid to prostaglandin. However, high levels of prostaglandin E evidently inhibit rather than promote inflammation. *Lymphokines are produced in a great profusion of types by lymphocytes; among their many effects are the inhibition of macrophage migration and an increase in capillary permeability. *Platelets and their factors also play an important part in acute inflammation. Adherence by platelets to damaged tissue or to antigen-antibody complex, or release of platelet-activating factor by degranulating mast cells, leads to the release of platelet prostaglandin E and ADP, which is a signal for mutual aggregation of the platelets. The platelets also release 5-

hydroxytryptamine, which causes effects similar to those of histamine.

Acute inflammation may be resolved by removal of the exudate and repair of any damaged tissue by *granulation and *fibrosis or by regeneration of the original tissue cells. However, these processes may be prolonged, leading to *chronic inflammation*. Chronic inflammation also describes a distinct process that tends to result from particular kinds of injury and infection, notably *autoimmune disease, persistent foreign bodies, and certain persistent infections, especially by such organisms as *Mycobacterium* spp. and protozoa of the genus *Leishmania*, which can survive phagocytosis by macrophages. Chronic inflammation is not exudative but is typified by an assembly of cells, mainly fibroblasts, lymphoid cells, and macrophages together with giant cells (*see* macrophage). This assembly frequently shows distinct organization and is known as a *granuloma.

influenza *See* avian influenza; cat flu; equine influenza; influenzavirus; swine influenza.

influenzavirus A genus of the *orthomyxovirus family. Some members can infect pigs, horses, or birds, and human influenzaviruses can cause infections in domestic animals.

infra- *Prefix denoting* below.

infrared radiation Electromagnetic radiation with wavelengths in the range $0.7\,\mu m$ to 1 mm; i.e. longer than that of red light but shorter than radiowaves. Infrared radiation is responsible for the transmission of radiant heat, and may be used in physiotherapy to warm tissues, reduce pain, and improve circulation. Infrared lamps are used to provide heat for newborns, especially chicks and piglets.

infraspinatus muscle The muscle lying in the infraspinous fossa of the *scapula. It inserts to the greater tubercle of the humerus and acts as a strong lateral collateral ligament to stabilize the shoulder joint.

infundibulum (*pl.* **infundibula**) Any funnel-shaped channel or passage, particularly the hollow conical stalk that extends downwards from the hypothalamus and is continuous with the posterior lobe of the pituitary gland. The infundibulum of the uterine tube is its outermost expanded portion.

infusion 1. A slow injection of a substance (e.g. saline) into a vein or subcutaneous tissue. **2.** The process whereby the active principles are extracted from plant material by steeping it in water heated to boiling point. After standing for some time the liquid is strained off. **3.** The solution obtained by this process. Their use in animals is restricted because of the large fluid volumes involved and the difficulty in making animals take them voluntarily.

ingestion The process by which food is taken into and stored in the alimentary canal. It includes *prehension, *mastication, and deglutition (*see* swallowing).

inguinal Relating to or affecting the groin (inguen).

inguinal canal One of a pair of passages lined with peritoneal membrane leading from the lower rear abdominal cavity through the abdominal muscles, through which the testes descend and, in some species, are retracted. Along the canal run the blood and lymph vessels, nerves, and *spermatic cord supplying the testis. In females, the canal is the course of the round ligament of the uterus when present, as, for example, in the bitch. Rabbits, some insectivores, and most rodents have a wide inguinal canal into which the testes are retracted when vulnerable to injury. Abnormal penetration of the abdominal organs into the inguinal canals constitutes an inguinal (or scrotal) *hernia.

inhalational anaesthetic A gas or volatile liquid used to produce general *anaesthesia. The most commonly used inhalational anaesthetics in veterinary practice are *halothane and *ether, with others (e.g. chloroform, *cyclopropane, *enflurane, *isoflurane, *methoxyflurane, and *nitrous oxide) used less commonly. They can be administered using open systems (e.g. jars, masks) or using anaesthetic circuits. The substances should be noninflammable and nonexplosive and, because most anaesthetic circuits use soda lime, compatibility with this absorber of carbon dioxide is important. Moreover, the agent should be nonirritant to mucous membranes, and since large volumes are used, it is important that there is negligible production of toxic metabolites. The depth of anaesthesia is proportional to the amount of anaesthetic reaching the brain: this is influenced by the concentration of anaesthetic in inspired gases, pulmonary ventilation, blood solubility of the gas, and pulmonary perfusion. The speed of induction depends on the blood solubility of the gas: high blood solubility gives slow induction and recovery, and ideally a gas with medium or low blood solubility should be used to give rapid induction and recovery.

inhibition (in physiology) The prevention or reduction of the functioning of an organ, muscle, etc., by the action of certain nerve impulses.

inhibitor A substance that prevents the occurrence of a given process or reaction.

injection The introduction into the body of drugs or other fluids by *syringe. The most common routes for injection are beneath the skin (*subcutaneous*), into a muscle (*intramuscular*), or into a vein (*intravenous*). Occasionally injections may be made into the peritoneal cavity (*intraperitoneal*) or into the pleural cavity (*intrapleural*) or less commonly directly into body organs, such as the rumen, or into the skin (*intradermal*). Care must be taken to maintain sterility of the syringe, the needle, and the solution to be injected, and it is important that the injection site is properly prepared by clipping the surface hair and adequately disinfecting the skin. Diseases may be transmitted from one animal to another by contaminated syringes.

inoculation *See* vaccination.

inotropic Describing the force of contraction of the heart. A *positive inotropic effect* occurs when the myocardium contracts more powerfully at the same filling pressure producing greater emptying of the heart, reduced venous pressure, reabsorption of oedema fluid, and a rise in blood pressure. A *negative inotropic effect* is the opposite. *Cardiac glycosides are drugs that produce a positive inotropic effect.

Insecta The largest class of the invertebrate phylum *Arthropoda. The insect body is divided into head, thorax, and abdomen. The head bears sensory antennae and complex mouthparts, which differ in structure according to the method of feeding. The thorax has three segments with three pairs of legs and usually two pairs of wings, while the segmented abdomen has no legs but may bear an ovipositor for laying eggs. In many insects the eggs hatch into larvae (e.g. caterpillars or maggots) that are quite unlike the adult. These form a pupa which undergoes metamorphosis to the adult. In other insects the eggs hatch into miniature adults, or *nymphs. The class includes numerous pests, disease vectors, and parasites of animals and humans, such as the *flea, *louse, and various flies (*see* fly).

insecticide An agent used to kill insects. Insecticides are used on animals to kill ectoparasites and in the environment to control insects. Insecticidal compounds include *organochlorine compounds and *organophosphorus compounds, as well as *pyrethroids, *derris, *benzyl benzoate, sulphur-containing compounds, carbamates, and *ivermectin. The compounds used should kill insects rapidly, have low toxicity to mammals and birds, and not give rise to toxic residues in the environment. Insecticides are applied in various forms, for example as dips, sprays, powders, pour-ons, impregnated ear tags, shampoos, impregnated collars, and impregnated strips. To protect against insects that spend only part of their time on the host, the product should have a repellant effect and persist on the animal for a time. To control insects in the environment, sprays or impregnated strips containing insecticides are used. Environmental contamination and persistence is a major problem with some compounds, notably organochlorines. Many insects have developed resistance to certain insecticides, and the insects' mobility can give rise to a rapid spread of resistance in the population over a wide area. Insect growth regulators (e.g. methoprene) are used to inhibit the maturation of larvae into adult insects, and may be combined with conventional insecticides.

insemination The introduction of *semen into the reproductive tract of the female. It can be either natural, i.e. during coitus, or achieved by artificial means (*see* artificial insemination). During coitus following *ejaculation, semen is deposited in the uterus in horses and pigs, whereas in sheep, cattle, and dogs the site of deposition is the cranial vagina.

insertion (in anatomy) The point of attachment of a muscle (e.g. to a bone) that is relatively movable when the muscle contracts. *Compare* origin.

instillation 1. The application of liquid medication drop by drop, as into the eye. **2.** The medication, such as eye drops, applied in this way.

instinct A complex innately determined pattern of behaviour that is characteristic of all normally reared individuals of the same species. Much instinctive behaviour takes the form of *fixed action patterns* – movements that, once started, are performed in a stereotyped way unaffected by external stimuli. Some complex instinctive behaviour, however, requires some learning by the animal before it is perfected.

insufficiency Inability of an organ or part, such as the heart or liver, to fulfil its normal function.

insulin A protein hormone secreted by the beta cells of the pancreatic islets (islets of Langerhans) in response to increased blood sugar. Insulin facilitates glucose transport through cell membranes in many tissues of the body. Inadequate insulin production results in sluggish glucose uptake by fat and muscle cells and can result in *diabetes mellitus. Insulin of animal origin has been used for many years to treat diabetes mellitus in humans and animals. It is available as a protamine zinc salt for intramuscular injection and as crystalline zinc insulin, which can be injected intravenously. Recently, human insulin derived from genetically engineered bacteria has become commercially available for human use. It is hoped that such preparations will result in fewer adverse reactions and refractory patients and better control of blood sugar.

insulinase An enzyme that hydrolyses *insulin and thus inactivates it. It is found in the liver and kidney.

insulin-like activity (ILA) *See* somatomedin.

insulin-like growth factor (IGF) *See* somatomedin.

insulinoma A tumour arising from insulin-secreting beta cells of the islets of Langerhans in the pancreas. The dog and cat are most commonly affected. Lesions may be solitary or multiple and may be *adenomas or *carcinomas. Insulinomas produce excess amounts of *insulin with resultant hypoglycaemia. This leads to convulsions, loss of consciousness, ataxia, and weakness. There is a dramatic improvement in signs following the intravenous administration of glucose. If the tumour is solitary, surgical excision is possible and will be curative, but multiple lesions or those that have metastasized (*see* metastasis) carry a poor prognosis.

integration The blending together of the *nerve impulses that arrive through the thousands of synapses at a nerve cell body. Impulses from some synapses cause *excitation, and from others *inhibition; the overall pattern decides whether an individual nerve cell is activated to transmit a message or not.

integument *See* skin.

intensive husbandry Systems of animal production that, broadly, use high inputs to achieve high outputs. They require accurate knowledge of the *nutrient requirements of animals and nutritive value of available feedstuffs (*see* nutrition) to enable the accurate formulation of *diets. Also, an understanding of the animal's biology allows *housing and *light requirements to be met and its maximum reproductive capabilities to be realized. An intensive system benefits from the use of genetically superior stock bred with the help of specially designed selection programmes.

Health problems associated with intensive systems are related to the large numbers of stock involved and high stocking density. Output and hence profitability can be seriously reduced by subclinical disease, hence preventive medicine is crucial. This may entail *vaccination programmes and the prophylactic administration of drugs (e.g. antibiotics) in the feed. Strict hygiene is necessary throughout, particularly between batches of stock. There are often recommended or even statutory conditions concerning the welfare of animals in intensive systems (*see* welfare codes), as well as other legal requirements regarding noise, smell, effluent disposal, etc. *See also* pig husbandry; poultry husbandry; turkey husbandry.

inter- *Prefix denoting* between. Examples: *intercostal* (between the ribs); *intertrochanteric* (between the trochanters).

intercalated Describing structures, tissues, etc., that are inserted or situated between other structures.

intercellular Situated or occurring between cells.

intercostal Situated between the ribs. The intercostal muscles fill the spaces between the ribs: the *external inter-*

costal muscles draw the ribs cranially during inspiration; the *internal intercostal muscles* draw the ribs caudally during expiration. Intercostal arteries, veins, and nerves lie in the intercostal spaces and supply adjacent structures.

intercurrent Describing a disease contracted by an animal that is already affected by another condition. For example, animals debilitated by parasite infestation are often prone to intercurrent infections.

interdigital cyst A *cyst that is similar in appearance to an *epidermal inclusion cyst except that it is usually surrounded by masses of inflammatory cells, indicating rupture into the surrounding tissues. It occurs between the digits.

interdigital cyst A deep-seated infection of dogs that causes a painful and discharging swelling between the toes. It is thought to be triggered by a reaction to coarse hairs penetrating the delicate web of skin between the toes. Treatment may involve bathing in warm saltwater, the administration of antibiotics, and surgical drainage or removal in severe cases. Other name: **interdigital pyoderma**.

interdigital necrobacillosis *See* foul-in-the-foot.

interferon Any of a number of proteins produced by the cells of an animal that inhibit the replication of viruses. They are involved in the animal's defence against viral infections, their antiviral effect being species specific. The production of interferon can also be elicited by nonviral materials, for example certain *nucleic acids.

interkinesis 1. The resting stage between the two divisions of *meiosis. 2. *See* interphase.

interleukin Any of a number of soluble factors (*lymphokines) that are produced by *lymphocytes and/or *macrophages and influence the behaviour of other similar cells. *Interleukin 1* (*IL1*) is produced by macrophages and acts on T-helper cells (*see* lymphocyte) to promote their differentiation and their secretion of interleukin 2. IL1 removes the need for macrophages in many immune responses (*see* immunity; lymphocyte).
Interleukin 2 (*IL2*) can stimulate activity in other T-cells, including their response to *antigens and the differentiation of cytotoxic T-cells (*see* lymphocyte). Other similar lymphokines have been described but their nomenclature has yet to be finalized.

internal capsule A large bundle of nerve fibres in each cerebral hemisphere of the brain. It comprises sensory fibres, coming mainly from the thalamus and running to the cerebral cortex, and fibres running from the cerebral cortex and descending to lower levels in the brain, many of which are involved in the control of motor activity. Fibres of the internal capsule mix with those of the *corpus callosum to form the *corona radiata. *See* corpus striatum.

interneurone A neurone in the central nervous system that acts as a link between the other neurones in a *reflex arc. It usually possesses numerous branching processes (dendrites) that make possible extensive and complex circuits and pathways within the brain and spinal cord.

internode A segment of *axon covered with a myelin sheath. Internodes are separated by nodes of Ranvier, where the sheath is absent.

interoceptor A sensory nerve ending in the internal organs of the body.

These are principally sensitive to pain. *See also* receptor.

interpeduncular Situated between the peduncles of the cerebrum.

interphase (interkinesis) The period when a cell is not undergoing division (mitosis), during which activities such as DNA synthesis occur.

intersex An organism having some of the characteristics of both sexes and therefore showing abnormalities of sexual development. The most extreme form is the *hermaphrodite, which has both ovarian and testicular tissue. The causes of intersexuality may be chromosomal, genic, or hormonal. *See also* freemartin.

interstice A small space in a tissue or between parts of the body.

interstitial cells (Leydig cells) The cells interspersed between the seminiferous tubules of the *testis. They secrete *androgens in response to stimulation by interstitial-cell-stimulating hormone from the adenohypophysis of the pituitary gland.

interstitial-cell-stimulating hormone *See* luteinizing hormone.

interstitial cell (Leydig cell) tumour A tumour arising from the interstitial cells of the testis. These occur mainly in the dog although other species may be affected. Small clinically inapparent lesions of this type affect about 20% of middle-aged to old dogs. Larger tumours usually form round discrete masses in the affected testicle; on pathological examination they display a light-brown to yellow coloration and often show cystic and haemorrhagic change. Both testes may be affected, and multiple lesions may occur in the same testis. The tumours are well encapsulated; however, large blood-filled

spaces develop in many cases and these often rupture to cause haemorrhage. Interstitial cells normally secrete male hormones (*androgens) but tumours of such cells are nonfunctional. Carcinomatous change, although infrequent, does occur and metastases may then be found, particularly in the regional lymph nodes. In the majority of cases, castration is curative.

interstitial myositis A condition in which muscle tissue is gradually replaced by adipose (fat) tissue without alteration in the gross shape of the muscle. The cause is unknown. Other names: **steatosis**; **muscular fibrosis**: **lipomatosis of muscle**.

intertrigo Inflammation of skin folds. It is caused by constant friction between opposing skin surfaces, especially where moisture favours the establishment of infection. Obesity may exacerbate the problem. Intertrigo is seen most dramatically in the heavily folded skin of the Sharpei dog. Facial fold intertrigo occurs in brachycephalic dog breeds, like the pug and Pekingese. The inflammation may be severe, the surface of the eye may be permanently damaged by friction from the facial folds. Intertrigo of the tail is seen in English bulldogs (*screw tail*). Local antisepsis is beneficial, although surgical reduction or removal of the folds is often necessary to prevent recurrence.

intervertebral disc The block of tissue connecting any two adjacent vertebrae in the spine. In young animals each disc consists of an outer *annulus fibrosus*, composed of collagen fibres and some fibrocartilage, and a central *nucleus pulposus* of semifluid gel, which is a remnant of the embryonic notochord. Structural changes occur as the animal matures, including loosening of the fibres in the annulus fibrosus and progressive conversion of

intestinal adenomatosis

the disc to fibrocartilage. These changes make the disc less flexible and can result in protrusion of the nucleus pulposus, particularly dorsally ('slipped disc'), leading to pressure on the spinal cord or spinal nerves. This is commonest in dogs. In certain breeds, for example dachshunds, these changes occur prematurely in cases of chondrodystrophia.

intestinal adenomatosis *See* adenomatosis.

intestinal (mesenteric) emphysema A rare condition of pigs in which small clear grape-like vesicles (about 1 cm in diameter) appear in the mesentery close to the intestine. They contain gas and burst easily on pressure. The cause is unknown.

intestine (gut) The part of the *alimentary tract extending from the stomach to the anus. Its wall consists of an inner tunica mucosa, a middle tunica muscularis, and an outer tunica serosa. The *small intestine*, comprising the *duodenum, jejunum, and *ileum, is where most of the digestion and absorption of food take place. To facilitate absorption the surface area of the mucosa is greatly increased by the presence of circular folds, from which project finger-like processes (*villi) and microscopic *microvilli. *Lieberkühn's (intestinal) glands are distributed in the mucosa (see illustration). The *large intestine* consists of the *caecum, *colon, and *rectum and is concerned with the absorption of water from digesta and, in nonruminant herbivores, with the breakdown of cellulose. Rhythmic contractions of the muscular layer in the wall (*see* peristalsis) propel the contents along the intestine towards the anus.

intima (tunica intima) The inner layer of the wall of an artery, vein, or lymphatic vessel. It comprises a lining of endothelial cells and an elastic membrane.

intra- *Prefix denoting* inside; within. Example: *intralobular* (within a lobule); *intrauterine* (within the uterus).

intracellular Situated or occurring inside a cell or cells.

intracranial Within the skull.

intracutaneous cornifying epithelioma A benign cystic skin tumour occurring mainly in the dog. It is usually a solitary well-circumscribed lesion, but in the Norwegian elkhound, a breed predisposed to such tumours, the lesions may be multiple or occur in succession. The tumour is a slightly raised firm nodule in the dermis of the neck or trunk, composed of single or multiple cavities lined with stratified cornifying squamous-cell epithelium and filled with

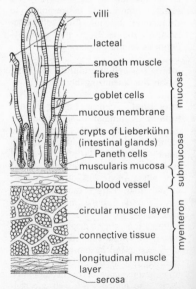

Longitudinal section through the ileum

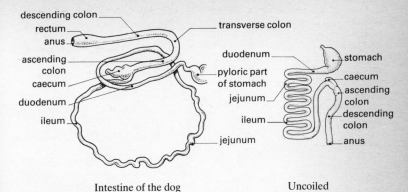

descending colon
rectum
anus
ascending colon
caecum
duodenum
ileum

transverse colon

duodenum
pyloric part of stomach
jejunum
ileum
jejunum

stomach
caecum
ascending colon
descending colon
anus

Intestine of the dog

Uncoiled

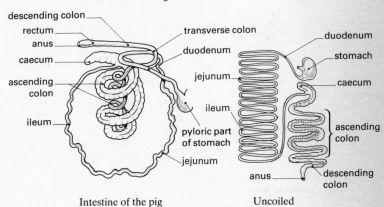

descending colon
rectum
anus
caecum
ascending colon
ileum

transverse colon
duodenum
jejunum
ileum
pyloric part of stomach
jejunum

duodenum
stomach
caecum
ascending colon
anus
descending colon

Intestine of the pig

Uncoiled

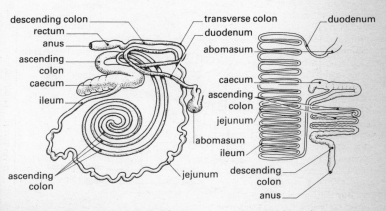

descending colon
rectum
anus
ascending colon
caecum
ileum
ascending colon
jejunum

transverse colon
duodenum
abomasum
caecum
ascending colon
jejunum
abomasum
ileum

duodenum
ascending colon
jejunum
descending colon
anus

The ruminant intestine (ox)

Uncoiled (sheep)

441

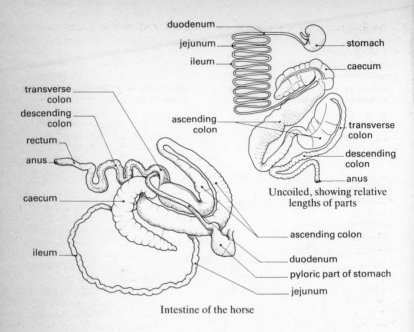

Intestine of the horse

Uncoiled, showing relative lengths of parts

Digestive tract of a turkey (uncoiled)

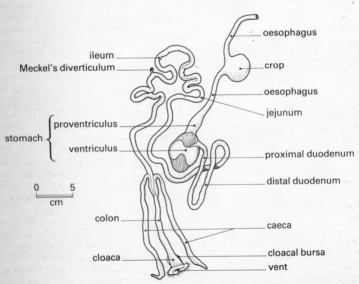

442

keratin. Often, a pore connects the cavity with the epidermal surface. Inflammation is common. Simple excision is curative, although in animals with a succession of growths the condition is extremely troublesome, requiring multiple excisions.

intradermal Within the skin. An *intradermal injection* is made into the skin, as in the testing of cattle for tuberculosis.

intraembryonic coelom The cavity that develops within the *mesoderm of the embryo. It communicates temporarily with the *extraembryonic coelom and subsequently forms the pericardial, pleural, and peritoneal cavities.

intramedullary Within the *medulla or inner part of an organ. *Intramedullary pinning* involves fixation of the fractured segments of a long bone by the insertion of a stainless steel pin within the shaft of the bone (*see* bone pinning).

intramuscular Within a muscle. An *intramuscular injection* is made into a muscle.

intraocular Within the eyeball. *Intraocular pressure* is the pressure of fluid within the eyeball.

intraperitoneal Within the peritoneal cavity. An *intraperitoneal injection* is made into the peritoneal cavity, particularly in fluid therapy.

intrathecal Within the *meninges of the spinal cord.

intratracheal Within the trachea. An *intratracheal tube* is inserted into the trachea for general anaesthesia.

intravenous Into or within a vein. An *intravenous injection* is made into a vein.

intrinsic factor A *glycoprotein secreted by gastric and/or duodenal mucosae and required for the absorption of dietary *vitamin B_{12} from the small intestine. Deficiency of this factor leads to *anaemia.

intrinsic muscle A muscle that is contained entirely within the organ or part it acts on. For example, there are intrinsic muscles of the tongue, whose contractions change the shape of the tongue.

intro- *Prefix denoting* in; into.

introitus (in anatomy) An entrance into a hollow organ or cavity.

intubation The insertion of a tube into the body. *Endotracheal intubation* involves the insertion of a tube, usually through the mouth, into the trachea. This may be performed during general anaesthesia in all species to administer anaesthetic gases and oxygen, to provide ventilation, and to ensure a patent airway. *Gastric intubation* is the insertion of a tube into the stomach, usually through the mouth or nose (*nasogastric intubation*). *See also* stomach tube.

intussusception The invagination or 'telescoping' of one part of the intestine into the lumen of an adjacent part. It probably results from abnormal peristalsis brought on by *enteritis or intestinal worms. The intestine becomes obstructed, with consequent abdominal pain and vomiting. Strangulation and occlusion of the blood supply to the affected part leads to gangrene and subsequent death of the animal. Instances of spontaneous healing and recovery have been recorded, but the usual treatment is attempted surgical correction of the intussusception or resection of the affected part.

Intussusception occasionally occurs due to unusually active peristalsis at death. It is seen at post-mortem examination, but the absence of swelling reveals that it occurred after and not before death.

invagination 1. The infolding of the wall of a solid structure to form a cavity. It occurs in some stages of embryonic development. **2.** *See* intussusception.

inversion 1. The turning inwards or inside-out of a part or organ. **2.** A chromosome mutation in which a block of genes within a chromosome are in reverse order, due to that section of the chromosome becoming inverted. The centromere may be included in the inverted segment (*pericentric inversion*) or not (*paracentric inversion*).

invertebrate 1. An animal without a backbone. The following are invertebrate groups of veterinary importance: insects (*see* Insecta), *ticks, *nematodes, *flukes, *protozoans, and *tapeworms. **2.** Not possessing a backbone.

in vitro Latin: describing biological phenomena, such as fertilization, that are made to occur outside the living body (traditionally in a test-tube).

in vitro fertilization (IVF) The fertilization of an *oocyte by a *spermatozoon outside the body of a living animal. Oocytes can be obtained from living or recently slaughtered animals and are cultured to reach a certain stage of development before being mixed with a culture containing capacitated spermatozoa. A high concentration of spermatozoa is necessary, the culture environment has to resemble that of the oviduct, and strict aseptic precautions need to be observed, with minimal temperature fluctuations. The resulting zygote or early embryo is then transferred to a recipient animal for development to term. Success rates in laboratory species are now quite high but it is still difficult to achieve repeatable successes in farm animals. The technique may be used to overcome infertility problems, such as blocked oviducts in valuable dams. Agriculturally, it has implications in the breeding of economically valuable dairy cattle since the technique potentially allows greater manipulation of the embryo (e.g. sexing and cloning) compared to *embryo transplantation alone.

in vivo Latin: describing biological phenomena that occur or are observed occurring within the bodies of living organisms.

involuntary muscle *See* smooth muscle.

involution The return of an organ to its normal size after enlargement, especially of the uterus after parturition. This is initiated during parturition by the increase in plasma *oestrogens, which sensitize the muscular wall, and effected by *oxytocin, which causes the muscle fibres to contract. In all domestic species, the uterus contracts by half its size within hours of completion of parturition. However, return of the *endometrium to the prepregnant state takes longer. Involution in the cow takes 35–40 days, and in the ewe 20–25 days; in both species this involves breakdown and voiding of the caruncular region of the endometrium and subsequent renewal and recovery. In mares involution is more rapid since there is no complex placental attachment involving caruncles.

iodide *See* iodophor.

iodine A nonmetallic element that is an important trace element (*see* essential element) for animals. It is normally present in the diet as iodide and is very efficiently taken up by the *thyroid gland, where it is used in the synthesis of the thyroid hormones *thyroxine and *triiodothyronine. Iodine deficiency causes decreased production of these hormones and results in enlargement of the thyroid gland (*goitre) and reproductive failure. Nuclear explosions and emissions from nuclear power stations produce short-lived radioactive isotopes of iodine (e.g. ^{127}I, ^{131}I) which are concentrated in the thyroid and thus provide a convenient way of monitoring exposure to such radioactivity. Symbol I.

iodophor A complex of iodine and a carrier molecule used as an *antiseptic or *disinfectant. The carrier is usually a detergent-type compound, which increases the penetration of the iodine. The iodine is then released from the carrier to act as a bactericidal, fungicidal, and virucidal agent. There is good activity in the presence of organic material. The most commonly used iodophor is *povidone-iodine, which is used as an antiseptic for wound cleaning and preoperatively to disinfect skin.

ionophores A group of antimicrobial agents obtained from various *Streptomyces* bacteria. They are used as *coccidiostats in poultry and as growth promoters in cattle. Those of veterinary importance include monensin, salinomycin, lasalocid, and narasin. Ionophores act on microorganisms by forming complexes with metal ions and disrupting mitochondrial function. They are poorly absorbed from the gastrointestinal tract and are given in the feed. In **poultry**, ionophores are used as coccidiostats and growth promoters in fattening birds. However, these agents kill coccidia at an early stage in their life cycle, thus preventing the host bird from developing immunity. Therefore, ionophores should not be used in breeding or laying birds. The drugs should be withdrawn at least three days prior to slaughter. In **cattle** monensin is used to modify rumen fermentation, causing increased propionate production, decreased methane production, and reduced protein degradation in the rumen, thereby improving the animal's feed conversion efficiency. Ionophores are particularly toxic in horses and donkeys and should never be given to these species, and in poultry overdosage causes depressed growth. Ionophores excepting lasalocid are incompatible with *tiamulin and the combination can cause growth depression and death.

ipsilateral (ipselateral, homolateral) On or affecting the same side of the body: applied particularly to paralysis (or other symptoms) occurring on the same side of the body as the brain lesion that caused them. *Compare* contralateral.

IPV *See* infectious bovine pustulovaginitis.

irid- (irido-) *Prefix denoting* the iris.

iridectomy The surgical excision of a portion of the iris of the eye. It is performed in dogs to control *glaucoma, and is usually restricted to the outer part of the iris (*peripheral iridectomy*). In humans iridectomy assists in the removal of a *cataract, but in the dog this tends to cause marked haemorrhage and so is often avoided.

iridovirus A family of DNA *viruses that have icosahedral *capsids and multiply in the cell cytoplasm (*see also* poxvirus). Members mostly infect insects or amphibians. The virus

iris

responsible for *African swine fever was originally classified in this family, but is now considered to have more affinity with the *poxviruses.

iris The anterior part of the vascular coat of the *eye that regulates the size of the opening (pupil) in front of the lens and thus the amount of light entering. The dilator pupillae muscle in the iris causes the pupil to enlarge and the constrictor pupillae causes it to constrict (*see* pupillary reflex). The iris is continuous posteriorly with the ciliary body.

iritis Inflammation of the iris. *See* periodic ophthalmia.

iron A metallic element that is an important trace element (*see* essential element), being used in the synthesis of *haemoglobin and *myoglobin as well as in many enzymes and *cytochromes. Iron is transported in blood plasma by the protein *transferrin and stored, mainly in the liver, in the protein *ferritin. Although most iron from the degradation of haemoglobin is recycled, dietary deficiency of iron leads to *anaemia. Dietary requirements are greatest for young and pregnant animals, or animals suffering prolonged haemorrhage. Milk contains relatively little iron, and suckling newborns housed without access to soil or pasture must receive dietary iron supplementation. This is especially important for young piglets (*see* piglet anaemia). Symbol Fe. *See also* haemosiderin.

iron dextran A *haematinic used in the treatment and prevention of anaemia. Iron dextran is injected intramuscularly and is absorbed over several days. The iron remains bound to the dextrans in plasma, reducing its toxicity, but is split from the sugar in reticuloendothelial cells to be made available for erythrocyte formation. Iron dextran is routinely administered to piglets at 2–3 days of age to prevent *piglet anaemia due to iron deficiency. There may be a reaction and staining at the site of injection.

iron poisoning A toxic condition that can occur in young pigs injected with an iron-dextran complex to prevent piglet anaemia. Deficiency of vitamin E and selenium in sows may cause their piglets to have an iron sensitivity, so that following the iron injection they exhibit laboured breathing and die rapidly. This can be avoided by injecting sows with vitamin E and sodium selenite in the week before farrowing. The injection of horses with iron-dextran is dangerous.

irrigation The washing out of wounds or cavities with large volumes of hot or cold watery solutions, often containing antiseptics. Irrigation may be employed in treating cases of uterine inflammation (*metritis) and in certain urinary bladder conditions, although antibiotics or other chemotherapeutic agents are now often used instead. It still has a place in the management of infected wounds.

isch- (ischo-) *Prefix denoting* suppression or deficiency.

ischaemia Inadequate blood supply to an organ or tissue, usually caused by the constriction or blockage of the blood vessels supplying it. This may be the result of a blood clot, inflammation, or external pressure. The affected area appears pale and surrounding tissues may be red and congested with blood. The tissue dies if the ischaemia is severe and lasts for more than 4–6 hours. Successful treatment depends on the prompt restoration of the circulation.

ischi- (ischio-) *Prefix denoting* the ischium.

ischium One of the bones that fuse to form the *os coxae in the adult pelvic girdle.

ischuria Retention or suppression of urine. Causes include deficiency or failure of urine production by the kidneys (*see* anuria), or retention of urine in the bladder, for example due to obstruction of the urethra.

islets of Langerhans (pancreatic islets) Small groups of cells, scattered through the substance of the *pancreas, that secrete the hormones *insulin and *glucagon. There are three main histological types of cell: alpha (α), beta (β), and D-cells (α_1). The alpha and beta cells produce glucagon and insulin, respectively.

isoagglutinin An *agglutinin, present in the blood, that reacts with blood group *antigens of other members of the same species.

isoagglutinogen A blood group *antigen (*see* agglutinogen), that is capable of eliciting and/or binding specific antibodies in members of the same species.

isoantibody An *antibody, present in an individual, that is specific for *antigens of other members of the same species.

isoantigen An *antigen, present in the tissues of an individual, that is capable of eliciting and/or binding specific *antibodies in other members of the same species.

isoenzyme (isozyme) A physically distinct form of a given enzyme. Isoenzymes catalyse the same reaction but have slight kinetic and immunological differences. Isoenzymes of dehydrogenases, oxidases, transaminases, phosphatases, and proteolytic enzymes are known to exist.

isoflurane A volatile liquid used as an *inhalational anaesthetic. Recently introduced and similar to *enflurane, it is noninflammable with low blood solubility giving very rapid induction and recovery from anaesthesia. It causes respiratory depression and potentiates the action of curare-type neuromuscular blockers. Hypotension is not as marked as with *halothane. Its expense precludes its widespread use in the veterinary field.

isograft (isogenic graft, syngraft) A *graft of tissue from one identical twin to another or between animals that are genetically identical.

isoimmunization *Immunization against *isoantigen. *See also* blood typing.

isoniazid (isonicotinic acid hydrazine) A drug sometimes used, in combination with other antibacterials (e.g. ethambutol and rifampicin), in the treatment of tuberculosis. It is effective against most *Mycobacterium* species and given orally, diffuses well throughout the body. Its metabolites are excreted in the urine. Toxicity to the central and peripheral nervous systems is the main side-effect, causing signs similar to pyridoxine (*see* vitamin B_6) deficiency. Occasionally there may be signs of hepatic toxicity.

isoprenaline (isoproterenol) A synthetic *catecholamine that acts at beta receptors of the sympathetic nervous system and causes increased heart rate, bronchodilatation, and vasodilatation in arterioles of skeletal muscle. This drug is rarely used but may be injected to increase myocardial contractions after defibrillation.

isopyrin *See* NSAID.

isoquinoline Any of a group of alkaloids obtained from crude *opium. They include the compounds *papav-

isotonic

erine and narcotine, which cause mild
sedation and smooth muscle relaxation. They were formerly used for
their constipating effect.

isotonic 1. Describing solutions that
have the same osmotic pressure. *See*
osmosis. **2.** Describing muscles that
have equal *tonicity.

isotope Any one of the different
forms of an element, possessing the
same number of protons (positively
charged particles) in the nucleus, and
thus the same atomic number, but
different numbers of neutrons. Isotopes therefore have different atomic
weights. Some isotopes are stable (e.g.
^{15}N) while others (e.g. ^{14}C) are radioactive and decay into other isotopes
or elements, emitting alpha, beta, or
gamma radiation. Some radioactive
isotopes may be produced artificially
by bombarding elements with neutrons. These are known as *nuclides*
and are used extensively in *radiotherapy for the treatment of cancer.

isoxsuprine An agent that causes
dilatation of peripheral blood vessels.
It is similar to the *sympathomimetic
amines and acts like a beta adrenergic agonist (*see* beta agonist),
although it also has a direct action on
vascular smooth muscle. Administered
orally, it is used in horses to treat
navicular disease and laminitis in an
attempt to improve vascular perfusion
of the lower limbs. It should not be
used in pregnant animals, since it
causes uterine relaxation. Tradename:
Oralject Circulon paste.

isozyme *See* isoenzyme.

isthmus A constricted or narrowed
part of an organ or tissue. The isthmus of the fauces is the narrowed
communication between the oral cavity and the oral part of the pharynx.
See also oviduct.

itching *See* pruritus.

-itis *Suffix denoting* inflammation of
an organ, tissue, etc. Examples:
arthritis (of a joint); *peritonitis* (of the
peritoneum).

ivermectin An *avermectin compound that is a potent anthelmintic
and ectoparasiticide. It acts by stimulating release of the inhibitory neurotransmitter gamma-aminobutyric acid
(GABA) and increasing its binding to
receptors. In nematodes, mites, and
insects this results in paralysis followed by death. Ivermectin has no
effect on tapeworms and flukes, which
do not use GABA as a neurotransmitter. In mammals GABA is confined to the central nervous system
(CNS), which ivermectin cannot readily penetrate. Ivermectin is available
for subcutaneous injection in cattle
and pigs and for oral administration
in horses and sheep. The drug persists
longer in tissues after injection, giving
greater efficacy against ectoparasites.
There is activity for up to 21 days in
cattle after injection, but only about 7
days in sheep after oral administration. Ivermectin should not be used
in lactating cattle because high levels
are found in the milk for long periods after administration.
In cattle, ivermectin has very good
efficacy against lungworms and gastrointestinal nematodes, including
inhibited larvae of *Ostertagia
ostertagi*, although efficacy against
Cooperia spp. and *Nematodirus helve-
tianus* is slightly less. It is also used
to kill sucking lice, mange mites, and
warble flies. In pigs, efficacy against
gastrointestinal nematodes, both
adults and larval stages, is good, as is
efficacy against sarcoptic mange mites
and lice. In sheep, ivermectin is effective against abomasal nematodes, but
has poorer efficacy against the intestinal nematodes *Cooperia* spp. and
Nematodirus spp. There is also good
efficacy against nasal bot larvae. In

horses ivermectin is efficacious against gastrointestinal parasites, including large and small strongylids, horse bot larvae, *Oxyuris equi*, and *Parascaris equorum*. The microfilariae of *Onchocerca cervicalis* in subcutaneous tissue are also killed. Ivermectin can also kill parasites in dogs and it is used to control microfilariae of the heartworm *Dirofilaria immitis*. However, in some breeds of dog the drug gains access to the CNS causing toxic signs, including depression, incoordination, convulsions, and paralysis. There have been reports of nematodes showing resistance to ivermectin, but there is no cross-resistance with other groups of anthelmintics.

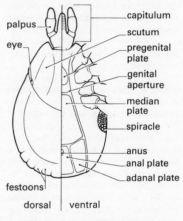

The anatomy of an ixodid tick

Labels on illustration:
palpus — capitulum
eye — scutum — pregenital plate — genital aperture — median plate — spiracle — anus — anal plate — adanal plate
festoons
dorsal | ventral

Ixodes A genus of hard *ticks containing over 50 species distributed worldwide and known as castor bean ticks or sheep ticks (see illustration). All are ectoparasites, especially of sheep, cattle, and dogs but will occasionally bite humans. The life cycle takes about three years to complete; the larva, nymph, and adult female are all bloodsuckers and each lives on a different host. They transmit a number of serious diseases, such as

*tick-borne fever in cattle and sheep, *louping ill in sheep and working dogs, *tick pyaemia in sheep, and the protozoan parasite *Babesia*, which causes redwater fever (*see* babesiosis) in cattle. The bite of some overseas species can cause *tick paralysis. These ticks are most common on rough grazing land; clearance of scrub, heather, bracken, etc., will assist in their control. Otherwise, control is by dipping animals in insecticides.

J

jaagsiekte *See* pulmonary adenomatosis.

Jacobson's organ *See* vomeronasal organ.

Japanese encephalitis A mosquito-transmitted disease of horses, pigs, and humans caused by a *flavivirus. It is characterized in horses by fever, loss of appetite, nervous signs, and death and in pigs by stillbirth. Many cases are subclinical, but almost half of those that develop nervous signs die. The virus is present throughout the Far East, but the incidence of the disease has been considerably reduced following the use of vaccines in horses and pigs and the control of *mosquitoes. *See* encephalitis.

jaundice The staining of tissues due to the accumulation in them of the *bile pigment bilirubin, a product of haemoglobin degradation. *Obstructive jaundice* occurs when the bile made in the liver fails to reach the intestine due to obstruction of the bile duct (e.g. by gallstones or parasites). *Haemolytic jaundice* occurs when there is excessive destruction of red cells in the blood (haemolysis), for example in certain protozoal diseases, such as *babesiosis, or as a result of *copper poisoning or *brassica poisoning. Medical name: **icterus**.

jaw Either of a pair of structures, the upper and lower jaws, that form the framework of the mouth. The upper jaw consists of the *maxilla and incisive bones; the lower jaw is formed by the *mandible. In mammals the jaws carry the teeth, whereas in birds they are surrounded by the hard keratinized epidermis of the beaks.

jejun- (jejuno-) *Prefix denoting* the jejunum.

jejunectomy Surgical removal of part of the jejunum. Total removal is not feasible because of the consequent maldigestion and malabsorption. For example, a horse cannot maintain its body weight if more than 50% of the jejunum has had to be removed. Jejunectomy is required if a length of jejunum is irreversibly damaged by the loss of its blood supply or by a foreign body.

jejunoileostomy Surgical creation of an opening to connect the jejunum and the ileum. This may be required to bypass a section of diseased jejunum if its removal is not possible.

jejunotomy Surgical incision into the lumen of the jejunum. The most common indication is for the removal of a foreign body causing an obstruction.

jejunum The part of the small *intestine between the duodenum and the ileum.

Jembrana disease A highly infectious fatal disease of cattle, recorded in Bali during 1964–67. The chief clinical features are fever, nasal discharge, anaemia, and dysentery. Lymph-node lesions and generalized haemorrhage and vasculitis are found at autopsy. The disease is generally considered to be associated with a rickettsia, and it remains confined to Bali.

Jerusalem cherry Either of two plants (*Solanum pseudocapsicum* or *S. capsicastrum*) belonging to the nightshade family and containing the toxic alkaloid solanine. *See* solanine poisoning.

jigger The sand flea or chigoe, *Tunga penetrans*, found in tropical America and Africa. The female burrows into the skin of humans and livestock, generally on the feet, causing a cyst to form around it. Intense itching occurs as the cyst enlarges to the size of a pea and scratching may cause secondary infections. *See also* flea.

jimsonweed poisoning *See* deadly nightshade poisoning.

Johne's disease (paratuberculosis) A disease of cattle (and to a lesser extent sheep and goats) characterized by chronic debilitation and weight loss and caused by the bacterium *Mycobacterium paratuberculosis*. It is widespread in Europe. Infection is by ingestion of contaminated water or food and the disease has a slow spread and a long incubation period of up to 18 months. In cattle the signs only appear in animals over 2 years of age. These include chronic diarrhoea, which has a 'pea soup' consistency, weight loss, and eventual emaciation. In sheep, weight loss and shedding of wool are the major signs, and the diarrhoea is less severe. Control of the disease depends upon prompt removal of affected animals from the herd/flock. Contamination of pasture and water supplies can be avoided by careful disposal of contaminated manure. There is no effective treatment, though vaccines are available in some countries.

usually permanent. It occurs, for example, where the bodies of adjacent vertebrae are joined by an intervertebral disc. In *synovial joints free movement occurs. The articulating surfaces of the bones are covered by articular cartilage and the bones are united by a joint capsule, which encloses the joint cavity and contains the synovial fluid.

joint ill *See* navel ill.

jugular Relating to or supplying the neck or throat.

junctional complex The group of specialized connections between epithelial cells close to their luminal surfaces. There are three components: the *zonula occludens; *zonula adherens; and *macula adherens. See illustration.

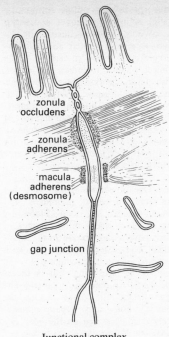

Junctional complex

K

joint (articulation) The region of contact between two or more bones. Three groups of joints are recognized on the basis of the nature of the intervening tissue. *Fibrous joints* are immovable and held together by fibrous connective tissue. These include the *sutures between the bones of the skull, a *syndesmosis, which occurs, for example, between the shafts of the metacarpal bones, and a *gomphosis*, which is the joint between a tooth and its alveolus in the jaw bone. *Cartilaginous joints* are joined by cartilage and slight movement may occur. Of these a *synchondrosis* is formed of hyaline cartilage and tends eventually to ossify. It occurs, for example, between the shaft and head of a long bone. A *symphysis is formed of fibrocartilage and is

kale poisoning *See* brassica poisoning.

kallidin A kinin that is produced in inflamed tissues and is active in promoting *inflammation.

kallikrein An enzyme responsible for the production of *kinins from their precursors (kininogens) in inflamed tissue (*see* inflammation).

Kalmia poisoning A toxic condition caused by ingestion of foliage from any of several species of evergreen shrub belonging to the genus *Kalmia* (mountain laurels), distributed throughout eastern North America. They include the alpine or bog laurel (*K. microphylla*), also known as the pale laurel or sheep laurel, and the calico bush or mountain laurel (*K.*

kanamycin

latifolia). The toxic principles are a resinoid (andromedotoxin) and a glycoside (arbutin), which cause salivation, severe abdominal pain, vomiting, weakness, convulsions, and death. Treatment is of the signs; the administration of *atropine may be beneficial.

kanamycin *See* aminoglycoside.

kaolin An aluminium silicate, obtained from certain clays, which acts as an *adsorbent. For therapeutic use it is available as a powder or combined with glycerin to form a paste, and is used in the treatment of diarrhoea to adsorb microbial toxins in the gastrointestinal tract and to form a protective layer over the gut mucosa. It has no activity against enterotoxins produced by *Escherichia coli*. Other forms include kaolin combined with pectin (kaogel), for use as an adsorbent in diarrhoea, and kaolin combined with morphine, to reduce gastrointestinal motility. Kaolin is also used as a dry powder in poultices over infected wounds to remove fluid and toxic material from the area. It has low toxicity but occasionally overuse can lead to malabsorption problems or the formation of granulomas in the gastrointestinal tract.

kary- (karyo-) *Prefix denoting* a cell nucleus.

karyokinesis Division of the nucleus of a cell, which occurs during cell division before division of the cytoplasm (*cytokinesis*). *See* mitosis.

karyotype The chromosomal complement of an organism, described in terms of chromosome number, size, shape, and staining patterns. The karyotype is most often shown as the chromosomes of the species arranged in their *homologous pairs. Most species have a unique karyotype.

kata (peste des petits ruminants; PPR) A disease of goats and sheep in West Africa caused by a *paramyxovirus related to the virus responsible for *rinderpest. The clinical picture resembles rinderpest, with fever, profuse nasal discharge, *necrotic stomatitis, diarrhoea, and usually death. Differential diagnosis requires laboratory examination of autopsy specimens. Newly purchased animals are usually quarantined for two weeks to avoid introducing the disease to a flock.

ked One of various small *flies that are ectoparasites of mammals and birds, feeding on their blood by means of a sharp biting proboscis. Keds have a short broad head, a flattened body, and strong legs with recurved claws for clinging to the host. Some have wings but in others the wings are reduced or absent. The eggs hatch into larvae within the female's body and pupate immediately once deposited on the host. *See also* New Forest fly; sheep ked.

Kennel Club A UK organization, founded in 1873, devoted to promoting the general improvement of dogs. It undertakes the classification of dog breeds and registration of pedigrees, besides promoting and staging dog shows and trials, including the prestigious annual Cruft's Dog Show. Address: 1–5 Clarges St., London W1Y 8AB.

kennel cough (infectious canine laryngotracheitis) A highly contagious condition, characterized by a hacking cough, that commonly spreads among dogs at boarding kennels, rescue homes, dog shows, and training classes. Infection remains localized to the upper respiratory tract and clinical signs are usually mild. It may be caused by one or more of several agents normally found in the upper respiratory tract, including the bacterium *Bordetella bronchiseptica*, canine *adenoviruses 1 and 2, canine *herpesvirus, canine *parainfluenzavirus, and *mycoplasmas. Mild cases of the disease are self-limiting and will clear if the dog is kept rested away from other dogs and given demulcents, such as glycerine and honey, to soothe the throat. More severe cases may require antibiotics, which are able to combat the bacteria and mycoplasmas, as well as cough suppressants and anti-inflammatory drugs. Vaccines are available to give protection against adenovirus, parainfluenzavirus, and *Bordetella bronchiseptica* infection, but do not offer complete protection against the disease.

kennel lameness A form of *rickets in dogs, predominantly due to vitamin D deficiency. It occurs in animals fed almost entirely on dog biscuits with no vitamin supplementation or access to sunlight. The condition is rare in pet dogs that are regularly exercised and thereby exposed to sunlight, which allows the skin to produce vitamin D.

kerat- (kerato-) *Prefix denoting* **1.** the cornea. Example: *keratopathy* (disease of). **2.** horny tissue, especially of the skin.

keratin A fibrous *protein that forms the horny tissues of the body, such as the outer layer of the skin, the claws, hoofs, horns, and hair.

keratinization (cornification) The process by which cells become horny due to the deposition of *keratin within them. It occurs in the *epidermis of the skin and associated structures (claws, hoofs, horns, and hair), where the cells lose their nuclei and are filled with keratin.

keratitis Inflammation of the *cornea of the eye. It may be due to chronic irritation by dust, barley awns, seeds, etc., lodged beneath the eyelid, or to a deficiency of tear production. It also occurs in cases of *New Forest disease in cattle, in *ovine keratoconjunctivitis, and in *malignant catarrhal fever of cattle. Dogs suffer a chronic superficial keratitis, known as *Uberreiter's syndrome. See also* canine viral hepatitis.

keratocele Herniation of the innermost layer of the cornea (Descemet's membrane), producing a bleblike outward pouching of the cornea. It may be a sequel to corneal ulceration, with weakness of the affected area allowing herniation to occur.

Ulceration is often accompanied by some exudation in the anterior chamber (anterior *staphyloma). The herniation may rupture, leading to leakage of aqueous humour with fistula formation and anterior uveitis. More seriously, the iris may be pulled towards the hernia site resulting in adhesion (anterior *synechia) or prolapse and incarceration of the iris portion in the hernia site.

Larger hernias result in loss of vitreous humour and possible lens prolapse, ending in *panophthalmitis. This condition is seen in dog breeds with prominent eyes that are subject to ulceration or abrasion of the cornea, for example Pekingese, boxers, and pugs.

Treatment should aim to minimize the severity of any initial ulceration; more severe corneal ulceration should be cauterized. Where chronic ulceration occurs, intraocular pressure may be relieved by anterior chamber *paracentesis (every 24–48 hours if necessary) to prevent corneal herniation. Large corneal ulcers may respond to conjunctival keratoplasty. Antibiotic coverage may be advisable, but use of corticosteroids is generally contraindicated.

keratoconjunctivitis Inflammation of both the cornea (*see* keratitis) and the conjunctiva (*see* conjunctivitis) in the eye. A common cause is bacterial infection, particularly in cattle (*see* New Forest disease) and sheep (*see* ovine keratoconjunctivitis). In growing broilers the eyes may be affected by ammonia fumes, due to, for instance, badly soiled litter, poor ventilation, high stocking density, or high humidity. The resultant keratoconjunctivitis leads to reduced performance in birds aged 2–4 weeks. Signs are ruffled feathers and closed eyes, giving a downcast appearance; there may be ulceration of the cornea.

keratome An instrument designed to cut the cornea of the eye. It consists of a handle and flat triangular blade, sharpened on both sides of the apex so that it will cut the cornea when thrust directly into the eye.

keratosis A skin disorder characterized by overgrowth of the horny *stratum corneum. Such disorders may result from prolonged irritation or from excessive exposure to sunlight. *See also* parakeratosis.

kerosene poisoning *See* fuel oil poisoning.

ketamine A dissociative anaesthetic that causes depression of the cerebral cortex with little effect on medullary centres, producing catalepsy, analgesia, loss of consciousness, and dissociation. Many reflexes are retained and muscle relaxation is poor or absent, but there is little respiratory depression and the cardiovascular system remains stable. Profuse salivation occurs, which can be counteracted by administering *atropine. Ketamine is safer and shorter acting than its analogue *phencyclidine. It can be administered intravenously, intramuscularly, or subcutaneously. Anaesthesia lasts 30–45 minutes and recovery normally takes up to 8 hours. Ketamine is metabolized in the liver and excreted by the kidneys, and anaesthesia is prolonged in animals with hepatic or renal insufficiency.

Ketamine is commonly used in combination with the sedative *xylazine to give better muscle relaxation, less twitching and reflex movement, and a smoother recovery. This combination can be administered to induce anaesthesia in dogs, horses, donkeys, sheep, goats, and cats. The xylazine should be given prior to induction of anaesthesia with ketamine in case there are problems with vomiting and bradycardia. Ketamine has a wide margin of safety and side-effects are uncommon.

ketoconazole *See* imidazoles.

ketogenesis The process by which the body synthesizes *ketone bodies. Abnormally high levels of ketogenesis lead to *ketosis, for example in animals suffering from starvation or *diabetes mellitus.

ketonaemia The presence of *ketone bodies in the blood, especially acetone, acetoacetate and β-hydroxybutyrate. Blood ketones, particularly β-hydroxybutyrate, provide an important diagnostic indicator of low energy status and negative energy balance, especially in lactating dairy cows. Ketonaemic animals have a characteristic sweet smell to the breath, which indicates either subclinical or clinical *ketosis. Ketonaemia occurs when there is insufficient blood glucose to fuel the crucial Krebs cycle, on which energy metabolism is based and which normally metabolizes the ketones. As a result, alternative pathways of energy metabolism are used, which leads to a build-up of ketones. A common exacerbating factor is fatty liver – a condition brought about by excessive mobilization of body fat. This impairs liver function and hence ketone metabolism. Ketonaemia is very common in diabetic dogs and also occurs in any animal that is ill-fed or starved. Even fish may be affected and tests have been developed to detect ketones in the mucus on their body surface to indicate when food is in short supply.

ketone body One of three substances – acetoacetate, β-hydroxybutyrate, and acetone – that are produced by the liver under certain conditions, particularly when blood glucose levels are low. There develops an excess of acetyl groups (produced, e.g., from the breakdown of *fatty acids) over oxaloacetate, an intermediate in the *Krebs cycle. Two molecules of acetyl CoA condense to form acetoacetyl CoA, the precursor of acetoacetate, β-hydroxybutyrate, and acetone. The ketone bodies (other than acetone) can be metabolized by other tissues and are a normal source of energy within the animal body. In ruminants the level of ketone bodies is substantially higher than in nonruminants because of the high level of metabolism of the *volatile fatty acids, acetate and butyrate. *See also* ketogenesis; ketonaemia; ketosis.

ketonuria The presence of *ketone bodies in the urine. It is a consequence of ketones in the blood (*ketonaemia) and indicates negative energy balance or an early stage in *ketosis. Testing for ketonuria enables the identification of animals likely to develop clinical ketosis so that extra dietary energy can be given. The collection of urine samples is not always easy and milk is normally used for diagnostic purposes. Special kits are available for simple on-the-spot testing.

ketose A simple sugar that contains a keto group ($-C=O$); for example, *fructose.

ketosis (acetonaemia) A metabolic disease, usually affecting dairy cows 4–6 weeks after calving, in which the level of glucose in the blood falls due to inadequate intake of metabolizable energy in the diet. A sweet smell (like peardrops) can be detected on the breath, caused by the presence of acetone and other ketone bodies in the blood (*see* ketonaemia). The liver may also be affected (*see* fatty liver). Initial signs are reduction in appetite and milk yield. Loss of bloom in the coat and reduction in bodyweight occur as the disease progresses and occasionally other nervous signs, such as muscle tremors, staggering gait, and head pressing, are seen. Diagnosis can be confirmed by demonstrating the levels of glucose and ketones in the blood using laboratory tests. The usual treatment is by injection of *corticosteroids. Prevention depends upon feeding a well-balanced ration containing adequate metabolizable energy. The milk or urine of animals at risk of developing ketosis can be tested for ketones using special 'on-the-spot' kits thereby giving early warning of the disease and enabling extra energy to be given. Ketosis can occur in any animal that is starved or affected by disease that causes loss of appetite and hence inadequate energy intake.

Key-Gaskell syndrome A form of *dysautonomia affecting cats. The cause is unknown and the disease has been reported in the UK only over the last few years. Signs include persistent dilation of the pupils of the eyes, vomiting, inappetence, and constipation. Only supportive treatment can be given to help alleviate the signs. The disease tends to cause slow debilitation, which may lead to death in some cases. Other names: **dilated pupil syndrome**; **feline dysautonomia**.

kidney Either of the paired principal organs of *excretion, responsible for

kidney worm

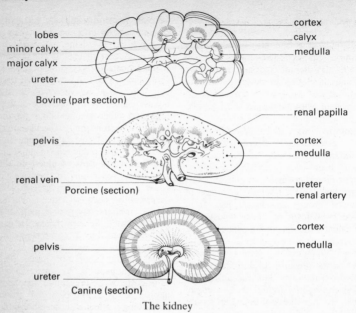

lobes
minor calyx
major calyx
ureter

cortex
calyx
medulla

Bovine (part section)

pelvis

renal papilla
cortex
medulla

renal vein

ureter
renal artery

Porcine (section)

pelvis

cortex
medulla

ureter

Canine (section)

The kidney

the removal of nitrogenous wastes, particularly urea, from the blood. The kidneys are situated in the dorsal abdomen on either side of the vertebral column in most species. However, in cattle the left kidney is displaced by the rumen to the right of the midline, so that it lies behind and a little below the right kidney. The renal artery enters the kidney and the renal vein and ureter leave it at the hilus.

The external form varies considerably between species: in mammals the kidney is typically bean-shaped, although the bovine kidney is lobated (see illustration). Beneath the tough fibrous external capsule is an outer cortex, which appears granular due to the presence of the renal *corpuscles. The inner medulla comprising the renal tubules has a striated appearance and is organized into distinct pyramid-shaped zones of tubules, the renal pyramids. The apices of these pyramids (the renal papillae) are each surrounded by a cup-shaped cavity (minor *calyx) that leads into the renal pelvis. Urine drains from the tubules into the pelvis and out of the kidney via the ureter. In the horse the renal pelvis has two long narrow diverticula, the *terminal recesses*. In the ox the ureter does not expand into a pelvis but divides into two *major calyces*, which receive the minor calyces. In the pig the major calyces arise from the renal pelvis. In birds each kidney is typically divided into several irregular lobes, which contain a large number of smaller lobules, each lobule being served by a branch of the ureter.

kidney worm 1. The common name for the pig hookworm, found in the kidney, *Stephanurus dentatus*. **2.** The giant kidney worm of the dog, *Dioctophyma renale (see* dioctophymosis).

kilo- *Prefix denoting* a thousand.

Kimberley horse disease A type of toxic hepatitis affecting horses in parts of Western Australia, caused by ingestion of plants of the genus *Crotalaria*, usually *C. retusa* or *C. crispata*. Affected animals lose appetite and weight. They often yawn and gallop or walk about aimlessly with the head held low, hence the term 'walkabout disease'. The effect is due to the presence in the plants of pyrrolizidine *alkaloids, which produce irreversible liver damage.

kin- (kine-) *Prefix denoting* movement.

kinaesthesia The sense that enables the individual to be aware of the position and movement of different parts of the body. This is achieved by means of *proprioceptors, which send impulses from muscles, joints, and tendons. Without this sense coordinated movement with the eyes closed would be impossible.

kinase An enzyme that catalyses the transfer of the terminal phosphate from ATP to another molecule. For example, hexokinase catalyses the reaction: glucose + ATP → glucose-6-phosphate + ADP. Sometimes the reverse reaction is more important, as in the case of pyruvate kinase, which catalyses the reaction: phosphoenolpyruvate + ADP → pyruvate + ATP.

-kinesis *Suffix denoting* movement.

kinin One of a group of polypeptides found in saliva, sweat, pancreatic juice, etc. that are powerful vasodilators. Their effects include the stimulation of smooth muscle, the relaxation of vascular smooth muscle, and the increase of blood capillary permeability. Kinins are not normally present in blood but are formed under certain conditions, for example when tissue is damaged or following pH or temperature changes in the blood. Kinins are produced in inflamed tissues by the enzyme kallikrein acting on precursor molecules called *kininogens*. *See also* bradykinin; kallidin.

kinky back A form of *spondylolisthesis causing *paraplegia in growing broilers. It involves displacement of the sixth thoracic vertebra, and affects birds aged 3–6 weeks, which collapse onto their hocks. It is usual to see a few cases in broiler flocks. There is both a hereditary factor and a link with very fast growth in the first 2 weeks. Although the condition has been experimentally prevented by drastic feed restriction in this early period, such a remedy is not commercially practicable.

Kirschner-Ehmer splint A type of *splint in which the fractured bone is fixed by means of a longitudinal external rod running between double-pin units on either side of the fracture site. Two pins are inserted transversely through the skin and soft tissues into the bone on each side of the fracture. The projecting shafts of each pair of pins are joined by a bar, forming a pin-unit, enabling the pin-units on each side of the fracture to be aligned and held in position by a longitudinal clamping rod. This method provides direct skeletal fixation and permits fracture manipulation without a full open *reduction. It also gives better fixation than a plaster cast, although the metalwork on the outside of the limb may be a drawback. Infection through the stab holes in the skin is largely avoided by permitting blood clots to form and adhere between the skin and the fixation pins. *See also* bone pinning.

Klebsiella A genus of nonmotile usually capsulated Gram-negative *bacteria, commonly found in soil and water and in the intestine and respiratory tract of humans and other animals. The capsulated (mucoid) types are often pathogenic. *K. pneumoniae* causes severe lobar pneumonia in humans, urogenital infections in animals, particularly *endometritis and *infertility in mares, and *mastitis in dairy cows. Infection is often derived from contaminated bedding, but stallions are also important sources of infection for the mare.

knee *See* stifle.

knee gall (knee thoroughpin) An inflammatory lesion of the 'knee' of the horse (*see* carpus), caused by irritation and trauma. The condition starts as an area of simple inflammation of the overlying skin, but progresses to ulceration and abscess formation. *Compare* thorough-pin.

knee spavin Osteoarthrosis of the carpal ('knee') joints of the horse. *See* arthritis.

knocked-up shoe A shoeing feature in which the inner branch of the horseshoe is hammered to a shape higher than wide to help prevent brushing.

knocked-up toe (interphalangeal dislocation) An injury, common in racing greyhounds, in which one of the small joints of the toe becomes dislocated, so that the toe nail tends to point up from the ground. In mild cases the dislocation can be put back into place and the nail cut short to prevent weight from being put on the foot. More severe cases may require surgical fixation or even amputation of the toe.

Koch's body *See* Theileria.

Krebs cycle (citric acid cycle; tricarboxylic acid cycle; TCA cycle) A cyclical series of biochemical reactions that is fundamental to the metabolism of aerobic organisms. The enzymes of the Krebs cycle are located in the matrix of the *mitochondrion; they catalyse the oxidation of acetyl groups (in the form of acetyl coenzyme A) to two molecules of CO_2, with the production of the equivalent of 12 molecules of *ATP per acetyl group. The acetyl CoA comes mainly from glucose (by *glycolysis), from the oxidation of fatty acids, or from the degradation of certain amino acids. The first step of the cycle is the condensation of acetyl CoA with oxaloacetate to form citrate. A deficiency in the level of oxaloacetate will lead to the conversion of excess acetyl CoA into *ketone bodies. The Krebs cycle can also serve as a source of intermediates for the synthesis of biomolecules, and is a central 'crossroads' in the complex system of metabolic pathways.

Kupffer cell A phagocytic cell in the lining of the sinusoids of the *liver (*see* macrophage). They are particularly concerned with the breakdown of haemoglobin following the phagocytosis of red blood cells.

kypho- *Prefix denoting* a hump.

kyphosis Abnormal upward (dorsal) curvature of the spine. It occurs when the body of one or more vertebrae collapse, and may be the result of congenital malformation, fracture, or pathological change. *Compare* lordosis; scoliosis.

L

labial Relating to the lips or to a labium.

labial necrosis of rabbits (Schmorl's disease) A fatal contagious disease of rabbits caused by *Fusobacterium necrophorum*, i.e. a form of *necrobacillosis. Swelling and discoloration of the upper lip spreads to involve the lower face and neck; there is toxaemia and progressive emaciation. On autopsy, a haemorrhagic exudate is present in the pleural and peritoneal cavities.

labile Describing a substance that is unstable and is rapidly modified in the environment or within the body.

labio- *Prefix denoting* the lip(s).

labium (*pl.* **labia**) The lip or any lip-like structure, especially the folds of skin surrounding the vulva.

labrum (*pl.* **labra**) A liplike structure occurring, for example, around the *acetabulum of the hip joint or the *glenoid cavity of the shoulder joint.

laburnum poisoning A toxic condition arising from the ingestion of laburnum (*Laburnum anagyroides*), grown as an ornamental shrub for its clusters of bright-yellow flowers. Horses and cattle may browse on shrubs growing wild or on branches pruned from cultivated plants. Free-range poultry may pick up the minute black seeds. The plant contains the alkaloid cytisine, which has a *nicotine-like action. It causes purgation, straining of the bowels, and coldness in the body's extremities. The animal appears narcotized and death is due to respiratory failure. Treatment is of the signs.

labyrinth *See* ear.

laceration A wound with torn and ragged edges.

lacertus (fibrosus) A band-like tendon of the biceps brachii muscle which spreads out into the antebrachial fascia.

lacrimal apparatus The structures that produce and remove fluid from

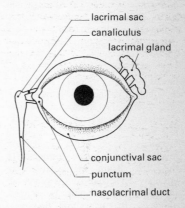

The lacrimal apparatus

the front of the eye (see illustration). The lacrimal gland secretes *tears into the conjunctival sac, from where the fluid drains through a small opening (punctum) at the inside of each eyelid into canaliculi. These convey fluid into the lacrimal sac to be discharged via the nasolacrimal duct to the nasal cavity.

lacrimal bone One of a pair of small bones of the face that form part of the orbit. *See* skull.

lacrimal gland The gland situated within the orbit that secretes tears. *See* lacrimal apparatus.

lact- (lacti-, lacto-) *Prefix denoting* 1. milk. 2. lactic acid.

lactalbumin One of the major proteins of milk and a component of the enzyme that synthesizes *lactose.

lactase The enzyme that hydrolyses *lactose to yield glucose and galactose. It is synthesized in the intestinal mucosa and is active in the intestinal lumen.

lactation The secretion of *milk by the *mammary glands. Changes in the mammary glands occur during pregnancy in readiness for lactation to commence following birth of the young. These changes are initiated and controlled by a group of hormones – the *lactogenic complex* – including *prolactin, *progesterone, and *oestrogens. Release of the milk (*letdown) is triggered by the suckling action of the young (or a milking machine) via a reflex mechanism involving the hormone *oxytocin. In the first hours of lactation an antibody-rich *colostrum is produced; thereafter, normal milk is secreted, although its composition may vary with the stage of lactation.

The frequency of suckling is a major factor in determining milk yield and the duration of lactation; as the offspring begin to utilize alternative sources of food, suckling declines, hence milk production falls off. The duration varies with species and with management techniques (see table). When the animal is systematically milked (*see* milking) as part of a production process, lactation is pro-

Duration of lactation in various domestic species

Species	Duration (days)*
Cow	3–205
Mare	120–180
Ewe	30–180
Doe	56–70
Sow	14–56
Bitch	20–56
Queen	20–56

*In species showing a wide range, duration depends on management

longed. In some species lactation is associated with reduced reproductive activity, i.e. lactational *anoestrus. Lactation may occur during *false pregnancy in the bitch.

lactation tetany A metabolic disease of mares involving incoordination, sweating, muscle tremors, rapid breathing, spasms of the diaphragm, and tetany. A number of factors can precipitate the condition: recent foaling or weaning of a foal; sudden access to lush pasture; or, in nonlactating horses, stress. Mild cases are responsive to calcium and magnesium salts administered intravenously. Severely affected mares often die within 24 hours.

lacteal A blind-ending lymphatic vessel that extends into a *villus of the small intestine. Digested fats are absorbed into the lacteals.

lactic acid An acid that is produced by the anaerobic metabolism of glucose. This happens in vigorously exercising muscle when oxygen supply to the tissues is limiting: *pyruvic acid is converted to lactic acid by the enzyme lactate dehydrogenase. A build-up of lactic acid may cause cramp if the exercise is prolonged. Lactic acid is also produced by fermentation in certain bacteria and is characteristic of soured milk.

lactiferous Describing tissues or structures that secrete or convey milk, for example the *lactiferous ducts* of the mammary gland.

lactiferous sinus The channel within the teat of the *mammary gland. Its glandular part receives lactiferous ducts from the gland substance and continues into the papillary part in the teat; this becomes the papillary duct, which opens to the surface.

Lactobacillus A genus of rod-shaped Gram-positive *bacteria that occur singly or in chains and prefer a *microaerophilic environment for growth. They are found in abundance as commensals on body surfaces, in the alimentary canal and urogenital tract of humans and animals, and in plants and certain types of food and agricultural products, especially dairy products. The lactobacilli are not important pathogens but they have been associated with gastric ulcers in the pig.

lactogenic Capable of causing the synthesis and/or secretion of milk. The *lactogenic complex* of hormones comprises all those hormones involved in the initiation and maintenance of lactation, especially *prolactin.

lactose (milk sugar) A *disaccharide comprising glucose and galactose; it is the main sugar of milk.

lactosuria The presence of milk sugar (*lactose) in urine. Although rare it can occur in milk-fed premature newborn animals or when inflammation of the intestine allows direct absorption of lactose. In lactating adults, lactose may be resorbed and subsequently excreted in the urine when milk has been retained overlong in the udder.

lacuna (*pl.* **lacunae**) (in anatomy) A small cavity or depression; for example, one of the spaces in compact bone in which a bone cell lies.

laevo- *Prefix. See* levo-.

laking The physical or chemical treatment of blood to abolish the structure of the red cells and thus form a homogeneous solution. Laking is an important preliminary step in the analysis of haemoglobin or enzymes present in red cells.

lamb dysentery A form of *dysentery affecting lambs in their first week of life and caused by the bacterium *Clostridium perfringens* type B. The bacterium is a normal inhabitant of the intestine, but overdistension of the stomach with milk favours its multiplication, leading to an acute fatal *enterotoxaemia with blood-stained diarrhoea. Pregnant ewes can be vaccinated in order to confer passive antitoxic immunity on the newborn lambs via the colostrum.

lambing sickness (moss ill) A metabolic disorder of ewes in late pregnancy or early lactation, similar to *milk fever in cows. The basic cause is an abnormally low concentration of calcium in the blood (*hypocalcaemia) brought on by the mineral demands of the developing foetus or the lactating mammary glands. Usually some kind of stress factor precipitates the disorder by inhibiting calcium absorption from the alimentary tract. Typical examples are changes of feed, or weather, or temporary interruption in feeding due to movement from field to field or transportation. Because the stress factor often applies to a group of sheep or a flock, outbreaks of the disorder have a similar pattern. After a brief period of excitability the affected animals go down as though paralysed, become comatose, and may die within a few hours. Treatment is by injection of *calcium borogluconate, and a good response to this confirms the diagnosis, although the disease can be confused with *pregnancy toxaemia.

lamella (*pl.* **lamellae**) **1.** A thin layer, membrane, scale, or plate-like tissue or part. In *bone tissue, lamellae are thin regular plates. In compact bone these can be arranged concentrically around a Haversian canal forming osteones (osteonic lamellae), between osteones (interstitial lamellae), or around the whole circumference of a

lamina

bone (circumferential lamellae). **2.** A *lamina.

lamina (*pl.* **laminae**) A thin membrane or layer of tissue. The lamina of a *vertebra is the thin platelike portion of the arch. The laminae (lamellae) of the horn of the equine *hoof interdigitate with those of the *corium. *See also* basal lamina.

laminectomy Surgical removal of the roof of the vertebral canal, i.e. the upper part of the arch of one or more vertebrae, to give access to the spinal cord. It is performed, for instance, to remove neoplasia or to allow decompression of the spinal cord.

laminitis Inflammation of a lamina or laminae, particularly the laminae of the *hoof in equine and bovine species. In **cattle** laminitis may be acute, chronic, or subclinical. All four feet or just fore- or hindfeet may be involved; often the inner front and outer hind claws appear most affected. The condition is painful and has an adverse effect on milk production, and may predispose to other conditions, such as bruising and ulceration of the sole; hoof deformity often results. In chronic cases the front wall of the hoof curves upwards so that the heels bear the weight. The aetiology is not fully understood but involves blood vessel damage. It may follow a toxaemia due to mastitis or metritis and there may be an association with high intakes of concentrates, especially high-carbohydrate concentrates. Treatment includes paring and dressing the affected feet, attention to the diet, and avoidance of very rough ground surfaces.

In **horses** laminitis may be acute or chronic, and varies greatly in its severity. In the worst cases the inflammation is sufficient to allow marked movement of the pedal bone within the hoof and it may prolapse through the sole. All four feet may be affected, but often one or two are worse than the others. The pain produced by the pedal bone rotation causes a characteristic stance, with the heels bearing the animal's weight. In severe cases the animal is unwilling to move, especially on hard surfaces, and may spend much time lying down. In chronic cases, laminitic rings can be seen on the hoof, the toe is long, the dorsal wall is concave in outline, and the sole may be convex. Again, the aetiology is complex and incompletely understood. *Carbohydrate overload can be important, and the condition is seen typically in fat ponies grazing on good pasture. Toxic factors can be involved and laminitis may follow metritis or colic if endotoxaemia is present. Treatment depends upon the severity and ranges from simple pain relief and gentle walking for exercise to dressing of the foot, resection of the dorsal hoof wall, and special shoeing procedures. The prognosis also depends on the severity and on the weight of the animal; the outlook is generally worse the larger the animal.

lampas Inflammation of the *palate, usually as part of a more general inflammation of the oral cavity (*see* stomatitis). It often accompanies inflammation of the tongue (*glossitis) and inflammation of the gums (*gingivitis). The lesions are painful and stop the animal eating. Possible causes include fungal infection and irritant chemicals. Treatment is difficult but may involve *emollients for pain relief. Accurate diagnosis is vital to ensure that the lesions are not due to a virus infection, such as *foot-and-mouth disease.

lamsiekte South African name for cattle *botulism caused by the ingestion of decomposing carcasses and bones contaminated with toxigenic strains of the bacterium *Clostridium *botulinum* type D. The animals' depraved appetite is due to grazing on phosphorus-deficient pastures, with consequent skeletal abnormalities (*styfziekte*).

lancet A broad two-edged surgical knife with a sharp point. It may be used for lancing abscesses, i.e. making a stab incision large enough to allow drainage.

lantana poisoning A toxic condition caused by ingestion of any of various ornamental woody shrubs or herbaceous plants of the tropical American genus *Lantana*. They contain poisonous triterpenes, and all parts of the plant are toxic, especially the leaves and green berries. The clinical signs of toxicity are anorexia, jaundice, secondary *photosensitization, and diarrhoea. The triterpenes cause degenerative changes in the heart, liver, and kidneys, and death is caused by hepatic and renal insufficiency and myocardial damage. Treatment is symptomatic.

laparo- *Prefix denoting* the abdomen.

laparoscope An *endoscope, also called peritoneoscope, used to visualize the abdominal organs. It is inserted through the abdominal body wall and peritoneum, and used, for example, to locate abnormalities, such as neoplasms, to facilitate the taking of biopsies, and to study the appearance of such organs as the ovaries. It can be used in the conscious animal (with or without sedation), under local anaesthesia, or in the generally anaesthetized animal. It must be sterilized before use and aseptic precautions taken during use.

laparotomy Surgical incision into the abdominal cavity. For example, an exploratory laparotomy is undertaken when an exact diagnosis has not been made but the cause is suspected to lie within the abdomen.

large intestine *See* intestine.

larkspur poisoning A toxic condition due to ingestion of various annual or herbaceous plants of the genus *Delphinium* (larkspurs). They contain polycyclic diterpenoid alkaloids (delphinine, delphinoidine, delphisine, and staphisagroine), which cause salivation, trembling, ataxia, bloat, and rapid weak pulse. The poisoning will terminate, favourably or unfavourably, within 24 hours. Treatment is symptomatic. *See also* aconite poisoning.

larva (*pl.* **larvae**) The preadult or immature stage hatching from the egg of some animal groups, e.g. insects and nematodes, which may be markedly different from the sexually mature adult and have a totally different way of life. For example, the larvae of some flies are parasites of animals and cause disease whereas the adults are free-living.

laryng- (laryngo-) *Prefix denoting* the larynx.

laryngeal paralysis Paralysis of the laryngeal muscles. This results in a loss of ability to control the *vocal folds (vocal cords), with consequent obstruction to the airflow on inspiration and hence noisy breathing. In **horses** the condition is most commonly caused by a lesion of the left recurrent laryngeal nerve, which results in laryngeal hemiplegia (*roaring). In many cases it is possible to detect a loss of muscle volume (due to atrophy) on palpating the larynx. In **dogs** laryngeal paralysis can cause collapse on exercise.

laryngitis Inflammation of the *larynx. Causes include irritant gases or smoke dust, and infectious diseases, such as *distemper in dogs, *infectious bovine rhinotracheitis, infectious canine laryngotracheitis (see kennel cough), *avian infectious laryngotracheitis, *strangles in horses, and *swine influenza. Coughing and difficulty in swallowing are characteristic signs, often with accompanying fever. In severe cases death can occur due to *laryngospasm. Apart from dealing with any underlying infection, treatment is with antibiotics and pain-relieving drugs. *Tracheotomy may be required in cases involving laryngospasm.

laryngopharynx The part of the *pharynx that communicates with the larynx via the laryngeal inlet. It extends from the tip of the epiglottis to the oesophagus.

laryngoscope An *endoscope designed for visualization of the larynx. It is used to aid positioning of an endotracheal tube in small animals, calves, goats, sheep, and pigs. A flexible fibrescope is used routinely for assessing laryngeal function in horses.

laryngospasm Spastic closure of the *larynx, obstructing the flow of air to the lungs. A possible cause is severe laryngitis. *Tracheotomy may be needed to prevent death due to asphyxia.

laryngotomy Surgical incision into the larynx. This may be done to remove foreign bodies, neoplasms, cysts, or part of the larynx itself. The laryngeal lumen is not sterile, therefore the incision, generally made in the ventral larynx, is left unsutured to allow drainage and subsequent healing.
In **horses** ventral laryngotomy is performed during the *Hobday operation* (laryngeal ventriculectomy) for laryngeal hemiplegia or paralysis (roarers or whistlers).

laryngotracheitis Inflammation of both the larynx (*laryngitis) and the trachea (*tracheitis). See also avian infectious laryngotracheitis; kennel cough (infectious canine laryngotracheitis).

larynx The organ connecting the pharynx with the trachea that serves as a valve in the airway and also as a sound-producing organ, especially in mammals. Essentially it comprises a cavity surrounded by a complex framework of cartilages: the epiglottis, thyroid, *arytenoid (paired), and *cricoid. These form joints with each other and can be moved by the laryngeal muscles. Stretched across the larynx between the vocal processes of the arytenoid cartilages and the thyroid cartilage are two *vocal ligaments. They are tightly wrapped by mucous membrane, forming the *vocal folds or true vocal cords. Movements of the highly mobile arytenoid cartilages cause the vocal folds to come together (adduct) or move apart (abduct), thereby changing the aperture of the *glottis. Cranial to the vocal folds, except in ruminants, are another pair of mucosal folds projecting across the larynx – the *vestibular folds* or *false vocal cords*. Beyond these, protecting the entrance from the pharynx, are the epiglottis and the membranous aryepiglottic folds. (See illustration.)
Closure of the laryngeal inlet during swallowing prevents food entering the airway. Closure of the glottis traps air in the airway caudal to it and increases intrathoracic pressure during coughing, etc. Vibration of the vocal folds causes production of sound, while variation in their tension affects the pitch of the sound produced. In birds the larynx functions primarily as a valve, sound being produced by the *syrinx, which is located further down the airway.

lasalocid See coccidiostat.

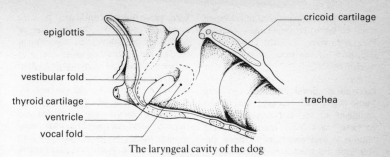

epiglottis

cricoid cartilage

vestibular fold

thyroid cartilage

ventricle

vocal fold

trachea

The laryngeal cavity of the dog

epiglottis

muscular process

arytenoid

tracheal cartilages

vocal process

thyroid

cricoid

The laryngeal cartilages of the dog

latency (virology) A stage in a viral infection during which the virus is not multiplying but residing in a specific tissue (usually nervous tissue) of the host. A subsequent stimulus to the animal may provoke multiplication of the latent virus, accompanied by its normal pathogenic effects. The physical state of the virus during latency is poorly understood, but it could be the whole *virion or the viral nucleic acid in an *episome-like state.

latent period (in neurology) The pause of a few milliseconds between the time that a nerve impulse reaches a muscle fibre and the time that the fibre starts to contract.

lateral 1. Situated at or relating to the side of an organ or organism. **2.** (in anatomy) Relating to the region

or parts of the body that are furthest from the *median plane.

lateral cartilages (cartilages of the distal phalanx) In the horse, plates of cartilage that extend either side of the distal phalanx above the border of the hoof, where they can be felt. In older life they can undergo ossification, producing the condition of *side-bones.

lateroversion A turning or displacement of an organ, for example the uterus (*uterine lateroversion*), to one side.

lathyrism A toxic condition arising from ingestion of seeds of the Indian pea or mutter pea (*Lathyrus sativus*) or other species of *Lathyrus*, which contain B-aminoproprionitrile and related compounds. This causes laryngeal paralysis, hepatitis, and lesions

latissimus dorsi muscle

of the skeleton due to interference with collagen cross-linkages. Poisoning only seems to occur when large quantities of the peas are eaten over a long period.

latissimus dorsi muscle A very broad flat muscle located behind the shoulder in the dorsal part of the thoracic wall. It inserts to the *humerus and contracts to draw the free limb backwards in locomotion.

laurel poisoning *See* cherry laurel poisoning; Kalmia poisoning.

lavage The use of water or a medicated solution to irrigate the surface or wash out the contents of tissues, organs, or cavities. It is required for exposed tissue during surgery to prevent desiccation. *Peritoneal lavage* involves irrigation of the peritoneal cavity with large volumes of fluid.

laxative An agent that increases intestinal motility and hence the rate of passage of intestinal contents. Many *purgatives given at low dose rates have a laxative effect. The main laxatives used in veterinary medicine are *liquid paraffin and white or yellow soft *paraffins. They are used to treat constipation and to aid the removal of foreign bodies from the intestinal tract.

layer A sexually mature female bird producing eggs for human consumption. *See* poultry husbandry.

LD$_{50}$ Lethal dose 50, or median lethal dose: the amount of a pharmacological or toxic substance that causes death in 50% of a group of experimental animals. For each LD$_{50}$ the species and weight of the animal and the route of administration is specified. LD$_{50}$s are used both in toxicology and in the bioassay of therapeutic compounds.

lead poisoning (plumbism) A toxic condition caused by the ingestion of lead. It is probably most common in cattle, but other species are also affected. Animals may ingest lead from discarded paint tins, from flaking lead paint on old woodwork, from putty, or as lead shot deposited on firing ranges or discarded by anglers. Land surrounding lead reclamation plants or spoil heaps of lead mines may be heavily contaminated, and acid rainwater is capable of dissolving lead salts or metallic lead. In **horses** and **dogs** lead poisoning is usually a chronic wasting disease with, in dogs especially, disturbance of the nervous system leading to whining, muscular twitching, and convulsions, which may be mistaken for *distemper. In **cattle** clinical signs are usually acute. The affected animal becomes dull, shows *colic, and may bellow. Some animals become blind, stagger sporadically, and develop muscular spasms and convulsions, during one of which the animal may die.

A single dose of 50 mg/kg will kill a calf, and a few ingested lead shot are fatal for a bird. Irrespective of its chemical form, about 98% of ingested lead is excreted in the faeces. The rest is absorbed, enters the bloodstream, and is excreted in bile, urine, and milk, or is stored in the liver and kidneys, especially the renal cortex. Diagnosis in the living animal is confirmed in some cases by an increased concentration of lead in the blood, and post mortem by a high lead concentration in the renal cortex. Magnesium sulphate and potassium iodide may be given, but the most rational treatment is daily intravenous injection of 75 mg/kg of sodium calcium edetate. This compound combines with absorbed lead to form a soluble complex which is excreted in bile and urine.

lecithin *See* phosphatidylcholine.

lecithinase An enzyme that hydrolyses lecithin. *See* phospholipase.

Legislation Affecting the Veterinary Profession in the United Kingdom A booklet published by the *Royal College of Veterinary Surgeons summarizing legislation relating to the veterinary profession and to animals, particularly veterinary practice, medicines, animal feedstuffs, artificial insemination, food hygiene, animal welfare, and wildlife.

leiomyoma A benign tumour of smooth muscle, seen in the genital tract, urinary bladder, and intestinal tract of most species, although the incidence is not high (*see also* fibroid). Histologically, leiomyomas consist of interlacing bundles of well-differentiated smooth muscle cells with minimal stroma. They are not encapsulated although a line of separation from adjacent tissue is apparent. Clinical manifestations follow from physical obstruction of normal function of the affected organ. Their complete surgical removal has a good prognosis.

leiomyosarcoma An uncommon malignant tumour of smooth muscle. The organs affected are mainly those involved with *leiomyoma, and the leiomyosarcoma may arise by malignant transformation of its benign counterpart. However, some leiomyosarcomas have also been reported in such organs as the kidney and ovary. There is a high risk of local recurrence after surgical excision, with the possibility of metastasis to other sites.

Leishmania A genus of protozoa that cause *leishmaniasis in humans, dogs, and occasionally other animals. *Leishmania* are related to *Trypanosoma* but the *flagellum is reduced or absent in most stages of the life cycle. They infect cells in the spleen, liver, lymph nodes, and other tissues of their mammalian hosts and are transmitted by *sandflies.

leishmaniasis A disease of humans and dogs occurring in tropical, subtropical, and warm-temperate regions of the Old and New Worlds. It is caused by various species of *Leishmania, notably *L. donovani*, *L. mexicana*, *L. brasiliensis*, *L. major*, and *L. tropica*. The disease is a *zoonosis, with reservoirs of infection persisting in dogs, wild canids, and small rodents, from which the parasite is transmitted to humans by sandflies. **Dogs** may be affected by both cutaneous and visceral forms of the disease, which affect skin tissues and internal organs respectively. It usually follows a chronic course and may be fatal. Human infections are treated with antimony compounds but canine infections respond less well and the drug is toxic. Control of the vector with insecticides is the most effective preventive strategy.

lemniscus (*pl.* **lemnisci**) A ribbon-like tract of nerve fibres in the central nervous system. The *medial lemniscus* is a major pathway conveying general sensory information mainly from the spinal cord to the thalamus in the brain. The *lateral lemniscus* is involved in auditory pathways.

lens 1. (in anatomy) The transparent avascular structure situated behind the pupil of the *eye and enclosed in a thin transparent capsule. In conjunction with the cornea, the lens refracts incoming light and focuses it onto the *retina. *See also* accommodation. **2.** (in optics) A piece of glass shaped to refract rays of light in a particular direction. *Convex lenses* converge the light and *concave lenses* diverge it.

lens dislocation Dislocation (luxation) of the crystalline lens of the eye.

It occurs when the supporting ligament of the lens breaks, either spontaneously or as a result of trauma. The condition occurs most commonly in terrier dogs as the result of an inherited defect, which results in subluxation and then luxation of the lens at about 4–5 years of age. The lens can displace downwards behind the iris, or downwards and forwards, with the lower half in front of the iris, or completely forward into the anterior chamber of the eye. In virtually all cases dislocation of the lens is followed by secondary *glaucoma, which leads to blindness.

lentiform nucleus *See* basal ganglia.

lept- (lepto-) *Prefix denoting* **1.** slender; thin. **2.** small. **3.** mild; slight.

leptocyte A thin *erythrocyte produced in many toxic disorders affecting the bone marrow, and sometimes in regenerative *anaemia. Because of their lack of thickness they may fold to give the appearance of *target cells or other abnormal morphology.

leptomeninges (*sing.* **leptomeninx**) The inner two fine *meninges: the *pia mater and the *arachnoid.

leptomeningitis Inflammation of the *leptomeninges, usually due to bacterial infection, for example *listeriosis in cattle, *strangles in horses, or *Streptococcus suis* type 2 in pigs. Infection may spread via the cerebrospinal fluid in the subarachnoid space. *See also* meningitis; meningoencephalitis.

Leptospira A genus of spiral-shaped Gram-negative *bacteria in the family Spirochaetaceae, widely distributed in fresh surface water, sewage, and the sea. They differ from the other *spirochaetes in their smallness, the fineness and closeness of their spiral coils, and their characteristic movement involving flexing and rapid rotation along the axis. There are two known species: *L. biflexa*, which includes all the nonpathogenic saprophytes, and *L. interrogans*, which includes all serotypes that cause disease in humans and animals (*see* leptospirosis). Over one hundred pathogenic serotypes affect animals, the most common being *icterohaemorrhagiae* in dogs, *canicola* in dogs and humans, *pomona* in pigs, cattle, and humans, and *hardjo* and *grippotyphosa* in cattle and other species. The main reservoirs of infection are rodents, but domestic animals, particularly dogs and pigs, also harbour the organisms. The leptospiras cannot survive for long in the environment without suitable moisture and temperature. In infected animals they spread through the blood and usually localize in the convoluted tubules of the kidney; spread to other hosts through urine may occur. Other sources of infection include milk, uterine discharges, and placenta.

leptospiral jaundice A disease of dogs due to infection with *Leptospira icterohaemorrhagiae*, a bacterium that causes severe damage to the liver and the linings of the blood vessels with consequent *jaundice; *L. canicola* infection can also cause jaundice. The organism is transmitted in urine, and is most commonly contracted from rodents' urine. The disease is usually fatal in dogs, and the bacterium can be transmitted to humans, in which it causes Weil's disease. It is therefore essential that all dogs are vaccinated, with annual boosters given subsequently. Other name: **canine leptospirosis**.

leptospirosis Disease caused by infection with various serotypes of the bacterium *Leptospira interrogans*. It can affect all the domestic species and humans and occurs throughout the world. In **cattle** *pomona* and *hardjo* are the commonest serotypes. Signs of disease can include jaundice, fever, and septicaemia in young calves and fever, inappetence, a rapid drop in milk yield, and abortion in adult cattle. Animals may remain carriers of the organism for long periods following recovery and excrete the organisms in urine. The disease is contagious and can result in outbreaks of illness, sometimes called the *milk drop syndrome*, in susceptible herds. Abortion 'storms' may also occur.

In **pigs** *canicola* and *pomona* are the commonest pathogenic serotypes, principally causing abortions and stillbirths. **Sheep** and **goats** are most often affected by *icterohaemorrhagiae* and *grippotyphosa*, with sometimes high mortality rates. Inappetence, jaundice, and the passage of dark-brown urine have been described in goats.

Leptospirosis is rare in **cats** but is common in **dogs**, with *icterohaemorrhagiae* and *canicola* the commonest serotypes. The former causes fever, jaundice, vomiting, and inappetence and the latter vomiting, depression, inappetence, and pain in the region of the kidneys. *Canicola* is the commonest cause of kidney failure in dogs (*see* leptospiral jaundice).

In humans the most important form of leptospirosis (also known as Weil's disease) is caused by *icterohaemorrhagiae* and is often contracted as the result of rat bites. Other *Leptospira* serotypes can infect humans and are nearly always derived from animal sources. For example, *hardjo* infection in farm workers has been associated with outbreaks of leptospirosis in dairy cattle. Canicola fever is a human syndrome associated with *canicola* infection, characterized by pyrexia, meningitis, kidney involvement, and sometimes jaundice. The condition is acquired by contact with the urine of infected animals (especially dogs, pigs and calves); swim-ming in urine-contaminated water is well known as a risk.

leptotene The first stage in the first prophase of *meiosis, in which the chromosomes become visible as single long threads.

lesion Any zone of tissue with impaired function as a result of damage by disease or injury. Apart from direct physical injury, examples of *primary lesions* include abscesses, ulcers, and tumours; *secondary lesions*, such as crusts and scars, are derived from primary lesions.

letdown (of milk) Release of milk from the mammary gland. Neurohumoral reflexes caused by suckling or similar stimuli, such as udder washing or milking, trigger the release of the pituitary hormone *oxytocin, which stimulates myoepithelial cells in the udder to eject the milk. This neurohumoral reflex is called *Ferguson's reflex*. See also milking.

lethal gene A gene having an *allele that, in the *homozygous state, causes the death of the organism. Such deaths frequently occur during embryonic or foetal development. Healthy offspring may act as *carriers of the lethal allele, which they possess in the *heterozygous state.

leuc- (leuco-, leuk-, leuko-) *Prefix denoting* **1.** lack of colour; white. **2.** leucocytes.

leucine An *amino acid. *See also* essential amino acid.

leucocyte (white blood cell) Any nucleated blood cell (corpuscle). In health there are three main divisions: *granulocytes (comprising *neutrophils, *eosinophils, and *basophils); *lymphocytes; and monocytes, which are the precursors of the *macrophages. They have various roles in protecting the body against foreign substances (*see* immunity) and in *inflammation and *hypersensitivity. In disease, a variety of other types may appear in the blood, notably immature forms of the normal cells. *See also* haemopoiesis.

leucocytosis An increase in the number of circulating white blood cells (leucocytes) in the blood. Leucocyte numbers are normally raised by the presence of pathogenic agents in the body. However, steroid hormones, noninfective inflammatory or degenerative disease, haemorrhage, and some physiological events also raise leucocyte counts. Leucocytosis may involve an excess of a particular type of white blood cell. Hence monocytosis involves an excess of *monocytes, and lymphocytosis an excess of *lymphocytes. Similarly, neutrophilia, eosinophilia, and basophilia refer to an excess of the corresponding cell type. Neutrophilia generally reflects pyogenic infection, necrosis, or acute inflammation. Eosinophilia is found in metazoan parasitism and in many hypersensitive disorders. Basophilia is rarely observed but is reported in a small proportion of dogs with mast cell tumours. Lymphocytosis is seen in protozoan parasitism, tuberculosis, and other chronic infections. It also occurs in a proportion of cases of *lymphosarcoma and is reported in herds of cattle infected with *enzootic bovine leukosis virus. However, lymphocytosis in an individual bovine does not by itself imply that the animal is clinically affected with leukosis. Corticosteroids affect leucocyte counts although the effects are complex, dose-dependent, and vary between species. Typically neutrophil and monocyte counts are raised by corticosteroids, and eosinophil and lymphocyte counts depressed. *Physiological leucocytosis* is caused by factors such as excitement or apprehension. In dogs and cats this takes the

form of slight neutrophilia and marked lymphocytosis. *See also* monocytosis.

leucoderma A patchy whiteness of the skin due to lack of the pigment melanin. *Vitiligo* is an inherited leucoderma and has been recorded in Asiatic cattle. Acquired leucoderma may result from nutritional deficiency, trauma, burns, or chemical agents. Leucoderma of the lips and nose may be a specific breed defect. In horses, prolonged contact of the lips with rubber bits may result in leucoderma at the points of contact. *See also* leucotrichia.

leucoma A dense white mark on the cornea of the eye, formed following the healing of a corneal ulcer. A deep corneal ulcer, one extending into the stroma of the cornea, gives rise to a considerable amount of scar tissue (fibroblasts), so producing the leucoma. The mark is most noticeable soon after the blood vessels supplying the healing ulcer have retracted, leaving the scar white. Eventually, the opacity may become less dense.

leucopenia A deficiency of *leucocytes in the circulating blood. All the leucocyte types may be affected, or only a single type, in which case the condition is more usually described by the name of the cell type concerned, for example lymphopenia, neutropenia, etc. Leucopenia occurs in many viral infections, most notably in feline panleucopenia, swine fever, canine distemper (in which lymphopenia is the characteristic change), and bovine virus diarrhoea. Bacterial endotoxins may also be associated with leucopenia. *Corticosteroids usually lower eosinophil and lymphocyte numbers while raising neutrophil numbers, and corticosteroid influence is presumed to be the reason for the lymphopenia and eosinopenia that accompany canine *hyperadrenocorticism. Eosinopenia occurs in various forms of stress, probably owing to the influence of adrenaline as well as corticosteroid hormones.

Any inflammatory condition involving a sudden influx of blood leucocytes into the tissues may result in temporary leucopenia if demand outstrips what the blood can supply. In severe chronic inflammation this situation may be prolonged. The leucopenia is then often characterized by marked neutropenia, in which a large proportion of neutrophils have juvenile appearance. This condition, the *degenerative left shift*, tends to carry a poor prognosis. *See also* pancytopenia.

leucoplakia Small white patches on mucous membranes, particularly in the mouth, vulva, or urinary bladder. They are seldom reported in animals.

leucosis (leukosis) Any condition in which there is an abnormal increase in the number of white blood cells. *See* avian leukosis; enzootic bovine leukosis; leucocytosis; leukaemia.

leucotrichia Whitening of the hair due to loss of the pigment melanin. The colour of hair is determined by the amount of melanin pigment produced by the *melanocytes. If these are congenitally absent or destroyed, for example by ionizing radiation, burns, or chemicals, leucotrichia is the result. Whitening of the hair is a manifestation of senility and is commonly seen first around the muzzle, eyes, and ears of aged animals. *See also* albinism.

leuk- *See* leuc-.

leukaemia Any of a group of malignant diseases in which there is over-production of white blood cells (*leucocytes) and hence an increased number of white cells in the circulating blood. Leukaemia is uncommon

in domestic animals; it has been occasionally reported accompanying *lymphosarcoma, and mast cell leukaemia is reported sporadically in cats. Leukaemias are classified according to the type of tissue or white cell involved: hence *lymphoid leukaemia involves the proliferation of cells derived from lymphoid tissue, particularly in the bone marrow (*see* lymphosarcoma); *myeloid leukaemia involves the nonlymphoid cells of the bone marrow. Monocytic (monocytes) and erythroid (erythrocytes) type leukaemias are also reported uncommonly in animals. Malignant cells carried by the blood invade the bone marrow and other organs, such as the lymph nodes, spleen, and liver. Large numbers of tumour cells are found in the circulating blood. The prognosis is invariably bleak. *See also* feline leukaemia.

leukoencephalomyelitis-arthritis A progressive nonfebrile disease of goats characterized by encephalitis, arthritis, mastitis, and pneumonitis and caused by a lentivirus. Many infected goats fail to develop clinical signs, although in some herds the disease prevalence can be high. Encephalitis is seen predominantly in kids between 2 and 4 months old, associated with nervous signs such as abnormal gait, ataxia, paralysis, and eventual death. In older animals arthritis, particularly of the carpal joints, is more common, although other fore- and hindlimb joints may be affected. The joint capsules are distended, although lameness may not be apparent. Nonsuppurative mastitis, with loss of milk yield, is an economically important sign of the disease in some nanny goats. Subclinical pneumonitis may occur in all age groups of infected animals and may predispose to other respiratory infections. Transmission is most common by infected colostrum and milk. There are no vaccines and control is by slaughter of all infected animals. *See also* maedi/visna.

leukosis *See* leucosis.

levamisole An *anthelmintic with a broad spectrum of activity against gastrointestinal nematodes and lungworms. It is used to treat parasitic infestations in cattle, sheep, pigs, and poultry. Soluble in water, levamisole is available for injection, oral administration, or as a pour-on. Pigs and poultry can be dosed with levamisole in the drinking water. It is absorbed rapidly and is excreted in the faeces and urine, with > 90% excreted within 24 hours. It acts as a ganglion stimulant, causing paralysis of parasites, although activity against immature forms of gastrointestinal parasites is less than that of either the *benzimidazoles or *ivermectin. Levamisole has no activity against inhibited *Ostertagia* larvae, nor against flukes and tapeworms. Some sheep parasites (e.g. *Haemonchus contortus, Trichostrongylus* spp., and *Ostertagia circumcincta*) have developed resistance to levamisole, and there is often cross-resistance to *morantel.

Levamisole should not be used in dogs, cats, and horses because of possible toxicity. Signs of toxicity include muscle tremors, salivation, pupillary constriction, bradycardia, and respiratory failure. Levamisole is also used as an immunostimulant: it is combined with clostridial vaccines for sheep to improve the immune reaction, and has also been used in the treatment of chronic infections.

levator 1. (in surgery) A surgical instrument used for levering up displaced bone fragments in a depressed fracture of the skull. **2.** (in anatomy) Any muscle that lifts the structure into which it is inserted; for example, the *levator palpebrae superioris* helps to lift the upper eyelid.

levo- (laevo-) *Prefix denoting* **1.** the left side. **2.** (in chemistry) levorotation.

lice *See* louse.

lichenification A skin condition in which there is marked thickening of all layers of the epidermis and the skin is much fissured, resembling lichen. In dogs it is often accompanied by hyperpigmentation. It frequently occurs as a response to prolonged friction or pressure; chronically pruritic animals may exhibit areas of lichenification.

licked back A condition caused by the presence of *warble fly larvae in the subcutaneous back fat of cattle. The tissue surrounding the larvae becomes gelatinous and greenish yellow in colour.

lick granuloma An area of chronic dermatitis, most often seen in cats and dogs, caused by prolonged licking and chewing of the skin. In dogs the lower anterior part of the limb, near to the carpus or tarsus, is commonly affected. Doberman pinschers may develop lick granuloma of the flank fold. The licking may be due to boredom, stress, or prolonged pruritus.

licking syndrome A clinical sign of salt (sodium chloride) deficiency in cattle (*see* sodium). The animals lick each other, drink urine, and may even eat soil and excavate cavities in hedgerows to obtain the mineral. About half the pastures in England are said to be sodium-deficient, and unless *salt licks are provided clinical signs are probable. If the licking behaviour becomes a vice it may persist after the deficiency is put right.

Lieberkühn's glands (crypts of Lieberkühn; intestinal glands) Simple tubular glands distributed throughout the walls of the small and large intestines and opening between the villi (*see* villus). Cells at the base of these glands are actively dividing and migrate outwards to the surface to replace those being continually lost. Included among these are the mucus-secreting *goblet cells. The majority of the cells within the crypts are undifferentiated and secrete water and ions into the lumen of the intestine. At the base of the crypts are a few *Paneth cells*, which may have a phagocytic function.

lien *See* spleen.

lien- (lieno-) *Prefix denoting* the spleen. Example: *lienopathy* (disease of).

ligament 1. A tough band of white fibrous connective tissue that links two bones together at a joint. Ligaments are inelastic but flexible; they strengthen the joint and limit its movements to certain directions. **2.** A sheet of peritoneum that supports or links together abdominal organs.

ligamentum arteriosum The fibrous remnant of the foetal *ductus arteriosus that joins the pulmonary trunk at its division with the aortic arch.

ligature Material, such as silk, catgut, or nylon, that is tied around a tubular structure to prevent passage of its luminal contents. Most commonly, ligatures are tied around blood vessels to restrict or stop bleeding during surgery or after injury. The material used must be sterile and may or may not be absorbable (*see* suture).

lighting *See* light requirements.

lightning stroke A high-energy electrical discharge that can cause sudden death or serious injury in animals, including humans. Grazing livestock are particularly at risk, especially animals sheltering under trees that have spreading root systems capable of conducting electricity over a wide area. Death is due to cardiac and respiratory arrest, and animals may show scorching; however, outward indications may be slight or absent. It is vital to eliminate other possible causes of sudden death.

light requirements The duration and timing of periods of light (photoperiods) needed by animals. The timing of reproduction in many animals is governed by photoperiod, which influences the endocrine system through the *pineal gland. Among farm livestock, control of photoperiod in laying hens has received most attention, hens usually housed in a completely controlled environment with entirely artificial lighting. Sexual maturity in pullets is achieved by approximately 22 weeks of age by maintaining the birds under artificial short days of 8 hours followed, at around 16 weeks of age, by increasing the light phase by half an hour a week to a maximum of 16 hours in every 24 hours to initiate egg production. In sheep the onset of sexual activity is triggered by the decreasing photoperiods of autumn, to an extent that is dependent upon breed. Attempts to vary this using artificial lighting patterns have met with only limited success and are too expensive to be justified economically. Mares respond to increasing daylight, and their breeding season can be brought forward by putting them under artificial light. Pigs and cattle do not appear to be affected dramatically by photoperiod, although there are definite seasonal patterns to their reproductive performance. Generally, light intensity and wavelength are of little importance.

lignocaine *See* local anaesthetic.

limberneck A form of *botulism, also known as *western duck disease*, that mainly affects water fowl, game birds, and broilers. The causative bacterium, *Clostridium botulinum*, does not cause infective disease but multiplies in putrefying organic matter, producing a potent toxin. Broilers can ingest this from a rotting carcass left in the broiler house; wild birds receive it from carcasses, dead maggots, and, especially water fowl, from rotting vegetation. Outbreaks in water fowl tend to occur in stagnant conditions in warm weather, and may cause high mortality. The characteristic sign is paralysis of the neck with the head resting on the ground. The wings and legs are also affected. Alternatively, birds may be listless, simply standing inactive for long periods. Death can occur in hours and there is no treatment. Control depends on prompt recovery of dead birds in commercial units, rigorous clean-out to reduce the bacterial population, and denying ducks and other birds access to stagnant water. In some outbreaks the toxin may be produced in the caeca of affected birds.

limbic system A complex system of nerve pathways in the brain involved with the expression of instinct and mood through the endocrine and motor nervous systems of the body. Among the brain regions involved are the *hippocampus and its connections and the *hypothalamus. The activities of the body that are governed are those concerned with self-preservation (e.g. searching for food, fighting) and preservation of the species (e.g. reproduction and the care of offspring), the expression of fear, rage, and pleasure, and the establishment of memory patterns.

lincomycin A lincosamide antibiotic that is mainly active against Gram-positive bacteria and is used as an alternative to penicillin in the treatment of bacterial infections. It penetrates well into bone and is therefore used in the treatment of *osteomyelitis in small animals. Expense precludes its use in large animals. Its mode of action is similar to the *macrolide antibiotics, the drug binding to bacterial ribosomes and causing inhibition of protein synthesis by disrupting peptide bond synthesis. Hence, microorganisms can show cross-resistance between macrolides and lincomycin. It is absorbed readily from the gastrointestinal tract and is nonirritant when injected intramuscularly.

linctus A syrupy liquid, usually made with sucrose, used as a soothing agent to decrease throat irritation and coughing.

lindane *See* organochlorines.

linea (*pl.* **lineae**) (in anatomy) A line, narrow streak, or stripe. The *linea alba* is a tendinous line, extending from the xiphoid process to the pubic symphysis, where the flat abdominal muscles are attached.

linear assessment *See* conformation.

line breeding A form of *inbreeding involving repeated crossing to one animal or its close descendants or relatives. This is done to produce homozygosity for desired traits shown by the particular animal.

lingual Relating to, situated close to, or resembling the tongue (lingua). The lingual surface of a tooth is the surface adjacent to the tongue.

Linguatula serrata An endoparasitic arthropod, known as the tongue worm because of its long wormlike limbless body but in fact related to the mites and ticks (*see* acarid). Tongue worms are found in the respiratory tract and nasal sinuses of dogs, attaching themselves by means of two pairs of mouth hooks and feeding on mucous and tissue secretions. The eggs are sneezed out and, when swallowed by a suitable intermediate host, such as a herbivorous mammal, hatch into larvae with four leglike appendages. The larvae are carried to the liver or lungs, where they develop within cysts into spine-covered larvae with four well-developed mouth hooks. These larvae may migrate into the body cavity of the intermediate host or may remain encysted until eaten by a dog. If the infestation is severe the intermediate host may suffer such loss of condition that it easily falls prey to predators or scavengers, including dogs.

lingula A lobule of the vermis of the *cerebellum.

liniment A preparation that is applied to skin as a counterirritant to improve the local blood supply and drainage from the area. It can be prepared in soaps, oils, or in alcohol or placed on lint or other surgical dressing. Some contain a *rubefacient.

linkage The situation in which two genes lie very close to each other on a chromosome and between which there is therefore very little likelihood of *crossing over. The alleles of genes showing linkage are thus very likely to be inherited in their parental combinations. The probability of new allelic combinations arising is proportional to the distance between the genes on the chromosome. Linkage can be exploited in breeding programmes, particularly where an allele that is useful but difficult to score is linked to an easily scored allele. Selection for the second allele will also produce selection for the first.

linoleic acid An *essential fatty acid with two double bonds (C18:2).

linolenic acid An *essential fatty acid with three double bonds (C18:3).

linseed poisoning A toxic condition due to ingestion of seeds (linseeds) of the cultivated flax (*Linum usitatissimum*). The seeds contain linimarin, a cyanogenetic glucoside, and the enzyme linimarase, which releases hydrocyanic acid from the glucoside. When gruel is made from powdered meal and allowed to stand, sufficient hydrocyanic acid is released to cause *cyanide poisoning. This can be prevented by boiling the gruel to destroy the linimarase or by diluting the meal with other nontoxic foodstuffs. Normal commercial processing of linseed to produce linseed meal destroys the enzyme and most of the linimarin.

lip 1. One of the folds of skin lined by mucous membrane bounding the entrance to the mouth. Upper and lower lips are joined on either side at the commissure of the lips. **2.** Any structure resembling a lip. *See also* labium.

lip- (lipo-) *Prefix denoting* **1.** fat. **2.** lipid.

lipaemia *See* hyperlipaemia.

lipase An enzyme that catalyses the hydrolysis of *triglycerides to yield a mixture of diglycerides, monoglycerides, and fatty acids. Pancreatic juice contains lipase to digest dietary *fat in the small intestine. Adipose tissue contains a hormonally controlled lipase that functions in the mobilization of depot fat.

lipid A group of compounds having a wide range of different structures but which are all insoluble in water and soluble in nonpolar organic solvents, such as chloroform, ether, benzene, etc. Lipids are broadly classified into two categories: *complex lipids*, which are esters of long-chain fatty acids and include the *glycerides (which constitute the *fats and *oils of animals and plants), *glycolipids, *phospholipids, and waxes; and *simple lipids*, which do not contain fatty acids and include the *steroids and *terpenes.

Lipids have a variety of functions in living organisms. Fats and oils are convenient and concentrated means of storing energy. Phospholipids and sterols, such as cholesterol, are major components of cell membranes. Waxes provide vital waterproofing for body surfaces. Terpenes include vitamins A, E, and K, while steroids include the adrenal hormones, sex hormones, and bile acids. Lipids can combine with proteins to form *lipoproteins, e.g. in cell membranes. In bacterial cell walls, lipids may associate with polysaccharides to form *lipopolysaccharides.

lipidosis (*pl.* **lipidoses**) Any disorder of lipid metabolism within the cells of the body. Lipidoses result from genetically determined enzyme deficiencies.

lipolysis The process by which the fat reserves in the white adipose tissue of the animal body are mobilized by hydrolysis to *fatty acids and *glycerol. These products are released into the bloodstream and used for energy generation by tissues, such as muscle. Lipolysis is under hormonal control.

lipoma A benign generally slow-growing tumour of fat cells (lipocytes), seen mainly in older dogs, especially obese bitches. They are uncommon in the cat, sheep, and pig and infrequent in other species. The growths may be single or multiple and arise in the subcutaneous fat of the flanks, chest, lower neck, axilla, and groin. They are round, ovoid, or discoid, well-circumscribed, and surrounded by a thin fibrous capsule. Lipomas are freely movable unless, as sometimes happens, they are attached to the underlying fascia and muscle. Fibrous septae may divide the tumour and be present to such an extent that the term *fibrolipoma* is justified.

Lipomas occurring behind the peritoneum, i.e. *retroperitoneal lipomas*, are described in horses and dogs and may become large. In horses they arise from the mesentery, tend to develop a *pedicle, and occasionally cause acute intestinal obstruction when the pedicle winds around a loop of bowel. In dogs their origin is mainly the omentum, the growths are not pedunculated, and they settle on the abdominal floor.

Lipomas do not recur after adequate excision except where infiltration between muscle bundles has occurred, making complete surgical removal difficult.

lipomatosis Excessive growth of fatty tissue to form tumour-like masses. It occurs especially in the peritoneal cavity (*see* peritoneum) of cattle; Channel Island breeds seem susceptible. Large masses accumulate in the mesenteries and omentum and may undergo necrosis because of defective blood supply; they can cause intestinal obstruction. The condition may be inherited.

lipopolysaccharide A complex molecule containing both a lipid and a polysaccharide component. Lipopolysaccharides are constituents of the cell walls of Gram-negative bacteria and are important in determining the antigenic properties of these bacteria.

lipoprotein A complex of *lipid and *protein. In organisms, lipoproteins occur chiefly in cell membranes and blood serum. Serum lipoproteins contain variable amounts of lipid (mainly *phospholipid, *triglyceride, and cholesterol) and are classed in three groups according to their density:

high-density lipoproteins (HDL); low-density lipoproteins (LDL); and *very low-density lipoproteins (VLDL).* As the amount of lipid relative to protein increases, the density decreases. These lipoproteins are involved in the transport of triglyceride around the body – between the gut, the liver, adipose tissue, and those tissues of the body that use fatty acids as a major fuel, for example cardiac muscle.

liposarcoma A rare malignant tumour of fat cells (lipocytes), affecting the same species and anatomical sites as its benign counterpart, the *lipoma. They are greyish in colour, firmer than lipomas, and often well vascularized, appearing as adherent masses causing ulceration of the skin. Because of their infiltrative growth, complete excision of liposarcomas is difficult so that there is a high risk of local recurrence and spread with the possibility of metastasis, particularly to the lungs.

liposome A microscopic spherical membrane-enclosed vesicle or sac (20–30 nm in diameter) made in the laboratory by the addition of an aqueous solution to a *phospholipid gel. Formed by the sonication of pure phospholipid, they enclose a volume of water but can be made to include other lipids, proteins, or other molecules. They are used to deliver relatively toxic drugs, antibodies, etc. to specific tissues of the body, thus maximizing the therapeutic effect while minimizing harmful side-effects on other tissues.

lipotrophin Either of two peptide hormones, produced in the mammalian adenohypophysis, that stimulate the mobilization of stored body fat and its transfer into the bloodstream.

lipotropic Describing an agent that enhances the metabolism of fat.

lipuria Fat in the urine. This can occur in any disease associated with a high concentration of serum lipid, for example *diabetes mellitus. A thin layer of fat globules is sometimes seen on the surface of centrifuged urine samples from diabetic patients.

liquid paraffin (mineral oil) A colourless odourless oily liquid consisting of a mixture of petroleum-derived hydrocarbons. It is nonirritant to skin and mucous membranes and is used as a laxative and as an emollient on skin; sterile liquid paraffin is used as a lubricant for introducing catheters and other surgical instruments. It is administered orally to treat constipation in small animals and horses, and to treat hair balls in cats. Long-term internal use reduces the absorption of fat-soluble vitamins, and the absorption of small amounts of liquid paraffin can cause *granuloma formation in the colon. Liquid paraffin is also applied topically to soften scabs and reduce skin irritation.

Listeria A genus of small rod-shaped aerobic Gram-positive *bacteria. Motility is conferred by flagella, which cover the entire cell surface; the cells have a tendency to form long filaments. There are three known species but only one, *L. monocytogenes,* is pathogenic to animals. The organism is widespread in nature and very resistant to physical and chemical agents. Infected materials, such as faeces and silage, can harbour the organism for many years. It is commonly isolated in the faeces and other tissues of healthy animals but stress or infections can precipitate *listeriosis. The organism infects a wide range of animals and birds, causing necrotic foci in the spleen, liver, and other organs, or small abscesses, particularly in the central nervous system. The organism gains access when susceptible hosts consume infected feed, particularly silage, and after initial bacteraemia it localizes in certain organs or causes septicaemia. The latter form is common in horses, fowls, and younger ruminants. In pregnant animals the organism localizes in the placenta, resulting in foetal death and abortion. Listeric abortions are common in cattle, sheep, and goats. When *L. monocytogenes* localizes in the central nervous system it causes a *meningoencephalitis, sometimes known as *circling disease. In humans *L. monocytogenes* can cause septicaemias, infection of newborns, abortions, and meningoencephalitis.

listeriosis An infectious disease caused by the bacterium *Listeria monocytogenes*. There are three main forms of the disease: inflammation of the brain and meninges (*meningoencephalitis), infectious *abortion, and *septicaemia. The disease principally affects cattle and sheep although most species, including humans, are susceptible. It is much less common in tropical and subtropical climates than in temperate climates. In cattle the principal form of the disease is meningoencephalitis, although the organism may cause sporadic abortion. Affected animals show such signs as lethargy, head pressing against fixed objects, abnormal positioning of the head, and aimless walking in circles (*see* circling disease). Raised body temperature is seen only in the very early stage of the disease, which usually lasts 1–2 weeks. Unless treated promptly, recovery is unlikely. In sheep the disease is often more acute although the signs are identical, and its occurrence is thought to be associated with feeding silage. Acute septicaemia is uncommon but can occur in lambs, foals, young pigs, and calves. Treatment with broad-spectrum antibiotics may be effective in the early stages, but the disease is usually unresponsive to therapy by the time signs appear.

lith- (litho-) *Prefix denoting* a calculus (stone). Example: *lithogenesis* (formation of).

-lith *Suffix denoting* a calculus (stone). Example: *faecalith* (a stony mass of faeces).

lithiasis (*pl.* **lithiases**) The formation of calculi (*see* calculus) or concretions within the body tissues or organs. This may occur in numerous sites, including the urinary tract (*see* urolithiasis), gall-bladder (*see* cholelithiasis), and intestine (*enterolithiasis*).

lithium A white alkali metal, found in small traces in the body. Lithium salts (e.g. lithium carbonate) are used in human medicine to treat depression and sleep disorders. Lithium ions pass across the blood–brain barrier into the cerebrospinal fluid and replace sodium at cell membranes. Acute toxicity produces seizures and death. Chronic toxicity causes renal damage with clinical signs of polydipsia and polyuria. There is also fluid and sodium retention.

lithotomy Surgical incision into a duct or organ to remove a stone (calculus), especially from the urinary bladder or urethra.

lithotrity The operation in which a stone (calculus) in the urinary bladder is crushed using an instrument (*lithotrite*) introduced via the urethra. It is rarely performed in animals.

lithuresis The passage of small stones (*gravel) in the urine. *See also* lithiasis.

litter 1. Material used to cover the floors of livestock houses or pens; the term usually refers to material for poultry and other birds, as opposed to *bedding for other stock. It acts as an insulator and absorbs liquid excreta. The material used is traditionally softwood shavings, but shredded newspaper is a suitable substitute. In *broiler production, litter must be maintained in a satisfactory condition: if too dry and dusty it may predispose stock to respiratory problems, whereas if too wet it forms an ideal environment for organisms such as flies and gastrointestinal parasites. **2.** The offspring of a single pregnancy; e.g. a litter of piglets.

liver The largest gland in the body that performs various vital functions, notably the synthesis, breakdown, and storage of key metabolic substances. Situated in the cranial part of the abdomen, mostly on the right side and in contact with the diaphragm, it is divided into lobes by fissures, although its form varies considerably between species (see illustration). The liver is attached to the diaphragm and ventral abdominal wall by the *falciform, coronary, and right and left triangular ligaments. The round ligament, which runs in the free edge of the falciform ligament, is the remnant of the foetal *umbilical vein. The lesser *omentum attaches the liver to the stomach. Blood vessels, nerves, and ducts enter and leave the liver through the *porta hepatis.

The glandular liver tissue is organized into lobules, each of which is arranged around a central vein. *Portal triads*, composed of an artery, vein, and duct, surround the lobules. Venous blood rich in nutrients absorbed from the gut reaches the liver via the hepatic portal vein; branches of both this and the hepatic artery run in the portal triads. Blood from the veins of the triads passes through the lobule via *sinusoids, between cords of liver cells (*hepatocytes), and drains into the central vein of the lobule and hence to the hepatic vein. Arterial capillaries and bile tubules also enter the lobules.

The liver has a number of important functions. It synthesizes *bile, which drains from the liver through various ducts to the duodenum (see bile duct). Many important steps in the metabolism of carbohydrates, fats, and proteins are performed by the liver. It regulates the amount of blood sugar, converting excess glucose to glycogen, which it stores. It removes excess amino acids by breaking them down into *urea or *uric acid, and it stores and metabolizes fat. The liver also synthesizes fibrinogen and prothrombin, essential blood-clotting substances, and the anticoagulant *heparin. It forms red blood cells in the foetus and is the site of production of plasma proteins. Moreover, it has an important role in the detoxification of poisonous substances (see Kupffer cell) and it is also the site of vitamin A synthesis; this vitamin is stored in the liver, together with vitamins B_{12}, D, and K.

liver abscess A chronic condition frequently seen at slaughter in cattle and less often in sheep. Multiple thick-walled abscesses containing yellowish or creamy pus are found, usually resulting from secondary infection of *liver necrosis lesions with *Corynebacterium pyogenes* or streptococci.

liver necrosis (hepatic necrobacillosis of ruminants) A form of *necrobacillosis (from *Fusobacterium necrophorum* infection) of growing cattle and occasionally lambs, characterized by multiple dry corklike necrotic foci in the liver. The organism occurs normally in the intestinal tract. In cattle, the disease is associated with the feeding of high-concentrate diets, and the primary lesion may be an almost inapparent area of inflammation in the rumen or reticulum, the bacteria reaching the liver by the

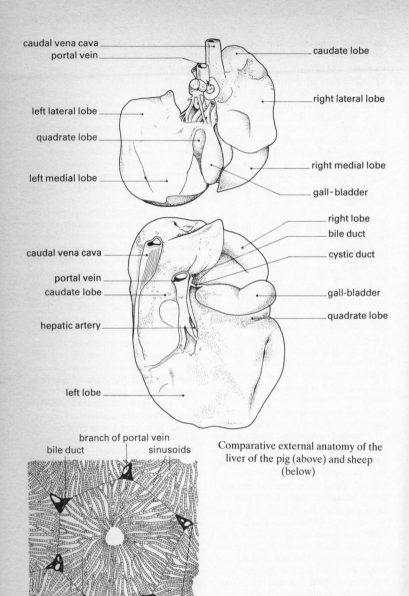

caudal vena cava
portal vein
caudate lobe
right lateral lobe
left lateral lobe
quadrate lobe
right medial lobe
left medial lobe
gall-bladder

right lobe
bile duct
cystic duct
caudal vena cava
portal vein
caudate lobe
gall-bladder
hepatic artery
quadrate lobe
left lobe

branch of portal vein
bile duct
sinusoids

central vein
lobule
liver cells
portal triad
branch of hepatic artery

Comparative external anatomy of the liver of the pig (above) and sheep (below)

The microscopic structure of the liver

hepatic portal vein. The condition is seen usually at slaughter, by which time an endogenous secondary infection with *Corynebacterium pyogenes* or streptococci has often converted the lesions to *liver abscesses.

lobe A major division of an organ or part of an organ, especially one having a rounded form and often separated from other lobes by fissures or bands of connective tissue. For example, the brain, liver, and lung are divided into lobes.

lobectomy The surgical excision of a lobe of an organ, such as the thyroid gland, lung, liver, or brain. Pulmonary lobectomy is indicated in dogs that have suffered torsion of a lung lobe or have a discrete pulmonary tumour.

Lobelia poisoning A toxic condition due to ingestion of any of various annual or perennial herbaceous plants of the genus *Lobelia*, found especially throughout the USA and southern Canada. They include *L. inflata* (asthmaweed, bladder pod, lobelia, eyebright, Indian tobacco), *L. cardinalis* (cardinal flower), and *L. dortmanna* (water lobelia). The plants contain toxic pyridine alkaloids (lobeline and lobelidine) with actions very similar to nicotine. The clinical signs are sweating, paralysis, vomiting, reduced body temperature, collapse, coma, and death. Treatment is of the signs.

lobule A subdivision of a part or organ that can be distinguished from the whole by boundaries, such as septa, that are visible with or without a microscope. For example, the *lobule of the liver* is a structural and functional unit seen in cross-section under a microscope as a column of cells drained by a central vein and bounded by a branch of the portal vein. The *lung lobule* is a practical subdivision of the lung tissue seen macroscopically in lung slices as outlined by incomplete septa of fibrous tissue. It is made up of three to five lung *acini.

local anaesthetic An agent used in local or regional *anaesthesia to reversibly block the conduction of sensory nerve impulses to the brain, without affecting consciousness or causing permanent nerve damage. All modern local anaesthetics have an aromatic group and an amino group linked by an ester or amide. Those containing an ester group are more rapidly metabolized than the amide-containing agents. All local anaesthetics act by stabilizing the neurone's cell membrane, thus preventing the influx of sodium and efflux of potassium ions and inhibiting the development of an *action potential. The order of loss of sensation is pain, cold, warmth, touch, and pressure. Local anaesthetics are used as water-soluble salts, usually the hydrochlorides, to improve their stability and solubility. Most cannot penetrate intact skin but are absorbed through mucous membranes (except procaine), and some agents are used in ear or eye drops. They may be injected, for example subcutaneously, intravenously below a tourniquet, or epidurally (*see* spinal anaesthesia). After entering the systemic circulation they are distributed rapidly throughout the body. Those with an ester linkage are hydrolysed by pseudocholinesterase enzymes in the liver and plasma, whereas those with an amide linkage are metabolized by liver enzymes. The duration of anaesthesia depends on the time the drug remains in contact with the nerve, which in turn depends on the volume injected, the rate of removal from the site, and the rate of metabolism. *Adrenaline, which causes local vasoconstriction, is often added to local anaesthetic solutions to reduce the rate of uptake.

locoweed poisoning

The main local anaesthetics used in veterinary practice can be categorized according to whether they have an ester or amide linkage.

Ester-containing agents *Procaine* is short-acting with effects lasting about 1 hour. It is poorly absorbed from mucous membranes but is rapidly metabolized. However, in horses it is poorly metabolized and there can be marked stimulation of the central nervous system (CNS). Procaine as a base is also used to produce antibiotic salts (e.g. procaine penicillin) and as a cardiac anti-arrhythmic agent. The use of *cocaine is restricted because of its addictive properties. It was formerly used topically in the eye. *Proparacaine* (*proxymetacaine*) is similar to procaine but is more potent and is more toxic. It is used topically, especially in the eye, where it is less irritant than other agents. *Amethocaine* is a good surface anaesthetic but is toxic if given parenterally. It is used in ear drops. *Benzocaine is almost insoluble and is used topically; parenteral use can produce *methaemoglobinaemia. *Butacaine* is used topically in the eye and does not cause clouding of the cornea. It is toxic when used parenterally.

Amide-containing agents *Lignocaine* (*lidocaine*) is the most commonly used local anaesthetic. It is 2–3 times more potent than procaine, with a rapid onset of action and effects lasting 1½–3 hours. It is absorbed from mucous membranes and can be injected. *Mepivacaine* is similar to lignocaine but less toxic, while *bupivacaine* has a longer duration of action (up to 4 hours); it is used for regional and epidural anaesthesia.

Toxicity of local anaesthetics is due to rapid systemic absorption. There is CNS stimulation with tremor and restlessness, and convulsions with high doses which may be followed by depression and respiratory failure. Most agents can cause arteriolarvasodilatation (except cocaine, which causes vasoconstriction), and act on the heart causing reduced conductivity, force, and rate of contractions. Local anaesthetics can be administered slowly intravenously to treat cardiac arrhythmias, but rapid injection may cause cardiac arrest.

locoweed poisoning *See* Astragalus poisoning.

loculus (*pl.* **loculi**) (in anatomy) A small space or cavity.

locus (*pl.* **loci**) **1.** (in anatomy) A region or site. The *locus ceruleus* is a small pigmented region in the floor of the fourth ventricle of the brain. **2.** (in genetics) The region of a chromosome occupied by a particular gene.

locust (black locust) poisoning A toxic condition caused by ingestion of foliage of a deciduous tree, *Robinia pseudoacacia*, distributed throughout the eastern and central USA and southern Canada. It contains a toxin that causes irritation of the gastrointestinal mucosa; clinical signs are weakness, posterior paralysis, nausea, weak irregular pulse, bloody diarrhoea, and death. Treatment is of the signs.

-logy (-ology) *Suffix denoting* field of study. Example: *cytology* (study of cells).

lonchocarpus *See* derris.

loperamide A drug with opioid effects that is used in the treatment of diarrhoea to reduce gastrointestinal motility. When used orally it is poorly absorbed. The side-effects usually associated with opioids (e.g. respiratory depression) are uncommon. Care should be taken when using this drug in cats.

lordosis Abnormal downward (ventral) curvature of the lower spine, which results in a markedly hollow back. It is seen most commonly in old horses that have been used for riding, although occasionally it is a feature of the animal's natural conformation. It is also a feature of certain breeds of pig.

lotion A liquid preparation used topically to give a soothing or antiseptic action on the skin. Lotions usually contain fats or oils, which penetrate and persist in the sebum layer. Drugs may be incorporated in lotions for ease of application.

louping ill An infectious disease of sheep, and occasionally of cattle, deer, dogs, and horses, characterized by fever and nervous signs. It is transmitted by ticks and caused by a *flavivirus. Louping ill is prevalent in Scotland and northern England, but similar diseases due to closely related viruses are found in Central Europe, Turkey, and Russia. Although ticks usually spread the disease, virus particles may enter via the lungs, carried on moisture droplets in the air. A fever develops after 2–3 days then subsides. This may be followed by complete recovery or, up to 2–3 weeks later, by invasion of the central nervous system by the virus. The infected animal then develops nervous signs, such as trembling and incoordination, and may collapse and die. The disease is named after the characteristic gait of affected animals. Recovered animals sometimes have persistent neurological disorders. In the UK the disease appears in the spring and autumn, coinciding with times of maximum tick activity. Control is by annual vaccination with a dead vaccine and dipping to prevent *tick infestation. Lambs of immune ewes are protected by antibody from the milk and should not be vaccinated before 4 months of age. Louping ill virus causes flulike symptoms in humans. Other name: **ovine encephalomyelitis.**

louse (*pl.* **lice**) A small wingless insect belonging either to the order Anoplura (sucking lice) or to the order Mallophaga (biting or bird lice). Sucking lice are ectoparasites of mammals, feeding on their blood using mouthparts specialized to form a snout-like proboscis for piercing and sucking. Biting lice are ectoparasites mainly of birds, feeding on feathers and skin debris and occasionally blood with the aid of biting mouthparts (*see* bird louse). A few infest pets and livestock, such as *Trichodectes canis* of dogs, *Felicola subrostratus* of cats, and *Damalinia* (*Boricola*) *bovis* of cattle. Both types lack eyes, have a flat transparent body which is resistant to crushing, and short, strong, clawed legs for attachment to the host's hair or feathers (see illustration). The eggs (nits) are glued to the hair or feathers and develop directly into blood-sucking nymphs resembling the adults. Transmission occurs by direct contact between hosts.

Lice are found worldwide and all are specific to a particular host or hosts. They cause intense skin irritation, and scratching can lead to secondary infections. A heavy infestation of sucking lice can cause *anaemia. The human louse, *Pediculus humanus*, can transmit diseases, such as typhus, and one of the dog lice, *Trichodectes canis*, may transmit the tapeworm *Dipylidium caninum*. Sheep and cattle lice cause their hosts to rub, damaging hides and wool; carcass quality may also be affected. Infestations can affect egg production in poultry. Lice may be controlled by dusting the animal's coat with a suitable *insecticide, and cattle, sheep, and dogs can be treated with dips. Dust baths containing insecticide can be provided for poultry and other domesticated birds, and bird houses and cages

Lugol's solution

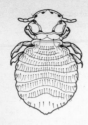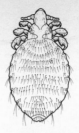

A biting louse, *Trichodectes canis* (left), and a sucking louse,
Linognathus setosus (right): both are parasites of the dog

should be dusted with a suitable *pediculicide.

Lugol's solution An aqueous solution containing 5% iodine and 10% potassium iodide, used as an *antiseptic and *disinfectant. It has activity against many microorganisms, including viruses, and activity is maintained in the presence of organic debris and tissue fluids. There is generally low tissue toxicity, but gastrointestinal irritation occurs after the ingestion of large volumes. Iodine solutions are used to disinfect skin prior to surgery and to clean wounds. For wounds and abrasions the solution should be diluted to a concentration of 0.5% iodine and 1% iodide.

lumbar Relating to the loin. The *lumbar plexus* is a plexus of nerves formed by the spinal nerves of the lumbar region. It supplies the hindlimb.

lumbo- *Prefix denoting* the lumbar region.

lumbosacral Relating to part of the spine composed of the lumbar vertebrae and the sacrum.

lumen (in anatomy) The space within a tubular or saclike part, such as a blood vessel, the intestine, or the stomach.

lumpy jaw *See* actinomycosis.

lumpy-skin disease (Neethling) An infectious pox disease of cattle characterized by fever and rash and caused by capripoxvirus (*see* poxvirus). The disease is enzootic in southern Africa but periodically spreads into Central and North Africa. It is transmitted by contact with an infected animal or by biting flies. Mortality is low but the animal's production is affected and the hide is damaged. Following an initial fever, skin lesions develop on the face and body, becoming more prominent then forming scabs; these may persist for many months as 'sitfasts', which eventually are shed leaving a deep scar. Inflammation and swelling of the lymph nodes also occurs. Channel Island breeds of cattle are particularly susceptible, although many animals have a natural resistance. Frequently less than 10% of a herd show clinical signs during an outbreak. Control is by vaccination using an attenuated live vaccine. Lumpy-skin disease is a *notifiable disease in the UK. *See also* pseudo lumpy-skin disease, sheep pox.

lumpy wool Strictly, a chronic form of *mycotic dermatitis in sheep, although the term is sometimes used to include all forms of mycotic dermatitis in sheep. It occurs mostly in

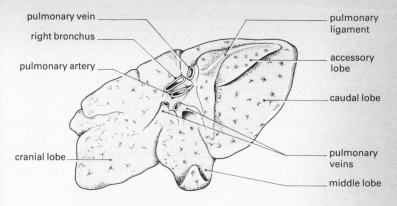

pulmonary vein

right bronchus

pulmonary artery

cranial lobe

pulmonary ligament

accessory lobe

caudal lobe

pulmonary veins

middle lobe

Right lung of dog, medial aspect

strong- or medium-woolled strains of merino sheep in Australia and is characterized by the progressive formation over the skin lesions of large hard conical masses of exudate with a horny tip, firmly anchored in the fleece. These scabs obstruct the process of shearing and reduce the value of the fleece. A single combined intramuscular injection of penicillin and streptomycin has been used to interrupt the progress of the causal infection (with the fungus *Dermatophilus congolensis*) and allow the scabs to be carried clear of the skin surface by the further growth of the wool before shearing. Control measures include dipping early after shearing and in drying conditions to avoid 'scald', and the selection of breeds or strains of sheep not prone to the disease.

lung One of the paired organs of respiration. They are situated in the thorax on either side of the space (*mediastinum) that contains the heart. Each lung is covered by a serous membrane (*pleura). In **mammals** the lungs are divided by fissures into lobes: the left lung into cranial and caudal lobes and the right lung

into cranial, middle (not in the horse), caudal, and accessory lobes. On the inner (medial) surface of each lung is a hilus, where the *pulmonary artery, *pulmonary vein, *bronchus, nerves, and lymphatic vessels enter or leave. (See illustration.) The bronchi communicate with the exterior via the *trachea, while in the lungs they divide into smaller *bronchioles; these terminate in alveoli (*see* alveolus), where gaseous exchange takes place. Air is drawn into the lungs and expelled by muscular movements of the rib cage and diaphragm.

In birds the lungs are relatively smaller, more compact, and unlobed. The bronchi give rise to a series of looped *parabronchi, in which gaseous exchange occurs. The bronchi also connect with the various *air sacs. In all groups the lungs also serve as cooling devices by allowing water to evaporate from the respiratory surfaces.

lungworm A *nematode that occurs as a parasite in the lungs, particularly a member of the family Metastrongylidae. These are slender worms with a reduced mouth capsule and commonly occur in the fine branches of the bronchial tubes, although some inhabit sites elsewhere in the body. They include the genera *Dictyocaulus*, which includes the lungworms responsible for *husk in cattle, and *Metastrongylus*, which includes the pig lungworm. *Filaroides osleri* inhabits the trachea and bronchi of dogs, and in cats the most common lungworm is *Aelurostrongylus abstrusus*. See also Syngamus.

lupinosis A toxic condition, characterized by hepatitis, caused by eating 'sweet' or 'bitter' lupins colonized by the fungus *Phomopsis leptostromiformis*. Proliferation of the fungus and consequent toxicity may be enhanced by rainfall or high humidity. The condition may occur wherever lupins are used as fodder. Most reports are from South Africa and Western Australia and involve sheep. Less commonly cattle, horses, or, on one occasion, pigs have been affected. Typically, listlessness and inappetence are followed by severe jaundice and death. Hepatogenous *photosensitization occurs but is not a constant feature. Animals surviving with permanent liver damage show a marked loss of weight.

lupin poisoning Poisoning caused by the ingestion of varieties of lupin (*Lupinus* spp.) containing toxic alkaloids ('bitter' lupins), which are concentrated in the seeds. It is clinically and aetiologically distinct from *lupinosis. All mammalian species are susceptible but under natural conditions the disease occurs mainly in sheep. Nervous signs may appear rapidly and include excitement, staggering, convulsions, and coma. Difficulties in breathing sometimes lead to death by asphyxiation. Some lupin species are *teratogenic to cattle.

lupus erythematosus See systemic lupus erythematosus.

lutein 1. The yellow pigment of the corpus luteum. **2.** See xanthophyll.

luteinizing hormone (LH; interstitial-cell-stimulating hormone; ICSH) A hormone (see gonadotrophin), produced by the adenohypophysis, that promotes ovulation and the formation and maintenance of the corpus luteum (and hence *progesterone secretion) in females, and the production of *testosterone by the interstitial cells of the testis in males.

luteo- Prefix denoting **1.** yellow. **2.** the corpus luteum.

luteolysis Regression of the *corpus luteum in the ovary that occurs as part of the *oestrous cycle in the absence of a pregnancy in the animal. Luteolysis is initiated by the hormone *prostaglandin $F_{2\alpha}$ secreted by the uterus, and is followed by a rapid fall in the circulating *progesterone concentration thereby allowing the oestrous cycle to continue and a return to oestrus. If pregnancy is established, luteolysis does not take place and the oestrous cycle is suspended. Luteolysis can be induced by the administration of prostaglandin $F_{2\alpha}$ to treat a persistent corpus luteum, which may be found in older cows.

luxating patella (slipping kneecap) A disorder where the kneecap has a tendency to dislocate from its normal position in the patellar groove on the front of the femur, usually in a medial direction, due to a weakness in the ligaments supporting the kneecap and/or the patellar groove being too shallow to hold the kneecap in place. The cause is most commonly hereditary, although it can be caused by an injury. Some animals may have the condition without showing any clinical signs, but most commonly the dog or cat will intermittently pick up the affected hindlimb as the kneecap slips out of place, and then walk normally again when it jumps back into position. Surgery is indicated for animals showing clinical signs to stabilize the kneecap, thus alleviating the signs and helping to prevent the development of arthritis in the joint. Dislocation of the patella of the **horse** is most commonly an upward fixation, with the strong arched medial patellar ligament caught over the medial trochlear ridge of the femur. The leg is consequently fixed in extension and normal movement cannot take place. The fixation can sometimes be relieved by backing the horse against a fixed object. Patellar fixation tends to recur unpredictably, and can be prevented by surgically cutting the medial patellar ligament.

luxation *See* dislocation.

Lyme disease (erythema chronicum migrans) A disease of humans and some domestic animals caused by the spirochaete bacterium *Borrelia burghdorferi* and transmitted by ticks from animals (especially deer and rodents). The disease has been described in the USA, Britain, and a number of other countries. Although rare, the untreated disease is serious and can be fatal. The name derives from a town in Connecticut, USA.

lymph The colourless or pale-yellow fluid present in the *lymphatic system. Lymph is derived from tissue fluid, which in turn is formed initially by *transudation from blood capillaries. Lymph and tissue fluid are thus similar in composition to plasma but have a lower protein content. Lymph also contains *lymphocytes and a few cells of the *macrophage system. Tissue fluid enters the lymphatic capillaries by passing between endothelial cells and also, probably, by *pinocytosis across the endothelial cells. During inflammation, lymph may also contain the products of exudation (*see* inflammation). The composition of lymph varies with the part of the body: lymph from the liver has a relatively high protein content; lymph from the *lacteals in the small intestine has a high fat content, especially following a feed.

lymphaden- (lymphadeno-) *Prefix denoting* lymph node(s).

lymphadenectomy The surgical excision of one or more lymph nodes. It is performed to obtain samples for diagnostic purposes or to remove lymph nodes containing tumour cells.

lymphadenitis Inflammation of a lymph node. This usually occurs in lymph nodes draining a site of infection; the affected node swells, possibly so much that it obstructs major organs. Lymphadenitis in the lymph glands draining the tonsil is common, and is frequently seen, without having caused clinical signs, after slaughter in pigs. Infection with *Mycobacterium tuberculosis* causes the disease *caseous lymphadenitis. Lymphadenitis is also a clinical sign of certain equine diseases, including *strangles, *glanders, and *melioidosis.

lymphagogue A substance that promotes the secretion of *lymph.

lymphangi- (lymphangio-) *Prefix denoting* a lymphatic vessel.

lymphangiectasis Dilatation of lymphatic vessels. It occurs, for example, as part of a malabsorption syndrome in dogs: dilated lymphatics in the intestinal mucosa leak lymph into the gut lumen, causing loss of metabolites into the faeces. The underlying cause is unknown.

lymphangiography *Radiography of the lymphatic vessels and lymph nodes after a contrast medium has been injected into them.

lymphangioma *See* angioma.

lymphangiosarcoma *See* angiosarcoma.

lymphangitis

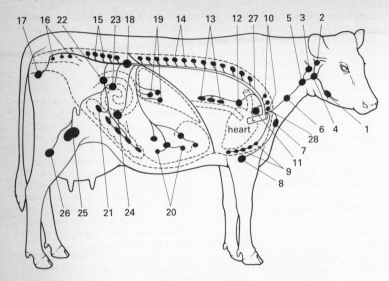

1 mandibular	11 cranial mediastinal	20 gastric
2 parotid	12 bronchial	21 mesenteric
3 lateral retropharyngeal	13 caudal mediastinal	22 hypogastric
4 medial pharyngeal	14 intercostal	23 medial iliac
5 cranial deep cervical	15 lumbar	24 subiliac
6 middle deep cervical	16 sacral	25 mammary
7 superficial cervical	17 anorectal	26 popliteal
8 axillary	18 renal	27 thoracic duct
9 sternal	19 hepatic	28 right lymphatic duct
10 caudal deep cervical		

Schematic diagram of the major lymph nodes of the cow

lymphangitis Inflammation of a lymphatic vessel. It commonly affects lymphatics draining a site of infection, such as an abscess. *Epizootic lymphangitis occurs in horses and is caused by a fungal infection. *Ulcerative lymphangitis also affects horses and is caused by a bacterial infection. Both are similar to and must be differentiated from the cutaneous form of *glanders.

lymphatic 1. A lymphatic vessel. **2.** Relating to or transporting lymph.

lymphatic system A network of *lymphatic vessels and *lymph nodes that serves to remove fluid and particles, including microorganisms, from the tissues in the form of *lymph, to filter it, and return it to the blood. It also transports *lymphocytes, proteins, and lipids to the blood. In birds the lymphatic system is basically similar to that of mammals but lymph nodes are largely absent, being replaced by a series of smaller *lymphatic nodules; additionally there occurs the *cloacal bursa. See illustration.

488

lymphatic vessels The vascular component of the *lymphatic system. They commence with fine blind-ended capillaries, which lie in intimate relation to blood capillaries. Their permeability varies in accordance with tissue needs and is especially high in *inflammation. The capillaries form afferent lymphatic vessels, which drain to *lymph nodes; efferent lymphatic vessels drain from the nodes. Larger lymphatic vessels have valves to ensure centripetal flow, and eventually lead to larger collecting ducts, which discharge into major veins (*see* right lymphatic duct; thoracic duct).

lymph node One of a number of spherical or bean-shaped organs found at intervals along the course of vessels of the *lymphatic system. Lymph nodes filter foreign particles from *lymph and hence prevent their entry into the bloodstream. Also, they are secondary *lymphoid organs, producing, and consisting largely of, *lymphocytes; these lie between the fibres of a meshlike reticular network, on which are also found *macrophages and dendritic cells.

In most species, *lymph arrives at the lymph node by afferent *lymphatics, which penetrate the outer cortex of the node and enter a subcapsular sinus. The lymph drains through further radially disposed sinuses, which converge on the inner medulla and join to form the single efferent lymphatic; this leaves the node at its stalk (hilus). This arrangement permits the continuous flow of lymph from cortex to medulla through the sinuses and facilitates maximum contact of the lymph with the macrophages and dendritic cells. Foreign particles, which are retained by the macrophages, are therefore filtered with high efficiency.

B-lymphocytes occur in the lymph node cortex in a number of follicles: each follicle has a centre rich in large lymphoblasts and possesses dendritic cells and fixed macrophages; smaller and more differentiated lymphocytes are present in the outer part of the follicle. B-lymphocytes are also found in the medulla between the sinuses. These B-cell areas are independent of *thymus gland control and will develop even in the total absence of a thymus. Between the cortex and medulla, T-lymphocytes occupy an incompletely defined region – the *paracortical area.* This area is thymus dependent and does not develop in animals whose thymus is removed at birth. In the pig, this arrangement of lymphoid tissues, and also the direction of the lymph flow, are reversed. Thus the porcine B-lymphocyte follicles are close to the hilus, at which the lymphatics enter.

The blood vascular system of lymph nodes has a unique structure – the *post-capillary venule* – which has a tall endothelium whose purpose is to convey T-lymphocytes from the blood into the lymph node. This ensures a continuous circulation of T-lymphocytes from the blood to the node via the venule and from the node back to the blood via the efferent lymphatic. For this reason the majority of circulatory lymphocytes are T-lymphocytes.

The filtering action of lymph nodes allows them to trap antigen and present it to lymphocytes, which react by producing *antibody and cell-mediated immune effects (*see* immunity; lymphocyte). Antigen is trapped principally by medullary macrophages and cortical dendritic cells. The latter only function well in the presence of specific antibody to the antigen, and are therefore highly active only in second or subsequent exposure to an antigen. The lymph nodes also produce memory cells, which are able to react swiftly on subsequent contact with the same antigen.

lymph nodule A small collection of lymphoid tissue (*compare* lymph node). Lymph nodules can occur separately or within the walls of other organs as solitary or larger aggregated nodules, for example in the mucosa of the small intestine as *gut-associated lymphoid tissue* (*GALT*), formerly termed Peyer's patches.

lympho- *Prefix denoting* lymph or the lymphatic system.

lymphocyte A type of white blood cell (leucocyte) present in the *bone marrow, *thymus, *lymph nodes, *spleen, *cloacal bursa (bursa of Fabricius), and other *lymphoid organs. Lymphocytes are, in vertebrates, the agents of active acquired *immunity. Unlike *granulocytes, they are able to divide indefinitely, the stimulus usually being contact with *antigen. Lymphocytes are first produced in the bone marrow but subsequently they mature and differentiate in the primary lymphoid organs, i.e. the thymus and, in birds, the cloacal bursa. Cells maturing in the thymus are *T-lymphocytes* (or *T-cells*), which then occupy definitive sites in the secondary lymphoid organs, such as the lymph nodes and spleen. T-lymphocytes undertake certain direct immune activities, including the destruction (cytotoxicity) of virus-infected cells or cells bearing foreign antigens. Other T-lymphocytes have regulatory functions: *T-helper cells* stimulate other lymphocytes to carry out their specific functions; *T-suppressor cells* limit the activity of other lymphocytes, thus controlling the intensity of immune reactions. A separate type of T-lymphocyte is responsible for Type IV *hypersensitivity.

Cells maturing in the cloacal bursa become *B-lymphocytes* (or *B-cells*) and are subsequently found in defined regions of the secondary lymphoid organs. Their function is to produce *antibodies, usually in collaboration with T-helper cells, which also aid in the differentiation of B-lymphocytes to mature plasma cells (*see* haemopoiesis). Mammals possess no cloacal bursa and an equivalent organ has not been identified, although its existence is presumed.

Receptors on the lymphocyte's cell membrane enable the cell to recognize specifically the antigen that physically binds to its receptors. Although a given lymphocyte bears only one type of receptor, the lymphocyte population of any individual collectively carries a vast array of receptors. According to the widely accepted *clonal selection theory*, antigen entering the body is likely to encounter lymphocytes bearing receptors that are preconstructed to fit its conformation. Contact between fitting receptor and antigen is the signal for cell division, which results in an expanded *clone of lymphocytes, all with the same receptor. These cells may then assume one of the roles appropriate to their type, or else become *memory cells*, which will respond to a second exposure to the antigen. When B-lymphocytes secrete antibody, its specificity is the same as that of the receptor. Recognition of foreign antigens by T-lymphocytes usually requires 'presentation' of the antigen in the presence of 'self' *histocompatibility antigens. This is evidently one reason why cells whose surfaces are rich in histocompatibility antigens, such as the *macrophages, are good presenters of antigen.

A class of lymphocytes without the properties of either T- or B-lymphocytes is the 'null cell' group; this contains the 'natural killer' cells, which are active against tumour cells.

lymphocytosis *See* leucocytosis.

lymphoedema The accumulation of lymph in tissues, producing swelling. Lymphoedema may result from obstruction to the flow of lymph through lymphatic vessels or lymph nodes, caused, for example, by a tumour or inflammation. Superficial lymphatic obstruction results in oedema of the tissues beneath the skin (*anasarca). Obstruction of a lymph node draining a limb results in oedema of the entire limb. Obstruction of the thoracic duct results in *ascites and the accumulation of fluid in the chest and peritoneal cavities. A form of generalized lymphoedema occurs in calves, due to congenital abnormality of the lymphatic vessels.

lymphoid Describing an organ or tissue in which *lymphocytes are produced. All lymphocyte populations originate from the bone marrow (*see* haemopoiesis). The *primary* lymphoid organs are the *thymus and, in birds, the *cloacal bursa (bursa of Fabricius). Lymphocytes in these organs give rise to, respectively, differentiated T-lymphocytes and B-lymphocytes. (The mammalian equivalent of the cloacal bursa has not yet been identified.) Populations of either cell type may also be found in the *secondary* lymphoid tissues or organs; namely the *lymph nodes, *spleen, *tonsils, and various other diffuse groups of cells, for example GALT (*see* lymph nodule).

lymphoid leukaemia A *leukaemia of bone-marrow origin arising from *lymphocytes. In many species, lymphoid leukaemia is thought to be associated with a virus (e.g. *feline leukaemia virus). There are two main divisions of this tumour type, according to the stage of differentiation. *Chronic lymphocytic leukaemia* occurs relatively frequently in the dog and cat as a slowly proliferating disease characterized by the laboratory finding of high numbers of mature lymphocytes in the peripheral blood and an ordered but increased proliferation within the bone marrow. The disease is commonly diagnosed as an incidental finding with no related clinical

signs. However, if left untreated, signs will develop but they tend to be varied and nonspecific. Treatment with cytotoxic drugs may control the proliferation and the prognosis may be fair to good in some cases. In some animals progression to the other form of leukaemia may suddenly occur.

Acute lymphoblastic leukaemia has a rapid clinical course, but again the signs are nonspecific, with fever, inappetence, weight loss, and joint pain; overwhelming infection, diffuse haemorrhage, and severe anaemia may occur in the terminal stages. The finding of large immature malignant lymphoblasts (*see* haemopoiesis) in the bone marrow and, less commonly, in the peripheral blood is diagnostic. Response to treatment with cytotoxic chemotherapy is poor and the prognosis grave. *Compare* myeloid leukaemia. *See also* lymphosarcoma.

lymphokine Any of a group of soluble glycoproteins, produced by activated *lymphocytes, that have various roles in promoting and regulating the activity of *lymphocytes and *macrophages. They include *interleukins, *interferon, and migration inhibition factor, which mediates Type IV *hypersensitivity.

lymphoma Any malignant tumour of lymph nodes, excluding *Hodgkin's disease. *See* lymphosarcoma.

lymphopenia *See* leucopenia.

lymphopoiesis The production of *lymphocytes. *See* haemopoiesis.

lymphosarcoma A malignant tumour derived from lymphoid tissue (i.e. lymph nodes, tonsils, thymus, spleen, etc.). Malignant change in lymphoid tissue of the bone marrow and circulating blood without the presence of solid tumours is described as *lymphoid leukaemia. Occasionally, leukaemia is associated with the other types of lymphosarcoma. In animals lymphosarcomas are classified by anatomical site and by the type of cell involved. *Multicentric lymphosarcoma* describes malignancy typically affecting lymph nodes on both sides of the body with some regional groups more obviously affected than others. The spleen is usually involved, with organs such as liver, kidney, lungs, heart, gastrointestinal tract, and bone marrow also affected. This form is recognized in all species. *Alimentary lymphosarcoma* principally involves the gastrointestinal tract and regional lymph nodes. This may be a regional form of multicentric lymphosarcoma and is seen mainly in the dog, cat, and horse. In *thymic lymphosarcoma* a large tumour replaces the thoracic thymus, with spread to mediastinal lymph nodes and other organs. This type is seen in all species but is uncommon in the horse. Other types include a renal form, seen in the cat, and a lymphoma-like lesion consisting of a large mass in one organ with secondary deposits (suggesting dissemination from that focus rather than a systemic neoplastic condition). Moreover some skin forms of lymphosarcoma are recorded, mainly in cattle and dogs.

Lymphosarcomas are probably the commonest tumours of cats and among the commonest in dogs, cattle, and horses. Malignant cells infiltrate affected organs, hence clinical signs relate to the organs involved. In cats lymphosarcoma is transmissible, being caused by a retrovirus (*see* feline leukaemia). While virus particles have been described in the dog, a causal relationship has not yet been established. In cattle, particularly in some parts of Europe, an association has been recorded between persistent lymphocytosis (*see* leucocytosis), overt lymphosarcoma, and a C-type retrovirus. Treatment of small animals with corticosteroids and other chemo-therapeutic agents has been attempted but with limited success.

lys- (lysi-, lyso-) *Prefix denoting* lysis; dissolution.

lysin An *antibody or *toxin that causes the destruction (lysis) of cells.

lysine An *amino acid. *See also* essential amino acid.

lysis The destruction of cells through damage or rupture of the plasma membrane, allowing escape of the cell contents. *See also* autolysis; lysozyme.

-lysis *Suffix denoting* 1. lysis; dissolution. 2. remission of symptoms.

lysogenic Producing *lysis.

lysogeny An interaction between a *bacteriophage and its host in which a latent form of the phage (*prophage*) exists within the bacterial cell, which is not destroyed. Under certain conditions (e.g. irradiation of the bacterium) the phage can develop into an active form, which reproduces itself and eventually destroys the bacterial cell.

lysosome A particle in the cytoplasm of cells that contains enzymes responsible for breaking down substances in the cell and is bounded by a single membrane. Lysosomes are especially abundant in liver and kidney cells. Foreign particles (e.g. bacteria) taken into the cell are broken down by the enzymes of the lysosomes. When the cell dies, these enzymes are released to break down the cell's components.

lysozyme An antibacterial enzyme occurring in tears, saliva, other body fluids, and egg white. It weakens the cell wall of certain bacteria by hydrolysing the proteoglycan component. It was the first enzyme to have its three-dimensional structure determined.

lyssavirus A genus of the *rhabdovirus family. It includes the *rabies virus.

M

maceration 1. The softening or removal of the soft parts of a solid by leaving it immersed in a liquid. 2. (in obstetrics) The natural breakdown of a dead foetus within the uterus.

macr- (macro-) *Prefix denoting* large size. Example: *macroglossia* (abnormally large tongue).

macrocyte An abnormally large red blood cell (*erythrocyte). Macrocytes may occur in regenerative *anaemia and in some defects of red cell maturation.

macrocytosis The presence in the circulation of an excessive number of large erythrocytes (*macrocytes). This tends to raise the mean volume of blood corpuscles above normal. Macrocytosis occurs as a result of accelerated erythrocyte formation by the bone marrow in response to haemolysis or haemorrhage. *Macrocytic anaemia* can also be induced by vitamin B_{12} or folic acid deprivation, although this is much rarer in animals than humans.

macroglia One of the two basic classes of *neuroglia (the non-nervous cells of the central nervous system), divided into *astrocytes and *oligodendrocytes. *Compare* microglia.

macroglobulin Immunoglobulin M (IgM). *See* antibody.

macroglobulinaemia An abnormally high concentration in the blood of macroglobulin, i.e. *globulin of molecular mass greater than 400 kDa. In domestic animals the condition is usually associated with neoplasia of lymphocytes or other plasma cells, and the globulin is found to resemble antibody immunoglobulin. *See* hypergammaglobulinaemia.

macroglossia An abnormally large tongue. The commonest cause in animals is inflammation (*glossitis), resulting from infection, insect stings, etc.

macrognathia Marked overgrowth of one jaw relative to the other. This leads to *prognathism*, in which one jaw is in front of the other, and consequent malocclusion of the teeth. The disorder is usually ascribed to an inherited skeletal defect and affects certain breeds of cattle and dogs. Sometimes it is so severe that newborn animals cannot suckle. In less severe cases in adult cattle, grazing is inefficient because the incisors overshoot the dental pad. *Compare* micrognathia.

macrolide antibiotics A group of closely related *antibiotics, which include erythromycin, oleandomycin, spiramycin, *tiamulin, and tylosin. They have high molecular weights (MW approximately 700), containing a macrocyclic lactone ring with sugar residues. Active against Gram-positive bacteria and mycoplasmas, they are bacteriostatic and act by binding to ribosomes, disrupting protein synthesis in microorganisms. After absorption the drugs are excreted in the urine and bile. Injectable preparations for intramuscular or intravenous use are available. Some microorganisms have become resistant to macrolides, and there is cross-resistance to other members of the group and also to *lincomycin. The macrolides are basic

macromolecule

drugs and are therefore active in tissues with an acidic pH (e.g. prostate). *Erythromycin* can be used as an alternative to penicillin G in cases where β-lactamase-producing organisms are present. It is also used for its activity against mycoplasmas in the treatment of mastitis in cattle and respiratory diseases in pigs and poultry. Because it is destroyed by acid, it is protected in coated tablets or as the stearate of lauryl sulphate for oral use. *Spiramycin* has a lower antibacterial activity than erythromycin but persists in tissues. It is used to treat *mycoplasmosis in poultry and spirochaetal diarrhoea in pigs (*see* spirochaetosis). *Tylosin*, which is not used in human medicine, is available for in-feed or in-water medication to control disease in pigs and poultry. It is also available for injection in cattle.

macromolecule A molecule with a high molecular weight, usually in the range $10^4 - 10^8$; it is built up by the linking of smaller molecules. Macromolecules found in living organisms include the *nucleic acids (DNA and RNA), *proteins, and *polysaccharides.

macrophage A large amoeboid white blood cell (*leucocyte) that can engulf (i.e. phagocytose) foreign particles in body tissues. It is the principal cell type in the *mononuclear phagocytic system*, a community of cells distributed widely throughout body organs. Macrophages appear in the blood as *monocytes, in connective tissue as *histiocytes, in the liver as *Kupffer cells, and also in the *spleen, *bone marrow, and *lymph nodes as fixed phagocytes. Macrophages differ from *neutrophils, which are also phagocytic, in being able to divide indefinitely. They may modify their appearance according to their state of activity; for example, they may appear like an epithelium when surrounding noxious foreign material, or they may

join together to form giant cells in an attempt to surround particles that cannot be phagocytosed.

The functions of macrophages are vital and include: the clearance of particles from body fluids by phagocytosis; the degradation of *haemoglobin from dead *erythrocytes and the manufacture of bilirubin and haemosiderin; the secretion of certain components of *complement; the secretion of the *prostaglandins, *interferon, and *interleukin 1; and the presentation of antigen to *lymphocytes. Dendritic macrophages (in lymph nodes) and Langerhans cells (in the skin) are antigen presenters but require the presence of antibody to do this efficiently.

macroscopic Visible to the naked eye. *Compare* microscopic.

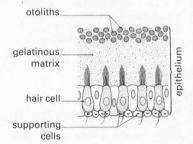

A macula of the inner ear

macula (*pl.* **maculae**) **1.** A small anatomical area that is distinguishable from the surrounding tissue. The macula of the *retina is the spot which surrounds the greatest concentration of cones. Maculae also occur in the saccule and utricle of the inner *ear (see illustration). Tilting of the head causes the otoliths to bend the hair cells, which send impulses to the brain via the vestibulocochlear nerve. **2.** *See* macule.

macula adherens (desmosome) An area of contact between two adjacent cells, occurring particularly in epithelia. The cell membranes at a desmosome are thickened and fine fibres (*tonofibrils*) extend from the desmosome into the cytoplasm. *See* junctional complex.

macule (macula) A circumscribed area of alteration in normal skin colour, with no elevation or depression of the affected area. Macules may result from increased or decreased pigmentation, and are to be distinguished from areas in which blood has escaped in the skin (*see* ecchymosis; petechia). The coat often obscures their presence.

maculopapular Describing a rash that consists of both *macules and *papules.

maedi/visna A progressive disease of sheep caused by a lentivirus and characterized by respiratory insufficiency (maedi) or nervous signs (visna). Transmission occurs by inhalation of viruses following contact between susceptible and infected sheep. Infection of lambs occurs after lambing by feeding on infected milk or contact with infected discharge from the vagina. This can be prevented by removing lambs at birth and rearing them on artificial food. Clinical signs of visna are rare in animals under 2 years of age, and those of maedi rare before 3 years of age. Visna is first seen as a stiff hindlimb gait in affected sheep, which develops into complete hindlimb paralysis, wasting, and death up to 1 year later. Except in Iceland visna is rare. Maedi is the more common clinical manifestation and appears as a progressive pneumonia, wasting, and death 6 months after the onset of clinical signs. Appetite is not affected in either condition. There is no vaccine and control is by serological identification of infected animals and their removal from the flock. Only a small percentage of infected animals show clinical signs. The disease was first diagnosed in the UK in 1978, although it had probably been present since 1973.

maggot The legless grub-like larva of a *fly. Maggots feed on plants, organic matter, or carrion but some, such as the *screw-worm flies, the African *tumbu fly, and occasionally bluebottles, are parasites of animals and humans producing the condition known as *myiasis.

magnesium A metallic element and a major mineral required in the diet. Most of the body's magnesium is associated with calcium and phosphorus in the skeleton, but the element is also required for the proper functioning of muscles and is an essential *cofactor for many enzymes, particularly those which use *ATP. Deficiency of magnesium in the diet results in abnormally low concentrations of the element in blood serum (*hypomagnesaemia) and eventual nervous signs, convulsions, and death. Signs of magnesium deficiency can have an acute onset in adult ruminants. Symbol Mg.

magnesium carbonate A white compound, which exists in either a light or a heavy form, depending on its density. It is used as an *antacid and *laxative in the treatment of gastrointestinal disorders.

magnesium hydroxide (magnesium hydrate) A white powder, insoluble in water, that is used as an *antacid and *laxative. The aqueous suspension of magnesium hydroxide (*milk of magnesia*) is a commonly used antacid with mild laxative properties.

magnesium sulphate A white soluble compound, also known as Epsom salts, in the form of the heptahydrate, $MgSO_4.7H_2O$. It is used as a *laxative or *purgative, to correct *hypomagnesaemia, and as an anti-inflammatory. When administered orally it acts along the length of the intestines, stimulating peristalsis and increasing the fluidity of the gastrointestinal contents. It is used in the treatment of poisoning to remove irritant substances from the gastrointestinal tract. Magnesium sulphate solution (5–25%) can be applied locally to abrasions and arthritic joints to reduce inflammation. Magnesium sulphate is administered intravenously in the treatment of hypomagnesaemic tetany in cattle and sheep. However, rapid intravenous injection can cause cardiac irregularities and death. Intravenous magnesium sulphate was formerly used in the treatment of tetanus and eclampsia for its anticonvulsant properties.

major histocompatibility complex *See* histocompatibility.

mal Disease or disorder.

mal- *Prefix denoting* disease, disorder, or abnormality.

malabsorption A state in which the absorption of one or more nutrients from the alimentary tract is impaired. Clinical signs depend on the degree of malabsorption and the nutrients involved. There are many causes, probably the most important being parasitic infestation of the intestine. Various types of *enteritis also cause malabsorption: for instance, rotavirus *diarrhoea in calves and *transmissible gastroenteritis in pigs both lead to atrophy of the mucosal villi and chronic malabsorption. An immune response to various antigens or allergens at the gut mucosal surface can also affect absorption.

A specific *malabsorption syndrome* occurs in poultry (*see* runting and stunting syndrome). Other malabsorption syndromes, especially in dogs,

involve deficiency of digestive enzymes. For instance, lactase deficiency prevents the complete digestion of milk. Even healthy animals may be affected by interactions between ingested substances that reduce the availability of certain nutrients. For example, phytic acid binds dietary calcium and magnesium (*see* phytin) and may reduce the amount of these minerals absorbed. The cause of malabsorption must be identified to enable effective treatment. Diagnosis may entail searching for parasite ova in the faeces, enzyme tests, and the identification of infectious agents.

malacia Abnormal softening of an organ or tissue, such as bone (*see* osteomalacia).

-malacia *Suffix denoting* abnormal softening of a tissue. Example: *keratomalacia* (of the cornea).

malar abscess *See* alveolar abscess.

malaria A disease of humans caused by protozoa of the genus *Plasmodium* and transmitted by mosquitoes. It is still one of the most important diseases of humans in tropical areas but has been eradicated from many temperate areas by the control of mosquitoes with insecticides. Other species of malaria parasite occur in primates and birds but they rarely cause disease. Malaria is characterized clinically by recurrent bouts of fever associated with fluctuating numbers of parasites in the blood. *See also* avian malaria.

malathion An organophosphorus compound that acts as an *anticholinesterase and is used as an insecticide. For signs of toxicity in domestic animals, and treatment, *see* organophosphorus compounds.

mal de Caderas A disease of horses occurring in South America and caused by a strain of *Trypanosoma evansi* (formerly called *T. equinum*). The parasite is transmitted by biting flies and vampire bats (*see* surra).

mal de playa Poisoning by the plant *Lantana camara*, which grows prolifically in some tropical pastures and when ingested can cause hepatogenous *photosensitization.

malformation Any variation from the normal physical structure, due either to congenital or developmental defects or to disease or injury.

malignant 1. Describing a tumour that invades and destroys the tissue in which it originates and can spread to other sites in the body, usually via the bloodstream or lymphatic system. If untreated, such tumours typically cause progressive deterioration and death. *See* cancer. **2.** Describing any disease that becomes progressively worse if untreated or is resistant to treatment and usually fatal, for example *malignant catarrhal fever of cattle and *malignant hyperthermia in pigs.

malignant catarrhal fever A fatal disease of cattle, buffalo, and deer characterized by mucopurulent nasal discharge and opacity of the cornea and caused in some cases by *herpesvirus. The disease appears in two clinically similar forms: one, caused by herpesvirus, is found in Africa and is associated with contact between calving wildebeest and cattle; the other is associated with contact between sheep and cattle, but the agent responsible for this has not been identified. Affected cattle develop eye and nasal discharge and a high and persistent fever. The discharges become mucopurulent (i.e. contain both mucus and pus), the epithelium of the nose and mouth is inflamed and sloughs off, and the nose is covered in a crust of dried

exudate. The cornea of both eyes appears white and the affected animal avoids light. Nervous signs develop and death follows in 5–12 days. Sheep and wildebeest do not show any clinical signs of disease, and there is no transmission of the disease between affected and susceptible cattle.

malignant hyperthermia A metabolic disorder of muscles that is triggered by the effects of stress on genetically susceptible animals, especially pigs suffering from *porcine stress syndrome (Hertztod disease). The exact cause of the condition is unknown but it appears to involve an inherited defect of intracellular calcium metabolism. Excessive calcium accumulation in mitochondria leads to uncoupling of oxidative phosphorylation pathways, with consequent consumption of *ATP and increased *glycolysis. The latter is probably responsible for the fever, and for the accumulation of lactate metabolites, which cause muscle rigidity. Several factors are known to precipitate the condition – physical activity, stress, climatic conditions and temperature, *vitamin D deficiency, and the inhalation of certain anaesthetics, notably halothane (*see* halothane challenge test). The condition is also associated with *vitamin E and *selenium deficiency; this may be related to the role played by these substances as antioxidants. The initial signs are muscle tremors, which progress to spasms. The body temperature rises rapidly, possibly as high as 45°C, and there is a dramatic increase in the heart and respiration rates. The results are often fatal. Post-mortem examination shows the damaged muscles oozing fluid (so-called 'watery pork' or *pale soft exudative muscle), and the affected meat's appeal to the consumer is reduced. Many species show a similar reaction to stress, especially wild animals when they are

malignant oedema

caught and handled. However, in pigs the condition is most likely in heavily muscled animals of the fast-growing breeds. There is no treatment but prevention consists in the avoidance of stress. Other name: **transport death**.

malignant oedema 1. A type of *gas gangrene affecting cattle, sheep, horses, and pigs, caused by infection of wounds and other injuries with the bacterium *Clostridium septicum*. Haemoglobin-tinged oedema is the most prominent local feature, but gas bubbles also occur. In the absence of antibiotic treatment, death occurs due to toxaemia or septicaemia. *See also* avian malignant oedema. **2.** A former term describing any form of gas gangrene in animals; *Cl. septicum* is often secondarily present in such conditions.

malignant theileriosis A severe often fatal tick-borne disease of sheep and goats occurring in northern Africa, southern and eastern Europe, the Middle East, and parts of Asia. It is caused by the protozoan parasite *Theileria lestoquardi* (*T. hirci*) and resembles *East Coast fever. *See also* theileriosis.

malleus The hammer-shaped *ossicle in the middle *ear. It is attached to the inner surface of the tympanic membrane and articulates with the incus.

Mallory's triple stain A histological stain consisting of water-soluble aniline blue or methyl blue, orange G, and oxalic acid. Before the stain is applied the tissue is mordanted, then treated with acid fuchsin and phosphomolybdic acid. Nuclei stain red, muscle red to orange, nervous tissue lilac, collagen dark blue, and mucus and connective tissue become blue.

Malpighian body *See* renal corpuscle.

maltase An enzyme that hydrolyses maltose to yield two molecules of glucose. It is found in the mucosa of the small intestine, along with *lactase and *sucrase.

maltose A disaccharide comprising two glucose residues linked by a 1-4 alpha bond. It is an intermediate in the digestion of amylose (*see* starch). *See also* amylase; maltase.

mamilla *See* papilla.

mamillary body One of the two paired rounded swellings on the undersurface of the *hypothalamus immediately behind the pituitary gland.

mammary gland The milk-producing gland in female mammals (see illustration). They occur in pairs on the ventral surface, their number varying according to species in relation to the number of offspring. The mare, ewe, and nanny goat each have two; the cow has four; the sow six or more pairs; and the bitch 4–6 pairs, depending on breed. In ruminants and the horse the mammary glands are collectively termed the *udder*. Each mammary gland consists of milk-secreting tissue divided into lobes, each of which drains via a *lactiferous duct towards the *papilla (teat) of the gland. Glandular activity and the release of milk from the gland are controlled by hormones produced in the pituitary gland (*see* lactation). All domestic mammals are liable to develop *mastitis – inflammation of the mammary gland. Other diseases include *mammary tumours and abscesses; injury, with the attendant risk of infection, is also common, especially in cattle and pigs.

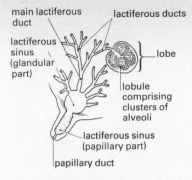

Principal features of one quarter
of the bovine mammary gland

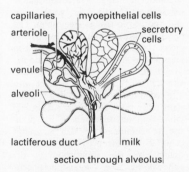

A cluster of mammary alveoli: the basic
milk-secreting unit of a gland lobule

mammary tumours Any of various
tumours arising in the mammary
gland or related structures. They
occur most commonly in the dog and
cat, but are rare in other domestic
species. In the dog *benign mixed
mammary tumours* are commonest.
These occur in middle-aged or older
bitches, are often multiple, and consist of firm well-circumscribed freely
movable nodules in one or more
mammary glands. Microscopically
they consist of a mixture of epithelial
and mesenchymal tissues. These
tumours grow more rapidly in the
immediate post-oestrus period and

may be under hormonal control. Surgical excision is curative. However, if
left untreated, a percentage will
undergo malignant change with rapid
growth, ulceration of the skin, and
infiltration of the surrounding tissues.
Local recurrence and metastasis to
regional lymph nodes and lungs are
common. Treatment other than surgery is of little benefit. Other benign
mammary tumours occurring in both
dogs and cats include *adenomas,
duct *papillomas, and fibroadenomas.
The papillomas consist of papillary
extensions from the mammary alveoli,
ductal system, or teat sinus and are
often cystic. Fibroadenomas are
found especially in the cat, in which
there is proliferation of ductular epithelium and a marked increase in
fibrous tissue. The latter change may
be related to progesterone stimulation.
*Carcinomas are much more common
than their benign counterparts, especially in the cat. They show rapid
growth, are poorly circumscribed, and
ulcerate through the skin, often with
secondary infection. Infiltration affects
adjacent glands, lymphatic vessels,
and blood vessels. Mammary carcinomas vary in type from tubular and
papillary *adenocarcinomas to solid
malignant growths. Metastasis to
regional lymph nodes and the lungs is
common, with approximately 40% of
all dogs so affected. In cats carcinomas are inclined to metastasize
early to form pulmonary secondaries
with a poor prognosis.

Manchester wasting disease *See*
enteque seco.

mandelic acid A urinary antiseptic,
available as ammonium mandelate or
calcium mandelate. The drug is given
orally and has an antibacterial action
in acidic urine (pH < 5.5). Both salts
can act as urinary acidifiers, but additional acidification using sodium acid
phosphate or ascorbic acid may be

necessary. Treatment should not be prolonged because mandelic acid is an irritant. *See also* hexamine.

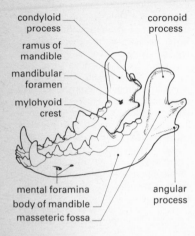

condyloid process
coronoid process
ramus of mandible
mandibular foramen
mylohyoid crest
mental foramina
body of mandible
masseteric fossa
angular process

Left and right mandibles of the dog, dorsal lateral aspect

mandible The bone of the lower jaw. It bears teeth in sockets (alveoli). On either side the head of the mandible forms a temporomandibular joint with the temporal bone of the cranium. At the apex of the lower jaw in the midline is the intermandibular joint; formed initially of fibrous and cartilaginous tissue, it undergoes ossification in early life in the horse and pig. See illustration.

mandibular glands One of the pairs of the major *salivary glands. Each lies deep and to the rear of the *mandible and is partially overlain by one of the *parotid glands. They have a duct, which opens on the sublingual *caruncle below the tongue.

manganese A metallic element and a trace element (*see* essential element) required in animal diets. It occurs in most tissues and functions as a enzyme *cofactor. Manganese defi-ciency is a factor in the development of *perosis in chicks, while in breeding hens it causes reduced hatchability, thinner shells, and head retraction in chicks. Ruminants are unlikely to suffer from a deficiency since most green crops contain adequate amounts. However, animals grazing on manganese-deficient pastures may develop such signs as impaired fertility, poor growth, and leg deformities. Lameness is a sign of deficiency in pigs. Symbol Mn.

mange Any of several intensely itchy skin diseases caused by parasitic *mites. The major forms are *demodectic mange, *sarcoptic mange (or scabies), *scaly leg, *sheep scab, and *notoedric mange (see table). The parasites spread from host to host by direct contact or by contact with infested woodwork, litter, or bedding. The mites are usually host specific, although stockpersons in contact with infested animals may develop a transient itchy rash. Diagnosis entails isolation and identification of the parasite in combings or skin scrapings using a microscope. The disease is treated by the application of organochlorine or organophosphorus *acaricides to affected animals and those in contact with them. Infested bedding or litter should be removed and destroyed, and buildings thoroughly cleaned. *See also* depluming mite; foot mange; otodectic mange.

mannosidosis A hereditary lethal disease involving deficiency of the enzyme alpha-mannosidase. It affects the nervous system and is characterized by ataxia, tremor, slow vertical nodding, and an aggressive tendency. This condition occurs predominantly in Angus cattle. Homozygotes (*see* homozygous) rarely live beyond 1 year of age, due to total deficiency of the enzyme; heterozygotes (*see* heterozygous) have half the normal amount of enzyme. Shortage of the enzyme

Mange mites and their hosts

Mite	Host
Psoroptes	Sheep (sheep scab), horse, cow, rabbit
Chorioptes	Horse (foot mange), cow, sheep, goat, rabbit
Sarcoptes	All species (sarcoptic mange)
Notoedres	Rabbit, cat (notoedric mange), dog
Otodectes	Dog, cat, fox, ferret (otodectic mange)
Demodex	All species (demodectic mange in some)
Cheyletiella	Rabbit, dog, fox, hare
Cnemidocoptes	Poultry (depluming scabies, scaly leg)

causes a lysosomal storage disease in foetal life, in which there is accumulation of metabolite in *lysosomes with consequent vacuole formation in neurones, macrophages, and cells of the lymph nodes, pancreas, and salivary gland. Postnatally this process continues in the brain, pancreas, and lymph nodes. Death may be due to paralysis or it may occur after a fit. Other name: **pseudolipidosis**.

manus The region of the forelimb corresponding to the human hand. It includes the *carpus, *metacarpus, and *digits (see illustration). *Compare* pes.

marasmus Extreme emaciation, especially in young animals.

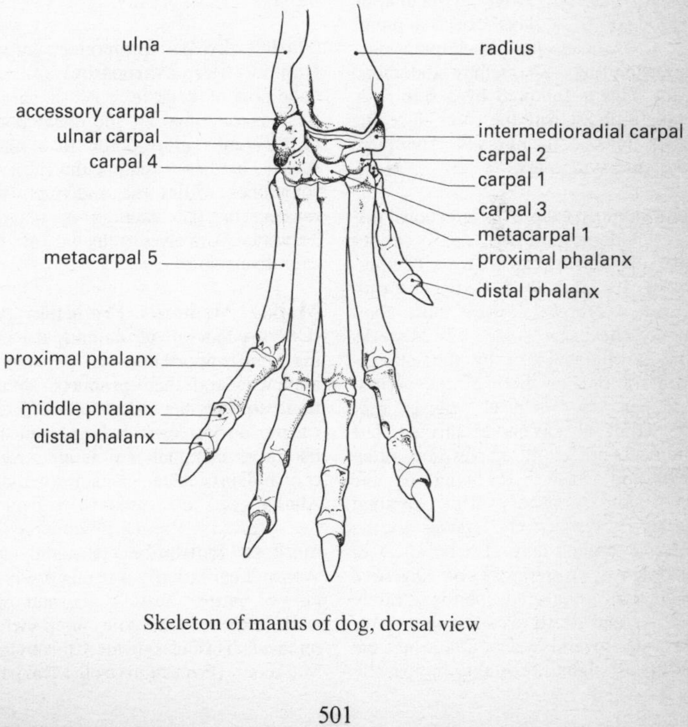

Skeleton of manus of dog, dorsal view

marble-bone disease *See* osteopetrosis.

marble spleen disease A disease of poultry, due to adenovirus infection that causes sudden death in pheasants and less severe signs in domestic fowls. There is enlargement of the spleen, and birds are asphyxiated due to a sudden accumulation of fluid in the lungs. There is no treatment or vaccine.

Marburg disease (green monkey disease) A disease of vervet (green) monkeys and humans caused by Marburg virus and characterized in humans by acute fever. Arthropods, such as ticks or mites, may be the natural reservoir of the virus and the source of infection for the monkeys. Laboratory workers exposed to the tissues of infected monkeys are particularly at risk. After an incubation period of 3–9 days, the symptoms are fever, headache, muscle pain, nausea, vomiting, and crampy abdominal pain. This is followed by a skin rash, and, in about half the cases, bleeding from mucous membranes. Treatment is of the symptoms.

Marek's disease An infectious disease of domestic fowls, and occasionally other birds, caused by a *herpesvirus. It takes two distinct forms. *Classical Marek's disease* most commonly affects birds aged 12–24 weeks and is characterized by the enlargement of one or more of the peripheral nerves. Clinical signs vary depending on the nerves affected. The brachial or sciatic nerves are often involved, causing drooping of the wing and lameness with eventual paralysis, respectively. Nerves to the internal organs may also be affected, leading to respiratory or digestive problems. Affected birds rarely recover and death occurs within a few days to several weeks following the onset of signs. Mortality is usually 10–20% of a susceptible flock. *Acute Marek's disease* involves widespread tumour invasion of body organs and tissues, may affect younger birds, and causes higher mortality (up to 60% or even more). In both forms of the disease, the complete virus lives in the cells lining the feather follicles and is transmitted on dander and fluff, which are inhaled by other birds. It can remain infective in poultry house dust for several months.

There is no treatment and control is the only option. Laying and breeding chicks are usually vaccinated when day-old and develop some immunity within 6–7 days. Broiler stock, which are destined for slaughter before the disease develops, are not usually vaccinated. Rigorous hygiene helps reduce the burden of infection and houses should be thoroughly cleaned and disinfected between batches of birds.

Marie's disease (pulmonary hypertrophic osteoarthropathy) A rare condition of dogs in which a painful swelling develops on the distal bones of the limbs in response to a mass, such as a tumour, within the chest, or sometimes within the abdomen. The reason for the swelling is unclear. Treatment involves removal of the causative mass.

Marine Mammals Protection Act (USA) A federal Act banning the taking and importation of all marine mammals and their products. Exceptions to the Act relate to porpoises caught during tuna fishing, and the taking of mammals by native American Indians, Aleut, and Eskimos in Alaska.

markets legislation (England and Wales) Legislation governing the welfare of cattle, sheep, goats, and pigs while exposed for sale or prior to removal. This is provided for by the Markets (Protection of Animals)

Orders (1964; amended 1965 and 1976). Under the Orders such animals must be fed and watered during and after the marketing process at least once in every 12-hour period. Animals must be penned so as to avoid injury and overcrowding, and a veterinary inspector may treat, cause to be treated, or cause to be removed for treatment any animal that is being caused or is likely to be caused unnecessary suffering.

markweed See Toxicodendron.

marrow See bone marrow.

masseter muscle A thick powerful muscle running from the *zygomatic arch to the ramus of the *mandible. It contracts to raise the mandible during mastication.

mast cell A tissue *leucocyte closely related to the blood *basophil, that has granular cytoplasm active in promoting *inflammation. Mediator substances (e.g. *histamine) are released from the granules during the process of 'degranulation'. Connective tissue mast cells probably have a bone marrow origin, while epithelial mast cells are thymus-derived and to some extent under thymic control. Mast cells bind IgE (see antibody) to their cell membrane and can then be degranulated by the action of specific antigen. This process is prominent in many helminth infestations and in inflammatory responses involving Type I *hypersensitivity. Mast cells can also be degranulated by activated *complement components.

mastication The process of chewing food.

mastitis Inflammation of the *mammary gland. The most common cause is bacterial or mycoplasmal infection. This infection may be ascending – via the teat canal – or haematogenous –

via the bloodstream. Mastitis occurs in all species and is most common around the time of parturition and early lactation. The principal signs are swelling and heat in the affected gland and changes in the milk, which may become watery or pus-like in consistency. In the early stages of the disease small clots in the milk may be the only sign. The milk contains an increased number of *neutrophils, a feature used to monitor the disease in the dairy industry (see cell count; California mastitis test). In certain cases bacterial *endotoxins may cause severe signs, such as anorexia, muscle weakness, vascular collapse, and death. When the blood supply to the gland is compromised, *gangrenous mastitis occurs.

Mastitis is of great economic importance in dairy cattle, in which the disease may be clinical, with overt signs, or subclinical, where inflammation is present but undetected. In clinical cases the affected teat and quarter become swollen and hard. The bacteria causing mastitis are loosely classified as either environmental organisms, such as *Escherichia coli, which are acquired from dirty bedding and equipment, or contagious organisms, such as Staphylococcus aureus and Streptococcus agalactiae, which are acquired from other infected cows and spread by poor hygiene at milking. Treatment entails regularly drawing off accumulated pus from the infected quarter and introducing a suitable *antibiotic via the teat canal. A systemic antibiotic may be required in severe cases. Prevention demands rigorous hygiene at milking, especially scrupulous attention to udder washing and *teat dipping. See also coliform mastitis; mycoplasmal mastitis; mycotic mastitis; nocardial mastitis; summer mastitis.

mastocytoma A skin tumour consisting of neoplastic *mast cells. It is one of the commonest skin tumours in the dog, occurs less frequently in the cat, and is comparatively rare in other species. In **dogs** there is a marked breed incidence, with boxers, Boston terriers, and Labradors most commonly affected. The lesions vary from well-circumscribed solitary subcutaneous nodules to multinodular poorly delineated masses that invade the skin and subcutaneous tissues. Well-differentiated lesions can be widely excised to give a high cure rate; less well-defined tumours are difficult to excise completely and often recur locally, with the possibility of metastasis to regional lymph nodes and internal organs. *Radiotherapy can prove beneficial in some cases.

Mastocytomas in **cats** are often multiple and involve the skin of the head and neck region. The lesions are generally smaller than those of the dog and consist of sheets of closely packed well-differentiated mast cells. A large number of such tumours show generalized involvement of other tissues, and mast cell *leukaemia is occasionally reported.

matrix (*pl.* **matrices** or **matrixes**) The substance of a tissue or organ in which more specialized structures are embedded; for example, the ground substance of connective tissue.

maturation The process of attaining full development. The term is applied particularly to the development of mature germ cells (ova and spermatozoa).

maxilla (*pl.* **maxillae** or **maxillas**) One of a pair of teeth-bearing bones that are the main components of the upper jaw. The body of the maxilla, which contains the maxillary sinus, contributes to the lateral wall of the nasal cavity and to the floor of the orbit in the *skull. Its palatine process contributes to the hard palate.

meat As defined in EEC regulations: *meat* is any part of a bovine, pig, sheep, goat, horse, ass, or mule that is fit for human consumption. A *carcass* is the whole body of a slaughtered meat animal after bleeding, evisceration, removal of the extremities at the carpus and tarsus, removal of the head and tail (and udder of a cow), and, with the exception of the pig, removal of the skin. *Offal* is fresh meat other than that of the carcass, even if it is naturally attached to the carcass (e.g. kidney). *See also* viscera.

meat- (meato-) *Prefix denoting* a meatus.

meat inspector A person who is legally authorized to inspect meat in a slaughterhouse. In the UK this may be a *veterinary surgeon, environmental health officer, or other authorized meat inspector. *See also* poultry meat inspector.

Meat (Sterilisation and Staining) Regulations (1982) (England and Wales) Legislation governing the movement of unfit meat (including poultry meat) from slaughterhouses, knacker meat, and imported meat that is unfit or not intended for human consumption. This may only be sent to a processor for sterilization or to certain other types of destination, unless it is sterilized before removal from the slaughterhouse, knacker's yard, or port of entry. Unfit carcass meat and certain types of offals that are not sterilized at the slaughterhouse or knacker's yard must be stained with the dye Black PN or Brilliant Black BN before removal. A movement permit issued by the local authority is needed before unfit red meat and knacker meat may be moved.

meatus (in anatomy) A passage or canal. The *external acoustic meatus* is the passage of the external *ear leading inwards to the tympanic membrane. The *nasal meatuses* are subdivisions of the nasal cavity produced by the projecting *nasal conchae.

mebendazole *See* benzimidazole.

mechanoreceptor A group of cells that respond to mechanical distortion, such as that caused by stretching or compressing a tissue, by generating a nerve impulse in a sensory nerve (*see* receptor). Touch receptors, *proprioceptors, and the receptors for hearing and balance all belong to this class.

Meckel's diverticulum A congenital disorder in which there is a pouch (*diverticulum) in the wall of the ileum resulting from an abnormal persistence of the vitellointestinal duct. It is reported in dogs and horses, and may give rise to intestinal obstruction. The condition was first reported in humans.

meclofenamic acid *See* NSAID.

meconium The first faecal material to be voided by the newborn, consisting primarily of cellular debris accumulated during foetal life and coloured dark green or black by *bile pigments. It is believed that the mother licking the anus of the young is important in stimulating expulsion of the meconium. If it becomes impacted it may be retained; this is a particular problem in colt foals.

media (tunica media) The middle layer of the wall of an artery, vein, or lymphatic vessel. It is usually the thickest of the three layers and contains smooth muscle tissue.

medial 1. Situated at or relating to the centre of an organ. 2. (in anatomy) Relating to the region or parts of the body nearest the median plane.

median (in anatomy) Situated in or towards the plane that divides the body into right and left halves.

median artery The continuation in the lower forelimb of the brachial artery. It continues into the manus to form the superficial *palmar arch.

median nerve One of the nerves of the forelimb extending from the *brachial plexus. It supplies motor fibres to some of the flexor muscles in the lower forelimb and carries sensory fibres from part of the manus.

mediastinum (*pl.* **mediastina**) A middle partition. In the thorax the mediastinum is the region between the two pleural cavities containing the heart, aorta, trachea, oesophagus, and thymus gland. The mediastinum of the testis is a cord of connective tissue running lengthways through its middle and containing the *rete testis.

Medicines Act (1968) (England and Wales) An Act of Parliament controlling medicinal products. These are substances or articles manufactured, sold, supplied, imported, or exported for use for medicinal purpose, including diagnosis, treatment, or prevention of disease; contraception; induction of anaesthesia; and interference with or prevention of normal physiological function. A *veterinary drug* is defined under the Act as a medicinal product that is intended for administration to animals (including birds, fish, and reptiles) but not for administration to humans. Regulations made under this Act provide for the safety, quality, and efficacy of such products through a licensing system.

Medicines (Medicated Animal Feeding Stuffs) Regulations (1985) (England and Wales) Statutes prescribing the form of written direction to be given by a veterinary surgeon for the purpose of the incorporation of a medicinal product in an animal feedstuff. The *British Veterinary Association publishes pads of the appropriate form, known as a *veterinary written direction* (*VWD*). These are valid for one supply only and for a period of 30 days from the date of signature by the veterinary surgeon.

Mediterranean fever (Mediterranean Coast fever) An important disease of cattle and water buffalo in North Africa, the Middle East, and Asia caused by the protozoan parasite *Theileria annulata*. Transmitted by ticks of the genus *Hyalomma*, the disease is characterized by fever, lymphnode enlargement, and anaemia and mortality rates may be high. The parasite's *piroplasms are predominantly round or oval, hence the specific name, and multiply in the host's red blood cells. Treatment is with tetracycline antibiotics or other specific antitheilerial drugs. Prevention entails tick control and/or vaccination using attenuated live vaccines.

medium (*pl. media*) 1. Any substance, usually a broth, agar, or gelatin, used for the *culture of microorganisms or tissue cells. An *assay medium* is used to determine the concentration of a growth factor or chemical by measuring the amount of growth it produces in a particular microorganism; all other nutrients are present in amounts adequate for growth. 2. *See* contrast medium.

medulla 1. The inner region of any organ or tissue when it is distinguishable from the outer region (the cortex), particularly the inner part of the kidney, adrenal glands, or lymph nodes. 2. *See* medulla oblongata. 3. The medulla spinalis. *See* spinal cord. 4. The *myelin layer of certain nerve fibres.

medulla oblongata The part of the *brainstem lying caudal to the pons

that is continuous caudally with the spinal cord. It contains pathways running to and from higher centres in the brain and various centres governing the cardiovascular and respiratory systems. Cranial nerves VI–XII originate from it.

medullary cavity The space in the shaft of a long bone that contains bone marrow. In birds the medullary cavity of some bones (e.g. humerus) contains an *air sac.

medulla spinalis *See* spinal cord.

medulloblastoma A tumour arising from undifferentiated cells found in the brain of neonates beneath the pia mater of the cerebellum; the cells are thought to be precursors of the cerebellar cortex. Such lesions have been reported in the cerebellum of calves, dogs, cats, and pigs and appear as soft bulging grey-red and rather circumscribed tumours. They compress or invade the fourth ventricle, infiltrate adjacent structures, and metastasize to other sites via the cerebrospinal pathways. There is little record of treatment of these tumours in domestic animals but, in general, prognosis would be poor.

mega- *Prefix denoting* 1. large size, or abnormal enlargement or distension. Example: *megacaecum* (of the caecum). 2. a million. Example: *megavolt* (a million volts).

megakaryoblast The earliest recognizable bone-marrow precursor cell of the line that gives rise to *platelets. It is larger than any other bone marrow precursor and has two nuclei. As differentiation proceeds the cell becomes multinucleate and is known as a *megakaryocyte*. This cell gives rise to platelets by fragmentation of its cytoplasm (*see* haemopoiesis).

megakaryocyte *See* megakaryoblast.

megal- (megalo-) *Prefix denoting* abnormal enlargement. Example: *megalomelia* (of limbs).

megalocephaly Abnormal enlargement of the head.

-megaly *Suffix denoting* abnormal enlargement. Example: *splenomegaly* (of spleen).

megestrol acetate A synthetic *progestogen given orally to dogs and cats to suppress or postpone oestrus. Postponement in bitches is achieved by treating animals during *anoestrus at least 1 week prior to expected prooestrus and continuing medication for up to 4 months. Oestrus usually occurs 2–3 months after withdrawal of treatment. In cats treatment should be started during *dioestrus or anoestrus. Oestrus recurs about 4 weeks after withdrawal of medication in the breeding season, longer at other times. To suppress oestrus in bitches and queens, higher doses are given over a short period, starting immediately signs of heat are noticed. If the animal has already been mated treatment will not affect conception. In bitches megestrol acetate is used to treat false pregnancies and oestrogen-dependent mammary tumours, while in male dogs it may be given to control undesirable behaviour, such as aggression, mounting, and urinating. In cats, the drug may act as an anti-inflammatory and sedative in cases of miliary eczema and eosinophilic granuloma. Tradenames: **Ovarid**; **Syntex Suppress**.
Melengestrol acetate is a similar progestogen used in feed or as an implant to prevent oestrus behaviour ('bulling') in heifers. This is used mainly in beef-fattening feedlots in North America.

meibomian gland adenoma A benign tumour arising from the meibomian glands – modified sebaceous glands of the eyelid margin. Although benign, they frequently cause physical irritation to the front of the eye with subsequent corneal ulceration. Surgical removal of the tumour and treatment for the ulcer is usually curative.

meibomian glands The tarsal glands. *See* tarsus.

meiosis (reduction division) (*pl.* **meioses**) A type of cell division that produces four daughter cells, each having half the number of chromosomes of the original cell. It occurs before the formation of spermatozoa and ova and the normal (*diploid) number of chromosomes is restored after fertilization. Meiosis also produces genetic variation in the daughter cells, brought about by the process of *crossing over. Meiosis consists of two successive divisions, each divided into four stages (*see* prophase; metaphase; anaphase; telophase). (See illustration.) *Compare* mitosis.

Meissner's plexus *See* submucosal plexus.

melaena Dark tarry faeces due to the presence of partly digested blood. It indicates gastrointestinal haemorrhage, for example from a bleeding ulcer.

melan- (melano-) *Prefix denoting* **1.** black coloration. **2.** melanin. Example: *melanaemia* (presence in the blood).

melanin Any of a group of polymers, derived from the amino acid tyrosine, that cause pigmentation of eyes, skin, and hair in vertebrates. Melanins are produced by specialized epidermal cells called *melanocytes*, and protect the skin from the harmful effects of ultraviolet radiation. Hereditary *albinism is caused by the absence of the enzyme tyrosinase, which is necessary for melanin production. *See also* melanoma.

melanism (melanosis) An unusually pronounced darkening of body tissues caused by excessive production of the pigment *melanin.

melanocyte A cell that produces the dark pigment *melanin. Melanocytes occur in the pigmented regions of the skin, in the choroid of the eye, and elsewhere.

melanocyte-stimulating hormone (MSH) A hormone, secreted by the intermediate part of the adenohypophysis, that controls skin colouring in amphibians and pigmentation of hair in some mammals. For example, stimulation of *melanocytes by MSH causes darkening of the skin in frogs. The snowshoe hare turns from white to brown when MSH is secreted in the summer months. Its role in other mammals is unclear.

melanocyte-stimulating-hormone-inhibiting hormone (MSHIH) A hormone, produced by nuclei in the hypothalamus of the snowshoe hare, that is released during the winter months to stop the production of melanocyte-stimulating hormone by the adenohypophysis, so causing the animal's coat to turn white for protective winter camouflage.

melanoma A tumour originating from the pigment-containing cells known as *melanocytes; consequently the mass is usually black-brown, although some tumours are nonpigmented (*amelanotic melanoma*). The commonly affected sites are the skin and the oral cavity. In humans the majority of melanomas are malignant, but in domestic animals there are significant differences. In dogs, melanomas of the skin tend to be benign whereas the majority of those of the

oral cavity are highly malignant. Melanomas are very common in older grey (i.e. white) horses and arise in the skin. Benign melanomas rarely cause problems unless secondarily damaged and infected. The malignant forms have a high tendency to metastasize to distant parts of the body and the prognosis must always be poor. Early surgical excision is the treatment of choice but the prognosis depends on the nature of the tumour.

melanuria The presence of dark pigment in the urine. The ingestion of various chemicals or poisons, such as phenols or coal-tar derivatives, may cause the condition.

melengestrol acetate *See* megestrol acetate.

melioidosis Disease due to infection with the bacterium *Pseudomonas pseudomallei*, which affects primarily rodents in tropical regions. The rodents constitute a reservoir for sporadic disease in other species. In farm animals this may be acute and fatal, or chronic with abscessation; treatment is never undertaken because of the extreme risk to humans. Melioidosis causes pneumonia, multiple abscesses, and septicaemia in humans, and is almost always fatal. *Compare* glanders.

membrane 1. A thin layer of tissue surrounding the whole or part of an organ or the layer of tissue lining a cavity, or separating adjacent structures or cavities. *See also* basement membrane; mucous membrane; serous membrane. **2.** The lipoprotein envelope surrounding a cell (*plasma* or *cell membrane*).

membrane bone A bone that develops by intramembranous *ossification. The bones of the face and the vault of the cranium are membrane bones.

menadione (menaphthone; vitamin K₃) A synthetic naphthaquinone with a potency about three times that of naturally occurring *vitamin K₁. It is used therapeutically in various blood coagulation disorders. However, for emergency treatment, for example in cases of *warfarin poisoning, vitamin K₁ is more effective than menadione because the latter must first be metabolized to its active form.

Mendelism The theory of heredity that forms the basis of classical *genetics, proposed by Gregor Mendel (1822–84) in 1866 and formulated in two laws (*Mendel's laws*). These deal with the inheritance of characters determined by 'factors' (now termed *alleles) that undergo segregation and independent assortment during sexual reproduction. The first law, or *law of segregation*, states that the members of a pair of alleles of any gene do not blend in the *zygote but segregate (separate) and pass into different gametes. Thus half the gametes will have a copy of one member, the rest will have a copy of the other member. If the organism is *heterozygous the members are different and so two sorts of gametes are produced, with equal frequency. The second law, or *law of independent assortment*, states that members of different pairs of alleles assort independently during gamete formation. This second law

applies only to genes on nonhomologous chromosomes, i.e. where there is no *linkage.

mening- (meningo-) *Prefix denoting* the meninges.

meninges (*sing.* **meninx**) The three connective tissue membranes that envelop the brain and spinal cord (see illustrations). The outermost *dura mater (pachymeninx) is separated by the subdural space from the

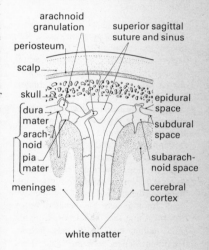

Section through the skull and brain to show meninges

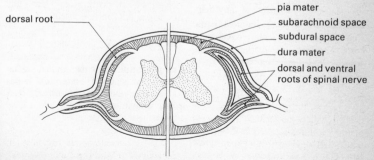

Transverse section through spinal cord of dog showing spinal meninges

middle *arachnoid mater; this is separated by the subarachnoid space, containing cerebrospinal fluid, from the innermost *pia mater. These inner two membranes are termed the *leptomeninges*.

meningioma A benign fibrous tumour arising from the *meninges, which envelop the brain and spinal cord. Meningiomas are uncommon in domestic animals, with greatest incidence in the dog and cat. See also brain tumours.

meningitis Inflammation of the *meninges, usually due to viral or bacterial infection. Inflammation of the inner two meninges (*leptomeningitis*) or of the outer dura mater (*pachymeningitis*) may be distinguished, although often all three meninges are involved. Meningitis is also a common complication of *encephalitis, producing *meningoencephalitis*. Various nervous signs may develop, including excitement, incoordination, painful cutaneous *hyperaesthesia, and bouts of depression, accompanied by elevated pulse and breathing rate and fever. Convulsions, coma, and death may follow. Treatment depends on the cause: bacterial meningitis may respond to appropriate antibiotics; viral meningitis cannot be treated with drugs, although rest and sedatives may help. Bacteria are a more frequent cause than viruses, and the commonest form of meningitis is that resulting from infections of the navel (omphalophlebitis) with streptococci and *Escherichia coli* in the newborn (*see* omphalitis). Other bacterial agents include *Listeria monocytogenes* (*circling disease), *Streptococcus equi* (*strangles), *Staphylococcus aureus* (producing *tick pyaemia of lambs), *Erysipelothrix rhusiopathiae* (causing

*swine erysipelas), *Haemophilus somnus* (*Haemophilus septicaemia of cattle), *Streptococcus suis* (causing *streptococcal meningitis of pigs), *Pasteurella haemolytica* and *P. multocida* in lambs (*see* pasteurellosis), *Mycobacterium tuberculosis* (*tuberculosis in calves), and *Cryptococcus neoformans*. The viruses of *malignant catarrhal fever and sporadic bovine encephalomyelitis (*see* encephalitis) may both cause meningitis in cattle, and meningitis often develops in cases of canine *distemper and *rabies.

meningoencephalitis Inflammation of the *meninges and brain. See also encephalitis; meningitis.

meniscus (*pl.* **menisci** or **meniscuses**) (in anatomy) A crescent-shaped structure, such as the fibrocartilaginous disc that divides the cavity of a synovial joint.

meniscus tear Splitting of the intra-articular cartilage (meniscus) of the *stifle joint, which occurs in cases of traumatic damage or stifle arthritis. In dogs the condition most commonly occurs in the posterior half of the medial meniscus and runs across the meniscus. It is not usual to find longitudinal splits (as in humans), and locking of the joint does not occur in dogs. The torn meniscus is usually identified at *arthrotomy and the damaged portion is excised.

mepivacaine See local anaesthetic.

mepyramine maleate An *antihistamine that acts at H_1 receptors. It has a shorter duration of action than *diphenhydramine, and its local anaesthetic and sedative effects are also less.

mercury A liquid metallic element, symbol Hg. Various inorganic mercury compounds have been used in animal treatment, including mercuric oxide (in eye ointment), mercuric chloride (as an antiseptic), and mercurous chloride (see calomel), as well as metallic mercury (as a purgative).

Mercury poisoning Both inorganic and organic mercury compounds can cause toxicity in animals. The inorganic compounds are absorbed through intact skin. Dogs and cats are very susceptible to toxicity because they can ingest mercury during grooming, while sheep and cattle are very susceptible to inhalation of mercury vapour. The soluble salts are absorbed from the gastrointestinal tract, but insoluble mercurous salts (e.g. calomel) are poorly absorbed unless there is damage to the gastrointestinal mucosa or conversion to more toxic mercuric salts. After absorption, mercury is distributed throughout the body and is stored in the liver and kidneys. Excretion into the urine is very slow. Acute toxicity causes severe gastroenteritis with haemorrhagic diarrhoea, circulatory collapse, and death or, in less acute cases, stomatitis and acute nephritis. Inhalation of mercury vapour leads to dyspnoea, coughing, oral and nasal ulceration, and nephritis. In more chronic cases of mercury poisoning there is gastroenteritis and nephritis accompanied by CNS signs. Sodium thiosulphate or *dimercaprol can be injected as antidotes, and dosing with egg whites or milk, or gastric lavage, can be tried to prevent further absorption of mercury from the gastrointestinal tract. *Spironolactone may protect against kidney damage due to mercuric chloride. Shock should be treated with fluid replacement therapy. See also organomercury poisoning.

merocrine (eccrine) Describing a type of *secretion in which the glandular cells remain intact during the process of secretion.

merogony (schizogony) A process of asexual division in protozoa whereby a single cell divides into many daughter cells (merozoites). The parent cell nucleus divides first forming a multi-nucleated cell (meront). The cytoplasm then divides liberating the merozoites.

meront (schizont) One of the stages that occurs during *merogony in protozoa.

mes- (meso-) Prefix denoting middle or medial.

mesaticephalic Describing a medium-shaped head, for example as in beagle dogs. Compare brachycephalic; dolichocephalic.

mesencephalon See midbrain.

mesenchyme An undifferentiated tissue of the early embryo that forms almost entirely from the *mesoderm. It is loosely organized with irregularly arranged cells and much extracellular matrix. Mesenchyme forms all the connective tissues and muscle tissues of the body.

mesentery A double-layered fold of *peritoneum attaching the intestine or other abdominal organs to the dorsal or ventral abdominal wall. It contains blood and lymph vessels and nerves supplying these organs.

mesocolon The fold of *peritoneum by which the colon is attached to the dorsal abdominal wall.

mesoderm The middle of the three *germ layers of the early embryo, which gives rise to the connective tissues, muscle tissues, and the kidneys and gonads and their ducts. Soon after its development the mesoderm within the embryo becomes divided into three paired columns: the paraxial (most medial); the intermediate;

and the *lateral plate* mesoderms. The paraxial mesoderm becomes segmented into the *somites. The lateral plate mesoderm splits into outer somatic and inner splanchnic layers when the *intraembryonic coelom forms. These layers are continuous with those of the extraembryonic mesoderm, which are separated by the *extraembryonic coelom.

mesometrium (*pl.* **mesometria**) The part of the *broad ligament of the uterus that attaches to the horns and body of the uterus.

mesonephric duct (Wolffian duct) The duct of the *mesonephros. In males it persists to form the epididymis and the ductus deferens. In females it normally disappears but may persist as a remnant (*Gartner's duct*).

mesonephros (*pl.* **mesonephroi**) The second area of kidney tissue to develop in the embryo, subsequent to the *pronephros. It forms a temporary embryonic kidney, which subsequently degenerates. Some of its tubules become incorporated into the testis to form the ductuli efferentes. In the female it normally disappears entirely but may occasionally form small remnants, termed the *epoophoron* and the *paroophoron*.

mesophilic Describing organisms, especially bacteria, that grow best at temperatures of about 25–45°C.

mesosalpinx (*pl.* **mesosalpinges**) The part of the *broad ligament of the uterus that attaches to the uterine tube.

mesosome A structure occurring in some bacterial cells, formed by infolding of the cell membrane. Mesosomes are associated with the DNA and play a part in cell division.

mesotendon The delicate connective tissue membrane that surrounds a tendon.

mesothelioma A rare tumour arising from the pleura, peritoneum, or pericardium. In humans, there is an established association between exposure to asbestos and the development of mesotheliomas, and evidence for a similar association in urban dogs has been reported. The tumour is reported in most domestic species, forming papillary growths, which may be multiple, and eliciting the production of copious amounts of serous fluid, which accumulates in the affected body cavity. Clinical signs are those associated with this fluid accumulation – difficulty in breathing or a pendulous abdomen. Diagnosis may be aided by the microscopic examination of drained fluid and the identification of malignant cells. Treatment has not been described in animals but drainage of the fluid may ease the clinical signs. Metastasis rarely occurs.

mesothelium (*pl.* **mesothelia**) The single layer of cells that lines *serous membranes. *Compare* endothelium; epithelium.

mesovarium The part of the *broad ligament of the uterus that attaches to the ovary.

messenger RNA A type of *RNA that carries the information of the *genetic code of the DNA from the cell nucleus to the ribosomes, where the code is translated into protein. *See* transcription; translation.

met- (meta-) *Prefix denoting* **1.** distal to; beyond; behind. **2.** change; transformation.

metabolic profile test A screening test involving a range of blood constituents that is used to diagnose various disorders, especially *production diseases in cattle, and to monitor the training of racehorses. The original concept, developed from human medicine, depended on the detection of excess or deficient concentrations of key substances in the blood that were used as indicators to give early warning of breakdown in energy, protein, mineral, or electrolyte (salt) status and enable recommendations for correction of the diet. The test has now been developed to investigate infertility and ill-thrift. It has also been used to survey large numbers of animals on a regional basis to indicate areas of incipient trace-element deficiencies. Using modern analytical apparatus coupled with computers, many tests can be included at the same time and results given rapidly.

In dairy herds, a test carried out just before calving will detect, for example, incipient magnesium deficiency, which precipitates *milk fever, especially on autumn pasture. Similarly, in mid-winter the early stages of *ketosis can be identified, usually implicating inadequacy of the forage. In horses undergoing training, muscle fatigue and overexercise may be diagnosed by detecting enzymes leaked from muscle.

metabolism The sum of the chemical reactions that occur within the body. The various compounds that take part in or are formed by these reactions are called *metabolites*. In animals, many metabolites are obtained by the digestion of food. The synthesis

(*anabolism*) and breakdown (*catabolism*) of most compounds occur by a number of reaction steps, the reaction sequence being termed a *metabolic pathway*. Some pathways (e.g. *glycolysis) are linear; others (e.g. the *Krebs cycle) are cyclic. The changes at each step in a pathway are usually small and are promoted by *enzymes, which act as biological catalysts.

metabolite A substance that takes part in the process of *metabolism. Metabolites are either produced during metabolism or are constituents of food taken into the body.

metabolizable energy The amount of ingested gross *energy available to the animal after deducting energy loss in the faeces and in the production of gases and urine. Its value for particular feedstuffs may be further refined by incorporating correction factors. Thus in poultry *true metabolizable energy* (*TME*) accounts for losses in the excreta of nondietary origin (i.e. endogenous losses), which include nonreabsorbed enzymes, sloughed-off mucosal cells, and microorganisms; *apparent metabolizable energy* (*AME*) does not account for these losses.

metacarpal Relating to the *metacarpus.

metacarpus (*pl.* **metacarpi**) The region of the *manus of the forelimb containing the metacarpal bones. The number and form of the metacarpals vary in relation to the digits present (see table). The base of each metacar-

Number and form of metacarpals in various animals

	Main metacarpals	Rudimentary metacarpals
Horse	Mc 3	Mc 2, 4 (splint bones)
Ruminants	Mc 3/4 (fused)	Mc 5
Pig	Mc 2–5	–
Carnivores	Mc 2–5	Mc 1

pal articulates with bones of the *carpus, while the distal head articulates with the proximal bones of the *phalanx. In birds the metacarpals are reduced (in common with the digits) and fused with the distal row of carpal bones forming the *carpometacarpus*.

metacentric A chromosome in which the centromere is at or near the centre of the chromosome.

metacercaria The encysted *cercaria larva in the life cycle of a *fluke. *See also* miracidium; redia; sporocyst.

metachromasia (metachromatism) **1.** The property of a dye of staining certain tissues or cells a colour that is different from that of the stain itself. **2.** The variation in colour produced in certain tissue elements that are stained with the same dye. **3.** Abnormal coloration of a tissue produced by a particular stain.

Metagonimus A genus of small *flukes, usually 1–2.5 mm long, parasitic in dogs, cats, and occasionally humans in the Far East. There are two intermediate hosts, a snail and a freshwater fish, and the primary host is infected by eating raw or inadequately cooked fish. Signs of infestation are usually mild but may include inflammation and ulceration of the intestinal lining, and diarrhoea.

metaldehyde poisoning A toxic condition caused by ingestion of polymerized acetaldehyde (or metaldehyde), a substance used for the destruction of slugs and snails in horticulture and agriculture. Metaldehyde is combined with bran to make it attractive to slugs and scattered as pellets over the ground. Dogs and cats may eat the pellets and cattle or sheep are poisoned by obtaining access to the product while it is stored in bags, often in food stores. The toxic dose is in the range 0.3–0.5 g/kg. Clinical signs are salivation, *hyperaesthesia, muscle tremors, and convulsions. *Emetics should be used in cats, dogs, and pigs; convulsions can be controlled by *pentobarbitone and *acetyl promazine (*see* phenothiazines). In cattle, calcium and magnesium injections are used as well as the sedative xylazine.

metamyelocyte A bone marrow precursor cell that differentiates without cell division into one of three cell types: a *neutrophil, an *eosinophil, or a *basophil. The staining reaction of the metamyelocyte granules indicates which line of differentiation is in progress. *See* haemopoiesis.

metanephros (*pl.* **metanephroi**) The third area of kidney tissue to develop in the embryo (i.e. subsequent to the *pronephros and *mesonephros) that forms the definitive kidney. It develops caudal to the mesonephros, and its duct (the future ureter) forms initially as an outgrowth from the terminal part of the *mesonephric duct.

metaphase The second stage of *mitosis and of each division of *meiosis, in which the chromosomes line up at the centre of the *spindle, with their centromeres attached to the spindle fibres.

metaphysis The growing end of the *diaphysis (shaft) of a long bone.

metaplasia An abnormal change in the nature of a tissue, especially a change in the differentiation of its cells to a type not normally present. For example, in *prostatic squamous metaplasia* the normally glandular cells of the *prostate change to a squamous cell type under the prolonged influence of *oestrogen.

Number and form of metatarsals in various animals

	Main metatarsals	Rudimentary metatarsals
Horse	Mt 3	Mt 2, 4 (splint bones)
Ruminants	Mt 3/4 (fused)	Mt 2
Pig	Mt 2–5	–
Carnivores	Mt 2–5	Mt 1
Fowl	Mt 2–4 (fused)	Mt 1

metastasis The process by which tumours spread to sites not directly connected with the primary mass to form secondary masses (*metastases*). This may occur by means of the lymphatic and/or blood vessels, or across body cavities. In the case of lymphatic spread, the draining lymph nodes are normally infiltrated by tumour cells; following vascular spread, secondary tumours may appear in virtually any organ. With spread through a body cavity, such as the abdomen or thorax, tumour cells may implant on the peritoneum to form tumour deposits. Metastasis of brain tumours may take place via the *subarachnoid space.

Metastrongylus A genus of parasitic nematodes (*see* lungworm), three species of which affect pigs. *M. apri* and *M. pudendotectus* are widespread; *M. salmi* is found in Zaïre and southeast Asia. The adult worms lodge in the larger airways of the lung. The eggs are coughed up, swallowed, and passed out with the faeces. They are then ingested by earthworms, in which the larvae develop to the infective stage. Pigs swallow the earthworms and thus become infested. The adult lungworms cause lung damage, which may lead to pneumonia, although lungworm disease mostly affects piglets. The larvae may also transmit the *swine fever virus. Pigs outdoors can be kept away from contaminated pasture after heavy rain, which brings earthworms to the surface; grazing should be rotated every

6 months. Treatment consists of dosing with a wormer, such as dichlorvos (*see* organophosphorus (OP) compounds), *piperazine, one of the *benzimidazoles, or *ivermectin (subcutaneous injection).

metatarsal Relating to the *metatarsus.

metatarsus (*pl.* **metatarsi**) The region of the *pes of the hindlimb containing the metatarsal bones. The number and form of metatarsals present vary according to the digits present (see table). The base of each metatarsal articulates with the distal bones of the *tarsus, while the distal head articulates with the proximal bones of the *phalanx. In birds the main metatarsals are fused with the distal row of tarsal bones forming the *tarsometatarsus*.

metencephalon The part of the brain comprising the *pons and *cerebellum.

-meter *Suffix denoting* an instrument for measuring.

methacycline *See* tetracyclines.

methaemoglobinaemia The presence in the blood of the pigment methaemoglobin, formed by the action of certain drugs and poisons on *haemoglobin. These toxic substances, such as methylene blue, acetaminophen, and benzocaine, usually act as oxidizing agents, changing the ferrous iron of haemoglobin to the ferric form.

Methaemoglobinaemia tends to occur with *Heinz body anaemia, since both result from toxic damage to haemoglobin. *See also* haemolytic anaemia.

methane A colourless odourless gas and the simplest hydrocarbon. It is an end-product of anaerobic metabolism in certain bacteria and is produced in considerable amounts in the rumen, from where it is discharged periodically by eructation, along with carbon dioxide. Methane also occurs in faecal gas.

methanol *See* methyl alcohol.

methicillin *See* penicillin.

methionine An *amino acid. *See also* essential amino acid.

methohexitone (*US* **methohexital**) *See* barbiturate.

methoxyflurane A volatile liquid used as an *inhalational anaesthetic for small animals. Noninflammable and nonexplosive, it has a low vapour pressure, hence the maximum concentration obtained at room temperature is about 3%, making induction slow but overdosage unlikely. Methoxyflurane gives good analgesia and muscle relaxation, and hypotension is usually not marked, making it a good anaesthetic for orthopaedic operations and in cases where the anaesthetic risk is high. There is respiratory depression, but recovery is slow and quiet. Methoxyflurane is extensively metabolized in the liver, forming products that include fluoride and oxalic acid, which can cause renal damage. However, this is less in dogs than in man.

methyl alcohol (methanol) A colourless inflammable liquid used as a solvent, antifreeze, and in chemical manufacturing. It is toxic, causing acidosis, stimulation then depression of the central nervous system, and neuritis, especially of the optic nerves with resulting blindness.

methylated spirit Any of various mixtures comprising chiefly ethanol (typically $\simeq 90\%$) plus *methyl alcohol. The addition of pyridine gives it an objectionable smell, and the dye methyl violet may be added to make it recognizable as unfit to drink. Volatile and highly inflammable, it is used topically, usually in the form of *surgical spirit, to clean and dry skin. It can also be used as a disinfectant for surgical instruments. It should not be used on damaged skin or mucous membranes. Acetone-free methylated spirit is used in the preparation of antiseptic iodine solutions.

The methyl alcohol in methylated spirit is toxic, causing visual impairment, acidosis, coma, and respiratory failure. Toxicity can occur after ingestion or absorption from broken skin or mucous membranes. Treatment involves correcting the acidosis with sodium lactate or sodium bicarbonate, administered intravenously. Nervous signs can be treated using *diazepam.

methyl benzoquate *See* coccidiostat.

methylene blue An oxidizing agent administered intravenously (as a 1–4% solution in saline) in the treatment of nitrate/nitrite and chlorate poisoning to reverse the effects of *methaemoglobinaemia. In chlorate poisoning treatment must be repeated until the chlorate ions are excreted in order to prevent further formation of methaemoglobin. In cats methylene blue can cause *haemolytic anaemia with Heinz body formation.

methyl green A basic dye used for colouring the stainable part of the cell nucleus (chromatin) and – with pyronin – for the differential staining of RNA and DNA, which give a red and a green colour respectively.

methyl testosterone *See* testosterone.

methyl violet (gentian violet) A dye used mainly for staining protozoa.

metiamide *See* antihistamine.

metoclopramide An *antiemetic that increases lower oesophageal sphincter tone, increases gastric contractions, and coordinates gastric emptying and duodenal motility. This re-establishes a more normal pattern of motility in the gastrointestinal tract. Available for injection or as tablets, the drug is well absorbed and is excreted rapidly in the urine and bile. It is used to prevent vomiting during travel, in parvovirus enteritis, peptic ulceration, gastric irritation, and during chemotherapy in dogs and cats. It should not be used if gastric emptying is blocked, for instance due to a foreign body, since metoclopramide can induce gastric rupture. Side-effects include depression, listlessness, and nervousness. Long-term therapy may produce constipation. The drug's effects can be antagonized by *atropine and opioid analgesics (*see* opiate). Tradename: **Emequell**.

metoestrus The stage of the *oestrous cycle following oestrus when the corpus luteum is forming and beginning to produce progesterone.

metomidate An *imidazole derivative that acts as a *hypnotic. It can be used in bait to capture wild birds or injected intramuscularly to immobilize birds. In pigs it is used intravenously after premedication with *azaperone. As metomidate is very acidic in solution and therefore irritant, it should be given slowly intravenously. Muscle relaxation occurs about 10 minutes after intramuscular administration, and recovery takes 2–4 hours. Analgesia is poor and there can be trembling, salivation, and apnoea. In horses metomidate combined with azaperone has been used to produce anaesthesia, although recovery can be very abrupt and may include violent motor activity. Intravenous metomidate causes haemolysis, especially if injected rapidly. Tradename: **Hypnodil.**

metoprolol *See* beta blockers.

metr- (metro-) *Prefix denoting* the uterus.

metritis Generalized inflammation of the *uterus (inflammation restricted to various parts of the uterine wall is termed *endometritis, *myometritis, or *perimetritis, depending on the site). Metritis may be acute or chronic, the latter often being a sequel to the former. Most infective agents causing inflammation are introduced via the vagina and infection is most common following copulation and parturition (i.e. when the cervix is open). The animal's hormone status influences the resistance of the uterus to infection; *oestrogens tend to promote the action of *leucocytes and enhance resistance, whereas a *progesterone-dominated uterus is more susceptible.

Acute cases of metritis are normally found in post-parturient animals (*see* post-parturient metritis), particularly following *retention of the placenta, although the condition can occur after an apparently normal birth. The signs are a foul-smelling brown discharge, lethargy, and depressed appetite; the animal may exhibit straining. In cases when uterine *involution does not occur, infection is easily established among the large amounts of blood, fluids, and foetal membranes present. Also after partial separation of the placenta, the *endometrium is easily invaded by bacteria, and bacterial toxins may be absorbed into the bloodstream (*toxaemia). In such cases the animal requires urgent antibiotic administration.

Chronic metritis is often a long-standing condition and has adverse effects on fertility. It is frequently characterized by a white discharge and a failure to conceive. Infection may be spread venereally, in which case the male also requires antibiotic treatment. Metritis is largely preventable by paying close attention to hygiene at parturition.

metritis-mastitis-agalactia syndrome See MMA.

metronidazole An antimicrobial drug used in the treatment of protozoal infections (such as trichomoniasis, giardiasis, and amoebiasis) and in anaerobic bacterial infections (e.g. gingivitis, abscesses, peritonitis, pyothorax, urinary tract infections, and foot infections). Although only slightly water-soluble, it is readily absorbed from the gastrointestinal tract after oral administration and distributes well throughout the tissues. It is metabolized and excreted in the bile and urine, with a half-life of approximately 5 hours. Metronidazole is selectively toxic to anaerobic organisms and anoxic cells, in which it acts as an electron acceptor, disrupts cellular DNA, and inhibits DNA synthesis. It is occasionally used in the treatment of cancer to sensitize hypoxic tumour cells to radiation. The drug is available for oral and topical use and as an intravenous injection. Side-effects due to neurotoxicity include ataxia, muscle spasms, tremors, and occasionally convulsions. Metronidazole should not be used in pregnant animals because of possible mutagenic or carcinogenic effects. Tradename: **Flagyl**.

metroposis Uterine haemorrhage, i.e. bleeding from the womb.

-metry *Suffix denoting* measuring or measurement.

Mexican poppy *See* blood root poisoning.

micelle A microscopic cluster of molecules. The products of fat digestion – monoglycerides and fatty acids – are absorbed from the gut via the lymphatic system, entering the gut wall in the form of micelles and passing into the lymphatic system as *chylomicrons. Formation of micelles is aided by emulsification, which is promoted by the *bile salts.

miconazole *See* imidazoles.

micr- (micro-) *Prefix denoting* **1.** small size. **2.** one millionth part.

microaerophilic Describing microorganisms that grow best at very low oxygen concentrations (i.e. below the atmospheric level).

microangiopathy 1. Thrombosis in the blood capillaries. It occurs in various diseases in which inflammatory lesions activate blood platelets and induce *disseminated intravascular coagulation. This can lead to anaemia and haemolysis; in young calves it is known as *microangiopathic haemolytic anaemia*. Thrombosis also occurs in the primitive capillaries of malignant tumours, where it precedes necrosis. **2.** Any condition involving damage to the walls of the blood capillaries.

microbe *See* microorganism.

microbiology The science of *microorganisms. Microbiology in relation to veterinary science is concerned mainly with the isolation and identification of the microorganisms that cause disease and with the study of symbiotic microorganisms that digest plant material in the gut of herbivores, especially in ruminants.

Micrococcus A genus of Gram-positive aerobic *bacteria, spherical or coccoid in shape, often arranged in irregular clusters or tetrads (formerly called *Gaffkya*). They are nonpathogenic free-living saprophytes, abundant in the environment and on the skin of animals.

microcyte An abnormally small *erythrocyte. Microcytes occur in iron-deficiency *anaemia and possibly also as a result of fragmentation of red cells.

microcytosis The presence in the blood of abnormally small red cells (microcytes). Microcytosis is most commonly associated with iron deficiency, both in humans and animals. It may also occur in cases where bone marrow function is impaired by lead poisoning or by dietary deficiency of copper.

microelectrode An extremely fine wire used as an electrode to measure the electrical activity in small areas of tissue. Microelectrodes can be used for recording the electrical changes that occur in the membranes of cells, such as those of nerve and muscle.

microfilaria (*pl.* **microfilariae**) A slender larval stage (immature embryo) produced by filarial nematodes and normally found in blood or lymph. Typically they are taken up by a blood-sucking intermediate host (e.g. mosquito) when it feeds on the primary host. The infective larval stage develops within the intermediate host, and enters the final host via the wound made by the intermediate host when it feeds. *See* Dirofilaria; Onchocerca.

microglia One of the types of *neuroglia (the non-nervous cells of the central nervous system), having a mainly scavenging function (*see* macrophage).

microglossia A condition in which the tongue is abnormally small.

micrognathia A condition in which one jaw is abnormally small. This occurs as a congenital developmental defect in sheep. The mandible may be reduced or completely absent, making suckling or eating difficult or impossible, with fatal consequences. *Compare* macrognathia.

micrograph (photomicrograph) A photograph of an object viewed through a microscope. An *electron micrograph* is photographed through an electron microscope; a *light micrograph* through a light microscope.

micrometer An instrument for making extremely fine measurements of thickness or length, often relying upon the movement of a screw thread and the principle of the *vernier.

microorganism (microbe) Any organism too small to be visible to the naked eye. Microorganisms include *bacteria, some *fungi, *mycoplasmas, *Protozoa, *rickettsiae, and *viruses.

microphthalmia A condition in which the eyeballs are abnormally small. It occurs as a congenital defect of piglets, an extreme form of which is complete absence of the eyes (*anophthalmus*).

micropipette An extremely fine tube from which minute volumes of liquid can be delivered or drawn up for examination. Using a micropipette it is possible to add or take away material from individual cells under the microscope.

microscope An instrument for producing a greatly magnified image of an object. *Light* or *optical microscopes* use light as a radiation source for viewing the specimen, and combinations of lenses to magnify the image; they give a resolution up to about 1000 times. The widely used *binocular microscope* consists of two microscopes coupled together, one for each eye, to give stereoscopic vision. *Operating microscopes* are based on the binocular microscope; the field of operation is illuminated through the objective lens by a light source within the microscope. Many models incorporate a beam splitter and a second set of eyepieces to enable the surgeon's assistant to view the operation, or employ a camera so that the operation can be viewed on a screen. *See also* electron microscope; ultramicroscope.

microscopic 1. What can be seen only with the use of a microscope. 2. Of, relating to, or using a microscope.

microsome A small particle consisting of a piece of *endoplasmic reticulum with ribosomes attached. Microsomes are formed when homogenized cells are centrifuged.

microsonation The use of ultrasound waves generated inside the body from an extremely small source, such as the tip of a needle or a bubble within the tissues. The technique is a specialized form of *ultrasonography, and is used to obtain a picture of the fine structure of neighbouring tissues.

Microsporum A genus of *dermatophyte fungi including about nine species that infect animals. *M. canis* is the usual cause of *ringworm in cats; less frequently it affects dogs, and it is readily transmitted to humans. *M. equinum* frequently infects horses in Britain but appears not to be distinguished from *M. canis* by some authorities, especially in the USA; it seems less common elsewhere and seldom infects other hosts. *M. gypseum*, a complex of three closely similar species, inhabits the soil and sporadically infects dogs, cats, horses, and occasionally other hosts. *M. nanum* is the cause of porcine ringworm in the USA but is apparently absent from Britain, where pigs are infected by *Trichophyton* spp.

The asexually sporing state, identifiable as a *Microsporum* species, is seen in normal laboratory cultures. But sexual spore-forming ('perfect') states of some species have been observed and classified in the ascomycete genus *Nannizzia*. The *Nannizzia* species that make up the *M. gypseum* complex are difficult to distinguish in their asexual form and as such are usually identified simply as *M. gypseum*.

microsurgery Surgery performed with the aid of an operating microscope, through which the tissues and instruments are viewed. This allows precise dissection and suturing of minute structures, such as fine nerves and blood vessels.

microtome An instrument for cutting extremely thin slices of material that can be examined under a microscope. The material is usually embedded in a suitable medium, such as paraffin wax. A common type of microtome is a steel knife.

microtubule A cellular organelle involved in stiffening certain regions of cytoplasm, thus determining cell shape. Microtubules are involved in the formation of the mitotic *spindle and are therefore necessary for cell division. They are also numerous in the axon of *neurones (nerve cells) and are involved in the flow of axoplasm.

microvillus (*pl.* **microvilli**) One of a number of microscopic hairlike structures (about 5 μm long) projecting from the surface of epithelial cells (*see* epithelium). They serve to increase the surface area of the cell and are seen on absorptive and secretory cells. In some regions (particularly the intestinal tract) microvilli form a dense covering on the free surface of the cells: this is called a *brush border*.

micturition (urination) The periodic discharge of urine from the urinary bladder through the urethra as a result of reflex contraction of the smooth muscle of the bladder. This reflex is triggered by distension of the bladder, and is accompanied by relaxation of the sphincter muscles around the urethra. The reflex can become modified by conscious control (housetraining), especially in dogs and cats.

midbrain 1. (in embryology) The middle portion of the embryonic brain that forms the adult midbrain. **2.** (in anatomy) The mesencephalon, i.e. the part of the *brainstem lying caudal to the *diencephalon and rostral to the *pons. Its dorsal part is the *tectum and its ventral part is the cerebral *peduncle. The midbrain contains the *aqueduct and is the origin for cranial nerves III and IV.

middle ear *See* ear.

midge Any of various species of *fly that are generally minute with short legs and long antennae. The females suck the blood of livestock and humans with the aid of a short, powerful proboscis. The eggs are laid in shallow waters or wet mud and hatch into aquatic or semi-aquatic larvae, which develop into aquatic air-breathing pupae. Biting midges, such as *Culicoides* spp., are found worldwide near water and are most active around dusk. Their bite produces a pricking sensation followed by severe irritation, which may develop into an allergic condition, such as *sweet itch in horses. They also transmit a number of filarial nematode worms and virus diseases, such as *bluetongue of sheep. Control of midges is difficult, but insect repellents give some protection to livestock, and the breeding grounds and known habitats can be sprayed with a suitable *insecticide.

midgut The middle portion of the embryonic gut, which gives rise to most of the small intestine and part of the large intestine. Early in development it is connected with the *yolk sac outside the embryo by the *vitellointestinal duct*, which passes through the *umbilicus.

miliary Describing or characterized by very small nodules or lesions, resembling millet seed.

miliary tuberculosis A disseminated usually terminal form of *tuberculosis in any species, resulting from the bacteraemia caused when an advanced lesion breaks down into the bloodstream. The small secondary *tubercles that develop simultaneously in susceptible organs throughout the body are so numerous that death occurs when they reach millet-seed size, as suggested by the term.

milk The secretion of the *mammary gland which provides the sole or major source of nourishment for young suckling mammals. The composition varies with the species (see table), but the chief constituent is water, dissolved in which are proteins (mainly caseinogen, *lactalbumin, and lactoglobulin), *lactose, minerals (especially calcium and phosphate), and a range of B vitamins. There is also a lipid fraction (cream) composed mainly of *triglycerides and fat-soluble vitamins, chiefly vitamin A. The milk produced immediately after parturition (*colostrum) is espe-

milk allergy

The composition of milk of various domestic animals

Species	Content (% by weight)						kJ per 100 g
	Dry matter	Total protein	Casein	Fat	Lactose	Minerals	
Cow	12.8	3.5	2.8	3.8	4.8	0.7	330
Goat	12.8	3.7	2.9	4.1	4.2	0.8	330
Ewe	16.8	5.4	4.3	6.2	4.3	0.9	450
Mare	10.7	2.5	1.6	1.6	6.1	0.5	230
Sow	20.4	6.3	4.4	7.7	5.6	0.8	560

cially rich in various components and also contains immunoglobulins, which are not present in ordinary milk. *See also* butterfat; lactation.

milk allergy A hypersensitive reaction caused by the entry of milk components into the circulation from an over-full mammary gland. The reaction is seen in cows and, less frequently, in mares. It is a form of Type I *hypersensitivity or anaphylaxis, and is usually relieved by emptying the gland.

milker's nodule *See* pseudocowpox.

milk fever A metabolic disease of dairy cows in their third or subsequent lactation caused by an abnormally low concentration of calcium in the blood (*see* hypocalcaemia). The clinical signs are muscle weakness, incoordination, and failure to rise after giving birth. Loss of consciousness and death follow unless treatment is given. Although usually occurring at the time of parturition, signs are sometimes seen at a later stage of lactation. The fall in blood calcium is the result of loss of calcium into the milk at the onset of lactation and a failure of the animal's metabolism to mobilize calcium reserves swiftly enough to replace it. If the disease occurs during the first

or second stages of labour then the process of calving ceases until treatment is given. This may result in the death of the calf. Treatment is by intravenous or subcutaneous injection of *calcium borogluconate. A range of measures can be taken to prevent the disease, including avoiding excessive *steaming up, attempting to improve the cow's capacity to mobilize calcium by giving low calcium/high phosphate diets for a few weeks prepartum, and giving prepartum injections of either *vitamin D or hydroxycholecalciferols. Also, autumn-calving cows should be fed silage at least 3 weeks before calving. Finally, stress at calving should be minimized. Other name: **parturient paresis.** *See also* downer cow syndrome.

milking The process of drawing milk from the *mammary glands, especially of dairy cows, either by hand or by *milking machine. Milk *let-down is controlled by the pituitary hormone *oxytocin, which causes the alveoli and small ducts of the *mammary gland to contract forcing milk into the lactiferous ducts and sinuses. Release of oxytocin is a conditioned reflex in response to familiar stimuli associated with milking, such as entering the milking parlour, washing the udder, feeding, or even the sound of the milking machine. If milking is delayed after milk letdown, emptying of the udder will be incomplete since the effects of oxytocin only last for a few minutes. Also milk letdown will be incomplete if the cows are stressed or the milking routine is markedly changed. The time taken to complete milking varies between individuals and is a function of the strength of milk letdown, rate of milking, and milk yield. The rate of milking is purely a function of the diameter of the papillary duct, which is a highly heritable trait; hence slow milkers cannot be induced to milk faster.

milking machine An apparatus for *milking cows, sheep, or goats. A metal teat cup containing a rubber liner is placed over each teat of the udder and a vacuum applied to draw off the milk. The vacuum is pulsed 45–70 times per minute by a pulsator; the teat would be damaged by a continuous vacuum. The milk is transferred to a receiving vessel via a pipeline or into a bucket. A vacuum regulator is incorporated into the system to ensure sufficient reserve vacuum to cope with the removal of teat cups and maintain a steady vacuum; this is important for minimizing udder damage and consequent *mastitis. After milking the system is thoroughly cleaned, either by circulating hot water containing cleaning solution or by washing through with acidified boiling water.

milk lameness A form of *osteoporosis that affects the bones of high-yielding dairy cows. It is brought about by the excessive resorption of bone to satisfy the mineral demands of milk production. The bone substance becomes excessively thin and porous. Phosphorus deficiency is often the cause, and *hypophosphataemia is a helpful diagnostic sign. However, protein deficiency may occur at the same time and this also causes bone thinning by restricting the synthesis

of bone matrix. The bones fracture easily and the joints become painful, which in turn upsets appetite and milk yield. Although dietary correction solves the problem any phosphorus supplements must be carefully selected to be free from fluorine contamination. Osteoporotic bone avidly takes up phosphorus and any fluorine present alongside. Fluorine toxicity induces another form of lameness.

milkspot liver A condition of pigs infested with *Ascaris suum* nematodes in which the liver shows whitish spots or streaks of fibrous tissue. These are associated with chronic inflammation caused by wandering parasite larvae. A similar condition can be caused in dogs by *Toxocara canis* or *T. cati*.

milk substitute Artificial milk used instead of natural dam's milk for rearing young mammals. A wide variety of formulations are available, usually supplied as a dry powder for reconstituting with water. The best milk substitutes are based on skimmed milk with added vegetable or animal fat since these form a good clot in the abomasum or stomach. *Zero milk powders* are based on whey products with additional protein from soya beans, fish meal, or single-cell protein, plus added fat as in skimmed milk powders. *See also* calf husbandry.

milk teeth *See* dentition.

milkweed poisoning A toxic condition arising from the ingestion of any of the various perennial herbaceous plants belonging to the genus *Asclepias*, distributed throughout North America. Their resinous sap contains a steroid glycoside, which causes mild to severe gastrointestinal irritation, staggering, violent muscle spasms, dyspnoea, increased temperature, rapid weak pulse, coma, respiratory paralysis, and death. Treatment is symptomatic.

milk yield The amount of *milk produced by a cow, sheep, goat, or other mammal in a given period (e.g. in one day or over one lactation cycle). In **dairy cows**, milk yield rises to a peak at about the 6th to 8th week of lactation. Thereafter it declines at a rate of about 2.5% per week until *drying off. In adult cows the total lactation yield is equal to approximately 200 times the peak yield; in heifers it is 220 times the peak yield. Milk yield is determined by various factors: season of calving – cows calving in the autumn give more milk because the decline following peak yield is arrested by turnout to grass in the spring; size of the cow – generally bigger cows have higher yields; age of the cow – maximum yield is reached in the third or fourth lactation; breed and genotype – milk yield is a heritable character; level of nutrition and body condition – cows need adequate nutrition or a reasonable level of body reserves to maintain high yields (*see* condition scoring); and health – ill health usually depresses milk yield. The average annual milk yield of dairy cows in the UK was 5186 litres in 1985/86. *See also* cattle husbandry.

milli- *Prefix denoting* one thousandth part.

mineralocorticoid *See* corticosteroid.

minerals *See* essential element.

mio- *Prefix denoting* 1. reduction or diminution. 2. rudimentary.

miosis (myosis) Constriction of the pupil of the eye. This occurs normally in bright light, but it may be induced by drugs (*miotics) or caused by damage to the sympathetic nerves of the head and neck, as in *Horner's syndrome.

miotic A drug that causes constriction of the pupil of the eye (miosis). *Parasympathomimetic drugs or *anticholinesterase drugs can be used to induce miosis. *Physostigmine, a reversible anticholinesterase, is used topically in the eye as a 0.5–1% solution and contracts the pupil for 12–24 hours, while *pilocarpine, a parasympathomimetic agent, is used topically at a concentration of 0.5–2% and miosis lasts for 12–24 hours. These drugs are used in the treatment of glaucoma to open the drainage angle in the eye and relieve intraocular pressure. Miotic drugs can be used after mydriasis (*see* mydriatic) to dilate and then constrict the pupil in order to break down adhesions between the iris and the cornea or lens.

miracidium (*pl.* **miracidia**) The first larval stage in the life cycle of a *fluke. It hatches from the egg, which passes out with the faeces of the primary host, and has a cylindrical body with cilia used for swimming. Before developing into a *sporocyst, it must find and enter the intermediate host, usually a snail. In some species the eggs are eaten by the snail and the miracidia hatch in the snail's gut. *See also* cercaria; redia.

miscarriage *See* abortion.

Misuse of Drugs Act (1971) *See* controlled drugs.

mite A small arachnid belonging to the order Acarina (*see* acarid), which also includes the *ticks. Mites are smaller than ticks but are otherwise similar although they lack the protective dorsal shield, the mouthparts are not modified for boring, and the legs often terminate in suckers for attachment or in sensory hairs. Many are bloodsucking ectoparasites of livestock, pets, and humans and are of considerable veterinary and economic importance. Their painful and irritating bites can cause loss of condition, while severe infestations of, for example, the *red mite (*Dermanyssus*), can cause anaemia and even death of poultry. Some, such as the scab mites (*Psoroptes*), the itch mite (*Sarcoptes*), and the follicle mite (*Demodex*) are responsible for often serious skin diseases, including *sheep scab and *mange (or scabies in humans). *Cnemidocoptes* is responsible for *scaly leg in poultry. Others, such as *Otodectes*, are found in the ears of dogs and cats, and the canine nasal mite inhabits the nasal passages of dogs.

Many mites live permanently on their hosts while others, such as *Dermanyssus*, feed only at night. Some are able to survive for several months without food if no suitable host is available thus making control difficult. In the harvest mite, *Trombicula*, only the larva is parasitic, the nymphs and adults being free living. Mites can be controlled by shearing or clipping the animal where appropriate and carefully dipping, spraying, washing, or shampooing with a solution of a suitable *acaricide. *Benzyl benzoate, organophosphorus, and sulphur preparations are commonly used to treat scaly leg and mange. However, resistance to a particular compound can develop. Beds, bedding, and animal houses must also be thoroughly cleaned and disinfected to ensure that all stages in the life cycle are eradicated.

mitochondrion (*pl.* **mitochondria**) A structure, occurring in varying numbers in the cytoplasm of every cell, that is the site of the cell's energy production. Mitochondria contain *ATP and the enzymes involved in the cell's metabolic activities; each is bounded by a double membrane, the inner being folded inwards to form projections (*cristae*).

mitogen Any substance that can cause cells to begin division (*mitosis).

mitosis (*pl.* **mitoses**) A type of cell division in which a single cell produces two genetically identical daughter cells. It is the way in which new body cells are produced for both growth and repair. Division of the nucleus (*karyokinesis*) takes place in four stages (*see* prophase; metaphase; anaphase; telophase) and is followed by division of the cytoplasm (*cytokinesis*) to form two daughter cells (see illustration). *Compare* meiosis.

mitral valve *See* bicuspid valve.

MMA (mastitis-metritis-agalactia syndrome) A syndrome affecting sows shortly after farrowing and involving inflammation of the udder (mastitis) and uterus (metritis), together with a lack of milk (agalactia). The incidence of MMA in a herd is variable: many sows may be affected over a short time or just an individual sow occasionally; it is very rare in outdoor units. Affected sows suckle their piglets normally for 12–24 hours after farrowing, but then show a decreased appetite and general lethargy with a raised body temperature. A vaginal discharge may be present, while the udder is usually hard and inflamed and the sow frequently lies on it, refusing access by piglets. Sow mortality is generally low but the agalactia leads to very high rates of piglet mortality due to *hypoglycaemia.

The causes are varied and include *endotoxins released by pathogenic bacteria, such as *Klebsiella* spp. and *Escherichia coli*. It is important to have clean farrowing pens; straw is better for bedding than wood shavings or sawdust as it is less easily contaminated. The condition is more common in old fat sows kept severely confined during pregnancy and fed on nutritionally inadequate diets. Stress factors seem to play a part, probably causing a hormonal imbalance. Treatment involves the use of antibiotics and hormones, such as *oxytocin and *corticosteroids, the aim being to establish lactation as soon as possible. Preventive measures involve reducing stress around the time of farrowing by moving sows into comfortable farrowing accommodation well before the expected date. Bran and/or oil can be given as a laxative, and sows should, if possible, be allowed some exercise in late pregnancy. Other name: **farrowing fever**.

Mokola virus A *rabies virus and member of the *lyssaviruses isolated from vertebrates.

molar Any of the rearmost teeth in the jaw. See dentition.

molluscicide An agent used to kill molluscs, particularly slugs and snails. Molluscicides are used in agriculture and horticulture to protect crops or to reduce populations of snails that act as intermediate hosts for parasites, for example the liver fluke (*Fasciola hepatica*) and the gastrointestinal nematode, *Strongyloides papillosus*. Copper sulphate, which is commonly used, persists for several months. Sheep are especially susceptible to *copper poisoning and should not be grazed on treated pasture for several months. Metaldehyde, which is used in slug bait, can cause poisoning in dogs and cats that consume the bait or in birds that consume dying molluscs (see metaldehyde poisoning). Methiocarb is also used as a molluscicide. Toxicity can occur in small animals, with signs including vomiting, diarrhoea, salivation, muscle tremors, miosis, convulsions, and bradycardia. Cases can be treated using *atropine.

molybdenosis (teart; peat scours) A toxic condition of grazing animals due to the ingestion of excessive amounts of molybdenum, which limits the absorption of copper in the presence of suphate. This occurs where the soil has a high molybdenum content (see teart soils) or where there is surface contamination by effluent from factories processing iron, aluminium, or oil. The main clinical sign is diarrhoea, which can be controlled by the administration of *copper, either orally or incorporated in licks.

molybdenum A metallic element that is a trace element (see essential element) required in animal diets. It functions as a *cofactor for certain enzymes, for example *xanthine oxidase. Ingestion of excessive amounts can give rise to the toxic condition *molybdenosis and can also lead to copper deficiency. Symbol Mo.

mon- (mono-) *Prefix denoting* one, single, or alone.

monensin See ionophore.

Moniezia A genus of large *tapeworms found worldwide and the commonest tapeworms of cattle and sheep. The adults live in the intestine, may reach 600 cm in length, and have broad proglottids, up to 2.6 cm wide. The intermediate host is an oribatid mite, which can occur in pastures. The mites are swallowed by grazing animals and the larval tapeworms emerge. The number of adults found in any individual is usually small and older stock develop resistance. However, infestations in lambs and calves may result in general debility and an impaired rate of growth. Treatment involves a course of *anthelmintics, and a grazing plan involving worm-free pastures will help in prevention.

Monilia A former name of the genus now known as *Candida*.

moniliasis A former term for disease caused by infection with yeasts now classified as species of *Candida*. *See* candidiasis.

monkshood poisoning *See* aconite poisoning.

monoblast A bone marrow precursor cell of the *monocyte line. *See* haemopoiesis.

monoclonal antibody A specific *antibody produced by one of numerous identical cells derived from a single parent cell. (The population of these cells comprises a *clone and each cell is said to be monoclonal.) The antibody-producing cells are specially prepared *lymphocytes, made by fusing a normal antibody-secreting lymphocyte with an actively dividing cell from a *myeloma, which also has a specific enzyme deficiency. The resultant hybrid cell (*hybridoma*) has the antibody-secreting properties of the lymphocyte and the multiplication potential of the myeloma. Under the particular culture conditions for hybridoma cells, unfused non-dividing lymphocytes and enzyme-deficient myeloma cells die and disappear from the culture: only the hybridoma cells survive and multiply. Single hybrid cells are cultured until they have multiplied to form a substantial clone of progeny cells. These monoclonal cultures are examined for the presence of antibody activity of interest. This may require the screening of many clones since the specificity of the secreted antibody is determined by the genes of the fused lymphocyte, and selection of the desired antibody is therefore a matter of chance. However, the chances of selection are improved if the antibody-secreting component of the hybridoma is taken from an animal immunized against the antigen in question (*see* lymphocyte). Hybridoma cells may be maintained in culture or in vivo.

Monoclonal antibodies are now widely used in diagnostic and research procedures where absolute specificity is required. Their potential as therapeutic agents, directed against specific antigens within the body, is also being explored.

monocular Relating to or used by one eye only. *Compare* binocular.

monocyte The blood-borne precursor of the *macrophage (*see* haemopoiesis).

monocytosis An abnormally high count of *monocytes in the blood. Like other forms of *leucocytosis, this condition tends to reflect infection or changes in hormone concentration. Most inflammatory diseases appear to raise the monocyte count at some period, but chronic infections, particularly tuberculosis and Johne's disease, are disorders associated with prolonged monocytosis. Corticosteroids influence monocyte counts, but the precise effect appears to vary with the species. *See also* avian monocytosis.

monophyletic Describing a number of individuals, species, etc., that have evolved from a single ancestral group. *Compare* polyphyletic.

monoplegia Paralysis of one side of the body or of one limb, usually caused by trauma to the nerve supplying the affected part. *Compare* hemiplegia; paraplegia.

monoploid *See* haploid.

monorchid An animal in which only one testis (testicle) develops. This is a rare condition, and results in reduced sperm density in the ejaculate compared to normal animals. The term is often used synonymously with *cryptorchid, in which the animal has two testicles but one (or both) may not have descended into the scrotum.

monosaccharide A simple sugar having the general formula $(CH_2O)_n$. Monosaccharides may have between three and nine carbon atoms, but the most common number is five or six. Monosaccharide sugars are classified according to the number of carbon atoms they possess. Thus *trioses* have three carbon atoms, *tetroses* four, *pentoses* five, and *hexoses* six. The most abundant monosaccharide is glucose (a hexose).

monosomy A condition in which there is one chromosome missing from the normal (*diploid) set. Such cells or individuals are described as monosomic. *Compare* trisomy.

monotocous Describing a species that normally produces a single foetus per pregnancy, for example cattle. *Compare* polytocous.

monozygotic twins *See* twins.

monster A foetus or newborn having gross deformities, often to the face and head. These may include *dicephalus* (duplication of the head), *diprosoplis* (duplication of the face), or *acephalia* (absence of the head). *Hydrocephalus is common, and there may be duplication and gross deformities to other parts of the body. Such deformities are not always immediately fatal, but postnatal survival is limited. The abnormalities are often due to changes in the chromosome complement of the individual. Other conditions that may occur in such individuals include *agnathia, brachygnathia, *chondrodysplasia, and *cleft palate.

moon blindness *See* periodic ophthalmia.

morantel A broad-spectrum anthelmintic, chemically related to *pyrantel, and available as the water-soluble morantel tartrate. It causes paralysis of nematodes and is administered orally to treat infestations of gastrointestinal nematode parasites. It is less efficacious against immature mucosal-dwelling parasites, and it has no activity against flukes, tapeworms, and lungworms, although lungworm larvae may be killed during passage through the gastrointestinal tract. Morantel is poorly absorbed from the gut and therefore has little host toxicity. It is available in a slow-release ruminal bolus (Paratect) to control gastrointestinal nematodes in cattle throughout the grazing season. Resistance of nematodes to morantel occurs, and cross-resistance with *levamisole is common.

Moraxella A genus of aerobic non-motile Gram-negative *bacteria, occurring singly, in pairs, or as short chains. They are strict parasites of the mucous membranes of animals, including humans. There are three known species: *M. lacunata* and *M. liquefaciens* cause conjunctivitis, arthritis, and endocarditis in humans; *M. bovis* causes *New Forest disease in cattle worldwide, the presence of flies helping to transmit infections from eye to eye.

morbid Diseased or abnormal; pathological.

morbidity 1. The state of being diseased. 2. The incidence of clinical cases of a disease in a given population. It is usually the number of clinically affected animals divided by the total number exposed to the same risk, expressed as a percentage.

morbillivirus A genus of the *paramyxovirus family. It includes the viruses responsible for *rinderpest in cattle and *distemper in dogs.

mordant (in microscopy) A substance, such as alum or phenol, used to fix a *stain in a tissue.

Morel's disease A suppurative disease of sheep reported from France and Kenya, clinically resembling *caseous lymphadenitis but caused by an unnamed Gram-positive micrococcoid bacterium.

moribund Dying.

morning glory poisoning A toxic condition caused by ingestion of seeds of the plant *Ipomoea purpurea*, which contain lysergic acid. The effects include disorientation, blurred vision, and dilated pupils and should be controlled by sedatives.

morphine A natural alkaloid that is a narcotic *analgesic. It is a *controlled drug, used as a painkiller, during anaesthesia, and to treat diarrhoea. Morphine is extracted from opium or from poppy straw because laboratory synthesis is difficult. It is a depressant of the central nervous system (CNS) that reduces the sensation of pain and produces sleep by acting at endorphin receptors on presynaptic neurones, thereby preventing the transmission of nerve impulses. Morphine is given orally or by intramuscular or subcutaneous injection, and begins to take effect after 15–30 minutes. It distributes well throughout the body and is metabolized by conjugation with glucuronide in the liver; excretion is in the urine. The actions of morphine on the cerebral cortex vary with species: in dogs, rabbits, birds, and humans there is CNS depression with analgesia and narcosis. In cattle, horses, and pigs CNS depression usually occurs, but there can be stimulation, particularly with high doses. In feline species high doses of morphine always cause CNS stimulation, with rage, mania, incoordination, and convulsions; lower doses may produce analgesia. In all species morphine causes depression of the respiratory centre, the cough centre, and the hypothalamus, thus reducing body temperature. There is stimulation then depression of the vomiting centre, and also vagal stimulation, leading to increased gastrointestinal peristalsis and defecation, followed by localized depression of peristalsis and an increase in sphincter tone, which causes constipation. Moreover, there is peripheral vasodilatation, which results in hypotension, and at high doses, spinal cord stimulation with convulsions.

Morphine is a potent analgesic and can be used in most species to reduce severe pain. It can also be used during anaesthesia to produce analgesia and permit a lighter plane of anaesthesia. Morphine is also given orally, usually in combination with kaolin, for its constipating effect in the treatment of diarrhoea. Overdosage with morphine causes profound coma, with respiratory depression, cyanosis, hypotension, a fall in body temperature, pulmonary oedema, and shock. The use of opiate antagonists (e.g. naloxone, nalorphine, and diprenorphine) can reverse the effects.

morpho- *Prefix denoting* form or structure.

morphogenesis The development of form and structure of the body and its parts.

morphology *See* anatomy.

-morphous *Suffix denoting* form or structure (of a specified kind).

mortality 1. The incidence of death in a population in a given period. 2. The case fatality rate: the incidence of death among animals affected by a particular disease or condition, expressed as a percentage.

Mortierella

Mortierella A genus of saprophytic fungi belonging to the order Mucorales of the class Zygomycetes, at least one of which (*M. wolfii*) can infect animals, causing *mucormycosis. *M. wolfii* is an important cause of *mycotic abortion in cattle.

morula (*pl.* **morulae**) An early stage of embryonic development formed as a result of *cleavage of the *zygote. It consists of a solid ball of cells and precedes formation of the *blastocyst.

mosaicism The phenomenon in which an organism consists of two genetically different cell types, both derived from the same *zygote. Such individuals arise by *mutation in a cell line during development. The most commonly encountered are *chromosome mosaics*, which have cell lines differing usually in chromosome number or, occasionally, in chromosome shape. Chromosome mosaics are usually aneuploid (*see* aneuploidy) in some of their cells and show, in a reduced form, the characteristics of organisms with aneuploidy affecting all their cells. Mosaics aneuploid for the sex chromosomes are most common. *See also* chimera.

mosquito A small, slender fly of the family Culicidae, distributed worldwide (see illustration). Mosquitoes have long legs and long narrow wings. The mouthparts form a long proboscis for piercing and sucking. Generally, the males feed on plant juices while the females suck the blood of birds and mammals; their saliva contains a powerful anticoagulant which prevents clotting of the host blood as they feed. The eggs are laid in water and hatch into actively swimming air-breathing larvae, which in turn develop into active pupae. Mosquitoes are abundant in the tropics throughout the year and in temperate regions in the summer. Most species are active after dark, shelter-

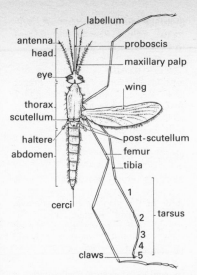

Anatomical details of a female mosquito
(*Anopheles maculipennis*)

ing in vegetation during the day. Their bite inflicts a painful wound, which can give rise to allergies. They transmit several serious diseases, such as *avian malaria, *dirofilariasis in dogs, *bluetongue in sheep, *equine encephalomyelitis, and malaria, yellow fever, and dengue in humans. Control measures can be aimed at the adults or the immature stages. The marshy areas favoured for breeding can be drained or the water sprayed with oil or paraffin thus preventing the eggs being laid or the larvae and pupae breathing; *insecticide sprays may also be used. Adults can be controlled by clearing vegetation or by spraying with insecticides. However, since mosquito populations can develop resistance to particular insecticides, the products used should be varied from time to time. Local populations can be eradicated by introducing natural parasites of mosquitoes, such as certain protozoans or bacteria. Less successful is the use of sterile male mosquitoes.

motile Being able to move spontaneously, without external aid: usually applied to a *microorganism or a cell (e.g. a spermatozoon).

motor cortex The region of the *cerebral cortex in the brain that is responsible for initiating nerve impulses that bring about voluntary activity in the muscles of the body. The motor cortex of the left cerebral hemisphere is responsible for muscular activity in the right side of the body.

motor nerve (efferent nerve) One of the nerves that carry impulses outwards from the central nervous system to bring about activity in a muscle or gland. *Compare* sensory nerve. *See also* motor neurone.

motor neurone (efferent neurone) A nerve cell that has its cell body in the brainstem or spinal cord and an axon that extends outwards in a cranial nerve or spinal nerve to reach an effector organ, such as a skeletal muscle. Such neurones are also termed *lower motor neurones*. An *upper motor neurone* has its cell body in the brain and an axon that forms synapses with lower motor neurones.

mould Any microscopic fungus that grows a visible matlike mass of *mycelium.

moulting 1. The periodic shedding of hair or fur in mammals, or of feathers in birds. **2.** The periodic shedding of the outer layer of the epidermis in reptiles, or of the cuticle in arthropods; also known as *ecdysis*.

mountain laurel *See* Kalmia poisoning.

mountain sickness A disorder of animals (including man) caused by the low oxygen availability at high altitudes. Livestock recently intro-duced to high altitudes suffer severely until adapted; some breeds, for example Friesian cattle, seem more susceptible than others. Mules are relatively unaffected and indigenous animals, such as llamas and alpacas, have evolved special types of haemoglobin with increased capacity for oxygen uptake. However, although cattle reared on high mountainsides adapt to the environment, they may suffer if an additional disorder, such as anaemia or low blood protein, is added to the metabolic burden. The lack of oxygen causes constriction of the pulmonary artery leading to hypoxic pulmonary hypotension. This results in *cor pulmonale*: characteristic clinical signs include overbreathing and rapid pulse with oedema of the brisket (hence 'brisket disease'). Advanced cases show accumulation of abdominal fluid (ascites) with diarrhoea. Long-term effects involve congestive heart failure with degenerative lesions in the liver and lung.

Movement of Animals (Records) Order (1960) (England and Wales) A Parliamentary Order requiring that farmers and others who move livestock must keep adequate up-to-date written records, which may be inspected by officers of the local authority or Ministry of Agriculture Fisheries and Food. The Order enables in-contact animals to be traced following an outbreak of contagious disease.

MSH *See* melanocyte-stimulating hormone.

MSHIH *See* melanocyte-stimulating-hormone-inhibiting hormone.

mucilage A highly viscous aqueous solution of various gums, such as acacia, calcium or sodium alginate, starch, and tragacanth. Mucilages can be used as carriers for insoluble drugs. They are also used as water-miscible bases for skin preparations, as binding agents in the manufacture of tablets, or as surgical lubricants, for example in obstetrics.

mucin A *glycoprotein and the principal constituent of *mucus.

muco- *Prefix denoting* 1. mucus. 2. mucous membrane.

mucolytic An agent that reduces the viscosity of mucus. Mucolytics are used in the treatment of respiratory disease to facilitate the removal of accumulations of debris and mucus from the airways. The principal agents are acetylcysteine and *bromhexine. Acetylcysteine is used as a 20% solution instilled into the airways or as an aerosol produced in a *nebulizer. It causes liquefaction of mucus and pus with no effect on blood or living tissue. Treatments should be repeated every 2–4 hours. There may be local irritation with some bronchoconstriction. Another mucolytic, trans-4-[(3,5-dibromo-2- hydroxybenzyl)amino]cyclohexanol hydrochloride monohydrate, is marketed as Sputolosin and is now available for injection or oral administration.

mucopolysaccharide An obsolete term for a *proteoglycan.

mucoprotein An obsolete term for a *glycoprotein.

mucopurulent Containing *mucus and *pus.

mucopus A mixture of *mucus and *pus.

Mucor A genus of saprophytic fungi that sometimes occur as opportunistic pathogens in cases of *mucormycosis.

mucormycosis Any disease caused by infection with a fungus belonging to the order Mucorales; i.e. a type of

*phycomycosis. These opportunistically pathogenic fungi include several species of the genera *Mucor, *Rhizopus, *Absidia, and *Mortierella, which occur worldwide as saprophytes in soil and moist rotting organic material. Sporadic infections have been reported in a wide variety of animal hosts, most often as nodular granulomatous lesions involving lymph nodes or visceral organs but rarely producing clinical signs until swellings become visible or the animal wastes.
In **cattle**, the host most affected, these fungi are important chiefly as a cause of *mycotic abortion. Infection by *Mortierella wolfii*, reported occasionally in Britain and elsewhere, is in parts of New Zealand the most prevalent cause of bovine mycotic placentitis, leading not only to abortion but often to a subsequent and often fatal infection of the maternal lungs. Saprophytic growth occurs in wet rotten hay and alkaline layers of silage. Less frequent in cattle are mucormycotic ulcers of the rumen and abomasum. Caseocalcareous lesions in lymph nodes of the respiratory or intestinal tract and, occasionally, other organs are sometimes seen in carcasses at the abattoir. Mucormycotic mastitis can occur but is rare. **Pigs** are occasionally subject to gastric ulceration or granulomatous nodular lesions caused by mucoraceous fungi. A few affected animals have been treated with antifungal drugs, such as *amphotericin B, but with little success.
The term *zygomycosis encompasses mucormycosis, and is increasingly being used in preference to the latter, especially in North America.

mucosa (*pl.* **mucosae** or **mucosas**) *See* mucous membrane.

mucosal disease An acute usually fatal disease of cattle characterized by ulceration of the intestine and caused by *pestivirus. Up to 1% of cattle may be persistent carriers of the virus responsible for *bovine virus diarrhoea (BVD). If these animals are infected with a second strain of the same virus, they develop mucosal disease. This involves extensive erosions of the intestine resulting in severe, often fatal, diarrhoea. There is no effective treatment.

mucous membrane (mucosa) The moist layer of tissue lining many hollow organs, such as the respiratory tract and alimentary canal. The mucous membrane consists of a surface layer of epithelium, which contains glands secreting *mucus, with underlying layers of connective tissue (lamina propria) and muscularis mucosae, which forms the inner boundary of the mucous membrane.

mucus A viscous fluid secreted by *mucous membranes in many parts of the body, including the mouth, bronchial passages, and gut. Mucus acts as a protective barrier over the surfaces of the membranes, as a lubricant, and as a carrier of enzymes. It consists chiefly of *glycoproteins, particularly *mucin*, which are responsible for its viscosity.

mulberry heart disease Degeneration of heart muscle in pigs caused by *selenium or *vitamin E deficiency. The disease, though sporadic, is acute with rapid onset and affects fast-growing pigs. Death occurs suddenly and may be precipitated by exercise. The characteristic heart lesion involves a distended pericardial sac containing fluid, and extensive haemorrhages in the myocardium. Prevention is by dietary supplementation of selenium or vitamin E.

multi- *Prefix denoting* many; several.

multiple vaccine A vaccine given in a single inoculation but conferring immunity against two or more diseases. Routine vaccination of dogs usually involves multiple vaccines and may include vaccines against *leptospirosis, *distemper, *canine adenovirus, and *canine parvovirus. *Compare* polyvalent vaccine.

multipolar (in neurology) Describing a neurone that has many processes radiating from the cell body. *Compare* bipolar; unipolar.

mummification The process whereby a foetus dies within the uterus, *autolysis occurs without putrefaction, and the remaining shrivelled mass of bones is usually enclosed in wrinkled brown skin. The cervix is thought to remain closed allowing no discharge and months usually pass before the mummified foetus is discovered. Such retention is the exception, since a dead foetus is usually dealt with in the manner of a foreign body with consequent expulsion of the uterine contents. The absence of microorganisms is thought to increase the chance of mummification. The process is known to occur in most domestic species.

murmur A noise, heard with the aid of a stethoscope, that is generated by turbulent blood flow within the heart or blood vessels. Turbulent flow is produced by damaged valves, septal defects, narrowed arteries, or arteriovenous communications. Murmurs may be classified as *systolic* or *diastolic* (heard during *systole or *diastole respectively), or *continuous* (heard throughout both systole and diastole).

muscarinic 1. Describing a division of receptors in the peripheral nervous system that are stimulated by the alkaloid muscarine. Muscarine acts at postganglionic receptors in the *parasympathetic nervous system, and causes vasodilatation, salivation, bronchoconstriction, gastrointestinal stimulation, and reduced heart rate. **2.**

Of muscarine or its pharmacological effects.

muscle A tissue whose cells have the ability to contract, producing movement or force. Muscles possess mechanisms for converting energy derived from chemical reactions into mechanical energy. The major functions of muscles are to produce movements of the body, to maintain the position of the body against the force of gravity, to produce movements of structures inside the body. There are three types of muscle: *striated muscle, attached to the skeleton; *smooth muscle, which is found in such tissues as the stomach, gut, and blood vessels; and *cardiac muscle, which forms the walls of the heart.

muscle relaxant An agent that produces relaxation of skeletal muscle. The *neuromuscular blocking drugs* act at the neuromuscular junction. They can be subdivided into *depolarizing* and *nondepolarizing* or *competitive* agents. The depolarizing agents, such as *suxamethonium (succinylcholine) and decamethonium, cause initial muscle twitching followed by, in most species, flaccid paralysis, or, in birds, spastic paralysis. These agents are used to improve muscle relaxation during surgery, and are administered in combination with anaesthetics since they have no analgesic properties themselves. They have been used with *dart syringes to capture wild animals but this is no longer recommended for humane reasons. They initially affect muscles controlling fine movements (e.g. facial muscles, neck muscles, muscles at the extremities) then swallowing muscles, abdominal muscles, intercostal muscles, and the diaphragm. Facilities for positive-pressure ventilation must be available. The nondepolarizing agents include d-tubocurarine, *gallamine triethiodide, and *pancuronium. Their actions can be reversed using *anticholinesterase

drugs (e.g. edrophonium and neo-stigmine).
Centrally acting muscle relaxants act on the central nervous system. The only drug used clinically in animals is *glyceryl guaiacolate.

muscle spindle A specialized receptor, sensitive to stretch, that is embedded between and parallel to the fibres of striated muscles. These receptors are important for coordinated muscular movement. *See also* stretch receptor.

muscular dystrophy Any of a group of diseases involving degeneration of muscles. Many are caused by deficiencies in the intake or metabolism of *selenium and/or *vitamin E, although *paralytic myoglobinuria is a severe form resulting from strenuous exercise or the ingestion of toxic substances. Muscular dystrophy is common in calves and lambs whose mothers receive selenium-deficient diets during gestation. The affected muscle is pale and may have white striations due to calcification of necrotic muscle fibres (*see* white muscle disease). Congenital muscular dystrophy may cause sudden death a few days after birth where there is extensive degeneration of the heart muscle. Surviving animals will remain affected if the dietary deficiency persists, and skeletal muscle becomes involved. Patients move stiffly, become recumbent, and eventually die because they stop eating. Diagnosis can be confirmed by determining the levels of the enzymes glutathione peroxidase (for selenium deficiency) and creatine phosphokinase (for evidence of muscle degeneration) in the blood. The feed of reproducing animals and their offspring should contain adequate levels of selenium and vitamin E but not exceeding 0.1 ppm selenium to avoid toxicity. Extremely careful mixing is vital to ensure uniformity of intake and avoid the risk of accidental poisoning.

Nutritional myopathy is a form of muscular dystrophy recognized in older animals. There are two possible causes. Firstly, certain additives used to preserve ensiled cereals destroy vitamin E. The resulting deficiency is only partially resolved by selenium supplementation. Secondly, some pastures are selenium deficient and induce deficiency in the grazing animals. Vitamin E and selenium have complementary metabolic roles in preventing the accumulation of toxic peroxides at the surfaces of cell membranes. Thus deficiency of one cannot be entirely counteracted by adding supplements of the other. Surveys using the glutathione peroxidase test show that selenium deficiency is widespread and that subclinical nutritional myopathy is a common limiting factor to optimal growth and production.

In **poultry**, muscular dystrophy is especially common in turkey poults. It typically occurs with diets low in cysteine and methionine (*see* amino acid) and can be treated and prevented by dietary vitamin E supplementation. The condition is often associated with *exudative diathesis.

muscularis A muscular layer of the wall of a hollow organ (such as the stomach) or a tubular structure (such as the intestine or ureter). The *muscularis mucosae* is the muscular layer of a mucous membrane complex, especially that of the stomach or intestine.

musculo- *Prefix denoting* muscle.

musculocutaneous nerve One of the nerves of the forelimb extending from the *brachial plexus. It carries motor fibres to the biceps brachii and brachialis muscles and sensory fibres from the medial side of the lower forelimb.

mushy chick disease *See* omphalitis.

mustard A compound obtained from the dried seeds of *Brassica alba* (white mustard) or *B. nigra* (black mustard). Mustard contains allyl isothiocyanate as well as other acids and oils. It is irritant to epithelial cells and acts as an *emetic when given orally and as a *rubefacient when applied to skin. *Nitrogen mustards*, a group of organic compounds developed from mustard gas (dichlorodiethyl sulphide), destroy lymphoid tissue and are used in the treatment of lymphoid neoplasia and leukaemia.

mustard poisoning *See* brassica poisoning.

mutant 1. An individual in which a mutation has occurred, especially when the effect of the mutation is visible. **2.** A characteristic showing the effects of a mutation.

mutation A change in the genetic material (*DNA) of a cell resulting in either new or rearranged hereditary determinants. A *point mutation* involves a change in one nucleotide of the DNA, which frequently produces a change in one allele of one gene; a *chromosome mutation* involves a change in the structure or number of the chromosomes. Mutations are rare in nature, and occur as a result of mistakes in the replication or distribution of the genes and chromosomes. The frequency of mutations may be increased by external factors (*mutagens*), but the process is always random and it cannot be directed. A mutation in developing sex cells (gametes) can be inherited; mutations in other cells (*somatic mutations*) are not inherited. *See also* deletion; inversion (def. 2); translocation.

mutter pea poisoning *See* lathyrism.

mutualism An interaction between two species in which both species benefit. (The term *symbiosis* is often used synonymously.)

muzzle 1. The snout: the rostral projecting portion of an animal's head. **2.** Apparatus designed to prevent an animal from biting or employed to ensure that an animal does not eat or drink for a period, for example in preparation for the administration of a general anaesthetic.

my- (myo-) *Prefix denoting* muscle.

myalgia (myodynia) Pain arising from muscle tissue.

myasthenia gravis A rare *autoimmune disease of dogs in which the muscles of the body rapidly become fatigued on exercise. It is due to a failure in the mechanism of the neuromuscular junction. Diagnosis can be confirmed by a rapid response to *neostigmine, which can also be given orally to treat the condition.

myc- (myco-, mycet(o)-) *Prefix denoting* a fungus.

mycelium (*pl.* **mycelia**) A network of intertwining often branching filaments (*hyphae) that forms the body of a fungus. *Aerial mycelia* may project above the surface on which the fungus is growing and include reproductive hyphae, which bear the spore-forming structures. The *vegetative mycelium* penetrates the substrate and anchors the fungus to the surface; it contains feeding hyphae. These may form part of a large complex firm or hard structure, such as the fruiting body of a mushroom, composed entirely of densely packed mycelial cells.

mycetoma A swelling caused by a localized chronic infection with a bacterium or a fungus and characterized by pus containing compact masses of the causal organism ('grains' or 'granules' up to 2–3 mm diameter), which is discharged through one or more sinus tracts formed when the lesion ruptures to the surface. Usually subcutaneous in origin and introduced via a wound, the infection very rarely disseminates but extends slowly and inexorably into adjacent tissues. Two main types of mycetoma are distinguished: *actinomycotic mycetomas*, caused by filamentous actinomycete bacteria; and *eumycotic mycetomas*, caused by mycelial *fungi. The former often respond to appropriate drug therapy, whereas surgical excision is the only likely cure for the latter and recurrence is common unless the mycetoma removed was small. The colour (white, yellow, red, brown, or black) and microscopic characteristics of grains often indicate the identity of the particular organism involved, which can then be firmly established by growth in culture. Mycetomas are prevalent in humans in some countries (e.g. regions of Africa), but reported cases in animals are few, mostly in dogs in the USA.

Mycobacterium A genus of aerobic or *microaerophilic pleomorphic non-motile Gram-positive *bacteria widely distributed in nature. They appear as straight or curved rods or as filaments, which break up into cocci or rods. Many live in the soil, water, and on plants or as animal saprophytes but a few are pathogenic to animals, including humans. They vary in their resistance to chemical and physical agents and their rate of growth; some produce pigments when exposed to light.
M. tuberculosis is the main cause of human *tuberculosis but can also affect animals. The infections are usually acquired by inhalation and the lesions are found in the lungs. Ingestion, particularly of infected milk, is also a source of infection of young

animals. *M. bovis* also causes tuberculosis, usually in cattle and other animals but also in humans, while *M. avium* causes the disease principally in birds and occasionally in pigs and cattle. *M. paratuberculosis* causes the chronic intestinal disease known as *Johne's disease in cattle, sheep, and goats, while *M. lepraemurium* causes a disease similar to human leprosy in cats and rats.

mycology The scientific study of fungi.

Mycoplasma (pleuropneumonia-like organism; PPLO) A genus of minute pleomorphic Gram-negative prokaryotic organisms, classified as bacteria but differing from other bacteria in not having a cell wall. They have cell diameters in the range 200–300 nm, and were long confused with the *viruses because they can pass through fine filters – they are frequent and troublesome contaminants of animal cell cultures. All are parasitic on plants or animals and a number are pathogenic (*see* mycoplasmosis).

The closely related genus, *Acholeplasma*, has no members of proven pathogenicity.

mycoplasmal arthritis Any of a group of related diseases, caused by infection with any species of *Mycoplasma*, in which the principal manifestations are *arthritis, *polyarthritis, or *synovitis. In cattle the most frequent cause of outbreaks is *M. bovis*, and the condition may be accompanied by mastitis (*see* mycoplasmal mastitis) or pneumonia. *M. capricola* has been incriminated in arthritis of goats. *M. hyosynoviae* causes arthritis with sudden lameness and joint swellings in young pigs; *M. hyorhinis* is also associated with porcine arthritis, sometimes together with *polyserositis (*see also* enzootic pneumonia of pigs). Mycoplasmal arthritis responds poorly to antibiotic therapy. *See also* infectious synovitis of poultry.

mycoplasmal mastitis An acute interstitial or suppurative *mastitis of cows, usually spreading to all four quarters of the udder and accompanied by fever and sometimes lameness. It is caused by *Mycoplasma bovis* and various other *Mycoplasma* species (including *M. alkalescens*, *M. bovigenitalium*, *M. bovirhinis*, *M. canadense*, and *M. californicum*). Both sporadic cases and outbreaks occur. None of the antibiotics commonly used for mastitis is very effective. *Compare* contagious agalactia.

mycoplasmosis Disease due to infection with a species of *Mycoplasma*. Mycoplasmosis in animals generally involves the respiratory tract, joints, serous membranes, or mammary gland. *Mycoplasma* species have an established causal role in *contagious bovine pleuropneumonia (*M. mycoides* subsp. *mycoides*), *contagious caprine pleuropneumonia (*M. mycoides* subsp. *capri*), *contagious agalactia of sheep and goats (*M. agalactiae*), *enzootic pneumonia of pigs (*M. hyopneumoniae*), *mycoplasmal arthritis (*M. hyosynoviae*), avian mycoplasmosis (*M. gallisepticum*), *infectious synovitis of poultry (*M. synoviae*), *mycoplasmal mastitis (*M. bovis*), and *air sacculitis in turkeys (*M. meleagridis*). A number of mycoplasmas are of low pathogenicity alone, but participate in a variety of microbial infections of which they are not the primary cause; others occur as harmless inhabitants of the mucous membranes, including that of the upper respiratory tract.

mycosis (*pl.* **mycoses**) Any disease caused by a fungal infection. Only a small minority of fungi are capable of infecting animals, and many of these are primarily saprophytes living in the

mycotic abortion

soil or rotting organic material. Very few fungi are primary pathogens capable of initiating and maintaining infection in an entirely healthy host (e.g. *coccidioidomycosis), and few mycoses are contagious (e.g. *dermatophytosis, *epizootic lymphangitis).

Mycoses can be classified broadly according to the usual site of infection: for example, *cutaneous mycoses*, which are most often caused in animals by *dermatophyte fungi; *subcutaneous mycoses*, which are usually caused when a fungus is implanted into a wound and develops at the site of inoculation (e.g. *sporotrichosis); and *systemic* (*deep* or *visceral*) *mycoses*. The latter may be caused by either primary pathogens from the soil, usually entering via the lungs (e.g. *histoplasmosis), or *opportunistic fungi that require some predisposing factor or defect in the host's normal resistance to enable them to establish infection (e.g. *aspergillosis).

mycotic abortion Abortion caused by a noncontagious fungal infection (mycosis) of the placenta, which sometimes spreads to the foetus. The disease occurs in many parts of the world, commonly in cattle, occasionally in horses, and rarely in other species. Many different placental mycoses are associated with abortion; by far the commonest is *aspergillosis, followed by *mucormycosis. The primary source of infection is mouldy fodder or bedding, and the disease is most prevalent among housed cattle. Ingested or inhaled fungal spores are thought to enter the bloodstream to be carried to the caruncles on the wall of the gravid uterus to which the placenta is attached. Here they germinate and develop into a *mycelium, which progressively invades the placenta. Most abortions occur in the last 3 months of pregnancy, often before the whole placenta is affected. In a minority of cases mycelial growth extends into the amniotic fluid, enters the lumen of the foetal stomach, and sometimes invades foetal tissues; occasionally, skin lesions are visible on the foetus. With the exception of *Mortierella wolfii*, fungal invasion appears to remain confined to the uterus and its contents, elicits no diagnostic signs before abortion, and is eliminated spontaneously soon after abortion. Diagnosis is made by microscopic demonstration of the mycelial invasion of affected tissues. Occurrence of the disease may be minimized by avoiding the use of mouldy material, particularly within buildings housing pregnant animals.

mycotic dermatitis A skin disease of ruminants caused by the filamentous bacterium *Dermatophilus congolensis* (*see* dermatophilosis). In sheep, the severity and persistence of lesions vary with the breed and country. Most prevalent in periods of prolonged wet weather, the disease is widespread among sheep in many parts of Britain, though relatively mild and affecting mostly close-woolled breeds. Exudate containing the bacteria accumulates at the base of the staple immediately above active lesions and binds it together as a firm mass. Chronic lesions build up over several months as large hard conical masses of this material; this is characteristic of *lumpy wool, the form of the disease seen mostly among some types of Merino sheep in Australia. When acute lesions resolve spontaneously, the exudate remains as a discrete layer moving outward from the skin as the fleece grows. Subsequent transient infections can produce a succession of layers. Moisture stimulates the release of motile infective zoospores from this material. The infection is then highly contagious among wet sheep, lambs often developing lesions initially on the face and ears, presumably as a result of contact with the dam when wet. Subsequent spread along the back and down the flanks appears to follow the pattern of greatest rain penetration and drainage through the fleece. The disease may spread through a flock unnoticed until severe enough to cause obvious wool loss or until shearing. An acute, often fatal, infection, extending over much of the body surface of lambs, occurs very rarely in Britain and has been reported in Australian outbreaks. The repeated application of potassium aluminium sulphate as a powder or dip has been advocated as a means of immobilizing the zoospores and controlling spread of the disease.

In **cattle**, affected animals develop a skin eruption with extensive exudation and scab formation. The disease is most severe in tropical Africa, where the incidence is highest during the rainy season due to the greater activity of ticks and small biting flies, which spread the disease. Deaths occur through debilitation and secondary bacterial infections, and the hides are damaged. A milder form occurs sporadically in temperate countries. Treatment with antibiotics administered systemically (penicillin, tetracycline) or topically (chloramphenicol) is possible, but usually impracticable in large cattle herds.

A similar disease, known as *rain scald, occurs in horses.

mycotic mastitis *Mastitis caused by a fungal infection. Yeasts, often *Candida* spp., are usually responsible, but several filamentous fungi, including species of Aspergillus and *Absidia*, occasionally cause a localized mammary infection. The most serious, albeit rare, form of yeast mastitis is caused by Cryptococcus neoformans (see cryptococcosis).

Affected cows show a dramatic and often permanent drop in milk yield, and the infection persists and spreads within a herd over a period of many months. Other yeast infections tend to be sporadic and self limiting, inflaming the gland for a week or so but resolving spontaneously over the ensuing month, although sometimes the yeast persists in the milk. Infections by filamentous fungi are often more severe and persistent, producing a marked induration (hardening) that may slowly resolve into localized nodular lesions.

The usual cause appears to be the accidental introduction into the mammary gland of fungal spores or yeast cells. Often the disease is identified after the injection of antibiotics via the teat canal. This may be due to contaminated preparations or inadequate hygiene during the procedure. Insufficient care and cleanliness in milking may have a similar result. The fungi often occur as saprophytes in the environment. For example, brewers grains can develop a dense population of these organisms if badly stored. In all types of mycotic mastitis specific treatment is of doubtful value.

mycotoxicosis Any of a diversity of toxic conditions caused by the ingestion of *mycotoxins produced by various *fungi. These toxins may be contained in a part of the fungus that is inadvertently eaten, as in *toadstool poisoning, *ergot poisoning, or *facial eczema; or they may be produced by fungal growth in or on crops before or after harvest, or in compound feeds during storage, as in *lupinosis, *fusariotoxicosis, and *aflatoxicosis. Mycotoxins are best discovered and quantified by specific chemical tests, for which adequate sampling is essential.

mycotoxin Any substance produced by a *fungus that causes disease (i.e. *mycotoxicosis) when eaten by an animal. Mycotoxins are among the many fungal products known as *secondary metabolites* – they have no obvious vital metabolic function for the organism. Production of any particular mycotoxin is often restricted to one or a few closely related species of *mould, and may occur only in a very limited range of conditions. *Compare* antibiotic.

mydriasis Marked dilatation (widening) of the pupil of the eye. Mydriasis accompanies some ocular abnormalities, especially those involving impaired vision, and is also seen in some diseases of the central nervous system. *See also* mydriatic.

mydriatic A drug that causes dilatation of the pupil in the eye (mydriasis). Mydriatics are used in diagnostic ophthalmology to allow examination of the eye, prior to surgery of the eye, to test for glaucoma, to treat anterior uveitis, and to reduce adhesions in the eye. The parasympatholytic agents *atropine, homatropine, and hyoscine act as mydriatics. Homatropine is preferred because of its shorter duration of action. When used topically in the eye homatropine causes mydriasis lasting for 1–2 days, whereas with atropine the effect can last for 1 week. Other agents include cyclopentolate and tropicamide, which are used topically in the eye. Tropicamide acts for 2–8 hours and cyclopentolate for 4–12 hours. Use of mydriatics causes blurred vision and with overdosage can cause reduced salivary secretion, thirst, ataxia, and stimulation of the central nervous system.

myel- (myelo-) *Prefix denoting* **1.** the spinal cord. **2.** bone marrow. **3.** myelin.

myelin A complex material formed of protein and *phospholipid that is laid down as a sheath around the *axons of certain neurones, known as *myelinated* (or *medullated*) *nerve fibres*. The material is produced and laid down in concentric layers by

*neurolemmal cells at regular intervals along the nerve fibre. Myelinated nerve fibres conduct impulses more rapidly than nonmyelinated fibres.

myelinated (medullated) nerve fibre Any nerve fibre that has a sheath of *myelin surrounding and insulating its axon.

myelination The process in which *myelin is laid down as an insulating layer around the axons of certain neurones.

myelitis 1. Inflammation of the bone marrow. When adjoining bone is also affected the term *osteomyelitis is used. **2.** An inflammatory disease of the spinal cord. It often has serious consequences and may lead to paralysis. *See also* encephalomyelitis.

myeloblast An early bone-marrow precursor cell that is the ancestor of all the *granulocyte series (*see* haemopoiesis).

myelocyte An early bone-marrow precursor cell in the *granulocyte series, more differentiated than the *myeloblast, in which characteristic neutrophilic, eosinophilic, or basophilic granulation is evident (*see* haemopoiesis).

myelofibrosis Replacement of the blood-forming elements in the bone marrow with fibrous tissue. It is seen occasionally in *myeloid leukaemia.

myelography A specialized radiographic technique for examining the vertebral column. Radiographs (*myelograms*) are taken of the spinal column after injection of a radio-opaque contrast material into the subarachnoid space under general anaesthesia. The contrast material passes along the subarachnoid space aided by gravity. The technique enables areas of cord compression to be seen; these can be due to space-occupying lesions (e.g. neoplasms) or intervertebral disc protrusions.

myeloid Like, derived from, or relating to bone marrow.

myeloid leukaemia A form of *leukaemia involving malignant transformation of one of the nonlymphocyte cell lines of the bone marrow, such as red blood cells, granulocytes (i.e. neutrophils, eosinophils, and basophils), monocytes, or platelets. It is rare in most species but is relatively more common in the cat, and in many species it is associated with a *retrovirus infection (e.g. *feline leukaemia virus).

Chronic myeloid leukaemia is a slowly proliferative disease characterized by the laboratory finding of large numbers of mature cells of the affected series. Clinically the disease may present as a chronic nonspecific illness, and in some cases is an incidental finding with no related clinical signs. Treatment is aimed at controlling the cell proliferation but the prognosis is guarded. *Acute myeloid leukaemia* has a rapid clinical course, again with nonspecific clinical signs, such as intermittent fever, inappetence, weight loss, joint pain, and muscular stiffness. Overwhelming infection, severe anaemia, or uncontrollable diffuse haemorrhage occur in the terminal stages. The finding of large numbers of immature neoplastic cells of the affected line in the bone marrow and, less commonly, in the peripheral blood is diagnostic. Response to treatment is poor and the prognosis is grave.

myeloid leukosis *See* avian leukosis.

myeloid tissue A tissue in the *bone marrow in which the various classes of blood cells are produced. *See also* haemopoiesis.

myeloma A malignant tumour of plasma cells, specifically activated B-*lymphocytes, usually with associated high blood levels of an immunoglobulin. It occurs as a rare tumour in most species, usually arising from within a bone, especially the vertebrae, pelvis, skull, and limb bones, and often at multiple sites. Clinical signs are due either to the local effects of a bone tumour, i.e. pain or fracture, or to the effects of high circulating levels of immunoglobulins, which produce a hyperviscosity syndrome involving bruising, nose bleeds, and gastrointestinal bleeding; severe neurological disorders may also occur. Treatment with cytotoxic drugs may achieve good periods of remission. Other names: **plasma cell tumour**; **plasmacytoma**.

myelomalacia A pathological softening of the structure of the spinal cord. This often occurs in *myelitis.

myeloproliferative Describing any of a wide group of diseases arising from any of the various components of the bone marrow. The term embraces the nonlymphoid dysplasias and neoplasias, including *myeloid leukaemia (acute and chronic), thrombocythaemia (platelet leukaemia), polycythaemia (red-cell leukaemia), myelodysplasia, and myelofibrosis.

myenteric plexus The nerve plexus of the *autonomic nervous system found within the *muscularis of tubular organs.

myiasis Parasitism of living tissue by *fly larvae. The best-known example is *strike, in which larvae of the *green-bottle fly hatch in wet soiled wool of sheep. Other examples include the parasitism of nasal passages by larvae of the *sheep nostril fly; parasitism of the intestine or urinary bladder of humans and other animals by the rat-tailed larvae of

myo-

Eristalis tenax; parasitism of the skin by *warble-fly larvae; and parasitism of the stomach and intestine by *horse bot larvae.

myo- *Prefix. See* my-.

myoblast A cell that develops into a muscle fibre.

myocardial infarction Death of a segment of heart muscle, which develops due to a sudden localized interruption in blood supply. Although of major importance and a frequent cause of death in humans, where it is associated with arteriosclerotic narrowing of the lumens of arteries, myocardial infarction is rare in domestic animals.

myocarditis Inflammation of the heart muscle (myocardium). It is nearly always secondary to other disease, which may be local or systemic. Local inflammation of the pericardium or endocardium may extend to the myocardium, while many systemic infections may spread via the blood to the myocardium and produce focal suppurative, necrotic, or even tuberculous lesions, depending on the organism involved. Focal lesions are found in association with bacterial infections by species of *Listeria*, *Shigella*, *Clostridium*, *Fusiformis*, and *Mycobacterium*; with viral infections, such as foot-and-mouth disease, bluetongue, Coxsackie, and canine parvovirus; and with parasitisms, such as cysticercosis and toxoplasmosis. The myocardium may also undergo a distinct and more diffuse form of inflammation, characterized by the appearance of mononuclear cells in the interstitial tissue. This is usually associated with inflammatory or hypersensitive disorders elsewhere. An eosinophilic myocarditis of unknown cause occurs in cattle.

myocardium The middle of the three layers forming the wall of the heart. Lying between the *endocardium and the *epicardium, it is composed of *cardiac muscle and forms the greater part of the heart wall, being thicker in the ventricles than in the atria.

myoclonia A disorder, characterized by spasmodic twitching, due to periodic involuntary contractions of skeletal muscle alternating with periods of relaxation.

myocyte A muscle cell.

myodynia *See* myalgia.

myoepithelium A tissue consisting of cells of epithelial origin having a contractile cytoplasm. Myoepithelial cells play an important role in the passage of substances into ducts. They occur, for example, in mammary glands and salivary glands.

myofibril One of numerous contractile filaments found within the cytoplasm of *striated muscle cells. When viewed under a microscope myofibrils show alternating bands of high and low refractive index, which give striated muscle its characteristic appearance.

myogenic Originating in muscle: applied to the inherent rhythmicity of contraction of some muscles (e.g. cardiac muscle), which does not depend on neural influences.

myoglobin A *porphyrin-containing protein, found in muscle cells. It acts as an oxygen reservoir within the muscle fibres by accepting oxygen from *haemoglobin. It is released into the blood when muscles are damaged (*see* paralytic myoglobinuria).

myoglobinuria The presence of *myoglobin in the urine. The urine appears dark-red and, to the naked eye, is indistinguishable from urine containing haemoglobin (*see* haemoglobinuria), although the two conditions can be differentiated by laboratory tests. Myoglobinuria is seen in conditions where there is sudden extensive damage to skeletal muscle in mature animals, such as *azoturia in horses and capture myopathy in wild animals. Probably because of the relatively low content of myoglobin in the skeletal muscles of calves and lambs, myoglobinuria is not a feature of *white muscle disease in these young animals. Serious kidney damage is a possible sequel to myoglobinuria: the presence of large casts of myoglobin in the renal tubules may cause anoxic death of the tubular cells.

myogram A recording of the activity of a muscle. *See* electromyography.

myograph An instrument for recording the activity of muscular tissues. *See* electromyography.

myoma A benign tumour of muscle. It may originate in smooth muscle (*see* leiomyoma) or in striated muscle (*see* rhabdomyoma).

myometritis Inflammation of the *myometrium – the muscular components of the uterine wall. This is usually part of a generalized *metritis (inflammation of the entire uterine wall from endometrial lining to the serosal layers). Most uterine infections are a result of pathogenic organisms entering via the vagina from the exterior and occur at oestrus (heat) or just after parturition when the cervix is open. Therefore myometritis rarely occurs without concurrent *endometritis. However, some organisms are spread in the bloodstream, for example those causing tuberculosis. These may cause *granulomata within the muscular septa of the myometrium,

usually as metastases from a primary lesion elsewhere.

myometrium (*pl.* **myometria**) The muscular layer of the wall of the *uterus. It is composed of smooth muscle that undergoes spontaneous contractions. The frequency and amplitude of these contractions is altered by the hormones *oestrogen and *progesterone, and by *oxytocin, especially during *parturition.

myopathy Any disorder or disease of muscle, especially skeletal or cardiac muscle. However, the term usually refers to noninflammatory disease (*compare* myositis). Myopathies may be of nutritional, toxic, exertional, or traumatic origin, and are common in domestic animals. Among the more important is *white muscle disease, a nutritional myopathy in ruminants associated with inadequate dietary levels of vitamin E and/or selenium. Similar dietary deficiencies are thought to be responsible for the pig diseases *mulberry heart and hepatosis dietica. The exertional myopathies include *azoturia (tying-up syndrome) in horses, *porcine stress syndrome, and capture myopathy in wild animals. Substances that exert a direct toxic effect on muscle include monensin (*see* ionophore), a common feed additive which may, if fed in excess, damage cardiac as well as skeletal muscles.

myosarcoma A malignant tumour of muscle. It may originate in smooth muscle (*see* leiomyosarcoma) or in striated muscle (*see* rhabdomyoma).

myosin The most abundant protein in muscle fibrils, having the important properties of elasticity and contractility. With *actin, it comprises the principal contractile element of muscles. *See* striated muscle.

myosis *See* miosis.

myositis Inflammation of muscle, usually with some degree of degeneration of the muscle fibres. It may occur as a primary pathological change in various bacterial infections and parasitic infestations, or secondary to other disease. The most common forms of *bacterial myositis* are caused by species of *Clostridium* and comprise *gas gangrene, which affects herbivores and pigs, *malignant oedema, and *blackleg, which affects cattle and sheep. Other, suppurative, forms of myositis occur usually following trauma that admits pathogenic organisms to muscle, although infection can also spread to muscle from adjacent sites. *Corynebacterium pyogenes*, *Streptococcus*, or *Staphylococcus* bacteria are most commonly involved. *Haemophilus agni* infection in lambs is an unusual suppurative myositis in that it is spread in the bloodstream. A type of granulomatous myositis may occur in response to *Staphylococcus aureus* and *Actinobacillus*. Treatment of bacterial myositis depends on antibiotic therapy to eliminate the causal infection. Clostridial myositis is often so rapidly fatal that treatment cannot be given. However it may be prevented by vaccinating against the relevant species of *Clostridium. Parasitic myositis* is found in connection with *Trichinella infestation and *cysticercosis.

Secondary myositis accompanies many systemic infections, including foot-and-mouth disease and toxoplasmosis. This may result, as in bacterial myositis, from the actual local activity of the organism, or may be due to acute viral and bacterial infections that primarily involve other tissues. In the latter case the muscle lesions are more degenerative than inflammatory (*Zenker's hyaline necrosis of the sarcoplasm*), the cause of which is not properly understood but is presumed to involve the toxins of microorganisms.

myotome Part of the *somite in the embryo that develops into some of the striated muscle of the body.

myotomy The dissection or surgical division of a muscle.

myotonia A defect of muscle characterized by a delay in relaxation after contraction. *Spastic paresis, a progressive inherited disease in Friesian cattle, is characterized by myotonia of the muscles extending the hindlimb. Myotonia also occurs as a progressive familial disease in chow dogs, and is a feature of a suspected inherited condition in goats.

myotonic Relating to muscle tone.

myringotomy (tympanotomy) Surgical incision of the eardrum to create an artificial opening, which relieves pressure and allows drainage of fluid from an inflamed middle ear (*otitis media).

myx- (myxo-) *Prefix denoting* mucus.

myxoedema Thickening and dryness of the skin and subcutaneous tissues found in certain patients with an underactive thyroid gland (*see* hypothyroidism).

myxoma A benign tumour arising from fibroblasts in connective tissue and characterized by the production of a mucin-like intercellular matrix. It is rare in domestic animals and behaves clinically in a similar manner to a *fibroma.

myxomatosis A virulent disease of European rabbits characterized by large swellings, particularly on the head, and caused by a myxomavirus (*see* poxvirus). The virus originated in South America where it causes only a mild disease in indigenous rabbits. It was introduced into Europe and Australia to control the rabbit populations, in which it causes a severe, usually fatal, disease. Mosquitoes and fleas transmit the virus, and are particularly efficient in spreading the disease in rabbit warrens. Large swellings develop over the body and the eyes may be completely closed by swelling of the surrounding tissue. Death may occur within 48 hours. Rabbits can be protected against the disease by vaccination with a live attenuated vaccine.

myxosarcoma The malignant counterpart of a *myxoma; it behaves clinically in a similar manner to a *fibrosarcoma.

N

NAD (nicotinamide adenine dinucleotide) The hydrogen acceptor for many *dehydrogenase enzymes in the metabolism of living organisms. Although often called a cofactor or coenzyme it is one of the substrates of the dehydrogenase; for example in the case of lactate dehydrogenase the reaction is: lactate $+$ NAD$^+$ $=$ pyruvate $+$ NADH $+$ H$^+$. The NADH has to be reoxidized, either by another enzyme or by the respiratory chain of the *mitochondrion. NAD is a derivative of the B vitamin, *nicotinic acid.

NADP (nicotinamide adenine dinucleotide phosphate) differs from NAD only in possessing an additional phosphate group. It functions in the same way as NAD, although anabolic reactions generally use NADPH (reduced NADP) as a hydrogen donor rather than NADH, for example in the synthesis of fatty acids.

NADP *See* NAD.

nafcillin *See* penicillin.

nagana (n'gana) The name given to African tsetse-transmitted bovine *trypanosomiasis. One of the most important cattle diseases in Africa, it may be caused by infection with *Trypanosoma vivax*, *T. congolense*, or often both together. The clinical syndrome is typically a chronic wasting disease with anaemia and a high mortality. Acute forms of the disease occasionally occur, notably due to *T. vivax* infection.

nail binding The condition in which a shoe nail is driven too close to the sensitive part of the horse's foot.

Nairobi sheep disease A noncontagious disease of sheep and goats characterized by fever, dysentery, and abortion and caused by a *bunyavirus. Its distribution follows that of the tick responsible for transmitting the disease, which is confined to East Africa. The incubation period is 4–15 days. Depending on the susceptibility of the infected animal the disease may be acute or mild and inapparent. Sheep and goats imported into an enzootic area are particularly susceptible while indigenous animals rarely show clinical signs. In the acute form a sudden high fever is followed by severe haemorrhagic diarrhoea and *mucopurulent nasal and eye discharges. The affected animal has difficulty breathing and collapses and dies within a few days. Control is by annual vaccination of nonindigenous sheep and goats with dead vaccine, coupled with control of the *ticks.

nalidixic acid A urinary tract antiseptic with greatest activity against Gram-negative bacteria, although it has little effect against *Pseudomonas* spp. It is thought to inhibit DNA synthesis in microorganisms. Administered orally, it is rapidly absorbed. Both nalidixic acid and an active metabolite, hydroxynalidixic acid, are excreted into the urine. The half-life is about 8 hours, which is increased in cases of renal failure. Variations in urinary pH have little effect on the drug's bactericidal activity. Possible side-effects include vomiting, hepatotoxicity, and some nervous signs, such as drowsiness and convulsions. Some microorganisms have developed resistance to nalidixic acid.

nandrolone *See* androgen.

nano- *Prefix denoting* **1.** extremely small size. **2.** one thousand-millionth part (10^{-9}).

naphthalene poisoning *See* phenol poisoning.

naproxen *See* NSAID.

narco- *Prefix denoting* narcosis; stupor.

narcosis A state of reversible *analgesia caused by the administration of *narcotic drugs.

narcotic An agent that causes depression of the central nervous system (CNS) and induces diminished or complete unconsciousness (i.e. narcosis). The main group of narcotic drugs are the opiate or narcotic analgesics, although other anaesthetic agents (e.g. barbiturates or *chloral hydrate) can produce narcosis. The opiate analgesics are used as premedicants prior to anaesthesia, as analgesics, and in combination with some tranquillizers to produce *neuroleptanalgesia. However, in feline species the opiates produce CNS stimulation rather than narcosis unless dosage is carefully controlled.

naris (*pl.* **nares**) Nostril: one of the paired openings into the nasal cavity. In the horse the upper part (*false nostril*) leads into the blind-ending diverticulum of the nostril.

nasal bone One of the paired narrow bones in the nose. *See* skull.

nasal bot fly *See* sheep nostril fly.

nasal cavity The space within the nose that lies between the floor of the cranium and the roof of the mouth. It is divided into two parts by the nasal septum. Each part communicates with the outside via a *naris (nostril) and with the nasopharynx via the *choana.

nasal concha (turbinate bone) Any of the scroll-like bones that project into the *nasal cavity. They include the dorsal, middle, ventral, and ethmoidal conchae.

nasal tumours Tumours of the nose. In dogs, intranasal tumours account for about 1–2% of all neoplasms; they occur less frequently in cats and are rare in other domestic animals. Initially there is discharge from one nostril, occasionally with blood. This may worsen into a bilateral discharge, and an external deformity may develop. Nearly all nasal tumours are malignant; just over half are adenocarcinomas (*see* carcinoma) and the rest are sarcomas. Diagnosis is based upon radiographic findings and may be confirmed by biopsy. The prognosis is generally poor; surgical treatment is usually unrewarding and the tumour will progress. Surgery followed by radiotherapy may be more effective.

naso- *Prefix denoting* the nose.

nasolacrimal Relating to the nose and the lacrimal (tear-producing) apparatus. The nasolacrimal duct drains the tears from the *lacrimal apparatus to the nasal cavity.

nasopharyngeal polyp A pedunculated growth of inflammatory origin arising from the auditory (Eustachian) tube or the middle ear. Although uncommon, they occur most frequently in young adult cats and may be associated with chronic respiratory viral infection. Clinical signs include a mucopurulent nasal discharge, respiratory embarrassment, swallowing difficulties, and middle ear disease. Surgical excision is the treatment of choice, but the prognosis is variable as recurrence is common unless the underlying cause is eliminated.

nasopharynx That part of the *pharynx lying behind the nasal cavity, with which it communicates via the *choanae. It lies above the soft palate and ends at the intrapharyngeal ostium. The auditory tube opens into its lateral wall. The nasopharynx forms part of the airway.

natamycin An antibiotic, isolated from *Streptomyces natiliensis*, used for the topical treatment of ringworm; it is also active against yeasts. Available as a powder, natamycin is reconstituted as a suspension in water. Treatment should be carried out indoors or at night because the drug is inactivated by ultraviolet light. The suspension can also be used to decontaminate the environment. Contact with some metals (e.g. copper) inactivates natamycin, and only galvanized containers should be used when preparing the suspension. The drug is toxic if given orally. Tradename: **Mycophyt**.

National Institutes of Health (NIH) Organizations within the US Department of Health and Human Services that control and distribute government grants for research in the biomedical sciences. Each institute has a particular area of interest, for example the National Cancer Institute and National Institute of Allergy and Infectious Diseases, and much of the comparative research carried out by veterinarians in the USA is funded by these bodies.

navel ill (omphalophlebitis) Inflammation of the umbilical veins caused by bacterial infection shortly after birth. It can occur in all domestic species but is of greatest economic importance in calves and lambs. The navel becomes swollen, hard, and painful; in many cases pus or brownish fluid can be expressed from the end. Various bacteria are involved, including the species *Escherichia coli* and *Corynebacterium pyogenes*, and *Fusobacterium*. Contamination is normally from environmental sources. Navel ill may lead to *septicaemia, liver abscessation, joint infection (*joint ill*), and *meningitis as a result of dissemination of the bacteria through the bloodstream. Treatment is usually by administration of antibiotics and local treatment of the navel. Prevention depends upon hygiene where parturition takes place. Dressing the navel of newborns with tincture of iodine is a useful safeguard.

navicular bone The distal *sesamoid bone in the horse.

navicular disease A condition of the horse's foot involving the navicular bone within the hoof. The pathological findings vary and include discoloration of the flexor surface of the navicular bone and of the associated portion of the deep digital flexor tendon; erosion of cartilage with rarefaction of underlying bone; and bone erosion with bony metaplasia. The possible causes are under debate, but among the factors proposed are poor conformation, trauma, and poor blood supply. These could result in bursitis, thrombosis, ischaemia, and bone remodelling. The condition is usually in the forefeet and tends to affect both sides, although one side may be worse than the other. It is more common in horses than ponies. The typical signs are chronic lameness with shortening of the stride, possibly with stumbling, wearing, and pointing of the toe. Eventually the shape of the foot alters as the heels contract and rise to avoid pressure on the frog. Diagnosis involves visual examination, response to hoof testers, and a palmar digital nerve block and radiography. Like the pathogenesis, treatment is also debatable. Regimes include rest and anti-inflammatory drugs early in the condition, corrective trimming and shoeing, *warfarin, *isoxsuprine hydrochloride, and *neurectomy. The prognosis must be guarded in all cases.

nebulizer An instrument used for applying a liquid in the form of a fine spray. *See* aerosol.

necro- *Prefix denoting* death or dissolution.

necrobacillosis Any of a group of infectious conditions affecting most domesticated animals (though not dogs and cats) and some wild species (reindeer and kangaroos), caused by the bacterium *Fusobacterium necrophorum* (formerly *Sphaerophorus necrophorus*; *Fusiformis necrophorus*). They are characterized by necrotic lesions in various sites in the body. The bacterium exists normally in the intestinal tract of many species, and the disease usually requires some initial damage to tissues or other precipitating factors, or concurrent infection by another bacterium. *F. necrophorum* is the primary pathogen in *calf diphtheria, *foul-in-the-foot of cattle, *liver necrosis and *liver abscess of ruminants, and rare cases of bovine *mastitis. It is associated, together with other bacteria, with *quittor and *fistulous withers (poll evil) in horses. In pigs, it is the principal infective agent found in various nonfatal

superficial necrotic conditions, which may follow fighting wounds and other injuries, including necrosis of the ears, tail, and scrotum, necrotic facial *cellulitis, snout, tongue, and jawbone necrosis, and 'bull nose' seen in ringed boars. Moreover, it is a secondary agent in the necrotizing enteritis of *swine dysentery. Labial necrosis, a disease causing losses in rabbits, is also a form of necrobacillosis. *F. necrophorum* plays a role, together with pyogenic bacteria, in a few conditions in which necrosis is not a prominent feature, notably *postparturient metritis of cattle and *foot abscess in sheep. The bacterium is susceptible to *sulphonamides and a number of antibiotics, and the first choice of treatment is frequently intravenous administration of a sulphonamide as a soluble sodium salt.

necrosis The death of some or all of the cells in an organ or tissue, caused by disease, physical or chemical injury, or interference with the blood supply (*see* gangrene). When the area of dead tissue is large enough to be visible to the naked eye it is often paler and softer than normal, and may be demarcated from the surrounding viable tissue by a zone of *hyperaemia.

Necrosis may assume a number of different morphological forms. *Focal necrosis* refers to randomly distributed small areas of necrosis in an organ system. *Coagulation necrosis* is caused by agents that rapidly abolish vital processes, including those responsible for the continued alteration of the tissue after its death. Ghostlike outlines of the dead cells remain, and the architecture of the dead tissue is retained. It is associated with acute tissue anoxia and also with the action of certain toxins. *Caseous necrosis* classically seen in lung tissue in cases of *tuberculosis, appears as friable cheese-like areas in which there is loss of the original architecture of the tissue. *Liquefactive necrosis* appears as a well-circumscribed area containing the partly or completely digested remains of necrotic tissue, which is reduced to a liquid or semiliquid. Abscesses represent areas of liquefactive necrosis formed by the proteolytic enzymes released from disintegrating leucocytes. *Zenker's necrosis* is death of striated muscle cells. It is characterized by coagulation of the proteins contained in these cells. *Fat necrosis* is a distinctive type of necrosis occurring in fat; the affected fat appears as hard gritty white lumps.

necrospermia The presence of dead spermatozoa in *semen. Up to 25% of spermatozoa in normal semen may be dead; semen containing more than this is likely to have low fertility.

necrotic enteritis 1. Any inflammatory condition of the intestines in which mucosal or submucosal necrosis occurs. Necrotic enteritis (necrotizing enteritis) is found, for example, in *swine dysentery, porcine intestinal *adenomatosis, *necrotic enteritis of chickens, and *Tyzzer's disease, and necrosis with ulceration is a feature of tuberculous *enteritis. **2.** A specific subacute or chronic enteritis of pigs caused by the bacterium *Salmonella choleraesuis*. Necrosis and caseation occur in the lymphoid follicles of the colon, leading to ulceration, and there may be necrotic foci in the liver. Soluble sulphonamide preparations given parenterally are effective in treatment. *Compare* swine fever.

necrotic enteritis of chickens A disease of domestic fowls, and also of ducks, caused by the proliferation and toxin production of *Clostridium perfringens* type C in the small intestine. The bacterium normally exists harmlessly in the large intestine and caecum. The small intestinal wall becomes thickened, necrotic, and haemorrhagic; clinical signs resemble those of *coccidiosis. Treatment is by medication of drinking water with antibiotics, including tetracyclines, bacitracin, avoparcin, and lincomycin.

necrotic stomatitis An ulcerative condition affecting the epithelium of the mouth in calves, lambs, and piglets. The lesions usually contain the bacterium *Fusobacterium necrophorum*, which is held principally responsible. Injury to the epithelium is probably an important predisposing factor, and the disease tends to be associated with poor hygiene. In calves the condition is known as *calf diphtheria and may involve the pharynx and larynx instead of or in addition to the mouth. Control depends on the isolation of animals showing signs and general attention to hygiene. Treatment with antibiotics or sulphonamides is effective.

needle A slender sharp-pointed instrument designed to pass through soft body tissues with minimum damage. Hollow needles are used to inject substances into the body (in hypodermic syringes), to obtain specimens of tissue (in a biopsy), or to withdraw fluid from a cavity (*see* aspiration). A surgical, or suture, needle is designed for sewing up operative or accidental wounds with *suture material. The cross-section of the needle tip is designed to suit the tissue in which it is to be used. For most tissues a round-bodied (non-traumatic) needle will make the smallest tract and give best results. But for skin a cutting (traumatic) triangular tip is required to make the small cuts required for penetration. Suture needles may have an eye through which the suture material is threaded, or the suture material may be swaged onto the needle, causing less tissue trauma.

negative-strand virus A *virus containing single-stranded RNA in which

Negri body

the viral RNA is not the messenger *RNA (mRNA) for the viral proteins but is complementary to it. Viral mRNA is transcribed from the viral RNA by a viral RNA replicase. See table at virus.

Negri body *See* inclusion body.

Neisseria A genus of nonmotile Gram-negative *bacteria usually arranged as *diplococci. Many species are nonpathogenic saprophytes of mucous membranes in humans and animals. However, *N. meningitidis* causes cerebrospinal meningitis in humans and *N. gonorrhoeae* causes gonorrhoea in humans.

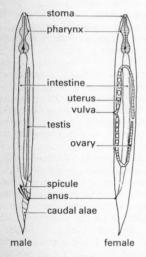

Structural features of a nematode

nematode (roundworm) An invertebrate belonging to the phylum Nematoda. Nematodes are found in virtually all habitats and include both free living and parasitic forms. Some of the latter cause disease in animals and humans, the adult parasites occurring in various sites in the body, such as the lungs (*see* lungworm),

intestine (e.g. *Haemonchus*), blood (e.g. *Dirofilaria*), and eyes (*see* eyeworm). They typically have a smooth cylindrical unsegmented body tapered at both ends and protected by an outer cuticle. The digestive system comprises a stoma (mouth), muscular pharynx, intestine, rectum, and anus. Parasitic forms often have a toothed and reinforced stoma for tearing at their host's tissues. Separate males and females occur and the females may be oviparous or ovoviviparous. Hatching of the eggs produces larvae that resemble the adults, and the larvae undergo generally four moults to develop into adults. The life cycle may be direct (e.g. *Ancylostoma*, *Ascaris*) or indirect (e.g. *Habronema*) involving intermediate hosts. Alternatively, the eggs may be taken up by a transport host (e.g. an earthworm, as in *Syngamus*). See illustration.

Nematodirus A genus of *nematodes containing *N. battus*, an important parasite of sheep and goats. The adults are found in the duodenum and lay large eggs (up to 200 μm in diameter), which are passed out with the faeces onto pasture. The larvae moult twice within the egg before hatching and climbing up a leaf blade to be ingested by a host. Infestation causes serious *parasitic gastroenteritis in lambs, normally in late spring and early summer (*N. baltus*) or later (other species of *Nematodirus*). The eggs can overwinter to establish infestation in lambs the following year. For details of treatment *see* ostertagiasis.

neo- *Prefix denoting* new or newly formed.

neocerebellum (pontocerebellum) The most recent part of the *cerebellum to evolve, occurring only in mammals. It receives input from the cerebrum via the pons and comprises much of the caudal lobe of the cerebellum and the hemispheres within the rostral lobe.

neocortex *See* neopallium.

neomycin *See* aminoglycoside.

neopallium (neocortex) A part of the *cerebral hemisphere that is the most recent to evolve. It is most highly developed in mammals, especially in humans, and is concerned with higher brain functions, including correlation, association, and learning.

neoplasm Any new or abnormal growth. A synonym for *tumour.

Neorickettsia A genus of *rickettsiae in the family Rickettsiaceae comprising a single species, *N. helminthoeca*. It has a life cycle involving the dog, salmon, and a trematode. Transmission occurs when animals, particularly dogs, eat raw trout or salmon containing the infected metacercariae of the trematode. The rickettsiae parasitize the white blood cells of the dog, causing a disease popularly known as *salmon poisoning.

neostigmine A reversible *anticholinesterase, used to reverse the action of competitive neuromuscular blocking drugs. It can be used to treat myasthenia gravis, and has been tried in the treatment of feline and canine dysautonomia (Key-Gaskell syndrome). It can be given orally and its effects last for 2–4 hours. Pyridostigmine, a similar compound, has also been used in cases of myasthenia gravis. It is active for 3–6 hours after oral administration.

Neotrombicula *See* trombiculosis.

nephr- (nephro-) *Prefix denoting* the kidney(s).

nephrectomy Surgical excision of a kidney. This is indicated where there is gross disease affecting primarily one kidney (e.g. renal tumour, gross pyelonephritis, etc.) with the second kidney either normal or much less affected.

nephritis Any inflammatory process occurring in the *kidney. Nephritis is common in domestic animals and occurs in a number of different forms. *Glomerulonephritis is an immune-mediated disease affecting the renal glomeruli and hence renal filtration. *Interstitial nephritis*, which may be acute or chronic, is characterized by inflammation of interstitial tissue in the kidney and is common in dogs. It is usually associated with blood-borne infection. Acute interstitial nephritis is associated with *Leptospira*, canine adenovirus, and canine herpesvirus infections; the chronic form may occur as a sequel to the acute form but in most cases the cause is unknown. *Pyelonephritis results from spread of infection from the bladder to the kidneys via the ureters. Any type of nephritis extensive enough to impair more than 70% of renal function will result in renal failure and the consequent development of *uraemia. Because of the functional interdependence of the different components in the kidney, pathological changes in one component will inevitably affect the rest of the kidney. So, any form of progressive renal disease eventually produces a small hard shrunken kidney, which is unable to function adequately.

nephroblastoma A tumour of the kidney arising from embryonic tissue and occurring in young animals, especially pigs, rabbits, rats, and birds; they occur rarely in dogs. In poultry, they may be associated with the leucosis virus (*see* avian leukosis). Treatment is by surgical excision, but the prognosis is guarded. In humans, this tumour accounts for 10–20% of childhood neoplasms. Other names: **embryonal nephroma; Wilm's tumour**.

nephrocalcinosis The deposition of calcium in the kidney. It occurs, for example, following the administration of excess vitamin D in the prevention of *milk fever in dairy cows. It also affects fish kept in relatively stagnant water containing excess carbon dioxide. This produces metabolic *acidosis in which calcium is mobilized and then precipitates in the abdominal organs, especially the kidney. The calcium deposits become fibrosed so that extensive *granulomas develop.

nephrogenic cord Either of the paired ridges of intermediate *mesoderm that run along the dorsal surface of the abdominal cavity in the embryo. They give rise to the kidney and associated ducts through a series of intermediate stages – *pronephros, *mesonephros, and *metanephros.

nephrolithiasis 1. The formation of a *calculus (*urolith*) within the kidney pelvis. *See* urolithiasis. **2.** Disease due to the presence of such a calculus.

nephron The functional excretory unit of the *kidney (see illustration). Blood, supplied by branches of the renal artery, is filtered through a knot of capillaries (*glomerulus) into the glomerular space, so that water, nitrogenous wastes, and many other substances (excluding colloids) pass into the renal tubule. Here most of the substances are reabsorbed back into the blood; the remaining fluid passes into the collecting tubules as *urine.

nephrosis Any pathological process occurring in the kidney, usually a noninflammatory condition (*compare* nephritis). *Tubular nephrosis* refers to damage to the cells lining the renal tubules. This is commonly due either

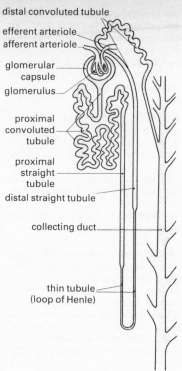

distal convoluted tubule
efferent arteriole
afferent arteriole
glomerular capsule
glomerulus
proximal convoluted tubule
proximal straight tubule
distal straight tubule
collecting duct
thin tubule (loop of Henle)

A single nephron

to anoxia (*ischaemic tubular nephrosis*) or to the action of poisonous substances (*toxic tubular nephrosis*). Important causes of ischaemic tubular necrosis are shock, haemoglobinuria, and myoglobinuria. Among the more common causes of toxic tubular nephrosis are poisoning by sulphonamides, ethylene glycol (antifreeze), oxalate, paraquat, mycotoxins, and the leaves and acorns of oak trees.

nephrotic syndrome A disorder that is characterized by *proteinuria, *hypoproteinaemia, *hyperlipaemia, and oedema. The nephrotic syndrome commonly accompanies disorders of the renal glomerulus where damage to the filtration mechanism allows leakage of blood proteins into the glomerular filtrate with ultimate protein loss in the urine. Protein deficiency develops and oedema occurs as an inevitable consequence of hypoproteinaemia (*see* oedema). The reasons for the hyperlipaemia are not understood, but it is thought that hyperlipaemia represents an attempt by the liver to compensate for the hypoproteinaemia. The nephrotic syndrome is common in animals with *glomerulonephritis and is also commonly seen when amyloid is deposited in the glomerulus (*see* amyloidosis).

nerve A bundle of *nerve fibres in the nervous system outside the brain and spinal cord. Most contain both sensory fibres, conveying impulses from sense organs to the *central nervous system, and motor fibres, conveying impulses from the *central nervous system to muscles and glands. Each fibre is surrounded by a fine connective tissue sheath (*endoneurium), and bundles of fibres are grouped together within a larger sheath (*perineurium). The entire nerve is surrounded by an outer sheath, the *epineurium.

nerve block A form of regional *analgesia in which a local anaesthetic solution is injected around the trunk of a nerve to abolish the conduction of impulses along the nerve trunk. Nerve blocking is employed mostly to provide an area of analgesia in which minor operations, such as dehorning or castration, can be performed painlessly or, in diagnosis, to desensitize a specific area in order to demonstrate that local pain is responsible for abnormal features shown by the animal. This latter procedure is particularly employed in horses to help localize the site of lameness.
A less frequent use of a nerve block is to inhibit muscle action at a specific site and to make local examination practicable. For example, blockade of the nerve branch supplying the muscle that closes the eyelid, the orbicularis oculi, will make examination of the eye possible where *blepharospasm has previously prevented it.

nerve cell *See* neurone.

nerve ending The final part of one of the branches of a nerve fibre, either where it contacts another *neurone at a synapse, or a muscle or gland cell at a neuromuscular or neuroglandular junction, or where it terminates in receptors, either freely or in association with specialized end organs.

nerve fibre The long fine process that extends from the cell body of a *neurone and carries nerve impulses. Bundles of nerve fibres running together form a *nerve. Each fibre consists of an *axon and a sheath, which in myelinated nerve fibres is a relatively thick layer containing the fatty insulating material *myelin.

nerve impulse The electrical activity in the membrane of a *neurone that – by its rapid spread from one region to the next – is the means by which information is transmitted within the nervous system along the axons of the neurones. The membrane of a resting nerve is charged (*polarized*) because of the different concentrations of ions inside and outside the cell. When a nerve impulse is triggered, a wave of *depolarization spreads, and ions flow across the membrane (*see* action potential). Until the nerve has undergone *repolarization no further nerve impulses can pass.

nervous system The principal control system of the body, conveying information throughout the body to coordinate bodily activities. The basic functional unit is the nerve cell, or *neurone, which transmits *nerve impulses to other cells. The nervous system may be divided into the *central nervous system (CNS), consisting of the brain and the spinal cord, and the *peripheral nervous system (PNS), consisting of the cranial nerves and spinal nerves and including the *autonomic nervous system (ANS).

nervus intermedius The smaller of the two roots of the *facial nerve. It consists of parasympathetic secretomotor fibres supplying various glands, and special sensory fibres for taste from the front two-thirds of the tongue.

neural crest The two bands of ectodermal tissue that flank the *neural plate of the early embryo and separate as the *neural tube is formed. They give rise to afferent neurones, neurones of the autonomic nervous system, and a variety of other cell types, notably in the facial and pharyngeal regions.

neural plate A strip of thickened ectoderm running along the dorsal surface of the early embryo. It folds to form the *neural tube.

neural tube The hollow tube of ectodermal origin in the embryo that is formed by folding of the *neural plate. It gives rise to the brain and spinal cord. Failure of normal formation of the neural tube produces a variety of defects.

neuraminic acid An amino *sugar of which *sialic acid is the N-acetylated derivative.

neuraminidase An enzyme that catalyses the removal of *sialic acid from the surface of cells.

neurectomy Surgical removal of part or all of a nerve. This is indicated where permanent abolition of all the sensory and/or motor functions of a particular nerve is required. It is most frequently performed to desensitize part of the foot of the **horse** where a chronic progressive disease is causing continuous pain and lameness. If the whole foot is rendered insensitive, there is a risk that the horse may damage it accidentally, and it is inadvisable to use such a horse for riding. In **cattle** neurectomy has been employed to overcome the features of 'spastic paresis'.

neurilemma (neurolemma) The sheath of the *axon of a nerve fibre. The neurilemma of a peripheral myelinated fibre contains *myelin laid down by Schwann cells.

neurilemmoma *See* neurofibroma.

neuritis Inflammation of a nerve or nerves, particularly the peripheral nerves.

neurobiotaxis The predisposition of a nerve cell to move towards the source of its stimuli during development.

neuroblast Any of the developing nerve cells of the embryo that give rise to functional nerve cells (neurones).

neuroblastoma A tumour arising from primitive neuroepithelial cells. They occur rarely in animals; in cattle they are usually benign, whereas in dogs they tend to be malignant. Anatomical sites affected include the adrenal gland medulla, abdominal autonomic ganglia, and the brain.

neurofibril One of the threads found in the cytoplasm of the cell body and axoplasm of a *neurone, as seen by the light microscope. *See* neurofilament.

neurofibroma A benign tumour arising from a nerve sheath, reported in most species of domestic animal. They usually involve peripheral nerves but can arise adjacent to nerve roots. If the brachial or lumbar sacral plexuses are involved then paralysis of the affected limb may occur. Peripheral neurofibromas cause few problems unless injured and ulcerated. Surgical excision must be extensive as recurrence is common. Other names: **neurilemmoma; neurinoma; perineural fibroblastoma; Schwannoma.**

neurofilament A fine thread of indefinite length as seen by light microscopy in the cytoplasm of the cell body and axoplasm of a *neurone (nerve cell). *See* neurofibril.

neurogenesis The growth and development of nerve cells.

neurogenic 1. Caused by disease or dysfunction of the nervous system. **2.** Arising in nervous tissue. **3.** Caused by nerve stimulation.

neuroglia (glia) The specialized connective tissue of the central nervous system. It is composed of different cells, including *oligodendrocytes, *astrocytes, ependymal cells (*see* ependyma), and *microglia, with various supportive and nutritive functions (see illustration). Neuroglial cells outnumber the neurones by between five and ten to one, and make up some 40% of the total volume of the brain and spinal cord.

neurohormone A hormone that is produced within specialized nerve cells and is secreted from the nerve endings into the circulation. The hormones produced and released by specialized nuclei in the hypothalamus (e.g. luteinizing-hormone releasing

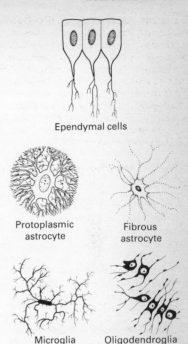

Ependymal cells

Protoplasmic astrocyte

Fibrous astrocyte

Microglia

Oligodendroglia

Types of neuroglia

hormone, somatostatin) are considered to be neurohormones. They are carried directly to the adenohypophysis via the hypothalamo-hypophyseal portal system. *Compare* neurotransmitter.

neurohypophysis (*pl.* **neurohypophyses**) The posterior part of the *pituitary gland, consisting of the infundibulum and the neural lobe.

neurolemmal cell (Schwann cell) A cell that lays down the *myelin sheath around the axon of a myelinated nerve fibre. Each cell is responsible for one segment of an axon, around which it twists as it grows, so that concentric layers of membrane envelop the axon. The gap between adjacent neurolemmal cells

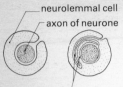

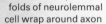

neurolemmal cell
axon of neurone

folds of neurolemmal cell wrap around axon

areas where myelin will form

Formation of myelin sheath by a neurolemmal cell

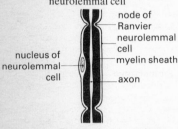

node of Ranvier
neurolemmal cell
myelin sheath
axon

nucleus of neurolemmal cell

Longitudinal section through a myelinated nerve fibre

forms a node of Ranvier. See illustration.

neuroleptanalgesia A state of immobilization in which an animal is not completely unconscious but is insensitive to painful stimuli. Neuroleptanalgesia is produced by administering a combination of a *tranquillizer and an *opiate analgesic (e.g. *Immobilon). The tranquillizer potentiates the action of the analgesic, producing a smooth recovery. This form of chemical restraint is easy to administer and the effects of the analgesic can be reversed. However, muscle relaxation is poor and it is unsuitable for major surgery. Neuroleptanalgesic agents should not be used in feline species because of the risk of nervous stimulation due to the opiate analgesics.

neurology The study of the structure, function, and diseases of the nervous system, including the brain, spinal cord, and all the peripheral nerves.

neuroma A painful proliferating mass that may develop at the end of severed nerves. It is not uncommon in horses following *neurectomy, but is not a true tumour.

neuromuscular junction The meeting point between the terminations of the fibre of a *neurone and the muscle fibres that it supplies. Each termination of the nerve fibre (*motor end-plate*) carries a number of small vesicles, which release *neurotransmitter substances to allow impulses to pass from the neurone to the muscle fibres across the intervening gap.

neurone (nerve cell) The basic functional unit of the nervous system. They are cells specialized to transmit electrical impulses (*see* nerve impulse) and so carry information from one part of the body to another (see illustration). Each neurone consists of a *cell body* (*perikaryon*) containing the nucleus, and a variable number of processes extending from the cell body. Of these the short branched *dendrites convey impulses towards the cell body, and a longer single *axon (which is normally unbranched except at the *nerve ending) carries impulses away from the cell body. The point of contact of one neurone with another is termed a *synapse. Structural types of neurones are: *pseudounipolar* (one single process soon dividing into two); *bipolar* (two processes); and *multipolar* (many processes). Functionally, neurones can be classed as *afferent* (or *sensory*), i.e. conveying information towards the central nervous system (CNS), *efferent* (or *motor*), i.e. conveying information away from the CNS, or *associative*, i.e. linking one part of the CNS with another.

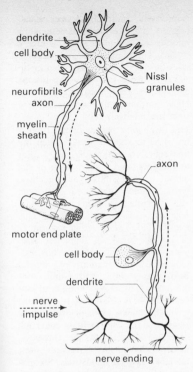

dendrite
cell body
Nissl granules
neurofibrils
axon
myelin sheath
axon
motor end plate
cell body
dendrite
nerve impulse
nerve ending

Types of neurone: motor (left) and sensory (right)

neuropathy Any disorder of the nervous system.

neurophysiology The study of the function of the nervous system.

neuropil Nerve tissue that is visible microscopically as a mass of interwoven and interconnected nerve endings, dendrites, and other neurone components, rather than an ordered array of axons.

neurosecretion Any substance produced within and secreted by a *neurone. Important examples are the hormone-releasing factors produced by

the cells of the *hypothalamus and released into blood vessels supplying the pituitary gland, on which they act.

neurotomy The surgical procedure of severing a nerve.

neurotoxin A poisonous substance that acts specifically on the nervous system.

neurotransmitter A chemical substance released from the synaptic vesicles in the terminations of nerve fibres to transmit impulses across *synapses to other *neurones, across *neuromuscular junctions to muscle cells, or across gaps to glandular cells. Within the central nervous system neurotransmitters are believed to include *acetylcholine, *noradrenaline, *dopa, *serotonin, *gamma-aminobutyric acid, and other substances. In the peripheral nervous system the principal neurotransmitter is acetylcholine, but noradrenaline is released from neurones of the sympathetic nervous system.

neurotrophic Relating to the growth and nutrition of neural tissue in the body.

neurotropic Growing towards or having an affinity for neural tissue. The term may be applied to viruses, chemicals, or toxins.

neutering *See* castration; spaying.

neutropenia *See* leucopenia.

neutrophil (polymorph) A mature phagocytic white blood cell (leucocyte) of the granulocytic series (*see* granulocyte). Neutrophils are the dominant circulating leucocyte in dogs, cats, and humans, but are outnumbered by *lymphocytes in ruminants. The granules in the cytoplasm contain enzymes to assist the digestion of phagocytosed material. Like other granulocytes, neutrophils develop in the bone marrow (*see* haemopoiesis), have a limited lifespan, and, in the mature state, are incapable of cell division. They are strongly attracted by several products of *inflammation, including materials released from dead cells or bacteria, and by activated *complement. Neutrophils, like *macrophages, fulfil the vital function of *phagocytosis. Unlike the latter, however, they act mainly in acutely inflamed tissue and are not directly interactive with cells of the immune system, although their phagocytic activity is promoted by *opsonins. Neutrophils die after carrying out their defensive function and consequently make up the main component of *pus. They also release some of their enzymes during inflammation and this may cause tissue damage.

neutrophilia *See* leucocytosis.

Newcastle disease (fowl pest) A highly infectious disease of poultry and other birds caused by a *paramyxovirus and characterized by respiratory and nervous signs, lowered production, and high mortality in the acute form. Newcastle disease occurs worldwide and affects virtually all birds, with the most severe outbreaks seen in domestic fowls and turkeys. All ages are affected. There is wide variation in the severity of outbreaks and nature of the clinical signs, and numerous strains of the virus have been identified. These range from 'Ulster', which produces no clinical signs, to 'Northampton '72', which can cause up to 100% mortality even in older birds. Strains of virus are classified as *lentogenic, mesogenic,* or *velogenic* in order of increasing virulence. Strains also vary in their preference or 'tropism' for different organ systems; marked *pneumotropism, neurotropism,* or *viscerotropism* causes,

respectively, severe respiratory signs, nervous signs, or visceral lesions in infected birds. For example, a highly virulent US strain known as velogenic viscerotropic Newcastle disease (VVND) tends to cause significant damage to the digestive tract and high mortality, although respiratory signs are relatively mild.

The incubation period ranges from a few days to about 2 weeks. Often the first sign is a period of uneasy calm in the flock, and a sharp drop in egg output in laying birds. Subsequently, birds become depressed, lethargic, and feverish, stop eating, and huddle together with feathers ruffled. This may be followed by either respiratory or nervous signs. In the latter case, wings tend to droop and there is progressive incoordination or ataxia. Birds may collapse and exhibit convulsions, or twitching of the head and neck. There is usually diarrhoea with greenish faeces. Where respiratory signs predominate, there is coughing, sneezing, gurgling in the throat, a nasal discharge, and, in severe cases, laboured gasping inhalations. Secondary infections, such as *colisepticaemia, often follow recovery in very young birds, as may twisting of the neck (torticollis). Signs of milder outbreaks in layers may be limited to a fall in egg production and shell quality. Apart from the strain of virus, the severity of outbreaks depends on the age and the vaccination status of the flock, and the presence of other infections. Outbreaks can spread rapidly to other flocks by wind-borne transmission in areas of high poultry population. Wild birds are also vectors, and a pigeon paramyxovirus is a subtype of Newcastle disease virus. The disease is also spread mechanically by boots, lorries, equipment, etc. and in contaminated feed. Imports of poultry products and of live cage birds, especially the parrot family, can introduce the virus.

There is no effective treatment; control depends on vaccination or slaughter. Both live and oil-based vaccines are available, and vaccination programmes must be tailored to suit local conditions, particularly the type and virulence of the viral strain likely to be encountered. In high-risk areas, chicks are often sprayed with a primary vaccine in the first few days of life, although maternal antibody can reduce the response. Subsequent vaccinations can be given in drinking water or – after some immunity has developed – as an aerosol. Immunity takes 3–8 days to develop (the longer period when administered in drinking water), peaks after 2–3 weeks, and declines subsequently. For protection in laying birds, an oil-based killed vaccine is injected just prior to lay. Some vaccines are combined with *infectious bronchitis vaccine. A slaughter policy and a ban on vaccines was introduced throughout the UK in 1981, but with the exception of Northern Ireland, this has since been discontinued. Currently (1987) only Hitchner B1 and killed vaccines are permitted in Great Britain.

Newcastle disease must be distinguished from infectious bronchitis, *avian infectious laryngotracheitis, *avian influenza, and *fowl cholera. The disease was first identified near Newcastle-upon-Tyne, England, in 1926. The term fowl pest is normally applied to Newcastle disease but also includes fowl plague (*see* avian influenza). Both are *notifiable diseases in the UK.

new duck disease *See* anatipestifer infection.

New Forest disease (infectious bovine keratoconjunctivitis) A disease affecting the eyes of cattle caused by the bacterium *Moraxella bovis*. Calves and young cattle are most frequently affected and the disease is prevalent during the summer and autumn, being spread by contact and by flies. The first sign is a copious watery discharge from the eye. As the disease progresses a white spot appears on the centre of the *cornea. This spot ulcerates and the animal keeps the eyelid closed. There is marked inflammation of the conjunctiva and in severe cases the whole cornea becomes discoloured and opaque, and the ulcer may rupture. Both eyes can be affected causing impaired mobility and loss of condition. Treatment with topical application or subconjunctival injection of antibiotics, such as cloxacillin or *chloramphenicol, should be commenced at the first sign of an eye spot otherwise blindness may result. US name: **pink-eye.**

New Forest fly (Forest fly) A bloodsucking *fly, *Hippobosca equina*, also called horse ked, that is ectoparasitic on cattle and horses in most warm countries but, in the UK, is mostly confined to the New Forest and parts of Dorset, Hampshire, and Wales. Although it has wings, it usually runs between the hairs of the host and is transferred from host to host by direct contact. The female deposits larvae in dry soil; these rapidly pupate and adults emerge in the summer. Once an adult has located a host it remains in position, commonly on the hind legs or under the tail. They may be controlled by the use of dips containing a suitable *insecticide.

Newmarket cough *See* equine influenza.

new wheat poisoning *See* avian monocytosis.

nexus (in anatomy) A connection or link. A nexus, or gap junction, between cells occurs where the intercellular space is very narrow and the adjacent cell membranes interlock. Substances may pass between the cells and electrical impulses can be conducted.

n'gana *See* nagana.

niacin *See* nicotinic acid.

nicking 1. The production of breaks in one strand of a DNA double helix. **2.** The surgical division of certain muscles under the tail of a horse to produce an artificially high tail carriage. The practice is illegal in the UK. *See* Docking and Nicking of Horses Act (1949).

niclosamide An *anthelmintic with activity against certain tapeworms, particularly *Dipylidium* and *Taenia* in dogs and cats, and *Moniezia* in cattle, sheep, and goats. It acts by inhibiting glucose metabolism; repeated dosing may be needed to clear infestations. Efficacy against *Echinococcus* is very poor. The drug is available in tablet form for small animals and as a drench for use in farm animals.

nicotinamide adenine dinucleotide *See* NAD.

nicotine poisoning A toxic condition due to ingestion of the alkaloid nicotine which is used as an anthelmintic in animals and as a plant pesticide. With the introduction of synthetic parasiticides the use of nicotine has decreased and poisoning is less common. Nicotine affects ganglia of the autonomic nervous system and signs include slowed breathing, narcosis, and death from respiratory failure. Nicotine is obtained from the tobacco plant (*Nicotiana* spp.), and the plant itself can produce skeletal deformities in the offspring of pregnant animals that have eaten it. The acute effects of nicotine are similar to those of cytisine, found in laburnum and broom, and to coniine, found in the spotted hemlock.

nicotinic 1. A class of receptors in the peripheral nervous system that are acted on by *acetylcholine and give rise to changes similar to those induced by the alkaloid nicotine. These changes include stimulation then depression of autonomic ganglia, the adrenal medulla, and neuromuscular junctions. **2.** Of nicotine or its physiological effects. **3.** Of *nicotinic acid.

nicotinic acid (niacin; nicotinamide) A *vitamin of the B-complex that is a constituent of the coenzymes *NAD (nicotinamide adenine dinucleotide) and NADP (NAD phosphate), which catalyse the transfer of hydrogen in the metabolism of proteins, fats, and carbohydrates. It is synthesized by microorganisms in the reticulorumen and large intestine and by conversion of the *essential amino acid tryptophan in animal tissues. This conversion is inefficient in most animals and is practically nonexistent in the cat. Rumen synthesis usually provides adequate supplies of the vitamin for ruminants, except those which are milk-fed and, possibly, very high-yielding dairy cows. In nonruminants coprophagia (ingestion of faeces) probably increases the utilization of nicotinic acid synthesized in the large intestine. Good natural sources are sunflower meal, fish meals, maize (corn) gluten, liver, and groundnut (peanut) meal. However, there are large variations in the nicotinic acid content of individual feeds, and biological availability is decreased by organic binding, especially in maize, rice, and wheat.
Nicotinic acid deficiency This is most likely to occur in animals given diets of low protein and/or high maize contents. Signs of deficiency are, initially, decreased appetite, decreased growth, and diarrhoea; later there may be dermatitis (pellagra), paralysis, stomatitis, and glossitis, which in severe cases causes blackening of the

tongue (*see* black tongue). Deficiency in pigs causes *necrotic enteritis, which may be complicated by *Salmonella cholerasuis* infection, and in fowls there is decreased egg production, decreased hatchability of eggs, and weak chicks with distorted legs. In dairy cattle supplements of nicotinic acid have been claimed to decrease the incidence of ketosis and to increase milk yields. For diagnosis and treatment *see* vitamin. Other names: **vitamin B₃; vitamin PP**.

nictitating membrane The third eyelid. *See* eyelid.

nidus (*pl.* **nidi** or **niduses**) A place in which pathogenic organisms, especially bacteria, lodge and multiply because of particularly favourable conditions; a focus of infection.

night blindness (nyctalopia) A reduced ability to see in dim light. It is one of the earliest clinical manifestations of *progressive retinal atrophy, an inherited disease of dogs; it also occurs as a syndrome in Appaloosa horses. Night blindness is also an early clinical manifestation of *vitamin A deficiency in all species, due to deficiency of the visual pigment rhodopsin. Although generally uncommon, night blindness associated with vitamin A deficiency is occasionally encountered in cattle housed and fed deficient diets over a prolonged period; young growing animals are the most vulnerable.

nightshade poisoning *See* deadly nightshade poisoning; solanine poisoning.

nigroid bodies (corpora nigra) Bodies forming part of the uveal tract of the horse. They can be seen on the pupillary margin of the iris. Their shape and number are variable but they are often more obvious on the upper than the lower margin. Their function is unknown.

nigropallidal encephalomalacia A condition of horses caused by ingestion of the poisonous yellow star thistle (*Centaurea solstitialis*) or Russian knapweed (*C. repens*), which grow commonly on waste areas, roadsides, etc. in western USA. The poison, apparently an alkaloid, irreversibly damages the central nervous system, inducing involuntary chewing movements and lip twitching. Then the mouth may be held permanently open so that the horse cannot eat and eventually dies from dehydration and starvation. Horses only graze the plant when forced through hunger. Euthanasia is recommended when clinical signs become advanced.

nikethamide *See* stimulant.

Nile blue An oxazine chloride, used for staining lipids and lipid pigments. *Nile blue A* (*Nile blue sulphate*), which stains fatty acids, changes from blue to purplish at pH 10–11.

ninhydrin reaction A histochemical test for proteins, in which ninhydrin (triketohydrindene hydrate) is boiled with the test solution and gives a blue colour in the presence of amino acids and proteins.

nipple *See* papilla.

Nissl granules Collections of dark-staining material seen in the cell bodies of neurones on light microscopic examination. They are composed of aggregations of rough *endoplasmic reticulum.

nit The egg of the sucking or biting *louse which is cemented to the host's hair and develops into a blood-sucking or biting nymph.

nitrate poisoning A toxic condition due to the ingestion of nitrites, or of nitrates, which are converted to nitrites in the alimentary tract, especially in ruminants. Small amounts are metabolized, but single large doses cause the conversion of haemoglobin to methaemoglobin and consequent interference with tissue oxygenation (*see* methaemoglobinaemia). Many plants may, in some circumstances, contain dangerous concentrations of nitrate; excessive application of nitrate fertilizer raises the nitrate concentration in streams and wells. Intravenous injection of a 4% solution of methylene blue is recommended for treating cases among cattle and sheep; it reduces the methaemoglobin to haemoglobin.

nitrite poisoning *See* nitrate poisoning.

nitrofurans A group of synthetic antibacterials, usually brilliant yellow in colour, that are effective against both Gram-positive and Gram-negative bacteria and against coccidia. They act by interfering with the carbohydrate metabolism. Resistance to nitrofurans develops relatively slowly, hence they are often used where other drugs have failed due to antibiotic resistance. *Nitrofurantoin* is well absorbed from the gastrointestinal tract and about 60% is excreted unchanged in high concentration in the urine, making it useful in the treatment of urinary tract infections. *Furazolidone*, *furaltadone*, and *nitrofurazone* are poorly absorbed and are thus given mainly for intestinal infections and in intramammary preparations to treat mastitis. Their relative cheapness allows them to be used routinely as coccidiostats and growth promoters added to feed, most commonly for pigs, poultry, and calves. Acute toxicity is usually caused by overdosage. In dogs this produces vomiting, while in other species signs of neurotoxicity occur, for example polyneuritis, tremors, convulsions, and spasticity. If the drug is withdrawn immediately animals can recover. Chronic toxicity, caused by long-term high dosage, produces depression of growth rate and a haemorrhagic syndrome. Signs are most frequently seen in calves.

nitrofurantoin *See* nitrofurans.

nitrofurazone *See* nitrofurans.

nitrogen A nonmetallic element and the most abundant gas in air (79%). Along with carbon, oxygen, and hydrogen, it is one of the principal elements of living organisms, occurring especially in *proteins and *nucleic acids. The nitrogen metabolism of organisms involves the reactions of *amino acids, *purines, *pyrimidines, and *porphyrins, and the element is excreted in the form of *urea or *uric acid. Symbol N.

nitrosamine A *carcinogen that acts by modifying the *DNA of a cell. Substituted nitrosamines are also carcinogenic and can be formed by the action of gastric acid on certain dietary components.

nitroscanate A broad-spectrum anthelmintic, available as film-coated tablets for use in dogs. It has good activity against canine roundworms and tapeworms, although activity against *Trichuris and Echinococcus is poorer. Vomiting is a common side-effect, but this does not reduce the efficacy of the drug. It should not be used in cats. Tradename: **Lopatol**.

nitrous oxide A noninflammable nonexplosive gas used in animal anaesthesia as an adjuvant with other *inhalational anaesthetics, at about 50–60% of the gas mixture, to increase analgesia. It cannot induce anaesthesia in animals when used alone due to its very low potency. The uptake of nitrous oxide into the bloodstream concentrates the remaining gases in the inhaled mixture. However, when nitrous oxide diffuses out of the blood the reverse happens and *hypoxia may occur unless supplementary oxygen is given during the recovery period. Nitrous oxide exchanges with nitrogen in the tissues and because of its greater solubility accumulates in gas-filled structures. It should not be used during anaesthesia if a gas-filled organ is present, for instance an intestinal blockage or gastric torsion. With adequate oxygenation nitrous oxide has low toxicity.

nitroxynil An anthelmintic used to treat infestations of flukes, particularly *Fasciola hepatica* (*see* fascioliasis). It acts by uncoupling oxidative phosphorylation in the parasite, and is effective against *F. hepatica* adults and immature stages over 6 weeks of age. It can be used orally or, preferably, injected subcutaneously, although the compound is yellow and may cause staining of wool at the injection site. Excretion of the drug is very slow, taking over a month. Toxicity due to overdosage causes increased metabolic rate with tremor, some hyperventilation, and hyperthermia. Nitroxynil is excreted in the milk and should not be used in lactating animals.

Nocardia A genus of aerobic non-motile Gram-positive *bacteria, commonly found in the soil. They grow primarily as mycelia but break up to form rods and cocci. Some produce various pigments. Most are nonpathogenic saprophytes, but some can be opportunistic pathogens in humans and various animals, causing ulcerative or granulomatous lesions. *N. farcinica* causes *bovine farcy. However, this organism has not been fully characterized and there is some doubt regarding its differences with

N. asteroides. The latter has been associated with bovine *mastitis and granulomatous lesions in the skin and lung of cats and dogs (*see* nocardiosis). The organism is a common commensal of the soil and causes disease after gaining entry through wounds, ingestion, and inhalation. Similar granulomatous and ulcerative lesions due to *N. asteroides* can also affect humans, particularly those suffering from neoplastic or immunosuppressive conditions.

nocardial mastitis An infrequent form of *mastitis in cows, usually granulomatous with suppuration, caused by *Nocardia asteroides*. The bacterium enters through soil contamination of the teat canal, sometimes attributable to faulty hygiene during intramammary medication. The udder becomes enlarged, with draining fistulous tracts. No treatment is effective.

nocardiosis Disease due to infection with bacteria of the genus *Nocardia*. *N. asteroides* and unnamed nocardioform bacteria are responsible for nocardiosis in dogs, which is characterized by superficial abscessation and interlocking sinuses, often of the thorax, with later lung involvement. Treatment is by a lengthy course of a sulphonamide or a tetracycline antibiotic. *See also* bovine farcy; nocardial mastitis.

node A small swelling or knot of tissue. *See* atrioventricular node; sinoatrial node.

node of Ranvier One of the gaps that occur at regular intervals in the *myelin sheath of myelinated nerve fibres, between adjacent *neurolemmal cells.

nodular necrosis (Roekl's granuloma) A condition of old cows in which greenish-yellow necrotic nodules, up to 2 cm in diameter, occur in muscles, particularly the tail muscles.

nodule A small swelling or aggregation of cells.

noradrenaline (norepinephrine) A *catecholamine, closely related to *adrenaline, that is the principal *neurotransmitter released from nerve endings of the sympathetic nervous system. It is also secreted by the medulla of the adrenal gland and functions as a hormone, with effects similar to those of adrenaline. Among these are the constriction of small blood vessels leading to a marked increase in blood pressure, increased blood flow through the coronary arteries and possibly a reflex slowing of the heart rate, increase in the rate and depth of breathing, and relaxation of the smooth muscle in intestinal walls. Noradrenaline is more concerned with maintaining normal body function than with preparing the body for emergencies. It may be administered intravenously to counter hypotension due to vasodilatation.

norepinephrine *See* noradrenaline.

normo- *Prefix denoting* normality.

normoblast A bone-marrow precursor cell of *erythrocytes (*see* haemopoiesis).

Northern fowl mite A small *mite, *Ornithonyssus sylvarium*, that is a widespread ectoparasite of poultry in the UK and many other countries. It causes scab formation and soiling of feathers. The entire life cycle is spent on the host.

nose The inlet to the air passages and the organ of *olfaction; it also filters, warms, and moistens inspired air en route to the lungs. The *external nose* or snout is the projection on the face; it consists of cartilages and, in the pig, the rostral bone, and is covered by skin. It leads into the *nasal cavity.

nosebleed (epistaxis) Haemorrhage from the nose. Strictly, epistaxis refers to haemorrhage originating from the nose itself, but the term 'nosebleed' is often used regardless of the source of the blood. Such blood may derive from anywhere in the nasopharynx, upper respiratory tract, or lungs, and it may also accompany diseases where there is generalized bleeding. Nosebleed (in the broader sense) occurs in *anthrax in cattle and sheep, *bracken poisoning in cattle, and guttural pouch mycosis in horses. Nosebleed is the usual presenting sign in exercise-induced pulmonary haemorrhage of racehorses, a condition characterized by bleeding into the lungs after strenuous exercise. Such blood is coughed up from the lungs (haemoptysis) and appears at the nostrils. Coughed up pulmonary blood coming from the nose is also a feature of thrombosis of the posterior vena cava in cattle.

nosode A homeopathic 'vaccine', which may also be used in treatment. It is prepared using minute quantities of the pathogen or agent causing the particular disease, and is administered according to the same principle as other homeopathic remedies. *See* homeopathy.

Nosopsyllus A genus of *fleas found throughout the world and containing the common rat flea, *Nosopsyllus fasciatus*, which transmits bubonic plague to humans.

nostril *See* naris.

nostril fly A *fly whose larvae are parasites of sheep or horses, such as the *sheep nostril fly (*Oestrus ovis*) and the horse nostril fly or Russian gadfly (*Rhinoestrus purpureus*). The larvae are deposited in and around the nostrils of their host, where they feed on nasal secretions.

Principal notifiable diseases in the UK

African horse sickness
African swine fever
anthrax
Aujeszky's disease
avian influenza (fowl plague)
brucellosis
contagious bovine pleuropneumonia
contagious caprine pleuropneumonia
contagious equine metritis
dourine
enzootic bovine leukosis
epizootic lymphangitis
equine infectious anaemia
equine viral encephalomyelitis
foot-and-mouth disease
glanders
Newcastle disease (fowl pest)
rabies
rinderpest (cattle plague)
sheep scab
sheep pox
swine fever (classical swine fever; hog cholera)
swine vesicular disease
Teschen/Talfan
tuberculosis
warble fly infestation

notifiable disease A disease that must be reported to the appropriate veterinary authority in order that speedy control and preventive action may be undertaken if necessary. In Britain the existence or suspected existence of such a disease must be notified by the owner of the animals or by a veterinary surgeon to the local Divisional Veterinary Officer of the Ministry of Agriculture or to the local police. Notifiable Diseases are listed in Orders made under the *Animal Health Act (1981) (see table). The Orders give the Minister power to impose movement restric-

tions in the event of an outbreak of disease and to order a particular method of disinfection to be used. The list of notifiable diseases varies for different countries, depending largely on the range of enzootic and epizootic diseases in a particular country, and the likely risk of diseases being imported. Animal diseases are categorized according to their importance internationally by the Office Internationale des Épizooties, 12 Rue de Prony, 75017 Paris, France.

notochord A longitudinal rod of mesodermal tissue below the *neural plate or *neural tube in the embryo. It becomes almost entirely obliterated by the development of the vertebrae, persisting only as the nucleus pulposus of each *intervertebral disc.

Notoedres A genus of *mites that are ectoparasitic on all carnivores, particularly cats, and responsible for *notoedric mange on the face and ears of their host. This condition is now rare in the UK.

notoedric mange A form of *mange affecting cats and rabbits and caused by the mite *Notoedres cati*, which resembles *Sarcoptes scabiei*. It causes intense itching, particularly of the head and neck, with much self-excoriation. Formerly very common, it is seldom seen now.

novobiocin An antibiotic, obtained from the actinomycetes *Streptomyces niveus* and *S. spheroides*, with a narrow spectrum of activity against Gram-positive bacteria; it is bacteriostatic. Novobiocin is used in intramammary preparations to treat bovine mastitis, and has also been incorporated in feed to control *Staphylococcus* infections in chickens and turkeys. However, its toxicity has limited its use; adverse reactions include skin rashes, pruritus, vomiting, diarrhoea, fever, and blood abnormalities. Novobiocin acts at the proximal tubules preventing renal secretion of acidic drugs in a similar way to *probenecid.

noxythiolin *See* growth promoter.

NSAID (nonsteroidal anti-inflammatory drug) Any of a large group of drugs with antipyretic, analgesic, and anti-inflammatory activity. Most of them are derived from organic acids and are classified according to their structure. They comprise the salicylates, fenamic acids, propionic acid derivatives, acetic acid derivatives, pyrazolones, and the oxicams. They are available for oral administration and some as injectable products. The NSAIDs act by inhibiting cyclo-oxygenase enzymes, which act as catalysts in the formation of prostaglandins – important mediators of inflammation. There is little effect on preformed tissue prostaglandins, and the activity against cyclo-oxygenase enzymes in different tissues can vary. This anti-inflammatory action is locally induced and produces a local analgesic effect by reducing prostaglandin levels. These drugs accumulate in areas of inflammation and can remain active for longer periods than suggested by the plasma *half-life. The antipyretic action of NSAIDs involves central inhibition of prostaglandin synthesis in the thermoregulatory zone of the hypothalamus, thereby raising the body temperature control setting. Other effects of NSAIDs include inhibition of phagocytosis by leucocytes, stabilization of lysosomal membranes, inhibition of parturition, and reduction in thromboxane production so reducing platelet aggregation. The half-lives and metabolism of the individual compounds vary among species. They are absorbed after oral administration, although some of the compounds bind to cellulose food material thus reducing absorption. Metabolism is usually in the liver and the drugs are excreted in the bile and urine.

Salicylates These include aspirin (acetylsalicylic acid) and sodium salicylate, which are used extensively in humans and dogs. Following absorption they are metabolized by conjugation to glucuronide in the liver. This mechanism is deficient in felines, and salicylates have a very long half-life in these species, with frequent dosing leading to accumulation of the drug and toxicity.

Pyrazolon derivatives These include phenylbutazone (PBZ), dipyrone, and isopyrin. PBZ is the most commonly used NSAID in veterinary therapy. It is metabolized in the liver to oxyphenbutazone, which is active, and gamma-hydroxyphenylbutazone. The half-life is long in cattle and humans, in which the metabolizing enzymes are less active than in dogs and horses. Excretion is increased in alkaline urine, and in animals with acidic urine the drug can be detected for several days. Dipyrone is used in combination with hyoscine (*see* atropine) as an anti-inflammatory and analgesic for the treatment of colic. Isopyrin is available combined with PBZ in an injectable preparation (Tomanol), which prolongs the activity of PBZ. The pyrazolons form highly alkaline solutions, which are irritant if injected intramuscularly.

Propionic acid derivatives These include ibuprofen and naproxen. Ibuprofen is available on the human market without a prescription but is not licensed for use in veterinary therapy and appears to be toxic in dogs because of its long half-life in this species. However, safe dosage schedules have been designed for dogs. Naproxen has good activity against cyclo-oxygenase enzymes in muscles and is effective in the treatment of myositis in horses.

Fenamic acids These include meclofenamic acid, which is used in the treatment of skeletal conditions in horses and ponies and is effective in reducing anaphylactic reactions in cattle, possibly by preventing the release of kinins and slow-reacting-substance of anaphylaxis.

Acetic acid derivatives In this group are paracetamol, phenacetin, and indomethacin. Paracetamol acts only centrally, unlike other NSAIDs, and therefore has good analgesic activity but less anti-inflammatory activity. Phenacetin is metabolized to paracetamol. Indomethacin has been found to produce toxic side-effects in animals and is not licensed for veterinary use.

Oxicams These NSAIDs (e.g. piroxicam and miloxicam) are currently used mainly in human therapy, but possible veterinary applications are being investigated.

Flunixin has good activity as an analgesic and anti-inflammatory in visceral and other soft-tissue conditions. It can be given by intramuscular injection and has a rapid onset of action, being used in the therapy of colic, respiratory conditions, and mastitis.

The NSAIDs are used as analgesics in the treatment of inflammatory conditions in animals, for example osteoarthritis, laminitis, joint inflammation, rheumatoid arthritis, myositis, and tendonitis. In racehorses these drugs are prohibited when the animals are competing but they can be used at low levels in eventing and showjumping horses. They are abused to mask lameness during examinations for soundness in horses. NSAIDs can also be given to reduce inflammation and pain postoperatively. Toxicity can occur with all these drugs and varies among species. Only drugs with a known half-life, metabolism, and toxicity for the particular species should be used. All the NSAIDs can cause gastrointestinal ulceration, particularly in the stomach and lower gastrointestinal tract. This effect varies with the drug and depends on the volume of secretion of the drug in bile. The fenamates have low toxicity, while ibuprofen, naproxen, and PBZ have medium toxicity. Higher toxicity is found with indomethacin and aspirin. PBZ may be more toxic in ponies than in horses and dogs, in which the drug is well tolerated. In ponies there is gastrointestinal tract ulceration followed by a protein-losing enteropathy. Long-term use of NSAIDs can cause renal damage. Overdosage with paracetamol causes acute centrilobular necrosis in the liver due to the build-up of a toxic metabolite. The effect of NSAIDs on prostaglandins can delay parturition in late pregnancy. In feline species metabolism of all NSAIDs is slow. Aspirin overdosage in cats causes a metabolic acidosis with dullness, hyperpnoea, tachypnoea, incoordination, and death.

nuchal ligament (ligamentum nuchae) The powerful structure formed of elastic tissue that assists the extensor muscles of the neck to support the weight of the head. Its cordlike (funicular) part extends from the skull to the vertebral spines at the withers. The sheet-like (lamellar) part extends from the funicular part of the spines of the cervical vertebrae.

nucle- (nucleo-) *Prefix denoting* a cell nucleus.

nuclease An enzyme that catalyses the hydrolysis of nucleic acids by cleaving a phosphodiester bond between adjacent nucleotides. Examples are *ribonuclease*, which acts on RNA, and *deoxyribonuclease*, which acts on DNA. *See also* *restriction endonuclease.

nucleic acid Either of the two types of *polynucleotides of cells and viruses – *DNA and *RNA.

nucleolus (*pl.* **nucleoli**) A dense spherical structure within the cell *nucleus that disappears during cell division. The nucleolus contains *RNA for the synthesis of *ribosomes and plays an important part in RNA and protein synthesis.

nucleoplasm (karyoplasm) The protoplasm making up the nucleus of a cell.

nucleoprotein A complex of nucleic acid and protein. *Ribosomes are nucleoproteins containing RNA; *chromosomes are nucleoproteins containing DNA.

nucleoside A molecule consisting of a nitrogen-containing base (a *purine or *pyrimidine) linked to a pentose sugar (*ribose or *deoxyribose). Examples are *adenosine, *guanosine, *cytidine, *thymidine, and uridine. *See also* nucleotide.

nucleotide A phosphorylated *nucleoside. *See* *DNA; *RNA.

nucleus (*pl.* **nuclei**) **1.** The part of a *cell that contains the genetic material, *DNA. The DNA, which is combined with protein, is normally dispersed throughout the nucleus as *chromatin. During cell division the chromatin becomes visible as *chromosomes. The nucleus also contains *RNA, most of which is located in the *nucleolus. The nucleus is separated from the cytoplasm by a double membrane, the *nuclear envelope*. **2.** An anatomically or functionally distinct mass of nerve cells within the brain or spinal cord.

nutrient Any substance that can be utilized by an animal to sustain its metabolic functions. Some nutrients are essential and must be provided in the *diet to promote optimum health and performance. These include the *essential amino acids, *vitamins, *essential elements, and *essential fatty acids. Water too is essential, as is a source of energy – *fat, *carbohydrates, and *protein all have energy-yielding potential. Furthermore, nutrient interconversions may take place in vivo, for example the synthesis of fat from carbohydrate.

nutrition All the processes by which an animal takes in and utilizes food, principally *ingestion, *digestion, and *absorption. Apart from studying the physiology of nutrition, animal nutritionists are also concerned with determining the *nutrient requirements of animals, characterizing the nutrient content of feedstuffs, and formulating *diets. The nutrient requirements of livestock are customarily divided into those for maintenance and those for production. *Maintenance requirements* are those needed to sustain the vital functions and prevent the depletion of body reserves. They thus vary, particularly according to the environmental conditions prevailing. *Production requirements* are those needed for growth, pregnancy, lactation, etc. and vary with the individual and the type and level of production. It is conventional to estimate requirements individually for each *nutrient, although interactions between them are often of considerable importance.

nutritional myopathy *See* muscular dystrophy.

nux vomica *See* strychnine poisoning.

nyct- (nycto-) *Prefix denoting* night or darkness.

nyctalopia *See* night blindness.

nymph An immature stage in the life cycle of certain insects, for example, grasshoppers, cockroaches, and dragonflies, which hatches from the egg and closely resembles the adult in structure except that the wings and reproductive organs are relatively undeveloped. There is no pupal stage and it develops directly into the adult via a series of moults.

nymphomania A syndrome affecting high-yielding dairy cows and associated with the presence of thin-walled *ovarian cysts. Most cases occur at or around peak lactation, and hereditary factors appear to be important in the incidence of this condition. Affected cows may show a thickening of the neck, relaxation of the pelvic ligaments, and a raised tail head. They have abnormally frequent and/or prolonged periods of oestrus, but some affected animals may be anoestrous. Bull-like behaviour is common. Rupture of the cysts, either manually via the rectum or by the administration of suitable drugs, may effect a return to normality.

nystagmus Rapid rhythmical movements of the eyes. It is commonly seen in the early stages of anaesthesia, and may occasionally occur due to malfunction of the central nervous system, particularly that involving the eighth cranial nerve.

nystatin An antibiotic with antifungal activity, isolated from *Streptomyces noursei*. It is incorporated in many skin and oral preparations for topical treatment of yeast infections, and acts by binding to fungal membranes, causing a change in permeability and leakage of intracellular material. Nystatin is nonirritant to skin and mucous membranes. However, it is not active against the dermatophytes causing ringworm.

O

oak poisoning *See* acorn poisoning.

oats A cereal grown extensively in Europe for its grain. It is used as an animal feedstuff following processing (i.e. grinding, rolling, or flaking). It is relatively high in fibre but its *protein quality is good compared to other cereals.

obesity Excessive deposition of fat in the body tissues, commonly due to high intake of energy-rich foods and/or inadequate exercise. It is a common disorder in ageing dogs; these tend to have a reduced rate of metabolism, which exacerbates the problem. Also, obesity often follows castration. Some breeds of dogs are almost naturally obese, for example dachshunds and Labradors, whereas hunting dogs and retrievers tend to stay lean. Cats are less prone, but caged birds often succumb to overindulgence and grow fat. As in man, obesity can follow changes in behaviour, particularly exercise routines, in which the pet owner may play an important role. Obesity reduces life expectancy and causes undue fatigue. Treatment involves careful dieting (*see* diet) and regular exercise.

obex The caudal curved margin of the fourth *ventricle of the brain where it becomes continuous with the central canal of the spinal cord.

obligate Describing an organism that is restricted to one particular way of life. For example, an *obligate parasite* cannot live without its host(s).

oblique abdominal muscle One of two sheets of muscle in each lateral abdominal wall. The superficial *external oblique abdominal muscle* runs caudoventrally; the deeper *internal* *oblique abdominal muscle* runs cranioventrally. Both insert to the *linea alba by means of an *aponeurosis, which contributes to the sheaths of the *rectus abdominis. Both muscles act to increase intra-abdominal pressure.

obstetrics The study and management of *parturition and the surrounding events; i.e. pregnancy, labour, and the immediate postparturient period (puerperium).

obturator nerve One of the nerves of the hindlimb extending from the *lumbar plexus. It runs medial to the ilium and through the obturator foramen in the *os coxae to supply the adductor muscles of the hip. In cattle it can be compressed against the ilium during parturition resulting in *obturator paralysis* in which the hindlimbs splay outwards.

obturator paralysis Paralysis of the adductor muscles of the hindlimbs caused by injury to the obturator nerve (and sometimes other pelvic nerves) due to the presence of a large foetus or pressure over a period of time in a case of *dystocia. The animal is usually bright and well but cannot use its hindlimbs and lies with them splayed out from the midline. The cow is most commonly affected. Treatment involves keeping the animal comfortable with dry bedding and on a nonslip surface. Turning the animal gently and some physiotherapy will aid recovery in most cases. The prognosis is poor if there is no improvement within 7 days. Occasionally other nerves can be involved, producing a similar condition.

occipital bone The bone forming the back (squamous part) and part of the base of the cranium (basilar part). Two occipital condyles form rounded surfaces that articulate with the first cervical vertebra (atlas) forming the atlanto-occipital joint. Between the condyles is the foramen magnum, the opening through which the spinal cord passes. *See* skull.

occiput The back of the head or skull.

occlusion 1. The closing or obstruction of a hollow organ or duct. **2.** The relationship between the contacting surfaces (*occlusal surfaces*) of the upper and lower teeth.

ochratoxicosis Disease caused by ingestion of ochratoxin A, which occurs principally in stored grain that is mouldy with strains of *Penicillium viridicatum* or *P. cyclopium*. The toxin is associated mainly with kidney disease in **pigs**; commonly recognized in Denmark and Sweden and also reported from the USA, this is apparently due to the prolonged use of feed containing small quantities of ochratoxin. Clinical signs include polyuria, polydipsia, and depression of growth; grossly the kidneys appear pale and enlarged. The renal pathology is not specific and diagnosis requires the support of demonstrable ochratoxin in feed and preferably in body tissues. A number of severe outbreaks of ochratoxicosis have occurred in **poultry**, in some cases with high mortality. There is decreased growth rate, poor feed conversion, kidney disease, and an *air sacculitis attributed to toxic immunosuppression.

oct- (octa-, octi-, octo-) *Prefix denoting* eight.

ocular Of or concerned with the eye or vision.

ocular tumours Any of various tumours of the eye. Although tumours of the eye itself (i.e. intraocular tumours) are uncommon in domestic animals, neoplasms of the eyelids are more frequent. In **dogs**, *melanomas arising from the iris or ciliary body are the most common intraocular tumour. They present as a black (occasionally unpigmented) mass associated with the iris; there may be secondary glaucoma. Removal of the whole eye is usually curative. *Lymphosarcoma may also involve the iris but is usually part of the more generalized disease. *Meibomian gland adenomas are not uncommon tumours of the eyelids in older dogs. In **cats**, both melanomas and lymphosarcomas occur in a similar pattern to dogs. *Squamous cell carcinomas of the eyelids and conjunctiva are not uncommon, especially in white cats. This tumour is locally aggressive but tends not to metastasize. Surgical resection or cryotherapy may be curative in early cases. Intraocular tumours are rare in **horses**, but tumours of the eyelids and conjunctiva are relatively common, especially fibrosarcoma (*see* equine sarcoid) and squamous cell carcinoma. Various types of treatment may be used, including surgical resection, cryotherapy, and local radiotherapy. In **cattle**, squamous cell carcinoma of the eyelids and conjunctiva is relatively common in certain parts of the world, especially the lower latitudes, and may cause appreciable economic losses. White-faced Herefords and Hereford crosses are most prone, and solar-induced dermatitis is considered to be a precancerous state. Early treatment may be curative, but prevention by selective breeding for pigmentation of the face is more important.

oculo- *Prefix denoting* the eye(s).

oculomotor Concerned with eye movements.

oculomotor nerve The third *cranial nerve (III). Its fibres supply many of the muscles that move the eye, and also the muscles that constrict the pupil and alter the focus of the lens.

odont- (odonto-) *Prefix denoting* a tooth.

odontoblast A cell of the *tooth germ and the *dental pulp concerned with the formation of *dentine.

odontoid process *See* dens.

odontoma A tumour arising from the tooth bud. They have been described in many species as rare tumours of the mouth.

odours (meat inspection) Any of various abnormal smells encountered during the examination of meat or carcasses. There are numerous causes, including: diet (e.g. fish meal fed to pigs too close to the date of slaughter); drugs administered to animals just before slaughter; products of a disordered metabolism (e.g. the smell of acetone in cows with *ketosis); sexual odours (e.g. in old boars or male goats); abscesses; putrefaction; gangrene; and other diseases (e.g. cheesy smell of muscle in blackleg).

-odynia *Suffix denoting* pain in (a specified part).

oedema The accumulation of excess fluid in a body cavity or tissue, popularly known as *dropsy*. Oedema is evidence of disturbance in the forces normally controlling the amount of fluid leaving and re-entering the bloodstream, and it commonly accompanies chronic congestive *heart failure, impairment in venous return to the heart, disturbances in lymphatic circulation, and conditions associated with *hypoproteinaemia. It may be generalized or localized. The terms *hydrothorax and *ascites are used for oedema in the thoracic and abdominal cavities respectively; severe generalized oedema is called *anasarca. In generalized oedema, the fluid's distribution is dictated by gravitational forces, and it accumulates especially in loose structures such as the brisket, in the middle of the lower jaw (bottle jaw), and around the extremities of the limbs. Oedema fluid is a transudate, formed passively and characteristically low in protein, in contrast to an exudate, which is an actively formed protein-rich fluid produced in inflammation.

oedema disease An infectious disease of young pigs caused by strains of *Escherichia coli*, characterized by oedema in various sites and neurological disturbances. The O serogroups mainly involved are 138, 139, and 141. In addition to the usual enterotoxins, these serogroups produce *EDP* (*oedema disease principle*), a toxin that damages blood vessels, including those of the brain. Recently weaned animals (8–12 weeks of age) in good condition are affected, and mortality may be high. Signs include ataxia, convulsions, paralysis, hoarse squealing, and oedema of the face and throat; death is sudden. Oedema of the stomach and mesentery is seen at post-mortem examination. Antibiotic treatment is used, with varying degrees of success. Other names: **bowel oedema**; **gut oedema**.

oesophag- (**oesophago-**) (*US* **esophag-, esophago-**) *Prefix denoting* the oesophagus. Example: *oesophagectomy* (surgical removal of).

oesophageal groove *See* reticular groove.

oesophageal obstruction *See* choke.

oesophagitis Inflammation of the oesophagus. Oesophagitis may occur in all species after ingestion of irritant chemicals, but in domestic animals it is probably most commonly seen as a feature of certain viral diseases of cattle, i.e. *bovine virus diarrhoea, and *bovine papular stomatitis.

Oesophagostomum A genus of *strongylid parasitic nematodes containing members that cause disease (*oesophagostomiasis*) in pigs and ruminants in most tropical countries. Important species include *O. radiatum* (in cattle), *O. venulosum* and *O. columbianum* (in sheep), and *O. dentatum* (in pigs). The adults inhabit the large intestine. Eggs are passed in the faeces and the larvae develop on herbage, where they await ingestion by a host. The larvae are found in the small and large intestine and take 8 weeks to develop into adults in the large intestine. Infestation causes loss of appetite, unthriftiness, anaemia, colitis, and diarrhoea. If severe it can cause necrotic enteritis. Peritonitis has been reported in goats. Treatment is with *benzimidazoles or ivermectin.

oesophagostomy An operation to create an opening into the oesophagus from the surface of the neck. In animals this is generally a temporary measure to allow force-feeding, which may be necessary in a debilitated animal or one in which grasping, chewing, or swallowing are difficult or impossible due to disease. Food or fluids can then be introduced to the oesophagus using a syringe or tube (*see* stomach tube).

oesophagotomy Surgical incision into the lumen of the oesophagus. This is most commonly performed to remove a foreign body firmly lodged in the oesophagus. Such obstruction generally occurs in small animals and in most cases involves a bone fragment. The incision may be into the cervical or thoracic parts of the oesophagus. The latter is more difficult as it involves entering the thoracic cavity, either between two ribs or after removal of one or more ribs. Access is limited and assisted ventilation under general anaesthesia is necessary.

oesophagus (*pl.* **oesophagi**) The muscular tube lined by mucous membrane that extends from the pharynx to the stomach. Waves of *peristalsis help to propel food towards the stomach after swallowing and in the opposite direction during vomiting or rumination. *See also* alimentary tract.

oestradiol The major female sex hormone produced by the ovary in many mammals. *See* oestrogen.

oestrogen Any of a group of female sex hormones, produced principally by the ovarian follicles, that promote the development of secondary sexual characteristics and control the *oestrous cycle. The oestrogens are *steroids, and the ovarian follicle has enzymes that catalyse the removal of carbon atom 18 from the steroid nucleus; 17-carbon steroids are generally oestrogenic in nature. *Oestradiol*, which has hydroxyl groups at the 3 and 17 positions, is the major oestrogen triggering the onset of *oestrus in many mammals. During pregnancy the foetal placenta can contribute to oestradiol production. *Oestrone* has a ketone group at the 17 position of the steroid nucleus. Its sulphate derivative is produced by the foetal placenta unit of many mammals and can be found in maternal plasma for the diagnosis of pregnancy and determination of foetal viability.

Therapeutic uses Both natural and synthetic oestrogens are used to treat a range of reproductive disorders. Oestradiol is not effective if given orally because of rapid liver metabolism, but it is used in implants. Various oestradiol esters (e.g. oestradiol benzoate, oestradiol valerate, oestradiol dipropionate) are available formulated in oil for injection. Absorption is slow and metabolism

varies: oestradiol benzoate is effective for 2–3 days and oestradiol dipropionate for 2–3 weeks. Ethinyl oestradiol is not inactivated in the liver and can be given orally.

Oestrogens can be used to induce heat in bitches; low doses over a prolonged period cause follicular development and ovulation. This does not occur in any other species. In cattle oestrogens are injected to treat uterine infections, induce abortion, and to expel the foetus in cases of foetal mummification. Oestrogens can also be used to prevent pregnancy after mismating in bitches. A single injection of oestradiol benzoate within 48 hours of mating prevents passage of fertilized ova to the uterus. There is a prolonged oestrus with increased bleeding after this treatment. False pregnancy in the bitch can be treated by oral dosing with a combination of ethinyl oestradiol and methyl testosterone, which reduces lactation and behavioural changes. In ovariohysterectomized bitches, urinary incontinence and alopecia can be treated with oestrogens. Prostatic hyperplasia and anal adenomas can be reduced in size with oestrogen therapy.

Oestrogens combined with other reproductive hormones have been used in implants as growth promoters in cattle, but these are now banned in EEC countries. The use of *stilbenes (synthetic oestrogens) is similarly illegal in food-producing animals, but they can be used therapeutically in small animals in some countries.

Side-effects with oestrogens can include abortion, formation of cystic ovaries, relaxation and oedema of the vulva and pelvic ligaments predisposing to prolapse of the rectum and vagina, bone marrow depression in dogs causing severe anaemia (injections for misalliance should be limited to one per season to try to reduce the risk of fatal anaemias), and feminization in male animals.

oestrogenic mycotoxicosis

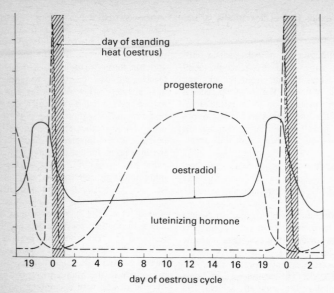

day of standing heat (oestrus)

progesterone

oestradiol

luteinizing hormone

| 19 | 0 | 2 | 4 | 6 | 8 | 10 | 12 | 14 | 16 | 19 | 0 | 2 |

day of oestrous cycle

The changing concentrations of oestrogens (oestradiol), progesterone, and gonadotrophins (luteinizing hormone) in peripheral blood during the bovine oestrous cycle

oestrogenic mycotoxicosis *See* fusariotoxicosis.

oestrogenism *See* vulvovaginitis.

oestrone One of the female sex hormones. *See* oestrogen.

oestrous cycle The cycle of reproductive activity exhibited by sexually mature nonpregnant female mammals (other than most primates, including humans, which undergo a menstrual cycle). The physiological and behavioural changes of the cycle are regulated by hormones, secreted by the pituitary gland and ovary. The cycle can be divided into phases (see illustration). *Pro-oestrus* involves the development of one or more *ovarian follicles under the influence of pituitary *gonadotrophins. These maturing follicles progressively secrete *oes-

trogens, which lead to *oestrus*, when the female becomes receptive to the male and *ovulation occurs. The next phase is *metoestrus*, during which the *corpus luteum develops from the ruptured ovarian follicle; this is succeeded by *dioestrus*, the longest phase, during which *progesterone produced by the mature corpus luteum exerts influence over the organs of the reproductive tract.

The length of the cycle depends on the species (see table). In *polyoestrous* mammals (e.g. cattle and pigs) the end of one cycle leads directly to the beginning of another. In *monoestrous* species (e.g. dog) a single cycle occurs two to three times per year each separated from the next by a lengthy *anoestrus phase, during which the oestrous cycle is suspended. *Seasonal polyoestrous* species (e.g. horse, sheep, and cat) exhibit a series of consecu-

Reproductive cycles of the principal domestic species

Species	Reproductive activity	Length of oestrous cycle (days)	Length of oestrus	Time of ovulation
Cow	Polyoestrous	21	18 hr	9 hr after end of oestrus
Ewe	Seasonally polyoestrous	17	29 hr	At end of standing oestrus
Sow	Polyoestrous	21	45 hr	24 hr before end of oestrus
Mare	Seasonally polyoestrous	21	4–5 days	24–28 hr before end of standing oestrus
Doe (goat)	Seasonally polyoestrous	20	40 hr	33 hr after beginning of oestrus
Bitch	Monoestrous (av. 7½ months between cycles)	Variable	Pro-oestrus 9 days (av.), oestrus 9 days (av.)	2nd–3rd day of oestrus
Queen	Seasonally polyoestrous	Variable (21 days is typical)	Pro-oestrus 1–3 days, oestrus 8 days	Reflex ovulator – induced 27 hr after coitus

tive oestrous cycles at particular times of the year.

oestrus (heat) The stage of the *oestrous cycle when the animal is receptive to the male and is willing to stand for mating. It occurs at the optimum time for fertilization when ovulation is imminent, and the behavioural signs (*see* oestrus detection) are triggered by the influence on the brain of the pre-ovulatory surge in plasma *oestrogens, following initial priming with *progesterone. For the duration of oestrus and its relation to the timing of ovulation, see table. *See also* oestrus synchronization.

Oestrus A genus of flies containing the *sheep nostril fly.

oestrus detection (heat detection) The identification of females demonstrating *oestrus (heat) and hence readiness to mate. Signs in most species include increased restlessness and excitement and reddening and swelling of the vulva. Oestrus detection is particularly important in animals destined for *artificial insemination; it is usually less critical where breeding females run with a breeding male. Correct timing of insemination is vital to ensure high *conception rates. In cattle the most obvious sign of oestrus is acceptance of mounting by other females, i.e. bulling behaviour. If cows are watched continually, about 95% of oestrus periods can be detected. However, since oestrus often occurs at night and is missed, the average oestrus detection rate is only 55–60%. Therefore, it is important that cows are observed for at least three 20-minute periods each day, when the cows are quiet and not distracted by other activities, such as milking or feeding. Successful detection is more likely if all observed occurrences of bulling are recorded, even if the cow is not served, so subsequent oestrus periods can be anticipated. Other signs of oestrus are a discharge of mucus from the vulva, lack of appetite, reduced milk production, and bellowing; these are useful indicators in cows housed in stalls with no opportunity to exhibit bulling behaviour. *See also* artificial insemination; oestrus synchronization.

In **pigs**, apart from reddening and swelling of the vulva, the sexually receptive sow will arch her back when it is pressed. A *teaser male can be employed for oestrus detection in cattle, pigs, mares, and sheep.

At oestrus the **mare** typically shows greater interest in the stallion and becomes more awkward to handle. In the presence of the stallion she may squat, raise the tail and pass urine, and 'wink' ('show') the clitoris. However, behaviour varies with individuals. There is slackening of the vulva and a slight discharge.

In the **bitch**, pro-oestrus is characterized by swelling of the vulva and a bloodstained vulval discharge, and frequently by a change of behaviour, with increased restlessness, thirst, and sexual interest. During oestrus itself the vulva remains swollen but the discharge becomes clear or straw-coloured.

In the **queen** pro-oestrus is characterized by increased friendliness and increased frequency of urination, sometimes with spraying like a tom-cat. During oestrus the queen emits loud calling noises to attract male cats, and often rolls about on the floor as if in great pain.

oestrus synchronization The manipulation of the *oestrus cycle so that all animals in a group exhibit *oestrus at the same time. The timing of insemination, birth, and weaning of the young are also synchronized, bringing considerable benefits. In **cattle** synchronization of oestrus can be especially useful for heifers, in which oestrus detection is often difficult; it also makes handling easier since all inseminations are performed on the same day and all heifers should enter the herd at about the same time. Two methods are available for cattle. A *PRID can be inserted into the vagina and left for 12 days; the cow comes into oestrus 2–3 days after removal of the PRID. Alternatively, injection of *prostaglandin $F_{2\alpha}$ or its synthetic analogues induces oestrus after 3–4 days but only if the cow is between day 5 and day 15 of her cycle. For this reason two injections of prostaglandin 11 days apart are needed for effective synchronization of a group of cows or heifers. Mares can be synchronized by the use of *prostaglandin $F_{2\alpha}$, and will come into oestrus 5 days after injection, if the drug is given 7 days after the end of oestrus. In **sheep** a *progesterone-soaked sponge is inserted into the vagina and left for 12–16 days. Ewes will come into oestrus 24–48 hours after sponge removal. In **pigs** a safe, reliable, and cost-effective artificial method has yet to be developed. In sows, synchronized weaning gives good synchrony of the subsequent oestrus. *See also* oestrus detection.

offal *See* meat.

offal 1. Waste products of the meat industry The evisceration and cutting of carcasses produces various types of offal, which are usually dried and ground to form a meal, for example meat meal or offal meat and bone meal. **2.** By-products of the milling industry, especially ones used as animal feedstuffs.

Official Veterinary Surgeon (OVS) (UK) A veterinary surgeon designated by the Minister and appointed by the local authority to carry out duties of inspection and supervision under the Poultry Meat (Hygiene) Regulations (1976) or Fresh Meat Export (Hygiene and Inspection) Regulations (1981).

-oid *Suffix denoting* like; resembling.

oil Any of various viscous liquids that are generally immiscible with water. Natural plant and animal oils are commonly *glycerides of fatty acids, although the *essential oils* of plant origin consist chiefly of *terpenes. Vegetable oils are an important dietary constituent for many animals and normally contain significant amounts of fat-soluble vitamins and *essential fatty acids. *Mineral oils* are mixtures of hydrocarbons (e.g. petroleum) and have no nutritional value although they are sometimes used medicinally, for example as laxatives. Various oils are used in therapy in tonics, bases for drugs, as vehicles for ointments, in dietary supplements, and for flavouring food.

olaquindox *See* growth promoter.

oleander poisoning Toxicity due to ingestion of the Mediterranean evergreen shrub, *Nerium oleander* (oleander), which is cultivated as an ornamental in the southern USA and elsewhere. It contains cardiac glycosides (oleandroside, nerioside, etc.) similar to digitoxin (*see* digitalis). The clinical signs are abdominal pain, vomiting, diarrhoea, increased pulse rate, weakness, and death. Treatment consists of *atropine administration and symptomatic therapy. *See also* foxglove poisoning.

oleandomycin *See* macrolide antibiotics.

oleo- *Prefix denoting* oil.

olfaction The sense of smell. Terrestrial vertebrates possess olfactory organs (such as the nose) containing olfactory cells that are sensitive to air-borne chemicals and are responsible for the sense of smell. Stimulation of these cells results in the transmission of nerve impulses to the brain via the *olfactory nerve. Fish and other aquatic animals have similar organs that are sensitive to water-borne chemicals.

olfactory bulb A large elliptical mass at the front of the brain that is the site of attachment of the *olfactory nerve and gives rise to the olfactory tracts, which run to the *piriform lobe and other parts.

olfactory nerve The first *cranial nerve (I). It comprises special sensory fibres that convey impulses concerned with the sense of smell from the mucous membrane in the upper part of the nasal cavity to the olfactory bulb of the brain.

olig- (oligo-) *Prefix denoting* **1.** few. **2.** a deficiency.

oligodendrocyte One of the cell types of the *neuroglia that is responsible for producing the *myelin sheaths of the neurones of the central nervous system. It is equivalent to the *neurolemmal cell of the peripheral nervous system.

oligodendroglioma A rare type of *brain tumour.

oligohydramnios The condition in which there is too little fluid in the amniotic cavity surrounding the developing foetus. *Compare* hydramnios.

oligospermia A condition in which there is an abnormally low number of spermatozoa in the semen, which can lead to *infertility. *See also* aspermia.

oliguria The production of an abnormally small volume of urine. It may be due to *shock, renal disease, dehydration (when highly concentrated urine is formed), or obstructive disease of the lower urinary tract (when the voiding of urine is impaired; *see* urolithiasis).

-ology *Suffix. See* -logy.

-oma *Suffix denoting* a tumour. Examples: *hepatoma* (of the liver); *lymphoma* (of the lymph nodes).

omasum (*pl.* **omasa**) The third of the four chambers of the ruminant *stomach, lying to the right of the midline in the cranial part of the abdomen. It is filled from the *reticulum via the reticulo-omasal orifice and empties into the *abomasum.

omental bursa The portion of the peritoneal cavity lying within the folded *omentum. It is continuous with the remainder of the peritoneal cavity via the omental (epiploic) foramen.

omentectomy Surgical removal of all or part of the *omentum. This may be necessary if, for example, the omentum is infected or develops a malignant growth.

omentopexy Surgical fixation of the omentum in a certain position. This can form part of the surgical treatment of left displacement of the abomasum in cattle. The displacement is corrected manually and the greater omentum is sutured to the parietal peritoneum. *See also* abomasopexy; pyloropexy.

omentum (*pl.* **omenta** or **omentums**) A double-layered fat-filled fold of *peritoneum attaching the stomach to other organs. The *greater omentum* attaches to the greater curvature of the stomach in monogastric species, and to the rumen, omasum, and greater curvature of the abomasum in ruminants. It is folded upon itself and attaches to other *mesenteries near the dorsal body wall. The *lesser omentum* forms an attachment between the lesser curvature of the stomach or abomasum and the liver.

omotransversarius A muscle that runs from the acromion and spine of the *scapula to the transverse process of the *atlas.

omphal- (omphalo-) *Prefix denoting* the umbilical cord.

omphalitis Inflammation of the navel (umbilicus) or *umbilical cord. In **mammals**, inflammation of the navel occurring shortly after birth is generally due to bacterial infection. *Omphalophlebitis* (i.e. inflammation of the umbilical veins) is a commoner condition in newborn farm animals, especially calves, and is associated with a variety of bacteria (*see* navel ill).

In **birds**, the *yolk sac is the main site of infection; *Staphylococcus aureus*, *Escherichia coli*, and various other bacteria may be involved, causing *mushy chick disease* (also called *yolk sac infection*). Chicks die on leaving the hatchery, with distended yolk sacs and occasionally with fluid oozing through the navel; the yolk sac may rupture internally. A similar condition is seen in turkey poults (*turkey omphalitis*): the navel is inflamed and fails to close. There is no adequate remedy except to empty, cleanse, and disinfect the hatchery.

omphalophlebitis *See* navel ill.

Onchocerca A genus of parasitic filarial nematodes (*see* filaria) that cause disease (*onchocerciasis) in cattle, horses, and humans and are found in most tropical countries, Australia, and North America. The adult female worms may reach 500 cm in length and are about 0.3–0.4 mm thick; males are shorter (20–70 cm). Distribution of the parasites is associated with rivers, the habitat of black flies (*Simulium* spp.), which act as main vectors. *O. gibsoni* occurs in cattle in Australia, Africa, Malaysia, and the Indian subcontinent. The adult worms are found in nodules in the brisket and outer surface of the hindlimbs. *O. lienalis* occurs in the gastrosplenic ligament. *O. gutturosa*, found in cattle in Britain and Africa, encysts in the ligamentum nuchae in the neck, especially at the point of attachment to the thoracic vertebrae. Infestation with *O. armillata*, found in some tropical countries, is thought to be more serious. The adult worms live in the aorta and its branches. *O. reticulata* occurs in the flexor tendons and suspensory ligaments of the fetlock and also in the knee of equines. These species are transmitted by *midges, which act as intermediate hosts. The larvae (*microfilariae) of most species occur in the skin. The skin-rasping blood-sucking vectors take up the microfilariae when feeding and transmit them to other host individuals. *O. volvulus* is responsible for disease in humans (river blindness).

onchocerciasis Disease due to infestation with parasitic nematodes of the genus *Onchocerca*. Species affected include cattle, horses and humans. The adult nematodes are encased in fibrous cysts or nodules in subcutaneous and connective tissues. The larvae (microfilariae) gather in skin and eye tissues causing papular itching skin sores. In horses the nodules in the neck may be referred to as *fistulous withers (poll evil), but these are not always onchocercal in origin. The microfilariae can be eliminated by using a suitable *anthelmintic while the nodules may be surgically removed. Control of the insect vectors helps prevent the disease. In humans, migration of the larvae to the eye can cause partial or total blindness (*river blindness*).

onco- *Prefix denoting* **1.** a tumour. **2.** volume.

oncogene A gene that induces cancer. *See* oncogenic virus.

oncogenic Describing an agent that is capable of causing or of facilitating the development of a neoplasm. Oncogenic agents act on target cells to produce a change in their genetic material, which results in uncontrolled proliferation of the transformed cells. Known oncogenic agents include physical factors, such as radiation, chemical substances (*see* carcinogen), and viruses. Important oncogenic viruses in domestic animals include the *papillomaviruses, responsible for warts, and the *oncoviruses (a subfamily of retroviruses), which are associated with *avian leukosis, *feline leukaemia, and *enzootic bovine leukosis. *See also* oncogene.

oncogenic virus A *virus that is able to induce tumours in animals or cause the transformation of cells grown in culture. Both DNA- and RNA-containing viruses are known to be oncogenic, including members of the *papovavirus, *adenovirus, and *herpesvirus families (DNA viruses) and the *oncovirus subfamily of the retroviruses (RNA viruses). Oncogenic viruses appear to induce tumours by

oncology

inserting part of their DNA (in the case of DNA viruses) or a DNA copy of their RNA (in the case of RNA viruses) into the DNA of their host cell, thus changing its genetic information and its growth behaviour. Viral antigens are commonly found in the transformed cells.

oncology The study and practice of treating tumours.

oncosphere (hexacanth) The initial larval stage of a *tapeworm, having six hooks for penetrating the intestinal wall of the intermediate host. It is then transported by the bloodstream or lymph to the muscles, liver, brain, etc., where it develops into the infective larval state (*see* bladderworm).

oncotic Characterized by a tumour or swelling.

oncovirus A subfamily of the *retrovirus family of RNA *viruses, members of which cause a variety of mammalian, avian, and human tumours.

Ondiri disease *See* bovine infectious petechial fever.

ontogeny The history of the development of an individual from the fertilized egg to maturity.

onych- (onycho-) *Prefix denoting* a claw or nail.

onychia Inflammation of the matrix of the claw.

onycholysis Abnormal loosening of the claws.

onychomycosis Any fungal infection of the claws or nails. It is rare in animals and is seen mostly as part of a more extensive *ringworm infection, for example *Microsporum canis* in cats (the infected claw may fluoresce under *Wood's light), or *Trichophyton mentagrophytes*, especially in dogs with a generalized infection. Prolonged *griseofulvin treatment may be necessary to eliminate infection, and in dogs amputation of the nail is recommended. Onychomycoses are not uncommon in humans, usually caused by *dermatophyte fungi (*tinea unguium*) or *Candida albicans*.

onychorrhexis Brittle nails. It occurs in all species of domestic animals and may be hereditary or related to poor nutrition.

oo- *Prefix denoting* an egg; ovum.

oocyst A spherical or ovoid microscopic nonmotile cyst formed during the life cycle of some protozoa following a sexual reproductive phase. In the *coccidia, oocysts have a tough wall and are passed in faeces from the host into the environment, in which they remain viable for many months. Within the oocyst *sporozoites are formed.

oocyte A cell in the ovary that undergoes *meiosis to form an *ovum. *Primary oocytes* are formed from oogonia in the foetal ovary, and are most numerous in late foetal life. However, only a fraction survive to sexual maturity and even fewer will be ovulated. The primary oocytes become surrounded by follicular cells to form *follicles. At ovulation the reduction division of meiosis is completed producing a *secondary oocyte* and a *polar body*. Fertilization of the egg stimulates the second meiotic division, which produces the haploid ovum and a second polar body.

oogenesis The process by which mature ova (egg cells) are produced in the ovary (see illustration). Primordial germ cells multiply to form *oogonia, which start their first meiotic division to become primary

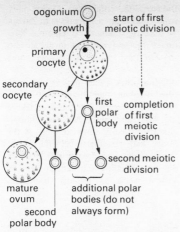

oogonium

growth

start of first meiotic division

primary oocyte

secondary oocyte

first polar body

completion of first meiotic division

second meiotic division

mature ovum

additional polar bodies (do not always form)

second polar body

Oogenesis

*oocytes in the foetus. This division is not completed until near the time of ovulation. The second meiotic division is only completed on fertilization. Each meiotic division is unequal, so that one large ovum is produced with much smaller polar bodies.

oogonium (*pl.* **oogonia**) A cell in the ovary that is the early precursor of an ovum (egg cell). In the young embryo, primordial germ cells migrate from the yolk sac to the site of the developing ovary, where they multiply to form oogonia. During embryonic and foetal life, these diploid cells commence the first reduction division of meiosis to form *oocytes, a full complement of which is formed before the birth of the animal.

oophor- (oophoro-) *Prefix denoting* the ovary.

oophorectomy *See* ovariectomy.

oophoritis (ovaritis) Inflammation of an ovary. The condition rarely occurs alone and is usually associated with *salpingitis (inflammation of the uterine tubes), pelvic *peritonitis, or both. Oopharitis may be acute or chronic and associated with a varying degree of abdominal pain and depression. The ovary is relatively resistant to infection, and the bloodstream is the more probable route for infective organisms. Tuberculosis occasionally causes metastatic *granulomata.

open joint A condition in which a joint cavity becomes open to the external environment. This facilitates the entry of pathogenic organisms to the joint, and an infective *arthritis is the likely outcome.

operon A unit of *DNA consisting of a *gene that codes for some recognizable product, and another portion of DNA that controls the switching on and off of that gene.

ophthalm- (ophthalmo-) *Prefix denoting* the eye.

ophthalmia (ophthalmitis) Inflammation of the eye. *Periodic ophthalmia is a disease of horses, mules, and asses characterized by recurring bouts of ophthalmia interspersed with periods of remission. *See also* conjunctivitis; retinitis; uveitis.

ophthalmic Concerned with the eye.

ophthalmitis *See* ophthalmia.

ophthalmology The study and treatment of eye diseases.

ophthalmoscope An instrument for examining the interior of the eye. It is designed so that the examiner, whose eye is shielded from extraneous light, looks down a beam of light directed through the pupil of the subject's eye. This illuminates the interior of the eye and makes its structures visible.
Lenses in the ophthalmoscope bring the structures under examination into

focus. A *direct ophthalmoscope* employs no lens in the light beam; it is used at a distance to examine for obstruction to the reflected light beam, or used close to to examine structures in detail, at the spot where the beam falls inside the eye. An *indirect ophthalmoscope* employs a condensing lens in the light beam and, unless corrected, gives an inverted image of the interior of the eye. It provides a wider field of vision but lower magnification than the direct ophthalmoscope.

-opia *Suffix denoting* a defect of the eye or of vision.

opiate A drug derived from *opium, such as *morphine, *codeine, and and the semisynthetic drug heroin. Often the term is also used to include synthetic drugs with morphine-like activity, referred to as *opioids*; these include *buprenorphine, diphenoxylate, *etorphine, *fentanyl, *pethidine, and *pentazocine.

opioid antagonist (narcotic antagonist) A drug that reverses the pharmacological effects of the morphine-type drugs (*see* opiate) by competitively binding to morphine receptors. The commonly used agents are naloxone, nalorphine, and *diprenorphine (the latter two are partial agonists).

opisth- (opistho-) *Prefix denoting* **1.** dorsal; posterior. **2.** backwards.

Opisthorchis A genus of *flukes, similar to *Dicrocoelium spp., occurring in eastern Europe and parts of southeast Asia. The adult flukes are parasites of the bile ducts of carnivorous mammals, although they may also infest pigs and humans (particularly *O. sinensis*). Heavy infestations are manifest as jaundice with cholangiohepatitis and biliary fibrosis. They are also associated with biliary adenomas and adenocarcinomas in

the cat. *O. tenuicollis* affects dogs, cats, and foxes in Europe and Russia; *O. sinensis* (Chinese or Oriental liver fluke) affects carnivores in Japan and the Far East.

opisthotonus (star gazing) A posture involving an involuntary spasmodic contraction of the muscles of the head and neck. Affected animals characteristically show arching of the body and extension of the neck. Opisthotonus is frequently seen in diseases affecting the central nervous system, such as tetanus, brainstem lesions, meningitis, and cerebrocortical necrosis.

opium A crude extract derived from the juice of the poppy *Papaver somniferum*, possessing analgesic activity. Crude opium contains more than 20 alkaloids, including *morphine and *codeine. Toxicity can occur in animals after eating the stems and seeds of *P. somniferum*: initial respiratory depression, sedation, and constipation are followed by central nervous stimulation, with tachypnoea, convulsions, and circulatory failure. It can be treated using the antagonists naloxone, nalorphine, or diprenorphine.

opportunistic Describing a pathogen that is capable of causing disease only in compromised hosts, i.e. ones whose innate defence mechanisms (e.g. immunity) are weakened, for example by a concurrent disease or defect. Some opportunists may cause infection exclusively in compromised hosts, while others (e.g. *Aspergillus fumigatus*) may be able to overcome the defences of a normal host if the inoculum size and circumstances of exposure are favourable.

opsonin Any agent, such as an *antibody, that promotes the *phagocytosis of *antigen. Antibody opsonins usually act in combination with *complement.

opsonization The coating of an antigenic particle with *opsonin.

opt- (opto-) *Prefix denoting* vision or the eye.

optic Concerned with the eye or vision.

optical activity The property possessed by some substances of rotating the plane of polarization of polarized light. A compound that rotates the plane to the left is described as *laevorotatory* (or l-); one that rotates the plane to the right is described as *dextrorotatory* (or d-). *See also* stereoisomers.

optic canal The opening (foramen) at the apex of the *orbit through which pass the *optic nerve and internal ophthalmic artery.

optic chiasma The X-shaped structure, located in the floor of the brain in front of the pituitary gland, that connects the *optic nerves and *optic tracts. Some of the optic nerve fibres cross through it to the opposite *optic tract (see illustration).

optic disc The circular area from which the optic nerve arises on the retina. It is devoid of light receptors and is hence otherwise termed the *blind spot*.

optic nerve The second *cranial nerve (II), which is responsible for transmitting visual information from the retina of the eye to the *optic chiasma.

optic tract The part of the optic pathway running from the *optic chiasma to the lateral *geniculate body of the thalamus in the brain. It transmits nerve impulses from the eyes.

oral 1. Relating to the mouth. **2.** Taken by mouth: applied to medicines, etc.

oral cavity (mouth) The space between the lips within the oral fissure. It consists of the cleft-like *oral vestibule* bounded by the lips, cheeks, teeth, and gums, and the oral cavity proper inside the teeth and gums. This is bounded above by the palate and below by the tongue. *See also* pharynx.

orbicularis oculi muscle A circular muscle within the eyelids surrounding the palpebral fissure. It acts to close the palpebral fissure during blinking.

orbicularis oris muscle A circular muscle within the lips surrounding the oral fissure. It acts to close the oral fissure.

orbit The pyramid-shaped cavity in the *skull containing the eye and related structures. In herbivores the orbits face more to the sides whereas in carnivores they typically face the front of the skull. A complete bony

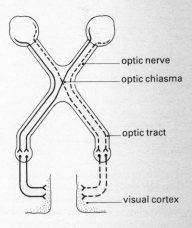

Optic pathways through
the optic chiasma

margin is present in herbivores, but in carnivores and the pig the margin is completed on its outer edge by the *orbital ligament*.

orbivirus A genus of the *reovirus family. Its members are known to infect bovine, ovine, canine, porcine, and equine hosts.

orchi- (orchido-, orchio-) *Prefix denoting* the testis or testicle.

orchidectomy Surgical removal of the *testis (*see* castration). Unilateral orchidectomy may be used on occasions to treat certain testicular tumours.

orchidotomy Surgical incision into the *testis. It may be performed to remove a tumour, for instance. *Compare* orchidectomy.

orchitis Inflammation of the *testis. It is usually the result of infection and/or trauma. The inflammatory process has deleterious effects on *spermatogenesis, and irreparable damage may be done to the seminiferous epithelium. In acute cases, the other testis may also be affected. Since the testis is encased in a tough fibrous capsule, little enlargement is possible, although necrosis may occur; however, the loose tissues of the scrotum may undergo considerable swelling. It is a relatively rare condition nowadays and may be treated by the systemic administration of antibiotics (if caused by infection), or warm poultices (in cases of trauma).

Oregon muscle disease (degenerative myopathy) A condition of turkeys and domestic fowls involving degeneration of the deep pectoral (breast) muscle, causing downgrading of carcasses. There is also green discoloration of the affected tissue. It mostly occurs in older birds, such as turkey breeders, but is also found in heavy fattening turkeys, broiler breeders, and even large roasters. No clinical signs appear in the live bird, thus precluding treatment, and it is hard to spot at meat inspection, sometimes only being revealed when the cooked bird is carved. The cause is inadequate blood supply to the muscle, exacerbated by excessive exertion. There is no treatment or prevention; birds rejected by inspectors can be trimmed and processed further.

orf An infectious pox disease of sheep and goats characterized by skin lesions and caused by parapoxvirus (*see* poxvirus). It can also be transmitted to humans. The disease occurs worldwide and can markedly affect production in some flocks, particularly in lactating ewes. The virus is transmitted by contact and enters the skin via abrasions. Infected lambs may spread the disease to the udder of their dams. The lesions occur mainly on the lips, developing from small pimples to pus-filled blisters, which eventually burst leaving a shallow ulcer. Scabs form over the ulcers, and wart-like growths may develop. Secondary bacterial infection can result in *mastitis, *dermatitis, and, where the foot is affected, lameness. Lesions uncomplicated by secondary infection usually heal in 3 weeks. Persistently infected animals become carriers of the virus, and virus may contaminate the environment. Vaccination with an attenuated live vaccine can help control the disease but will not eliminate it. Secondary infections may require antibiotics. Immunity to orf is poor and animals can be reinfected. In humans, orf may cause a skin eruption on the hands and forearms and even inflammation of the lymph nodes. Other names: **contagious pustular dermatitis**; **contagious ecthyma**.

organ A part of the body, composed of more than one tissue, that forms a structural unit responsible for a particular function (or functions). Examples are the heart, lungs, and liver.

organelle A structure within a cell that is specialized for a particular function. Examples of organelles are the nucleus, endoplasmic reticulum, Golgi apparatus, lysosomes, and mitochondria.

organic 1. Relating to any or all of the organs of the body. **2.** Describing chemical compounds containing carbon.

organo- *Prefix denoting* organ or organic. Examples: *organogenesis* (formation of); *organopathy* (disease of).

organochlorine poisoning A toxic condition caused by ingestion of any of a wide range of organochlorine compounds. Being fat-soluble, lindane or other organochlorines can penetrate unbroken skin and enter the body, where they are stored in body fat. Cats are particularly susceptible, perhaps because they clean their coats by licking and can therefore ingest substantial amounts. Affected animals show *hyperaesthesia, muscle tremors, teeth grinding, *nystagmus, tetanic spasms, and epileptiform convulsions. These signs may persist for long periods before death occurs. Low doses or long-term exposure to organochlorines produces chronic toxicity, with increased liver metabolism of drugs and hormones, infertility, poor growth, lowered egg production, production of thin-shelled eggs, and possible carcinogenicity. Poisoning has occurred in fasted animals due to the mobilization of organochlorine compounds from body fat. Also, carcasses of pigeons or other birds poisoned by organochlorine-dressed seeds are potentially hazardous to animals, such as dogs and cats, that consume them.

organochlorines (chlorinated hydrocarbons) A group of agents widely used as pesticides for both crops and livestock. The group includes the chlorinated ethane derivatives (e.g. DDT, TDE), the cyclodienes (e.g. aldrin, dieldrin, heptachlor) and the hexachlorocyclohexanes (e.g. BHC, lindane, and toxaphene – *see* benzene hexachloride). All these compounds have low water-solubility but high fat-solubility. When applied to the skin in fats, oils, or lipid solvents they are absorbed; absorption is poor if used in powders or aqueous suspensions. The compounds are stored in adipose tissue and are excreted very slowly. Degradation of organochlorines in the environment is very slow and animals are likely to accumulate the compounds over long periods. Along a food chain there is a concentrating effect, with carnivores accumulating high levels of organochlorines in their tissues, leading to toxicity (*see* organochlorine poisoning).

DDT was banned in the USA in 1972 and aldrin and dieldrin in 1974, with other countries later following suit. Benzene hexachloride (BHC) is still used to kill external parasites in certain species, but the risk of toxicity is now considered too high for the treatment of sheep scab with BHC. Insects can become resistant to the effects of organochlorine insecticides.

organ of Corti (spiral organ) *See* cochlea.

organomercury poisoning A toxic condition caused by ingestion of methyl-, ethyl-, and phenyl-mercury compounds, which are used as antifungal dressings for cereal seeds. The accidental incorporation of dressed seed in animal feed has caused poisoning. Organomercury compounds may also be derived from inorganic industrial pollutants. Methylmercury compounds are con-

organophosphorus (OP) compounds

centrated in food chains, with high levels in fish. Toxicity has occurred in humans and cats after eating contaminated fish. The clinical signs are those attributable to *gastroenteritis and *nephritis, and may be chronic when ingestion of low doses continues for some time. Treatment may include the use of *dimercaprol. The nervous system may be affected, with blindness, incoordination, and paralysis, in which case the prognosis is grave. *See also* mercury.

organophosphorus (OP) compounds A group of compounds used widely as insecticides for both crops and livestock, and as anthelmintics. OP compounds bind to the enzyme cholinesterase at nerve endings (*see* anticholinesterase). This binding is reversible initially but subsequently becomes irreversible, requiring the synthesis of new cholinesterase enzyme to overcome the blockade. This accounts for their insecticidal and anthelmintic activity, but also for possible toxic effects in animals. Compared to *organochlorines, their persistence in the environment is much less. They are used in dips, powders, sprays, pour-ons, or administered orally. OP insecticides for crops and environmental use include parathion, malathion, dimpylate, diazinon, and fenthion. To control external animal parasites, such as lice, ticks, keds, blowflies, and mites, especially those causing sheep scab, dipping or spraying is used. The compounds used in these preparations include bromophos, carbophenothion, ethion, chlorfenvinphos, diazinon, phosalone, and propetamphos. Persistence on the coat is much lower than with organochlorine compounds, and protection against reinfestation may last only 1–2 weeks, although some (e.g. diazinon) can persist for 6–8 weeks.
The high lipid-solubility of OP compounds enables their use in pour-on preparations to control internal parasites, such as warble flies in cattle and deer. Similar preparations are also used to control ectoparasites in pigs. Pour-ons may contain coumaphos, fenthion, fenchlorphos, trichlorophon, or phosmet. OP preparations are also administered orally to control nostril fly infestations in sheep and bots in horses, and for the treatment of demodectic mange in dogs. To prevent toxicity, orally administered products are formulated in plastic pellets for slow release over a long period. Products used include dichlorvos (in horses), dichlorvos and ronnel (in dogs), and fenchlorphos, dichlorvos, famophos, trichlorophon, or ruelene (in sheep).

Organophosphorus poisoning Animals exposed to high levels of OP compounds can suffer acute toxicity. Signs include miosis, bronchoconstriction, salivation, vomiting, bradycardia, muscle tremors, weakness, paralysis, ataxia, and death. Treatment is with *atropine, which antagonizes the action of OP compounds at muscarinic receptors. High doses of atropine are required to counteract effects on the central nervous system. Cholinesterase reactivators – the oximes, e.g. pralidoxime or obidoxime chloride – can be used intravenously to relieve paralysis and weakness. In severe cases, repeated treatment with atropine may be necessary. Chronic toxicity with long-term use of OP compounds can involve neurotoxicity and myopathies. Animals can become conditioned to constant low levels of OP compounds.

origin (in anatomy) **1.** The point of attachment of a muscle that remains relatively fixed during contraction of the muscle. *Compare* insertion. **2.** The point at which a nerve or blood vessel branches from a main nerve or blood vessel.

ornithine *See* amino acid; urea.

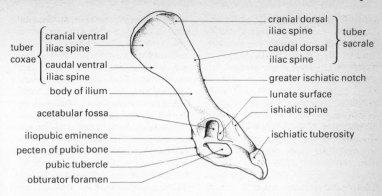

Left os coxae of the dog, lateral aspect

Ornithodoros A genus of soft *ticks found in warm countries, especially in Africa. They are ectoparasites of domestic animals and humans and inflict very painful bites. *O. moubata* and *O. erraticus* are principal vectors of the virus responsible for *African swine fever. The adults of the related *Otobius megnini*, the American spinose ear tick, are not parasitic but the spine-covered larvae and nymphs inhabit the ears of horses, etc. causing intense irritation.

ornithosis The term for disease caused by *Chlamydia psittaci* in non-*psittacine birds, otherwise identical with *psittacosis. Occasional outbreaks are recognized in turkeys and ducks, and the infection is enzootic in feral pigeons in the UK.

oro- *Prefix denoting* the mouth.

oropharynx *See* fauces.

ortho- *Prefix denoting* **1.** straight. **2.** normal.

orthomyxovirus A family of RNA *viruses that have enveloped helical *capsids and contain segmented nega-

tive-strand RNA. The most important genus is *influenzavirus.

Orthopedic Foundation for Animals A non-profit-making US organization concerned with promoting awareness of and research in orthopaedic diseases of animals. One of its major roles is to run the *hip dysplasia registry and diagnostic service to provide information about this condition in dogs of all breeds. Address: University of Missouri, Columbia, MO 65211.

os 1. (*pl.* **ossa**) A bone. The *os coxae* is the bone of the pelvic girdle, composed of the ilium, ischium, and pubis; in the dog it additionally comprises the acetabular bone (see illustration). The *os penis* is the ossified part of the *corpus cavernosum in carnivores. **2.** (*pl.* **ora**) The mouth or a mouthlike part.

oscilloscope A cathode-ray tube designed to display electronically a wave form corresponding to the electrical data fed into it. Oscilloscopes are used to provide a continuous record of many different measurements, such as the activity of the heart and brain. *See* electrocardiography, electroencephalography.

-osis *Suffix denoting* **1.** a diseased condition. Examples: *nephrosis* (of the kidney). **2.** any condition. Example: *narcosis* (of stupor). **3.** an increase or excess. Example: *leucocytosis* (of leucocytes).

osmium tetroxide (osmic acid) A colourless or faintly yellowish compound used to stain fats or as a *fixative in the preparation of tissues for microscopical study. Osmium tetroxide evaporates readily, the vapour having a toxic action on the eyes, skin, and respiratory tract.

osmoreceptor A group of cells in the *hypothalamus that monitors blood concentration. Should this increase abnormally, as in dehydration, the osmoreceptors send nerve impulses to the *neurohypophysis, which then increases the rate of release of *vasopressin. Loss of water from the body in the urine is thus restricted until the blood concentration returns to normal.

osmosis The passage of a solvent from a less concentrated to a more concentrated solution through a *semipermeable membrane. This tends to equalize the concentrations of the two solutions. In living organisms the solvent is water and cell membranes function as semipermeable membranes, and the process of osmosis plays an important role in controlling the distribution of water. The *osmotic pressure* of a solution is the pressure by which water is drawn into it through the semipermeable membrane; the more concentrated the solution (i.e. the more solute molecules it contains), the greater its osmotic pressure. *See also* hypertonic; hypotonic; isotonic.

ossicle A small bone. The *auditory ossicles* are three small bones (the malleus, incus, and stapes) in the middle *ear. They transmit sound from the external ear to the internal ear.

ossification (osteogenesis) The formation of *bone, which takes place by the action of *osteoblasts (bone-forming cells). A meshwork of collagen fibres is deposited, followed by the production of a matrix of cementing polysaccharide. Finally the cement is impregnated with minute crystals of calcium salts. The osteoblasts become enclosed within the matrix as *osteocytes (bone cells). In *endochondral ossification* the bone replaces cartilage. This process starts fairly early in foetal life. *Intramembranous ossification*, in which the bone forms within a membrane of connective tissue, occurs, for example, in the flat bones of the skull. This also commences in early foetal life.

ost- (oste-, osteo-) *Prefix denoting* bone. Examples: *osteocarcinoma* (carcinoma of); *osteonecrosis* (death of).

osteitis Inflammation of *bone, particularly the solid cortical (outer) bone tissue. It commonly originates from an inflammatory focus in the periosteum (*see* periostitis) and may spread to involve the medullary cavity (*see* osteomyelitis). The condition is marked by swelling and tenderness of the bone and overlying tissue. The inflammation may be acute, chronic, or suppurative, and is usually associated with primary or secondary bacterial infection. Sterile osteitis may be seen in traumatic tearing of ligamentous insertions in equine limbs. In cattle and sheep, foot lesions (e.g. *foot rot) may extend to produce osteitis from a periostitis. Similarly, puncture wounds and polyarthritis associated with secondary bacterial infection (e.g. with *Corynebacterium pyogenes*) may progress to osteal involvement. Mandibular bone infection by *Actinomyces bovis* is responsible for the osteitis known as 'lumpy jaw', which occurs chiefly in cattle (*see* actinomycosis).

Treatment depends on the presence and duration of infection. Early osteitis responds well to broad-spectrum antibiotics, although achieving sufficiently high local levels of antibiotic may be problematic, especially if there is much bone necrosis or excessive fibrous reaction. Surgical amputation of affected digits may be necessary. Other sites may require drainage after trephining (*see* trephine) the affected bone, followed by antibiotic wound packing and, eventually, bone grafting to effect a mechanically sound repair.

osteo- *Prefix. See* ost-.

osteoblast A cell that is responsible for the formation of *bone. See* ossification.

osteochondritis dissicans A disease syndrome affecting immature joints and characterized by local separation of the articular cartilage from the adjacent bone support, leading to the formation of a cartilage flap. The defect may become filled with irregular fibrocartilage; separated or fractured fragments of bone associated with the flap may form small bony ossicles known as joint 'mice'. The syndrome is most commonly identified in the elbow, shoulder, stifle, and hock joints of young (4–8-month-old) male dogs of the larger breeds (e.g. German shepherd dogs, Labrador/retrievers). It may also occur in pigs, affecting the humeral and femoral medial condyles at 5–7 months of age. In horses, foals aged from a few weeks up to 2 years may suffer lesions of the medial aspects of the femur and tibial bones; the articular processes of the cervical vertebrae may also be affected, and this may form part of the *wobbler syndrome. The cause is unknown, although trauma to immature joint cartilage in young animals has been suggested. Other factors that have been implicated but not proven are elevated production of the hormone *calcitonin due to a high plane of nutrition, and local bone necrosis.

osteochondroma (osteochondromatosis) A solitary or multiple mixed cartilaginous and bony proliferation arising from chondral *ossification centres (e.g. the cartilaginous portions of ribs, tracheal rings, various flat bones, including the scapulae, and the skull). The clinical signs are pain, swelling, and locomotor disturbance, which are related to the size and shape of the lesions. In **cats** multiple osteochondroma-like lesions affecting the long bones, vertebrae, scapulae, and skull are characteristic of hypervitaminosis caused by excess dietary vitamin A, especially following an exclusively liver diet.

osteoclasia (osteoclasis) 1. The absorption or destruction of bone by osteoclasts. It occurs during the remodelling of bone (as part of normal growth or at the site of a healing fracture) or in certain pathological conditions (*see* osteolysis). 2. The deliberate breaking of a malformed or malunited bone, for instance in the resetting of an improperly aligned fracture.

osteoclast A large multinucleated cell that breaks down calcified *bone matrix. Osteoclasts are found in depressions (*erosion lacunae*) on a surface of bone tissue.

osteocyte A *bone cell. It is formed from an *osteoblast that has become surrounded by bone tissue and lies within a small depression (lacuna). Cytoplasmic processes of the osteocyte extend from the lacuna through canaliculi to make contact with the processes of other osteocytes and with blood capillaries, thereby providing a mechanism for nutrition of the osteocytes.

osteodystrophy Defective bone development. It is caused by a variety of disorders and agents, predominantly nutritional in origin. These include nutrient deficiencies and imbalances, such as *vitamin A and D interactions, copper deficiency (*see* hypocuprosis), or inadequate dietary protein. Intensively reared animals may be more prone where rapid growth induced by high feed intake coupled with unsuitable floors leads to weight-bearing problems for immature bones. Various poisons also cause osteodystrophy, for instance lead and fluorine, as well as certain poisonous plants, for example *Solanum malacoxylon* and *Trisetum flavescens*. Phosphorus-deficient animals are very susceptible to fluorine toxicity and to osteodystrophy. Congenital defects may also cause the disorder. These include *osteogenesis imperfecta* in Charolais cattle and *osteopetrosis in Aberdeen Angus calves. A further cause may be infection, for example *atrophic rhinitis in pigs. Preventive measures depend on accurate diagnosis of the cause or causes. *See also* osteomalacia; osteoporosis; rickets.

osteogenesis *See* ossification.

osteolysis The dissolution of bone. It may occur in association with tumours or space-occupying lesions, which cause pressure necrosis of adjacent thin bones (e.g. nasal tumours); as a result of severe bone infection and inflammation (*see* osteomyelitis); or due to hormonal influences, such as secondary *hyperparathyroidism. Radiographically the condition is seen as a loss of bone density.

osteoma A benign tumour of bone that occurs infrequently in domestic animals. In the dog and the horse they tend to involve the flat bones of the skull and mandible. Adequate surgical excision can be curative but recurrence is common.

osteomalacia A bone disorder affecting mature animals. Like *rickets in young growing animals, it is caused by a deficiency of phosphorus and/or vitamin D. This results in a failure to calcify the ground substance of bone. It occurs in cattle grazing on phosphorus-deficient pastures; sheep suffer in the same way, but may be less severely affected. A similar disorder afflicts animals housed indoors without access to sunlight or supplementary vitamin D. Another cause is shortage of bone mineral due to the metabolic mineral demand of pregnancy and lactation. This commonly occurs in sows after a long lactation if their food is not supplemented adequately with calcium and phosphorus. Various clinical signs appear, resembling those of *phosphorus deficiency and including depraved appetite (*see* pica). The bones and joints become painful and the animal walks stiffly. Spontaneous fractures are common. Treatment is difficult because established lesions resist repair. A balanced intake of minerals with adequate vitamin D prevents the condition.

osteomyelitis Inflammation of the medullary cavity and marrow of bone. It often involves the adjacent bony cortex but should be differentiated from primary inflammation of the cortex *(osteitis). Most commonly a bacterial infection is implicated, but viruses, fungi and parasitic agents can also infect the marrow. The infection may be blood-borne (e.g. following septic arthritis) or arise from exogenous sources, such as puncture wounds, gunshot wounds, open fractures, or surgical repair of fractures where the operation site is contaminated. Necrotic bone fragments buried in poorly vascularized tissue is a common feature. Treatment typically combines surgical excision of necrotic bone with long courses of broad-spectrum antibiotic therapy.

In **poultry**, osteomyelitis is caused by *Escherichia coli* infection and occurs in growing birds. The bacteria cause abscesses within bones in the region of the growth plates. If the leg bones are affected there is lameness, while involvement of the vertebral column results in crooked necks or paralysis (*compare* spondylolisthesis). If the wing joints are affected there may be no clear signs. Cases are usually sporadic in a flock and serious outbreaks are uncommon. There is no reliable treatment, although antibiotics can be used for major outbreaks. *Compare* synovitis.

osteone One of the cylindrical units of which compact *bone is made. It consists of a central canal (*Haversian canal*) containing blood vessels, surrounded by a variable number of lamellae of bone matrix enclosing lacunae, which contain bone cells (*osteocytes). The lacunae are linked together and to the central canal by canaliculi, to form a *Haversian system*.

osteopetrosis (marble-bone disease) A disease involving overcalcification of the skeleton. *Congenital osteopetrosis* is an inherited defect found in some Aberdeen Angus calves. These are born with shortened long bones containing no marrow cavity, apparently due to defective remodelling during foetal development. *Nutritional osteopetrosis* occurs in bulls kept at stud and fed excessive calcium. This inhibits the secretion of the hormone *calcitonin so that bone mineral is laid down but not resorbed. In practice, the condition often results when bulls are fed diets designed to meet the mineral needs of lactating dairy cows.

Osteopetrosis in domestic fowls, involving thickening of the long bones, is caused by an RNA tumour virus. It is one of the unusual forms of the *avian leukosis complex and is of negligible economic importance.

osteophagia A clinical sign of mineral deficiency in which cattle or sheep chew and eat the bones of dead animals. It occurs in areas deficient in phosphorus and represents an extreme example of depraved appetite (*see* pica). It was initially described in South Africa, where *botulism became a secondary feature. The carcasses of dead animals putrefied and the botulism bacteria, *Clostridium botulinum*, proliferated producing botulinum toxin. Thus animals chewing the bones died of botulism.

osteophyte A knoblike or spurlike projection of bone found at sites of cartilage degeneration. These sites include the articular cartilage of joints, sites of attachment of tendons and ligaments, and the bodies of vertebrae adjacent to intervertebral disc deformity or displacement. Osteophytes are common in older animals. Joint osteophytes are most common in cattle and horses, while vertebral osteophytes often occur in long-backed dog breeds (e.g. dachshunds, basset hounds) or other breeds (e.g. boxers, German shepherd dogs) in association with chronic *spondylitis. However, the spinal lesions are sometimes incidental autopsy findings. The only possible treatment is surgical excision, which is often impractical.

osteoporosis A disease of bones involving excessive removal of mineral to compensate for a dietary deficiency. Some rarefaction of bone is inevitable to supply the mineral needs of lactation in dairy cows. However if these reserves are not replaced the bone becomes brittle, porous, and liable to spontaneous fracture (*see* milk lameness). Prevention entails ensuring adequate supplies of mineral for the needs of the animal. Osteoporosis differs in pathology from other osteodystrophies, such as *osteomalacia and *rickets; it refers simply to removal of bone substance without overgrowth of osteoid or fibrous tissue.

osteosarcoma A malignant tumour of *bone, derived from osteoblasts or osteoclasts. It is the most common primary bone tumour in dogs, affecting mainly large or giant breeds (e.g. Great Danes, Irish wolfhounds, St Bernards, German shepherd dogs, golden retrievers); it is uncommon or rare in other domestic species. The most commonly affected sites are the metaphyseal regions (*see* metaphysis) of the long bones, especially the humerus, radius, femur, and tibia. The stresses on these growth areas in young rapidly growing dogs may predispose to malignant transformation.

An osteosarcoma causes local destruction of normal bone and produces an expanding painful mass and acute lameness. Radiography reveals areas of bone lysis and bone production with palisading of new bone laid down by the periosteum, which is elevated by the expanding tumour. Nearly all such tumours will have produced metastatic deposits in the lung or liver by the time they are first diagnosed; these metastases may not be detectable radiographically. The prognosis is very poor and treatment is aimed largely at relieving the acute pain. This may be achieved by analgesic drugs initially but the pain soon becomes refractory. Amputation of the affected limb or local radiotherapy may give a better quality of life until metastatic disease becomes overpowering.

Extraskeletal osteosarcomas can arise in a variety of tissues but are generally rare.

osteosclerosis A condition of bone in which there is localized or more generalized ossification of the spongy bone matrix, thereby obliterating the marrow cavity. The condition may occur as a result of accidental or *iatrogenic vitamin D poisoning and consequent ossification of soft tissues; similar poisoning may occur in herbivores grazing such plants as *Solanum malacoxylon* and *Trisetum flavescens* (yellow oat). Osteosclerosis of vertebral bodies has been recorded in association with thyroid C-cell tumours in bulls.

A congenital form of osteosclerosis has been reported as a genetic defect (an autosomal recessive trait) in Aberdeen Angus, Hereford, and Simmental cattle. The calves are premature or stillborn and small; they have normal-shaped bones with no marrow cavities, compact vertebrae, and narrow channels for the cranial nerves in the skull, which leads to optic nerve hypoplasia. Osteosclerosis is also thought to be a variant form of *osteopetrosis in the rabbit, dog (e.g. dachshund), sheep, and pig.

Ostertagia A genus of *nematodes (roundworms) that parasitize the alimentary tract of cattle and sheep. Infestations cause *parasitic gastroenteritis or *ostertagiasis in their hosts. In cattle, *O. ostertagi* is one of the most pathogenic and economically important species; in sheep the main species involved is *O. circumcincta*. The life cycle is simple but can involve a period of dormancy within the host. Eggs are passed in the faeces and after about 24 hours the minute larvae hatch. The speed of development of the larvae depends on temperature, and hence season. Eggs passed in the spring develop more slowly than those passed in early summer. They pass through two larval stages before migrating onto herbage as infective larvae. These can overwinter and cause heavy infestations in young stock in the spring.

The number of infective larvae on herbage reaches a peak in July–August for cattle and sheep. The ingested larvae migrate to the abomasum, enter the gastric glands, and develop into adults, which emerge to lie on the surface of the stomach lining. The period from infestation to adult egg-laying worm is normally 21 days.

ostertagiasis A disease of cattle and sheep in temperate areas caused by nematode worms of the genus *Ostertagia*. The worms are found in the abomasum, where they interfere with the secretion of digestive juices, causing diarrhoea, loss of appetite, and poor growth. The disease is mainly a problem for young stock, adults acquiring fairly good immunity to the worms, and is more likely with high stocking rates and overgrazing. Ostertagiasis occurs in two forms, depending on the season. *Type 1 ostertagiasis* occurs in young stock from late summer to the end of the grazing season. It follows on from the peak level of infective larvae on pasture and is characterized by dark-green diarrhoea, general unthriftiness, and high output of parasite eggs from the host animal. The larvae that develop from these eggs may give rise to *Type 2 ostertagiasis*, also known as 'winter ostertagiasis' or 'winter scours'. The fourth-stage larvae settle in the lining of the abomasum and remain dormant until late winter before developing further. In ewes, host immunity to the worms is reduced before lambing and dormant larvae emerge causing a significant increase (*periparturient rise*) in the output of worm eggs, the infective larvae from which can be picked up by the lambs.

Control is by rotation of grazing, so that susceptible animals are not grazed on heavily infested pasture, if possible, in conjunction with anthelmintic treatment. For *Type 1 ostertagiasis* most currently available anthelmintics are suitable, but for *Type 2 ostertagiasis* an agent that is more active against the dormant larvae is needed. For both cattle and sheep fenbendazole, oxfendazole, albendazole, levamisole, febantel, thiophanate, thiabendazole, and ivermectin will achieve this. *See also* parasitic gastroenteritis.

ostium (*pl.* **ostia**) (in anatomy) An opening. The *ostium abdominale* is the opening of the uterine tube into the abdominal cavity.

-ostomy *Suffix. See* -stomy.

ot- (oto-) *Prefix denoting* the ear. Example: *ototomy* (surgical incision of).

otic Relating to the ear.

otitis Inflammation of the *ear. Otitis externa* – inflammation of the external ear – is particularly common in the dog and cat, and may involve one or more of the following: congenital narrowing, tortuosity, or malformation of the external auditory meatus (auditory canal), with or without excessive hair growth (e.g. in miniature poodles, cocker spaniels); excessive wax secretion; foreign bodies (e.g. grass awns); inflammatory polyps (especially in cats); or neoplasms (benign adenomas, ceruminous carcinomas, squamous cell carcinomas in cats). Moreover, bacteria (e.g. *Pseudomonas* spp., *Proteus* spp.) and yeasts (e.g. *Pityrosporum canis*) that are common in normal ears can multiply excessively in inflamed conditions. In canine breeds with pendulous ears (e.g. Afghan hounds), Gram-negative bacteria are commonly isolated in otitis externa; Gram-positive bacteria, often in association with fungal agents, are a feature of dogs with tortuous inflamed canals (e.g. poodles). In cats, and to a lesser extent dogs,

Otodectes

ear mites (*Otodectes cynotis*) are important in initiating inflammation, especially by causing the animal to scratch itself. Affected animals exhibit head shaking, scratching of the ears (with obvious pain in advanced cases), and, less commonly, head tilting. Diagnosis is usually made with the aid of an *auriscope. Treatment consists of cleansing and lavage with mild antiseptic agents, followed by instillations of antibiotic/fungicidal preparations. Recurrent cases, or cases where excessive distortion of the auditory canal has occurred, often require surgical resection of the lateral wall of the auditory canal or complete ablation of the vertical canal to ensure drainage and resolution.

Otitis media is inflammation of the tympanic cavity within the temporal bone. This usually results from an ascending bacterial infection via the *auditory tube (in pigs and sheep) or extension of otitis externa via a perforated eardrum (dogs and cats). Otitis media is often an intermediate stage in the development of otitis interna (see below). The inflammatory exudate is initially serofibrinous, becoming more purulent and chronic; it may induce bone lysis and spread to the inner ear and, more rarely, the nearby brainstem. Clinically, there is discharge from the affected ear with pain on palpation, and occasionally involvement of the temporomandibular joint causing pain on opening the mouth. Also affected may be the facial nerve, leading to *facial paralysis, and sympathetic nerves near the tympanic bulla, causing *Horner's syndrome. In the cat, inflammatory *polyps may expand outward through the eardrum from the middle ear, or via peduncles down the auditory tube into the nasopharynx, or produce pressure effects on the inner ear, manifested as loss of balance. Diagnosis of otitis media is made using a combination of auriscopic examina-

tion, radiography, and possibly exploratory surgery. Treatment of uncomplicated conditions consists of *myringotomy and irrigation of the middle ear with sterile saline or mild antiseptic, followed by pulsed antibiotic therapy. In cats, care should be taken in irrigation, and in the choice of drugs since this species is highly susceptible to ototoxic drugs (e.g. streptomycin, neomycin, chlorhexidine). Polyps should be removed by *curettage.

Otitis interna (*labyrinthitis*) is inflammation of the inner ear (or labyrinth), which accommodates the cochlea and semicircular canals. The commonest cause is extension of inflammation/ infection from otitis media. The condition is usually unilateral and causes dramatic neurological signs, such as head tilting with the affected side downwards, circling towards the affected side, falling towards the affected side on walking, and *nystagmus. *Deafness, especially if unilateral, is difficult to detect. Treatment may be attempted using lavage and surgery to ensure drainage, together with long courses of broad-spectrum antibiotics. Where excessive granulation tissue has formed, treatment is rarely completely successful and although balance may be regained, head tilt may become a permanent feature.

Otodectes A genus of *mites that are ectoparasites of cats and dogs. They inhabit the external ear canal, causing intense irritation, over-production of wax, and inflammation leading to auricular or *otodectic mange. This condition is very resistant to treatment because of the associated yeast and bacterial growth in the ear.

otodectic mange (auricular mange; ear mange) A form of *mange, caused by infestation of the external auditory meatus of the ear by the parasitic mite *Otodectes cynotis*, which can affect cats, dogs, ferrets, and foxes. It may spread from the ear to the face and tail tip. More severe clinical signs are seen in dogs than cats, with head shaking and scratching. It may lead to bacterial *otitis externa, middle-ear disease, and *haematoma of the pinna. Diagnosis is confirmed by examination of the ear canal with an auriscope to reveal the mobile grey-white mites. Treatment is by the application of ear drops containing an *acaricide; dogs and cats in contact with the patient should also be treated.

otolith (otoconium) One of the small particles consisting of calcium carbonate and protein that are embedded in the gelatinous mass covering the surface of the *maculae in the utricle and saccule of the inner *ear. Movements of the otoliths as a result of head movements cause stimulation of the hair cells of the maculae.

-otomy *Suffix. See* -tomy.

ouabain A water-soluble *cardiac glycoside, obtained from the seed of *Stropanthus gratus*, with a rapid onset of action and short half-life. It is administered intravenously for emergency treatment of heart failure, producing effects similar to *digitalis.

outbreeding *See* crossbreeding.

ovalbumin A *glycoprotein of egg white that serves as the major source of protein for the developing chick embryo.

oval window The fenestra vestibuli. *See* ear.

ovari- (ovario-) *Prefix denoting* the ovary.

ovarian cyst A cavernous or fluid-filled swelling on or within the ovary. They are common in the cow and seen infrequently in sows and mares. There is little information on their incidence or importance in other species. In the cow, three major types of ovarian cyst occur: *follicular cysts* (*cystic Graafian follicles*), in which the follicle fails to ovulate and grows greater than 2.5 cm in diameter and there is no corpus luteum; *luteal cysts* (*luteinized cysts*), in which the follicle fails to ovulate but there is some luteinization of follicular cells; and *cystic corpora lutea*, in which there is an exaggerated fluid-filled cavity within the corpus luteum. These are of no clinical significance, whereas follicular and luteal cysts are considered pathological.

Infertility due to the endocrine imbalance resulting from follicular and luteal cysts is common in high-yielding dairy cows, particularly in the autumn and winter. Cows with ovarian cysts often show signs of *hyperoestrogenism, such as prolonged absence of oestrus (anoestrus), nymphomania, or virilism (masculinization). The cause is thought to be a deficiency of *luteinizing hormone prior to ovulation. There is also a hereditary factor, so cows with cystic ovarian disease and bulls that pass this trait on to their offspring should be culled. Normal use of *oestrogens, such as diethylstilboestrol (DES), or oestrogenic pasture do not increase the incidence of cystic ovarian disease, although the condition has been induced by very high doses. Treatment traditionally entails the manual rupture of the cysts during rectal palpation and/or the administration of luteinizing hormone. There is increasing use of *progesterone or *progestogens and *prostaglandins. None of these treatments is very convincing, however, since a high percentage of cows with cystic ovaries resume normal cyclical activity with no treatment. There are risks with manual rupture, including haemorrhage and bursal adhesions.

ovarian follicle One of the structures in the *ovary in which the *oocytes mature. The primordial follicle consists of a small primary oocyte enveloped by a single layer of flattened epithelial cells. An animal has its full complement of these by the late foetal stage. Under the influence of pituitary *gonadotrophin, these follicles mature progressively from puberty onwards into *primary follicles*, which are enveloped by a single layer of cuboidal or columnar epithelial cells, *secondary follicles*, with a stratified epithelium, and finally *tertiary* or *Graafian follicles. These undergo *ovulation, releasing an oocyte from the follicle; the remainder of the follicle then develops into a *corpus luteum. As the follicles enlarge they become surrounded by specialized ovarian stroma (*theca). Maturing follicles secrete *oestrogens and small amounts of *androgens.

ovarian tumours Any of various tumours affecting the ovary. Although uncommon, ovarian tumours occur most frequently in bitches and mares, with *granulosa theca cell tumours having the highest incidence.

ovariectomy (oophorectomy) Surgical removal of one or both ovaries, i.e. unilateral or bilateral ovariectomy. This forms part of the routine *spaying operation in dogs and cats (*see also* ovariohysterectomy). The other common indication is ovarian neoplasia.

ovariohysterectomy Surgical removal of both the ovaries and uterus. This is most commonly performed to 'neuter' female dogs and cats (*see* spaying) or to treat *pyometra (filling of the uterus with purulent material); this condition, which is most common in bitches, can be acutely life-threatening and the treatment is coupled with supportive therapy. Possible risks and side-effects of ovariohysterectomy include haemorrhage, infection, and hormonal imbalances that may contribute to weight gain, skin disorders, and urinary incontinence. Technically the operation is easier to perform in the young animal before its first season. However, some workers feel that hormonal imbalances and, especially, urinary incontinence are less likely if ovariohysterectomy is performed after the first season.

ovariotomy Surgical incision into the ovary. This may be performed to attempt removal of a neoplasia without removing the whole ovary, to inspect the cut surfaces of the ovary, or as part of an experimental procedure.

ovary The female gonad, in which the oocytes mature in the *ovarian follicles. The ovary comprises an outer cortex containing the follicles, and an inner medulla containing the main blood vessels, which enter at the *hilus (see illustration). In mammals the ovary is paired and is situated in the dorsal part of the abdomen, caudal to the kidneys. In birds only the left ovary normally develops. *See also* reproductive system.

overgrown foot A condition in which the horn of the wall of the *hoof grows without normal compensatory wear along the lower edge, leading to an overlong hoof. It may result in curling upwards of the toe region and consequent inability to walk, and predispose to tendon disease (sprains and contractions) and splitting of the hoof wall. Horses, cattle, and sheep are chiefly affected, particularly where animals are subject to very soft conditions underfoot, where their movements are restricted, or where regular shoeing or foot trim-

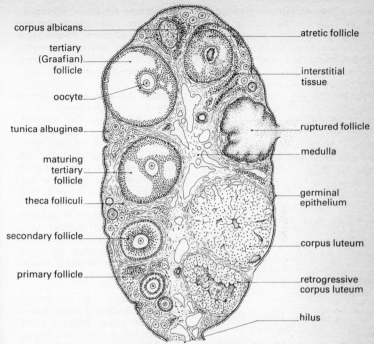

corpus albicans

tertiary (Graafian) follicle

oocyte

tunica albuginea

maturing tertiary follicle

theca folliculi

secondary follicle

primary follicle

atretic follicle

interstitial tissue

ruptured follicle

medulla

germinal epithelium

corpus luteum

retrogressive corpus luteum

hilus

Section through a mammalian ovary showing a composite of the structures formed during the oestrous cycle

ming is neglected. The condition is common in exotic hoofed species kept in confined spaces in zoos.

over-reaching An abnormality of gait, seen in some horses, in which the toe of the hindfoot strikes the forefoot of the same side. Any injury caused is generally to the heel, and there may even be loosening of the front shoe. Over-reaching boots can help prevent tissue damage, and corrective shoeing may be beneficial. *Compare* forging.

ovi- (ovo-) *Prefix denoting* an egg; ovum.

oviduct In birds, the tubular part of the female reproductive system. Generally only the left oviduct develops, but cystic remnants may occur on the right. The oviduct consists of a funnel-shaped *infundibulum*, which receives the egg shed from the ovary; the *magnum*, which forms much of the albumen; the *isthmus*, which forms the shell membranes; the *uterus*, which forms the shell; and the *vagina*, through which the egg passes to the cloaca. In mammals the oviduct is referred to as the *uterine tube.

ovine encephalomyelitis *See* louping ill.

ovine enzootic abortion *See* enzootic ovine abortion.

ovine epididymitis *See* ram epididymitis.

ovine interdigital dermatitis A milder form of *foot rot of sheep, caused by *Bacteroides nodosus* strains of low virulence. Moist areas of low-grade inflammation affect the skin of the interdigital spaces of one or more feet, causing lameness. Treatment is by removal to dry ground and topical application of antibiotic sprays. Other name: **nonprogressive foot rot.**

ovine keratoconjunctivitis (pink eye; heather blindness) An eye disease of sheep and goats involving inflammation of the conjunctiva (*conjunctivitis), which progresses to corneal ulcers and blindness. The condition occurs worldwide and is contagious, being associated with a number of microorganisms, although *Chlamydia psittaci ovis* and *Mycoplasma conjunctivae* are the most commonly isolated pathogens. In North America a *polyarthritis has also been associated with the condition in feedlot lambs. Economic losses are largely the result of misadventure (e.g. drowning) following blindness in young lambs. Treatment consists in the topical application of broad-spectrum antibiotics (e.g. oxytetracycline) or the use of phenarthridine compounds, such as ethidium bromide (*see* homidium bromide). Development of immunity is poor and the pathogens may persist after treatment, providing a reservoir of infection in a flock. Outbreaks of disease are common following the introduction of new stock to an infected flock. Transmission is probably via contact, and trough-fed sheep are particularly at risk.

oviparous Describing an animal in which fertilized eggs are laid or spawned by the mother and hatch outside her body. It occurs in most animals except marsupial and placental mammals. *Compare* ovoviviparous; viviparous.

ovoviviparous Describing an animal in which fertilized eggs develop and hatch in the oviduct of the mother. It occurs in many invertebrates and in some fish and reptiles (e.g. the viper). *Compare* oviparous; viviparous.

ovulation The process by which an oocyte is released from a mature *ovarian follicle and shed from the ovary. Ovulation is triggered by a surge in the level of pituitary *gonadotrophin hormones in the blood, which provokes structural changes in the follicle. It occurs around the time of *oestrus, when the female is ready to accept the male (see table), thus maximizing the chances of successful mating. The number of follicles ovulating at each ovulation varies with species: in cattle a single egg is generally released; in sheep the number is 1–3, whereas in pigs 11–24 are shed.
In certain mammals, for example cats, rabbits, and ferrets, ovulation is induced by coitus. Nervous stimuli associated with copulation trigger the release of the gonadotrophins that activate ovulation.

ovum (egg cell) (*pl.* **ova**) The mature female sex cell (female gamete) that is released from the ovary at ovulation. Strictly it is formed only after a secondary *oocyte has undergone the final stage of meiosis, and in some species this does not occur until the oocyte has been activated by fertilization. An ovum is normally spherical with a nucleus and a variable amount of yolk enclosed in a vitelline membrane. In birds and other egg-laying animals the very large ovum has a further surrounding layer of albumen, more membranes, and a protective hard outer shell (*see* egg).

ovum transplantation 1. The collection of a recently fertilized ovum (i.e. *zygote) from a donor animal and its transfer into the oviduct or uterus of a recipient animal of the same species for development to term. **2.** The collection of *oocytes from the ovary of a living or recently slaughtered animal for subsequent fertilization and transfer into recipients (*see* in vitro fertilization). *Compare* embryo transplantation.

oxalate poisoning A toxic condition caused by the ingestion of sorrel (*Rumex acetosa*), sheep's sorrel (*R. acetosella*), docks (*Rumex* spp.), the cultivated rhubarb (*Rheum rhaponticum*) or unwilted sugar-beet tops. It is thought that the oxalate content of these plants, if ingested and absorbed from the alimentary tract, interferes with calcium metabolism. It may cause hypocalcaemia with clinical signs resembling those of *milk fever, but death is usually due to the obstruction of kidney tubules by crystals of calcium oxalate. Animals not previously exposed to plants containing oxalate are especially susceptible, but exposure to sublethal amounts is believed to encourage adaptive changes in ruminal microorganisms and increase the efficiency with which they detoxify the oxalate. Care should be taken that sugar-beet tops are properly wilted before animals have access to them. Additional protection can be provided by a light dusting of the tops with powdered limestone.

oxalic acid (ethanedioic acid) The first member of the alkanedioic (dicarboxylic) acid series. In pure form it is a crystalline solid, slightly soluble in water. It is strongly acidic and very poisonous, occurring in many plants, for example rhubarb (*see* oxalate poisoning). Its ability to form complexes with calcium ions is exploited to prevent blood clotting.

oxfendazole *See* benzimidazole.

oxibendazole *See* benzimidazole.

oxidase An *oxidoreductase enzyme that uses molecular oxygen as hydrogen acceptor, for example xanthine oxidase, which catalyses the reaction: xanthine + O_2 = uric acid + H_2O_2.

oxidoreductase One of a group of enzymes that catalyse oxidation-reduction reactions. *See* dehydrogenase; oxidase.

oxyclozanide An anthelmintic used in cattle and sheep to treat fluke infestations. It acts by uncoupling oxidative phosphorylation in flukes, and, at the normal dose rate, is active against adult liver flukes (*Fasciola hepatica*); three times the normal dose rate is effective against immature flukes over 8 weeks of age. It is available as a drench, or as granules for incorporating into feedstuffs; it is also combined with *levamisole as a fluke and worm drench. After absorption, oxyclozanide is conjugated with glucuronide in the liver and excreted in the bile. High concentrations are found in the liver, kidneys, and intestine, with tissue residues detected for 14 days after administration. There may be transient diarrhoea and a reduced milk yield. With overdosage, signs of toxicity include hyperventilation, hyperthermia, and metabolic disturbances.

oxygen A colourless odourless nonmetallic element that, in its molecular form, is present in air (21% by volume). Along with carbon, hydrogen, and nitrogen it is one of the principal constituents of living things. Atmospheric oxygen is essential for the metabolism of *aerobic organisms, being used to oxidize glucose and other energy sources to produce *ATP and yielding carbon dioxide and water. In higher vertebrates, oxygen is absorbed into the blood from air in the lungs, and transported in the blood bound to *haemoglobin. Symbol O. *See* respiration.

oxygen debt

Oxygen is used as the carrier gas for *inhalational anaesthetics. It is administered using a mask or through an endotracheal tube (*see* endotracheal anaesthesia). Oxygen therapy to increase the amount of oxygen circulating in the blood can be performed by placing animals, especially small animals, in an *oxygen tent*, in which the atmosphere contains a high concentration of oxygen. This is indicated in some respiratory diseases, pulmonary haemorrhage, and heart disease, and in neonates. Overdosage with oxygen produces respiratory depression, alveolar oedema, pulmonary congestion, hyaline membrane formation, intra-alveolar haemorrhage, central nervous system disturbances with convulsions, and death.

oxygen debt (oxygen deficit) The physiological state that exists in a normally aerobic animal when insufficient oxygen is available for metabolic requirements (e.g. during strenuous activity). To meet the body's increased demand for energy, pyruvate (derived from glucose) is converted in the absence of oxygen to lactic acid, which accumulates in tissues. The oxygen required to oxidize this lactic acid is equivalent to the oxygen debt. This 'repayment' of the debt occurs after the exertion stops and sufficient oxygen is again available.

oxyhaemoglobin The oxygenated form of *haemoglobin. When fully oxygenated, each of the four haem residues in the vertebrate haemoglobin molecule binds one molecule of oxygen.

oxyphenbutazone *See* NSAID.

oxytetracycline *See* tetracyclines.

oxytocic 1. A drug that induces or accelerates parturition by stimulating the muscles of the uterus to contract.

See also oxytocin. **2.** Describing such a drug.

oxytocin A peptide hormone secreted from the neurohypophysis of the pituitary gland in response to stimulation of the mammary glands, preparation for milking, or clitoral or vaginal stimulation. The hormone causes contraction of oestrogen-primed uterine myometrium (e.g. during parturition), and of the myoepithelial cells of the mammary gland resulting in milk letdown. No physiological role for oxytocin has been found in males.
Preparations of oxytocin, either extracted from pituitary tissue or synthesized, can be used therapeutically. They are injected intramuscularly or intravenously and are inactivated rapidly by the liver and kidneys, with a plasma half-life of about 2 minutes. Oxytocin can be used to induce parturition in the mare but should be used only when the cervix is dilating. It can also be used in cases of uterine inertia in all species but only where there is no blockage to foetal expulsion. The action of oxytocin on myometrial tissue depends on the prevailing progesterone to oestrogen ratio. To exert its effects there must be falling progesterone and rising oestrogen levels. After parturition oxytocin can be used to induce uterine involution thus preventing uterine prolapse, and in the treatment of postpartum haemorrhage. Oxytocin can also be used to treat agalactia, usually in pigs.

Oxytropis *See* Astragalus poisoning.

Oxyuris A genus of parasitic nematodes (*see* pinworm), which includes *O. equi*, found in the caecum and colon of horses. The adult female worms migrate to the perianal region to lay eggs, and this causes intense irritation; the eggs are infective within 4–5 days, and can survive for several weeks in moist conditions.

Infestation is established by eating contaminated fodder or licking the perianal region. The parasite occurs in temperate regions, mainly Europe and North America. Affected animals can be treated with thiabendazole, mebendazole (*see* benzimidazole), or *pyrantel.

ozaena A disease of the nasal passages resulting in an odorous mucopurulent discharge. It is associated with *cleft palate conditions in young animals or buccal fistula formation in adults; occasionally it occurs as a sequel to a malar abscess in the dog (*see* alveolar abscess). Moreover, the condition may accompany *atrophic rhinitis in pigs, mycotic rhinitis (caused by fungi, e.g. *Aspergillus* spp.) in dogs, and necrotic neoplasms (e.g. turbinate carcinomas). Treatment consists in surgical excision of the affected part (*rhinotomy*) with drainage and broad-spectrum antibacterial or antifungal therapy.

ozone A colourless gas formed from molecular *oxygen in the upper atmosphere of the earth by the action of ultraviolet light. The ozone layer screens the earth's surface from most of the solar ultraviolet light, which is harmful to living organisms.

P

Pacheco's parrot disease A disease of *psittacine birds caused by a highly contagious *herpesvirus infection, with signs similar to those of *psittacosis. The liver shows multifocal necrosis and infiltration, and liver cells contain characteristic intranuclear inclusion bodies. The birds' droppings are infective. Control is by disinfection of aviaries; conures, which can be symptomless carriers of

the virus, are removed. Other name: **psittacine inclusion body hepatitis**.

pachy- *Prefix denoting* **1.** thickening of a part or parts. **2.** the dura mater.

pachydermia Excessive thickening of the skin. This can be a normal feature in certain species (e.g. elephants and whales). Alternatively, localized or generalized disease may result in apparent skin thickening (e.g. due to underlying neoplasia or inflammatory reactions), or in real increases in thickness as a result of neoplastic infiltration or fibrous reaction (e.g. scars).

pachyglossia Thickening of the tongue. It may result from bacterial infection, the best example being wooden tongue in cattle (*see* actinobacillosis). In the dog and cat, pachyglossia due to neoplasia (e.g. *squamous cell carcinoma in the cat, *rhabdomyoma in the dog) is seen uncommonly.

pachymeningitis Inflammation and thickening of the *dura mater, one of the membranes (meninges) that cover the brain and spinal cord. It may occur as part of the reaction to infection by specific *neurotropic agents, such as *Listeria monocytogenes*, *Haemophilus suis*, or viruses (canine *distemper). Spread of infection from abscesses or other lesions in the vertebral canal causes a similar response. Dural ossification or *ossifying pachymeningitis* may occur in older members of the larger dog breeds (e.g. Labradors, German shepherd dogs). At autopsy, lesions are often seen in the lumbar region of the spinal cord, and range from multiple discrete plaques on the dural surface to areas of rigid intradural ossification extending over several segments of the cord. The more extensive formations are often concurrent with *spondylitis and degenerative joint changes, usually associated with a history of impaired mobility.

pachytene The third stage of the first prophase of *meiosis, in which *crossing over begins.

Pacinian corpuscle One of several types of encapsulated nerve endings found in the skin. The membranous capsule is arranged in 'onion-skin' layers. They are believed to be sensitive to touch, pressure, and vibration.

packed cell volume (haematocrit) The proportion of the blood volume occupied by cells. *See also* cell count.

palaeo- (*US* paleo-) *Prefix denoting* 1. ancient. 2. primitive.

palaeopathology The study of disease in specimens or bodies preserved from ancient times. In veterinary species such studies have been mostly confined to dental and bone examinations as incidental to other archaeological investigations. Human palaeopathology has obtained considerable information from Egyptian mummies and desiccated or petrified bodies (e.g. Scandinavian peatbog dwellers).

palatability The attractiveness of food; the degree to which animals will consume it voluntarily. It is related essentially to the smell, taste, and texture of the food, but also to its *nutrient content – unbalanced *diets may reduce feed intake. Palatability may be influenced adversely by certain substances, for example tannins in some legume seeds. Also, unpleasant odours and flavours may arise due to poor storage conditions: food may become mouldy, and fats and high-fat feedstuffs rancid. Dry and dusty diets often have low palatability with consequent low feed intake and high wastage. Good palatability of *creep feed during and

immediately following *weaning is particularly important. This may be achieved by the addition of, for example, fat or molasses and the use of specific flavouring agents.

palate The roof of the *oral cavity, which separates it from the nasal cavity and nasopharynx. It is lined by mucous membrane and consists of two parts: the *hard palate* in front, which contains bone; and the *soft palate* behind containing only soft tissue, including muscles to control its position.

palatine bone Either of the paired L-shaped bones that contribute to the wall of the nasal cavity and the hard palate. *See* skull.

palato- *Prefix denoting* 1. the palate. 2. the palatine bone.

pale laurel *See* Kalmia poisoning.

pale soft exudative muscle (PSE) A condition affecting the meat in some pig carcasses after slaughter. It is accompanied by excessive water loss, and the meat's appeal to the consumer is reduced. Its development is associated with biochemical changes in muscle leading to protein denaturation. Its incidence is related to genetic selection for leanness, and it is triggered by acute pre-slaughter stress. Stress susceptibility, and hence the risk of PSE meat, can be indicated by the *halothane test.

pali- (palin-) *Prefix denoting* repetition or recurrence.

palindromic Recurrent or relapsing: describing diseases or clinical signs, for example bouts of fever, that recur or get worse.

palium The outer wall of the *cerebral hemisphere as it appears in the early stages of evolution of the mammalian brain. In the modern brain the term is applied either to the cerebral hemisphere or more specifically to the cerebral cortex. In evolutionary terms, the oldest parts of the cerebral hemisphere are the *archipallium*, which consists of the *hippocampus and its connections, and the *palaeopallium*, which comprises the piriform lobe and is olfactory in function. *See also* neopallium.

pallidum (globus pallidus) *See* basal ganglia.

palmar Relating to the back of the *manus (front foot).

palmar arch An arterial *anastomosis in the palmar part of the *manus. The *superficial palmar arch* is closely related to the flexor tendons and supplies superficial branches to the digits (*palmar common digital arteries*). The *deep palmar arch* is closely related to the bones and supplies deep branches to the digits (*palmar metacarpal arteries*).

palpation The process of using the hand or fingers to determine the outline, consistency, and/or movement of parts of the body. It is used to detect abnormal swellings or enlargement of organs. *Abdominal palpation* is useful in small animals in the examination of the abdominal organs or to indicate the presence of fluid within the peritoneal cavity (*see* ascites). Abdominal palpation in large animals gives rather less information. Ruminal movements can be discerned by prolonged palpation of the left sublumbar region and gaseous distension of the gut or peritoneum can be ascertained. *Lymph-node palpation* forms part of a routine clinical examination in all species. Superficial lymph nodes (e.g. submandibular) can be palpated in normal animals, and an increase in size indicates infection,

inflammation, or neoplasia in the areas draining to the lymph node.
Rectal palpation involves inserting the hand, or in the case of small species, a single finger, into the rectum via the anus. It is used extensively in bovine and equine practice for the diagnosis of alimentary tract and reproductive tract disorders. Pregnancy diagnosis and investigation of infertility involve rectal palpation of the ovaries and uterus. In small animals the most common conditions diagnosed in this way include rectal diseases and canine prostatic disease.

palpebral Relating to the eyelid (palpebra).

pan- (pant(o)-) *Prefix denoting* all; every: hence affecting all parts of an organ or the body; generalized.

pancreas A large gland situated in the dorsal part of the abdomen. In the domestic mammals it consists of a body, left lobe, and right lobe; the latter lies alongside the descending part of the duodenum (see illustration). In birds the pancreas is elongated and divided into dorsal, ventral, and splenic lobes. The pancreas consists of *acini, which secrete *pancreatic juice; this is rich in digestive enzymes and passes to the duodenum via the *pancreatic ducts. The pancreatic *islets secrete the hormones *insulin and *glucagon into the bloodstream.

pancreatic duct The duct that carries pancreatic juice from the *pancreas to the duodenum. It unites with the *bile duct and opens into the duodenum at the major duodenal papilla. An *accessory pancreatic duct* may also be present; this discharges at the minor duodenal papilla. The occurrence of these ducts varies in domestic mammals (see table). In birds, two or three pancreatic ducts are present.

pancreatic juice

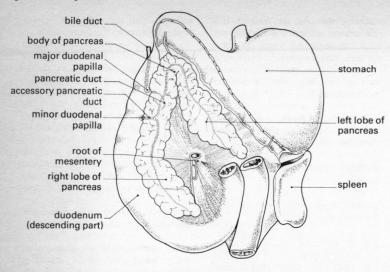

The pancreas and its relations in the dog

Occurrence of pancreatic ducts in various species

Species	Pancreatic duct	Accessory pancreatic duct
Horse	+	+
Ox	−	+
Sheep, goat	+	−
Pig	−	+
Dog	+	+
Cat	+	+

pancreatic juice Digestive juice secreted by the *pancreas and conveyed via a duct system to the duodenum, which it enters either alone or mixed with *bile. Pancreatic juice is secreted in response to a variety of stimuli. The hormone *secretin stimulates the production by pancreatic cells of a watery alkaline fluid, while another hormone, *cholecystokinin, stimulates the secretion into this fluid of a wide range of proenzymes and enzymes, such as trypsinogen (*see* trypsin), chymotrypsinogen (*see* chymotrypsin), procarboxypeptidase, α-*amylase, *lipase, *lecithinases, and *nucleases. With its high concentration of hydrogencarbonate (bicarbonate) ions, pancreatic juice (together with bile) neutralizes the acid digesta from the stomach and provides an optimum environment (pH 7–9) for the pancreatic enzymes to catalyse the breakdown of protein, fats, and carbohydrates. Pancreatic juice acts as a buffer in the large intestine. This is particularly important in those herbivores, for example horses, in which the large intestine is the chief site for the microbial fermentation of plant material and the production of short-chain fatty acids.

pancreatitis Inflammation of the *pancreas. The condition is not uncommon in the dog and occasionally occurs in the cat, but is rarely identified as a clinical entity in other species, although in pigs and cattle suppurative *peritonitis may extend to involve the pancreas. Acute or chronic pancreatitis may occur. *Acute pancreatitis* can be of two types: a mild acutely oedematous interstitial form, which is common in middle-aged obese and sedentary bitches; and a less common but usually fatal haemorrhagic or necrotizing form, which mainly affects male dogs. Clinical signs are similar in both types but are more severe in the necrotizing form. Variable but constant vomiting occurs with lethargy, anorexia, and thirst. Abdominal pain may be obvious, and is invariably elicited on abdominal *palpation. In the necrotic form blood may be present in vomit and in the diarrhoeic faeces. Diagnosis may be difficult and is usually based on a summation of clinical findings, such as elevated serum amylase and lipase levels. Transient or more permanent *diabetes mellitus may be present, indicated by blood sugar levels. Therapy for acute necrotizing pancreatitis is often unsuccessful since the condition is rapidly progressive, and generalized peritonitis is often well-established at presentation. In the milder form, treatment consists in reducing pancreatic secretion by initially withholding food and subsequently avoiding fatty food. Fluid and electrolyte therapy is used to prevent dehydration, and broad-spectrum antibiotics are advocated to prevent infection. The causes

of acute pancreatitis are unknown, although several factors have been suggested, such as high-fat diet, viral infections (e.g. *parvovirus) with or without autoimmune reactions, heredity (in dogs with necrotizing pancreatitis), pancreatic-duct occlusion, or drugs (e.g. corticosteroids). An acute pancreatitis in the cat has been associated with generalized *Toxoplasma gondii* infection.

Chronic pancreatitis may occur as a relapsing manifestation of acute pancreatitis, particularly in the dog. More common, especially in cats, is a chronic interstitial pancreatitis characterized by low-grade but constant inflammation leading to anatomical and functional destruction of the pancreas. Clinical signs are often rather vague, and affected animals may present late in the disease with jaundice and weight loss. Frequently, diabetes mellitus, as a result of loss of islets of Langerhans, is the main sign. Abdominal palpation may reveal a distorted hard pancreas, resulting from successive healing episodes. Again, the causes are often obscure; occasionally, biliary or gastrointestinal obstruction is implicated, necessitating corrective surgical intervention. Most cases are regarded as *idiopathic and are treated by fluid and electrolyte support during crises, with dietary management in the long-term.

pancuronium A competitive neuromuscular blocking drug that acts in a manner similar to tubocurarine (*see* curare) and *gallamine triethiodide. It is five times more potent than tubocurarine but has a slower onset of action. It is used during anaesthesia to achieve muscle relaxation, although positive-pressure ventilation is necessary and there is blockade of parasympathetic receptors at the heart leading to tachycardia. Its effects can be antagonized using *anticholinesterase drugs (e.g. *neostigmine or *edrophonium) with *atropine.

pancytopenia An abnormally low count of all types of blood cell. The only veterinary disease to be characterized by pancytopenia is feline pancytopenia, otherwise known as *feline viral enteritis or feline panleucopenia.

pandemic A term used in human medicine to describe a widespread epidemic. The equivalent term in veterinary medicine is *panzootic.

panhysterectomy Surgical removal of the entire uterus. *See* hysterectomy.

panniculitis A rare inflammatory condition of the subcutaneous fat involving the formation of small palpable nodules in the skin. First described in humans it has been reported in horses, dogs, and cats. It is a manifestation of several diseases of widely differing aetiology. For example, it may occur in infectious diseases, nutritional deficiency, pancreatic disease, and immunological disorders.

pannus 1. A subepithelial infiltration of the cornea of the eye by vascular or fibrovascular tissue, producing an opaque area in the cornea. Common in German shepherd dogs and some collies, it appears initially in the lower outer corner of the eye and is usually self-limiting, affecting one-quarter to one-third of the cornea. Rarely it spreads over the entire surface, causing blindness. The cause is unknown, possibly a hypersensitivity or autoimmune reaction. Surgical excision of the cornea followed by topical *corticosteroid application together with antibiotic/antimycotic therapy gives the best results. Other names: **pseudopterygium**; **chronic superficial keratitis**.
2. An inflammatory exudate overlying the inner lining of a joint. It is associated with fibrinous or purulent *arthritis in farm animals (especially pigs and cattle), and with canine autoimmune arthritis. The fibrinous exudate becomes organized and adheres to the articular cartilage, and its collagenolytic activity causes destruction and erosion of the articular surface. Joint movement may be restricted, resulting in fibrous *ankylosis of the joint. Therapy is often ineffective since the lesion is typically well established when diagnosed. In the early stages, *corticosteroid therapy, combined with antibiotic where a bacterial infection is suspected, may ameliorate the adhesions and pannus formation.

panophthalmitis Inflammation of the entire tissues of the eye, often with spread to orbital structures. It is usually caused by infection with pyogenic organisms following, for example, penetration by foreign bodies, or more generalized disease (e.g. *feline infectious peritonitis, streptococcal infections in dogs following trauma, *listeriosis in cattle and sheep, *malignant catarrhal fever in cattle). The affected eye swells with purulent fluid and the cornea becomes opaque and vascularized. If left untreated the eye degenerates and atrophies; rupture of the eyeball is unusual. Treatment is aimed at achieving a high concentration of antimicrobial drugs in the affected tissue; surgical removal of the eyeball is often mandatory. Other name: **purulent uveitis**.

panosteitis *See* canine panosteitis.

pantothenic acid A *vitamin of the B-complex that is a constituent of *coenzyme A, which is required in the body for acyl group transfer in energy metabolism and in the synthesis of fatty acids, cholesterol, steroid hormones, and the neurotransmitter acetylcholine. It is synthesized by microorganisms in the reticulorumen and intestines and is found, usually as a constituent of coenzyme A, in many plant and animal tissues. Good natural sources include yeast, liver, egg yolk, milk, groundnuts (peanuts), sunflower meal, soya-bean meal, legumes, bran, animal protein meals, and molasses.

Pantothenic acid deficiency Deficiencies are rare because of the vitamin's wide distribution. Initial deficiency signs are poor appetite and decreased growth; later there is dermatitis, especially near body orifices and on the feet, depigmentation, and loss of hair or feathers. Pigs may also suffer diarrhoea with intestinal ulceration, decreased litter sizes and increased neonatal mortality, and a characteristic goose-stepping gait. Fowls may produce eggs of decreased hatchability. In fish, deficiency signs include decreased growth, swollen gills, and dermatitis. For diagnosis and treatment *see* vitamin. Other names: **vitamin B₃; vitamin B₅; d-calpan; d-panthenol; anti-grey hair factor; chick antidermatitis factor**.

pantropic Describing a virus or other agent that replicates and/or exerts its pathogenic effects on several tissues of the host, with no affinity for a particular tissue. *Compare* neurotropic.

panzootic 1. Distributed globally or widely throughout a region. **2.** A widespread *epizootic disease.

papaverine An alkaloid, derived from opium, that relaxes smooth muscle. High doses given parenterally cause dilatation of arterioles. Papaverine has been used to treat cardiovascular conditions, but is not used extensively in veterinary medicine. Side-effects include tachycardia, drowsiness, gastrointestinal disturbances, and possibly hepatic toxicity.

papilla (*pl.* **papillae**) **1.** The nipple or teat. One papilla is associated with each *mammary gland. The sow usually has 14, the bitch 10, the cow 4,

and the mare, ewe, and goat 2. At the tip of each papilla opens the papillary duct(s): in ruminants there is only one, in the mare 2, in the sow usually 2, and in the bitch 6–12. Each papillary duct leads from a *lactiferous sinus. **2.** Any small nipple-shaped protuberance. Several different kinds of papillae occur on the *tongue and may be associated with taste buds. The major and minor duodenal papillae occur where the bile duct and accessory pancreatic duct open into the duodenum.

papilloma A small raised benign tumour, usually arising from the epidermis of the skin. It may be single or multiple. Viral papillomas are caused by one of various *papovaviruses and are common in dogs, cattle, and horses, occurring primarily in young animals and particularly on the lips, mouth, teats, and udder. They may, however, be found on any part of the skin. In cattle, papillomas may also occur in the oesophagus, oesophageal groove, and reticulum, where they can cause digestive disturbance, and in the urinary bladder. The bovine papovavirus may also cause *fibropapillomas* of the genitalia, a venereal disease.

Usually whitish grey and varying from 3 mm to several centimetres in diameter, papillomas are generally of little significance, but they may be cosmetically undesirable or sufficiently extensive to be harmful. Spread is by direct contact with infected animals, the virus entering the skin where it is abraded. Usually no treatment is necessary since immunity develops with age and regression occurs spontaneously. However, they may be removed surgically if necessary, and an autogenous *vaccine may be prepared from papilloma tissue. Other names: **verruca; wart**.

papillomavirus A genus of the *papovavirus family. Its members are notable for causing warts. Bovine papillomavirus has been of particular experimental interest and there is considerable evidence linking it with certain human cancers.

papovavirus A family of DNA *viruses that have a naked icosahedral *capsid and contain circular DNA. The name derives from *pa*(pilloma) *po*(lyoma) *va*(cuolating) *virus*, i.e. the three main members of the family. Apart from the *papillomaviruses, members are not important disease agents. However, laboratory studies of them, particularly polyoma and SV40 (Simian Virus 40), have contributed greatly to the understanding of virus mutliplication and virus–cell interactions.

papule A solid elevated skin lesion that is less than 1 cm in diameter. Papules may be single or, more usually, multiple, and result from cellular infiltrations, metabolic deposits, fluid beneath the epidermis, or local *hypertrophy of the epidermis. Papules are seen in insect hypersensitivity (e.g. *sweet itch) and contact *allergy. *Compare* nodule; pustule.

papulo- *Prefix denoting* a papule or pimple.

para- *Prefix denoting* **1.** beside or near. Example: *paranasal* (near the nasal cavity). **2.** resembling. **3.** abnormal.

parabronchus (tertiary bronchus) (*pl.* **parabronchi**) One of a series of looped airways connecting the secondary bronchi in the avian lung. The parabronchi have extensions (atria), which lead into funnel-shaped infundibula and air capillaries, where gaseous exchange takes place.

paracentesis The process of tapping fluid from a body cavity using a needle or cannula. In veterinary practice abdominal paracentesis is most frequently performed. Paracentesis is used to determine the type of fluid present, for example transudate or exudate in cases of *ascites. In all species, an increased white cell count is indicative of *peritonitis, and pathogenic bacteria may be seen on a smear or cultured from the fluid. Inadvertent puncture of the gut, spleen, or bladder may occur in any species and the technique should not be performed by untrained personnel. Aseptic precautions are necessary, and the needle or cannula should be inserted in the ventral midline. *Compare* aspiration; enterocentesis.

paracetamol *See* NSAID.

paradental disease *See* periodontal disease.

paraffin 1. A mixture of hydrocarbons obtained from the distillation of petroleum. It is available as hard paraffin, *liquid paraffin, yellow soft paraffin (yellow petroleum jelly), or bleached as white soft paraffin (white petroleum jelly). Both soft paraffins are known commonly as Vaseline. *Hard paraffin* is a wax-like substance used to thicken ointments. The wax can also be used topically to treat chronic inflammation and soften scar tissue. It is melted and applied in layers onto skin, causing localized vasodilatation, and can be peeled off after approximately 20 minutes. *Soft paraffins* are used as the basis for ointments and in wound dressings. They are not absorbed and are nonirritant, keeping skin surfaces moist and allowing the easy removal of wound dressings or protecting skin from irritant aqueous solutions (e.g. tear scalding). They are also used in eye ointments. Many ointments combine hard and soft paraffins. **2.** Alkane: a saturated hydrocarbon with the general formula C_nH_{2n+2}.

paraffin poisoning *See* fuel oil poisoning.

Parafilaria A genus of parasitic *nematodes found in cattle and horses, mainly in tropical regions. *P. multipapillosa* affects horses; *P. bovicola* infests cattle in India, the Mediterranean region, and the Philippines. The adults live in subcutaneous or intermuscular connective tissue, forming nodules within the hide. They pierce their host's skin to deposit eggs, causing *summer bleeding*. Flies (e.g. *Musca*) feed at these sites and take up the eggs, which develop within the fly before migrating to the fly's proboscis to await a suitable host. Affected animals can be treated with ivermectin, and fly control is useful.

paragonimiasis Disease caused by infestation with *flukes of the genus *Paragonimus*, which inhabit the lungs and occasionally the central nervous system of various mammals, including the pig, cat, dog, goat, ox, and humans. Infestation occurs in the USA, southern Africa, and the Far East. Mammals become infested after eating a crustacean containing the infective cercarial form of the parasite. The signs are mild except when the central nervous system is involved.

Paragonimus A genus of large *flukes that are parasitic in the lungs of dogs, cats, pigs, and humans and found in the Americas and the Far East. It causes the disease *paragonimiasis, with signs resembling those of chronic bronchitis. There are two intermediate hosts, a snail and a crab or crayfish; the primary host is infected by eating raw or inadequately cooked seafood.

parainfluenzavirus A genus of the *paramyxovirus family. Its members cause disease, especially in domestic fowls (e.g. *Newcastle disease virus) although members infecting bovine, ovine, and canine hosts are known.

parakeratosis An abnormality of the outermost horny layer of the skin (stratum corneum) in which prominent nuclei are retained in flattened cells, instead of the normal thin layer of non-nucleated laminar *keratin. It is a common nonspecific reaction, often associated with healing inflammatory reactions or other pathological processes that have upset the normal metabolism and turnover of keratin-producing cells (keratinocytes).

Hereditary and congenital parakeratosis due to *zinc deficiency have been described in Holstein-Friesian cattle. Dietary zinc deficiency, complicated by phytic acid binding of zinc (e.g. with soya-bean protein extracts), high calcium/low free fatty acid levels, and the presence of bacterial or viral pathogens, has been identified as the cause of parakeratosis in pigs. Affected pigs show reddening of the skin, progressing to eruptions and scab formation. Dietary zinc supplementation corrects the condition.

paralysis (*pl.* **paralyses**) Loss of voluntary muscle control resulting in partial or complete loss of movement of the affected part of the body. The loss or impairment of function is usually the result of nerve lesion(s). Paralysis is a sign of many different diseases, and such conditions may be classified as acute/nonprogressive, acute/progressive, or chronic/progressive. Motor paralysis does not automatically imply sensory impairment also. Generally, types of paralysis are classified according to the level of the nervous system at which damage or failure of the descending motor pathway occurs, i.e. cerebral, spinal, or peripheral. Paralysis also shows varying degrees of spasticity (*see* spastic) or flaccidity (*see* flaccid).

paralysis

Types of neuropathies resulting in paralysis

Type	Examples of conditions/diseases
Congenital	Giant axonal neuropathy of German shepherd dogs (autosomal recessive) Central and peripheral neuropathy of boxer dogs Hypertrophic neuropathy in Tibetan mastiffs (inherited) Afghan hound hereditary myelopathy Poodle demyelinating myelopathy Lysosomal storage disease (leukodystrophy) in cats and dogs Spinal dysraphism in Weimaraner dogs
Metabolic/toxic/nutritional	Tick paralysis in dogs, humans, etc. Diabetic neuropathy in dogs and cats Swayback in lambs Arsanilic acid poisoning in pigs Organophosphorus poisoning in all species Lead poisoning in calves Hypervitaminosis A in cats Chastek paralysis in foxes, mink, and cats
Trauma	Brachial paralysis in dogs and horses (road accidents, etc.) Radial paralysis in dogs Femoral and obturator-sciatic nerve paralysis in horses (trauma, foaling) and cattle and sheep (parturition) Degenerative intervertebral disc disease in dogs (Pekingese, dachshund)
Inflammatory/immune-mediated	Polyneuritis of coonhound paralysis in dogs Polyradiculo-neuropathy/-neuritis in dogs and cats Cauda equina neuritis in horses Discospondylitis in dogs and pigs Distemper myelitis in dogs Polioencephalomyelitis in cats Feline infectious peritonitis Toxoplasmosis in dogs and cats Leukoencephalomyelitis-arthritis in goats Rabies Marek's disease in fowls

Type	Examples of conditions/diseases
Idiopathic	Feline dysautonomia (Key-Gaskell syndrome)
	Idiopathic facial paralysis in dogs and horses
	Distal denervating disease in dogs
	Cranial nerve disease in dogs, cats, and horses (associated with vestibular disease)
	Scotty cramp in Scottish terriers
	Wobbler syndrome (cervical vertebral osteoarthropathy) in horses and large-breed dogs
	Stringhalt in horses
Neoplastic	Primary nerve or nerve sheath tumours (e.g. neurofibromas, meningiomas)
	Metastatic infiltration (e.g. lymphosarcoma metastasis in cats, dogs, and cattle)
	Paraneoplastic syndrome in dogs (neurotoxic factors?)
Other	Aortoiliac thrombosis in horses and cats

Cerebral paralysis is associated with disease or damage to the brain, brain-stem, or cranial nerves, and generally results in *quadriplegia or *hemiplegia characterized by flaccid paralysis with pain sensation maintained. Such central involvement is seen in *encephalitis (e.g. rabies, canine distemper), cranial fractures with nervous tissue involvement, brain haemorrhages or haematomas, and brain tumours (e.g. gliomas, astrocytomas).

Spinal paralysis is probably the most common type of paralysis encountered in domestic animals, particularly in dogs and cats involved in road traffic accidents. Fractures and/or haematomas leading to spinal cord compression or anoxia are common sequelae to such accidents. Pathological fractures, especially of the thoracolumbar region, may be associated with *discospondylitis in pigs especially. Spinal intervertebral disc protrusion in canine breeds, such as Pekingese, dachshunds, Sealyhams, and some spaniel families, leads to acute or chronic spinal cord compression and varying degrees of paralysis, depending on the sections of cord or nerve outflows affected (see below). Secondary cervical spinal cord or nerve involvement may be seen in the *wobbler syndrome in horses and breeds of large dog (e.g. Great Danes). Most spinal paralyses are acquired conditions although some congenital abnormalities (e.g. spinal dysraphism in Weimaraner dogs) do occur.

Patterns of sensory perception and motor dysfunction can be used to allocate cord lesions to one or more of four categories: damage above the level of the brachial plexus; damage between the brachial and lumbar nerve outflows; damage at the level of lumbar nerve outflow; and damage caudal to the lumbar outflows. The assessment of spinal paralysis cases depends on the unilateral or bilateral nature of involvement, the severity of clinical signs, and the speed of development of paralysis. Diagnosis is aided by the use of radiography and *myelography to localize sites of lesions.

Peripheral paralysis arises due to injury or disease of nerve trunks or nerve endings in muscle fibres. The causes are extremely varied and extensive (see table). Among the commonest is damage to the brachial plexus or suprascapular or radial nerves (especially in horses, dogs, and cats) resulting from collisions or stake wounds. Diseases of muscle (myopathies) are generally characterized by weakness and fatigue rather than true paralysis, but they may occur secondarily to primary nerve disease. *Botulism, caused by *Clostridium botulinum* toxin, is characterized by paralysis due to blockage of the release of *acetylcholine at neuromuscular junctions.

Generally the prognosis for all forms of paralysis is poor. There is no effective treatment for the more severe cerebral and spinal lesions unless specific causal agents can be identified and treated appropriately. With traumatic damage some compensation or motor recovery may occur with time but this is not predictable.

paralytic myoglobinuria A severe form of *muscular dystrophy in which *myoglobin released from damaged muscle cells escapes into the urine giving it a dark red-brown colour. Extensive and severe muscle lesions cause severe stiffness. There are various causes. In horses, forced exercise after a period of rest, especially when coupled with excess energy intake, may precipitate the condition, as may strenuous exercise in greyhounds, or even a bout of fighting in aggressive dogs. In very rare cases, the same applies to cattle exercising after release onto pasture following winter housing. Various substances (*ionophores) increase the permeability of cell membranes. These include the feed additive monensin sodium, which may trigger the condition if consumed in undiluted form or mixed in the wrong concentration. Also, certain plants, for example coyotilla (*Karwinskia humboldtiana*) and sennas (*Cassia* spp.), contain myotoxins, which have similar effects. The muscle lesions result from the rapid breakdown of glycogen, contained in muscle fibres, to lactic acid. If this accumulates and is not removed by the blood then toxic levels build up locally and muscle cells die. The released myoglobin appears in the urine. Exessive myoglobin production can also lead to renal damage. The gluteal muscles of the rump are especially affected, presumably because of their relatively high glycogen content. Clinical signs include profuse sweating and stiffness, progressing to severe pain and distress. The affected muscles harden. Recovery follows quickly if the animal is rested before the lesions become severe. The disease was formerly common in draught horses rested over the weekend and overexerted on the Monday, hence the alternative name, 'Monday morning disease'.

paramesonephric duct (Müllerian duct) Either of the paired ducts that develop adjacent to the *mesonephric ducts in the embryo. In the female they develop into the uterine tubes, uterus, and part of the vagina. In the male they degenerate, usually completely, although they may persist as a remnant (*uterus masculinus*).

parameter (in medicine) A measurement of some factor, such as blood pressure, pulse rate, or haemoglobin level, that may have a bearing on the condition being investigated.

parametritis Inflammation of the *parametrium. *See also* metritis.

parametrium (*pl.* **parametria**) The connective tissue and smooth muscle within the mesometrial part of the *broad ligament of the uterus.

paramyxovirus An important family of RNA *viruses that have enveloped helical *capsids and contain segmented negative-strand RNA. It includes the genera *morbillivirus, *parainfluenzavirus, and *pneumovirus.

paranasal sinus One of the several air-filled cavities, lined by mucous membrane, within some of the bones of the skull. They open into the nasal cavity and are named according to the bones in which they lie, principally the frontal, maxilla, sphenoid, and ethmoid bones. The *maxillary sinus* has a close relationship to the teeth of the upper jaw; in the horse it is divided by a septum into rostral and caudal maxillary sinuses, and in the ox it extends into the palatine and lacrimal bones. The *sphenoidal sinus* in the horse extends into the palatine bone as the *sphenopalatine sinus*. The *ethmoidal sinus* contains, in the horse, large extensions within the nasal conchae, the *conchal sinuses*. In the ox the *frontal sinus* is very large and extends into the cornual process when this is present.

paraphimosis A condition in which the penis protrudes from the preputial sheath and cannot be retracted. It usually affects young male **dogs** following coitus, trauma, or masturbation where the erect penis fails to detumesce and a narrow preputial orifice or the inward-rolled hairy tip of the prepuce prevents retraction. The exteriorized penis becomes congested and traumatized, and inflammation is frequently exacerbated by the dog licking the penis. Necrosis of the penis may occur quickly and treatment should seek to return the penis, either manually, using lubricants, or surgically, by enlarging the preputial orifice. Where necrosis has occurred partial penile amputation may be necessary.

In **bulls**, paraphimosis may occur as a result of tumours (e.g. *fibropapilloma) or following scarring and distortion with preputial lacerations. In **horses** the condition may arise from a variety of traumatic lesions (e.g. fence post injuries, kicks from mares during service), neoplasia (*squamous cell carcinoma), or parasitic granulomas (e.g. *Habronema spp. larval lesions); postcastration infections may also involve the prepuce causing paraphimosis. In all instances in large animal species, surgical reduction of the constriction with or without penile amputation is usually necessary.

paraplegia *Paralysis of both hindlimbs.

paraprotein Protein that appears in the blood as the result of a pathological process.

paraquat poisoning A toxic condition caused by ingestion of paraquat or related bipyridyl compounds, such as diquat, which are widely used as herbicides. Pastures treated with the recommended dilution are innocuous to grazing animals although it is a wise precaution to keep animals away for a few days after spraying. However ingestion of the undiluted or partially diluted herbicide causes an irreversible proliferative bronchiolitis and alveolitis in the lungs, which is

Parascaris

almost invariably fatal in animals and humans.

Parascaris A genus of *nematodes containing *P. equorum*, a parasite of horses that is mainly a problem for foals in their first year. The adult worms are found in the small intestine where, in large numbers, they can cause enteritis; there may also be diarrhoea and flatulence. In very heavy infestations the migration of the larvae may cause coughing. The adult worms lay eggs, which are passed out with the faeces onto pasture or straw. The eggs can survive for several years and, being very sticky, can adhere to the host's udder or coat. The larvae develop within the egg but do not hatch until the egg is swallowed by a suitable host. After entering the bloodstream through the stomach wall the larva passes to the liver, where it changes to a third-stage larva, and then to the lungs, where it becomes a fourth-stage larva. These migrate up the windpipe to be swallowed and return to the small intestine, where they mature to adult worms, some three months after the initial infestation. *Pyrantel tartrate as a drench, mebendazole (*see* benzimidazole), or *ivermectin in the feed can be used to treat affected animals.

parasite An organism that lives in (*endoparasite*) or on (*ectoparasite*) another living organism (the *host). The parasite obtains food and/or shelter from its host and contributes nothing to its host's welfare. Indeed, parasites often affect the health of their host: this may range from mild irritation to chronic debilitation or even death. Parasites of domestic animals include viruses, bacteria, protozoa, nematodes, tapeworms, flukes, mites, ticks, insects, and fungi.

parasitic bronchitis A condition of sheep, cattle, and horses caused by *lungworms. It is mainly a problem in calves in their first grazing season (*see* husk); older animals acquire immunity. The condition is characterized by coughing and shallow breathing, and affected animals stand with head and neck outstretched. These signs are caused by the host reaction to the migration of larval worms through the lungs and by adult worms residing in the trachea and bronchi.

parasitic gastroenteritis (PGE) Inflammation of the alimentary tract due to infestation with parasitic worms, usually *nematodes (roundworms). *Tapeworms and *flukes are occasionally involved. PGE occurs in all host species but is of most importance in ruminants, particularly cattle and sheep. Small numbers of worms in the alimentary tract do not usually cause signs of disease. Moderate numbers can cause reduced weight gain, but large numbers need to be present before typical signs are seen. These usually include diarrhoea, loss of weight, and dehydration. Some intestinal nematodes (e.g. *Haemonchus) suck blood and may cause *anaemia. Animals develop immunity to the nematodes, consequently disease is most often seen in young animals. However, immunity may break down under heavy challenge or in times of extreme stress. Moreover, PGE may predispose animals to other diseases (*see* pasteurellosis).

The principal causative agents vary according to host species and geographical region. In **cattle** *Ostertagia ostertagi* predominates in temperate climates whereas in tropical and subtropical regions *Haemonchus placei*, *Oesophagostomum radiatum*, and *Strongyloides papillosus* may all cause disease. In **sheep** *Ostertagia circumcincta*, *Haemonchus contortus*, *Trichostrongylus vitrinus*, *T. axei*, *T. colubriformis*, and *Cooperia curticei* inhabit the abomasum and small

parasympathomimetic

intestine and may cause disease. *Nematodirus battus* causes losses among lambs in the UK. *Hookworms cause disease in many regions, particularly in Africa, the Indian subcontinent, and Indonesia, where *Gaigeria pachyscelis* can cause heavy mortality. Both *Oesophagostomum venulosum* and *Oe. columbianum*, which inhabit the large intestine, tend to be confined to warm-temperate and tropical regions.

Gastrointestinal roundworms in **horses** include *Strongylus*, trichonemes, and *Habronema* (*see* habronemiasis). Other common parasites include *Oxyuris equi* and *Parascaris equorum*. *Hyostronglyus, Strongyloides ransomi, Oesophagostomum dentatum*, and *Trichuris suis* are commonly occurring species in pigs. Infestation with *Ascaris suum* is also widespread. **Dogs and cats** are affected by *Toxocara* and *Toxascaris*, the adults of which inhabit the intestine following migration of the larvae through the bloodstream, liver, and lungs. They are extremely common throughout the world. Puppies and kittens are often born infested with worms that have migrated from the tissues of the dam across the placenta and entered the foetal lungs, later moving to the intestine. Other intestinal parasites of dogs include the hookworms *Ancylostoma* (in tropical countries) and *Uncinaria* (in temperate areas). In **poultry** *Acuaria uncinata* and the gizzard worm *Amidostomum* cause disease in water fowl, such as ducks and geese.

In all cases diagnosis of PGE depends upon relating clinical signs of disease with the demonstration of large numbers of parasite eggs in the faeces. Treatment consists in administering a suitable *anthelmintic. Prevention entails avoiding the exposure of animals to environments heavily contaminated with infective eggs or larvae. For example, grazing animals should be provided with worm-free pasture wherever practicable. This, coupled with the routine prophylactic use of anthelmintics, will prevent the build-up of high parasite numbers.

parasiticide An agent used to kill parasites. Examples include *anthelmintics, *acaricides, and *insecticides.

parasitology The study and science of parasites.

parasympathetic nervous system One of the two divisions of the *autonomic nervous system. Its fibres are contained within cranial nerves III, VII, IX, and X and the sacral spinal nerves, and are distributed to most organs within the body. The system works in balance with the *sympathetic nervous system, the actions of which it frequently opposes. See illustration.

parasympatholytic An agent that opposes the effects of the *parasympathetic nervous system by preventing acetylcholine from acting as a neurotransmitter. There may be some effect at *nicotinic sites at ganglia and neuromuscular junctions but this is usually at high doses and activity is low. The major parasympatholytic drugs are *atropine and hyoscine, and the semisynthetic compound homatropine. For actions and therapeutic usages *see* atropine.

parasympathomimetic A drug that stimulates the *parasympathetic nervous system by mimicking the action of acetylcholine on muscarinic receptors at the parasympathetic neuroeffector junction. Acetylcholine itself is not used, but synthetic choline esters have been used therapeutically. These include methacholine, which causes marked cardiovascular effects, and bethanechol and carbachol, which act mainly on the urinary bladder and intestines. They were formerly used to

parathyroid glands

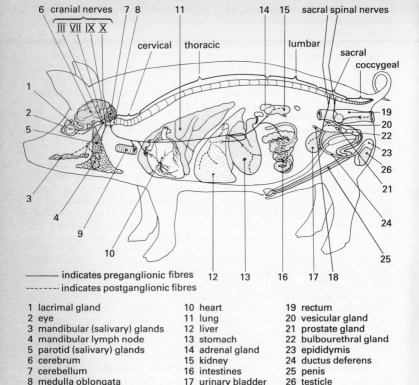

6 cranial nerves 7 8 11 14 15 sacral spinal nerves

III VII IX X

cervical thoracic lumbar

sacral
coccygeal

1
2
5
3
4
9
10

19
20
22
23
26
21

24

25

——— indicates preganglionic fibres
- - - - - indicates postganglionic fibres

12 13 16 17 18

1 lacrimal gland	10 heart	19 rectum
2 eye	11 lung	20 vesicular gland
3 mandibular (salivary) glands	12 liver	21 prostate gland
4 mandibular lymph node	13 stomach	22 bulbourethral gland
5 parotid (salivary) glands	14 adrenal gland	23 epididymis
6 cerebrum	15 kidney	24 ductus deferens
7 cerebellum	16 intestines	25 penis
8 medulla oblongata	17 urinary bladder	26 testicle
9 trachea	18 ureter	

Parasympathetic division of the autonomic nervous system in a pig

treat intestinal impaction or bladder atony but safer agents are now used instead. Various natural alkaloids (e.g. muscarine, pilocarpine, and arecoline) are parasympathomimetics: *pilocarpine is used to treat glaucoma, and *arecoline has been used as a purgative and taeniacide in dogs. Overdosage with parasympathomimetics is treated with *atropine.

parathyroid glands Two pairs of *endocrine glands situated close to, or embedded within, the *thyroid gland in higher vertebrates. They are stimulated to produce *parathyroid hormone by a decrease in blood calcium.

parathyroid hormone (PTH; parathormone) A protein hormone secreted by the parathyroid glands in response to decreased blood calcium. It is the major hormone controlling calcium homeostasis. PTH increases blood calcium by activating cellular mechanisms of the intestine to increase calcium absorption from food; by promoting increased calcium resorption in the kidney, as well as transformation of the *vitamin D metabolite, 25-hydroxycholecalciferol, to the more active 1,25-dihydroxy-cholecalciferol; and by increasing the transfer of calcium from bone to the blood.

paratuberculosis *See* Johne's disease.

parbendazole *See* benzimidazole.

parenchyma The functional tissue of an organ, as opposed to the supporting tissue (*stroma*).

parenteral Administered by any way other than by mouth: applied, for example, to the introduction of drugs or other agents into the body by injection.

paresis Muscular weakness of neural origin. It is usually regarded as a state of partial or incomplete *paralysis, resulting in a deficit of voluntary movement.
Paresis may result from lesions at any level of the descending motor innervation pathway from the brain. It is most commonly associated with serious diseases of the central nervous system; less commonly the peripheral nerves are involved. *Monoparesis* refers to single limb involvement; *hemiparesis* describes paralysis of two limbs on one side of the body; and *tetraparesis*, or *quadriparesis*, indicates involvement of all four limbs. *Paraparesis* refers to weakness of both hindlimbs.

paries (*pl.* **parietes**) **1.** The enveloping or surrounding part of an organ or other structure. **2.** The wall of a cavity.

parietal 1. Of or relating to the inner walls of a body cavity, as opposed to the contents: applied particularly to the membranes lining a cavity (*see* peritoneum; pleura). **2.** Of or relating to the parietal bone. The parietal lobe

of the cerebral hemisphere is located below the *parietal bone.

parietal bone Either of the paired bones forming the top and side of the cranium. *See* skull.

parity The state of an animal in terms of the number of previous parturitions it has had. For example, nulliparous is none, primiparous is one, and multiparous is several.

paronychia Inflammation of the bed of the nail or claw, usually involving bacterial or fungal infection but with a number of disparate causes. For example, paronychia is common in sporting dog breeds as a result of chronic *hookworm dermatitis. The soft tissues around the *corium are swollen, often hairless, and painful. Treatment may involve removal of the nail or claw to permit proper drainage and healing. *Antibiotic therapy may be prescribed. If all the claws are affected it may indicate autoimmune disease or systemic disease.

paroophoron *See* mesonephros.

parotid gland The largest of the *salivary glands. It is irregular in shape and is located near to the external acoustic meatus of the ear and the mandible. Its duct runs forward and empties into the vestibule of the *oral cavity.

parotitis Inflammation of the *parotid gland. It results in local swelling and tenderness just behind the ramus of the mandible and below the ear.

parthenogenesis The development of offspring from unfertilized eggs. It occurs normally in certain plants and simple animals, for example aphids and worms. In mammals it can be artificially induced, but has not been

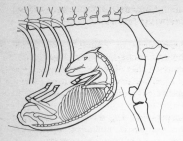

Foetus near term

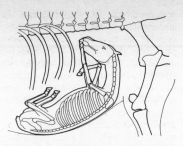

Changes in posture prior to first stage of labour

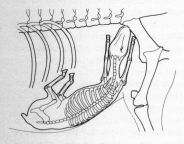

First stage of labour: head and forelimbs extend and rotate ready for delivery

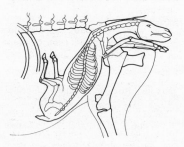

Second stage of labour: head and neck of foetus enter the birth canal; distal part of body is still in ventral position

Movements of the foetus during parturition in the mare

found to proceed beyond the early stages of development. Parthenogenetically produced offspring are genetically identical to the parent.

parturient paresis *See* milk fever.

parturition (birth) The delivery of viable offspring at the end of *pregnancy. It is thought to be initiated by the foetus in response to stress. *Adrenocorticotrophic hormone (or ACTH), secreted by the adenohypophysis of the pituitary gland of the foetus, causes increased secretion of foetal *corticosteroids, which act on the uterus resulting in the production

of *prostaglandins from the endometrium. These prostaglandins cause a drop in circulating *progesterone, which maintains the uterus in a quiescent state throughout pregnancy, and allow the rising concentration of placental oestrogens to sensitize the uterus in readiness for muscular contractions. Uterine contractions increase in the last few days of gestation and result in the *presentation of the foetus or foetuses ready for delivery (see illustration).

In the first stage of labour, the cervix, which is sealed throughout pregnancy, becomes softened and dilated under the influence of oestrogens and other hormones. In the second stage of labour, the uterine contractions increase in frequency and strength, propelling the foetus partly through the cervix. This stimulates the release of *oxytocin from the neurohypophysis of the pituitary gland of the mother; oxytocin and uterine prostaglandins cause further uterine contractions, and the presence of the foetus in the pelvis initiates powerful contractions of the abdominal muscles, resulting in the expulsion of the foetus along the vagina and through the vulva.

In monotocous species, after a short period during which the dam tends to her offspring, the third stage of labour begins. During this phase the foetal placenta separates from the wall of the uterus and forms a mass in the pelvic area, which stimulates further abdominal contractions and straining resulting in expulsion of the foetal membranes. In polytocous species the foetal membranes are shed between the delivery of each offspring. After parturition, the uterus returns to its prepregnant state (*see* involution).

Delivery of the foetus involves rupture of the umbilical cord, release from the foetal membranes, the initiation of active breathing, and the acquisition of a fully competent pulmonary circulation. Suckling should be commenced as soon as possible to gain the maximum benefit from the maternal *colostrum.

Death of offspring before, during, or immediately after birth can be caused by various factors. These include protracted birth (resulting in asphyxia); abnormal presentation and consequent difficult birth (*dystocia); metabolic disturbance of the mother (e.g. *pregnancy toxaemia); inadequate maternal care; failure to suckle or lack of milk (*see* agalactia); congenital and genetic abnormalities; and disease in the newborn (e.g. *anae-

mia; *diarrhoea). *See also* calving; farrowing; foaling.

parvovirus A family of DNA *viruses distinguished by having single-stranded DNA. Several members are of veterinary importance, especially the *canine parvovirus.

paspalum staggers A nervous syndrome, usually affecting cattle but occasionally sheep and horses, caused by ingestion of ergots (sclerotia) of the fungus *Claviceps paspali*, which parasitizes grasses of the genus *Paspalum*. Apparently the signs are due to *mycotoxins, not the alkaloids also present in the sclerotia. This form of ergotism has occurred in several countries where *Paspalum* spp. are grown in pasture, including New Zealand, Australia, and South Africa. In the USA it is common in cattle grazing Dallis grass (*P. dilatatum* – incorrectly called 'Dallas' grass). Affected animals are hyperexcitable, tremble, and have an uncoordinated gait intensified by forced movements, when they may fall and undergo convulsions. Clinically similar outbreaks occur on some ryegrass and Bermuda grass swards free of *C. paspali* infection. *See also* ergot poisoning. *Compare* Bermuda grass staggers; ryegrass staggers.

pastern 1. The joint between the proximal and distal phalanges (*see* phalanx) in the digit, especially of the horse. **2.** The region surrounding this joint in the horse.

Pasteurella A genus of nonmotile pleomorphic Gram-negative *bacteria that are facultatively anaerobic and live as commensals or parasites in animals. Some are pathogenic. In **cattle** *P. multocida* and *P. haemolytica* are normally carried as commensals in the oropharynx, but certain predisposing factors allow the bacteria to multiply in the lower respiratory tract. These include poor weather and housing conditions and transport (as in *transit fever). Primary infections by viruses or mycoplasmas also predispose to pneumonic pasteurellosis. Certain biotypes and serotypes of *P. multocida* cause *haemorrhagic septicaemia in cattle, buffaloes, sheep, and goats. In **sheep** and **goats** bronchopneumonias due to both *P. multocida* and *P. haemolytica* occur, often in association with viral infections, particularly *parainfluenza-type 3 virus.

In **poultry** *P. multocida* is a common secondary invader to respiratory viral infections, such as *avian infectious laryngotracheitis. It also causes *fowl cholera in domestic fowls, ducks, geese, and turkeys. *P. anatipestifer* causes a septicaemia (*see* anatipestifer infection) in ducks. *P. multocida* infection in **rabbits** causes a septicaemic pneumonia, generally known as snuffles, whereas the same pathogen in **pigs** plays a role in the pathogenesis of *atrophic rhinitis, in conjunction with *Bordetella bronchiseptica* and viral infections. The pneumonias that follow other viral infections in pigs are also usually due to *P. multocida*. In humans wound infections following animal bites are often due to *P. multocida*. *P. pneumotropica* causes pneumonias in mice and has also been associated with wound infections following cat bites in humans.

pasteurellosis Disease due to infection with bacteria of the genus *Pasteurella*.

pasteurization A method of heat-treating milk to improve its storage qualities and destroy pathogenic bacteria. Milk is heated to 65°C for 30 minutes or to 72°C for 15 minutes followed by rapid cooling to below 10°C. The method was devised by the French microbiologist Louis Pasteur (1822–95). It delays souring but not to the same extend as *ultrahigh temperature (UHT) treatment.

patch test A skin test used to identify the causal allergen(s) in cases of *allergic contact dermatitis. A nonallergenic cotton square is impregnated with a sample of an individual test allergen in solution. Several squares may be used to test different allergens, and one square is moistened only with the solvent to serve as the control. The squares are taped into position on a close-clipped area of unaffected skin and removed for examination after 72 hours. Each site is compared to the control site; a positive reaction is an area of erythema (redness) with papule formation in the absence of a reaction at the control site. Patch tests are often not very practical in animals because of the difficulty in maintaining the patches in position. Also, false positives are common.

patella (*pl.* **patellae** or **patellas**) The largest *sesamoid bone. It occurs in the tendon of the quadriceps femoris muscle and articulates with the trochlea of the femur. In most species it is attached to the tibial tuberosity by a single patellar ligament, although there are three in horses and cattle.

patent ductus arteriosus A condition in which the *ductus arteriosus, a foetal blood vessel connecting the pulmonary artery to the ascending arch of the aorta, persists after birth. This results in recirculation of arterial blood (shunting) from the aorta through the lungs, thereby diminishing cardiac output to the rest of the circulation (see illustration). The ductus normally degenerates and closes at or soon after birth, leaving a ligamentous structure in species such as the dog and cat. In these species a persistent patent ductus arteriosus is regarded as a congenital defect. There is evidence that the condition is

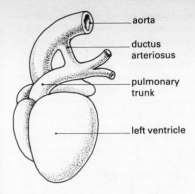

aorta

ductus arteriosus

pulmonary trunk

left ventricle

Site of patent ductus arteriosus as seen from left side of canine heart

inherited as a polygenic trait in the miniature poodle, Pomeranian, and Shetland sheepdog. Where the shunting of blood is mainly from the aorta to the pulmonary arteries it results in cardiac insufficiency and left-sided heart failure, apparent in young pups. A more slowly induced cardiac failure becomes apparent in 4–5-year-old adults, due to the shunting of blood from right (pulmonary artery) to left because of a persistent foetal pulmonary vascular formation. Turbulent flow in the ductus may also predispose to *thrombus formation. A diagnostic finding is a variably pitched continuous ('machinery') murmur on cardiac *auscultation. Radiographic examination using intravenous contrast media (angiocardiography) is also an important diagnostic procedure. Surgical ligation is feasible, depending on the size of the vessel, in the left-to-right ductus. Surgery is not an option in a right-to-left shunt since ablation in these cases precipitates right-sided heart failure and death.

In the sheep and horse it is normal to find persistence of a patent ductus arteriosus at up to 2 weeks of age without apparently any ill-effects. Diagnosis of the condition in these species is largely by ausculation and electrocardiophonography – a technique in which the heart sounds are recorded simultaneously with an electrocardiogram. Most causes of patent ductus arteriosus in large animals are discovered only at autopsy.

path- (patho-) *Prefix denoting* disease.

pathogen A microorganism, such as a bacterium, that parasitizes an animal (or plant) and produces a disease.

pathogenic Capable of causing disease. The term is applied to a parasitic microorganism (especially a bacterium) in relation to its host.

pathognomonic A clinical sign (or group of signs) that is characteristic of or unique to a particular disease and allows positive diagnosis of that disease. For example, the diamond-shaped skin lesions in *swine erysipelas are pathognomonic.

pathology The study of the structural and functional changes in tissues and organs that are caused by or result in disease. There are various specialities within the field. *Clinical pathology* is the study of clinical cases, their diagnostic features, and the effects of treatment regimes. *Comparative pathology* is the study of similarities and differences between diseases in various animal species. *Experimental pathology* is the study of artificially induced disease or the use of natural or induced model systems (in vivo or in vitro) to simulate disease processes.

-pathy *Suffix denoting* **1**. disease. Example: *nephropathy* (of the kidney). **2**. therapy. Example: *osteopathy* (by manipulation).

peach *See* cherry laurel poisoning.

peat scours *See* molybdenosis.

peck order A social hierarchy found in bird flocks, including domestic poultry. A linear hierarchy is the common form, in which one individual is dominant over another, which in turn is dominant over another bird, and so on. However, other more complex hierarchies have been identified. Hierarchies take time to develop, as they require the ability of individuals to recognize each other. Hence, they may not be of much relevance in broiler production. The peck order may be of importance in *pullet rearing, and the disruption of well-established hierarchies by transferring pullets from large groups into battery cages containing only a few randomly mixed individuals may improve subsequent performance. The bullying of a smaller individual by a larger one, particularly if feeder space is limited, is a less sophisticated behavioural pattern.

pectoral Relating to or describing the thoracic region (chest).

pectoral girdle *See* shoulder girdle.

pectoral muscles The muscles of the chest wall that attach the forelimb to the trunk. They consist of the superficial pectoral and deep pectoral muscles. In birds they are particularly well developed for flight.

pedicle 1. The part of the arch of a *vertebra attaching to the body of the vertebra. **2.** The narrow neck of tissue connecting some tumours to the normal tissue from which they have developed. **3.** (in plastic surgery) A narrow folded tube of skin that, initially, remains attached to its original site after being grafted. Pedicles are typically employed for defects where there has been considerable tissue loss. Firstly, two sides of the donor area are dissected free and the pedicle is formed into a tube attached at both ends. The donor site is closed by sutures. Secondly, after a period to ensure the establishment of a good blood supply to the pedicle, one end is separated and reattached to one side of the recipient site. Thirdly, again after an interval sufficient to ensure a good blood supply at the reattached end, the second end is separated, and the pedicle is split open and positioned on the prepared recipient site. This technique can reform quite sizeable defects but must be carefully planned from the outset. *See also* skin graft.

pediculicide An agent that kills lice. Various compounds are available, in the form of dips, sprays, and dusting powders, or for injection. Compounds with efficacy against lice include *amitraz, the carbamates, *derris, *ivermectin, the organochlorine compounds and *organophosphorus compounds, *pyrethroids, and organic sulphur compounds.

Pediculoides (Pyemotes) A genus of *mites widely distributed in stored cereal products whose bite causes allergic dermatitis (grain itch) in humans.

pediculosis Infestation with lice of the genus *Pediculus*. *See* louse.

Pediculus A genus of *louse containing a single species, the human louse, *Pediculus humanus*. There are two varieties, the head louse and the slightly larger body louse. The former lives in the hair of the head, while the latter is found more commonly in underwear, laying its eggs either in clothing or on body hairs. Both cause intense itching, and scratching can lead to secondary infections. They also transmit diseases, such as relapsing fever, trench fever, and typhus.

pedigree 1. The record of the ancestry of an animal. The pedigree allows some determination of the genetic constitution of the animal, and assists the selection of individuals for breeding. Official pedigrees are usually subject to the regulations of the relevant breed society and recorded in a central register. **2.** Describing an animal with such a pedigree.

peduncle A narrow process or stalklike structure, serving as a support or a connection. For example, the *middle cerebellar peduncle* connects the pons and cerebellum.

pellagra A nutritional disease of pigs, poultry, cats, and humans due to *nicotinic acid (niacin) deficiency. A similar disease in dogs is called canine pellagra or *black tongue. The clinical signs involve redness of the mouth progressing to ulceration, emaciation, and death. In pigs, there are necrotic lesions of the intestine accompanied by severe diarrhoea. Most animals synthesize their own nicotinic acid using the amino acid tryptophan as a precursor. However, this is impossible when tryptophan is in short supply, as occurs in diets based on maize or flaked maize. Supplements of the vitamin are then required.

pellicle A thin layer of skin, membrane, or any other substance.

pelvis (*pl.* **pelves** or **pelvises**) **1.** The bony structure formed by the paired *os coxae and the *sacrum. **2.** The region of the body lying caudal to the abdomen in the vicinity of the bony pelvis; it contains the pelvic cavity. **3.** Any basin-shaped structure; for example, the renal pelvis is the expanded origin of the ureter within the *kidney.

pemphigus One of various uncommon autoimmune skin diseases, recorded in cats, dogs, horses, and humans, in which the body produces antibodies against the basal membrane of the epidermis and the bridges between cells, resulting in tissue damage and blister formation. The thin epidermis of the skin is quickly sloughed off and ulcers may form. In some variants the mucous membranes are also involved. Pemphigus ranges from mild to severe and life-endangering. Corticosteroid therapy under the direction of a veterinary surgeon can be used but may need to be continued throughout the animal's life. A course of injections of a gold salt can also provide significant therapeutic benefit for many months.

pendulous crop A condition of turkeys and domestic fowls involving abnormal enlargement and protrusion of the *crop. The cause is unknown, although the condition has been variously linked to genetic factors, *Marek's disease, yeast infections, and excess water intake. It may affect scattered individuals or occur as outbreaks in a flock. There is no effective treatment.

-penia *Suffix denoting* lack or deficiency. Example: *neutropenia* (of neutrophils).

penicillamine A *chelating agent that has been used to treat copper and lead poisoning. It is also used to treat cystine urinary calculi and rheumatoid arthritis. L-penicillamine antagonizes pyridoxine (vitamin B_6), hence the less antagonistic D-form should be used clinically. It is absorbed from the gastrointestinal tract and is rapidly excreted in the urine. Supplementation with pyridoxine is recommended with long-term use of penicillamine. D-penicillamine is relatively nontoxic, although blood abnormalities may occasionally occur;

these regress when treatment is halted.

penicillin Any of a group of *antibiotics derived from moulds of the genus *Penicillium,* or their synthetic derivatives. Natural penicillin was identified first by Alexander Fleming in 1928, in cultures of *P. notatum* (*P. chrysogenum*), and by 1940 Florey, Chain, and Abrahams had pioneered its use in the therapy of bacterial diseases. By changing the constituents of the mould's growth medium, different natural penicillins can be produced, with benzylpenicillin (penicillin G) being the most active. Semisynthetic penicillins can be made by varying the side chain of 6-aminopenicillanic acid, obtained from cultures of *P. chrysogenum.* All penicillins contain a thiazolidine ring connected to a beta-lactam ring with a side chain; the beta-lactam ring is necessary for antibacterial activity, and the side chain determines the spectrum of activity and pharmacological properties. Penicillins act by preventing cross-linking of peptidoglycans in the cell wall of bacteria. This alters the permeability of the bacterial cell wall and causes lysis of the organism. This action is greatest in rapidly multiplying cells.

Penicillins can be injected or administered topically or orally (except benzylpenicillin, which is destroyed by acid in the stomach). They are absorbed rapidly and distribute widely throughout the body, although they are actively secreted from the cerebrospinal fluid and have poor penetration into skeletal and cardiac muscle, eyes, joints, pericardial and pleural fluid, and abscesses. They are excreted unchanged in the urine. The half-life of penicillins is typically short (e.g. benzylpenicillin is about 90 minutes), but it can be prolonged by administering *probenecid to prevent renal secretion, or by employing suspensions or less soluble organic salts of the drug. These are slowly absorbed from the injection site. For example, procaine penicillin has activity for 24 hours, benzathine penicillin acts for up to 72 hours, and benethamine penicillin can act for 120 hours. Various mixtures of these salts are available. Many organisms (e.g. *Staphylococcus* spp.) are resistant to the action of natural penicillins because they produce the enzyme beta-lactamase, which opens the beta-lactam ring and destroys the drugs' bactericidal action. However, synthetic penicillins that are unaffected by beta-lactamase are available.

Penicillin G and *penicillin V* are the natural penicillins available. Both have a narrow spectrum of activity against Gram-positive bacteria and are broken down by beta-lactamases. Penicillin G is poorly absorbed after oral administration, penicillin V absorption is better. These antibiotics have good activity at low concentrations against sensitive organisms (e.g. *Streptococcus* spp.) and are still the drug of choice in the treatment of streptococcal and certain other bacterial infections. Combination with streptomycin or other *aminoglycoside antibiotics increases the spectrum of activity to include Gram-negative organisms and produces synergism, with more effective killing of microorganisms.

Methicillin, oxacillin, cloxacillin, dicloxacillin, floxacillin, and *nafcillin* are semisynthetic penicillins that have activity against Gram-positive organisms and are resistant to breakdown by beta-lactamases. Methicillin and nafcillin are poorly absorbed following oral administration, but the others are well absorbed. Nafcillin and cloxacillin are incorporated in intramammary preparations for the treatment of mastitis.

Ampicillin and *amoxycillin* have a broad spectrum of activity against both Gram-positive and Gram-negative organisms but are inactivated by beta-lactamase. Both are absorbed well after oral administration, with amoxycillin producing higher plasma concentrations than ampicillin. Their antibacterial activity is inferior to that of penicillin G. They are used in the treatment of a wide range of bacterial infections in all animals.

Carbenicillin, ticarcillin, mezlocillin, azlocillin, and *piperacillin* have a broad spectrum of activity including good efficacy against *Pseudomonas* spp. and *Proteus* spp. However, they are poorly absorbed following oral administration and are inactivated by beta-lactamases. Carbenicillin is available for use in human medicine.

Combinations of penicillins (e.g. ampicillin and cloxacillin) can increase their activity and protect against inactivation by beta-lactamase. Amoxycillin is used in combination with *clavulanic acid to protect against degradation by beta-lactamases.

The penicillins are generally nontoxic and very high doses are tolerated in most species. However, hypersensitivity reactions occur in humans and occasionally in animals, with urticaria and anaphylactoid reactions. Procaine penicillin at high dose rates can cause restlessness, hyperexcitability, mydriasis, and convulsions due to the procaine. Procaine penicillin may occasionally cause abortion in pigs. In rodents (e.g. hamsters, rats, guinea pigs) penicillins can cause changes in the gastrointestinal flora leading to overgrowth of *Clostridia spp. and severe gastroenteritis.

penicillinase An enzyme that inactivates *penicillin by hydrolysing its four-membered lactam ring. The gene for this enzyme is carried on some resistance transfer *plasmids, and renders certain bacterial strains resistant to penicillin.

Penicillium A genus of over 300 species of *fungi, typically blue-green

*moulds, common in the environment but only rarely affecting animals. A wide range of *mycotoxins and several antibiotics, notably *penicillin and *griseofulvin, are produced by species of *Penicillium.*

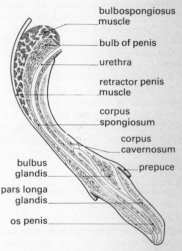

Section through the canine penis

penis The male organ of copulation that carries the *urethra, through which urine and semen are discharged. It is most highly developed in mammals, comprising the root, body, and *glans penis, and is enclosed by the *prepuce (see illustration). Attachment to the ischium is by the paired crus penis; this continues into the *corpus cavernosum, which is formed of erectile tissue. The urethra is enclosed within the *corpus spongiosum, which is also erectile. Mechanisms of *erection differ among domestic species. *See also* phallus.

pent- (penta-) *Prefix denoting* five.

pentazocine A synthetic opioid *analgesic used in dogs and occasionally in horses. It was developed to produce analgesia without the addictive properties associated with *morphine, and as a partial agonist it has both agonistic and antagonistic activity at opioid receptors. It produces analgesia, sedation, and respiratory depression comparable to morphine. However, unlike morphine, there is an increase in blood pressure and heart rate, and vomiting in the dog is much less common. The respiratory depression and other effects can be antagonized by naloxone or nalorphine. Pentazocine is well absorbed after oral administration or following subcutaneous or intramuscular injection. In dogs it is effective for 3–4 hours. It should not be used in cats. Being less addictive than morphine in humans, it is not a controlled drug. Tradename: **Fortral**.

pentobarbitone (*US* **pentobarbital**) *See* barbiturate.

pentose A *monosaccharide with five carbon atoms: for example, ribose and xylose.

People's Dispensary for Sick Animals (PDSA) A British charity whose aim is to provide free medical or surgical treatment to animals belonging to persons who appear to the society to be unable to afford the service of a veterinary surgeon. Address: PDSA House, South Street, Dorking, Surrey.

pepsin One of a group of endopeptidase enzymes (*see* peptidase) that hydrolyses food proteins and peptides in the stomach. They also act to coagulate milk in young animals. They are secreted in the form of *pepsinogens* by the chief cells of the gastric mucosa, and converted to pepsins by gastric hydrochloric acid. They are unusual among enzymes in having pH optima in the range 1.8–3.5.

peptic 1. Relating to pepsin. **2.** Relating to digestion, with particular reference to the stomach.

peptic ulcer *See* gastric ulcer.

peptidase One of a group of enzymes that hydrolyse the *peptide bonds of proteins and peptides. They are divided into *exopeptidases*, which sequentially cleave single *amino acids from one end of the peptide chain (e.g. carboxypeptidase, aminopeptidase), and *endopeptidases*, which cleave peptides internally, often showing specificity for the adjacent amino acid (e.g. *chymotrypsin, *pepsin, *trypsin). Peptidases catalyse the digestion of protein in the alimentary tract, while within cells they convert proteins from one form (usually inactive) to another (active) form by limited *proteolysis.

peptide A molecule consisting of two or more *amino acids joined by *peptide bonds. The bond is hydrolysed by *peptidases, enzymes that are important in the digestion of *proteins. *Dipeptides* contain two amino acids, *tripeptides* three, and so on. *Polypeptides contain more than ten and usually 100–300. Naturally occurring *oligopeptides* (of less than ten amino acids) include the tripeptide glutathione and the pituitary hormones vasopressin and oxytocin, which are octapeptides.

peptide bond The chemical bond formed by the reaction between adjacent carboxyl ($-COOH$) and amino ($-NH_2$) groups with the elimination of water. Such bonds join adjacent amino acids in *peptides and *polypeptides.

peptone A large protein fragment produced by the action of enzymes on proteins in the first stages of protein digestion. Peptones are often used as a constituent of microbiological culture media.

peracute Extremely acute; describing a disease with a dramatic and sudden onset of clinical signs, such as *paraquat poisoning in dogs.

percussion A technique, used as an aid to diagnosis, that involves detecting changes in the vibrations produced when a part of the body wall is struck a short sharp blow. It is employed particularly over the thorax: loss of resonance occurs in cases of consolidative pneumonia, exudative pleurisy, and diaphragmatic rupture when abdominal contents enter the thoracic cavity, whereas increased resonance occurs in pneumothorax. It is also useful in detecting enlargement of heart size.

The strength of the blow required varies with the thickness of the thoracic wall: a tap by a single digit suffices in dogs and cats; a blow by the fist is needed in cattle and horses.

percutaneous Through the skin: often applied to the route of administration of drugs in ointments, etc., which are absorbed through the skin.

perforation An opening or an aperture in a tissue or membrane. It may be caused by a pathological process or trauma (e.g. perforation of the mediastinal pleura in cats associated with *pyothorax, or perforation of the stomach or bowel wall following ulceration, or surgery (e.g. *trephine of a bony cavity to release fluid and relieve pressure, or puncture of an abscess to allow drainage).

performance testing A method of evaluating the genetic worth of an animal and thus its *breeding value by measuring its performance (e.g. milk yield, liveweight gain). The greater the *heritability of the charac-

ter concerned, the greater the accuracy of this method.

Performing Animals (Regulation) Act (1925) (England and Wales) An Act of Parliament regulating the exhibition and training of performing animals. Trainers must have a certificate of registration from the local authority. A magistrates' court may prohibit or restrict the exhibition of performing animals where it has been proved that such training or exhibition has been accompanied by cruelty.

perfusion 1. The passage of fluid through a tissue, for example the passage of blood through the lung to pick up oxygen from the air in the alveoli and to release carbon dioxide. If perfusion is impaired insufficient gas exchange takes place. **2.** The deliberate introduction of fluid into a tissue, usually by injection into the blood vessels supplying the tissue.

peri- *Prefix denoting* near, around, or enclosing. Examples: *pericardial* (around the heart); *peritonsillar* (around a tonsil).

perianal gland tumour A tumour, common in dogs, arising from the perianal glands – modified sebaceous glands located around the anus but which may also occur in the perineum, tail gland area, and groin. Such tumours are common in older entire male dogs; they are thought to be testosterone dependent and are usually benign. In bitches they are rare but usually malignant. Both the benign and malignant forms are similar in appearance: they may be solitary or multiple and are often hyperaemic, ulcerated, and bleed readily. Histological examination is essential as treatments and prognoses of the two forms differ markedly. The treatment of choice for the benign tumours is surgical excision, with cryotherapy if complete removal is not possible. Castration of male dogs is usually recommended to remove the hormonal influence. Testosterone antagonists (e.g. oestrogens or delmadinone acetate) may produce temporary partial remission and represent an alternative to surgery in poor anaesthetic risk patients. These tumours are sensitive to radiotherapy and cure rates of up to 70% have been achieved. Malignant perianal gland tumours respond poorly to testosterone antagonists and early surgical excision with cryosurgery is more effective. However, they commonly recur and metastasize, and the prognosis is poor.

pericard- (pericardio-) *Prefix denoting* the pericardium.

pericarditis Inflammation of the *pericardium, the membranous sac enclosing the heart. Bacterial pericarditis is not uncommon in pigs, sheep, and cattle; it is less common in equines and uncommon in dogs and cats. In **pigs** and **sheep** the most common cause is spread of inflammation from initial *pneumonia/*pleurisy followed by secondary bacterial infection. For example, in pigs pericarditis may follow enzootic pneumonia, *Glasser's disease, or *Pasteurella* spp. pneumonia. The affected pericardium usually adheres to adjacent pleura and lung tissue, initially by fibrinous strands but later, following organization of effusion within the pericardium, by fibrous adhesions, which limit the movements of heart and lung tissue. This produces dyspnoea and cardiac *tamponade, leading in turn to cardiac failure. Agents such as *Corynebacterium pyogenes* may superpopulate the inflamed tissue, producing a more purulent reaction within the pericardial sace.

In **cattle**, in addition to spread of inflammation and infection from a pre-existing pneumonia (e.g. *pasteurellosis), a purulent pericarditis may result from *traumatic reticulitis/pericarditis, in which a sharp foreign body (e.g. piece of wire) penetrates the anterior wall of the reticulum and punctures the diaphragm and pericardium. Reticular contents are introduced into the pericardium, and fibrinous or more often purulent effusion results. Adhesions of reticulum, diaphragm, and pericardium develop, and organization of purulent exudate within the pericardium leads to cardiac tamponade and heart failure. Diagnosis in the early stages is difficult, and many affected animals first present with cardiac failure and advanced lesions. Surgical removal of the foreign body may be attempted but the prognosis is guarded. In **calves**, a generalized septicaemia resulting from coliform infections (*see* colibacillosis) can cause pericarditis.

In the **horse**, pericarditis may be associated with severe *Streptococcus* infection as part of *strangles; *polyarthritis may also be present. In these instances, the reaction is usually serofibrinous and adhesion following organization of the effusion again causes cardiac embarrassment and heart failure.

Bacterial pericarditis is uncommon in **dogs** and **cats.** However, cats may show a suppurative pericarditis associated with *empyema; *Pasteurella* organisms can often be isolated. Tuberculous pericarditis may occur in both dogs and cats as a result of extension from lung lesions. Similarly, soft granulomatous lesions may be seen on the external pericardium as a result of infection by *Nocardia asteroides.

In all species, but particularly the dog and cat, extension from lung carcinomas, pleural tumours (e.g. mesotheliomas), and other thoracic neoplasms (e.g. osteosarcomas of ribs) may result in pericardial involvement, either as part of the neoplastic process or following inflammation associated with tumour necrosis.

Diagnosis is usually made on the identification of abnormal and muffled sounds on *auscultation. Haematological examination yields information on reactions to infective agents and is very useful in cases of bovine traumatic reticulitis. In dogs and cats, radiography may be beneficial. Treatment is of the cause, but is often difficult because of late diagnosis. Broad-spectrum antibiotics may be effective providing the effusion is not too great and adhesions are minimal. Diuretics may be helpful in large animal species.

pericardium (*pl.* **pericardia**) The membrane surrounding the heart, consisting of two portions. The outer *fibrous pericardium* completely encloses the heart and is attached to the large blood vessels emerging from the heart. The internal *serous pericardium* is a closed sac of *serous membrane. Its inner visceral layer (*epicardium) forms the outer layer of the wall of the heart and its outer parietal layer lines the fibrous pericardium. Between the two layers lies the *pericardial cavity* containing a very small amount of fluid; this prevents friction between the two surfaces as the heart beats.

pericardotomy (**pericardiotomy**) Surgical incision into the pericardium. This forms part of any heart surgery but may be used in its own right in cases of excess pericardial fluid, especially if due to severe *pericarditis.

perichondritis Inflammation of the *perichondrium. It occurs as part of the complex disease process known as *chondrodysplasia, in which the growth of cartilage is defective.

perichondrium (*pl.* **perichondria**) The dense layer of fibrous connective tissue that covers the surface of *cartilage.

pericystitis Inflammation of the tissues surrounding the urinary bladder. It most commonly develops due to the spread of inflammation from other abdominal or adjacent pelvic organs or structures.

pericyte The undifferentiated cell type surrounding the smallest blood vessels (terminal arterioles, venules, and capillaries). Its function is uncertain.

perihepatitis Inflammation of the liver capsule and surrounding peritoneal tissue. Acute inflammation is often manifest as a fibrinous coating of the liver capsule, known as 'frosted liver'. More chronic or subacute reactions tend to be manifest as granulation or fibrous tissue, frequently with adhesions to adjacent structures.

perilymph The fluid that fills the bony labyrinth of the internal *ear and surrounds the membranous labyrinth.

perimetritis Inflammation of the *perimetrium around the uterus. *Compare* parametritis. *See also* metritis.

perimetrium (*pl.* **perimetria**) The outer connective tissue layer (tunica serosa) of the *uterus.

perimysium The fibrous sheath that surrounds each bundle of *muscle fibres.

perinephritis Inflammation of the peritoneum and associated fascia surrounding or adjacent to the kidney. It usually arises as a sequel to lesions of the kidney. Inflammation may spread secondarily from the kidney following inflammatory and infective lesions in the renal cortex (e.g. purulent *nephritis).

perineum The region of the body surrounding the anal and urogenital openings.

perineurium The sheath of connective tissue that surrounds individual bundles of nerve fibres within a large *nerve.

periodic acid-Schiff (PAS) reaction A test for the presence of glycoproteins, polysaccharides, certain mucopolysaccharides, glycolipids, and certain fatty acids in tissue sections. The tissue is treated with periodic acid, followed by Schiff's reagent. A positive reaction is the development of a red or magenta coloration.

periodic ophthalmia (moon blindness) An intermittent but recurrent eye inflammation affecting horses and mules worldwide, particularly in North America. Blindness results from repeated attacks of anterior *uveitis (mainly affecting the iris), which occur unpredictably with increasing severity and increasing involvement of the retina, lens, and ultimately the optic nerve. The disease has acute phases (lasting several days to a week), which may lead directly to severe lesions culminating in blindness; however, often there are interspersed quiescent phases followed by recurrences of varying severity. In the quiescent phases, inflammatory changes continue but do not manifest themselves clinically.

In the acute phases, clinical signs include fever, depression, excessive tear production, and marked *blepharospasm; *photophobia is a marked feature. There may be congestion of the sclera and conjunctiva with corneal oedema. Ophthalmoscopic examination shows a thickened inflamed iris, and there may be adhesions to the adjacent cornea (*synechiae); focal depigmentation may be seen on the retina near the optic disc. In the quiescent phase(s) the effects of previous acute inflammation are evident – corneal opacities (due to oedema or fibrosis and vascularization), thickening and pigmentation of the iris or iris atrophy, multiple synechiae, and retinal scarring or detachment. *Cataracts and *glaucoma are rare complications in long-established cases. Eventual blindness is caused by one or a combination of the following: corneal opacity, retinitis (with or without detachment), cataract, or optic neuritis.

The cause is not certain, but is generally thought to involve *hypersensitivity to exogenous antigen. The most frequent implicated agents are *Leptospira* spp. (especially *L. pomona*) and larval forms of the nematode worm *Onchocerca cervicalis*. Periodic ophthalmia can occur months or years after *Leptospira* infection, and these cases are associated with high titres of antibody to *L. pomona*. Similarly, a reaction to dead aberrant microfilariae of *O. cervicalis* in the conjuctiva and uveal tissues has been implicated. It is suggested that both agents result in a chronic autoimmune uveitis.

Topical administration of *atropine to relax the ciliary muscles of the eye, together with topical and systemic *corticosteroids and prostaglandin inhibitors (acetylsalicylic acid, phenylbutazone, or flunixin meglumine) are claimed to be effective in both acute and quiescent stages. During acute phases, placing the affected horse in a darkened stall is beneficial. Where *Onchocerca* infestation is suspected then anthelminthic therapy and prophylaxis (e.g. diethylcarbamazine) may be given, but not during acute phases. Midge or other vectors of the nematode should be controlled. Other name: **equine recurrent uveitis.**

periodontal Denoting or relating to the tissues surrounding the teeth.

periodontal disease A chronic infection of tissues surrounding the neck and root of the tooth, usually preceded by *gingivitis or gingival recession brought about by *dental plaque or *tartar. It is mostly seen in dogs, and also in sheep (*see* broken mouth). The breath becomes foul and mastication is difficult or painful. In longstanding cases there may be suppuration and formation of discharging fistulae, with osteitis and absorption of alveolar bone; the tooth, although sound, loosens and is shed. Treatment is by extraction of loosened teeth, attention to remaining plaque or tartar, and administration of antibiotics to clear the infection.

periodontal membrane (periodontal ligament) The *ligament around a tooth by which it is attached to the bone of the *alveolus.

periople A thin layer of soft light-coloured horn over the proximal (coronary) border of the equine *hoof. It widens at the heels forming the *bulbs.*

periosteum (*pl.* **periostea**) The layer of dense connective tissue that covers the surface of a bone except at the articular surfaces. The outer layer of the periosteum is extremely dense and contains a large number of blood vessels. The inner layer is more cellular in appearance and contains cells that can transform into *osteoblasts. The periosteum provides attachment for muscles, tendons, and ligaments.

periostitis Inflammation of the membranous covering (periosteum) of bones. 'Open' periostitis is associated with wounding (punctures or compound fractures) and is often accompanied by infection (*Corynebacterium pyogenes* in farm species; *Streptococcus* or *Staphylococcus* in dogs and cats). 'Closed' periostitis may result from traumatic blows to bones with resultant *haematoma formation,

which usually remains sterile and resolves with exostosis formation; alternatively, the tearing of a ligament or tendon may cause inflammation with pain and swelling. These latter lesions are best treated by cold applications and pressure bandaging. Periostitis arising from infection in adjacent soft tissue is not uncommon; it may occur, for example, with foot rot in cattle, necrotic stomatitis in calves, and paranasal sinus infections in horses and dogs. *Alveolar periostitis (periodontitis)* occurs in all species, with carnivores especially affected (*see* periodontal disease). Secondary periostitis is frequently seen in cases of *actinomycosis ('lumpy jaw') in cattle, and also in periodontal infection by *Corynebacterium pyogenes* and *Actinobacillus lignieresi.* Neoplasms may cause secondary periostitis as a result of pressure necrosis and local invasion, and periostitis may accompany certain forms of osteopathy and osteodystrophy, particularly in dogs.

peripheral nervous system (PNS) That part of the nervous system located in the peripheral or outer parts of the body and consisting of the *cranial nerves and the *spinal nerves. The peripheral nervous system is responsible for transmitting sensory information to the *central nervous system and motor information from the central nervous system to effector organs. It includes the *autonomic nervous system.

peristalsis A wavelike sequence of involuntary muscular contraction and relaxation that passes along the alimentary tract and other tubular structures, such as the ureters, thus propelling their contents. The longitudinal layer of musculature in the gut wall is particularly involved, and coordination of the process occurs through local nerve plexuses in the wall of the gut under the influence of parasympathetic (excitatory) and sympathetic

peritendineum

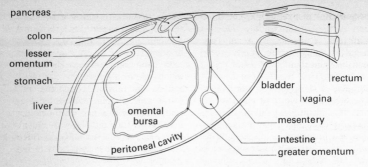

pancreas

colon

lesser omentum

stomach

liver

omental bursa

peritoneal cavity

bladder

vagina

rectum

mesentery

intestine

greater omentum

Stylized diagram showing the general arrangement of the peritoneum

(inhibitory) nerves. During *rumination in ruminants, the bolus is passed up the oesophagus to the mouth by reverse peristalsis (*antiperistalsis*).

peritendineum The fibrous covering of a tendon.

peritoneum The *serous membrane of the abdominal cavity (see illustration). The parietal peritoneum lines the walls of the abdomen and the visceral peritoneum covers the abdominal organs. *See also* mesentery; omentum.

peritonitis Inflammation of the *peritoneum, usually due to an infective agent. Domestic species have widely differing resistance to such agents: the horse is especially susceptible, the dog comparatively resistant, while other species show a relative ability to localize the infection. Peritonitis can be caused by penetration of the body or internal organ by a nonsterile foreign object, by infection passing from the alimentary tract, urogenital tract, or other abdominal organ, or by blood-borne infection. The nature of the inflammation depends on the infective agent. *Acute peritonitis* is characterized by serofibrinous or purulent exudates, with the risk of adhesion of the peritoneal surfaces. *Chronic peritonitis*, which may develop

in tuberculosis and actinobacillosis, involves a granulomatous inflammation.

The clinical effects of peritonitis are produced by various combinations of abdominal distension, toxaemia, and shock. The affected animal has fever, abdominal pain, and inappetence. Dogs and cats frequently vomit, cattle show depressed ruminal activity and loss of milk, while horses, in which peritonitis is commonly fatal, show loss of intestinal movement and colic. In all species the leucocyte counts of both blood and peritoneal fluid are raised, and the fluid exudate may be detectable in small animals by radiography. Death is usually due to circulatory collapse. Treatment may involve surgical removal of a foreign body or the repair of a ruptured organ. The maintenance of circulating fluid volumes (*see* fluid replacement therapy) and antibacterial therapy are essential. The latter may include peritoneal drainage and *lavage with antibiotics. *See also* feline infectious peritonitis.

periureteritis Inflammation of the tissues surrounding or adjacent to a ureter. This is rarely seen as an isolated phenomenon and is likely to accompany a more generalized abdominal condition.

permethrin *See* pyrethroids.

pernicious Describing diseases that are highly dangerous and likely to be fatal unless treated.

peroneal Relating to or supplying the outer (fibular) side of the leg.

peroneal nerve One of three nerves in the hindlimb. The *common peroneal nerve* is a terminal branch of the *sciatic nerve, and divides into the superficial peroneal nerve, which mainly carries sensory fibres from the cranial parts of the leg and pes, and the *deep peroneal nerve*, which carries motor fibres to muscles that flex the hock and extend the digits.

perosis (chondrodystrophy; slipped tendon) A leg deformity, seen in domestic fowls, turkey poults, and ducklings, in which the gastrocnemius tendon slips off the hock joint, causing lameness. It is caused by deformity of the hock joint, but the underlying cause is uncertain. In chicks and poults it is sometimes linked to *manganese deficiency or to deficiencies of B-complex vitamins or zinc. Some cases of *twisted leg result in slipped tendon.

peroxidase One of a class of *enzymes that catalyse the detoxification of peroxides, which are highly reactive and toxic to living organisms. The simplest is *catalase, the enzyme that catalyses the breakdown of hydrogen peroxide to water and oxygen. *See also* glutathione.

peroxisome A small structure within a cell that is similar to a *lysosome but contains different enzymes, some of which may take part in reactions involving hydrogen peroxide.

Perthes' disease (avascular necrosis of the femoral head) A disease causing hindlimb lameness in small breeds of dog due to arthritis in the hip joint following a failure of the blood supply to the head of the femur. Although this may be due to injury, it has been shown conclusively that, in some cases at least, the condition is hereditary. While mild cases may recover with time and rest, an *excision arthroplasty to surgically remove the head of the femur is often necessary. Both parents of affected offspring are likely to be carriers of the disease and neither should be bred from again. Other name: **Legg-Calve-Perthes' disease**.

pervious urachus A congenital failure of the *urachus to close, resulting in leakage of urine from the umbilicus. It is most common in foals. This condition often requires surgical repair. Occasionally umbilical infection may track along the urachus to involve the abdominal cavity and organs, such as the kidneys.

pes (*pl.* **pedes**) **1.** The region of the hindlimb corresponding to the human foot (see illustration). It includes the *tarsus, *metatarsus, and *digits. *Compare* manus. **2.** A part resembling a foot.

pessary A plug or cylinder of cocoa butter or other soft material containing a drug that is fitted into the uterus for the treatment of uterine disorders. *See also* suppository.

peste des petits ruminants *See* kata.

pesticide Any of various compounds used to control pests in the environment or on animals. They include *acaricides, *molluscicides, *rodenticides, *fungicides, and *insecticides. Many can cause toxicity to livestock, pets, and other animals if ill-used.

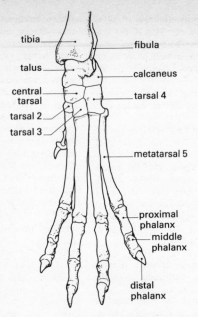

tibia
fibula
talus
calcaneus
central tarsal
tarsal 4
tarsal 2
tarsal 3
metatarsal 5
proximal phalanx
middle phalanx
distal phalanx

Dorsal view of skeleton of pes of dog

pesticide poisoning *See* metaldehyde poisoning; organochlorine poisoning; organophosphorus (OP) compounds.

pestivirus A genus of the *togavirus family. An important veterinary example is the European *swine fever virus.

Pet Animals Act (1951) (England and Wales) An Act of Parliament controlling the keeping of pet shops. The keeper of a pet shop requires a licence from the local authority. When considering the granting of such a licence, the local authority must consider the need for ensuring that the animals will be properly fed, watered, and housed, and that young mammals will not be sold at too early an age. There must be adequate measures to protect the animals from fire and the spread of infection. The

Act forbids the sale of animals in any street or public place, or the sale of pets to children under 12 years old. An amendment to this Act, passed in 1983, prohibits the sale of animals as pets from stalls and barrows in a market.

petechia (*pl.* **petechiae**) A small round flat dark-red spot caused by bleeding into the skin or beneath the mucous membrane.

pethidine (meperidine) A synthetic opioid (*see* opiate) used as an analgesic and spasmolytic in the treatment of spasmodic colic in horses, and as an analgesic in dogs. It is a less potent analgesic than *morphine, although the onset of analgesia is more rapid; respiratory depression and sedation are similar to the effects of morphine. Administration is by intramuscular or subcutaneous injection. The duration of action in horses is about 1–2 hours, and in dogs up to 4 hours. Side-effects are similar to those found with morphine, but toxicity can cause central nervous stimulation, with muscle tremors, excitation, and convulsions. This may be due to normeperidine, a metabolite produced in the liver. Opioid antagonists (e.g. naloxone or nalorphine) can be used to reverse these effects. After injection there may be local irritation with fibrosis of tissue. Meperidine is safer than morphine in cats but should be used at low doses. It is a controlled drug. US name: **demerol**.

Petri dish A flat shallow circular glass or plastic dish with a pillbox-like lid, used to hold solid agar or gelatin media for culturing bacteria.

-pexy *Suffix denoting* surgical fixation.

Peyer's patches *See* lymph nodule.

pH A measure of the concentration of hydrogen ions in a solution, and therefore of its acidity or alkalinity. It is defined as $-\log_{10}c$, where c is the concentration of hydrogen ions in moles per cubic decimetre. A neutral solution has a pH of 7 (at 25°C); a pH below 7 indicates an acid solution, and a pH above 7 indicates an alkaline solution.

phaeochromocytoma (pheochromo-cytoma) A tumour of the medulla of the *adrenal gland. It is rare, with the greatest incidence in older cattle and horses. When hormonally active, phaeochromocytomas secrete *adrenalin and related hormones, causing the clinical signs of severe *hypertension, i.e. tremors, weakness, venous distension, sweating, fast heart-rate, and evidence of cardiac failure.

phag- (phago-) *Prefix denoting* **1.** eating. **2.** phagocytes.

phage *See* bacteriophage.

phagocyte A cell with the ability to perform *phagocytosis.

phagocytosis The process whereby certain body cells, notably *macrophages and *neutrophils, engulf and destroy invading foreign particles. The cell membrane of the phagocytosing cell (*phagocyte*) invaginates to capture and engulf the particle. Proteolytic and other enzymes are introduced into the vicinity of the particle to digest it. A potent feature of phagocytosis is the 'respiratory burst', a sudden acceleration of *glycolysis by the phagocyte with the production of oxygen metabolites, including hydrogen peroxide, that are highly active in destroying bacteria. However, microorganisms show widely varied susceptibility to phagocytosis. Free-living and parasitic amoeboid protozoa (e.g. *Entamoeba*) feed by phagocytosis.

phalanx (*pl.* **phalanges**) One of the bones of the *digits. In mammals, the first digit (when present) contains proximal and distal phalanges. Each remaining digit contains proximal, middle, and distal phalanges. In the manus of birds usually two are present in the alular digit (*see* alula), two in the major digit, and one in the minor digit. In the avian pes there are usually two in the first digit, three in the second, four in the third, and five in the fourth.

phalaris poisoning A toxic condition that can occur in sheep grazing on the grass *Phalaris tuberosa*. The grass contains the alkaloid N-N-dimethyltryptamine and its derivatives. Poisoning may be acute, in which case affected sheep collapse suddenly and then either recover or die from cardiac failure. The more persistent chronic form is characterized by ataxia and weakness. There is no known treatment.

phallus (*pl.* **phalli** or **phalluses**) The male organ of copulation in birds, located at the ventral margin of the vent (*see* cloaca). In the domestic fowl, turkey, and many other species it is relatively small and nonprotrusible. However, in certain species, for example ducks and geese, it is relatively large on erection and protrusible, with a spiral seminal groove to aid transfer of semen on insertion into the vent of the female.

phantom pregnancy *See* false pregnancy.

pharmaco- *Prefix denoting* drugs.

pharmacodynamics The science of the relationship of the dynamic concentrations of a drug with its physiological and biochemical effects.

pharmacokinetics The study of the rate and method of movement of drugs within the body. This includes the processes of absorption from the site of administration, distribution throughout the body, availability and localization in various tissues, drug metabolism, binding, and excretion.

pharmacology The study of the properties of drugs and their effects on living organisms. *Clinical pharmacology* is concerned with the effects of drugs in treating disease.

pharmacopoeia A catalogue containing information on drugs, including their method of preparation, assays of purity and strength, formulae, and dosage rates. There are various works published by medical authorities; the *British Pharmacopoeia*, published under the auspices of the General Medical Council and the Medicines Commission, describes all officially listed drugs. *Extra Pharmacopoeia*,

published by the Pharmaceutical Society of Great Britain, includes drugs not on the official list. The *Pharmacopoeia Internationalis* (International Pharmacopoeia), published under the auspices of the World Health Organization, provides international standards for drug preparation.

pharyng- (pharyngo-) *Prefix denoting* the pharynx. Example: *pharyngopathy* (disease of).

pharyngeal arch (branchial or **visceral arch)** Any of the paired series of ridges of tissue on each side of the primitive pharynx of the embryo that correspond to the gill arches of fish. Each arch contains a rod of cartilage, a cranial nerve, and an artery. Adjacent pharyngeal arches are demarcated by a *pharyngeal cleft externally and by a *pharyngeal pouch internally.

pharyngeal cleft (branchial or **visceral cleft)** Any of the paired series of grooves on the external surface of the primitive pharynx of the embryo that demarcate the *pharyngeal arches externally. They correspond to the gills of fish. In higher vertebrates they subsequently disappear, except for the first pharyngeal cleft, which persists as the external acoustic meatus.

pharyngeal pouch (branchial or **visceral pouch)** Any of the paired series of pouches that extend from the cavity of the primitive pharynx in the embryo and demarcate the *pharyngeal arches internally. They give rise to the auditory tube and tympanic cavity, the parathyroid glands, the thymus, and the C cells of the thyroid gland.

pharyngitis Inflammation of the pharynx. The upper alimentary tract (i.e. oropharynx and buccal cavity) may also be involved, as may the

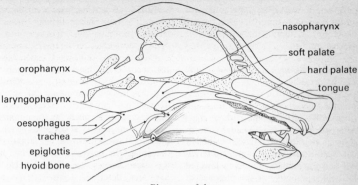

Pharynx of dog

nasopharynx. Pharyngitis is often an extension of oral or upper respiratory tract disease. Examples include *distemper, *tonsillitis, and *kennel cough in dogs; feline viral rhinotracheitis and calicivirus infections (*see* cat flu); *infectious bovine rhinotracheitis or *actinobacillosis in cattle; *anthrax and *Aujeszky's disease in pigs; and *strangles and various equine respiratory virus infections in horses. Foreign bodies – bones, splinters of wood, and needles (in dogs and cats); root crops, especially turnips (in cattle, sheep, and goats); and straw or hay boluses (in horses) – may become impacted and cause localized trauma. Damage from drenching guns is not uncommon in sheep and may include perforation of the pharynx with resultant *cellulitis as well as trauma and inflammation. Pigs possess a pharyngeal diverticulum dorsal to the oesophagus and this may become impacted with food, thereby causing dysphagia and starvation.

Young thoroughbred racehorses (aged under 5 years) can develop a chronic pharyngitis associated with lymphoid hyperplasia of the pharyngeal mucosa. The lesion may be exaggerated and form nodular lymphoid masses, which resemble neoplasia and may cause dyspnoea. The cause is unknown but the condition is thought to be a benign immunoreactive hyperplasia, similar to adenoids in children. Equine guttural pouch infections (*see* guttural pouch diphtheria) may also involve the pharynx.

pharynx (*pl.* **pharynges** or **pharynxes**) A muscular tube, lined by mucous membrane, that extends from the base of the skull to the oesophagus (see illustration). It is divided into the *nasopharynx, *fauces (oropharynx), and *laryngopharynx. The pharynx conveys food from the mouth to the oesophagus and acts as an air passage connecting the nasal cavity and mouth to the larynx.

phenacetin *See* NSAID.

phencyclidine A dissociative *anaesthetic now rarely used. It can be given by intravenous, intramuscular, or subcutaneous injection, and produces catalepsy, analgesia, and dissociation from the environment. However, many reflexes remain and muscle relaxation is poor. The use of this drug in humans was discontinued because of prolonged recovery periods, convulsions, and hallucinations. In pigs anaesthetic deaths have occurred. The drug is useful for primates, although supplies are limited

phenobarbitone

because of the drug's potential for abuse. The similar compound, *ketamine, is more widely used in the veterinary field.

phenobarbitone (*US* **phenobarbital**) *See* barbiturate.

phenol 1. Carbolic acid: a strong and inexpensive disinfectant with a characteristic pine odour. At low concentrations it is bacteriostatic, but higher concentrations (1–2%) are bactericidal and fungicidal. Activity is lowered by cold, alkalinity, or the presence of lipids and soaps. It is thought to act by denaturing protein and is able to penetrate skin, causing inflammation and local precipitation of protein with necrosis.

Phenol is toxic, especially in cats. If absorbed through the skin or taken orally it causes necrosis of the gastrointestinal mucosa with vomiting and diarrhoea. There is also depression of the CNS and cardiovascular system, leading to a fall in blood pressure and heart rate and death.

2. Any of a group of organic compounds, including phenol itself, that contain a hydroxyl group bound directly to a carbon atom in a benzene ring. Phenols are used as disinfectants and as bactericidal agents in sheep dips. High concentrations are required for good efficacy. The substituted phenols, such as *cresol, chlorocresol, and *hexachlorophane, are more potent and less toxic than phenol.

phenolphthalein A dye, almost insoluble in water but soluble in alcohol, used as an acid-base indicator. It is colourless below pH 8.5 and deep red above pH 9. It has ben used in animals as a laxative or purgative.

phenol poisoning A toxic condition caused by ingestion of creosote or other phenol-containing tar products, which are widely used as wood preservatives. Poisoning has occurred in animals that have licked newly treated timber, by ingestion from open containers, and after application of tar to the skin as a ringworm treatment. Pigs have been poisoned by pitch, which is used for roofing and flooring and can be picked up as debris from clay-pigeon (skeet) shooting. Ingestion of phenolic compounds causes anorexia, abdominal pain, muscular weakness, and laboured breathing. In calves a thickening of the skin known as *hyperkeratosis has been described. This is particularly related to the use of wood preservatives containing chlorinated naphthalenes.

phenothiazines A group of compounds used as *tranquillizers, *antiemetics, and *antihistamines. Chlorpromazine is the prototype of the group. The compounds differ in their potency, duration of action, side-effects, and adverse reactions. They act as antagonists at dopamine receptors in the central nervous system (CNS), reducing sensory awareness and motor activity. High doses produce a state of *catalepsy. The effects of phenothiazines are quite variable between individual animals. They depress activity of the hypothalamus causing a fall in body temperature, and also depress the chemoreceptor trigger zone in the medulla preventing centrally induced vomiting. Moreover, they act as *alpha$_1$ blockers, causing a fall in blood pressure. There may be some *parasympatholytic or *spasmolytic action. Some phenothiazines act as antagonists at H$_1$-receptors (*see* antihistamine), preventing histamine-induced inflammatory reactions. There is also smooth muscle relaxation and an anti-arrhythmic action on the heart. When injected they cause local analgesia, and by acting as membrane-stabilizing agents they potentiate the effects of local anaesthetics.

The most commonly used phenothiazine in veterinary therapy is acetylpromazine (Acepromazine); others include chlorpromazine (Largactil), promazine (Sparine), and trifluromazine (Nortran). Usually in the form of the maleate hydrochloride salt, they are available for injection or oral administration. The onset of action is typically 5–10 minutes after intravenous injection, 20 minutes after intramuscular injection, and 30–60 minutes after oral administration. Their effects vary between individuals. Increasing the dose prolongs the duration of action but does not produce greater sedation; excitement during administration reduces the response. The duration of action is several hours. Phenothiazines are metabolized in the liver, although the mechanism and rate differ among species and for different compounds. Excretion in the urine and faeces can occur for long periods (over a week) after administration.

Phenothiazines are used in combination with analgesics to induce *neuroleptanalgesia, and as premedicants prior to anaesthesia in healthy patients to reduce the amount of induction agent required and minimize recovery excitement. Their tranquillizing action can be exploited to facilitate handling of animals and, in dogs, to prevent motion sickness. For heat exhaustion both the hypothermic and tranquillizing effects are useful. In the treatment of shock following the replacement of circulating fluid, the alpha blocking properties of phenothiazines reduce vasoconstriction, thus aiding tissue perfusion and reducing the risk of irreversible shock. Phenothiazines should not be used in animals with a history of epileptiform seizures. They are also contraindicated for anaesthesia for epidural procedures and in hypovolaemic animals. Relaxation of smooth muscle with phenothiazines causes penile protrusion in male animals, which can be complicated by damage to the penis and paraphimosis in entire animals; therefore phenothiazines should be avoided. Rapid intravenous injection of phenothiazines can cause excitement.

phenotype The total of all the measurable attributes of an organism. The phenotype reflects the *genotype but is produced by the interaction between the genotype and the environment. Different environments may produce different phenotypes from the same genotype, and in some cases the same phenotype may develop from different genotypes.

phenylalanine An *essential amino acid, which can act as the precursor of tyrosine. See also amino acid.

phenylbutazone (PBZ) See NSAID.

phenytoin sodium An anticonvulsant drug used to control epileptiform seizures in animals. It acts as a membrane-stabilizing agent, modifying the movement of sodium, potassium, and calcium ions across membranes. Phenytoin causes depression of the motor cortex in the brain, with less effect on the sensory cortex. Sedative effects and ataxia are less compared to the other anticonvulsants, *phenobarbitone and *primidone, which may be used in combination with it. Phenytoin is administered orally, absorbed from the intestines, and metabolized in the liver. The half-life in dogs is 3–6 hours although this is shorter if the drug is given with phenobarbitone and also after administration of several doses of phenytoin itself. Excretion of the drug is faster in young animals, which require higher doses. Toxicity causes ataxia, blurred vision, and nystagmus; with long-term treatment side-effects may include excessive eating, drinking, and urination, hyperglycaemia, glycosuria, gingival hypertrophy, and folic acid deficiency anaemia. Gastrointestinal disorders and nervousness may occur at the start of therapy, and allergic reactions are occasionally reported. Phenytoin is not recommended for use in cats. Tradename: **Epanutin**.

pheromone (ectohormone) A chemical substance emitted by an organism into the environment as a specific signal to another organism, usually of the same species. Pheromones play an important role in the social behaviour of certain animals, notably mammals and insects. They are used to attract mates, to mark trails, and to promote social cohesion and coordination in colonies. Pheromones are usually highly volatile organic acids or alcohols and can be effective at minute concentrations.

phimosis A condition in which there is an abnormally small preputial opening, thus preventing retraction of the *prepuce over the glans penis. The condition may potentially occur in all species as a congenital malformation. In dogs, phimosis can affect small or toy breeds (e.g. Yorkshire terriers, toy poodles). The dog is unable to protrude an erect penis and therefore erection causes pain and excoriation of the penis. Urine often accumulates in the prepuce and predisposes to balanoposthitis (*see* balanitis). Correction can be achieved by surgical enlargement of the preputial orifice. Less commonly, phimosis may occur in bulls where scar tissue resulting from trauma or prolapse of the prepuce may cause adhesions or stenosis. Correction is usually by circumcision. A comparable congenital malformation in the female may result in atresia of the vagina but this is rare in domestic animals.

phleb- (phlebo-) *Prefix denoting* a vein or veins. Example: *phlebectopia* (abnormal position of).

phlebitis Inflammation of veins. It may be caused by extension of a local tissue inflammation or, less commonly, blood-borne infection. It may also result from infection due to injection or penetration of irritant substances in the region of a vein. Inflammation of the venous endothelium leads to thrombosis and hence to *thrombophlebitis.

phlebotomy Surgical puncture or opening of a vein, in order to remove blood or to infuse blood, fluids, or drugs.

phon- (phono-) *Prefix denoting* sound or voice.

phonation The production of vocal sounds. In mammals the organ of phonation is the *larynx; in birds it is the *syrinx.

-phoria *Suffix denoting* an abnormal deviation of the eyes or turning of the visual axis.

phosphagen Creatine phosphate (*see* creatine).

phosphataemia The presence of phosphates in the blood.

phosphatase An *enzyme that catalyses the hydrolysis of *phosphate esters. For example glucose-6-phosphatase catalyses the reaction: glucose-6-phosphate $\rightarrow$ glucose + phosphate. They are classified as acid- or alkaline-phosphatases, depending on their pH optimum. Phosphatases are important in the absorption and metabolism of carbohydrates, nucleotides, and phospholipids. Alkaline phosphatase is essential in the calcification of bone.

phosphate One of several anionic forms of phosphoric acid (which is strictly termed *ortho*-phosphoric acid, and hence *ortho*-phosphate), often referred to as 'inorganic phosphate'. The main physiologically important anions are $H_2PO_4^-$ and HPO_4^{2-}. These act as *buffers in blood and other biological fluids. Most free phosphate in animals occurs as a component of *hydroxyapatite in bones and teeth. Combined phosphate is found in many important *esters *phosphomonoesters* (such as glucose-1-phosphate, glucose-6-phosphate, phosphoenolpyruvate), *phosphodiesters* (e.g. *phospholipids and *nucleic acids), and *anhydrides* or *pyrophosphates* (e.g. *ATP, ADP). Some proteins, the *phosphoproteins*, have phosphate esterified to serine, threonine, or tyrosine amino acids, either in large amounts (e.g. caseinogen) or in small amounts (e.g. glycogen *phosphorylase). The addition of a phosphate group (phosphorylation) is important in controlling the activity of certain enzymes. Deficiency of phosphate in the diet lowers phosphate concentration in blood serum and can cause stunted growth and *rickets in young animals; cows may show reduced milk yield and low fertility (*see* hypophosphataemia).

phosphatidic acid (phosphatide) A *glyceride in which two of the three hydroxyl groups of glycerol are esterified with long-chain *fatty acids while the third is esterified with *phosphate. Phosphatidic acid is the parent compound of the *phospholipids.

phosphatidylcholine (lecithin) One of a group of *phospholipids containing *choline.

phosphatidylinositol A *phospholipid found in cell membranes in which the *phosphatidic acid is esterified to inositol.

phosphatidylserine A *phospholipid containing the *amino acid serine.

phosphocreatine Creatine phosphate (*see* creatine).

phosphodiester A diester (*see* ester) of phosphoric acid found principally in *nucleic acids and *phospholipids. The individual *nucleotides of the nucleic acids are joined by phosphodiester bonds; these define the polarity of the nucleic acid chain, which has a 3'- and a 5'- end.

phosphofructokinase An enzyme that catalyses the conversion of fructose-6-phosphate to fructose-1,6-diphosphate. This is one of the controlling reactions of *glycolysis.

phospholipase An *enzyme that catalyses the hydrolysis of a *phospholipid. *Phospholipase A* releases one of the two *fatty acids from the remaining lysophospholipid residue; *phospholipase C* yields a diglyceride and the phosphorylated head group; and *phospholipase D* cleaves the head group to yield *phosphatidic acid. These changes radically alter the properties of the phospholipid and thus affect its role in cell membrane structure and function. A membrane-bound phospholipase C is involved in the action of certain hormones (e.g. *bradykinin) that bind to receptors on the cell membrane.

phospholipid One of a group of lipids having both a phosphate group and one or more fatty acids. With their hydrophilic polar phosphate group and long hydrophobic hydrocarbon 'tail', phospholipids readily form membrane-like structures in water. They are a major component of cell membranes, and interact noncovalently with membrane proteins. *See also* phospholipase.

phosphorus A nonmetallic element that occurs in organisms in the form of *phosphate and its derivatives.

phosphorylase

phosphorylase An enzyme that catalyses *phosphorolysis*, i.e. the cleavage of a bond by the introduction of a phosphate group. Many enzymes of this type are found in cells, but the term phosphorylase usually applies to glycogen phosphorylase, which cleaves *glycogen to glucose 1-phosphate (*see* glycogenolysis).

phot- (photo-) *Prefix denoting* light.

photodynamic Describing a substance that, following ingestion, accumulates in the skin where it is activated by sunlight and causes tissue damage. The agent's molecules become activated and pass their excess energy to other molecules, including tryptophan and tyrosine, in the cells of the skin and conjunctiva. The consequent rapid oxidation causes inflammation and necrosis of tissues. Examples of photodynamic agents include hypericin, found in the leaves of St John's wort (*Hypericum perforatum*), and fagopyrin, found in buckwheat (*Fagopyrum esculentum*). *See* photosensitization.

photomicrograph An enlarged photograph taken through an optical or electron microscope.

photophobia An abnormal sensitivity to or intolerance of light. Most clinical cases are associated with diseases of the cornea and anterior uvea (iris and ciliary body), although any painful or inflammatory eye condition (e.g. foreign body lodgment, *conjunctivitis, irritant vapours) may affect light sensitivity. Corneal ulceration and *keratitis can cause severe photophobia, as may anterior *uveitis. Photophobia may also be seen as part of a more generalized primary *photosensitization reaction resulting from the absorption of *photodynamic agents. Treatment is of the cause; housing affected animals in darkness is beneficial.

photophthalmia Inflammation of the eye caused by exposure to intense light. Ultraviolet radiation may cause corneal lesions with photophthalmia in range cattle exposed to high levels of solar radiation. Polar bears and hill sheep in snowy areas are reported to be similarly affected (*see* snow blindness), although some authorities have suggested that frost damage may be responsible for the keratitis seen in affected sheep.

photosensitization (light sensitization) A local or generalized reaction to bright sunlight resulting in inflammation and itching, which can be severe. In *primary photosensitization* the ingestion of *photodynamic substances (i.e. substances that accumulate in skin and are activated by sunlight) sensitizes the skin, which then reacts when exposed to bright sunlight. Some wild plants, such as St John's wort and buckwheat, contain photodynamic substances, and certain drugs and chemicals are also photodynamic, for example the anthelmintic phenothiazine sulphoxide, which can cause keratitis in recently dosed calves exposed to excessive sunlight. *Secondary sensitization* or *hepatogenous photosensitization* occurs when the liver is sufficiently damaged to prevent the excretion of phylloerythrin, a product of chlorophyll degradation. This accumulates in tissues, including the skin, where it is photodynamic. Ragwort (*Senecio jacobaea*) causes chronic liver disease in cattle and horses and may also cause photosensitization. Also, sheep and cattle ingesting spores of the fungus *Pithomyces chartarum*, which grows on dead leaf litter at the base of grass pastures in New Zealand, Australia, and parts of South America, become sensitized and develop *facial eczema. *Inherited* or *congenital photosensitization*, seen in cattle, pigs, and humans, is caused by deficiency of the enzyme uroporphyrinogen III cosynthase, which results in failure of haem synthesis and excessive production of uroporphyrin and coproporphyrin. These are photodynamic pigments that stain bones and teeth, consequently the condition is known as 'pink tooth'.

Light penetrating the sensitized skin triggers the liberation of *vasoactive substances, such as histamine. These disrupt blood and lymph vessels causing *oedema, inflammation (dermatitis), and intense itchiness. The results vary from mild *erythema with subsequent scaling to widespread loss of skin, shock, and subsequent death. The sensitized subject suffers dermatitis only when bright sunlight is able to penetrate the skin sufficiently deeply. Signs are therefore usually seen only in short-coated animals, in relatively hairless regions, such as the ear, lips, nose, and udder, or where the skin and hair contain little pigment. This is strikingly demonstrated in Friesian cattle that have become photosensitized: the white areas of the body will be severely affected while the black areas may be spared. Affected animals must be immediately removed from bright sunlight. Treatment will depend upon the extent of the danger. *Antihistamines and *corticosteroid therapy may be prescribed, supplemented with local *astringent application. The nature of the photosensitivity should be investigated to determine if the factor(s) involved can be removed to prevent recurrence.

photosynthesis The process whereby green plants and some bacteria manufacture carbohydrates from carbon dioxide and water, using energy absorbed from sunlight by the green pigment chlorophyll. In green plants this complex process may be summarized thus:

$$6CO_2 + 6H_2O \rightarrow C_6H_{12}O_6 + 6O_2.$$

phren- (phreno-) *Prefix denoting* **1.** the mind or brain. **2.** the diaphragm. **3.** the phrenic nerve.

phrenic nerve The nerve that stimulates the muscle of the diaphragm to contract during inspiration. It is formed by branches from the fifth, sixth, and seventh cervical spinal nerves in the neck, and runs through the thorax to the diaphragm.

phthisis Any disease involving wasting away or *atrophy of all or part of the body. The term is rarely used in veterinary science. *Phthisis bulbi* describes a shrunken, disorganized, and distorted eye that is the end-stage of severe *ophthalmia. In dogs it may be an end-stage of *glaucoma.

phycomycosis Any of a diverse and extensive group of diseases caused by infection with *fungi, traditionally placed in the class Phycomycetes, that grow in the tissues as a *mycelium composed of wide *hyphae (up to about 15 μm), often haphazardly branched, twisted, swollen, or collapsing, with very few cross-walls. The class is not recognized in modern taxonomy. It contained, among others, the fungi responsible for *pythiosis and *zygomycosis. The term is still used to designate any *mycosis in which the infected tissue contains mycelium characteristic of a 'phycomycete' but which cannot be identified more precisely.

phylogenesis The evolutionary history of a species or individual.

phylogeny The evolutionary history of a type of organism or of related organisms.

physi- (physio-) *Prefix denoting* **1.** physiology. **2.** physical.

physiological saline A liquid medium in which animal tissues may be kept alive for a few hours without pathological changes or distortion of the cells taking place, for example, for experiments. Such fluids are salt solutions that are isotonic with and have the same pH as the body fluids of the animal concerned. An example is *Ringer's solution.

physiological solution A solution used to maintain cells and tissues in a functional state. Such solutions are normally *isotonic with tissue fluids and contain mainly inorganic salts, such as NaCl, KCl, NaHCO$_3$, etc. An example is *Ringer's solution. Physiological saline is 0.9% (0.15 M) NaCl and is the simplest physiological solution.

physiology The science of the function of living organisms and of their component parts.

physo- *Prefix denoting* air or gas.

physostigmine (eserine) A reversible *anticholinesterase used topically in the eye to cause pupillary constriction and reduce intraocular pressure in glaucoma. It is an alkaloid obtained from the Calabar bean of *Physostigma venenosum*, and was once used in West Africa as a poison in witchcraft. It has been tried in the treatment of feline and canine dysautonomia (Key-Gaskell syndrome), and is used intravenously as an antidote in poisoning by *atropine or related drugs. In contrast to most other anticholinesterases, it is able to cross the blood–brain barrier.

phyt- (phyto-) *Prefix denoting* plants; of plant origin.

phytin The calcium or magnesium salt of phytic acid (inositol hexaphosphate), which occurs in plants, especially cereals. Phytic acid is important in nutrition because it binds dietary calcium and magnesium, making it less available to the animal.

pia mater The innermost of the three *meninges. It envelops the outer surface of the brain and spinal cord, following the various indentations and irregularities, and is highly vascular, giving rise to blood vessels that supply the central nervous system. It is linked to the *arachnoid by numerous fine strands; these cross the intervening subarachnoid space, which contains cerebrospinal fluid.

pica (depraved appetite) The ingestion of materials not normally considered to be food. Most cases are the result of dietary deficiencies, which force the animal to satisfy its craving by eating unusual items. In particular, mineral and trace-element deficiencies, especially of *sodium, *phosphorus, and *cobalt, can result in animals eating soil, bones, or bark from trees or drinking urine. Also, *gastritis or abdominal pain frequently provokes animals to consume their own hair or wool. Dogs and cats may eat grass and even poisonous plants. The consequences are often detrimental, for example, obstruction of the gut due to hair balls. Boredom and lack of exercise can cause behavioural vices and pica (*see* cannibalism; feather pecking; tail-biting). In all cases, treatment and prevention depends on the diagnosis and removal of the cause.

picked-up nail The injury occurring in horses when a nail or similar sharp metal object penetrates the horn of the hoof and produces lameness. The effect may be immediate if the nail damages an important structure, such as the bone in the hoof; but more often is delayed and results from the build-up of pus between the horn of the sole and the underlying sensitive tissue. Treatment consists of removing all the under-run horn and subsequently protecting the foot until the horn regrows. Administration of tetanus antitoxin is necessary if tetanus toxoid has not been given previously.

pico- *Prefix denoting* one million-millionth (10^{-12}).

picornavirus An important family of RNA *viruses that have naked icosahedral *capsids and positive-strand RNA. It includes the genera *aphthovirus, *enterovirus, and *rhinovirus. Most members show a high specificity towards their particular host species.

picrotoxin A powerful CNS stimulant obtained from the seeds of *Anamirta cocculus* ('fishberries'), formerly used as a fish poison. Picrotoxin contains picrotoxinin, which causes clonic convulsions with accompanying salivation, hypertension, and vomiting. It antagonizes the inhibitory neurotransmitter *gamma-aminobutyric acid. Picrotoxin has been used as an analeptic by intravenous injection. Overdosage or toxicity can be treated by sedation using barbiturates or diazepam, similar to the treatment of *strychnine poisoning.

pig An omnivorous mammal belonging to the Old World family *Suidae* (order *Artiodactyla*). The European wild boar, *Sus scrofa*, is assumed to be one ancestor of the modern domestic pig, which is reared worldwide for its meat and hide. Several subspecies have been identified, including *Sus scrofa scrofa*, *Sus scrofa pallustris* (the turbary pig of southeast Europe), and the smaller *Sus scrofa vittatus* from the Far East. Pigs from different subspecies readily interbreed and classification presents problems. In addition, a wide variety of breeds and strains have emerged due to artificial selection for specific characteristics. The current commercial trend is towards hybridization with selection

for well-defined biological traits, such as growth rate. *See also* pig husbandry.

pigeonberry *See* pokeweed poisoning.

pigeon pox *See* fowl pox.

pig health scheme A scheme intended to reduce disease in pig units. Such schemes comprise both disease diagnosis and advice on control and eradication as part of the overall management of the unit, and extend into such areas as herd replacement policy and breeding strategy. In Britain they are run by the Meat and Livestock Commission and many commercial breeding companies.

pig husbandry All aspects of the management of a pig herd, whether it be the production of *weaners, *porkers, *cutters, *baconers, or *heavy hogs, or the running of a breeding herd. One or more categories of pig may be reared on the same unit. *Intensive pig production* involves obtaining the fastest possible growth rates consistent with economic and health considerations. Nutritional inputs may represent up to 75% of the costs of producing the meat animal, and successfully meeting the specific requirements of the pig for energy, protein, amino acids, minerals, vitamins, and essential fatty acids with the available feed resources is fundamental to optimum performance (*see* nutrition). *Housing, especially temperature control and ventilation, is also of vital importance. Young pigs in particular are susceptible to cold. *Extensive pig production* systems, where the breeding herd is maintained outdoors, are becoming popular. To be successful, such enterprises need a freely-drained soil, a relatively dry climate, and a hardy sow bred for outdoor conditions and good mothering ability. The young pigs from such enterprises tend to be fattened under more intensive conditions.

Herd health always needs careful monitoring, particularly under intensive conditions where animals are confined in large numbers. Improvements to herd performance may be achieved by breeding policy. Thus *food conversion ratio and carcass quality, which are comparatively heritable traits, may be improved by using quality hybrid pigs bred specifically for those characteristics. Less heritable traits, e.g. reproductive performance, may be improved by crossbreeding (*see* breeding). Crucial factors in assessing the economic performance of a pig herd are, for the meat enterprise, daily liveweight gain and food intake (from which food conversion ratio may be calculated), and time taken to reach a specific slaughter weight. For the breeding herd, litters per sow per year and numbers of pigs reared per litter (i.e. pigs reared per sow per year) are of vital importance.

piglet A young pig, usually from birth until weaning age; occasionally referred to as pigling.

piglet anaemia A common blood disorder of young piglets resulting from iron deficiency. Sow's milk contains insufficient iron and the initial deposits of iron in a piglet's liver are only enough to last 2–3 weeks after birth. Newborn piglets have haemoglobin levels of 90–110 g per litre of blood, but this commonly falls to 40–50 g per litre at 2–3 weeks. Piglets grow very rapidly, quadrupling their weight in 3 weeks, thus extra iron is vital to supply the rapid increase in blood volume. Once the piglets are anaemic they fail to thrive and may become too weak to consume creep feed. Treatment and prevention depend on iron supplementation. Various iron dextran solutions are customarily given by intramuscular injection, but these have undesirable side effects, including abscesses at the injection site and residual green stains in the ham. An alternative is to feed iron supplements to the mother sow. These pass through into her faeces and are consumed by the suckling piglets, presumably via faecal contamination of the teats.

piglet hypoglycaemia (baby pig disease) A condition affecting piglets up to 1 week of age caused by low blood glucose levels resulting from inadequate intake of milk. This may be due to failure to suckle, lack of milk (*see* agalactia), or other piglet disease. Affected piglets are dull with a subnormal temperature; later they convulse, become unconscious, and die. Treatment consists of fluid therapy with glucose solutions, nursing, and, where necessary, fostering.

pig pox An infectious disease of pigs characterized by pustules on the belly and groin and caused by a suipoxvirus (*see* poxvirus). The disease is distributed worldwide but is rarely diagnosed in the UK. Transmission is associated with the presence of pig *lice, which introduce the virus when feeding on their host. In consequence, the lesions are usually seen in those sites favoured by the lice. Small swellings develop, which become vesicles, then pustules, and eventually scabs. Lesions are seen particularly in young pigs, and secondary complications may result in severe skin infections and even mortality. Control is by improving the husbandry and eliminating the lice infestation.

pili (fimbriae) (*sing.* **pilus, fimbria**) Hairlike processes present on the surface of certain bacteria. They are thought to be involved in the adhesion of bacteria to other cells and in transfer of DNA during *conjugation.

pilo- *Prefix denoting* hair.

pilocarpine A natural alkaloid, obtained from the leaves of certain shrubs (*Pilocarpus* spp.), that acts as a *parasympathomimetic agent. It is used in the treatment of glaucoma and alternately with *mydriatics to break down adhesions between the iris and lens. A 0.5–4% aqueous solution is applied to the eye causing pupillary constriction and a transient rise then a fall in intraocular pressure. This effect lasts for 12–24 hours. Pilocarpine is tolerated well in the eye.

pilomatricoma (pilomatrixoma) A benign tumour arising from the germinal cells at the base of a hair follicle. They are seen as uncommon skin tumours in dogs and are rare in other species. Clinically this tumour presents as a well-circumscribed mass, usually on the trunk. Following surgical excision, the prognosis is good. Other name: **hair matrix tumour**. *Compare* trichoepithelioma.

pilus A hair. *See also* pili.

pimel- (pimelo-) *Prefix denoting* fat; fatty.

pineal gland (pineal body; epiphysis cerebri) A small endocrine gland situated in the roof of the third ventricle in the brain. It secretes various hormones, including melatonin, and is thought to be involved in the seasonal regulation of reproductive activity by responding to changes in light.

pinealoma A tumour arising from the *pineal gland. These rare tumours have been reported in dogs, horses, and cattle; the clinical signs are those associated with a space-occupying mass in the brain (*see* brain tumours).

pining (pine) A colloquial and ill-defined term meaning ill-thrift in either sheep or calves. The term usually applies to *cobalt deficiency in sheep, but it also describes the clinical signs of *copper deficiency in calves.

pink-eye *See* New Forest disease.

pinna *See* auricle.

pinocytosis The intake of small droplets of fluid by a cell by cytoplasmic engulfment. It occurs in many white blood cells and in certain kidney and liver cells. *Compare* phagocytosis.

pinworm (threadworm) Any of various threadlike parasitic *nematodes of the family Oxyuridae that infest the intestines of vertebrates, especially *Enterobius vermicularis*, which is found in the large intestine in humans. *See also* Oxyuris.

piperazine An *anthelmintic with activity against ascarids and nodular worms. It is less effective against hookworms, whipworms, and strongyles. Piperazine is used extensively in the veterinary field, especially in dogs, because it is inexpensive. Various piperazine salts are available (e.g. hydrochloride, citrate, adipate, phosphate, and sulphate), all equally effective. Only parasites dwelling in the gastrointestinal tract are affected. Piperazine is given orally as tablets or as a powder; the adipate salt is given in a syrup. All expelled worms should be removed because eggs within the parasites remain viable. Toxicity is low but with overdosage there can be vomiting and signs of neurotoxicity, including incoordination and muscle tremors.

piriform lobe A part of each cerebral hemisphere situated at the base of the brain. It receives impulses concerned with the sense of smell.

piriform neurones

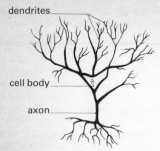

A piriform neurone (Purkinje cell)

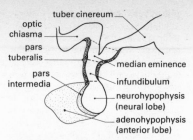

Principal anatomical features of the pituitary gland

piriform neurones (Purkinje cells)
Nerve cells found in great numbers in the cortex of the cerebellum in the brain. The cell body is flask-shaped, with numerous dendrites branching from the neck and extending fanwise among other cells towards the surface, and has a long axon that runs from the base deep into the cerebellum (see illustration).

piroplasm The form in which protozoan parasites of the genera *Theileria* and *Babesia* occur in their hosts' red blood cells. It is used colloquially as a collective noun for these two groups of organisms, and the term 'piroplasmosis' is sometimes used as a synonym for *babesiosis.

piroplasmosis *See* babesiosis.

pit (in anatomy) A hollow or depression, such as any of the depressions on the surface of an embryo marking the site of future organs.

pitch poisoning *See* phenol poisoning.

pituitary gland (hypophysis) The master endocrine gland: a small body attached by a thin stalk (infundibulum) to the *hypothalamus at the base of the brain. The anterior *adenohypophysis secretes *thyroid-stimulating hormone, *adrenocorticotrophic hormone, *follicle-stimulating hormone, *luteinizing hormone, *somatotrophin, *prolactin, *lipotrophins, and *melanocyte-stimulating hormone. The secretion of all these hormones is regulated by specific hormone-releasing factors produced by the hypothalamus and conveyed to the pituitary gland by the hypothalamo-hypophyseal portal system. The posterior *neurohypophysis is where the hormones *oxytocin and *vasopressin are stored and released. These are synthesized in the hypothalamus and transported, in conjunction with the carrier protein neurophysin, to the neurohypophysis. See illustration.

pityriasis The shedding from the skin of branlike scales. *Pityriasis rosea* is an acute uncommon skin eruption of young pigs (usually less than 8 weeks old), of unknown cause. Although the condition superficially resembles dermatophytosis, there is no evidence to suggest a causal relationship. It may affect a whole litter, but the dam is unaffected. Initially there may be transient anorexia followed by the appearance of papules noticeable on the comparatively hairless abdomen. These enlarge and coalesce to form mosaics of raised tortuous purple lines, about 1 cm across, covered by scales and scabs. Pityriasis rosea is a self-limiting disease and no treatment will affect its course, which is usually

3 weeks. If there is secondary bacterial infection antibiotics may be prescribed. Affected animals should be isolated. Although it superficially resembles the disease of the same name in man, it is apparently not related to it and cannot be transmitted to man.

A number of other skin diseases are characterized by pityriasis, resulting from an increased rate of exfoliation of surface squamae (keratinocytes). It is particularly marked in seborrhoeic dermatitis and ectoparasitic disease. *See also* Cheyletiella.

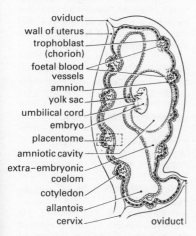

oviduct
wall of uterus
trophoblast (chorion)
foetal blood vessels
amnion
yolk sac
umbilical cord
embryo
placentome
amniotic cavity
extra-embryonic coelom
cotyledon
allantois
cervix
oviduct

Diagram of a gravid uterus of the sheep showing the arrangement of placental membranes and placentomes

placenta (*pl.* **placentas** or **placentae**) The organ, occurring in all mammals except monotremes and marsupials, that attaches the foetus to the wall of the uterus (see illustration). Essentially it is formed by the close association of the epithelium (endometrium) of the uterus and the foetal membranes (chorion and allantois). The placenta varies considerably in its form. The association between material and foetal membranes is simple and diffuse in the horse and pig. In ruminants there are more complex areas of attachment, the *placentomes*, where foetal cotyledons and maternal caruncles interdigitate. Zones of attachment occur in carnivores. The close proximity of maternal and foetal circulations allows the exchange of nutrients, waste products, and respiratory gases. Additionally, the placenta secretes hormones, which help maintain pregnancy and bring about *parturition. The placenta is normally expelled shortly after parturition, but it may occasionally be retained, especially in cattle (*see* retention of placenta).

placentome One of the units attaching the foetus in the *placenta of ruminants. It includes uterine tissue (*caruncle) and foetal tissue (*cotyledon).

placode Any of the thickened areas of ectoderm in the embryo that develop into the cranial nerve ganglia or special sense organs, such as the eye, ear, or olfactory mucosa.

plague 1. Any disastrous widespread infection or infestation. **2.** One of a number of specific diseases, including cattle plague (also known as *rinderpest), fowl plague (*see* avian influenza), and *bubonic plague.

plane An imaginary line of section dividing the body when in the anatomical (standing) position. The three principal descriptive planes are frontal, sagittal, and transverse (see illustration).

plantar Relating to the back of the *pes (hindfoot).

plantar necrosis A necrotic condition affecting the ball of the foot of poultry. It is closely associated with *bumblefoot.

649

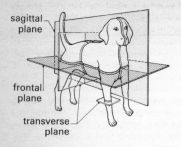

sagittal plane

frontal plane

transverse plane

The three principal descriptive planes

plantigrade Walking on the entire sole of the foot: a habit of humans and certain animals, e.g. rabbits and bears. *Compare* digitigrade.

plaque (virology) A hole in a mono-layer of cultured animal cells (*see* cell culture) caused by the growth of a single infectious *virion. *See also* plaque assay; plaque-forming unit.

plaque assay The usual method for measuring the *infectivity of a *virus preparation. A suitable dilution of virus is applied to a monolayer host *cell culture in the presence of an agent (e.g. a specific antiserum) which prevents horizontal spread of virus in the monolayer. After a suitable period of time for the virus under study (typically 1–7 days), the cells are fixed and stained and the number of holes or *plaques counted. From this number and the dilution of virus used, the *titre of the virus may be calculated. *See also* plaque-forming unit.

plaque-forming unit (pfu) The amount of *virus preparation suffi-cient to cause a single *plaque under the conditions of the *plaque assay for that particular virus.

-plasia *Suffix denoting* formation; development. Example: *hyperplasia* (excessive tissue formation).

plasm- (plasmo-) *Prefix denoting* **1.** blood plasma. **2.** protoplasm or cyto-plasm.

plasma The fluid component of *blood in which the blood cells and platelets are suspended. Plasma is obtained as a clear yellow-to-white liquid when blood is collected into an *anticoagulant and the cells are removed by centrifugation. It consists of a solution of various inorganic salts of sodium, potassium, calcium, etc., with a high concentration of pro-tein and a variety of trace substances. *Compare* serum.

plasma cell A mature B-*lymphocyte that is committed to the production of *antibodies. *See also* haemopoiesis.

plasmacytoma *See* myeloma.

plasmalogen A *phospholipid deriva-tive in which one of the fatty acids is replaced by an unsaturated alcohol.

plasma substitute (plasma volume expander) Any of various solutions that have osmotic characteristics and viscosity similar to blood plasma which can be infused intravenously to replace plasma, for example in cases of haemorrhagic shock. Apart from freeze-dried plasma, there are syn-thetic plasma substitutes, based on solutions of polysaccharides (e.g. *dextrans) or polypeptides (e.g. *Haemaccel).

plasmid An independently replicating circular piece of *DNA, usually found in cells outside the nucleus but in some cases capable of integrating into *chromosomes. Some plasmids, especially bacterial plasmids, can move between cells of the same or other species, transferring genetic material. This may, for example, include genes for *drug resistance. Plasmids are also used in *genetic engineering to transfer genes from one species to another. *See also* R-factor.

plasmin (fibrinolysin) An enzyme that digests the protein fibrin, thus serving to dissolve blood clots (*see* fibrinolysis). Plasmin is formed from its inactive plasma precursor, *plasminogen, by the action of various activators. Its principal substrate is fibrin, but in excess it will digest fibrinogen and other clotting proteins, a condition known as *hyperplasminaemia*, which is associated with paradoxical bleeding. The precise mechanism of activation remains uncertain.

plasminogen A plasma protein that is the inert precursor of *plasmin (*see* fibrinolysis). It is closely associated with *fibrinogen and is thus uniquely placed in fibrin gels to initiate their dissolution when activated to form plasmin. Vascular endothelium contains very high levels of plasminogen activator, which presumably plays a protective role in maintaining the patency of vessels following the deposition of fibrin upon their walls as part of the normal repair processes.

Plasmodium A genus of protozoa in the group *Apicomplexa that live inside red blood cells in mammals and birds and are transmitted between animals by mosquitoes. Four species, the most important of which is *P. falciparum*, cause human *malaria. The parasite multiplies in liver cells before infecting red blood cells, in which it undergoes a series of synchronous multiplications. The waves of parasite populations are associated with bouts of fever. *See also* avian malaria.

plaster of Paris The hemihydrate of calcium sulphate, $2CaSO_4.H_2O$, pre-

pared by heating the mineral gypsum and ground to a fine powder. The addition of water produces a porous mass that sets hard in a few minutes. It is commonly incorporated into bandages to form *casts for fractured limbs.

plastic surgery The branch of surgery dealing with the correction or reconstruction of deformities or defects, either for therapeutic or cosmetic reasons. Plastic surgery is employed most commonly to correct skin defects, as in the reformation of areas of tissue loss. It is also used for the correction of nasal fractures, the elevation of depressed fractures of the paranasal sinuses, and for other structural defects.

-plasty *Suffix denoting* plastic surgery.

platelet (thrombocyte) A small blood cell that is important in blood clotting (*coagulation), *thrombosis, and *inflammation. The role of platelets in coagulation involves not only stopping bleeding after trauma, but also maintaining the general integrity of blood vessels in the face of wear imposed by blood pressure. Platelets are formed by the fragmentation of megakaryocyte cytoplasm in the bone marrow (*see* haemopoiesis). They lack a nucleus, but possess granules containing a variety of enzymes, ADP, and 5-hydroxytryptamine (5-HT). Their cytoplasm also contains a contractile protein, *thrombasthenin*, and their cell membrane a phospholipid known as *platelet factor 3*.

When platelets contact a damaged area in a blood vessel they first adhere to it and then initiate the so-called 'platelet release reaction', giving out ADP, 5-HT, and other cell contents. The formation of *thrombin, a blood coagulation factor, also causes this release. ADP encourages the aggregation of platelets, during which further ADP is formed as part of a self-promoting response; the resultant aggregation is then irreversible. However, low concentrations of ADP can induce reversible adhesion without causing the platelet release reaction. The adhered platelets serve to plug the damaged blood vessel. At this stage the components of the blood coagulation system are activated by platelet factor 3, with the production of thrombin (and thus the further stimulation of platelet aggregation) and ultimately the formation of *fibrin, the principal noncellular component of blood clots. *Prostaglandins and thromboxane are also manufactured by activated platelets. In addition to mediating inflammation, these substances promote platelet release reactions and aggregation.

plating 1. Bone plating: a technique for the fixation of fractures and correction of bone malformations in which a metal or carbon-fibre plate is screwed onto the bone surface to act as a clamp. It is important to employ plates and screws of the same composition to avoid the damaging effects of electrolysis on bone. Many different designs of plates and screws have been developed for various anatomical sites and fracture types. The standard technique requires the use of at least two points of fixation on each side of the fracture and for each screw to penetrate both cortices of the bone. Plates with specially shaped screw-holes cause the fractured ends of the bone to be impacted as the screws are tightened. Detailed engineering of plates and screws has made the A/O system popular in small animal surgery. It aims to provide very rigid fixation and firm apposition of the bone ends so that healing occurs directly without marked callus formation. Its main disadvantage is the high cost of the special instruments employed and of

the plates and screws. Very occasionally, failure will occur at the fracture site after a time. It is imperative that strict asepsis is employed in all bone plating operations. **2.** (in microbiology) The technique of culturing bacteria on plates of nutrient substrate, such as nutrient-enriched agar gel.

platy- *Prefix denoting* broad or flat.

Platyhelminthes An invertebrate phylum comprising the flatworms. They have simple flattened bodies, no coelom, and a rudimentary nervous system. Most are hermaphrodite and their eggs give rise to one or more larval stages. There are three classes: the Turbellaria, which are mostly free-living, and the Trematoda (*flukes) and Cestoda (*tapeworms), which are all parasitic. Parasitic flatworms often have complex life cycles involving several hosts, and many are important pathogens in veterinary and human medicine.

Platynosomum A genus of *flukes that are parasites of carnivores and which cause lizard poisoning in cats. There are three intermediate hosts in the life cycle: a snail, a crustacean, and a frog or lizard.

-plegia *Suffix denoting* paralysis.

pleio- (pleo-) *Prefix denoting* **1.** multiple. **2.** excessive.

pleiotropy A situation in which a single gene is responsible for more than one effect in the *phenotype. The mutation of such a gene will therefore have multiple effects.

pleomorphism The condition in which an individual assumes a number of different forms during its life cycle. The malarial parasite (*Plasmodium*) displays pleomorphism.

pleur- (pleuro-) *Prefix denoting* **1.** the pleura. **2.** the side of the body.

pleura (*pl.* **pleurae** or **pleuras**) A *serous membrane in the thorax. The *parietal pleura* lines the inner surface of the thoracic walls, the diaphragm, and the surfaces of the mediastinum. The *pulmonary pleura* covers the lungs. Parietal and pulmonary pleurae are separated by the *pleural cavity.

pleural cavity The space between the parietal and pulmonary *pleurae, which normally contains a small amount of fluid to lubricate the adjacent layers and allow breathing movements. An abnormally large pleural cavity indicates the entry of fluid from outside.

pleurisy (pleuritis) Inflammation of the *pleura. It occurs in all species, usually due to *pneumonia in the underlying lung. The inflammation may be localized or diffuse, acute or chronic, and is usually accompanied by an exudative response. The exudate commonly forms adhesions between the lung tissue and parietal pleura, thereby limiting respiratory movements of the lung over the pleura. Excessive exudation results in *hydrothorax or *pyothorax.
Pleurisy is common in pigs, sheep, and cattle, often as an extension of a viral or mycoplasmal pneumonia combined with a secondary haematogenous bacterial infection (e.g. *Corynebacterium, *Pasteurella). In pigs, *Haemophilus* spp. may cause a *polyserositis with pleurisy as part of *Glasser's disease. Pleurisy also occurs in horses, especially after the stress of haulage over long distances, being fairly common in North America. Equines and dogs may develop pleurisy and pyothorax as an extension of bacterial pneumonia (e.g. *Streptococcus, *Pseudomonas, Pasteurella* spp., and *Escherichia coli*). A severe pleurisy without pneumonia

may be seen in rurally located working dogs following infection by *Nocardia or *Actinomyces spp. Pleurisy as a result of *Mycobacterium infection is uncommon in the UK nowadays but may occur in cattle, dogs and cats. The virus responsible for *feline infectious peritonitis causes pleurisy in cats; this species may also develop a chylous pleurisy due to a damaged or ruptured thoracic duct.
Clinical signs are *tachypnoea, *dyspnoea, and often *tachycardia with secondary heart failure, depending on the severity of pleural effusion. Lung sounds are often muffled on auscultation, and fluid lines or diffuse opacity may be seen on radiography. Treatment is of the underlying cause.

pleurocentesis (pleuracentesis; thoracentesis; thoracocentesis) The *aspiration of material from the *pleural cavity by means of a hollow needle inserted through the chest wall. The material aspirated may be fluid exudate, pus (in cases of pyothorax), air (in cases of *pneumothorax), or blood (in cases of *haemothorax). Pleurocentesis is both a diagnostic and a therapeutic technique.

pleuropneumonia Any inflammatory disease of the lungs and pleura together producing a combination of *pneumonia and *pleurisy. It usually follows a severe pneumonia, which may involve the adjacent pleura (pulmonary or/and parietal) directly by extension or as a secondary inflammatory reaction. This situation is often seen in *Pasteurella spp. pneumonia in sheep, cattle, and pigs. Less commonly, initial pleurisy (pleuritis) may predispose to secondary lung inflammation; this may occur in pigs with *Haemophilus* spp. infections. In most farm animals the initial pneumonia is the result of a viral or mycoplasmal infection, which becomes colonized by bacteria (e.g.

Corynebacterium pyogenes in sheep and cattle; *Pasteurella* spp. in sheep, cattle, and pigs; streptococci and *Corynebacterium equi* in horses). In dogs *Bordetella bronchiseptica*, streptococci, staphylococci, and coliform bacteria are common, while in the cat, although less common, bacteria such as *Pasteurella* spp. and coliforms can be isolated.

In the pig, *Pasteurella* spp. can complicate *enzootic pneumonia (caused by *Mycoplasma hyopneumoniae*), leading to pleuritis and often abscessation. *Pasteurella multocida* is most commonly implicated. Sometimes a more acute and severe pneumonia is seen, associated with stress from overcrowding, rough handling, or poor housing, possibly with an intercurrent subclinical virus infection. There is a fibrinous or necrotizing pneumonia with a severe serofibrinous pleurisy. Massive endotoxin production usually has a fatal outcome, although if pigs survive they are chronically ill with adhesive pleurisy, pericarditis, and sometimes polyarthritis. *See also* contagious bovine pleuropneumonia; contagious caprine pleuropneumonia; contagious porcine pleuropneumonia.

pleuropneumonia-like organism (PPLO) *See* Mycoplasma.

plexus A network of nerves or blood vessels. *See* brachial plexus.

plication A surgical technique in which the size of a hollow organ is reduced by taking tucks or folds in the walls.

plochteach A form of hepatogenous *photosensitization that affects young lambs on hill grazings in the north and west of Scotland. Animals are affected at about the time they start eating significant amounts of grass. Extensive feeding trials with bog asphodel (*Narthecium ossifragum*) have failed to implicate the plant in

causing plochteach, although it is reputed to be the cause of *alveld, a similar disease of sheep in Norway.

plumbism *See* lead poisoning.

PML (Product on the Merchants' List) (UK) A drug that can be sold by an agricultural merchant, without prescription or pharmacist's supervision, to a farmer or other person who has in his or her charge or maintains animals for business purposes. The drugs must be sold in unopened containers supplied by the manufacturer or assembler of the drugs, and the container and package must be labelled with the symbol 'PML'. Veterinarians may dispense PML drugs for administration to animals or herds under their care.

PMSG (pregnant mare's serum gonadotrophin) A polypeptide hormone secreted in mares during pregnancy at the junction of the placenta and endometrial cups. It stimulates the formation of a secondary wave of follicles in the ovary, which luteinize and form additional corpora lutea. The progesterone secreted by these corpora lutea maintains pregnancy between days 40 and 140 of gestation. After this time PMSG decreases and the corpora lutea atrophy, the placenta producing the progesterone necessary to maintain pregnancy.

Preparations of PMSG are used to manipulate breeding cycles in other species. The hormone is available as a freeze-dried powder, which is reconstituted in water and injected intramuscularly or subcutaneously. PMSG is used to induce follicular development: in all animals (except the bitch and mare) maximum follicular development occurs 2–5 days after PMSG administration. It is used in sows after early weaning to reduce time to conception. In sheep it is used to stimulate follicular development early in the breeding season and after treatment with *progestogens. It is ineffective in mares. Administration of PMSG can be used to increase the number of ovulating follicles (superovulation) for ovum transplantation. The response is variable and repeated doses may cause a reduced effect on the ovaries and occasionally an anaphylactic reaction. Tradename: **Foligon**.

pneum- (pneumo-) *Prefix denoting* **1.** the presence of air or gas. Example: *pneumocolon* (within the colon). **2.** the lung(s). Example: *pneumogastric* (relating to the lungs and stomach). **3.** respiration.

pneumat- (pneumato-) *Prefix denoting* **1.** the presence of air or gas. **2.** respiration.

pneumatization The presence of air-filled cavities in bone, such as the paranasal sinuses of the skull. In birds much of the skeleton may be pneumatized.

pneumaturia The presence of air or gas in the urine. This is uncommon in domestic animals. It may result from congenital malformations of the urethra, vagina, and rectum in females, gas-producing bacteria in cases of *cystitis, and in *diabetes mellitus, when the high sugar content of urine may predispose to further fermentation and gas production if there is coexistent bacterial cystitis.

pneumocephalus The presence of air or gas in the intracranial cavity. This condition does not occur spontaneously in domestic animals. The most likely cause is the entry of air via penetrating wounds to the cranium or ethmoid region in shooting, blunt trauma, or road traffic accidents. Alternatively, air may aspirate into the cranium from the nasal passages following pressure necrosis or rarefaction of ethmoid bones by aggressive

tumours, such as carcinomas or fibrosarcomas in dogs. Air may be introduced into the cranial cavity during cranial ventriculography, a contrast-radiographic technique; this is not widely used but may be useful for confirming the presence of *hydrocephalus in dogs.

pneumococcus A group of encapsulated Gram-positive *bacteria occurring as ovoid cocci arranged in pairs or short chains. They are now regarded as a single species in the genus *Streptococcus, i.e. *S. pneumoniae*. They cause serious pneumonias in humans and some animals (monkeys and rats) and uterine infections in guinea pigs.

pneumocyte One of the types of cell lining the alveoli of the lungs. *Type I pneumocytes* (*squamous alveolar epithelial cells*) are very thin and flat and allow respiratory exchange to occur. *Type II pneumocytes* (*great alveolar epithelial cells*) are cuboidal and contain spherical lamellar bodies, which are the source of *surfactant.

pneumomediastinum The presence of air or gas in the *mediastinum of the thorax. It may arise following deep penetrating neck wounds, especially if the trachea or oesophagus is punctured or ruptured (e.g. in foreign body obstructions or misguided venepuncture attempts); it may also arise following bronchial rupture associated with blunt trauma (e.g. impacts) where air fills the pulmonary hilus and then the mediastinum.

pneumon- (pneumono-) *Prefix denoting* the lung(s).

pneumonia Inflammation of the lungs, particularly where the air sacs (*alveoli) fill with pus so that air is excluded and the lung solidifies (*see* consolidation). There may be involvement of the bronchial tree (bronchopneumonia) or pleura (pleuropneumonia). Pneumonia can also be described in terms of the pathological changes that occur – catarrhal, suppurative, haemorrhagic, fibrinous, or necrotizing – and can range from inapparent to severe and from acute to chronic. Typical signs are rapid deep breathing, coughing, and elevated body temperature. Food intake may be reduced and growth rates depressed.

Pneumonia has various causes. Virus infections give rise to *calf pneumonia and the typical bronchopneumonia occurring in *distemper. Mycoplasmas are responsible for *contagious bovine pleuropneumonia, *contagious caprine pleuropneumonia, and *enzootic pneumonia of pigs. Infection with bacteria is a further cause, particularly those of the genus *Pasteurella* (*see* pasteurellosis); these may cause pneumonia in cattle (*see* transit fever) and sheep (*see* enzootic pneumonia of sheep). *Haemophilus pleuropneumonia* is responsible for *contagious porcine pneumonia. Fungal infection, such as *aspergillosis, or allergic reactions, for example farmer's lung (*see* allergic alveolitis), are further possibilities, and pneumonia is a characteristic sign of infestation with *lungworms. Other causes include accidental aspiration of fluids, for example milk, into the lungs, or the improper administration of therapeutic agents, for instance via a stomach tube mistakenly passed down the trachea instead of the oesophagus. The aspiration of toxic dips, sprays, or powders may also give rise to pneumonia. Secondary and mixed infections often complicate the picture, and infectious organisms may reach the lungs not only via the bronchial tree but also via the bloodstream.

Poor ventilation is often a major contributory factor, causing increased ammonia levels as well as an increase in the concentration of pathogens in the environment. The ammonia damages the cilia lining the airways in the lungs, thus decreasing the efficiency with which the airways are cleared of inhaled particles. Often, groups of animals housed together are affected. Control consists of improving ventilation. Vaccines are available to protect against particular infections in certain species. Antibiotics and drugs designed to improve respiratory function can be given to treat clinical cases. *See also* pneumonitis.

pneumonitis Inflammation of the functional tissues (parenchyma) of the lungs. The term has had several different interpretations, and is often regarded as being synonymous with *pneumonia. Most modern pathologists regard pneumonitis as describing inflammatory cellular proliferation and infiltration of alveolar septa rather than exudation into the alveolar lumen. Some, however, have regarded pneumonitis as a more chronic proliferative lesion compared with pneumonia – an acute exudative inflammation. Others, including human pathologists, have referred to pneumonitis as an acute localized inflammation of the lungs with an attendant toxaemia.

Clinicians tend to use the term to describe an interstitial pneumonia. This may have various causes. *Chemical aspiration pneumonitis* has been described in dogs following aspiration of gastric juice. Such inhalation may occur during anaesthetic induction where there is a full stomach or severe vomiting episodes. The low pH produces tissue necrosis and localized inflammation, resulting in a respiratory shock syndrome. Treatment includes positive-pressure ventilation where damage is severe and widespread, tracheo-bronchial lavage with physiological saline, and oxygen administration. *Corticosteroids and intravenous fluids are helpful for shock.

Allergic pneumonitis has been described in dogs as part of a heartworm (*Dirofilaria immitis*) infestation. Microfilariae (larvae) lodge in interalveolar septa and provoke an allergic reaction, which is compounded by death of the microfilariae. Affected dogs have a cough and may exhibit *haemoptysis. There is usually an eosinophilia (*see* leucocytosis) on haematological examination. Radiography reveals mixed alveolar-interstitial lung opacities. Administration of corticosteroids results in regression of these lesions and reveals the more characteristic vascular lesions of heartworm disease. Standard therapy for heartworm disease is beneficial. The pneumonitis is thought to be a mixture of immediate and delayed-type *hypersensitivity to the microfilariae.

Pneumonitis due to a hypersensitivity reaction also occurs in *allergic alveolitis in cattle (bovine farmer's lung). This is due to the inhalation of spores. *See also* feline pneumonitis.

pneumopericardium The presence of air or gas in the *pericardium. This is rare in domestic animals, but may occur as a complication following spontaneous *pneumomediastinum or *pneumothorax. Gas production may occur as a sequel to an initial hydropericardium or pericarditis in sheep or cattle involving infection with gas-producing *Clostridium* bacteria. More likely, however, is the iatrogenic instillation of air following attempts at drainage of pericardial fluid or blood.

pneumoperitoneum The presence of air or gas in the peritoneal cavity, i.e. the abdomen. The most likely cause in dogs, cats, small ruminants, and horses is the iatrogenic distension of the abdomen with sterile air prior to a fibre-optic laparoscopy (*see* laparoscope) for diagnostic purposes. This technique is gaining in popular-ity in North America and is commonplace in human fields. Spontaneous pneumoperitoneum is rare. Putrefying bacterial fermentation in the abdominal cavity after death may result in distension of the abdomen, particularly where the cadaver has been exposed to high ambient temperatures or not refrigerated. Enterotoxaemias in cattle and to a lesser extent sheep, caused by *Clostridium perfringens* types B and C, may progress to severe peritonitis with gas production, thereby producing pneumoperitoneum.

pneumothorax The presence of air or gas in the pleural cavities. This results in the loss or reduction of negative pressure so that the lungs partially or completely collapse and cannot be inflated by normal respiratory inspiration. Pneumothorax may be spontaneous or due to injury (traumatic); it may also be induced for surgical or therapeutic reasons under carefully controlled conditions. Traumatic pneumothorax is most common. Causes include penetrating stake wounds or rib fractures following road traffic accidents. Pneumothorax also occurs where sudden severe abdominal compression has resulted in diaphragmatic rupture; the abdominal viscera may be forced into the thoracic cavity. Spontaneous pneumothorax may be a sequel to a severe destructive lung condition causing rupture of pulmonary parenchyma at the pleural surface, such as the rupture of emphysematous bullae in cats, horses, and cattle. Other similar ruptures may be associated with parasitic cysts (e.g. aberrant fluke cysts in bovine lungs) or spontaneous bullae or lung cysts of unknown (possibly congenital) origin in dogs and cats. Pneumothorax may develop secondarily to *pneumomediastinum (mediastinal emphysema).

Affected animals may show obvious signs of trauma such as wounding and rib fractures, but *tachypnoea may be the only clinical sign where trauma is less obvious. There is increased resonance on chest percussion and radiographic examination confirms unilateral or bilateral pneumothorax. Treatment involves rest and sedation with repair of obvious physical damage. Mild pneumothorax with partial lung collapse often resolves spontaneously; more severe forms may require the withdrawal of air using a syringe and three-way tap valve or an underwater air trap. Severe lung damage, such as lung lobe rupture, may need thoracotomy to effect repair.

pneumovirus A genus of the *paramyxovirus family. An important veterinary example is bovine respiratory syncytial virus, which causes *pneumonia in cattle.

-pnoea (US **-pnea**) *Suffix denoting* a condition of breathing. Example: *dyspnoea* (breathlessness).

pod- *Prefix denoting* the foot.

-poiesis *Suffix denoting* formation; production. Example: *haemopoiesis* (of blood cells).

poikilo- *Prefix denoting* variation; irregularity.

poikilocyte An irregularly shaped red blood cell (erythrocyte). Poikilocytes may be spherical, oval, thin, spiked, or tailed, and arise during excessive red cell breakdown (*see* haemolytic anaemia) or accelerated blood-cell formation by the bone marrow. A commonly encountered poikilocyte is the so-called '*target cell*' characterized by central and peripheral zones of cytoplasmic opacity with an intervening ring of pale cytoplasm. Target cells occur in many canine blood disorders, including *canine autoimmune

haemolytic anaemia and *lead poisoning.

poikilocytosis The presence of *poikilocytes in the blood.

poikilothermic Cold-blooded: describing an animal whose internal body temperature varies passively with that of the external environment. All animals except birds and mammals are poikilothermic. Although unable to maintain a constant body temperature, they can respond to compensate for very low or very high temperatures. For example, the tissue composition (especially cell osmotic pressure) can change to regulate the blood flow to peripheral tissues and thus increase heat loss or heat absorption. Also, the animal may actively seek sun or shade. In very hot climates, cold-blooded animals may undergo *aestivation to escape the heat. *Compare* homoiothermic.

points of the horse The external features of a horse used for descriptive purposes, especially in certification.

poison A substance that when ingested, inhaled, or applied to the skin causes disease and, possibly, death. *See* poisoning.

poison elder *See* Toxicodendron.

poisoning Any disease caused by the ingestion or inhalation of toxic substances, for example plant or fungal poisons, chemical agents in the environment, or wrongly administered therapeutic agents. The amount of a particular substance causing illness or death varies with the species of animal: detoxification and excretion of the substance are determined by the presence or absence of appropriate enzymes in the tissues of the affected animal. Poisoning often occurs when an animal's normal food is in short supply or unavailable, forcing the animal to seek alternative food. However, a poison may be inadvertently incorporated in prepared feedstuffs or excessive amounts of a pesticide or parasiticide applied to an animal. In an outbreak of poisoning, the agent responsible must be identified so that, besides treatment of the clinical signs, a specific antidote may be administered where appropriate.

poison ivy *See* Toxicodendron.

poison laurel *See* Kalmia poisoning.

poison oak *See* Toxicodendron.

poison sumac *See* Toxicodendron.

poison vine *See* Toxicodendron.

pokeweed poisoning A toxic condition due to ingestion of the perennial herbaceous plant *Phytolacca americana* (pokeweed), which is distributed throughout the eastern USA and is also known as pigeonberry, pokeroot, or scoke. The toxic principles – saponins and insoluble oxalates – cause ulceration and haemorrhage in the oral and gastrointestinal mucosa. The clinical signs are violent vomiting, purging, spasms and convulsions, and death due to respiratory paralysis. Treatment consists of protectors and symptomatic therapy.

polar body One of the small cells produced during the formation of an ovum from an *oocyte that does not develop into a functional egg cell. A primary oocyte divides to form a secondary oocyte and *first polar body*. A secondary oocyte divides to form an ovum and the *second polar body*.

pole (in anatomy) The extremity of the axis of the body, an organ, or a cell.

poli- (polio-) *Prefix denoting* the grey matter of the nervous system.

polioencephalomalacia *See* cerebrocortical necrosis.

poliomyelitis 1. Any inflammation of the spinal cord involving principally the grey matter. Although rarely encountered in domestic animals, it is a pathological feature of *Teschen/ Talfan disease of pigs, the spinal lesions being most prominent in the dorsal horns of the grey matter. **2.** (human medicine) Infantile paralysis (Heine-Medin's disease): an enterovirus infection characterized by degenerative changes in the anterior horns of the grey matter.

poll The uppermost part of the head.

'poll evil' Inflammation of the bursa between the *nuchal ligament and the atlas/axis vertebrae of the horse. It characteristically produces a chronic fistulating skin lesion in the poll region (i.e. top of the head), which discharges pus. The cause is probably a skin puncture wound allowing infection with *Brucella or *Actinomyces organisms. In the Americas and tropical countries, infestation by the filarial worm *Onchocerca cervicalis has been implicated in the primary lesion. Treatment consists of *antibiotic administration, possibly coupled with surgical drainage of the lesion. *See also* fistulous withers.

poly- *Prefix denoting* **1.** many; multiple. **2.** excessive. **3.** generalized; affecting many parts.

polyamine An organic molecule having two or more amino groups and which is thus positively charged. Several members of the group are found associated with *nucleic acids. Polyamines have an unpleasant smell and some, for example putrescine and ptomaine, are found in rotting flesh.

polyarteritis

Important causal agents of polyarthritis in farm animals and horses

Causal organism	Pig	Ocurrence in:		
		Cow	Sheep	Horse
Streptococcus spp.	S. suis; S. parasuis +++	S. pyogenes; S. pneumoniae ++	++	S. equisimilis ++
Staphylococcus spp.	S. aureus +	S. aureus +	S. aureus +	–
Erysipelothrix rhusiopathiae	+++	–	+++ (lambs)	–
Haemophilus spp.	H. suis; H. parasuis +++	–	H. agni ++	–
Escherichia coli	+	+++ (calves)	+	+ (foals)
Corynebacterium pyogenes*	++	+++	+	–
Salmonella spp.	++	++	–	+
Actinobacillus spp.	A. suis +	–	–	A. equuli +
Mycoplasma spp.	M. hyorhinus; M. hyosynoviae +++	M. mycoides; M. bovis +	+ (experimental)	–

+++ common
++   does occur
+   uncommon
* Usually a secondary effect, often where there is abscess formation elsewhere in the body with C. pyogenes infection.

polyarteritis See arteritis.

polyarthritis (pl. **polyarthritides**) *Arthritis of several or all joints of an individual. It may be of noninfectious or infectious origin; traumatic and degenerative lesions, sometimes associated with relative immaturity or nutritional factors, are seen in horses, especially racing thoroughbreds. Most polyarthritides result from bloodborne spread of microorganisms. The large limb joints are preferentially affected and involvement tends to be bilateral. Polyarthritis is not uncommonly associated with neonatal bacterial infections in farm animals and equine species, and is known as *joint ill. Also, it may be only part of a disease syndrome involving other body systems (e.g. *Glasser's disease in pigs).

Infectious polyarthritis This is seen mainly in farm animal species and less commonly in horses, usually as a result of bacterial infections. The important causative agents in these species are shown in the table. *Erysipelothrix rhusiopathiae is a common cause of polyarthritis in pigs of all ages (especially animals aged 2–12 months), in lambs, and in some avian species. In pigs, joint involvement often follows the acute form of *swine erysipelas. Chronic infection results in *endocarditis and/or arthritis. However, vaccination against the acute disease appears to enhance susceptibility to polyarthritis. In lambs polyarthritis as a result of *E. rhusiopathiae* infection is seen following infected docking or castration wounds, and less commonly following navel infections. *Osteomyelitis is common and affected joints become ankylosed (*see* ankylosis) as a result of chronic reactions.

Streptococcus suis causes a polyarthritis and meningitis in young pigs (*see* streptococcal meningitis). Lambs are less commonly affected by streptococcal polyarthritis and the clinical course is usually short and fatal as a result of acute *septicaemia. In septicaemic *colibacillosis in calves (caused by *Escherichia coli*) localization of bacteria in joints and/or meninges is common. Usually the major limb joints are acutely affected, although chronic polyarthritis may develop. This chronic situation may be coincident with development of interstitial *nephritis. *Haemophilus agni* can cause an acute haemorrhagic septicaemia in lambs, which usually results in death in less than 24 hours; lambs surviving 24 hours or more develop polyarthritis and meningitis. In pigs *H. suis* or *H. parasuis* are responsible for the polyserositis-polyarthritis syndrome known as Glasser's disease.

An important cause of polyarthritis in pigs, goats, and sheep, and cattle to a lesser extent, is infection by *Mycoplasma* organisms (*see* mycoplasmal arthritis). In pigs especially, mycoplasmal polyarthritis may complicate enzootic *pneumonia or *atrophic rhinitis. *M. hyorhinis* causes a polyserositis-polyarthritis disease in piglets aged 3–10 weeks, and *M. hyosynoviae* causes polyarthritis in older pigs. Both organisms reside in nasal passages and are thought to be transmitted from sows to piglets during the suckling period or as a result of aerosol transmission. Management stresses are thought to be important in outbreaks. Both acute and more chronic forms can develop, the latter with involvement of joint surfaces, cartilage erosions, *pannus formation, and joint contractures developing over a period of months. Many animals become chronically lame and fail to gain weight. A septicaemia-polyarthritis syndrome has been recorded in goats in North America, Sweden, and Australia following infection by *M. mycoides mycoides* and *M. capricolum*. Following an acute septicaemia with fever (and a drop in milk yield in adult milking goats) an acute polyarthritis develops over 2–3 days. The outcome is usually fatal. A similar acute disease but with serositis and meningitis also has been induced in sheep experimentally. *M. mycoides* may cause polyarthritis in calves when used as a vaccine against *contagious bovine pleuropneumonia, and *M. bovis* is thought to be associated with sporadic outbreaks of polyarthritis in North America and Australia. Most animals recover in one or two months but chronic cases end up being culled.

Chlamydia psittaci causes polyarthritis, encephalitis, and conjunctivitis (*see* ovine keratoconjunctivitis) in sheep, calves, and, less commonly, in foals, following enteritis. The infection is common in intensive sheep units in the USA but may also occur in unweaned lambs on pasture. There is a high morbidity but low mortality in sheep. Affected lambs are depressed, reluctant to move, anorexic, and have joint stiffness. Only a few affected lambs become permanently lame. Rarely, pneumonia and encephalomyelitis may be seen. In calves the disease is severe, with high mortality. Affected calves show fever, anorexia, weakness, and joint swelling developing over 2–3 days. Death occurs after 2–14 days.

*Calicivirus infection in kittens is said to be a possible cause of acute polyarthritis, and in goats a retrovirus is responsible for *leukoencephalomyelitis-arthritis, with neurological and respiratory complications, although arthritis is usually the main clinical feature. Rarely, polyarthritis may be complicated by or caused by the presence of fungal organisms, for example *Coccidioides immitis* and *Blastomyces dermatitidis* in dogs.

Treatment of bacterial and related infections with broad-spectrum antibiotics (oxytetracycline, tylosin, lincomycin) may be effective if given early in the disease, but polyarthritis, especially in neonates, is an indication of a widespread serious septicaemia, often of a peracute and fatal nature. Fungal pathogens require the additional use of an antimycotic or fungistatic.

Noninfectious polyarthritis This occurs mainly in dogs and cats, and is divided into erosive (deforming) and nonerosive types. Most are thought to be immunologically mediated. A form of erosive polyarthritis resembling *rheumatoid arthritis occurs in miniature and toy breeds of dog, particularly Shetland sheepdogs. Affected dogs have recurrent episodes of anorexia, depression, and fever, with generalized or shifting lameness caused by inflammation of joints, especially the carpal, tarsal, elbow, and stifle joints. The joint lesions are seen to involve thickening of the joint capsule with enlargement of synovial villi and erosion of cartilage commencing at the joint margins. The erosion of articular cartilage and subchondral bone may be severe with deformity and luxations (dislocations) of the affected joints. Fibrous ankylosis of joints may occur. The condition is progressive and treatment often not effective; *corticosteroids (parenteral and intra-articular) may give only temporary remission. Other therapeutic agents, including antihistamines, gold preparations, and cytotoxic drugs, have been used but with no great success.

Polyarthritis of greyhounds is an erosive polyarthritis of young greyhounds aged 3–30 months. It has been recorded in North America and Australia. The condition is manifest as a mild or severe lameness with swelling of limb joints, distal to and including the elbow and stifle (rarely the shoulder, hip, and atlanto-occipital joint). Lesions are seen initially as swelling of joints with excess joint fluid, haemorrhage, and fibrous tags, followed by articular erosions and pannus formation, although erosions are less severe than in rheumatoid arthritis. The aetiology is unknown but is not obviously immune-mediated.

*Feline progressive arthritis may occur in an acute erosive form or a more chronic proliferative disease, usually in male cats aged 18 months to 5 years.

Nonerosive polyarthritis of noninfectious origin may occur as a true primary disease or secondary to another systemic disease. It is usually immunologically mediated. Secondary polyarthritis of this type is usually part of the *systemic lupus erythematosus syndrome in the dog, or associated with chronic enteropathies (e.g. ulcerative colitis) or infections (e.g. endocarditis, salmonellosis). Treatment of these nonerosive polyarthritides with *corticosteroids or other immunosuppressives is said to be effective. Broad-spectrum antibiotics and fungicides should also be contemplated where appropriate.

polycythaemia An abnormally high concentration of cells in the blood. The term usually refers in practice to red blood cells. *Relative polycythaemia* is often seen as a concentration of cells caused by a decrease in circulating fluid volume as, for instance, in dehydration. It is also common when animals are excited (particularly horses) as a result of splenic contraction and mobilization of extra red cells.

Absolute polycythaemia describes a disease of blood-forming tissue in which red cells are produced in excess. *Polycythaemia vera*, reported very infrequently in dogs and cats, is a form of *primary absolute polycythaemia* in which multiplication of primitive red cells in the bone marrow is uncontrolled and irreversible. This leads to permanent and progressive overpopulation of the blood with red cells. *Secondary absolute polycythaemia*, a much commoner condition, may result from some insufficiency of respiration or circulation in which the tissues are chronically short of oxygen. In this case the polycythaemia is an attempt at compensation and is reversed by removal of the primary cause. Secondary absolute polycythaemia is also occasionally found in conjunction with tumours secreting *erythropoietin, a hormone-like agent that arises in the kidney and stimulates red cell production. Polycythaemia vera has been treated by repeated bleeding or by drugs that directly suppress bone marrow activity. Treatment of other forms of polycythaemia depends on correcting the primary disorder.

polydipsia Excessive drinking. The increased uptake of water causes a decrease in plasma volume and excess loss of water in urine, faeces, and sweat. Usual causes include lesions of the hypothalamus and excess intake of sodium.

polygene One of a number of genes that together control a single characteristic in an individual. Each polygene has only a slight effect and the expression of a set of polygenes is the result of their combined interaction. Characteristics controlled by polygenes are usually of a quantitative nature, e.g. height or milk yield.

polymer A molecule formed by the linking together (*polymerization*) of simpler units (*monomers*). Those comprising only one type of monomer are termed *homopolymers*; those comprising more than one type are *heteropolymers*. Three types of polymer are biologically very important – *polysaccharides, *polynucleotides, and *polypeptides. In these the number of monomers can vary from about a hundred to several million. *See also* macromolecule.

polymerase An enzyme that catalyses the combination of small molecules to form *macromolecules. *DNA polymerase* is responsible for the synthesis of *DNA from its component nucleotides; while *RNA polymerase* is responsible for the synthesis of *RNA.

polymorph **(polymorphonuclear leucocyte)** *See* neutrophil.

polymorphism (in genetics) A condition in which a chromosome or a genetic character occurs in more than one form, resulting in the coexistence of more than one morphological type in the same population at frequencies such that the rarest cannot be maintained only by mutation.

polymyxin One of a group of five antibiotics, obtained from strains of the bacterium *Bacillus polymyxa*. Polymyxin B and polymyxin E, also known as colistin, are available commercially and are used frequently in topical preparations to kill Gram-negative bacteria. They are highly ionized and combine with the bacterial cell membrane, causing disruption of the cells. Resistance is uncommon. They are poorly absorbed from the gastrointestinal tract, and parenteral use is limited because of toxicity, although it may be warranted in severe infections with *Pseudomonas* spp. Signs of toxicity are found only after systemic use, with nephrotoxicity (tubular swelling), neurotoxicity, and histamine release from mast cells. These signs are reversible if administration of the drug is stopped.

polyneuritis Inflammation of many nerves simultaneously. Polyneuritis may be seen as a transient phenomenon or as a component of a generalized inflammation of the central nervous system culminating in *encephalitis. Many infectious agents, particularly viruses, reach the central nervous system by invasion of peripheral nerves following initial skin or connective tissue penetration. For example, the *rabies virus and herpes simplex virus gain access by ascension via nerves and cause an incidental neuritis while in transit. Similarly, the Aujeszky's disease (pseudorabies) virus in pigs, sheep, cattle, dogs, and rabbits ascends to the brain via sensory nerve fibres and incidentally causes neuritis. Other viruses may not have nerve affinity but cause neuritis because of the close proximity of nerve fibres to degenerating mesenchymal tissue (e.g. adenovirus type I in *canine infectious hepatitis). Bacterial infections are less commonly associated with neuritis, although *Listeria monocytogenes* is known to gain access to the brain via the trigeminal cranial nerve from dental and buccal roots, causing localized neuritis.

The classic example of polyneuritis accompanied by acute febrile episodes is the Guillain-Barré syndrome in humans. The veterinary equivalent to this condition is thought to occur in the dog as *coonhound paralysis and in the horse as *cauda equina neuritis.

A chronic progressive polyneuritis has been recorded in dogs and cats. It is similar to the acute disease but is insidious in onset and progression. Spinal reflexes may become progressively lost with atrophy of muscles. There may be unilateral or bilateral involvement. Mild to moderate lymphocytic and plasma-cell infiltrations are seen in sensory nerve branches; nerve roots are rarely involved.

polynucleotide A macromolecule consisting of *nucleotides linked by *phosphodiester bonds. Two types are found in nature, *DNA and *RNA. They are commonly in the form of a chain, with a 3'- and a 5'- terminus, although in certain cases they are circularized and show no terminus.

polyoestrous Describing an animal that has several consecutive *oestrous cycles per year. Some are seasonally polyoestrous and cycle within a specific part of the year, for example sheep and goats; others, such as the cow and pig, can cycle at any time of year.

polyp A non-neoplastic papillary growth arising in epithelial tissue. Polyps usually arise following inflammation and only cause clinical problems if there is haemorrhaging following injury or if they become secondarily infected and ulcerating. They are most commonly found in the nasopharynx (especially in cats), vagina (bitch and mare), and bladder (dogs and cattle – *see* polypoid cystitis). Unlike in humans, rectal polyps are rare in domestic animals. Treatment is by surgical excision. *Compare* papilloma.

polypectomy Surgical removal of a *polyp.

polypeptide A *peptide comprising ten or more *amino acids. Polypeptides that constitute *proteins usually contain 100–300 amino acids. The properties of a polypeptide are determined by the type and sequence of its amino acids.

polyphagia Excessive overeating.

polyphyletic Describing a number of individuals, species, etc., that have envolved from more than one ancestral group. *Compare* monophyletic.

polyploid Describing cells, tissues, or individuals in which there are three or more complete sets of chromosomes. *Compare* diploid; haploid.

polypoid Having the appearance of a *polyp.

polypoid cystitis A chronic inflammatory condition of the urinary bladder (*see* cystitis) seen in cattle, especially ones grazing bracken-infested pastures, and in dogs. Multiple haemorrhagic polyps are present on the epithelial lining of the bladder and result in *haematuria. Such polyps must be distinguished from transitional cell carcinomas (*see* bladder tumours), which carry a poor prognosis. *See also* bracken poisoning.

polyribosome *See* polysome.

polysaccharide A macromolecule comprising long chains of *monosaccharides. The molecules of a particular polysaccharide vary in chain length, but show a characteristic statistical distribution of lengths. Polysaccharides are used by living organisms for energy storage (e.g. *glycogen, *starch) or for structural purposes (e.g. *mucopolysaccharides, *cellulose).

polyserositis Generalized inflammation of *serous membranes with accompanying serous effusions. Often the condition is part of a syndrome that includes *polyarthritis. The pig is most commonly affected.

Glasser's disease of pigs comprises a polyserositis, polyarthritis, and frequently a fibrinous meningitis, caused by *Haemophilus suis* or *H. parasuis*. The disease has been recorded in the UK, Australia, the USA, and Canada in pigs aged from 2 weeks to 4 months, although the peak incidence is in pigs that have been stressed by weaning or transportation. Often the best pigs of a group are affected and mortality exceeds 50% without treatment. Affected pigs develop an acute fever with dyspnoea and tachycardia. Swollen joints and lameness are seen in acute cases. Where meningoencephalitis develops, muscle tremors and incoordination are seen. Death occurs after 1–2 days. Lesions are seen in the meninges, joints, peritoneum, pleura, and pericardium, with fibrinous or serofibrinous effusions. Large limb joints have increased synovial fluid, which is often cloudy because of increased leucocyte content. The causal bacteria are found as commensals in the upper respiratory tract and therefore carrier animals are present in groups. Treatment may not be effective in peracute cases, although sulphadimidine, streptomycin, or oxytetracycline are recommended for treatment of in-contact and at-risk pigs.

Mycoplasmal polyserositis (i.e. caused by mycoplasma organisms) is often part of a polyarthritis-polyserositis syndrome in pigs, goats, sheep, and cattle, although the polyserositis element is most marked in pigs. *Mycoplasma hyorhinis* is a commensal of the nasal passages of most pigs, and it is thought that transmission from sows to young pigs (aged 3–10 weeks) occurs via direct contact and aerosols. The organism colonizes existing pneumonias or becomes significant in stressed individuals. After an incubation of 3–4 days affected pigs show lethargy, anorexia, and loss of weight with or without fever. During the ensuing acute phase (lasting

10–14 days) the organism localizes in serosal cavities and joints, producing swollen joints and abdominal tenderness. Survival beyond this stage leads to a subacute stage with swollen joints; this may eventually resolve after 2–3 months although viable organisms can still be recovered from joints at this time. Therapy with antibiotics (lincomycin or tylosin) may be effective in the acute phase. Prevention is assisted by the avoidance of stress and minimizing contact with infected pigs.

A polyserositis in pigs has been caused by infection with *Streptococcus suis* (Group D), but this is not a major problem.

polysome (polyribosome) A structure that occurs in the cytoplasm of cells and consists of a group of *ribosomes linked together by *messenger RNA molecules: formed during protein synthesis.

polyspermy (polyspermia) The penetration of more than one sperm into the ovum. Polyspermy causes the formation of a genetically abnormal embryo, which usually soon dies. It is more likely with ageing eggs and is one reason why the optimum timing of insemination is so important.

polytocous Describing a species that normally produces more than one foetus per pregnancy, for example pigs. *Compare* monotocous.

polyuria The production of abnormally large quantities of urine. The condition may be a physiological one, resulting from raised intakes of water, or it may be associated with pathological conditions involving *diuresis. In solute diuresis, in which solute levels in the filtrate are raised, there is usually renal disease; examples of such conditions include primary renal failure (e.g. acute or chronic *glomer-

ulonephritis, nephrotic syndrome, acute tubular necrosis), disorders of renal tubular reabsorption, *diabetes mellitus, and some hepatic failures. Water diuresis (i.e. increased water output) of a pathological type usually involves abnormal *vasopressin (antidiuretic hormone) metabolism (e.g. *diabetes insipidus). *Polydipsia is invariably associated with polyuria. The combination of polyuria and polydipsia, particularly in the presence of other clinical findings, such as anorexia and depression, is an indicator of serious clinical disease.

polyvalent vaccine A single vaccine that confers immunity against a range of different serotypes of the same disease-causing organism. For example, *foot-and-mouth disease vaccines usually contain antigens of up to four related virus types. *Compare* multiple vaccine.

pons A prominent swelling of the *brainstem lying between the midbrain and the medulla oblongata. It contains nerve fibres running to and from higher centres, and also fibres running transversely prior to entering the cerebellum via the middle cerebellar peduncle. These fibres form the bridge-like elevation of the pons. The pons is the origin of the fifth cranial nerve.

poorness (meat inspection) A condition affecting many carcasses, especially of very young and old animals (e.g. calves, cows, ewes, and sows). It is the result of a physiological state, not disease, and can be caused by, for example in cows, a shortage of food or overmilking. The carcass has a marked shortage of fat (which, however, is of normal consistency) and the flesh is darker than normal; the carcass sets well. It is important not to confuse poorness with *emaciation.

popliteal Relating to the region behind the *stifle joint.

popliteus A muscle behind the *stifle joint that acts to flex the joint.

porcine contagious pleuropneumonia *See* contagious porcine pleuropneumonia.

porcine intestinal adenomatosis *See* adenomatosis.

porcine parvovirus infection A contagious disease of pigs characterized by stillbirths, mummified foetuses, embryonic deaths, and infertility (*SMEDI) and caused by strains of *parvovirus. Infection with parvovirus has also been associated with poor growth and pneumonia. Porcine parvovirus is distributed worldwide, with antibody to the virus present in over 50% of the national herd in countries where serological surveys have been carried out. The virus is transmitted by ingestion or in the semen of an infected boar. In infected herds in which the young gilts are reared with the sows, immunity develops before the first pregnancy and clinical disease is rarely seen. When the gilts are reared in isolation, their first contact with parvovirus may be at service or soon after. Parvovirus can cross the placenta up to 80 days after conception in nonimmune gilts, causing abortion or stillbirths or resulting in the birth of piglets persistently infected with the virus. However, the only apparent sign may be small litters in the gilts. A killed vaccine has been shown to be effective in infected herds where infection in the gilts prior to mating cannot be guaranteed. The immune status of the herd can be ascertained by examining serum samples from representative groups for evidence of parvovirus antibody. However, the immune status of the herd may vary considerably between years.

porcine streptococcal meningitis *See* streptococcal meningitis.

porcine stress syndrome (PSS; Hertztod disease) An inherited condition of pigs involving increased susceptibility to stress. Affected animals may respond to stress by developing *pale soft exudative (PSE) muscle and, in more severe cases, the often fatal disorder called *malignant hyperthermia. The condition is controlled by a *recessive allele, known as the 'halothane gene' – homozygotes (*see* homozygous) suffer malignant hyperthermia as a result of the *halothane challenge test, which can be used to detect susceptible strains or individuals. The condition is common in many European breeds, particularly Piétrain and Poland China (up to 100%); occurrence is low in British and Danish landrace pigs and rare in large whites. Prevalence is increasing due to the association of desirable carcass traits with the PSS gene – the conformation score of loin and ham is high in halothane-positive pigs. The degree and length of stress determine which manifestation of the syndrome occurs. Mild stress prior to slaughter will cause PSE pork, resulting in poor quality meat and considerable economic loss. More severe stress will cause rapid death (in 4–6 minutes) as a result of malignant hyperthermia. Levels of the enzyme creatine kinase are high in susceptible animals and can be used diagnostically. Detection of heterozygotes is only possible through blood typing. Great care to reduce stress is needed with susceptible animals. High temperatures and humidity, excessive exercise, and pre-slaughter handling are among the most important causes of stress.

A special case of the syndrome is *back-muscle necrosis*, affecting pigs of 75–100 kg in weight. This is an acute condition lasting about 2 weeks, with swelling and pain over the back muscles (e.g. longissimus dorsi), followed by atrophy of affected muscles. In pigs that have suffered several episodes the muscle fibres may be fragmented with evidence of necrosis. The pathological changes and precipitating factors are similar to those of malignant hyperthermia.

pore A small opening; for example, *sweat pores* are the openings of the sweat glands on the surface of the skin; nuclear pores are gaps in the membranes surrounding the nucleus of a cell.

porker A meat pig that has reached pork weight, or one that is destined to do so. In Britain the final liveweight is 55–70 kg depending upon local market demands. This is usually achieved at between 110 and 125 days of age.

porphin A molecule consisting of four pyrrole units linked in a ring. *See* porphyrin.

porphyria Any of several inherited conditions in which there is accumulation of *porphyrins in blood and other tissues. The porphyrins, most commonly uroporphyrin, protoporphyrin, and coproporphyrin, accumulate where there is abnormal or failure of *haem synthesis arising from deficiency of the enzymes haem synthetase or cosynthetase. These enzymes are required for iron and magnesium chelation in the haem synthesis pathway. The porphyrins are *photodynamic agents, which cause *photosensitization in affected animals. Porphyria has been recorded in cats and pigs, but most recorded cases are bovine.

In *congenital erythropoietic porphyria of cattle* (and Siamese cats) porphyrins accumulate following deficiency of uroporphyrinogen III cosynthetase. The disease is inherited as a simple recessive trait in short-

horn, Ayrshire, Holstein, and Jamaican breeds of cattle, but has also been seen in cross-bred cattle. Deposition of reddish-brown porphyrin pigment in bones and teeth (dentine) is seen, hence the colloquial name of *pink tooth*. Pigmentation of other tissues, especially lungs, spleen, and kidneys, also occurs. Fresh urine is amber and darkens on exposure to ultraviolet light. Urine and tissues from affected animals, especially bones and teeth, fluoresce in ultraviolet light. Exposure to even moderate levels of sunlight causes photosensitization. There is also mild to moderate anaemia, and although the block in haem synthesis is rarely complete, affected cattle become more anaemic if exposed to sunlight. Other name: **osteohaemochromatosis.**

Bovine erythropoietic protoporphyria results in the accumulation of protoporphyrin III following a deficiency of haem synthetase (ferrochelatase). The disease is inherited as a recessive trait and has only been seen in females to date. Photodermatitis is the major clinical manifestation; there is no pigmentation of tissues and no urinary excretion of porphyrins.

In **Siamese cats** excessive accumulation of uroporphyrinogen, coproporphyrinogen, and protoporphyrin occurs in blood and other tissues, and they are excreted in faeces. The condition has been recorded as an inherited familial one.

In **pigs** porphyria is known to be inherited as a dominant trait but the exact defect remains unknown. Some aspects of the porcine condition mimic the bovine erythropoietic porphyria; photosensitization does not occur.

There is no effective treatment for these diseases; control by breeding selection is advised.

porphyrin One of a class of organic compounds comprising a *porphin molecule linked with various side-chain groups. Porphyrins are ubiquitous in organisms and form chelates with iron (as in *haemoglobin, *myoglobin, and most *cytochromes), copper (*cytochrome oxidase), magnesium (*chlorophyll), and cobalt (*vitamin B_{12}). Proteins containing porphyrins, such as *protoporphyrin IX, are called *haemoproteins*.

porphyrinuria The presence in the urine of porphyrins – intermediate compounds in *haemoglobin synthesis that accumulate in blood and other tissues in various similar inherited disorders (*see* porphyria).

porta The aperture in an organ through which its associated vessels pass. Such an opening occurs in the liver (*porta hepatis*).

portacaval shunt (portacaval anastomosis) A connection between the *portal vein and caudal vena cava that allows blood carried by the portal vein (from the stomach, intestine, etc.) to bypass the liver. It can occur as a developmental abnormality, particularly in dogs, and is associated with an abnormally small liver and biochemical disturbances. In moderately affected cases, surgical closure of the shunt can be performed. Portacaval shunt can also occur in advanced cases of liver cirrhosis, and surgical construction of such a shunt has been attempted to overcome *portal hypertension resulting from cirrhosis, although this is of limited value.

portal 1. Relating to the portal vein. 2. relating to a porta.

portal hypertension Abnormally increased blood pressure in the portal venous system (*see* portal system). It is usually associated with *ascites and is often indicative of serious liver disease. This condition is usually classified according to the location of the

inciting lesion. *Prehepatic portal hypertension* is relatively uncommon and involves compression or destruction of the vena cava (e.g. by thrombosis in cattle or due to neoplastic metastasis or direct spread from pancreatic carcinoma in dogs), or congenital malformations of vessels resulting in arteriovenous shunting between the portal veins or cranial mesenteric vein and the caudal vena cava or renal veins. These portosystemic shunts or anastomoses are most common in dogs.

Intrahepatic portal hypertension is associated with any diffuse liver disease that reduces effective hepatic vascular perfusion. Lipidosis, chronic active *hepatitis, diffuse hepatic fibrosis (*cirrhosis), metastatic neoplasia, biliary obstruction, thromboses, and intrahepatic arteriovenous fistulae have all been incriminated. In the dog and cat nodular hyperplasia combined with fibrotic scarring (often referred to as 'cirrhosis') or chronic active hepatitis (in dogs especially) may result in portal hypertension. In cattle insidious hepatic fibrosis following chronic venous congestion or diffuse hepatotoxicity (e.g. pyrrolizidine alkaloids in *ragwort poisoning; dimethylnitrosamine in rotten fishmeal) may predispose to portal hypertension. In horses chronic ragwort ingestion has similar effects. Portal hypertension is commonly seen in pigs with liver disease resulting from *aflatoxicosis and also in cases of hepatosis dietetica.

Posthepatic portal hypertension is usually associated with congestive heart failure, which is common in dogs, or constrictive pericarditis with cardiac tamponade (e.g. in cattle following *traumatic reticulitis). In cattle, thrombosis of the caudal vena cava or hepatic vein may also result in portal hypertension.

portal system A vein or group of veins that terminates at both ends in

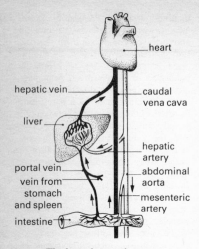

The hepatic portal system

a capillary bed. The *hepatic portal system* consists of the *portal vein and its tributaries (see illustration). Blood is drained from the spleen, stomach, pancreas, and small and large intestines into veins that join to form the portal vein leading to the liver. Here the portal vein branches, ending in many small capillaries called *sinusoids. The system enables transport of nutrients absorbed from the intestine to the cells of the liver. The *hypophyseal portal system* consists of a capillary plexus in the *hypothalamus, connected by portal veins to a capillary plexus in the *adenohypophysis. It transports substances produced in the hypothalamus to the pituitary gland.

Birds have a *renal portal system* (see illustration). Blood from the caudal mesenteric, internal iliac, and external iliac veins can flow into the caudal vena cava via the common iliac vein. Closure of the renal portal valve diverts blood flow into the kidney tissue, where it mixes with blood in the peritubular capillary sinuses. This is of importance in the excretion of uric acid by tubular secretion.

portal vein (hepatic portal vein) A vein of the hepatic *portal system, formed in a variable manner by the confluence of the cranial mesenteric, caudal mesenteric, and splenic veins. It enters the porta of the liver and divides into left and right branches.

posology The science of the dosage of medicines.

post- *Prefix denoting* following; after. Example: *postnatal* (after birth).

posterior Situated at or near the back of the body or an organ. In quadrupeds the use of this term is restricted to certain structures in the head, e.g. the posterior chamber of the eye. *Compare* anterior.

postero- *Prefix denoting* posterior. Example: *posterolateral* (behind and at the side of).

postganglionic Describing a neurone in a nerve pathway that starts at a ganglion and ends at the muscle or gland that it supplies. In the sympathetic nervous system, postganglionic fibres are *adrenergic, unlike those in the parasympathetic system, which are *cholinergic. *Compare* preganglionic.

posthitis Inflammation of the *prepuce. In domestic animals this often occurs in combination with inflammation of the glans penis (*balanitis), resulting in *balanoposthitis*. Posthitis can affect young male **dogs** at around puberty and thereafter. A purulent or bloody preputial discharge may occur and the prepuce is often red with small ulcerations; the adjacent glans penis may be involved. The condition is localized and often causes no inconvenience to the dog. *Staphylococcus* bacteria can be isolated from

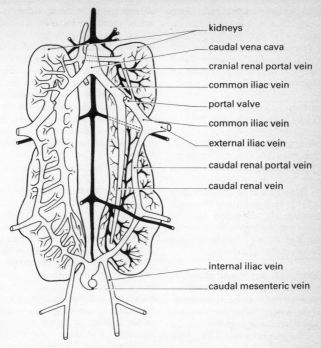

kidneys
caudal vena cava
cranial renal portal vein
common iliac vein
portal valve
common iliac vein
external iliac vein
caudal renal portal vein
caudal renal vein

internal iliac vein
caudal mesenteric vein

The renal portal system of fowl

the pus. The discharge may clear up spontaneously, but more persistent conditions are treated with broad-spectrum antibiotics administered parenterally or locally. Antiseptics may exacerbate the condition.

In **horses**, traumatic lesions caused by kicks from badly controlled mares during mating may result in localized inflammation. An added complication may be *paraphimosis, and surgical correction, including penile amputation, may be necessary if the condition is sufficiently severe and long-standing to cause *ischaemia. Pustules and ulcers on the prepuce are a feature of the viral disease *equine coital exanthema, and in tropical countries, preputial inflammation may be associated with *dourine and *habronemiasis.

An ulcerative posthitis of unknown aetiology is known to affect **bulls**. Ulcers are found near the preputial orifice and remain localized. More severe pustules and ulcers with sero-mucoid discharge are associated with *infectious bovine rhinotracheitis in bulls. The lesions often heal in 2 weeks but result in a latent infection, which may be triggered by stress or administration of corticosteroids. *See also* enzootic posthitis.

postoperative Describing an event, syndrome, or phenomenon occurring after an operation. The *post-operative recovery stage* is the period immediately after a surgical procedure or operation; patients, particularly those recovering from general anaesthesia, may exhibit violent recovery movements (e.g. in horses), or there may be *shock following excessive blood or tissue loss (e.g. in amputations or prolonged procedures).

postpartum Relating to the period of a few days immediately after birth.

postparturient fever A febrile condition occurring after farrowing (pigs) or whelping (dogs) and usually due to infection and inflammation of the uterus. Retention of a placenta may be involved. In severe cases the surgical removal of the uterus may be needed. Otherwise, combinations of *prostaglandins or *oxytocin and *antibiotics may be indicated.

postparturient haemoglobinuria A condition in cattle, usually occurring 2–3 weeks after calving and characterized by general weakness, jaundice, and sometimes haemoglobin in the urine (*haemoglobinuria). The animals are found to be anaemic, and the condition is attributed to haemolysis caused by phosphate deficiency. Treatment consists in phosphate injections.

postparturient metritis Inflammation of the uterus (*metritis) following parturition. In cattle, *retention of the placenta due to uterine inertia prevents normal involution of the uterus. In the absence of manual cleansing or hormonal treatment, this predisposes to the entry of bacteria, frequently a mixed infection with *Corynebacterium pyogenes and *Fusobacterium necrophorum. Yellowish foetid pus collects in the vagina and is discharged from the vulva; the cow shows systemic toxic illness. Treatment is by uterine irrigation with iodine-containing antiseptics, and intrauterine or systemic administration of antibiotics.

potassium A metallic element and one of the major minerals required in animal diets. Most potassium in the body is located within the cells, potassium ions (K^+) being the principal intracellular cations (*compare* sodium). They are required for the maintenance of fluid and ionic balances, the transmission of nerve impulses, and muscle function. Most diets provide potassium in excess of requirements; the surplus is excreted, mainly in the urine. *See also* hyperkalaemia; hypokalaemia.

potassium permanganate A purple crystalline compound used in aqueous solution as an *antiseptic and *disinfectant. Dilute solutions are used on wounds for their antiseptic and deodorant properties. Stronger solutions (5%) have astringent properties and can be used to suppress formation of excess granulation tissue; they have been used to harden greyhounds' feet. Potassium permanganate causes brown staining of tissue; this can be removed using dilute oxalic acid or sulphurous acid. Potassium permanganate crystals are used with *formalin to produce formaldehyde gas for the fumigation of buildings.

potato poisoning *See* solanine poisoning.

potentiation (pharmacology) The phenomenon in which the combined effect of two drugs is greater than the sum of their individual effects.

Potomac horse fever *See* equine ehrlichiosis.

pouch (in anatomy) A small sac-like structure, especially occurring as an outgrowth of a larger structure.

poultice (fomentation) A preparation of hot moist material spread between layers of gauze and applied to an area of the body surface to soothe pain or draw pus. A poultice may be prepared from a mixture of kaolin and glycerine, or from cooked cereals.

poultry A general term for domestic fowls (chickens), which is sometimes used to include all domestic birds, i.e. fowls, ducks, geese, turkeys, and guinea-fowl. Domestic chickens are assumed to have descended from one, or possibly more, species of jungle fowl (genus *Gallus*) of southeast Asia. A long history of breeding for show purposes explains the diversity of forms, but since the early part of the 20th century, the emphasis has been on selecting breeds and crosses for the production of meat and eggs for human consumption. Consequently breeding strategy is now dominated by relatively few strains, particularly since the need to breed for local climatic conditions has been removed due to the almost universal practice of housing commercial flocks under similar environmental conditions worldwide (*see* poultry husbandry). The *broiler industry is based upon such breeds as the Cornish and Plymouth Rock; white layers were developed from Leghorns, and brown layers from such breeds as Rhode Island Red. Modern breeding programmes are very sophisticated and produce hybrids following multiple crosses between strains.

poultry husbandry All aspects of the production of domestic fowls (chickens). *Broiler husbandry* is concerned with the rapid production of meat birds, usually on intensive units where the number of birds can be up to several hundred thousand. The control of all aspects of the birds' performance is unsurpassed. Optimum nutritional and environmental conditions have been precisely calculated to achieve maximum biological and economic output. Due to the numbers involved, and to the extremely low

financial margins, minimizing disease is crucial.

Egg production can be divided into two discrete phases: *pullet rearing* and *layer production*. The onset of sexual maturity is controlled by artificial lighting regimes (egg laying in the wild state is induced by increasing daylength). Thus a gradual change from 8 hours light per 24 hours (the usual pullet rearing photoperiod) to 16 hours light per 24 hours will promote laying. Therefore, the actual age at point of lay can be varied, but is usually around 20 weeks of age. Egg colour is genetically determined; in Britain the overwhelming demand is for brown eggs, but white in N. America. Hens are normally kept in lay for around 52 weeks, producing up to 300 eggs per hen; thereafter, declining numbers of eggs and deteriorating shell quality necessitate restocking. Occasionally a shorter second laying cycle may proceed following an artificially induced halt to production through a procedure known as forced moulting. In intensive systems, birds are housed in battery cages (*see* battery systems); disquiet over possible adverse effects on the animals' welfare has led to renewed interest in the more expensive 'free-range' production which must involve a degree of access outdoors. *Breeder production* follows a similar pattern to layer production except that the presence of a sexually mature male is essential to produce fertilized eggs for hatching (*see* incubation). Birds are therefore kept on floors rather than in battery cages (*see* housing).

poultry litter Dried or ensiled poultry excreta used as a feedstuff for ruminants. If obtained from broiler houses it will be mixed with shavings, straw, or other *litter or *bedding. Poultry litter is usually used as a source of nonprotein nitrogen, containing 250–300 g crude protein/kg dry matter. The high proportion of urates makes it unsuitable for nonruminants. A major associated health hazard is the risk of spreading *Salmonella* organisms or *botulism to the recipient animal or stockmen; drying or ensiling the litter considerably reduces this risk.

poultry meat inspector A person who is authorized to inspect poultry in a licenced poultry slaughterhouse. In the UK this may be a veterinary surgeon who has attended a special course and is designated *Official Veterinary Surgeon (OVS), or a person who has passed the poultry meat inspection examination.

Poultry Meat (Hygiene) Regulations (1976) (England and Wales) Statutes requiring poultry processing plants to be licensed by the local authority. Poultry slaughtered are subject to ante-mortem and post-mortem inspection by poultry meat inspectors acting under the supervision of an *Official Veterinary Surgeon. 'Farm-gate' sales are exempt from these regulations.

povidone-iodine An antiseptic *iodophor combining iodine and polyvinyl pyrrolidone, an organic carrier molecule that improves the penetration of the iodine. It is used on skin prior to surgery, as an antiseptic for wounds, and in teat dips and sprays. Active in the presence of organic material, it is generally bactericidal and has activity against viruses, although some organisms (e.g. *Mycobacterium tuberculosis*) are resistant. It is nonirritant to skin, although wound healing may be delayed slightly, and continual use carries a risk of contact dermatitis.

pox 1. Any of various infectious diseases characterized by a skin rash. *See* buffalopox; cowpox; fowl pox; goat pox; horsepox; pig pox; pseudocowpox; sheep pox. **2.** A rash

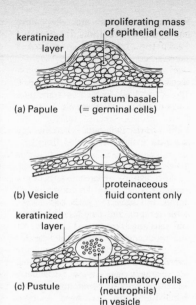

(a) Papule

(b) Vesicle

(c) Pustule

The development of pox lesions in the skin

of pimples that become filled with fluid (e.g pus), as in the pox diseases (see illustration).

poxvirus A family of DNA *viruses, causing disease in most domesticated and wild mammals and birds. They are the largest of all viruses and multiply in the cytoplasm of the host cell, whereas most other animal DNA viruses multiply in the cell nucleus (*see also* iridovirus). The sizes of both the *virion, which has a complex enveloped brick-shaped *capsid, and the viral DNA approach those of the smallest bacteria. They are classified into six main groups: the *orthopoxviruses* are the largest group, causing *cowpox, *buffalopox, catpox, *vaccinia infections, mousepox (*ectromelia), and formerly smallpox; the *parapoxviruses* cause *orf in sheep and goats, *pseudocowpox, and *bovine papular stomatitis in cattle;

the *capripoxviruses* are the most important economically and cause *sheep pox, *goat pox, and *lumpy-skin disease (Neethling) of cattle; the *avipoxviruses* cause disease in most species of bird; *suipoxvirus* causes *pig pox; and *leporipoxvirus* causes *myxomatosis in rabbits.

PPR (peste des petits ruminants) *See* kata.

praziquantel An anthelmintic with specific activity against tapeworms, particularly against mature and immature stages of *Taenia* spp., *Echinococcus* spp., and *Dipylidium* in dogs and cats, and against all tapeworms in pigeons and ornamental fowl. Available as tablets for oral administration or as an oil-based injection for intramuscular or subcutaneous use, it is rapidly absorbed and distributed throughout the body. Animals do not need to be deprived of food before administration. Praziquantel has several modes of action, including disruption of carbohydrate metabolism, and the tapeworms undergo severe contraction of the entire strobila, increased motility, and malfunctioning of the suckers. Toxicity is very low but overdosage may cause diarrhoea. The drug's expense has limited its use.

prazosine *See* hypotensive agent.

pre- *Prefix denoting* **1.** before; preceding. **2.** (in anatomy) in front of; anterior to. Example: *precardiac* (in front of the heart).

precancerous Describing a tissue or condition that is not yet truly malignant but which may progress to being so. For example, solar dermatitis of unpigmented areas of skin, such as ears, eyelids, and nose, can affect cats, cattle, and horses and is a well-recognized precancerous state that often progresses to *squamous cell carcinoma. Other names: **atypia**; **severe dysplasia**.

precipitation 1. The formation of an insoluble deposit (precipitate) from soluble interactants. **2.** The formation of an insoluble complex as the result of a specific interaction between soluble *antigen and *antibody. The complex is visible as a precipitate, and this feature is the basis of various assays and diagnostic techniques, such as *immunoelectrophoresis. *Compare* agglutination.

precipitin An *antibody that combines with an *antigen to cause *precipitation.

predisposition A tendency to be affected by a particular disease. Such a tendency may be hereditary or due to such factors as low nutritional status, compromised immunological competence, or stress (e.g. caused by transportation or overcrowding).

prednisolone *See* corticosteroid.

prednisone *See* corticosteroid.

preganglionic Describing fibres in a nerve pathway that end in a ganglion, where they form synapses with *postganglionic fibres that continue the pathway to the effector organ, muscle, or gland.

pregnancy The period spent by the mammalian conceptus in the female genital tract. The mean duration of pregnancy (*gestation period*) varies according to species (see table). Following fertilization of the egg(s) in the uterine tube, the developing embryo(s) move into the uterus some 2–3 days later. *Implantation of the embryo leads to the formation of the *placenta, via which respiration and exchange of nutrients and other metabolites between the maternal and embryonic blood takes place. The

pregnancy test

Gestation periods of various domestic species

Species	Length (days)
Horse	335–345
Ox	279–282
Sheep	148–150
Goat	150
Pig	114–115
Dog	63
Cat	60

presence of a viable embryo in the uterus prevents regression of the corpus luteum (*luteolysis) and suspends the *oestrous cycle, so that the animal does not return to oestrus during pregnancy. Maintenance of pregnancy requires the continued production of *progesterone, initially by the corpus luteum and later by the placenta. Progesterone suppresses contractile activity of the uterine musculature, and a sharp decline in its concentration towards the end of pregnancy signals the start of *parturition.

Most losses during pregnancy involve the death of embryos in the early stages, probably most often because they exhibit abnormalities. Foetal loss is generally much less, and may be due to inadequate function of the placenta or overcrowding in the uterus. In monotocous species (i.e. involving a single conceptus) loss of the embryo or foetus terminates the pregnancy and the dam returns to heat in due course. *See also* abortion; pregnancy test.

pregnancy test Any of various methods of diagnosing pregnancy. Accurate pregnancy diagnosis is necessary especially in farm animals, to maximize productivity of breeding stock and identify nonpregnant animals so they may be remated, culled, or treated for infertility. The most useful and popular tests are those that are accurate, relatively simple to perform, inexpensive, and can be performed at an early stage (although a confirmatory test may be needed later in case of foetal mortality). The oldest method is close observation of the recently inseminated female at the time of the next expected *oestrus; if no signs of oestrus are apparent, pregnancy is assumed. The presence of a vasectomized male (*see* vasectomy) gives a more reliable result. In large animals, such as cows and mares, rectal *palpation of the reproductive tract is a common method and gives accurate results in quite early pregnancy. In small animals, such as bitches and queens, abdominal palpation of the uterus can be performed, although this may be difficult in a very obese animal.

Many tests rely on detecting hormonal changes in the body fluids of a pregnant animal. These include *progesterone tests* on blood and milk, which are used in the cow, sow, and mare; a pregnant animal has a higher level of *progesterone than a nonpregnant one at a particular stage of the reproductive cycle. Good records relating to oestrus and insemination need to be kept so that the test is performed at the most appropriate time (a requirement for all pregnancy tests). *Radioimmunoassay of progesterone has now been largely replaced by immunological methods (e.g. *enzyme-linked immunosorbent assay), which give the results faster and can be incorporated in kits for use on the farm. In the mare, blood samples may be analysed for the presence of *PMSG (pregnant mare's serum gonadotrophin), which is present in high levels in early pregnancy. The *Cuboni test may also be used. In cows and sows, milk or blood samples may be analysed for the presence of *oestrone sulphate, which is a foetal not maternal hormone; this makes the test very accurate. In sows, research is underway to develop this test to predict numbers of foetuses, not just the existence of a pregnancy. Ultrasonic scanning can be used to demonstrate an audible difference in the blood circulation in a pregnant animal, or to present a visual image on a screen and so indicate the number of foetuses present; this latter technique is becoming increasingly popular for ewes.

pregnancy toxaemia (twin-lamb disease) A metabolic disorder, especially of ewes, occurring towards the end of pregnancy. Ewes carrying twins or triplets are especially affected and the disorder may be precipitated by stress factors, such as an interruption in food supply due to bad weather. The primary cause is a fall in blood glucose followed by severe *ketosis and *acidosis. Brain function is affected and the ewe behaves abnormally, staggering and swaying. Eventually blindness and collapse followed by unconsciousness and death occur. Treatment with intravenous glucose is not always effective, though administration of *adrenocorticotrophic hormone (ACTH) may be of help. Delivery of the lambs by Caesarean section may be the best alternative. Prevention involves keeping the ewes on a modest plane of nutrition in early pregnancy and maintaining food intake in the latter stages.

pregnant mare's serum gonadotrophin See PMSG.

prehension The intake of food achieved mainly by the lips and the tongue.

Preliminary Investigation Committee A committee of the Council of the *Royal College of Veterinary Surgeons that has the statutory duty of conducting a preliminary investigation into every disciplinary case against a veterinarian (i.e. a case in which it is alleged that a person is liable to have

his name removed from the *Register of Veterinary Surgeons or to have his registration suspended), and of deciding whether the case should be referred to the *Disciplinary Committee.

premature birth A birth that occurs before the end of the normal *gestation period. The offspring are usually of low birthweight and may require special postnatal care. Mortality is higher in premature offspring. See abortion; parturition.

premedication Preliminary medication administered to assist in the action of or to prevent an undesirable effect of drugs to be given subsequently. Premedication is employed especially prior to administration of a general anaesthetic.

pre-milking See pre-partum milking.

premolar Any of the teeth on each side of each jaw behind the canine and in front of the molars in the permanent *dentition.

premunition *Immunity to an infective organism that persists only while the organism is present in the body in an inactive state.

prenarcotization The administration of a narcotic or sedative prior to general or local anaesthesia. Such agents are often employed to restrain animals, thus frequently reducing the amount of anaesthetic subsequently required.

pre-partum milking Removal of milk from a heifer or cow a few days before calving. This should only be done where there are signs of discomfort because the udder is filled with milk. Typical signs are a distended hard tense udder, and a paddling gait of the hindlimbs; the animal tends to look around at its hindquarters. Once

prepotency

started, pre-partum milking should be continued until calving and the calf should be given *colostrum from another cow.

prepotency The ability of an animal to produce young like itself. This probably reflects either homozygosity (*see* homozygous) for dominant *alleles or a high *heritability of the trait concerned. *See also* proven sire.

prepubic tendon rupture Rupture of the prepubic tendon, which provides much of the support to the caudal ventral abdomen. It may result from external trauma, from the predisposition of certain individuals, or from excessive intra-abdominal pressure, such as may occur in *hydramnios or *hydrallantois. It is particularly important in pregnant animals, making the gravid uterus lie in a much more ventral position than normal with the increased risk of difficult birth (dystocia).

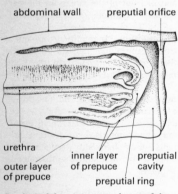

abdominal wall   preputial orifice

urethra

outer layer of prepuce   inner layer of prepuce   preputial cavity

preputial ring

Section of the prepuce and part of the penis of the horse

prepuce The fold of skin enclosing the free part of the *penis. It consists of an outer layer and an inner layer; the latter is continuous with the skin covering the surface of the penis and

is separated from it by the preputial cavity. In the horse the internal layer has an additional fold producing the preputial ring (see illustration). In the pig there is a preputial *diverticulum.

presby- (presbyo-) *Prefix denoting* old age.

prescription The written order given by a practitioner to a pharmacist for the supply or compounding of medicines required in the treatment of a case. Traditionally the prescription was written in Latin, but this practice is no longer regularly observed.

Prescription Only Medicine (POM) (UK) A drug that may only be sold or supplied by a veterinarian for administration to an animal or herd under his care.

presentation The orientation of a foetus prior to delivery at birth. It is described in terms of the vertical or horizontal axes. In monotocous species, for example cattle (and sheep), the foetus normally adopts an *anterior presentation*, in which the head and legs are directed towards the cervix. In polytocous species, such as pigs, both anterior and *posterior presentations* are considered normal, whereas posterior presentation in monotocous species is associated with difficult birth (*dystocia). In a *transverse presentation* the foetus lies across the cervix and therefore cannot engage in the cervix for normal parturition. *Breech presentation* occurs where the tail of the foetus is presented and there is bilateral flexion of the hip joints of the foetus, thus obstructing delivery.

pressor An agent that raises blood pressure.

pressoreceptor *See* baroreceptor.

presternal calcification (putty brisket) A condition of cattle in which fat in the brisket undergoes necrosis due to pressure when the animal is lying down. It is manifested by white putty-like masses; older lesions become calcified.

presymptomatic Describing or relating to the early stages of a disease before the typical clinical signs appear.

presystole The period in the cardiac cycle just preceding systole.

prevalence A general term describing the commonality of a disease or condition in a group of animals. *Compare* incidence.

priapism A persistent nonsexual *erection of the penis. It may occur in horses following the use of certain sedatives or anaesthetics. Occasionally the condition may last for several days, resulting in the formation of an oedematous cuff so that the penis cannot be retracted into the prepuce. *See also* paraphimosis; phimosis.

prickle cells Cells with cytoplasmic processes that form intercellular bridges. The germinative layer of the *epidermis is sometimes called the prickle cell layer.

prickly poppy *See* blood root poisoning.

PRID (progesterone-releasing intravaginal device) A plastic coil used to introduce the hormones *progestrone and, usually, *oestrogen, to the vagina of a heifer or cow in order to influence the animal's *oestrus cycle. *See* oestrus synchronization.

primidone A drug, chemically similar to phenobarbitone (*see* barbiturate), used in the control of epileptiform convulsions and fits in dogs. It is available for oral administration and is absorbed rapidly; about 20–25% is metabolized to phenobarbitone, which is believed to account for about 90% of the biological activity. There is depression of the central nervous system, so reducing the excessive electrical activity in the brain that results in seizures. Several days of therapy are required before effective concentrations of the drug accumulate in the body; therapy is then maintained to control fits. Primidone acts as a sedative although this effect can subside as therapy continues. Accumulation of the drug causes ataxia, which should be monitored by the owner so the dosage can be adjusted. Side-effects include polydipsia, polyuria, irritability, and restlessness. This drug may be used in combination with other anticonvulsants (e.g. phenytoin sodium). Tradename: **Mysoline.**

primitive streak A linear region of the early embryo that proliferates rapidly to produce the mesodermal cells, which spread outwards between the layers of ectoderm and endoderm.

primordial (in embryology) Describing cells or tissues that are formed in the early stages of embryonic development.

prion *See* slow virus.

pro- *Prefix denoting* **1.** before; preceding. **2.** a precursor. **3.** in front of.

probang A strong flexible rod designed to pass through the mouth and down the oesophagus. It can be used to apply medication, but the most common use is to relieve choke (oesophageal blockage) in adult cattle. A gag is inserted between the teeth and the probang is advanced in an attempt to loosen and then push the obstructive material into the rumen. *See also* stomach tube.

probenecid A drug that influences the rate of excretion of various compounds from the kidneys and is used to prolong the action of antibiotics. It is a lipid-soluble benzoic acid derivative that acts by inhibiting the transport of organic acids across epithelial barriers. It prevents the proximal tubular secretion of penicillin and related antibiotics into the kidney tubules thereby increasing plasma concentrations and half-lives of these drugs. It also increases uric acid excretion. Probenecid is given orally and is active for 5–8 hours. It may also be used to prevent detection of drugs in the urine of racing animals.

procainamide A procaine derivative used to treat cardiac arrhythmias. It acts directly on the heart, decreasing excitability, increasing the refractory period, slowing the rate of conduction, and reducing spontaneous depolarization. There may also be hypotension. The drug is injected (intramuscularly or intravenously) in emergency situations but for long-term therapy oral treatment is used. It is metabolized in the liver to N-acetyl-procainamide, which has mild antiarrhythmic properties. Excretion is via the kidneys, with about 50% of the procainamide excreted unchanged in the urine. Procainamide is used to treat ventricular tachycardias and arrhythmias induced by cardiac glycosides. It is of no value in the treatment of atrial fibrillation. Frequent dosing is required and the incidence of toxicity is high. Toxic signs include myocardial depression, ventricular tachycardia, ventricular fibrillation, hypotension, gastrointestinal disturbances, hypersensitivity reactions (fever and blood dyscrasias), and nervous signs (incoordination and convulsions).

procaine *See* local anaesthetic.

process (in anatomy) A thin prominence or protuberance; for example, any of the processes of a vertebra.

proct- (procto-) *Prefix denoting* the anus and/or rectum.

proctitis Inflammation of the anus and adjacent rectum. Although comparatively rare in animals it can occur in pigs given antibiotics that alter the anal flora so enabling fungi to multiply freely. Anal pruritus (itching) in dogs and cats carrying a heavy burden of intestinal worms may be accompanied by proctitis.

proctocele (rectocele; rectal prolapse) The protrusion of one or more layers of the rectal wall through the anus. Prolapse of the mucosa only is described as *incomplete*; eversion of all the layers is termed *complete*. The prolapse commonly follows persistent straining during attempts to defecate, and is frequently associated with chronic diarrhoea or weakness due to parasitic infestation or vitamin deficiency. The protruding tissue may become congested and ulcerated, or even necrotic. The primary cause must be identified and corrected. Manual reduction under anaesthesia may suffice, but in severe cases amputation may be advisable.

proctocolitis Inflammation of both the colon and rectum. It is unusual in domestic animals. However, *swine dysentery due to *Treponema hyodysenteriae*, which primarily affects the colon, may spread to involve the upper region of the rectal mucosa.

proctodeum (*pl.* **proctodea**) An ectoderm-lined depression in the embryo located in the region of the future anus. It is separated by the cloacal membrane from the terminal part of the hindgut (*cloaca). *Compare* stomatodeum.

proctoscope An *endoscope used to visualize the lining of the rectum. A rigid scope is often used for the diagnosis of rectal inflammation, neoplasia, diverticuli, or strictures.

proctotomy Surgical incision into the rectum. This may be necessary for surgical correction of strictures, diverticuli, or rectovaginal fistulae or for the removal of neoplasms.

prodromal 1. Relating to the period of time between the appearance of the first clinical signs of an infectious disease and the development of a full-blown rash or fever. **2.** Describing premonitory clinical signs. Such signs frequently give forewarning of disease and allow early treatment. *Compare* presymptomatic.

prodrug An inactive or weakly active compound that, following administration, is metabolized within the body to a pharmacologically active form.

production disease One of various livestock diseases caused by the stresses of high production. Animals bred for high productivity, for example, high-yielding dairy cows, will be subject to production disease unless dietary inputs match their production output. Similarly, hitherto hidden trace-element deficiencies can be revealed as production disease when even modest improvements in animal production are made. All the main metabolic systems of the body may be affected, including those linked to energy, protein, minerals, and sodium. Breakdown in any of these leads to either well-defined clinical problems, such as *milk fever, *grass tetany, and *ketosis, or to incipient difficulties that limit production but have no clear clinical signs. Typical of the latter are trace-element deficiencies of copper, selenium, iodine, zinc, and cobalt. These may be confirmed by a *metabolic profile test. Lack of suffi-

cient drinking water may lead to reduced milk yields and behavioural abnormalities (*see* dehydration). Shortage of salt (sodium chloride) leads to unusual behaviour, with excessive licking of soil (pica) and drinking of urine.

Product on the Merchants' List *See* PML.

proenzyme (zymogen) The inactive form in which some enzymes are synthesized and secreted, particularly by the pancreas. This prevents self-digestion of tissues, which can happen in certain diseases, such as *pancreatitis. Activation usually occurs by limited *proteolysis of the proenzyme to yield the active form of the enzyme. For example, the proenzyme trypsinogen is converted to *trypsin by the enzyme enterokinase.

proerythroblast A bone-marrow precursor cell of the red blood cell series, i.e. normoblasts, reticulocytes, and erythrocytes (*see* haemopoiesis).

profunda Describing blood vessels that are deeply embedded in the tissues they supply.

progeny testing A method of evaluating an animal for breeding purposes by measuring the performance of its offspring. Progeny testing is appropriate when selecting for characters of low *heritability, and is used to determine the *breeding value of an individual. There is obviously a time lapse between the initial choice of an animal and the availability of young for testing. However, progeny testing is widely used to assess breeding sires, especially those used for artificial insemination.

progesterone A steroid hormone secreted by the *corpus luteum and placenta, that promotes the maintenance of pregnancy and also prepares

progestin

the reproductive tract for pregnancy during the *dioestrous phase of the *oestrous cycle. Progesterone causes asynchronous muscular activity of the myometrium; this activity becomes synchronized as the progesterone level in the blood drops at the time of *parturition.

progestin *See* progestogen.

progestogen (progestin) One of a group of naturally occurring or synthetic steroids, including *progesterone, that prepare for and maintain pregnancy. Synthetic steroids with an action similar to progesterone are used to manipulate the reproductive cycles of veterinary species and for certain therapeutic applications. They include allyl trenbolone, flugestone acetate, medroxyprogesterone acetate, *megestrol acetate, melengestrol acetate, and proligestone. They mimic the presence of a corpus luteum and cause feedback at the pituitary, so preventing the surge of gonadotrophins necessary for ovulation. These synthetic progestogens can be given orally, injected in oil, or used in intravaginal devices. They have a longer duration of action and are cheaper than natural progesterone.

In sheep and cattle progestogens are used in intravaginal devices to synchronize oestrus; on removal of the device the animal comes into oestrus. In cattle natural progesterone is used because of the risk of synthetic hormones in milk. In horses, dogs, and cats progestogens are used to suppress oestrus and the associated behavioural signs. In mares progestogens can be used to delay the foal heat immediately after parturition (allyl trenbolone is the only effective progestogen in the mare). Progestogens are also used to try to prevent early embryonic death in pregnant mares, to treat cystic ovaries, to treat anoestrus in cows, to treat miliary eczema and rodent ulcers in cats, to treat false pregnancy in the bitch, and to suppress aggressive behaviour in male dogs.

proglottis (*pl.* **proglottids** or **proglottides**) One of the segments of a *tapeworm. They are differentiated in the neck region behind the head (scolex) and each proglottis contains a complete set of both male and female reproductive organs. The male organs develop before the female organs, and the most mature or gravid segments at the rear of the tapeworm have a uterus containing fertilized eggs. In most species the terminal segments break off and are discharged with the faeces.

prognosis (*pl.* **prognoses**) An assessment of the future course and probable outcome of a patient's disease.

progressive retinal atrophy (PRA) A progressive hereditary disease of dogs affecting the retina of both eyes. The disease exists in two forms: *generalized PRA*, which extends across the whole of the retina, initially causing poor night vision but eventually resulting in total blindness; and *central PRA*, which only affects the central area of the retina, causing a problem with near vision that tends to be worse in bright light but does not usually progress to total blindness. The disease can be recognized in its early stages by ophthalmoscopic examination of the eye by an experienced veterinary ophthalmologist. There is no cure for the disease, but it can be controlled by only breeding from animals that have been examined and found to be free of the disease. The form of PRA and earliest age at which diagnosis can be performed vary with breed (see table).

prohormone A precursor of a *hormone. Biochemical alterations to a prohormone will result in the release

Progressive retinal atrophy: form and earliest age for diagnosis in various breeds

Breed	Type	Approximate earliest age for diagnosis
cairn terrier	generalized	3 months
cocker spaniel	generalized	1 year
elkhound	generalized	1 year
miniature long-haired dachshund	generalized	3 months
miniature and toy poodles	generalized	2 years
Irish setter	generalized	3 months
Tibetan terrier	generalized	9 months
Cardigan corgi	generalized or central	3 months
English springer spaniel	generalized or central	1 year
briard	central	1 year
Border collie	central	2 years
rough and smooth collies	central	1 year
Shetland sheepdog	central	1 year
golden and Labrador retrievers	central	18 months

of the more active metabolite. An example is *proinsulin.

proinsulin A *prohormone, produced by the islet cells of the pancreas, from which *insulin is formed by cleavage of a 30 amino acid connecting (C) peptide.

projectile syringe A reinforced syringe designed to be fired from a special gun or crossbow. It is mostly employed to administer sedatives or narcotics to wild animals. See dart syringe.

prolactin A hormone synthesized and stored in the adenohypophysis. In mammals it stimulates the mammary glands to produce milk (see lactation) and the corpus luteum of the ovary to secrete *progesterone. In birds prolactin stimulates secretion of crop milk by the crop glands.

prolapse Downward or outward displacement of an organ or part from

its normal position. It may be the result of weakness in the supporting tissues, or follow unusually heavy loading or stress. See proctocele; prolapsed oviduct; prolapsed uterus.

prolapsed oviduct Downward displacement of the oviduct (uterine tube) towards the uterus. This is very rare except in **domestic fowls**. It is more frequently seen in heavy layers, associated with some inflammatory condition of the genital tract, or with the presence of a large egg or obstruction causing straining. The prolapse forms a dark-red protrusion from the vent; other birds may peck at it, and the affected bird should be removed from the flock immediately. The prolapse should be washed gently with warm water containing antiseptic, and replaced while holding the bird upside down.

prolapsed uterus Outward displacement of the uterus through the vagina. It may occur in any species but is most common in dairy cows, less so in ewes and sows. Prolapse of the uterus can only occur within a few hours of parturition, when the cervix is open and the muscles of the uterus, cervix, and vagina lack tone. The condition often occurs after a difficult or prolonged birth, perhaps when traction has been applied to the foetus. Replacement of the uterus involves removing any placental remnants and debris from the lining of the uterus (endometrium), washing the endometrium gently with warm water, and gently pushing the uterus back into position through the vagina. The process is made easier if assistants hold the prolapsed uterus up on a tray or sling, and, if the animal is recumbent, by elevation of its hindquarters. The administration of *oxytocin and antibiotics is usually beneficial. Prognosis is good if a clean uninjured uterus is promptly replaced. In cases of prolonged prolapse *shock often occurs and requires treatment. A severely traumatized uterus may necessitate amputation to save the animal.

proline See amino acid.

promazine See phenothiazines.

promethazine See antihistamine.

prominence (in anatomy) A projection, such as a projection on a bone.

promontory (in anatomy) A projecting part of an organ or other structure. The promontory of the sacrum is the downward projection of its base.

promyelocyte A bone-marrow precursor of the *granulocyte white cell series. It is more differentiated than the *myeloblast but less so than the *myelocyte, and is the first stage to display granules, although the neutrophilic, eosinophilic, and basophilic staining reactions cannot yet be distinguished.

pronephros (pl. **pronephroi**) The first kidney tissue that develops in the embryo. It is nonfunctional and soon disappears. Compare mesonephros; metanephros.

pronucleus (pl. **pronuclei**) The nucleus of either the ovum or the spermatozoon after fertilization but before the fusion of nuclear material. The pronuclei are larger than the normal nucleus and have a diffuse appearance.

pro-oestrus The stage in the *oestrous cycle prior to oestrus during which the follicle(s) are approaching maturity. There is a rise in the level of circulating *oestrogens produced by the follicles. A vulval swelling becomes evident in some species and in bitches there is a bloodstained discharge, but the animal will not yet stand for the male.

proparacaine (proxymetacaine) See local anaesthetic.

properdin (protein P) A serum protein involved in the activation of complement by the alternative pathway (see complement). It stabilizes the complex of C3b with protein B and in this way promotes the further generation of C3b from C3. This amplifies the effects of complement activation.

prophage The state (lysogeny) of a *temperate phage when its *DNA is integrated into the DNA of the host bacterium. Certain stimuli, for example ultraviolet light, can induce the prophage to *virulent (or lytic) multiplication.

prophase The first stage of *mitosis and of each division of *meiosis, in which the chromosomes become visible under the microscope. The first prophase of meiosis takes place in five stages (*leptotene, *zygotene, *pachytene, diplotene, and *diakinesis).

prophylactic A drug or other agent used for the prevention of disease i.e. prophylaxis.

prophylaxis Treatment that prevents disease, for example vaccination or the routine administration of antimicrobials or anthelmintics.

propionic acid (propanoic acid) One of the *volatile fatty acids produced by the rumen microflora and absorbed directly from the rumen into the bloodstream of the animal. The propionate (propanoate) is carried to the liver where it is converted to glucose; this represents a significant source of energy for ruminants.

propranolol See beta blockers.

proprietary name Tradename or brand name: the name under which a product is patented and marketed by a particular manufacturer. According to convention, the initial letter of a proprietary name is capitalized.

proprioceptor A specialized sensory nerve ending (see receptor) that monitors changes in the body brought about by movement and muscular activity. Proprioceptors located in muscles and tendons transmit information that is used to coordinate muscular activity (see stretch receptor tendon organ). See also mechanoreceptor.

propylene glycol A clear viscous liquid used as a solvent for drugs and as a preservative in drug solutions. It is miscible with water and can be given orally or injected. It is also used in topical lotions and ointments.

prosencephalon The embryonic *forebrain.

prostaglandin One of a group of compounds, synthesized in the body from the polyunsaturated fatty acid, arachidonic acid, that have a wide range of localized and systemic effects. They occur in many tissues. Six classes are distinguished – A, B, C, D, E, and F – with prostaglandins E_2 and $F_{2\alpha}$ being most important. Some have hormone-like activity. Their effects include the contraction or relaxation of smooth muscle; the regulation of blood flow or alteration of blood pressure; the induction of labour or abortion (see parturition); and the mediation of *inflammation. These effects show species variation.

Prostaglandin $F_{2\alpha}$ (*dinoprost) and its synthetic analogues (e.g. cloprostenol, fluprostenol, fenprostalene, alfaprostol, luprostiol, and tiaprost) are used in the control of reproductive functions in animals. Dinoprost is injected intramuscularly and has a short duration of action. The synthetic analogues are slightly longer-acting and are injected either subcutaneously or deeply intramuscularly. Prostaglandin $F_{2\alpha}$ causes luteolysis of a responsive corpus luteum in cattle, sheep, goats, pigs, and horses, and is used to synchronize oestrus: after luteolysis the animal comes into oestrus within a fixed time, although in mares this time can be quite variable. Prostaglandins can also be used to induce abortion: in cattle they are effective up to day 120 of pregnancy, with some action up to day 150; in mares pregnancy should be terminated before day 40 since after this time the endometrial cups have formed and although the foetus is lost the mare will not come in season immediately. Induction of parturition using prostaglandins is possible in mares, sows, goats, and cattle. This does not require the presence of a live foetus (compare corticosteroids). In cattle parturition occurs within 48 hours of injection, in pigs about 24 hours after injection, and in mares within 2–3 hours of injection. Prostaglandins are also used in the therapy of luteal cysts and pyometra in cattle, and prolonged dioestrus in mares. In bitches there is only transient luteolysis after prostaglandin treatment, and the drugs are toxic to dogs.

Side-effects caused by prostaglandins include sweating, restlessness, increased heart rate, increased respiratory rate, and bronchoconstriction. These side-effects are more noticeable with dinoprost compared to the synthetic analogues. Horses are particularly susceptible, showing marked side-effects with dinoprost. Injection of prostaglandins should be carried out with care, using antiseptics on the injection site. Prostaglandins cause localized inflammation and vasoconstriction, and an area of necrosis with infection can develop. Care should also be taken when handling these drugs. They can cause abortion in pregnant women, and inhalation or absorption through the skin causes bronchoconstriction, which can be life-threatening in asthmatics.

prostatectomy Surgical removal of the prostate gland. This is indicated particularly for the management of prostatic neoplasms, and occasionally for gross prostatic hyperplasia and prostatic cysts and abscesses. In dogs, the occurrence of urinary incontinence after prostatectomy is a major drawback to this procedure.

prostate gland One of the accessory male genital glands that produces the seminal plasma for *semen. It may consist of a body and/or a disseminate part. The body is a compact region lying just caudal to the urinary bladder, and is found in all domestic mammals except sheep and goat. In the horse and in carnivores it is divided into left and right lobes with an intervening isthmus. Enlargement may interfere with urination and defecation, especially in older dogs, and may necessitate a *prostatectomy. The disseminate part occurs in all domestic species other than the horse and carnivores. It consists of lobules scattered around the pelvic part of the urethra.

prostatic carcinoma An uncommon malignant tumour of the prostate gland, occurring in older male dogs. Clinically it causes problems with defecation and urination, pain, haematuria, and occasionally hindlimb incoordination. These tumours are felt as irregular, usually unilateral, firm masses when the inside of the rectum is palpated. Radiographically there may be evidence of local bony reaction and metastases to the local lymph nodes, pelvic bones, or lumbar vertebrae. As such tumours are usually at an advanced stage when diagnosed, treatment is often ineffective and the prognosis is grave.

prostatic hyperplasia A non-neoplastic proliferative condition of the prostate gland, producing prostatic enlargement. The condition is common in older entire male dogs and is thought to be due to an imbalance between oestrogens and androgens. In the dog prostatic enlargement compresses the rectum causing problems with defecation, whereas in the human male prostatic hyperplasia tends to occlude the urethra and leads to difficulty in urinating. Canine prostatic hyperplasia may be treated either by testosterone antagonists or, more permanently, by castration.

prostatitis Inflammation of the *prostate gland. This is usually due to infection, for example by *Streptococcus* bacteria in dogs, resulting in enlargement of the gland and dysfunction of the genitourinary tract. There is associated pain and possible

protein

incontinence. Treatment is with antibiotics. *Compare* prostatic carcinoma; prostatic hyperplasia.

protamine One of a group of basic proteins that form complexes with nucleic acids and which occur especially in association with the *DNA in spermatozoa. It is also combined with *insulin to form a complex, which – when injected – is absorbed much more slowly than ordinary insulin.

protease *See* proteolytic enzyme.

Protection of Animals (Cruelty to Dogs) Act (1933) (England and Wales) An Act of Parliament enabling a magistrates' court to disqualify from keeping dogs a person convicted of cruelty to them.

Protection of Animals Acts (England and Wales) Legislation, passed between 1911 and 1964, intended to prevent cruelty to animals and to alleviate their suffering. The Act of 1911 lists actions that constitute cruelty, which is an offence punishable on conviction by fine or imprisonment.

Protection of Animals (Anaesthetics) Acts (1954, 1964) (England and Wales) Acts of Parliament prohibiting the carrying out of any operation (with or without instruments) involving interference with the sensitive tissues or the bone structure of an animal unless an anaesthetic is used in such a way as to prevent any pain to the animal during the operation. There are certain exceptions under the Act, including: the making of injections or extractions by means of a hollow needle; and experiment duly authorized under the Animals (Scientific Procedures) Act 1986; the rendering in an emergency of first-aid for the purpose of saving life or relieving pain; the castration of a male animal before it has reached a specified age (namely: bull, 2 months; sheep, 3 months; goat, 2 months; pig, 2 months); the docking of the tail of a puppy or the amputation of the dew claws of a puppy before its eyes are open.

protein Any of a large group of *macromolecules found in all living organisms. They have molecular weights ranging from 6000 to several million. Protein molecules consist of one or several *polypeptide chains of *amino acids linked in a sequence (the *primary structure*) that is characteristic for a particular protein. This sequence is determined by the nucleotide sequence of the *gene for the protein. The polypeptide(s) may undergo coiling or pleating, the nature and extent of which is described as the *secondary structure*. The three-dimensional shape of the coiled or pleated polypeptides is called the *tertiary structure*. *Quaternary structure* specifies the structural relationship of the component polypeptides. *Simple* proteins contain only amino acid residues; *conjugated* proteins contain additional components, for example *glycoproteins, metalloproteins, and haemoproteins.

Proteins perform a host of key functional roles in living organisms. Of prime importance are the biological catalysts – the *enzymes. *Antibodies help combat infection; *haemoglobin is just one of the many carrier proteins; and *keratin and *collagen are important structural proteins. The interaction of actin and myosin proteins in muscle brings about muscle contraction; and blood *coagulation or clotting involves the fibrous protein fibrin.

Protein is one of the major components of the animal diet and is the source of amino acids, especially the *essential amino acids. *See also* protein quality.

protein equivalent A statutory declaration required for *compound feeds containing *urea, equal to the urea nitrogen content multiplied by 6.25.

protein quality The degree to which a *diet or feedstuff satisfies the protein requirements of an animal. Requirements vary with species and type of production. In **nonruminants**, dietary protein must supply the *essential amino acids (EAAs) both quantitatively and qualitatively; consequently the relative proportions of EAAs are fundamental to protein quality. In **ruminants** dietary protein undergoes considerable microbial breakdown in the rumen, and microbial synthesis of amino acids normally provides sufficient EAAs for the animal. The ruminant thus has two sources of protein: dietary protein that escapes rumen fermentation (*undegradable protein*; *UDP*) and protein of microbial origin produced in the rumen from true protein or nonprotein nitrogen (*rumen degradable protein*; *RDP*). Only ruminants with a high protein turnover, such as dairy cows in early lactation, ewes in late pregnancy, or rapidly growing young animals, need substantial amounts of UDP in the diet.

proteinuria The presence of protein in urine. Protein is not normally lost in urine in detectable amounts and proteinuria indicates protein leakage through the glomeruli as a result of kidney disease or leakage of protein elsewhere in the urinary system due to inflammation, for example, *cystitis. Substantial protein loss occurs in *glomerulonephritis and renal *amyloidosis. Detection of protein in urine, especially albumen (albuminuria), can be achieved by simple dipstick tests and is therefore a useful diagnostic indicator.

proteoglycan (mucopolysaccharide) A *polysaccharide typically containing amino sugar residues (e.g. *glucosamine) and a small percentage of *amino acids. They are major components of connective tissue, e.g. *chondroitin sulphate. *Compare* glycoprotein.

proteolysis The enzymatic hydrolysis of a protein. It is catalysed by *peptidase enzymes, and occurs, for example, in the digestion of dietary proteins in the gut. Limited proteolysis is of physiological importance in a number of areas, such as blood clotting and hormone secretion.

proteolytic enzyme (protease) An enzyme that catalyses *proteolysis. *See* peptidase.

Proteus A genus of motile rod-shaped facultatively anaerobic *bacteria, widely distributed and commonly found in the faeces of animals. They do not form spores and exist as saprophytes in decomposing organic matter, in the soil, and on plants, often due to faecal or sewage contamination. Unlike *Escherichia coli* and *Salmonella*, they can metabolize *urea. *P. mirabilis* and *P. vulgaris* cause septic infections in humans and some animals, usually in wounds and burns. They have also been associated with *otitis externa in the dog and urinary infections in humans and animals, particularly bitches.

prothrombin (Factor II) A *coagulation factor and the soluble plasma precursor of *thrombin. It is synthesized in liver parenchymal cells by a process dependent upon *vitamin K. An abnormally low level of prothrombin factor in the blood (*hypoprothrombinaemia*) has been described in a number of species (including cattle, domestic fowls, rats, mice, and dogs) following the ingestion of chemicals (e.g. warfarin) that antagonize the action of vitamin K.

proto- *Prefix denoting* **1.** first. **2.** primitive; early. **3.** a precursor.

protoplasm The material of which living cells are made, which includes the cytoplasm and nucleus.

protoplast A bacterial or plant cell without its cell wall.

protoporphyrin IX The most commonly occurring *porphyrin found in nature. It is a constituent of haemoglobin, myoglobin, most of the cytochromes, and the commoner chlorophylls.

protothecosis Disease due to infection with unicellular algae belonging to the genus *Prototheca*. Three species are known – *P. zopfii*, *P. wickerhamii*, and *P. stagnora* – all resembling green algae of the genus *Chlorella* but lacking chlorophyll and therefore colourless. All three occur as saprophytes in the environment but only the first two are known to infect animals (including humans); these occur widely in sewage, water courses, and in the faeces of pigs and cattle.

The commonest form of protothecosis is probably bovine *mastitis, producing a dramatic fall in milk yield but not always marked inflammation or hardening of the infected quarters. *Prototheca* can be isolated readily in routine culture of the udder secretion, but it has frequently been mistaken for a *yeast. Absence of budding and the internal division of cell contents into endospores are notable differentiating characteristics. Within the udder the organism is markedly more invasive and persistent than yeasts in *mycotic mastitis, sometimes infecting regional lymph nodes and able to remain dormant through a dry period to produce clinical disease in the fol-

lowing lactation. While not directly contagious, poor hygiene may produce numerous cases within a herd.

In **dogs**, protothecosis is usually a severe disseminated disease with lesions scattered through a variety of tissues and organs. The presenting signs differ according to the distribution of infection. In nearly all of about 20 reported cases there was evidence that the colon was affected, producing intermittent bloody diarrhoea, and involvement of the eye was also common. In cats, only localized cutaneous lesions have been reported.

The manner of infection is uncertain and no predisposing factors in animals have been identified. In humans there is evidence that the disease occurs when the normal defence mechanisms are impaired. Treatment has very rarely proved successful; one human infection was cured by the complete excision of the localized cutaneous lesions, and the effective use of a combination of amphotericin B and tetracycline has been reported.

Protozoa A vast subkingdom of single-celled organisms that generally lack chlorophyll and thus cannot photosynthesize. Almost all are microscopic. The single cell is divided into a cytoplasm, or cell matrix, and a nucleus; sometimes there is more than one nucleus. Within the cytoplasm or associated with the cell membrane are a variety of organelles with digestive, excretory, locomotory, and other functions. About 65 000 species have been described, most of which are free-living. Of the remainder, many are harmless parasites or commensals, or beneficial symbionts. However, a few cause important diseases of humans (e.g. *malaria) or animals (e.g. *babesiosis, *coccidiosis, *trypanosomiasis).

proud flesh Excessive *granulation tissue that tends to develop at the site of skin wounds that are unable to close over because the skin is bound by subcutaneous tissue. Such lesions develop especially on horse's legs where there has been some skin loss, and cause long delay in the ultimate healing of the wound. In all cases there is surface contamination because the wounds are open. Control of the excessive granulation can be difficult; many different methods have been employed, including excision and pressure bandaging, the use of *astringents, and the application of radiotherapy in the form of gold seeding.

proven sire A sire that has been shown by testing to be likely to produce some predictable desired effect on the genotype and thus performance of its young. *See also* contemporary comparison.

proventriculus (*pl.* **proventriculi**) The more cranial part of the avian *stomach, which produces digestive secretions. *See also* alimentary tract.

provirus The state of a *retrovirus after oncogenic transformation of its host cell. A *DNA copy of the viral *RNA, made with the aid of a *reverse transcriptase enzyme, is integrated into the cell DNA, thus changing the cell's genetic constitution and causing it to become cancerous. This occurs, for example, with Rous sarcoma virus of chickens. *See also* oncogenic virus.

provitamin A precursor of a *vitamin. *See* vitamin A; vitamin D.

proximal (in anatomy) Situated close to the origin or point of attachment or close to the median line of the body. *Compare* distal.

Prunus *See* cherry laurel poisoning.

pruritus Itchiness. The most common cause of pruritus in domestic animals is infestation with ectoparasites, such as *fleas, *ticks, and mites (*see* mange). Other causes are *allergy, inflammation, and certain infections. Pruritus provokes scratching and self-excoriation, which in turn stimulates further pruritus; an itch–scratch cycle is thus initiated which may cause extensive skin damage. Treatment involves removal of the cause.

pruritus pyrexia haemorrhage syndrome An obscure disease of cattle, only recently recognized in the UK, in which adult cows develop *fever (pyrexia), malaise, and usually marked itching (pruritus), which often leads to excoriation of the skin. Extensive haemorrhage throughout the carcass is found at post-mortem examination. The disease is sporadic with only a few animals in a herd affected. The cause is unknown but the disease has been linked to the use of certain silage additives.

pseud- (**pseudo-**) *Prefix denoting* superficial resemblance to; false.

pseudocowpox An infectious disease of cattle caused by a parapoxvirus (*see* poxvirus) and characterized by lesions on the teats. It is distributed worldwide, and can become a serious problem in lactating cattle. Horseshoe-shaped scabs develop at the site of the primary lesion, and these are frequently pulled off during milking, encouraging the spread of the virus and resulting in secondary infection. Affected cows can be difficult to milk, and *mastitis may be an additional complication. No vaccines are available and antibiotic cream may be necessary to facilitate healing. Infection may spread to humans and cause *milker's nodules*. Other name: **paravaccinia.** *Compare* bovine herpes mamillitis, cowpox.

pseudotuberculosis

pseudocyesis *See* false pregnancy.

pseudocyst A false cyst: a fluid-filled space without a proper wall or lining, within an organ or tissue. It occurs occasionally in connective tissue due to the localized accumulation of fluid.

pseudohaemophilia *See* von Willebrand's disease.

pseudohypertrophy An increase in the size of an organ without any increase in its functional components. This is caused by excessive growth of cells that have only a packing or supporting role.

pseudoleukaemia Any condition in which there is enlargement of several lymph nodes and/or the spleen, but without any blood abnormality. *Compare* leukaemia.

pseudo lumpy-skin disease A benign disease of cattle caused by a *herpesvirus and characterized by mild fever and a variable number of skin nodules. The disease, thought to be transmitted by insects, has been reported in North America and Africa but is probably more widespread. The incubation period is 5–9 days, and is followed by the development of a mild fever and the appearance of firm nodules on the face, back, and under the tail. The nodules usually subside after 7 days, leaving at first a scab and then a small circular hairless area. The hair regrows and there is no scar formation. Other name: **lumpy-skin disease (Allerton).** *See also* lumpy-skin disease (Neethling).

Pseudomonas A genus of aerobic rod-shaped motile Gram-negative *bacteria, widely distributed in nature. Some can grow anaerobically if nitrates are present. The organisms are common inhabitants of the soil, water, and animal body surfaces.

Most of them are nonpathogenic saprophytes but some are pathogenic to animals. Certain species produce pigments, such as pyocanin and fluorescein. *P. aeruginosa* causes localized infections or septicaemias and has been associated with *mastitis and *infertility in cattle, pneumonias in pigs, *otitis externa in dogs, and haemorrhagic *pneumonias in mink and chinchillas. Sheep in Australia suffer from a condition known as *green wool caused by *P. aeruginosa* multiplying in great numbers in wetted fleece. *P. mallei* causes *glanders in horses and other equines, while *P. pseudomallei* causes *melioidosis, a disease similar to glanders affecting many animals and humans.

pseudopodium (*pl.* **pseudopodia**) A temporary and constantly changing extension of the body of an amoeba or a cell, such as a phagocyte. Pseudopodia engulf bacteria and other particles and are responsible for the movements of the cell.

pseudorabies *See* Aujeszky's disease.

pseudotuberculosis A *tuberculosis-like infectious condition characterized by the progressive formation of multiple granulomatous lesions in internal organs. It is caused by the bacterium *Yersinia pseudotuberculosis* and affects guinea pigs and other laboratory animals, wild mammals and birds, and occasionally domestic ruminants. Infected laboratory animal colonies are best destroyed and started afresh with clean stock. The bacterium is also responsible for a form of necrotizing enteritis, sometimes accompanied by mesenteric lymphadenitis, in children and adolescents. *Compare* Johne's disease.

Outbreaks in **poultry** are caused by *Yersinia pseudotuberculosis* and tend to be more common in turkeys than in domestic fowls. The signs are diarrhoea, ruffled feathers, weight loss, weakness, and dejection. Mortality can reach 80%. Some birds may die without showing signs. Post-mortem examination may show enlargement and/or yellowish lesions on the spleen, liver, and other organs. Heavy doses of antibiotics can sometimes help during outbreaks, but control essentially relies on rigorous hygiene. *See also* avian pasteurellosis.

psittacine 1. A bird of the parrot tribe, which includes parrots, parakeets, macaws, cockatoos, cockatiels, lorikeets, budgerigars, and lovebirds. **2.** Describing such birds and their diseases.

psittacosis (parrot disease) A fatal contagious disease of *psittacine cage birds caused by *Chlamydia psittaci*. Affected birds develop oculonasal discharge and diarrhoea; the liver and spleen are enlarged. Lengthy treatment with chlortetracycline (*see* tetracyclines) is required to effect a cure. The disease is transmissible to humans by inhalation of dried faecal material, and causes headache, bleeding from the nose, shivering, fever, and complications involving the lungs. Untreated, it can be fatal (*compare* bird fancier's disease). Psittacosis is not notifiable, but the Importation of Birds, Poultry, and Hatching Eggs Order (1979) provides for licensed importation and quarantine of susceptible exotic birds. *See also* ornithosis.

psoas Either of two muscles in the sublumbar region – the psoas major and psoas minor. The psoas major joins with the iliacus, which originates from the ilium, and they insert jointly to the femur as the *iliopsoas*, the main flexor of the hip.

Psoroptes A genus of ectoparasitic *mites found especially on sheep but also on horses and cattle, and known as scab mites because they are responsible for the extremely conta-

gious condition called *sheep scab. The mites have an oval body and legs bearing so-called suckers. The entire life cycle takes about two weeks and is spent on the host. The mites penetrate the skin, usually on the back, feeding on blood from the wounds and causing the formation of pustules and hard scabs. An infestation results in general loss of condition and causes acute irritation so that an affected sheep scratches and bites, thereby damaging the fleece.

psoroptic mange *Mange caused by parasitic mites of the genus *Psoroptes*. *See also* sheep scab.

psychro- *Prefix denoting* cold.

Pthirus A genus of *louse containing the crab or pubic louse of humans, *Pthirus pubis*, found mainly on the hairs of the pubic and anal regions but occasionally on the hairs of the face, eyelashes, or armpits and causing intense itching. Adults have a short broad grey body and long legs. Transmission occurs by direct, usually sexual, contact.

ptomaine A nonspecific term applied to the products of *protein degradation, usually during the putrefaction of meat. The products are *amines, including putrescine, cadaverine, and neurine, and are responsible for the unpleasant taste and smell of decayed food.

ptosis Drooping of a structure, particularly the upper eyelid. This may result from a lesion of the *oculomotor nerve (cranial nerve III). Drooping of the lower eyelid is a common congenital defect in certain breeds of dog, and requires surgical correction to protect the cornea from drying.

-ptosis *Suffix denoting* a lowered position of an organ or part; prolapse.

ptyal- (ptyalo-) *Prefix denoting* saliva. Example: *ptyalorrhoea* (excessive flow of).

ptyalin Salivary *amylase.

puberty The stage in an animal's life when it reaches sexual maturity and is capable of successful mating.
In the female, puberty is marked by the first *oestrus, accompanied by swelling of the external genitalia and a readiness to be mounted and mated. In the male, puberty is more difficult to pinpoint but is usually marked by secondary sexual changes, such as the development of a mature physical conformation or libido. The age of onset of puberty varies between species and also within a species, according to breed, nutritional status, housing or stocking density, and season of the year.

pubis One of the bones that in adults fuses to form the pelvic girdle, or *os coxae.

puerperium The period following parturition during which the reproductive system returns to a state consistent with normal fertility.

Pulex A genus of *fleas found throughout the world and containing the human flea, *Pulex irritans*, a common parasite of humans but also found on other animals such as pigs. It is capable of jumping up to 30 cm horizontally and 20 cm vertically. Its bite causes intense irritation, and scratching may result in secondary infections. It transmits plague and murine typhus.

pulicide An agent used to kill fleas. Various products are available in powders, washes, sprays, and flea collars, and for oral administration. The compounds used include *organophosphorus compounds, carbamates, *organochlorine compounds,

*pyrethroids, *derris, and sulphur-containing compounds. Frequent usage of some of these can result in toxicity, especially in cats.

pullet An immature female bird, usually a chicken, from hatching until sexual maturity.

pullet disease *See* avian monocytosis.

pullorum disease (bacillary white diarrhoea) A highly infectious disease of poultry and other birds caused by the bacterium *Salmonella pullorum*, causing variable mortality in young chicks. The main economic loss is in domestic fowls, although turkeys, ducks, game birds, and wild birds can be infected. The disease can be transmitted via the egg (i.e. vertically) or from bird to bird (i.e. horizontally). It has been virtually eradicated from commercial flocks in Europe and the USA by blood testing of breeders, but backyard and hobby flocks remain a reservoir of infection. In domestic fowls, signs of disease are usually seen in birds under 3 weeks old. If the infection is egg-transmitted the first cases tend to be found dead without warning shortly after hatching. The outbreak spreads rapidly, with peak mortality in about 1 week. Chicks appear depressed, refuse to eat, and may seem somewhat unsteady; they huddle together, close their eyes, and emit a continous dull cheeping. There may be white diarrhoea and a pasted vent but these are not always seen. Mortality ranges from a few percent to over 50%. If the flock is infected after hatching (horizontal transmission), the outbreak tends to peak at 2–3 weeks, the mortality is comparatively low, and signs last longer. A more chronic condition, seen particularly in broilers up to 6 weeks, involves lameness due to bacterial invasion of the joints. There is also poor growth and feathering, with mortality of up to 5%. Many of these chronic cases have been linked with a variant *S. pullorum* strain.

The severity and rate of spread of outbreaks is influenced by standards of hygiene and environmental conditions, such as stocking density, ventilation, and brooding management. Very exceptionally, adult flocks may show clinical signs, with mortality of up to 20%; such outbreaks are usually triggered by the introduction of a highly infective source, such as contaminated feed. Normally, infected adult flocks act as carriers, having recovered from an outbreak as chicks or having acquired chronic infection when older. The ovaries become a primary site of infection: up to 40% of eggs from carrier breeders are infected, hatching into chicks that carry heavy bacterial contamination on their down. These rapidly cross-infect other chicks by inhalation of down particles. The disease is also transmitted in droppings, both within flocks and between flocks, for example on drinkers, feeders, boots, etc. Contaminated equipment on farms and in hatcheries should be fumigated with formaldehyde. Treatment with dietary furazolidone (*see* nitrofurans) can be effective, but carriers persist. A vaccine is available in some countries. In Britain regular blood tests are performed on commercial breeding stock under the (voluntary) Poultry Health Scheme. Vaccination is not allowed and infected breeders must be destroyed. The hobby sector does not participate. *See also* avian salmonellosis.

pulmo- (pulmon(o)-) *Prefix denoting* the lung(s).

pulmonary Relating to, associated with, or affecting the lungs.

pulmonary adenomatosis (of sheep) A disease of sheep characterized by emaciation, respiratory distress, and death and caused by a *retrovirus. Transmission is by close contact between susceptible and infected animals. Clinical signs are not usually seen before 3 years of age and manifest themselves as reduced exercise tolerance and weight loss. Infected animals tend to lag behind the rest of the flock and when lifted by their hindlimbs large quantities of fluid drain from the lungs through the nose. On post mortem the lungs are consolidated and grey; secondary bacterial infection is common. There is no vaccine and removal of all infected animals from the flock, or even total flock replacement, is recommended. Other name: **jaagsiekte.**

pulmonary artery Either of a pair of arteries – left and right pulmonary arteries – that arises from the pulmonary trunk to supply their respective lungs with deoxygenated blood. In the foetus the left pulmonary artery is joined at its origin to the aorta by the *ductus arteriosus, which after birth becomes the ligamentum arteriosum. *See* pulmonary circulation.

pulmonary circulation The system of blood vessels that transports blood between the heart and lungs. Deoxygenated blood passes from the right ventricle via the *pulmonary trunk and *pulmonary arteries to the lungs. Gaseous exchange occurs in the alveolar capillaries, with oxygen entering and carbon dioxide leaving the circulation. The oxygenated blood then leaves the lungs and returns via the pulmonary veins to the left atrium of the heart. *See also* systemic circulation.

pulmonary emphysema *See* emphysema.

pulmonary oedema Abnormal accumulation of fluid in the tissues of the lung. It may occur terminally as a result of heart failure, or following changes in blood osmolarity as, for example, in protein deficiency. Also, anaphylactic reactions (*see* anaphylaxis) may increase vascular permeability and allow fluid into the lungs. It may also occur secondarily to pneumonia, in which the lung consolidates with inflammatory exudate and oedemal fluid. In all cases the reduction in the functional capacity of the lungs' air spaces and passages leads to respiratory distress and overbreathing. Treatment depends on identifying and correcting the cause.

pulmonary trunk The artery that arises from the right ventricle of the heart and conveys deoxygenated blood towards the lungs.

pulmonary vein One of several veins that returns oxygenated blood from the lungs to the left atrium of the heart. *See* pulmonary circulation.

pulp A soft mass of tissue: for example, of the spleen (splenic pulp) or the *dental pulp of a tooth.

pulpy kidney disease (overeating disease) An acute fatal *enterotoxaemia that can affect lambs aged 3–8 weeks and, later, during fattening. It is caused by the bacterium *Clostridium perfringens* type D, which is a normal inhabitant of the intestine. However, factors such as overeating and the abrupt introduction of high-protein concentrates favour the bacterium's multiplication. The clinical signs are not characteristic, and the post-mortem softening of the kidneys indicated by the name of the disease occurs only irregularly. Effective vaccines are available and can be given either to ewes or young lambs.

pulse A series of pressure waves within an artery caused by the contractions of the left ventricle and corresponding with the heart rate. It is

Average resting pulse rate for various domestic species

Species	Rate/minute
Horse	28–40
Ox	36–60
Sheep, goat	70–80
Pig	70–120
Dog	70–120
Cat	120–140
Fowl	128–140

easily detected in superficially located arteries, for example the femoral artery in the dog and cat and the facial artery and radial artery in large animals. Average pulse rates at rest in the various domestic species are shown in the table. The pulse rate increases as a result of exercise and in various emotional states, such as fear. Examining the pulse is an important part of clinical examination: various diseases result in changes not only in the rate, which increases (e.g. in fever), but also in the character, which is often much weaker in such conditions as shock. *See also* bradycardia; tachycardia.

punctum (*pl.* **puncta**) (in anatomy) A point or small area, especially the *puncta lacrimalia* – the two openings of the tear ducts in the inner corners of the upper and lower eyelids (*see* lacrimal apparatus).

pupil The opening in the centre of the *iris through which light passes to the lens of the eye. The pupil is circular in many species, for example the dog, transversely oval in cattle and horses, and vertically slit-like in the cat.

pupillary reflex (light reflex) The reflex change in the size of the pupil according to the amount of light entering the eye. Bright light reaching the retina stimulates nerves of the

Pupipara

*parasympathetic nervous system, which cause the pupil to contract. In dim light the pupil opens, due to stimulation of the *sympathetic nervous system. *See also* iris.

Pupipara A group of *flies, including the *sheep ked and *New Forest fly, so called because the eggs hatch into larvae within the female's body and pupate almost immediately after they are deposited.

purgation The use of drugs or other *purgative substances to empty the gut. Purgation can be used to treat animals that have ingested poison, but must be avoided if there is any possibility of obstruction as fatal gut rupture could occur.

purgative (cathartic) An agent that increases intestinal motility causing rapid expulsion of contents from the large intestine. Purgatives are used to eliminate material, such as stones, bones, etc., from the intestinal tract; they were also used formerly to remove tapeworms. Bulk purgatives, which incorporate substances such as saline, agar, bran, carboxymethylcellulose, and magnesium carbonate, oxide, or sulphate, act by increasing the volume of fluid in the intestinal tract and thus stimulating peristalsis. Purgatives that act by causing intestinal irritation include phenolphthalein, anthracene compounds, and vegetable oils. *Parasympathomimetic drugs (e.g. bethanechol, carbachol, and arecoline) have also been used as purgatives.

purine An organic nitrogenous base comprising fused five- and six-membered rings that gives rise to biologically important derivatives, notably *adenine and *guanine. These occur in *nucleotides and nucleic acids (DNA and RNA). The degradation of purines leads to the production of *uric acid.

Purkinje cells *See* piriform neurones.

Purkinje fibres The specialized conducting muscle fibres of the heart that form the *atrioventricular bundle.

purpura Bleeding into the skin from the capillaries. It is seen as diffuse blotches, which are initially red then gradually change to purple and then to yellow/brown as the blood breaks down and is resorbed. Severe purpura involving extensive subcutaneous haemorrhage is known as *purpura haemorrhagica*. A common cause is deficiency of blood platelets (*thrombocytopenia); the platelets normally seal tiny ruptures in the capillaries. Other causes of failure of the blood coagulation mechanism include certain poisons (e.g. *warfarin). Purpura may also be caused by a defect in the capillaries, for example due to damage by certain virus infections. Treatment involves removing the causative agent. In severe cases blood transfusion may be necessary. *See also* ecchymosis; petechia.

purpura haemorrhagica *See* purpura.

purulent Forming, consisting of, or containing *pus.

pus A fluid product of *inflammation variably composed of dead *phagocytes, exudate, and tissue debris. Living or dead organisms may also be present. The colour and consistency vary depending on the contents, but pus is frequently white to yellow or pale green and of creamy texture.

pustule A small pus-containing blister on the skin.

putamen Part of the lentiform nucleus in the cerebrum of the brain. *See* basal ganglia.

putrescine *See* polyamine.

py- (pyo-) *Prefix denoting* pus; a purulent condition.

pyaemia Invasion of the blood by pus-forming organisms. The process may begin with any suppurative inflammatory process that is not adequately contained by the body. Pyaemia is usually associated with the formation of multiple secondary *abscesses throughout the tissues. *Compare* septicaemia; toxaemia.

pyel- (pyelo-) *Prefix denoting* the pelvis of the kidney. Example: *pyelectasis* (dilatation of).

pyelitis Inflammation of the kidney pelvis. Causes include irritation by urinary stones and extension of infection from the bladder. However, uncomplicated pyelitis is rare because it usually involves inflammation of the renal medulla as well (*see* pyelonephritis).

pyelogram A radiograph of the pelvis of the kidney. *See* pyelography.

pyelography *Radiography of the pelvis of the kidney. The radiograph (*pyelogram*) may reveal the presence of radio-opaque calculi (stones) without contrast medium, but generally a contrast material is used to outline the pelvis. A contrast medium that passes rapidly from the blood to the urine after intravenous injection is often used, giving an *intravenous* or an *excretion pyelogram*.

pyelonephritis Infection of the *kidney pelvis, usually due to bacteria ascending the ureter from an infected bladder or other lower part of the urinary tract. In cows, pyelonephritis is caused by the bacterium *Corynebacterium renale* and is accompanied by lumbar pain, straining, and wasting. Antibiotic treatment

rarely effects a permanent cure because of reinfection, but the temporary improvement in body condition allows sale of the animal for slaughter. Related bacteria have been associated with the condition (*C. cystitidis*; *C. pilosum*), and *C. suis* is recognized as causing a similar infection in sows.

pyelotomy Surgical incision into the pelvis of the kidney. This is rarely performed in animals but in dogs kidney stones have been removed through such an incision.

pykno- *Prefix denoting* thickness or density.

pyknosis The process in which the cell nucleus is thickened into a dense mass, which occurs when cells die.

pyl- (pyle-) *Prefix denoting* the portal vein.

pylor- (pyloro-) *Prefix denoting* the pylorus. Example: *pyloroduodenal* (of the pylorus and duodenum).

pyloropexy Surgical fixation of the pylorus of the abomasum in a certain position. This can form part of the surgical treatment of left displacement of the abomasum in cattle. The displacement is corrected manually and the pylorus is sutured to the parietal peritoneum. *See also* abomasopexy; omentopexy.

pylorospasm Spasm of the outlet of the stomach (pylorus). This presents as intermittent vomiting or abdominal pain, especially after eating. It may be relieved by the administration of *atropine or by partially sectioning the intestinal wall at the pylorus (*pyloromyotomy*).

pylorus (*pl.* **pylori**) The region of the stomach where it joins the duodenum. The aperture of the opening into the duodenum is regulated by the *pyloric sphincter*. In the pig a prominence, the *torus pyloricus*, projects from the wall and decreases the size of the orifice. It is thought to enable complete closure of the orifice.

pyo- *Prefix. See* py-.

pyocele The accumulation of pus in a body cavity.

pyogenic Causing the production of *pus. The term is usually applied to certain species of bacteria.

pyometra A condition characterized by the progressive accumulation of pus in the uterus. It frequently occurs as a sequel to *metritis, and if left untreated may lead to *pyosalpinx, pyosalpingitis, and eventual death. It is relatively common in maiden bitches over 5 years old and is frequently associated with ovarian dysfunction, such as hypersecretion of *progesterone and a concurrent persistence of luteal tissue in the ovary. The signs are lethargy, fever, and depressed appetite with increased water consumption and urination. The most common type is *open pyometra*, where the cervix is partly dilated and a vaginal discharge (varying from bloodstained to purulent) is apparent. Cases of *closed pyometra* are more difficult to diagnose as there is no visible discharge. Treatment may involve injections of *prostaglandin $F_{2\alpha}$ (to cause luteal regression and uterine evacuation), but often the only satisfactory solution is *ovariohysterectomy. The condition is relatively uncommon in other domestic species.

pyometritis A condition in which infection of the uterus leads to the accumulation of pus inside it. *See also* metritis; pyometra.

pyosalpinx A condition in which pus accumulates in the oviducts. *See also* salpingitis.

pyosis The formation and/or discharge of *pus.

pyothorax The presence of *pus within the thoracic cavity. It may be due to a penetrating wound or to the spread of infection from the lungs through the pleura, and often causes respiratory embarrassment. *See also* feline pyothorax.

pyramid 1. One of the conical masses (renal pyramids) that comprises the medulla of the *kidney. **2.** Either of two elevations on the base of the medulla oblongata produced by the descending fibres of the *pyramidal tract.

pyramidal cell A type of neurone found in the *cerebral cortex, with a pyramid-shaped cell body, a branched dendrite extending from the apex towards the brain surface, several dendrites extending horizontally from the base, and a long axon running into the white matter of the cerebral hemisphere (see illustration).

pyramidal disease (Buttress foot) An abnormality of the horse's foot due to new bone growth around the extensor process of the distal *phalanx. This produces an enlargement at the coronary band in the mid-dorsal region. The resultant pain can cause a shortening of the stride and a tendency to land on the heel of the foot. Corrective shoeing and neurectomy may be used to alleviate the condition.

pyramidal tract A collection of nerve fibres descending from the cerebral cortex through the brainstem and including the *pyramids of the medulla oblongata, within which many fibres cross to the opposite side to form the *lateral corticospinal tract*; those descending on the same side of the spinal cord form the *ventral corticospinal tract*. The pyramidal tract is involved in the control of voluntary muscle activity.

pyrantel A broad-spectrum anthelmintic with activity against gastrointestinal nematodes (roundworms) in cattle, sheep, horses, pigs, and small animals. Available as a paste or in pellet form, it has good efficacy against adult parasites but is less effective against larval forms in the mucosa. It has no activity against flukes and tapeworms. Pyrantel acts as a depolarizing muscle relaxant in parasites and to a slight extent in the host. It is poorly absorbed from the gastrointestinal tract and therefore has little activity against tissue parasites and lungworms. Some parasites are resistant to pyrantel, and there is resistance to its analogue *morantel, and cross-resistance to *levamisole. Pyrantel is used particularly in horses to kill ascarids, strongylids, and *Oxyuris*. It is also used in dogs. Host toxicity can occur rarely in debilitated animals or with overdosage. Tradename: **Strongid P**.

pyret- (pyreto-) *Prefix denoting* fever.

pyrethroids A group of synthetic compounds used to kill ectoparasitic insects and as insect repellants. They are chemically similar to the naturally occurring pyrethrins, obtained from the dried flower heads of *Chrysanthemum cinerariaefolium*. Both synthetic and natural compounds have insecticidal activity, although the latter are unstable in the environment, being inactivated by light, moisture, and air. The synthetic pyrethroids (e.g. permethrin and cypermethrin) are more stable. They are absorbed through the insect's cuticle and cause neurotoxicity, with rapid knock-down,

although some insects can recover. Pyrethroids are available as pour-on preparations, impregnated ear tags, and powders. The compounds are lipid-soluble and spread throughout the lipid layer of the skin from the site of administration, remaining there for long periods. Pyrethroids are relatively nontoxic to mammals and birds and are metabolized by tissue esterases. They are toxic to fish.

pyrexia *See* fever.

pyridoxine *See* vitamin B$_6$.

pyrimethamine *See* coccidiostat.

pyrimidine An organic nitrogenous base, comprising a six-membered ring, that gives rise to a group of biologically important derivatives, notably *cytosine, *uracil, and *thymine. These occur in *nucleotides and nucleic acids (DNA and RNA).

pyrogenic Describing a substance or agent (*pyrogen*) that causes fever.

pyruvic acid (2-oxopropanoic acid) An organic acid that is a key substance in the metabolism of living organisms, being the end-product of *glycolysis. It can be converted to lactate during anaerobic metabolism, to acetyl coenzyme A in order to enter the *Krebs cycle, and to oxaloacetate to initiate the process of *gluconeogenesis. It also arises from the *amino acid alanine by *transamination or *deamination.

pythiosis A disease, primarily of horses, caused by infection with a fungus of the genus *Pythium* (belonging to the class Oomycetes; now transferred from the Fungi to the Protista in some modern systems of classification). The fungal *mycelium previously named as *Hyphomyces destruens* and isolated from cases of *equine phycomycosis, has now been identified as *P. insidiosum*; it is apparently the commonest cause of that condition. The disease occurs principally on the skin of the legs and ventral parts of the chest and abdomen of the horse, producing ulcerative granulomas up to 45 cm in diameter. Infection can occur on other parts of the body but lesions on the head or nostrils are more often due to *basidiobolomycosis or *conidiobolomycosis. *Pythium* spp. are semi-aquatic organisms, usually associated with plant material and spreading by the discharge of motile zoospores into water. Early lesions of equine pythiosis are often associated with wounds, thought to be the point of entry for the infective spores.

In addition to the usual diagnostic procedures for a *phycomycosis, a precipitin test for equine pythiosis has been developed. Excision of all diseased tissue is curative but not always possible because of the site. *Amphotericin B has been used with variable success, and a specific vaccine for immunotherapy has been found effective. *P. insidiosum* infection has been specifically identified in the USA, South America, and Australia, and may account for a proportion of equine phycomycosis wherever the disease occurs. The pathogen has also been shown to cause gastrointestinal phycomycosis in dogs in Gulf states of the USA.

pyuria The presence of *pus in the urine. This may originate from the kidneys, the urinary bladder, or the associated accessory glands.

Q

Q fever An infectious disease of domestic animals and humans caused by the rickettsia *Coxiella burnetti*. The disease was first described in abattoir workers in Australia but is now worldwide. In animals the disease is fairly mild or inapparent, although there may be abortions in sheep, goats, and cattle. In humans the organism causes a serious influenza-like syndrome. The organism is very resistant to physical and chemical agents, and the main sources of infections for humans and other animals are the expelled placenta and other uterine discharges of aborted sheep and cattle, and unpasteurized milk. Cows and goats may become chronically infected, with the organism residing principally in the udder. The disease is diagnosed by demonstrating the rickettsia in placental or other smears stained with such stains as Macchiavello or modified Ziehl-Neelsen. The organisms are partially susceptible to tetracyclines and chloramphenicol, with relapses occurring in treated individuals. In enzootic areas, the use of inactivated vaccines and the isolation of aborting animals are useful control measures. Humans should avoid consuming unpasteurized milk.

quadratus Describing a four-sided muscle, such as the *quadratus lumborum*, which is one of the sublumbar muscles close to the *psoas muscles, and the *quadratus femoris*, which lies just caudal to the hip joint and produces extension and lateral rotation of the thigh.

quadri- *Prefix denoting* four. Example: *quadrilateral* (having four sides).

quadriceps femoris The large muscle on the front of the thigh that inserts to the *patella and extends the *stifle joint. It has four components: the *vastus lateralis*; *vastus medialis*; *vastus intermedius*; and *rectus femoris* (see illustration).

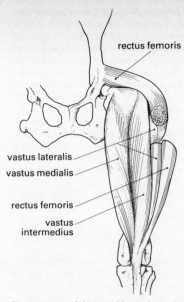

Components of the quadriceps femoris

quadriplegia (tetraplegia) Paralysis of all four limbs. This usually indicates a dysfunction or lesion of the brain or spinal cord, for example destruction of the cerebellar cortex (as in certain congenital diseases), accidental injury to the upper spinal cord, or *encephalitis. Treatment and prognosis depend on the cause.

quarantine A period of isolation imposed on an animal to prevent the spread of disease to other animals or to protect it from disease. Quarantine is usually imposed on animals entering a country or establishment so that any diseases they may be carrying or incubating can be identified. They may also be vaccinated against diseases in their new environment. Quarantine may also be applied to imported animal products. The duration of quarantine depends on the incubation period of specific diseases.

For *rabies the quarantine period is 6 months and for *equine infectious anaemia it is 2 months, while for the majority of other infectious diseases it is 3 weeks.

Queensland itch *See* sweet itch.

quidding A condition seen in horses in which food taken into the mouth and chewed is not swallowed but instead falls out of the mouth. It can result from disease or injuries of the teeth, gums, tongue, or other parts of the mouth.

quiescent Describing a disease that is in an inactive or undetectable phase.

quinalbarbitone (*US* **quinalbarbital**) *See* barbiturate.

quinapyramine (antrycide) A trypanocidal drug with activity against *Trypanosoma congolense*, *T. evansi*, *T. vivax*, *T. equiperdum*, and *T. equinum*. There is some activity against *T. brucei*. Two salts of quinapyramine are available: the sulphate, which is rapidly absorbed but has little prophylactic effect; and the chloride, which has slower absorption but gives prophylaxis. Usually, three parts sulphate and two parts chloride are combined in a single injection for therapy and prophylaxis. The drug is thought to act by inhibiting trypanosomal growth and cell division, and gives protection against infection in high-risk areas for about 2–3 months; repeated injections are given at 2-monthly intervals. The prophylactic effect can be increased by using *suramin concurrently. Subcutaneous injections can cause localized persistent reactions; in horses there may be sloughing of skin, and intramuscular injection at several sites may prevent this. Overdosage causes toxicity, with sweating, increased salivation, muscle tremors, increased respiratory rate,

quinidine sulphate

and, in severe cases, cardiac irregularities and death. Some strains of trypanosomes are now resistant to quinapyramine.

quinidine sulphate A drug used to treat cardiac arrhythmias. It is obtained from cinchona trees, along with the other alkaloids, quinine, cinchonine, and cinchonidine. Quinidine was initially used as an antimalarial but was found to have antipyretic, anti-arrhythmic, and oxytocic properties. It acts directly on cardiac cells, reducing cell excitability, increasing the refractory period between contractions, slowing the rate of conduction of impulses, and reducing spontaneous depolarization. It simultaneously inhibits vagal activity by blocking muscarinic receptors, causing an increase in heart rate. It can be administered orally, although it is unpalatable, or by slow intravenous injection. The half-life is short and slow-release preparations are available. Quinidine is used in small animals and horses to treat atrial and atrioventricular fibrillation, although *digitalization or the use of *beta blockers may also be required. It has also been used to correct ventricular tachycardia or ventricular premature beats. Toxicity can cause gastrointestinal disturbances, with vomiting and diarrhoea. Overdosage can produce incoordination, myocardial depression, atrioventricular block, ventricular fibrillation, and convulsions.

quinine *See* quinidine sulphate.

quinuronium sulphate A complex urea-based compound used to treat *babesiosis. It is available for subcutaneous injection as a 5% solution, although this should be diluted to 0.5% for the treatment of dogs. Cattle given a single injection show clinical improvement in 24–48 hours, but not all the parasites may be eliminated, necessitating another injection after 48 hours. Repeated treatments should be avoided because animals can become sensitized to the drug. Quinuronium inhibits cholinesterase, and side-effects include sweating, salivation, diarrhoea, respiratory distress, and occasionally cardiovascular shock. These can be counteracted using atropine. Quinuronium can be administered in conjunction with inoculation of parasites to enable the development of immunity in cattle. Safer drugs are now being developed to treat babesiosis and for prophylaxis (*see* imidocarb, amicarbalide). Tradenames: **Acaprin**; **Acapron**; **Babesan**; **Diveronel**; **Ludobal**; **Pirevan**; **Piropan**.

quittor A chronic condition involving infection of the lateral cartilages of the horse's foot. The infection may enter through a wound in the sole of the foot or close to the coronary band. The consequent lameness is mild or severe, typically accompanied by one or more sinuses from the cartilage discharging in the coronary band region. There are varying degrees of associated swelling, heat, and pain. Treatment entails radical surgical excision of the affected cartilage.

R

rabbit syphilis A venereally transmitted infection of rabbits caused by the spirochaete bacterium *Treponema paraluiscuniculi* (*T. cuniculi*). It is characterized by erosions of the genitalia and surrounding region, and sometimes of the head. These persist longer in the female than in the male. The agent cannot infect humans.

rabies A usually fatal disease of mammals caused by a *rhabdovirus and characterized by severe nervous signs. Only the UK, Australia, New Zealand, Sweden, and Portugal are free of the disease. Rabies is maintained in wild mammals, notably foxes in Europe, skunks in North America, bats in South America, and wolves and wild and feral dogs in Africa and Asia. The disease is transmitted by the bite of an infected animal although aerosol transmission is possible. The incubation period is between 2 weeks and 1 year depending on the site of entry of the virus. Initially a fever develops together with a slight change in temperament. The disease appears in two classical forms, furious and dumb, although the virus is excreted in the saliva before the onset of frank clinical signs. In the *furious form*, typically seen in carnivores, the affected animal becomes very aggressive, salivates, and bites indiscriminately at other animals or inanimate objects. Convulsions, coma, and death usually follow in 3–10 days. In the *dumb form*, also seen in carnivores but more typical in herbivores, a change in voice is first noticed. Cattle bellow persistently, and strain unproductively. First the lower jaw becomes paralysed, and the affected animal has difficulty in swallowing; saliva drools from the mouth. The paralysis progresses followed by collapse, coma, and death. Horses show a wide range of clinical signs, including mild colic, lameness, depression, excitement, etc. Some animals, including dogs but particularly bats, may have mild or inapparent infection, but continue to excrete rabies virus.

Control in enzootic countries is by vaccination and destruction of stray dogs. In the UK control is by strict *quarantine regulations coupled with the vaccination of imported carnivores. While the UK is free of rabies it is against the law to vaccinate dogs, except those being taken abroad. Humans are susceptible to rabies, and if bitten by a suspected carrier, a person must receive an immediate course of vaccination and rabies antiserum. The disease is virtually always fatal once clinical signs develop. Rabies is a *notifiable disease in the UK and North America.

Rabies Act (1974) (England and Wales) An Act of Parliament repealed by the Animal Health Act (1981).

Rabies (Importation of Dogs, Cats and Other Mammals) Order (1974) (England and Wales) A Parliamentary Order, amended in 1977, that regulates the importation of all mammals that might bring rabies into the UK and lays down quarantine regulations for them. The Order empowers magistrates to fine persons who land animals illegally and to order the destruction of the animals. The *Rabies (Control) Order* (1974) contains provisions for the containment and eradication of any rabies outbreak that might occur outside quarantine premises.

racemose Resembling a bunch of grapes. The term is applied particularly to a compound gland whose secretory part consists of a number of small sacs.

rachi- (rachio-) *Prefix denoting* the spine.

radial Relating to or associated with the radius (a bone in the forelimb).

radial artery A branch of the *median artery in the lower forelimb. It runs in close relation to the radius and finally forms the deep *palmar arch in the manus.

radial nerve One of the nerves of the forelimb, extending from the *brachial plexus. It curves around the shaft of the humerus, carrying motor fibres to the extensor muscles of the elbow, carpus, and digits, and sensory fibres from parts of the front of the lower forelimb and manus. Fracture of the humerus can result in *radial paralysis.

radial paralysis Paralysis and lack of sensation affecting the muscles and skin of the forelimb supplied by the *radial nerve. In *high radial paralysis* all the muscles supplied by the nerve are affected, including the *triceps group, so that the elbow cannot be extended, and also the extensors of the carpus and the digits. As a result the paw is dragged along the floor on its dorsal surface and the limb is unable to bear any weight. Skin sensation is lost, both to this part of the paw and to the dorsal and lateral aspects of the forearm and the paw. This injury occurs commonly in small animals following road accidents, or in large animals following lengthy anaesthesia or lateral recumbency with the affected limb under the body. *Low radial paralysis* occurs when the nerve is damaged below the branches supplying the triceps muscles. Lack of sensation is similar, the animal is unable to extend the carpus and digits, and the paw 'knuckles' readily. This injury is also often related to road accidents, especially those involving fractures of the shaft of the humerus. Treatment is difficult and, in most situations, is dependent on the degree of damage to the nerve and its ability to regenerate.

radiation sickness A condition induced by excessive exposure to ionizing radiation (e.g. X-rays or radiation from radioisotopes). Radiation stops the normal regeneration of cells in the intestinal mucosa and animals lose their appetite and suffer from gastroenteritis. Also, the production of white blood cells in the bone marrow and lymph nodes is suppressed and immunity to infection is therefore compromised. Strict rules limit the exposure of humans to radiation, and animals sharing the same environment should never suffer from radiation sickness unless due to accidental exposure. Treatment is not normally feasible, although antihistamines are said to give temporary relief.

radicle (in anatomy) **1.** A small *root. **2.** The initial fibre of a nerve or the origin of a vein.

radiculitis Inflammation of the root of a nerve.

radio- *Prefix denoting* **1.** radiation. **2.** radioactive substances.

radiograph An image produced on a film by X-rays: an X-ray picture. *See* radiography.

radiography The technique of examining a body or structure by directing X-rays through it to produce images (*radiographs* or *radiograms*) on photographic plates or fluorescent screens (*see* fluoroscope). Tissues with high density (i.e. *radio-opaque* tissues), such as bone, absorb the X-rays to a greater extent than soft tissues, such as muscle; gases are virtually 'transparent' to X-rays, i.e. *radiolucent*. The radiograph is similar to a photographic negative; after developing, radiolucent tissues (e.g. air-filled lungs) appear dark, whereas radio-opaque tissues (e.g. bone) appear white. *Contrast media may be employed in more specialized investigations, e.g. *myelography or *pyelography. Radiography is used primarily in the diagnosis of bone fractures and lesions, gastrointestinal blockages, tumours, and stones (calculi) in the kidney, urinary bladder, or gall-bladder. Powerful (and costly) equipment is required for the radiography of deep internal structures in large animals; low-powered apparatus is suitable for small animals and for the limbs, head, and neck of large animals. *See also* radiology; X-rays.

radioimmunoassay A technique for identifying and measuring the concentration of antibodies in blood, in which a radioactive *tracer is used to label the antibodies. The tracer is injected into the animal and is incorporated into certain antigens; for example, radioactive iodine is incorporated into insulin. The labelled antigens form complexes with specific antibodies, where these are present. A blood sample is subsequently analysed (e.g. by *chromatography or *electrophoresis) and the labelled complexes detected and quantified by the presence and amount of radioactivity they emit.

radioisotope An *isotope of an element that emits alpha, beta, or gamma radiation during its decay into another element. Artificial radioisotopes, produced by bombarding elements with beams of neutrons, are used as *tracers and as sources of radiation in *radiotherapy.

radiology The study and use of radiation and radioactive substances. This includes the use of diagnostic X-rays in *radiography, the therapeutic use of ionizing radiation to treat disease (*see* radiotherapy), and the experimental and diagnostic use of radioisotopes introduced into the body.

radiotherapy The use of ionizing radiation for the treatment of disease, particularly tumours. Although its availability is limited in veterinary medicine, radiotherapy is effective against certain tumours. Radioactive implants may be used for the control of equine *sarcoids, while local application of radioactive isotopes to *squamous cell carcinomas in horses and cattle can produce remission. In dogs and cats, radiation produced by cobalt units or powerful X-ray machines is used to treat various tumours, with varying degrees of success.

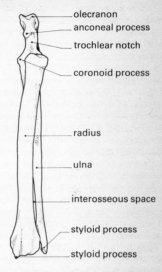

Left radius and ulna of the dog
(cranial aspect)

radius (*pl.* **radii**) One of the bones of the forearm (see illustration). The head of the radius contributes to the *elbow joint, while its lower end articulates with the bones of the *carpus forming the *radiocarpal joint*. It also forms upper and lower *radioulnar joints* with the *ulna when this is fully developed as a separate bone, as in carnivores and the pig.

rafoxanide An anthelmintic used for the routine treatment of fluke infestations in sheep and cattle. It also has good activity against the nematode *Haemonchus contortus*, and against larval stages of the *sheep nostril fly, *Oestrus ovis*. Administered orally and absorbed from the gastrointestinal tract, rafoxanide is eliminated unchanged from the body with a half-life of approximately 5–10 days. It

ragwort poisoning

kills adult liver flukes (*Fasciola hepatica*) and immature flukes over 4–6 weeks of age. Toxicity is low, although high doses in sheep may cause ocular damage. Rafoxanide should not be used in lactating animals if the milk is to be sold for human consumption.

ragwort poisoning A toxic condition caused by ingestion of the common ragwort (*Senecio jacobaea*) or other ragworts, such as the marsh ragwort (*S. aquaticus*) or Oxford ragwort (*S. squalidus*), or groundsels. In Britain this condition mainly affects cattle and horses, although sheep and poultry are occasionally affected. Toxicity is due to the presence in the plant of pyrrolizidine *alkaloids, which also occur in plants of the genus *Crotalaria*. In Britain, many pastures are contaminated with ragwort, noticeable by its yellow flowers in late summer. The plant is not particularly palatable to grazing animals so poisoning is not common provided the amount of grass in the pasture is not reduced, for instance by drought or overstocking.

However, problems do arise if pastures contaminated with ragwort are conserved as hay, silage, or grass cubes. Animals fed on this material ingest the alkaloids, which cause progressive and irreversible pathological changes in the cells and blood vessels of the liver. The walls of the central veins of the liver lobules become fibrosed producing a lesion described as veno-occlusive disease. The condition worsens even if further access to contaminated food is prevented. Clinical signs are variable. Some animals lose their appetite, develop diarrhoea and straining, and show impaired coordination. Cattle develop maniacal convulsions ('*mad staggers*') whereas in horses a more depressive form occurs ('*sleepy staggers*'). In some areas, grazing cattle develop a more chronic form of the disease characterized by loss of condition and abdominal distension due to the collection of fluid in the abdominal cavity.

There is no treatment and preventive measures are the sole option. The amount of ragwort in pastures may be reduced by frequent cutting or the use of selective weedkillers. Above all, the incorporation of ragwort into conserved forage must be avoided because the alkaloids are not destroyed by the heating that occurs during conservation.

rain scald A skin condition of horses in temperate climates, associated with exposure to prolonged wet weather. It involves infection with the filamentous actinomycete *Dermatophilus congolensis*, which causes lesions over the most exposed areas, notably the rump and back, extending downward following the natural pattern of water drainage. Exudate from the lesions solidifies into a series of hard round or oval scabs (typically 1–2 cm across), binding the coat at its base into a series of tufts; this is often more evident to the touch. Removal of the scab from an active lesion reveals pus and a raw area of skin. If the animal is kept dry the condition resolves spontaneously, the lesions drying and the scabs detaching the coat as they come away from the skin. Similar lesions may occur on other parts of the body, especially when these are subject to repeated and prolonged wetting; for example the face and lower limbs of horses grazing wet pasture. Local treatment with antibiotics, such as *chloramphenicol, may be beneficial; systemic antibiotic treatment has been used to treat severe generalized infections.

rale An abnormal *sound arising from the lower respiratory tract, due to some pathological condition interfering with the normal flow of air. Such sounds may be classified as *dry* or *moist* (*see also* rhonchus) and as *inspiratory* or *expiratory*.

ram epididymitis (ovine epididymitis) A disease of sheep, occurring worldwide but especially important in Australia and New Zealand, caused by the bacterium *Brucella ovis*. It is characterized by *epididymitis, scrotal swelling, and infertility in the ram, and occasionally placental lesions and abortion in ewes. The semen is infective and transmission is venereal. Vaccines are available, but infected rams are best culled. *See also* brucellosis.

ramus (*pl.* **rami**) **1.** A branch, especially of a nerve fibre or blood vessel. **2.** A process projecting from a bone, e.g. the ramus of the *mandible.

ranitidine An *antihistamine that acts as a reversible competitive antagonist of histamine at H_2 receptors. It has similar actions to but greater potency than *cimetidine. Tradename: **Zantac**.

ranula A small cyst found beneath the tongue and due to blockage of a salivary duct. The condition most commonly affects the sublingual gland, which may become obstructed by trauma or inflammation. The condition often resolves spontaneously but, if persistent or troublesome, a simple incision releases the contained saliva. Recurrence may indicate surgical restructuring of the salivary duct.

rape poisoning Any of various toxic conditions arising from the ingestion of rape (*Brassica napus*), which is cultivated in cool temperate regions as a forage crop and for its oilseeds. Rape has been incriminated in four distinct toxic syndromes. Firstly, cattle grazing on rape pasture have developed a respiratory syndrome, of which the clinical signs are increased heart rate, jaundice, dyspnoea, and paresis of the

gastrointestinal tract. Affected animals are shown to have oedema and emphysema of the lungs, a pale friable liver, and gastrointestinal irritation. Secondly, there is a nervous syndrome (or *rape blindness*) in which animals become blind and aggressive. Recovery usually takes 2–3 months after removal from rape pasture. Thirdly, there is the haemolytic anaemia and haemoglobinuria ('redwater disease') characteristic of other forms of *brassica poisoning; the mucous membranes are jaundiced, the liver has moderate to severe necrosis, and the kidneys are congested. Finally, fowls on rape pasture can suffer a haemorrhagic syndrome in which the blood does not clot.

raphe A line, ridge, seam, or crease in a tissue or organ, especially the line marking the junction of two embryologically distinct parts that have fused to form a single structure in the adult. For example, the scrotal raphe is the ridge in the middle of the scrotum.

rarefaction Thinning of bony tissue due to withdrawal of its mineral content. Various conditions lead to rarefaction of bone, including mineral deficiency (especially of phosphate) and vitamin D deficiency. High-yielding dairy cattle are susceptible to rarefaction of bones because of the high mineral demands of milk production.

rash A temporary skin eruption, usually typified by red inflamed spots (*papules), which may occur on any part of the skin but is usually observed on hairless areas. It may be due, for example, to allergic dermatitis or contact sensitivity.

rat-bite fever (sodokosis) A disease of humans, contracted by the bite of a rat, due to infection by either the bacterium *Spirillum minus*, which causes ulceration of the skin and recurrent fever, or by the bacterium *Streptobacillus moniliformis*, which causes inflammation of the skin, muscular pains, and vomiting. Both infections respond well to penicillin.

ration *See* diet.

rattlebox Any of various toxic North American plants belonging to either of the genera *Crotalaria* (*see* ragwort poisoning) or *Sesbania*. The latter are found in Gulf coastal states. They contain a toxic saponin that causes gastrointestinal haemorrhage; clinical signs are haemorrhagic diarrhoea, rapid respiration, fast irregular pulse, subnormal temperature, coma, and death. Treatment is of the clinical signs.

rattleweed A North American toxic plant belonging to the genus *Crotalaria* (*see* ragwort poisoning).

RCVS *See* Royal College of Veterinary Surgeons.

reagin *Antibody that is able to bind to *mast cells and thus mediate Type I *hypersensitivity.

receptor 1. (in physiology) A sensory nerve ending or a cell or group of cells specialized to detect changes and trigger impulses in the sensory nervous system. Receptors either simply detect touch, as in the skin, or chemical substances, as in the nose and tongue, or sound or light, as in the ear and eye. *See* exteroceptor; interoceptor; mechanoreceptor; proprioceptor. **2.** (in virology) A molecule at the cell surface, usually a membrane *glycolipid or *glycoprotein, to which a particular *virus can bind specifically to initiate its infective cycle.

recess (in anatomy) A hollow chamber or a depression in an organ or other part.

recessive Describing an *allele that, in combination with a *dominant allele, shows no effect.

recombinant DNA *DNA formed by joining DNA strands from different sources. Typically, a DNA fragment, containing a desired gene for instance, is inserted into an existing strand using a *plasmid as a vehicle. This technique is commonly used in *genetic engineering.

recombination The rearrangement of genes that can occur when gametes are formed during meiosis. This is caused by the interchange of DNA segments between homologous pairs of chromosomes (*crossing over*) and results in offspring with combinations of characters that differ from either parent.

recruitment (in physiology) The phenomenon whereby an increase in the strength of a stimulus or repetition of the stimulus will cause increasing numbers of nerve cells to respond.

rect- (recto-) *Prefix denoting* the rectum.

rectum The terminal part of the large intestine. In mammals it succeeds the descending colon (small colon in the horse) and leads to the anal canal (*see* anus). In birds it is the main portion of the large intestine, succeeding the caeca and terminating in the cloaca. *See also* alimentary tract.

rectus (*pl.* **recti**) Any of several straight muscles. Rectus muscles are among the extrinsic muscles of the *eye. The *rectus femoris* forms part of the *quadriceps femoris. *See also* rectus abdominis.

rectus abdominis One of a pair of long flat muscles on either side of the *linea alba in the thoracic and abdominal walls. They contract to flex the vertebral column and to increase intra-abdominal pressure. Both their surfaces are covered by external and internal sheaths, formed by the *aponeuroses of the other abdominal muscles. These sheaths are important surgically in closing abdominal incisions.

recurrent (in anatomy) Describing a structure, such as a nerve or blood vessel, that turns back on its course, forming a loop.

recurrent laryngeal nerve A branch of the *vagus nerve. On the right side it arises in the caudal part of the neck and curves around the right subclavian artery. On the left side it arises within the thorax and curves around the ligamentum arteriosum before re-entering the neck. On both sides it runs cranially in the groove between trachea and oesophagus, supplying branches to both. At the larynx it supplies all the laryngeal muscles, except the cricothyroid, and supplies sensation to the mucosa of the glottis and lower regions.

red blood cell *See* erythrocyte.

redia (*pl.* **rediae**) An intermediate larval stage in the life cycle of a *fluke. It typically has a long sac-like body, small mouth, and a short intestine, and develops from germinal cells within the inert *sporocyst in the intermediate host. It gives rise asexually either to more rediae or to the final larval stage, the *cercaria. *See also* miracidium.

redleg syndrome A disease of domestic and edible frogs that occurs especially after periods of stress and malnutrition. Its immediate cause appears to be a skin infection with *Pseudomonas or *Proteus bacteria, which causes ulceration and haemorrhage of the legs and abdomen. Oxy-

tetracycline appears to be an effective treatment, although prevention by proper care and feeding, is preferable.

red maple poisoning A toxic condition of horses due to the consumption of a large volume of fresh, wilted, or dried leaves of the red maple (*Acer rubrum*), a broad-leaved deciduous tree found in the USA, primarily east of the Mississippi. The toxic principle is not known, but it causes *methaemoglobinaemia, Heinz body anaemia, and haemolysis. The animal exhibits icterus and cyanosis, and acquires a brownish coloration of the blood and urine. Treatment is symptomatic but is usually unrewarding.

red mite A bloodsucking mite, *Dermanyssus gallinae*, that is one of the principal ectoparasites of poultry. Domestic fowls and turkeys are chiefly affected, although other birds are susceptible. The mite can also cause irritation to humans and other mammals. Visible to the naked eye, the mites live in cracks and crevices and only move onto their host to feed, usually at night. Immediately after a blood meal the mites appear bright red, becoming dark brown and eventually greyish white as digestion proceeds. The eggs are laid in crevices and hatch after 2 days into minute mites. In summer the life cycle can be completed very quickly (1 week) and heavy infestations develop rapidly. Tell-tale signs of infestation are reddish-black spots of mite excrement on woodwork or on eggs. However, care must be taken to distinguish the mite from other, nonparasitic, mites that may inhabit feed or litter.
Red-mite infestation can affect egg output, cause unthriftiness in young birds, and force brooding hens to desert the nest. In severe cases there may be anaemia and even death. Control centres on eradicating the mite from poultry houses. This is best undertaken when birds have been

reduction

removed. All fittings and nest boxes should be dismantled and cleaned, all litter removed for burning, and the house vacuum-cleaned. Various pesticides can be used for space spraying, including pyrethrum, malathion, dichlorvos, and gamma-benzene hexachloride (BHC). Certain products can be used with the birds in situ, for example in battery units, but recommendations must be strictly followed.

reduction (in surgery) The restoration of a displaced organ or part of the body to its normal anatomical position by manipulation or surgery. The fragments of a broken bone are reduced before a splint is applied; a dislocated joint is reduced to its normal seating; or a hernia is reduced when the displaced organ or tissue is returned to its normal position. Other examples are the straightening of an intussusception in the intestine, the return of a prolapsed uterus or anus, or the respositioning of a torsioned uterus or stomach.

reduction division The first division of *meiosis, in which the chromosome number is halved. The term is sometimes used as a synonym for the whole of meiosis.

reduplication Doubling or splitting of the normal heart sounds heard on auscultation. It usually occurs when the ventricles contract asynchronously owing to partial block of the conducting fibres in the heart muscle. Other causes include *Dirofilaria* infection in the dog and pulmonary *emphysema in the horse.

redwater fever *See* babesiosis.

reflex An automatic or involuntary activity brought about by relatively simple nervous connections, without consciousness being necessarily involved (*see* reflex arc). Thus a painful stimulus to the foot will produce

the reflex of withdrawing the limb before the brain has time to receive the information and send a message to the mucles involved.

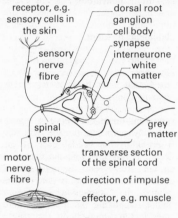

A reflex arc

reflex arc The nervous circuit involved in a *reflex. At its simplest it comprises a receptor organ linked to a sensory neurone, which in turn is linked at a synapse in the central nervous system with a motor neurone, which supplies the effector organ, for example a muscle or gland (see illustration). Thus in a simple reflex arc, such as the patellar reflex (or 'knee jerk'), only two neurones are involved, but in other reflexes several additional *interneurones may also take part.

reflux A backflow of liquid, against its normal direction of movement.

refractory Unyielding or resistant: applied to a disease or condition that fails to respond to therapy.

refractory period (in neurology) The time needed for *repolarization of a nerve cell that has just transmitted a nerve impulse or of a muscle fibre that has just contracted. During the refractory period a normal stimulus will not bring about excitation of the cell.

regional anaesthesia *See* anaesthesia.

Registered Animal Nursing Auxiliary (RANA) *See* veterinary nurse.

Register of Veterinary Surgeons A list, maintained by the *Royal College of Veterinary Surgeons under the Veterinary Surgeons Act 1966, of persons who may use the title *veterinary surgeon. The Register has three categories of members of the College. The *General List* contains the names of those persons who gained their qualification at a UK or Irish university or at a university or veterinary school within the EEC. The *Commonwealth List* comprises the names of those whose qualifications were obtained at the Universities of Guelph, Murdoch, Saskatchewan, Melbourne, Queensland, Sydney, or Massey or whose basic qualifications were obtained elsewhere in the Commonwealth and were supplemented by passing the statutory examination for membership of the Royal College. The *Foreign List* contains the names of those whose qualifications were obtained at the University of Pretoria or whose basic qualifications were obtained in a foreign country and were supplemented by successfully taking the statutory examination for membership of the Royal College.

regurgitation 1. The return of undigested material from the stomach to the mouth (*see* rumination; vomiting). **2.** The flowing back of a liquid in a direction opposite to the normal one, as when blood surges back through a defective valve in the heart.

relapse The return of disease signs after apparent recovery, or the wors-

ening of an apparently recovering patient's condition during the course of an illness.

relative breeding value *See* breeding value.

relaxant An agent that reduces tension, usually of muscles. Certain muscle relaxants act on skeletal muscle (e.g. *suxamethonium, *curare), others act on smooth muscle as *spasmolytics, *vasodilators, or *bronchodilators (e.g. *atropine and *clenbuterol).

relaxation (in physiology) The diminution of tension in a muscle, which occurs when it ceases to contract: the state of a resting muscle.

relaxin A hormone, produced by the ovary prior to parturition, that causes changes in connective tissue proteins resulting in slackening of the pelvic ligaments and an increase in the diameter of the birth canal.

remission The temporary abatement of clinical signs during the course of a disease.

renal Relating to or affecting the kidneys.

renal artery Either of the pair of large arteries that arises from the abdominal aorta to supply the kidneys.

renal corpuscle Part of a *nephron in the kidney comprising the *glomerulus and the surrounding glomerular capsule.

renal tubule The tubular portion of a *nephron in the kidney through which water and various dissolved substances are reabsorbed back into the blood.

renin

renin An enzyme that is released from the juxtaglomerular complex of kidney in response to a fall in blood pressure and causes the formation of angiotensin I from its precursor. *See* angiotensin II.

rennin An endopeptidase enzyme (*see* peptidase) that is secreted by the gastric mucosa of young animals to catalyse the clotting of milk in the stomach. In the presence of calcium ions, rennin hydrolyses caseinogen to para-*casein. An extract (*rennet*) prepared from calf's stomach and containing rennin is important in the manufacture of cheese.

reovirus A family and genus of RNA *viruses, distinguished by having double-stranded RNA (all other RNA viruses are single-stranded). The reoviruses have an enveloped icosahedral *capsid containing segmented RNA. There are three main genera: the *orbiviruses, reoviruses, and *rotaviruses. Some are important pathogens of dogs and cats.

replication The process by which *DNA makes copies of itself when the cell divides. The two strands of the DNA molecule unwind and each strand directs the synthesis of a new strand complementary to itself (see illustration).

repolarization The process in which the membrane of an excitable cell, i.e. nerve or muscle, returns to its normal electrically charged state after an *action potential, during which a temporary change in the molecular structure of the membrane allows a surge of ions across the membrane. During repolarization ions diffuse back to restore the charge and the cell becomes ready to transmit further impulses. *See* refractory period.

reproductive system The group of organs concerned with reproduction.

In male **mammals** these include the *testis (gonad), the *epididymis, *ductus deferens, and *urethra (ducts), the *ampulla of the ductus deferens, *seminal vesicles, and *prostate and *bulbourethral glands (accessory glands), and the *penis (copulatory organ). The female equivalents are the *ovary, *uterine tube, *uterus, *vagina, and *vestibule; the female accessory glands are limited to the *vestibular glands. In **birds** the male system includes the testis, epididymis, ductus deferens, *cloaca, and *phallus. The female system includes a single ovary, oviduct, and the cloaca. See illustration.

resection Surgical removal of part of an organ or other body structure. The term is commonly applied to the soft palate, external ear, or parts of the gut.

reserpine An alkaloid, obtained from the roots of the shrubs *Rauwolfia serpentina* and *R. vomitoria*, used as a rodenticide. Reserpine depletes storage granules of noradrenaline at sympathetic nerve endings and acts on serotonin stores in the central nervous system. Species vary in their susceptibility, with rodents, dogs, and horses more susceptible than cats and poultry. Signs of toxicity in dogs are dullness, diarrhoea, and respiratory and circulatory failure; horses experience violent colic. In poultry reserpine has been used as a tranquillizer and hypotensive agent. Direct-acting *sympathomimetic drugs (e.g. metaraminol or amphetamines) should be used to treat toxicity, combined with long-term nursing (fluids, warmth, etc.), since reserpine has a prolonged action. Tradename: **Betakil**.

residual volume The volume of air that remains in the lungs after maximal expiration. This volume is increased in *emphysema.

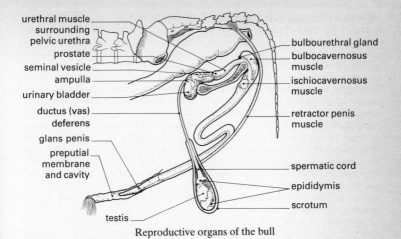

urethral muscle surrounding pelvic urethra
prostate
seminal vesicle
ampulla
urinary bladder
ductus (vas) deferens
glans penis
preputial membrane and cavity
testis

bulbourethral gland
bulbocavernosus muscle
ischiocavernosus muscle
retractor penis muscle
spermatic cord
epididymis
scrotum

Reproductive organs of the bull

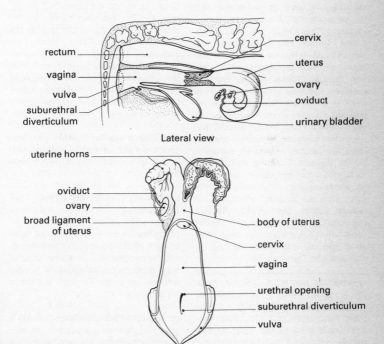

rectum
vagina
vulva
suburethral diverticulum

cervix
uterus
ovary
oviduct
urinary bladder

Lateral view

uterine horns
oviduct
ovary
broad ligament of uterus

body of uterus
cervix
vagina
urethral opening
suburethral diverticulum
vulva

Dorsal view with vagina and right horn of the uterus opened
Reproductive tract of the cow

713

resistance The degree of *immunity displayed by the body. *See also* drug resistance.

resolution 1. The stage during which inflammation gradually disappears. **2.** The degree to which individual details can be distinguished by the eye, as through a *microscope or from a *radiograph.

resorption Loss of substance through physiological or pathological means; for example, the loss of an early embryo by absorption of the embryonic tissues into the maternal tissues. In this case there is little loss of tissue remnants to the exterior.

respiration 1. The process of gaseous exchange between an organism and its environment. *External respiration* involves *breathing, in which air passes into and out of the lungs; oxygen diffuses from the alveoli of the lungs into the capillaries, while carbon dioxide diffuses in the opposite direction. *Internal respiration* involves gaseous exchange between the blood and the tissues. Blood transports the gases between the lungs and the tissues; its carrying capacity, particularly for oxygen, is greatly increased by the pigment *haemoglobin. **2.** The metabolic processes inside living cells by which organic compounds are broken down to simpler substances to release energy (*see* ATP). Aerobic organisms utilize oxygen to oxidize foodstuffs to carbon dioxide and water (*aerobic respiration*) via *glycolysis and the *Krebs cycle.

respiratory centre A collective term for a group of centres within the brainstem controlling respiration. The main inspiratory and expiratory centres are located in the reticular formation of the *medulla oblongata. They are stimulated alternately by the levels of carbon dioxide and, to a lesser extent, oxygen in the blood and

excite the muscles of inspiration and expiration respectively. Additional centres, for example the *apneustic centre* and the *pneumotaxic centre*, govern the character of breathing.

respiratory chain (electron transport chain) A sequence of biochemical reduction-oxidation reactions that forms the final stage of aerobic cellular *respiration. It results in the transfer of electrons or hydrogen atoms derived from the *Krebs cycle to molecular oxygen, with the formation of water. At the same time it conserves energy from food (or in plants from light) in the form of *ATP. The chain comprises a series of electron carriers that undergo reversible reduction-oxidation reactions, accepting electrons and donating them to the next carrier in the chain. This process is coupled to the formation of ATP, which is exchanged for ADP across the membrane of the mitochondria, in which the components of the respiratory chain are located. An electron transport chain also takes part in photosynthesis in green plants.

respiratory quotient (RQ) The ratio of the volume of carbon dioxide produced to the volume of oxygen utilized.

respiratory syncytial virus *See* pneumovirus.

response The way in which the body or part of the body reacts to a *stimulus. For example, a nerve impulse may produce the response of a contraction in a muscle that the nerve supplies.

restriction endonuclease One of a group of *deoxyribonuclease enzymes found in bacteria that hydrolyse *DNA only at a particular sequence of *nucleotides. These enzymes are used in the isolation and manipulation of specific DNA fragments in *genetic engineering.

resuscitation The process of restoring an animal from apparent death or unconsciousness, due either to cessation of breathing (*apnoea) or *cardiac arrest.

Resuscitation involving some form of *artificial respiration is most often employed during general *anaesthesia when the action of the anaesthetic on the respiratory centres in the brain causes impairment or cessation of breathing.

Cardiac arrest can be treated by cardiac massage, involving manual compression of the thoracic wall directly over each side of the heart. This should be started promptly, and combined with active artificial respiration if the animal is under general anaesthesia. If no heartbeat returns within 2 minutes, emergency *thoracotomy is required in order to facilitate direct cardiac massage. If this fails, adrenaline can be injected into the heart. Coupled with cardiac massage, this may re-establish cardiac contractions, or it may result in the initiation of ineffective cardiac *fibrillation. In this case, an electrical defibrillator (*see* defibrillation) may restore a normal heart rhythm. If circulatory function is not restored within 4 minutes, the likelihood of severe brain damage is high. The state of tissue oxygenation can be judged approximately by noting the colour of mucosae, for example the tongue.

rete A network of blood vessels, nerve fibres, or other strands of interlacing tissue in the structure of an organ. The *rete testis* is a network of tubules conducting sperm from the seminiferous tubules of the *testis to the ductuli efferentes.

retention of placenta Failure of the placenta (afterbirth or 'cleansing') to be expelled normally at or shortly after *parturition (birth). There is an increased risk of *metritis and/or uterine necrosis if the afterbirth is not expelled at the normal time, which varies with species. Since most animals eat the afterbirth of their young at the time of birth or shortly afterwards it may be difficult to determine if any remains attached to the uterus. Careful observation is necessary to diagnose quickly and treat promptly and hence avoid complications.

The afterbirth of the **cow** should be expelled within 12 hours of parturition; retention occurs in about 7% of deliveries. Treatment by manual removal is rapidly becoming unpopular because of the increased risk of metritis, abscess formation, and uterine perforation. Normal care and observation coupled with antibiotic therapy is now the preferred course of action. Preventive measures include good nutrition during pregnancy, avoidance of stress and bacterial infections, and maintainance of good hygiene at parturition.

In the **bitch**, expulsion of the afterbirth should occur within 15 minutes of each pup being delivered. Persistence of the normal green/black postparturient vaginal discharge beyond 12 hours indicates that some or all of the afterbirth has been retained. Metritis, uterine necrosis and *toxaemia may result if the bitch if left untreated. *Oxytocin administered by injection and followed by gentle manual removal through the vagina is usually successful. If unsuccessful, surgical removal may be necessary. In either case antibiotic therapy to prevent infection is recommended.

In the **mare**, the foetal membranes are normally expelled very soon after foaling. If the membranes are still retained 4 hours after foaling, a close watch should be kept on the mare for any sign of illness or depression. The diffuse attachment of the placenta to the endometrium allows acute *metritis to develop very quickly following the retention of even a small area of foetal membrane. For this reason the membranes should be examined for missing sections, even when expelled apparently normally. Acute metritis can lead to *septicaemia, in turn causing acute *laminitis. Therapy should be commenced if clinical signs appear.

reticular fibres Microscopic almost nonelastic branching fibres of *connective tissue that join together to form a delicate supportive meshwork around blood vessels, muscle fibres, glands, and nerves. They are composed of a collagen-like protein (*reticulin*) and are particularly common in lymph nodes, the spleen, liver, kidneys, and muscles.

reticular formation A network of nerve fibres and nuclei in the *brainstem that makes connections with the spinal cord, cerebellum, cerebrum, and cranial nerves.

reticular groove (oesophageal groove) A groove in the right wall of the *reticulum in the ruminant stomach, that closes reflexly during suckling to form a canal. This directs milk from the end of the oesophagus (cardia) to the omasal groove and into the abomasum, thus bypassing the reticulorumen. It forms the first part of the ventricular groove, which also comprises the omasal and abomasal grooves. Reflex closure of the groove depends on receptors, located chiefly in the pharynx and upper oesophagus, that are sensitive to fluid and certain chemicals. The motor components of the reflex involve the vagus nerve.

The reflex is chiefly of importance in the young ruminant, before it develops fermentative digestive in the reticulorumen. It is activated in the young in response to the taking of milk or other fluids to satisfy hunger.

Water drunk to satisfy thirst does not activate the reflex and so enters the rumen. The reflex may occasionally be exhibited by adult ruminants, for instance when liquid medication is administered. In cattle sodium bicarbonate and in sheep copper sulphate solution activate the reflex very effectively.

reticulocyte An immature *erythrocyte. Reticulocytes differentiate from normoblasts and mature into erythrocytes (*see* haemopoiesis). In regenerative *anaemia they may enter the circulation in appreciable numbers.

reticuloendothelial system The mononuclear phagocyte system; *see* macrophage.

reticuloendotheliosis An abnormality in the *reticuloendothelial system. In veterinary medicine the term has been widely used to describe a particular disorder of bone-marrow function in cats, *feline reticuloendotheliosis*. This is considered to form part of the complex of feline myeloproliferative disorders, the majority of which are associated with *feline leukaemia virus. Reticuloendotheliosis in cats is characterized by the presence in the blood of leucocytes with a 'primitive' or undifferentiated appearance.

reticulum 1. The most forward chamber of the ruminant *stomach, lying almost in the midline in the front of the abdomen, in contact with the liver and diaphragm (see illustration). The reticulum communicates freely with the *rumen via the *ruminoreticular orifice*, which is bounded by the *ruminoreticular fold*; for this reason, reticulum and rumen are sometimes jointly referred to as the *reticulorumen*. The oesophagus opens into the reticulum at the cardia, located at the top of the *reticular groove; this extends down to the reticulo-omasal orifice and opens into

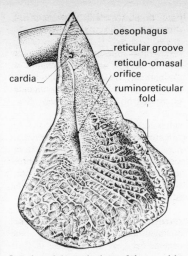

Interior of the reticulum of the ox with reticular groove, seen from left

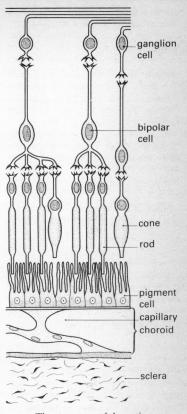

The structure of the retina

the omasum. Closure of this groove effectively bypasses the reticulum and rumen. The lining of the reticulum is raised into folds, about 1 cm high, forming a honeycomb pattern over the surface. Foreign bodies, such as nails and wire, are often swallowed by cattle and commonly lodge in the reticulum; they may perforate the reticular wall, the diaphragm, or even the pericardium. **2.** A network of tubules or blood vessels. *See* endoplasmic reticulum; sarcoplasmic reticulum.

retin- (retino-) *Prefix denoting* the retina.

retina The light-sensitive layer that lines the interior of the *eye, consisting of an outer pigment layer and an inner nervous layer. This contains specialized neuroepithelial cells, the rods and cones, which are sensitive to dim and bright light respectively. The greatest concentration of cones occurs in the *macula of the retina. Light incident on the rods and cones causes nerve impulses to be transmitted via the bipolar cells to the ganglion layer; this contains large neurones whose axons converge within the retina at the *optic disc, forming the *optic nerve (see illustration).

retinal (retinene) The aldehyde of retinol (*vitamin A). *See also* rhodopsin.

retinal atrophy Degeneration of the light-receptive cells of the retina. Nutritional deficiency, especially of vitamin A, may be an underlying cause. *Progressive retinal atrophy is

retinene

an important inherited disease in certain breeds of dog.

retinene *See* retinal.

retinitis Inflammation of the *retina. It occurs in a variety of infectious disease, such as *toxoplasmosis, canine *distemper, and bacterial *septicaemia. Fibrosis of the lesions causes scarring, but provided the scars are small vision is not noticeably impaired.

retinol *See* vitamin A.

retinopathy Any disease of the retina, usually of a degenerative character.

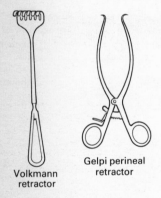

Volkmann retractor

Gelpi perineal retractor

Examples of retractors

retractor A surgical instrument used to expose the operative site by holding overlying tissue away from the area. There are many different types and sizes of retractor; some are hand-held, for instance Lagenbeck or Volkmann retractors, others are self-retaining, such as Gelpi or Weitlaner retractors (see illustration).

retro- *Prefix denoting* at the back or behind. Examples: *retrobulbar* (at the

back of the eyeball); *retroperitoneal* (behind the peritoneum).

retrograde Going backwards, or moving in the opposite direction to the normal. Damage to the axon of a neurone results in retrograde changes in the cell body and dendrites.

retropharyngeal abscess An *abscess of the retropharyngeal lymph node at the back of the throat. It may arise from the spread of infection in cases of *pharyngitis or *tonsillitis, or occur in horses suffering from *strangles.

retrovirus A family of RNA *viruses distinguished by possessing the enzyme *reverse transcriptase in their *virion. This enzyme transcribes the single-stranded RNA molecules of the virus, first into an RNA-DNA hybrid and then into a double-stranded DNA molecule; this can then integrate into the DNA of the host cell, establishing the *provirus state. There are three subfamilies: the lentiviruses, spumiviruses, and *oncoviruses, the last of which exhibit *oncogenic behaviour. The family includes the *feline leukaemia virus and the human AIDS virus.

reverse transcriptase A *polymerase enzyme that uses an *RNA molecule as a template for the synthesis of a *DNA molecule. Such enzymes are known only in the *retroviruses, where they are present in the *virion and bring about the production of a DNA copy of the viral RNA.

R-factor A *plasmid carrying one or more genes conferring resistance to certain drugs. *See also* drug resistance.

rhabdomyoma A benign tumour of striated muscle origin. This and its malignant counterpart (*rhabdomyosarcoma*) are rare in domestic species, although their incidence is greater in juvenile animals. They have been reported arising in skeletal muscles, in the heart, and in the urinary bladder. Due to their diffuse and infiltrative nature, surgical resection of these tumours must be radical, and the prognosis for the malignant form is poor.

rhabdomyosarcoma *See* rhabdomyoma.

rhabdovirus A family of RNA *viruses characterized by having a *virion with a bullet-shaped envelope and which contain segmented negative-stranded RNA. The two main genera are the *lyssaviruses and *vesiculoviruses, which include, respectively, the viruses responsible for *rabies and *vesicular stomatitis.

rheo- *Prefix denoting* **1.** a flow of liquid. **2.** an electric current.

rheumatism Any disorder involving inflammation or pain in the joints or muscles. It cannot be properly applied to animals because of the lack of subjective symptomatology.

rheumatoid arthritis A form of *arthritis in which there is inflammation of a joint or joints with progressive erosion of the articular cartilages and adjacent bone. Eventually it leads to lameness or severe deformity. It is believed to be an *autoimmune disease. The disease occurs rarely in dogs and cats, although it is an important cause of disability in humans. *See also* polyarthritis.

rhin- (rhino-) *Prefix denoting* the nose.

rhinencephalon The part of the *cerebrum in the brain that originally evolved in connection with the sense of smell. The basal part is still olfactory in function and includes the *olfactory bulb, olfactory tracts, and *piriform lobe. The limbic part, which includes the *hippocampus and its connections (i.e. the *limbic system), has lost its olfactory function and become associated with emotion and memory.

rhinitis Inflammation of the mucous membrane of the nose. There are various acute forms of rhinitis caused by virus infections, including feline rhinotracheitis (*see* cat flu) and *infectious bovine rhinotracheitis. Rhinitis also occurs in horses suffering from *strangles. *Atrophic rhinitis is an important cause of economic loss in pigs. Mycotic rhinitis is caused by fungi, such as *Aspergillus* spp. (*see* aspergillosis).

rhinopneumonitis Inflammation of the lungs (*pneumonitis) and the nose or nasal passages. *See also* equine rhinopneumonitis.

rhinosporidiosis A chronic infection of humans, horses, mules, cattle, goats, dogs, and waterfowl characterized by the formation of polyps on the mucous membranes, usually around the eyes and interior of the nose and nasopharynx but also at other sites. It is caused by the fungus *Rhinosporidium seeberi*, and diagnosis is made by microscopic examination of the polyps, which contain giant sporangia (200–400 μm in diameter) filled with thousands of endospores. Treatment consists of surgical removal of the polyps and cauterization of their bases.

rhinotracheitis Inflammation of the nose and trachea. *See also* cat flu; infectious bovine rhinotracheitis; turkey rhinotracheitis.

rhinovirus A genus of the *picornavirus family. It includes viruses that infect horses and cattle.

Rhipicephalus

Rhipicephalus A genus of hard *ticks found in Africa and southern Europe. They are ectoparasites of humans but mainly attack domestic animals, transmitting many diseases, such as *louping-ill in sheep, *East Coast fever, *babesiosis, and *Nairobi sheep disease, as well as bacterial diseases.

rhiz- (rhizo-) *Prefix denoting* a root.

Rhizopus A genus of saprophytic fungi, some of which are opportunistic pathogens causing forms of *mucormycosis.

Rhodococcus equi *See* Corynebacterium.

rhododendron poisoning A toxic condition caused by the ingestion of leaves and stems of *Rhododendron ponticum*, an evergreen flowering shrub commonly found in gardens and ornamental woodlands. Most cases occur in the winter months when grazing is in short supply or unobtainable due to snow cover and animals may gain access by breaking through fences. The toxicity is due to andromedotoxin, also known as grayanotoxin, which causes vomiting, colic, staggering gait, respiratory depression, and death. Cattle and goats may survive as a result of projectile vomiting, which is characteristic of rhododendron poisoning in these species. In addition to treatment of the clinical signs, the administration of 3 mg/kg of morphine may be curative.

rhodopsin (visual purple) A light-sensitive pigment occurring in the *rods of the vertebrate eye. It comprises a protein (*opsin*) combined with *retinal*, the aldehyde of retinol (*vitamin A). Bleaching of the pigment initiates the transmission of a nerve impulse to the brain. The great sensitivity of rhodopsin allows vision in dim light (night vision).

rhombencephalon The embryonic *hindbrain.

rhomboid Any of three muscles in the back (*rhomboideus thoracis*, *rhomboideus cervicis*, and *rhomboideus capitis*) that attach to the scapula.

rhonchus (*pl.* **rhonchi**) An abnormal harsh dry *sound arising from the lower respiratory tract (*see also* rale). It is caused by partial obstruction of the airway.

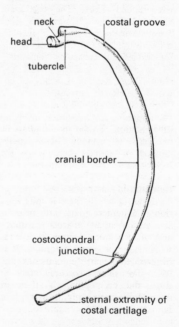

Right rib and costal cartilage of the horse (medial view)

rib A curved bar of bone forming part of the skeleton of the thorax that protects the heart and lungs and produces the movements necessary for

Number of ribs in various domestic species

Species	Total no. of pairs of ribs	True ribs	False ribs
Horse	18	8	10
Ox	13	8	5
Sheep	13	8	5
Pig	14 (15)	7	7
Dog, cat	13	9	4

respiration. The head and tubercle of each rib form joints with the vertebral column (see illustration). *True ribs* are joined directly to the sternum by their costal cartilages; in *false ribs* the costal cartilages either end freely (floating ribs) or unite together into the costal arch. The number of ribs present differs in various species (see table). In birds each rib consists of two portions – the *vertebral rib* and the the *sternal rib*. Anatomical name: **costa**.

riboflavin *See* vitamin B₂.

ribonuclease An enzyme, located in the *lysosomes of cells, that splits RNA at specific places in the molecule.

ribonucleic acid *See* RNA.

ribose A pentose sugar (i.e. one with five carbon atoms) that is a component of *RNA and several coenzymes.

ribosome A particle, consisting of RNA and protein, that occurs in cells and is the site of protein synthesis in the cell (*see* translation). Ribosomes are either attached to the *endoplasmic reticulum or free in the cytoplasm as *polysomes.

ricin *See* castor seed poisoning.

rickets A bone disease of young animals caused by deficiency of *vitamin D and/or *phosphorus. The main defect involves failure to mineralize

growing *bone so that the growthplate cartilages persist and the bone matrix (osteoid) remains uncalcified, and even unresorbed. Affected bones become distorted. Although vitamin D deficiency may be significant in animals not exposed to sunlight, phosphorus deficiency is the usual cause in animals at pasture. Lameness occurs, with enlargement of the ends of long bones. Bone abnormalities can be diagnosed by radiography, and analysis of the blood reveals abnormally low concentrations of both calcium and phosphorus (the Ca × P index falls below 30). Levels of the enzyme alkaline phosphatase increase due to its escape from the bone cells. Prevention and treatment are both successfully undertaken using vitamin D and phosphorus supplementation. An inherited form of rickets is said to occur in pigs, in which there is a congenital failure to absorb calcium from the intestine. *Compare* osteomalacia.

rickettsia (*pl.* **rickettsiae** or **rickettsias**) One of a group of obligate intracellular parasitic microorganisms, once regarded as intermediate in their properties between bacteria and viruses but now classified as *bacteria in the order Rickettsiales. They possess cytoplasmic membranes and cell walls as well as both DNA and RNA. The order includes 17 genera in three families: Rickettsiaceae, Bartonellaceae, and Anaplasmataceae. Most of the rickettsiae that infect domestic animals are known to parasitize *ticks, with the exception of

Neorickettsia helminthoeca, which has a complicated life cycle involving a trematode, salmon, and dogs (*see* salmon poisoning). The following genera are of veterinary importance: *Anaplasma*, *Haemobartonella* (or *Bartonella*), *Cowdria*, *Coxiella*, *Cytoecetes*, *Ehrlichia*, *Eperythrozoon*, and *Neorickettsia*. Various *Rickettsia* species are responsible for the *spotted fever group of diseases.

rickettsialpox *See* spotted fever.

ridge (in anatomy) A crest or a long narrow protuberance, e.g. on a bone.

Riding Establishments Acts (1964, 1970) (England and Wales) Acts of Parliament that require the keeper of a riding establishment to hold a licence (renewable annually). The Act defines such an establishment as a place where horses are kept to be let out on hire for riding or to be used in providing riding instruction in return for payment. The Act exempts army and police riding schools from having to be licensed, as well as university facilities for instructing veterinary students. Before a licence is granted, the premises must be inspected by a veterinary surgeon or practitioner who is authorized by the local authority and who is a member of the panel of inspectors maintained by the Royal College of Veterinary Surgeons and British Veterinary Association. A veterinarian may only join this panel if he or she has been qualified for five years and is in regular attendance on horses.

rifampicin (rifampin) One of the rifamycin group of antibiotics, derived from the bacterium *Streptomyces mediterranei*. It inhibits DNA-dependent RNA polymerase in microorganisms, preventing polynucleotide chain formation during RNA synthesis. It is active against Gram-positive and some Gram-negative bacteria.

However, bacterial resistance develops rapidly. The drug is given orally and, after absorption, high concentrations are found in the bile. It is used in combination with other antimicrobial agents (e.g. *isoniazid) in the treatment of tuberculosis. Side-effects are unlikely, but jaundice, hepatotoxicity, and gastrointestinal disturbances can occur. Rifampicin also has antiviral activity and its usefulness in treating viral diseases is being investigated, along with other members of the rifamycin group.

Rift Valley fever An infectious disease of sheep, goats, cattle, other ruminants, and humans characterized by fever, hepatitis, and abortion and caused by a *bunyavirus. It is prevalent in Africa south of the Sahara, but occasionally spreads into northern Africa. Young animals are particularly susceptible and may die within 24 hours of developing a fever. Adult animals have a transient fever following an incubation period of 1–4 days, and then develop diarrhoea which may involve blood loss. Pregnant animals abort. Periods of up to 20 years may elapse between major outbreaks of disease; these are usually associated with increased numbers of mosquitoes, which harbour the virus. The livers of animals which have died of Rift Valley fever have clearly visible areas of diseased tissue. Control is by vaccination of nonpregnant animals with live attenuated vaccine. The disease in humans causes symptoms resembling those of influenza and can sometimes be fatal.

rig *See* cryptorchid.

right lymphatic duct One of the principal *lymphatic vessels. It occurs on the right side and terminates in the great veins near the commencement of the cranial vena cava. In some cases it may be absent.

rigor 1. An abrupt attack of shivering in the early stages of a *fever. 2. *See* rigor mortis.

rigor mortis The stiffening of a body that occurs some hours after death. It starts to disappear after about 24 hours.

rima (in anatomy) A cleft. The *rima glottidis* is the space between the vocal margins of the *glottis.

rinderpest A contagious disease of cattle and pigs caused by a *morbillivirus and characterized by fever, erosions of the gum and lip membranes, and diarrhoea. It is endemic in Central Africa and Asia and frequently spreads into North Africa and the Middle East. Transmission is by direct contact between infected and susceptible animals. Fully susceptible animals develop a high fever after an incubation period as short as 3 days, and may die before showing any other clinical signs. The incubation period can be as long as 15 days in animals with some natural resistance. Three days after the onset of fever, small necrotic lesions develop on the inside of the lips, the gums, and hard palate. These lesions increase in size and the animals have a foul odour on their breath. Diarrhoea, usually severe, develops 2 days later and the fever subsides. Blood and shreds of intestinal lining may be seen in the diarrhoea and the animal strains, partially prolapsing the rectal mucosa. The affected animal quickly becomes dehydrated, collapses, and dies within 2 weeks of the onset of clinical signs. In endemic areas animals have a higher natural resistance, and the disease tends to be correspondingly milder. Infection with rinderpest virus reduces animals' resistance to other diseases and death may occur as a result of these secondary infections. Immunity following infection is lifelong. Control is by vaccination with a live attenuated vaccine and strict importation control of animals from enzootic areas. Rinderpest is a notifiable disease in the UK. Other name: **cattle plague**.

ringbone A condition of horses caused by bony outgrowths (exostoses) around the phalangeal bones (*see* phalanx). *High ringbone* can involve the distal first phalanx, the proximal interphalangeal (pastern) joint, and/or the proximal part of the middle phalanx. *Low ringbone* can involve the distal portion of the middle phalanx, the distal interphalangeal (coffin) joint, and/or the proximal part of the distal phalanx (pedal bone). It arises due to *periostitis, which in turn may be caused by pulling of the collateral ligaments or tendons or direct trauma. Ringbone is more common in the front feet than the hind feet, and the degree of lameness varies greatly. If the joint surface is involved (*articular ringbone*), there is likely to be more lameness and pain than if the new bone forms around the joint (*periarticular ringbone*). When the new bone is away from the joint (*nonarticular* or *false ringbone*) the lameness is even less; however, mechanical lameness may occur especially with low nonarticular ringbone. Diagnosis includes the use of radiography and nerve and articular blockade. Treatment regimes are varied, and may include rest (possibly enforced with a cast), sodium hyaluronate, polysulphated glycosaminoglycan, and, for high ringbone, surgical *arthrodesis. The prognosis is variable.

Ringer's solution A clear colourless *physiological saline solution, first formulated by the British physiologist Sydney Ringer (1835–1910). It consists of sodium chloride, potassium chloride, sodium bicarbonate, and calcium chloride prepared with recently boiled pure water.

ringwomb A condition in the ewe in which the cervix dilates not at all or only very slightly just prior to term of pregnancy, thereby preventing birth from taking place. In cases where there is slight dilatation, foetal membranes may protrude from the vulva. If no action is taken the foetus will die and decompose inside the ewe. Manual dilatation of the cervix or *Caesarean section are often the only means of saving the lamb(s).

ringworm A disease resulting from a contagious infection of the nonliving *keratin of the surface layer of the skin, hair, feathers, or nails by any of the *dermatophyte fungi. The condition is so called because of a tendency to produce circular lesions. Wild and domesticated mammals, humans, and, less commonly, birds are affected. Individual hairs become infected when the fungal *mycelium growing on the skin enters a hair follicle and extends downwards over the hair base towards its root. Further growth of that hair is then invaded, the hair emerging from the follicle covered with a layer of infective spores. Microscopic demonstration of this characteristic fungal invasion is the most reliable method of diagnosis, but the dermatophyte must be isolated in culture to be precisely identified. Sometimes infected hairs are shed, or so weakened that they break near the skin surface producing a bald patch giving the 'moth-eaten' appearance (from which the term *tinea was derived). There may be inflammation of the skin, exudation, and the formation of a scab or crust. Secondary bacterial infection can occur. The severity and duration of the disease depends upon the sensitivity of the host to metabolites liberated by the fungus and the responsiveness of the host's immune system to the infection. In some species, notably cats and rodents, infected carriers show hardly any visible sign of disease but are able to transmit their infection to humans or to other animals.

Ringworm is transmitted by direct contact with infected animals or with equipment, walls, fittings, etc., contaminated by dermatophyte spores in material shed from the infected areas of skin or hair. Spores in this material sometimes survive for several years in dry conditions and can resist mild disinfectant procedures. Contaminated buildings require vigorous cleaning; disinfection with superheated steam is effective. People in contact with infected animals should take precautions, such as promptly and thoroughly washing exposed skin and contaminated clothing with soap, detergent, or disinfectant.

Acute cases of ringworm tend to recover slowly without treatment owing to the immune response of the host. However, treatment is advisable, and the antifungal antibiotic *griseofulvin given in the feed is usually curative. If treatment is sufficiently prolonged, recovery follows, although the fungus remains in the hair for some time; the host's immune response usually prevents reinfection. Healthy but nonimmune animals are protected from infection only while receiving griseofulvin. Topical antifungal agents must penetrate surface crusts and keratin to be effective. Prevention of ringworm by vaccination, especially of cattle, has been extensively practised in the USSR and some eastern European countries, with apparent success.

ritual slaughter Special procedures for the slaughter of animals consistent with the law of certain religious faiths, particularly Judaism and Islam. In the UK, provisions in the Slaughter of Animals Act and Slaughter of Poultry Act allow Jews and Muslims to slaughter animals without prestunning; in practice, this applies to cattle, sheep, and goats. Meat slaughtered according to Jewish law is termed *kosher*; that slaughtered in accord with Islamic law is termed *halal*.

RNA (ribonucleic acid) A *polynucleotide that occurs in cells and is concerned with protein synthesis. In some viruses, RNA is also the hereditary material. RNA comprises the sugar *ribose and the bases adenine, cytosine, guanine, and uracil (*compare* DNA). *Messenger RNA* (*mRNA*) is responsible for carrying the genetic code transcribed from DNA to specialized sites (*ribosomes), where the information is translated into protein composition (*see also* transcription; translation). *Ribosomal RNA* (*rRNA*) is present in ribosomes; it is single-stranded but helical regions are formed by base pairing within the strand. *Transfer RNA* (*tRNA*) is involved in the assembly of *amino acids in a protein chain at a ribosome. Each species of tRNA is specific for a particular amino acid and bears a triplet of bases complementary with a triplet on mRNA.

roaring (whistling) A condition typically of large horses and characterized by an abnormal inspiratory noise during exercise. There may be an associated exercise intolerance. It is due to atrophy and paralysis of the laryngeal muscles resulting from a lesion of the left recurrent laryngeal nerve. The cause of this neuropathy is unknown; changes have been found in the foetus but there is conflicting evidence on the possible inherited nature of the condition. The paralysis may be complete or partial (paresis). With complete paralysis the affected arytenoid cartilage and vocal fold collapse into the laryngeal lumen (*see* larynx), especially during inspiration due to a negative pressure effect. If the arytenoid is not abducted, the vocal fold is relaxed and the ventricle of the lar-

ynx fills with air, producing further narrowing of the airway.
Diagnosis is confirmed by laryngeal asymmetry seen by endoscopy. There is no cure for the neuropathy but two surgical procedures alleviate the noise and any exercise intolerance: *ventriculectomy* (*Hobday operation*), i.e. removal of the ventricle of the larynx, or *arytenoid lateralization* (*tieback* or *Marks operation*). The latter carries a better prognosis but also additional risks of inhalational problems. Other names: **idiopathic laryngeal hemiplegia**; **idiopathic laryngeal paralysis**.

roaster A meat-type chicken, less common than the *broiler, and reared more slowly to a greater liveweight. In Britain they are of only local significance.

Robertsonian translocation A type of chromosomal *translocation very similar to *centric fusion.

Rocky Mountain spotted fever (RMSF) *See* spotted fever.

rod One of the two types of light-sensitive cells in the *retina of the eye (*compare* cone). They are sensitive to dim light and contain a pigment (*rhodopsin), which is broken down in the light and regenerated in the dark.

rodenticide A toxic agent used to kill rodents, particularly rodent pests. These agents are usually incorporated in baits. Many are toxic to other animals, including birds and fish, and recommendations for their use should be strictly adhered to. Commonly used rodenticides include *warfarin and other coumarin derivatives, fluoroacetates, *reserpine, *alpha-chloralose, *ANTU, thallium, and zinc phosphide.

rodent ulcer *See* eosinophilic granuloma complex.

Romanowsky stains A group of stains used for microscopical examination of blood cells, consisting of variable mixtures of thiazine dyes, such as azure B, with eosin. Romanowsky stains give characteristic staining patterns, on the basis of which blood cells are classified (*see* cell count). The group includes the stains of Leishmann, Wright, May-Grunwald, Giemsa, etc.

Romney Marsh disease *See* struck.

root 1. (in neurology) A bundle of nerve fibres at its emergence from the spinal cord. Each *spinal nerve has two roots: a ventral root containing motor nerve fibres and a dorsal root containing sensory fibres. The roots merge outside the cord to form mixed nerves. **2.** (in dentistry) The part of a *tooth that is not covered by enamel and is normally attached to the alveolar bone by periodontal fibres. **3.** The origin of any structure, i.e. the point at which it diverges from another structure. Anatomical name: **radix**.

rostellum (*pl.* **rostella**) A small muscular projection on the head (*scolex) of certain tapeworms that usually has numerous hooks used for attachment to the host's intestinal wall.

rostral Relating to the nose or the front-end of the head. It is applied to structures within the head; the equivalent term *cranial is applied to structures elsewhere in the body.

rostrum (*pl.* **rostra**) (in anatomy) A beaklike projection, such as that on the corpus callosum in the brain.

rotavirus A genus of the *reovirus family. It includes *viruses that cause gastrointestinal disease in bovine and equine hosts.

rotenone A naturally occurring insecticide and the active principle in derris, derived from rhizomes and roots of some leguminous plants. It is a white crystalline powder and is reconstituted in oil or spirit for the treatment of demodectic mange in dogs. It is also used to treat ear mite infestations. Its effects are not persistent, and treatment should be repeated at weekly intervals. Rotenone is unlikely to cause toxicity to mammals, although there can be transient vomiting in cats and dogs after treatment. It is extremely toxic to fish.

Rothera's test A method of testing urine (or milk) for the presence of ketones, i.e. acetone or acetoacetic acid – a sign of ketosis or diabetes mellitus. Strong ammonia is added to a sample of urine saturated with ammonium sulphate crystals and containing a small quantity of sodium nitroprusside. A purple colour confirms the presence of acetone or acetoacetic acid.

roughage A feedstuff with a high fibre content and high dry matter content, such as *straw or *hay. It sometimes also refers to other high-fibre feedstuffs, such as *silage and kale, which are more correctly termed succulents. *See* dietary fibre.

rouleau (*pl.* **rouleaux**) A cylindrical aggregate of red blood cells (erythrocytes) in which the red cells appear like coins in a pile. Rouleaux are formed spontaneously in blood (especially horse blood) in vitro. *See also* erythrocyte sedimentation rate.

round heart disease A condition of domestic fowls involving abnormality of the heart and characterized by sudden death. It mainly affects laying hens aged 6–12 months (and often younger) and is chiefly associated with Leghorn-related strains. Warning signs are uncommon, and death typically occurs after sudden activity.

Mortality can range up to 50%. The heart becomes enlarged, barrel-shaped, and discoloured. The condition principally affects birds on deep litter, and some toxic factor may be involved, but there is not thought to be an infectious agent. Other names: **barrel heart**; **egg heart**.

roundworm A common name for *nematode.

Royal College of Veterinary Surgeons (RCVS) The body that regulates the veterinary profession in the UK. It is established by Royal Charters and by the *Veterinary Surgeons Act (1966). The governing Council of the RCVS comprises members elected by the profession or appointed by the Privy Council and certain universities, and the College is administered by the Registrar, deputy Registrars, and other staff. For its functions *see* Veterinary Surgeons Act (1966). Address: 32 Belgrave Square, London, SW1X 8QP.

Royal Society for the Prevention of Cruelty to Animals (RSPCA) A British charity founded in 1824 for the purpose of preventing cruelty to animals. The Society now has a force of over 200 inspectors who investigate complaints of cruelty to animals. Veterinary advice and treatment schemes provide skilled attention for injured and sick animals at RSPCA clinics or through vouchers, issued by the branches, enabling an animal and its owner to attend the surgeries of private veterinary surgeons. Many stray and unwanted animals are temporarily accommodated at RSPCA welfare centres and often placed in new homes. Headquarters: RSPCA, Causeway, Horsham, West Sussex, RH12 1HG.

-rrhaphy *Suffix denoting* surgical sewing; suturing.

-rrhexis *Suffix denoting* splitting or rupture of a part.

-rrhoea (*US* **-rrhea**) *Suffix denoting* a flow or discharge from an organ or part.

Rubarth's disease *See* canine viral hepatitis.

rubber jaw (renal hyperparathyroidism) A sign of chronic kidney disease in dogs in which the teeth can be sprung towards each other due to softening of the mandible. Kidney disease results in an accumulation of phosphate in the blood, causing a compensatory drop in blood calcium levels. The *parathyroid glands attempt to compensate for this by mobilizing calcium from the skeleton, so that bones become demineralized; this is most evident in the bones of the skull. Although a diet with restricted phosphate levels and high calcium levels may help the condition, the underlying renal damage is usually beyond cure.

rubberweed poisoning *See* Hymenoxus poisoning.

rubefacient An agent that causes localized inflammation of the skin. Such agents include locally applied heat, camphor, iodine, turpentine, and ammonia. The rationale for their use is that the local inflammation increases the blood supply and influx of leucocytes to the area, helping combat infection and stimulating the removal of waste products.

rumen The largest chamber of the ruminant *stomach (see illustration). Occupying the left half of the abdominal cavity and extending well into the right half, the rumen is divided internally into dorsal and ventral sacs by pillars; these divisions are marked externally by right and left longitudinal and caudal grooves. The ventral

rumenitis

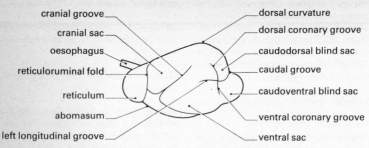

Left (parietal) surface

cranial groove — dorsal curvature
cranial sac — dorsal coronary groove
oesophagus — caudodorsal blind sac
reticuloruminal fold — caudal groove
reticulum — caudoventral blind sac
abomasum — ventral coronary groove
left longitudinal groove — ventral sac

External features of the reticulorumen in a sheep's stomach

sac is particularly large in the sheep and goat. To the rear, the dorsal and ventral sacs lead to the caudodorsal and caudoventral blind sacs respectively; these are demarcated by dorsal and ventral coronary grooves and pillars. At the front, again both dorsal and ventral sacs end blindly – in the cranial sac and ruminal recess respectively; these are demarcated by the cranial groove and pillar. At the front the rumen opens into the *reticulum via the ruminoreticular orifice, which is bounded by the ruminoreticular fold. Hence, rumen and reticulum are sometimes jointly termed the *ruminoreticulum* or *reticulorumen*. The lining of the rumen is mostly dark, except over the pillars, and is covered by large papillae.

Rhythmic contractions of the wall of the ruminoreticulum mix ingested food with the watery rumen contents. The bacteria and protozoa in the rumen digest the food; most importantly, they break down celluloses and hemicelluloses of plant origin (*see* digestion). Fibrous food can be regurgitated for mastication (*see* rumination). From the rumen, food passes to the omasum via the reticulo-omasal orifice. The gas that accumulates as a result of microbial *fermentation in the rumen is lost by *eructation. Failure of the mechanism results in ruminal tympany or *bloat.

rumenitis Inflammation of the wall of the rumen. It usually occurs as a sequel to acute or chronic *indigestion and ruminal acidosis. The rumen papillae become hypertrophied and swollen, and the epithelial and subepithelial tissues show signs of necrosis, vesicle formation, and oedema. Colonies of bacteria (e.g. *Fusobacterium necrophorum*) may become established in the wall. In chronic cases there is depigmentation, loss of papillae, ulceration, and often *parakeratosis. Affected animals are more prone to develop liver abscesses, due to infective thromboembolism arising from the ruminal blood vessels. Treatment is of the underlying cause.

rumenostomy Surgical creation of an opening into the rumen, usually through the skin and abdominal wall. The opening may be permanent (usually for experimental purposes) or temporary; an indwelling *cannula may be used to maintain patency of the opening. The most common clinical indication is for the relief of chronic *bloat. *Compare* rumenotomy.

rumenotomy Surgical incision into the rumen. Generally performed in the conscious animal under local *analgesia, it involves an incision in

728

the left sublumbar fossa and may require sedation. Rumenotomy is most commonly undertaken to remove foreign bodies, usually wire, from the reticulum: the object is removed by inserting the hand through the rumen into the reticulum. *Compare* rumenostomy.

ruminal tympany *See* bloat.

rumination (cudding) The process in ruminants whereby contents of the reticulorumen are regurgitated for remastication. This assists fermentative *digestion in the rumen by reducing the particle size of the rumen contents and by stimulating salivation. The process involves contractions of the reticulum coupled with relaxation of the cardia and a powerful inspiratory movement with the glottis closed. This causes a sharp fall in intrathoracic pressure and the aspiration of material into the thoracic oesophagus. The *bolus is conveyed to the mouth by antiperistalsis (*see* peristalsis). The cud is chewed for about 40 seconds, with the addition of saliva. *Eructation may occur during this time without interrupting the chewing. Then the bolus is swallowed and returns to the reticulorumen, to be followed, a few seconds later, by the regurgitation of another bolus. This sequence may be repeated for several minutes, or even several hours if the animal is undisturbed. The mechanical events are coordinated by neural reflexes, and the chief stimulus is the presence of fibrous material in the reticulorumen. The more roughage in the diet the greater the time the animal devotes to rumination. A dairy cow at pasture may spend up to 10 out of every 24 hours ruminating, involving almost 30 000 individual jaw movements.

runt The smallest pig of a litter, which typically fails to thrive due to the dominance of its siblings.

runting and stunting syndrome (helicopter chicks) A disease of broiler chicks of uncertain cause, known as *malabsorption syndrome* in the USA. Other meat birds, such as turkeys and guineafowl, may also be affected. In broilers it is of worldwide economic importance. A high proportion of flocks are affected, with morbidity usually ranging up to a few percent. From 5 days of age, a number of thin undersized birds become apparent in the flock; these fall progressively further behind the other birds but remain quite active, although they have little economic value and are candidates for culling. A characteristic feature is the poor feathering, which sticks out at odd angles on the back in a 'helicopter' effect. Acute forms of the disease cause significant mortality in chicks aged 5–10 days. The condition is thought to be due to a virus or viruses that interfere with intestinal absorption and also cause degeneration of the pancreas. There is no treatment or vaccine. Meticulous hygiene and clean-out and disinfection is recommended.

rupture 1. *See* hernia. **2.** The bursting apart or open of an organ or tissue, such as the liver or spleen. This commonly results from trauma and rapidly leads to fatal haemorrhage.

ruptured gastrocnemius tendon (green leg) A condition of domestic fowls in which the tendon of the gastrocnemius muscle in the leg ruptures. It chiefly affects older broilers being fattened to roaster or capon weights, typically achieved at 12 weeks of age or more, and causes downgrading of carcasses. The area just above the hock around the damaged tendon becomes swollen and discoloured. There may be a hereditary factor, and nutrition is also implicated – the problem can be alleviated by feeding rations lower in protein than conventional broiler feeds. Severe cases of *viral tenosynovitis may also lead to the condition.

ryegrass poisoning *See* facial eczema.

ryegrass staggers A nervous disease, clinically similar to *paspalum staggers, important in New Zealand and reported elsewhere. It affects mainly sheep and cattle (also horses and farmed deer) that are grazing pastures in which perennial ryegrass (*Lolium perenne*) is dominant. Many strains of the grass are inhabited by a commensal fungus, which in New Zealand is strongly associated with both the occurrence of the disease and the presence of neurotoxins (lolitrems) in the herbage.

S

sac A pouch or baglike structure. Sacs can enclose natural cavities in the body, e.g. in the lungs (*see* alveolus) or in the *rumen, or they can be pathological, as in a hernia.

sacchar- (saccharo-) *Prefix denoting* sugar.

saccharide A carbohydrate. *See also* disaccharide; monosaccharide; polysaccharide.

saccule The smaller of two membranous sacs lying within the vestibule of the bony labyrinth of the internal *ear and forming part of the membranous labyrinth. It is filled with fluid (endolymph) and contains a *macula, which responds to gravity and relays information to the brain about the position of the head.

sacral Relating to the *sacrum. The *sacral plexus* is a network of nerves formed by the spinal nerves of the sacral region. It supplies branches to the hindlimb, pelvic region, and perineum. Together with the lumbar plexus it forms the *lumbosacral plexus*.

sacro- *Prefix denoting* the sacrum. Examples: *sacrococcygeal* (relating to the sacrum and coccyx); *sacrodynia* (pain in); *sacroiliac* (relating to the sacrum and ilium).

sacrum (*pl.* **sacra**) The rigid part of the vertebral column that articulates cranially with the last lumbar vertebra, caudally with the first coccygeal vertebra, and laterally with the ilium. It is formed by the fusion of the sacral vertebrae, which usually number five in the horse and ox, four in the sheep and pig, and three in the dog and cat.

saddle galls Skin lesions occurring under the saddle in riding horses due to improper fitting of the saddle. New lesions may take the form of ulcers, where both the hair and skin have been lost through repeated pressure and chafing. Older lesions become covered with dry leathery hairless skin, which may be undermined by pus. The term 'sitfast' is often applied because they are difficult to separate from underlying tissue. Galls may develop over the spinous processes or, more commonly, to either side of the midline where the arch of the saddle tree sits. Rest from work is an essential part of treatment, combined with local hygiene and the complete excision of chronic lesions. Post-treatment care is important, with regular cleaning of the skin of the back after work. The saddle may require alteration, with possible reshaping of the saddle tree.

saddle sores Abrasions of the skin and underlying tissue caused by pressure and rubbing from the saddle. They are caused by ill-fitting tack and/or poor conformation and condition. Complete rest from work is essential to allow healing, and padding (*numnah*) should be subsequently placed under the saddle. *See also* saddle galls.

Saffan Tradename for an injectable anaesthetic combining two steroid drugs – alphaxalone and alphadolone acetate – solubilized in an aqueous formulation containing polyoxyethylated castor oil (cremophor). Alphadolone has less anaesthetic activity than alphaxalone but is included to improve the solubility. Saffan is used as an anaesthetic in cats and can be given intravenously or into a well-perfused muscle. Induction is rapid after intravenous injection and anaesthesia lasts 10–15 minutes. When used intramuscularly the onset of anaesthesia takes about 6 minutes. Recovery is rapid, and supplementary doses can be given during anaesthesia without increasing the recovery time. During anaesthesia there is a fall in blood pressure and mild tachycardia. Occasionally, respiratory embarrassment occurs during induction; this may be an allergic reaction, and positive-pressure ventilation should be given. In some cats sneezing and transient paw and ear oedema is seen. This usually regresses, but in rare cases necrosis of the extremities is found 8–10 days after anaesthesia. The reason for this is unknown. Saffan can also be used as an anaesthetic in rabbits and monkeys, but it should not be used in dogs because the solubilizing agent causes histamine release and an anaphylactoid reaction.

sagittal Describing the dorsoventral plane that extends down the long axis of the body in the anatomical (standing) position. The *mid-sagittal* (median) plane divides the body into right and left halves (see illustration at plane).

salazopyrin (sulphasalazine) A *sulphonamide used in the treatment of ulcerative colitis, regional enteritis, and granulomatous colitis in dogs. After oral administration it is broken down in the gut to form sulphapyridine, which is absorbed, and 5-aminosalicylate, which acts as an anti-inflammatory in the intestines. Long-term therapy may be required and hypersensitivity reactions, with urticaria, vomiting, and anaemia, can develop. Salazopyrin should not be used in cats.

salicylanilides A group of compounds, having a similar ring structure, that includes the anthelmintics *oxyclozanide, *rafoxanide, closantel, and brotianide. *Nitroxynil is not a salicylanilide but is closely related. They are all effective against flukes acting in the same manner, uncoupling oxidative phosphorylation. Differences in their *pharmacokinetics are due to halogen substitutions on the ring structure.

salicylate *See* NSAID.

salinomycin *See* coccidiostat.

saliva A watery alkaline secretion delivered into the mouth by various *salivary glands. The primary secretion is actively produced in the acini of the glands but is modified during passage through the ducts. Saliva moistens and lubricates food for chewing and *swallowing, assists *taste by acting as a solvent, protects the teeth and oral mucosa, and assists in evaporative heat loss during panting. It contains the enzyme *lysozyme, and in pigs, but not in other common domestic species, an *amylase is present. In calves a lipase has been reported. Saliva's bicarbonate and phosphate ions are impor-

salivary gland

tant chemical buffers, especially in the reticulorumen.

Secretion of saliva is triggered by parasympathetic nerves as a reflex response to the sight, smell, taste, and mechanical stimulus of food and also, by conditioning, to associated stimuli. Sympathetic nervous stimulation may cause a small amount of salivary secretion. In ruminants the mechanical stimulus of the contents of the reticulorumen causes saliva to be secreted continuously, especially from the parotid glands. The amount is increased by eating and by *rumination.

salivary gland One of several glands that produce *saliva. There are four main pairs: the *parotids, *mandibulars, monostomatic *sublinguals, and polystomatic sublinguals. Minor salivary glands include the labial, lingual, palatine, and buccal, which in carnivores are grouped together to form the *zygomatic gland.

Salmonella A genus of rod-shaped aerobic or facultatively anaerobic *bacteria that cause serious systemic or enteric diseases in animals, including humans, and abortions in domestic animals. Most are motile. They primarily inhabit the intestine but can survive outside the host for prolonged periods, being commonly found in surface and sea water, sewage, and some food products. A number of species cause *salmonellosis in humans and animals following ingestion of contaminated food or water. Some salmonellae affect only certain host species while others can infect a whole range of animals. *S. dublin* and *S. typhimurium* are the most common serotypes for bovine *salmonellosis, although many animals harbour *S. dublin* without any clinical signs. *S. typhimurium* is the commonest cause of equine salmonellosis while *S. abortus-equi* causes abortions. In pigs *S. choleraesuis*, *S. typhimurium*, and *S.*

dublin are the most common serotypes. *S. gallinarum* and *S. pullorum* affect only poultry, causing *fowl typhoid and *pullorum disease respectively.

salmonellosis Disease caused by infection with bacteria of the genus *Salmonella. The species of this large genus are differentiated into *serotypes according to their serological reactions.

Most cases of salmonellosis in animals and humans are caused by a relatively small number of common serotypes. Infection is usually by ingestion of water or feed contaminated with faeces from infected animals. Clinical signs include diarrhoea, ranging from simple loose faeces to very severe dysentery, fever, and varying degrees of malaise. Pregnant animals may abort and *septicaemia is not uncommon. Pneumonia and joint infections are occasionally seen. Animal species vary in their susceptibility: cattle, sheep, and horses are generally more likely to show clinical illness than pigs, poultry, and dogs. Stress, intercurrent illness, or debility make animals more susceptible. Recovered animals often shed the pathogens in faeces for some time after recovery. Symptomless carriers can develop clinical signs if subject to stress and debility.

In **cattle** *S. typhimurium* and *S. dublin* are the most important serotypes. The former causes diarrhoea, dysentery, and occasionally abortion in adult cattle, and diarrhoea, dysentery, and septicaemia in calves. *S. dublin* causes abortion in adult cows and septicaemia and diarrhoea in calves. However, many animals harbour *S. dublin* without clinical signs. In **sheep** *S. abortus ovis* causes abortion in ewes, while *S. typhimurium* can cause enteritis and septicaemia in lambs and ewes. Exotic serotypes are becoming more important in the UK, imported feedstuffs being the source in many cases. *S. choleraesuis* causes severe diarrhoea in **pigs**. Although now rare in the UK it is common in the Far East, where it is an important cause of food poisoning in humans. In **poultry** *S. pullorum* causes *pullorum disease, which can be transmitted via the egg. *S. gallinarum* causes *fowl typhoid, a cause of heavy losses in growing birds. Poultry may be infected by many types of *Salmonella*, often as symptomless carriers. *S. typhimurium*, *S. virchow*, and many other serotypes are commonly incriminated in cases of human food poisoning caused by poorly cooked frozen chicken (*see* avian salmonellosis). In **horses**, *S. typhimurium* is the most frequent cause of equine salmonellosis, and food poisoning caused by contaminated horse meat is well known in Europe. *S. abortus equi* causes abortions in mares. **Dogs** and **cats** are occasionally infected with *Salmonella* but clinical disease, which usually comprises diarrhoea, is uncommon. Tortoises and terrapins may be infected with salmonella. Humans can become infected with *Salmonella* either by direct contact with infected livestock or by the consumption of meat, milk, or milk products contaminated with the organism. Vegetables fertilized with contaminated manure are also a possible source.

Treatment is usually by administration of antibiotics and fluid therapy to counteract dehydration caused by diarrhoea. Prevention depends upon isolating infected animals and disinfecting contaminated premises. The application of contaminated manure on pasture can be an important method of spreading the disease. To minimize this risk, manure should be stored for at least 4 weeks before spreading, and animals kept off treated pasture for 4 weeks. Young stock and pregnant animals should be denied access to treated pasture for at least 6 months.

salmon poisoning (canine rickettsiosis) A disease of dogs, foxes, coyotes, and bears, caused by the rickettsia *Neorickettsia helminthoeca*. This is acquired through eating the flesh of salmonid fish containing an encysted stage of the parasitic *fluke *Nanophyetus salmincola*, which inhabits the intestine of canines and is the vector for the rickettsia. The disease occurs only in the USA (in Oregon, North California, and Washington). The fluke's invertebrate host is a small snail (*Goniobasis plicifera* var. *silicula*), from which fish (species of salmon and trout) become infected. Dogs acquire both the parasite and the rickettsia it carries by catching and eating fish from streams that flow into the Pacific. The rickettsiae parasitize the white blood cells of their host, causing fever, vomiting, dysentery, and, unless treated with tetracyclines or a sulphonamide, death. *See also* Elokomin fluke fever.

salping- (salpingo-) *Prefix denoting* **1.** the uterine tube (oviduct). **2.** the auditory tube (meatus).

salpingectomy Surgical removal or cutting of an oviduct.

salpingitis Inflammation of the oviducts. In **poultry** it is caused by infection of the oviduct with strains of the bacterium *Escherichia coli* and other agents. Normal functioning of the oviduct may be impaired, leading to internal laying and hence possibly fatal peritonitis. The infection may, moreover, be transmitted through the egg in breeding hens. Hormonal activity at sexual maturity may be a trigger since salpingitis usually sets in at point-of-lay.

salt lick A block of salt provided for cattle or sheep to lick in order to supplement their intake of salt; it may also contain iodine and other *essential elements. Salt licks are useful for grazing animals, especially where little or no compound feed is given and salt deficiency is possible. Intake is extremely variable and depends upon individual animal preference and an adequate supply of drinking water. *See also* feed block.

salt poisoning A toxic condition that occurs when animals, particularly pigs and poultry, are given a ration with a high sodium chloride content and are deprived of their normal water supply. Excess salt may be eaten due to errors in mixing a compound ration, from feeding pickling brine or bakery waste, or by access to fields contaminated with brine. Affected animals show thirst, salivation, diarrhoea, and gasping breathing. In poultry there is loss of fluid from the beak, while pigs display staggering and circling. More than 0.3% sodium chloride in the stomach contents discovered post mortem should cause suspicion of salt poisoning. An adequate water supply should be restored at the earliest opportunity, although the sudden restoration of unlimited water can itself precipitate the neurological signs of acute brain swelling.

sand colic *Colic of horses due to accumulation of sand in the caecum and colon. It occurs commonly where horses are fed food contaminated with soil or sand, or when grazing on sandy soil. The condition may also arise in sodium-deficient horses, which lick sand to obtain salt. Mild but persistent abdominal pain may be accompanied by bouts of diarrhoea. The sand can often be detected if faeces are shaken with water in a test tube; sand falls to the bottom. The sand intake should be reduced, and feeding bulk laxatives, such as bran or hemicellulose, frequently gives a good response.

sandcrack A condition of the horse's *hoof in which a crack appears at the

weight-bearing surface and extends upwards, or originates at the coronary band. If the crack extends into the sensitive laminae, usually in the quarter or heel of the foot, lameness is likely. Haemorrhage may occur and infection is often present. Treatment includes corrective trimming and grooving, possibly with the use of an epoxy resin or acrylic to repair the hoof wall defects. The prognosis is generally favourable.

sandfly A tiny compact *fly of the genus *Phlebotomus* and *Lutzomyia* having a hairy body and wings, long slender legs, and short piercing mouthparts. The females are blood-sucking ectoparasites of animals and humans and deliver a very painful and irritating bite to which the host may develop an allergy. Sandflies also transmit such diseases as dermal and visceral *leishmaniasis and, in humans, Oroya fever (bartonellosis) and sandfly fever (papataci). The adults are short-lived and are common in nearly all warmer regions, being active on warm still nights. During the day they shelter in cool moist places, where they lay their eggs. Control of sandflies is difficult as they are too small for the satisfactory use of nets. Screens treated with insect repellent can be used, and the breeding sites sprayed with a suitable *insecticide.

sangui- (sanguino-) *Prefix denoting* blood.

sanguineous 1. Containing, stained, or covered with blood. **2.** (of tissues) Containing more than the normal quantity of blood.

saphenous nerve A branch of the *femoral nerve that carries motor fibres to the sartorius muscle and sensory fibres from the inner side of the leg and part of the pes.

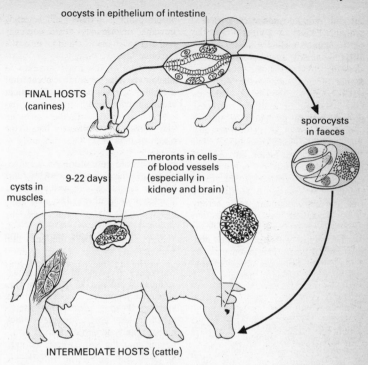

oocysts in epithelium of intestine

FINAL HOSTS
(canines)

sporocysts
in faeces

meronts in cells
of blood vessels
(especially in
kidney and brain)

cysts in
muscles

9-22 days

INTERMEDIATE HOSTS (cattle)

Life cycle of *Sarcocystis cruzi* of cattle

sapr- (sapro-) *Prefix denoting* **1.** putrefaction. **2.** decaying matter.

saprophyte Any free-living organism that lives and feeds on the dead and putrefying tissues of animals or plants. *Compare* parasite.

sarc- (sarco-) *Prefix denoting* **1.** flesh or fleshy tissue. **2.** muscle.

Sarcocystis A genus of protozoa in the group *Apicomplexa (see illustration). They undergo an obligatory two-host life cycle involving a carnivore and a herbivore, often in a predator/prey relationship. In the predator host (definitive host), for example dogs, cats, or raptorial birds, the parasite multiplies in the intestine and resistant cysts are passed in the faeces. These infect prey animals (the intermediate hosts), for instance sheep, cattle, or rodents, and invade their tissues forming resistant cysts in muscle and brain. Predator animals become infected by ingesting these cyst-containing tissues. There is a large number of different species of *Sarcocystis* with a well-defined host specificity. While very common throughout the world they rarely cause disease, but fatal illness and abortions can occur with some species in the intermediate hosts, notably in cattle and sheep.

sarcoid A skin tumour of horses – probably caused by a virus – and the most common equine tumour, usually affecting middle-aged animals. Sites subjected to trauma are most commonly affected, such as the legs, ventral abdomen, and head. Sarcoids may be single or multiple, verrucose (up to 6 cm in diamater) or smooth and sessile (up to 25 cm in diameter). The available evidence indicates that a virus is a causal factor. Sarcoids are locally invasive but do not metastasize. Surgical excision is the usual therapy but recurrence at the same site is very common; radiotherapy and vaccination by BCG injection have also been used. A significant number regress with age but this may take several years. The lesion must be distinguished from the unrelated sarcoid and sarcoidosis of humans.

sarcoidosis A skin cancer, occurring only in horses, in which tumours appear commonly on the legs, head, and prepuce. The tumours resemble *sarcomas histologically although they do not metastasize or invade other tissues. They may be treated by surgical removal but tend to recur; radiation and local BCG vaccine injection have been used as additional treatments. Virus infection has been proposed as the cause.

In human medicine sarcoidosis is a generalized disease of unknown cause in which chronic inflammatory foci or granulomas are formed in lymphoid and other organs.

sarcolemma The cell membrane that encloses a muscle cell (muscle fibre).

sarcoma Any malignant tumour of connective tissue (*see* cancer). Sarcomas may occur in any part of the body because they arise in the tissues that make up an organ rather than being restricted to a particular organ. *See* angiosarcoma; chondrosarcoma; fibrosarcoma; liposarcoma; lymphosarcoma; myosarcoma; osteosarcoma; rhabdomyosarcoma; and synoviosarcoma.

sarcomere One of the basic contractile units of which *striated muscle fibres are composed.

sarcoplasm (myoplasm) The cytoplasm of muscle cells.

sarcoplasmic reticulum An arrangement of membranous vesicles and tubules found in the cytoplasm of striated muscle fibres. The sarcoplasmic reticulum plays an important role in the transmission of nervous excitation to the contractile parts of the fibres.

Sarcoptes A genus of *mites which includes *S. scabiei*, the itch mite. This is relatively minute with an oval body and legs bearing suckers for attachment to the host. *Sarcoptes* attack humans and domestic animals, burrowing into the skin (where the eggs are laid) and causing intense itching leading to *sarcoptic mange in livestock and dogs (or scabies in humans). The whole 3-week life cycle is spent on the host.

sarcoptic mange (scabies) A skin disease caused by the itch mite *Sarcoptes scabiei* and affecting sheep, cattle, pigs, goats, equids, camels, dogs, and humans. Each host species has its own host-specific variety of itch mite. For example, *S. scabiei* var. *ovis* parasitizes sheep. Signs of infestation first appear on parts of the body that most often come into contact with other animals or infected surfaces, especially the head and other relatively hairless areas; spread to other parts of the body is rapid. The disease is particularly common in intensively housed young pigs. Scabies is very itchy so there is much self-excoriation with consequent damage to the coat and skin and loss of condition; severely infested animals may die. *See also* mange.

sarcostyle A bundle of muscle fibrils.

sartorius muscle A long flat muscle in the cranial part of the thigh. It acts to flex the hip.

sawdust liver (focal necrosis of the liver) A condition of the bovine liver in which small areas of necrosis, which are bacterial in origin and resemble sawdust, are scattered throughout the liver substance.

scabies *See* sarcoptic mange.

scad (scald) Colloquial name for a condition of lameness in sheep which occurs after exposure to frozen or cold ground. Mechanical damage by hard stubble has a similar effect. Inflammation between the digits occurs and lameness ensues. The physical damage may allow the entrance of such bacteria as *Fusobacterium* or *Corynebacterium*. Recovery usually follows spontaneously after a change of pasture or the return of better conditions underfoot. Footbaths of 5% formaldehyde may assist healing. Other name: **ovine interdigital dermatitis**. *Compare* foot rot.

scala One of the spiral canals in the *cochlea.

scald *See* scad.

scalpel A small pointed surgical knife used in dissection or by surgeons for cutting tissues. It has a straight handle with either a fixed blade or, more commonly, detachable disposable blades of different shapes and sizes.

scaly leg A condition of poultry characterized by scalelike lesions of the legs and feet caused by tiny burrowing mites (*Cnemidocoptes mutans*). The female mites produce live young in the burrows, and the condition progresses from initial reddening of the shanks to a state in which the chalky debris from the burrowing mites raises the scales of the toes and shanks. Transmission is by physical contact, favoured especially when the birds are perching side-by-side. The infestation causes discomfort and unthriftiness, and in more severe cases deformities of the legs and feet. Affected flocks should be treated by dipping the feet and scaly part of the legs of each bird in 0.1% gamma-*benzene hexachloride (BHC) emulsion or oil solution. Small numbers of birds can be treated by removing the crusts with soap and water and applying a suitable *acaricide.

scaphoid The large central bone of the *tarsus or hock.

scapul- (scapulo-) *Prefix denoting* the scapula.

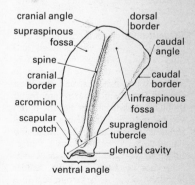

Left scapula of dog (lateral aspect)

scapula One of the bones of the shoulder girdle. In mammals the scapula is typically broad and flat, providing a surface for the attachment of muscles that flex the fore-limb. The head of the humerus articulates with the socket formed by the glenoid cavity of the scapula (see illustration). In birds the scapula forms joints with the furcula, comprising fused left and right clavicles, and the coracoid. However, in mammals the *clavicle is much reduced or absent and the coracoid is represented by the coracoid process of the scapula.

scar *See* cicatrix.

scarification The process of making a number of scratches in the skin to allow a substance to penetrate the body. It was employed as the means of administering smallpox vaccine.

Schiff's reagent Aqueous fuchsin solution decolorized with sulphur dioxide. A blue coloration develops in the presence of aldehydes.

-schisis *Suffix denoting* a cleft or split.

schisto- *Prefix denoting* a fissure; split.

Schistosoma A genus of *flukes that parasitize humans, cattle, dogs, and other animals and are widespread in Asia, especially the Far East, and in Africa, South America, and the West Indies. The mature flukes are found in blood vessels of the hepatic-portal system and cause the disease *schistosomiasis (bilharziasis). In India and Bangladesh, *S. nasalis* causes *infectious nasal granulomas in cattle. Schistosomes have a long slender body and occur in large numbers in a host. The sexes are separate but are always found together, the male having a special gynaecophoric groove in which the female is permanently held. The spiked eggs can cause inflammation, bleeding, and anaemia as they penetrate the intestine or bladder to

pass out with the urine or faeces of the host. The *miracidium larva enters a water or mud snail as an intermediate host. Eventually a free-swimming *cercaria larva emerges to infect the primary host via drinking water or by penetrating the skin of the host.

schistosomiasis (bilharziasis) Disease caused by infestation with parasitic flukes of the genus *Schistosoma. The mature adult worms, 1–3 cm long, are found in male-female pairs in the portal and mesenteric blood vessels. Infestation of domestic animals and humans occurs in much of Africa and parts of the Middle and Far East. The cercaria larvae penetrate the skin of a mammalian host, are carried to the lungs and liver, and eventually mature in the blood vessels. Clinical signs are either an acute haemorrhagic enteritis with diarrhoea, dehydration, and loss of appetite, or else a chronic hepatitis caused by an immune reaction to the parasites' eggs involving *granuloma formation, anaemia, and loss of blood proteins. Diagnosis is by examination of the faeces for the eggs. Treatment is by suitable anthelmintics, such as trichlorophon. Control depends on reducing the numbers of snail intermediate hosts.

schiz- (schizo-) *Prefix denoting* a split or division.

schizogony *See* merogony.

schizont *See* meront.

Schmorl's disease *See* labial necrosis of rabbits.

Schwann cell *See* neurolemmal cell.

Schwannoma *See* neurofibroma.

sciatica Pain felt in the thigh and leg due to a lesion of the *sciatic nerve.

The cause in animals is usually constriction of the foramen through which the sciatic nerve emerges from the vertebral column.

sciatic nerve The largest nerve originating from the *sacral plexus. It runs in the caudal part of the thigh supplying biceps femoris, semimembranosus, and semitendinosus muscles, and finally divides into the common *peroneal and *tibial nerves.

sciatic paralysis Paralysis and loss of sensation affecting the hindlimb due to a lesion of the *sciatic nerve. The condition is uncommon, but can result from gross trauma causing fracture of the pelvis and damage to the nerve trunk. The degree of nerve damage can be assessed best by *electromyography, and cases that do not have total denervation may improve slowly. The clinical features include loss of all muscle action below the stifle and in the caudal region of the thigh, and loss of sensation below the stifle, except for the small area on the medial side supplied by the *saphenous nerve, which runs to the medial toe. The pedal reflex is lost and the patellar reflex is uncontrolled.

scintigram *See* scintillascope.

scintillascope A instrument used to record the distribution of a radioactive *tracer in the body or part of the body. The tracer particles emit high-energy radiation, which causes material in the instrument to emit a fluorescent flash. These flashes are recorded photographically or electronically to produce a *scintigram*. By scanning the body, section by section, a 'map' of the radioactivity in its various parts is built up. This can be useful both for experimental purposes and for diagnosis, especially of cancer.

scirrhous cord A condition in which the spermatic cord enlarges following castration due to the deposition of fibrous connective tissue. In extreme cases the hard swelling may even extend up the *inguinal canal and into the abdominal cavity. Frequently, the castration wound fails to heal and a purulent discharge (usually as a result of *Staphylococcus* infection) is apparent, while the animal may exhibit a general stiffness. Treatment involves surgical removal of the infected portion and antibiotic administration.

scler- (sclero-) *Prefix denoting* **1.** hardening or thickening. **2.** the sclera. **3.** sclerosis.

sclera (*pl.* **scleras** or **sclerae**) Part of the fibrous coat of the *eye. It is tough white tissue and is continuous anteriorly with the cornea.

scleritis Inflammation of the *sclera of the eye. It usually occurs as part of a more general inflammation of the eyeball (*see* ophthalmia).

sclerosis Hardening of tissue, usually due to scarring (fibrosis) after inflammation. For example, *atherosclerosis involves hardening of the walls of the arteries.

sclerotium (*pl.* **sclerotia**) A hard blackened elongated mass of fungal cells that destroys and replaces the seeds or grains of maturing grasses and cereals. It contains the ergot alkaloids responsible for *ergot poisoning.

sclerotome **1.** A surgical knife used for incising the *sclera. **2.** (in embryology) the part of the *somite that develops into the skeletal tissues of the body (e.g. vertebrae, ribs).

scoke *See* pokeweed poisoning.

scolex (*pl.* **scolices**) The head of a tapeworm, which bears suckers and usually hooks for attachment to the host's intestinal wall.

scoliosis Deformity of the spine resulting in lateral (sideways) deviation. It occurs rarely in animals, except for the severe developmental defect of *schistosomus reflexus*, which occurs occasionally in cattle.

-scope *Suffix denoting* an instrument for observing or examining. Example: *gastroscope* (instrument for examining the stomach).

Scottie cramp An inherited condition of Scottish terriers and West Highland white terriers in which sudden bouts of muscle spasm occur when the dog is exercising. Muscle relaxant drugs, such as *diazepam, may help to alleviate the signs.

scouring *See* diarrhoea.

scouring rush A plant of the genus *Equisetum* (horsetails) that causes toxicity following ingestion (*see* bracken poisoning).

scrapie A disease of sheep and goats characterized by progressive degeneration of the central nervous system and caused by a subviral agent. Following an incubation of 18 months to 5 years the affected sheep appears excitable and develops a high-stepping gait. Intense irritation of the skin may cause the animal to mutilate itself. Incoordination, collapse, and death inevitably ensue. Control is by slaughter of all affected animals and their lambs or even complete replacement of the flock. Scrapie is enzootic in the UK and is present in most of the sheep-rearing countries of the world.

screw-worm fly One of various metallic-greenish-blue blowflies, including the Old World screw-worm fly (*Chrysomya* spp.) of Africa, southern Asia, and parts of the Far East, which attacks sheep, and *Callitroga* spp. of North and South America, which attacks cattle, pigs, horses, and humans. The eggs are usually laid in or close to wounds and sores or in discharges from the host's orifices, and hatch into strongly spined larvae with prominent bands of spines. The larvae cause irritation and loss of condition; they are voracious feeders and rapidly reach maturity, whereupon they leave the host to pupate in the soil. Prevention entails employing one of the many suitable *insecticides as a dip or spray; some insecticides can also be used as a dressing for the wounds.

scrotum (*pl.* **scrota** or **scrotums**) The skin-covered sac that holds the testes and epididymides outside the abdominal cavity in mammals. It thus allows the production and storage of spermatozoa at a temperature lower than that inside the abdomen. Contraction of the muscular tunica dartos draws the scrotum nearer the abdomen and enables some degree of temperature control. Internally the scrotum is divided into two by the *scrotal septum*, indicated externally by the *scrotal raphe*.

scrub typhus (tsutsugamushi; mite disease) A zoonotic rickettsial disease of humans caused by *Rickettsia tsutsugamushi*. Infection is transmitted from the reservoir hosts, wild rodents, by trombiculid mites (e.g. *Leptotrombidium deliense*), whose larvae ('chiggers') burrow into the skin of animals or humans to feed. It occurs throughout southeast Asia, in northern Australia, and some Pacific islands. Symptoms include headache, chills, high temperature, a widespread rash, a cough, and delirium. A small ulcer forms at the site of the bite.

Treatment is with tetracycline antibiotics.

season *See* oestrous cycle; oestrus.

seaweed Any of various marine algae. Occasionally seaweed is fed to cattle and horses but it has a low nutritive value. Extracts of seaweed are sometimes used as a source of iodine and other trace elements.

sebaceous cyst A non-neoplastic lesion of a sebaceous gland. These *cysts are not uncommon in dogs and present as solitary masses from which sebaceous material may be squeezed. They should be differentiated from true tumours and usually do not represent a clinical problem unless secondarily infected.

sebaceous gland Any of the single or branched glands in the *skin that produce an oily substance, *sebum. They open into hair follicles and their secretion is produced by the disintegration of their cells.

sebaceous gland tumour A benign or malignant tumour of a sebaceous gland. The benign form (adenoma) is commonly seen in older dogs, especially cocker spaniels and poodles. They may be solitary or multiple and are often of various sizes. Unless ulcerated, bleeding, or secondarily infected they rarely cause clinical problems. Surgical excision is usually curative. The malignant form (adenocarcinoma) is rare in all species. They tend to be invasive and ulcerating and the prognosis should be guarded as they frequently metastasize.

seborrhoea Excessive secretion of sebum by the *sebaceous glands. It is a poorly understood condition, common in dogs but less common in other species, characterized by a strong rancid odour from the coat and a scaly (exfoliative) dermatitis. Sometimes the coat is quite greasy. It may be secondary to a number of diseases. For example, itchy seborrhoea may follow ectoparasitism. However, the cause of the seborrhoea itself has not been determined. Treatment depends on the associated condition.

sebum The oily substance secreted by the *sebaceous glands of the skin and reaching the surface through small ducts that lead into the hair follicles. Sebum provides a thin film of fat over the skin, which reduces evaporation of water and also has an antibacterial effect.

secondary infection The invasion of an existing infective lesion by another, different, infective agent, which continues or compounds the primary pathological process. The invading organisms in secondary infection are commonly bacteria from the diseased individual's own mucous membranes, skin, or intestine; they reach the existing lesion by direct contamination or via blood or lymph. The secondary invader may be of low intrinsic pathogenicity, or may have disease potential of its own.

Secondary infection plays an important part in pneumonias, where a primary viral or mycoplasmal infection may be complicated by secondary bacteria (e.g. *canine distemper, *enzootic pneumonia of pigs); in the chronic necrotizing or granulomatous infections, such as *necrobacillosis and *tuberculosis, where progressing lesions may undergo haematogenous secondary infection with pyogenic bacteria; and in ulcerative enteric conditions, such as *swine dysentery and *necrotic enteritis. The presence of secondary infection multiplies the problems of clinical and laboratory diagnosis, and of selecting appropriate antibiotics or other treatment.

secretin A hormone secreted by the epithelium of the duodenum in response to the presence of acidified food from the stomach. It stimulates the secretion of a virtually enzyme-free alkaline watery fluid from the pancreas (*see* pancreatic juice) and of bile from the liver. Secretin was the first substance to be described as a hormone (in 1902).

secretion 1. The process by which a gland produces a substance that it discharges either for use by the body or to be lost by the body. The principal methods of secretion – *apocrine, *holocrine, and *merocrine – are illustrated in the diagram. **2.** The substance that is produced by a gland.

secretory immunoglobulin Immunoglobulins in body secretions, predominantly of the IgA class (*see* antibody).

section 1. (in surgery) The act of cutting (the cut or division made is also called a section). For example, an *abdominal section* is performed for surgical exploration of the abdomen. A *transverse section* is a cut made at right angles to a structure's long axis. *See also* Caesarean section. **2.** (in microscopy) A thin slice of the specimen to be examined under a microscope.

sedative A drug that causes depression of the central nervous system and a consequent reduction in responsiveness to stimuli. High doses of sedatives can produce *anaesthesia. Many sedatives are used as anaesthetics or as premedicants prior to anaesthesia to facilitate handling of animals. Commonly used sedatives include some *barbiturates and *xylazine.

sedimentation rate The rate of settlement of *macromolecules when subjected to high-speed centrifugation,

usually in an *ultracentrifuge. It is measured in Svedbergs (symbol S) and is often used as an estimate of the size of large molecules and cell organelles.

seed dressings *See* organomercury poisoning.

seedy cut (seedy belly) *Melanism (darkening of tissues) in the mammary glands of pigs. It only occurs in pure- or crossbred black pigs or in pigs with some black hairs.

seedy toe A condition of the *hoof of the horse in which separation of the laminae is visible at the white line of the sole. It is commonest at the toe but may occur at other points around the circumference. The separation may allow the entrance of infection, with likely consequent lameness, and this infection may track between the laminae to erupt as a discharging sinus at the coronary band. It is particularly common in cases of chronic *laminitis. Treatment consists of the removal of diseased tissue and, where necessary, antibiosis or poulticing.

segment (in anatomy) A portion of a tissue or organ, usually distinguishable from other portions by lines of demarcation. *See also* somite.

selection The process whereby certain individuals breed more successfully than others and so increase the frequency of their genes in the population. Selection in wild populations is the result of environmental forces, such as climate, disease, and competition. According to classical Darwinian theory, this *natural selection* acts on the variability in populations and eventually leads to the evolution of new species.

In farm livestock, artificial selection is employed to change the genetic make-up of a population (e.g. a herd or flock) over several generations in a desired way. Mating is closely controlled, with only certain chosen individuals used as sires and dams. The suitability of individuals, which may be expressed as their *breeding value, can be assessed in various ways. These include reference to their existing *pedigree, *performance testing, testing the performance of other family members (usually half-sibs), and *progeny testing.

selenium A metalloid element and an *essential (trace) element required by animals in their diets. In the body it is a constituent of the enzyme *glutathione peroxidase, which protects red blood cells against harmful peroxides. *Vitamin E, which prevents the formation of peroxides, complements the metabolic role of selenium, although neither can be replaced by the other. Symbol Se.
Selenium deficiency This is of most importance in cattle and sheep, although it can occur in poultry, horses, and pigs. Dogs and cats are rarely affected. Dietary deficiency is usually associated with inadequate levels of the element in the soil, and selenium-deficient areas are well recognized in New Zealand, Australia, and parts of the USA. In recent years they have become increasingly important in the UK; this may be related to reduced feeding of proprietary feeds (which often contain fish meal or other selenium-rich animal protein) and increased reliance on home-grown feedstuffs. Heavy use of fertilizer, rapid plant growth, and the presence of large amounts of legumes all reduce the selenium content of pasture.
In ruminants, the major disease caused by selenium and/or vitamin E deficiency is *white muscle disease. *Paralytic myoglobinuria in cattle may also be related to the same deficiency. In pigs, liver necrosis and *mulberry heart disease are due to the same cause, as are *crazy chick

disease and exudative diathesis in poultry (*see* vitamin E).
Selenium-responsive or *selenium-related conditions* comprise a group of diseases that may be associated with deficient selenium levels but for which there is little direct proof. In cattle and sheep these include ill-thrift and reproductive problems; in pigs they include agalactia and infertility in adults, and skin conditions and weakness in newborns.
In all cases, treatment is by subcutaneous or intramuscular injection of vitamin E and potassium selenite. Deficiency disease can be prevented by supplementing the diet with selenium and vitamin E, the oral administration of slow-release boluses, or prophylactic injections. *See also* Astragalus poisoning.

selenium poisoning *See* Astragalus poisoning.

sella turcica The 'Turkish saddle'; the region in the middle of the floor of the cranial cavity consisting of the *hypophyseal fossa*, which accommodates the pituitary gland, and the more caudal elevation, the *dorsum sellae*.

semen The fluid ejaculated from the penis at sexual climax, consisting of spermatozoa mixed with seminal plasma produced by the accessory glands – the paired seminal vesicles, the prostate, and bulbourethral glands. This plasma contains nutrients to provide energy for the swimming sperms, and also prostaglandins, which enhance the muscle contractions of the female genital tract and so assist the sperms' progress. Semen can be collected by various methods for use in *artificial insemination, most commonly by using a *teaser or dummy in conjunction with an artificial vagina, or by electroejaculation (*see* ejaculation). Semen samples require careful handling, and chilling or freezing usually requires dilution and the addition of protective agents. Criteria routinely assessed include the concentration of spermatozoa (*see* sperm count) and the proportion of actively mobile spermatozoa. The cells are also examined for abnormalities.

semi- *Prefix denoting* half.

semicircular canals Three bony canals and their ducts that form part of the membranous labyrinth of the internal *ear and are concerned with balance. They lie within the petrous part of the temporal bone of the skull and are termed *anterior*, *posterior*, and *lateral semicircular canals*. Each duct contains endolymph and is surrounded by perilymph, and at its end has an enlargement (*ampulla*), which is lined by a specialized epithelium (*crista*). When the head moves the endolymph stimulates cells in the cristae, which send nerve impulses to the brain.

semilunar valve Either of the two valves of the heart situated at the origin of the aorta (*aortic valve*) and pulmonary trunk (*pulmonic valve*). Each consists of three flaps (*valvulae*), which allow blood to flow from the heart but prevent it flowing back.

semimembranosus muscle A large fleshy muscle lying in the caudal part of the thigh. It acts to extend the hip and stifle joints.

seminal vesicle One of the accessory male genital glands of the horse that produce the seminal plasma (*see* semen). It is paired and lies on the lateral side of the terminal part of the *ductus deferens, terminally discharging either with or alongside it into the urethra on the lateral side of the *colliculus seminalis. In ruminants and the pig it is termed the *vesicle gland* and is a compact lobulated structure.

seminiferous tubule One of the long convoluted tubules of the *testis. It is lined by specialized seminiferous epithelium, which contains both spermatogenic cells and *sustentacular cells.

seminoma A tumour arising from the epithelial cells of the seminiferous tubules of the testicle. Seminomas are seen mainly in middle-aged dogs, in which they represent about one-third of all testicular tumours. A similar proportion is found in *cryptorchid testicles. They usually affect only one testicle and are solitary, although a few affect both and are multiple. The normal consequence is clinical enlargement of the testicle. Although histologically seminomas have a malignant appearance, *metastasis is found in only a small proportion of cases – in the regional lymph nodes and, occasionally, in the lungs or visceral organs. Those arising in cryptorchid testicles are inclined to be more dangerous since the tumours are generally larger at diagnosis, by which time intra-abdominal spread may have taken place. Hormonal upset is not normally seen in affected animals and castration is usually curative. Seminomas are uncommon in other species.

semipermeable membrane A membrane, e.g. cell membrane, that allows the passage of some molecules but not others, depending on their size, shape, and molecular charge.

semitendinosus muscle A thick muscle lying in the caudal part of the thigh. It acts to extend the hip, stifle, and hock joints. If the limb is free it acts to flex the stifle joint.

Sendai virus A *paramyxovirus that has been widely used experimentally in developing *monoclonal antibody technology. When inactivated (e.g. by ultraviolet light) the virus can promote the fusion of two different cells to form a heterokaryon. Fused lymphocyte-tumour cells (hybridomas) are used for the production of monoclonal antibodies.

Senkobo disease An African name for *mycotic dermatitis in cattle, usually accompanied by skin infestation with the mange mite *Demodex bovis*.

senna A purgative obtained from the leaves of *Cassia acutifolia* or *C. angustifolia*. The active principles are senna glycosides, and when given orally to nonruminants they produce purging after several hours. Lower doses have a laxative effect. *See* anthraquinones.

sense organ A collection of specialized cells that is capable of responding to a particular stimulus from either outside or inside the body, and transmitting impulses in the nervous system (*see* receptor). Sense organs can detect light (the eyes), heat, pain, and touch (the skin), smell (the nose), and taste (the taste buds).

sensitization A state of active *immunization. The term is used particularly for the process whereby previous exposure to a particular *antigen renders an individual susceptible to a *hypersensitivity reaction when the antigen is subsequently encountered, as in an *allergy. *See also* desensitization.

sensory Relating to the input division of the nervous system, which carries information from *receptors throughout the body to the central nervous system.

sensory nerve (afferent nerve) A nerve that carries information inwards, from an outlying part of the body towards the central nervous system. *Compare* motor nerve. *See also* sensory neurone.

sensory neurone (afferent neurone) A nerve cell that has its cell body located in a *ganglion, a peripheral process extending from some point in the body (e.g. skin, muscle, tendon, or internal organ), and a central process that connects to the central nervous system. *Compare* motor neurone.

sepsis (*pl.* **sepses**) The putrefactive destruction of tissues by pathogenic microorganisms, especially bacteria or their toxins. The term is used generally to indicate wound infection. *Compare* asepsis.

sept- (septi-) *Prefix denoting* **1.** seven. **2.** (*or* **septo-**) a septum, especially the nasal septum. **3.** sepsis.

septic The presence of *sepsis.

septicaemia The presence of pathogenic bacteria in the circulating blood accompanied by signs of disease. (The term is sometimes used to mean *bacteraemia.) It is a potentially fatal condition, especially in patients with low body reserves, for example neonates, aged animals, or those with coexisting debilitating disease. Infection may enter the blood from any area of the body. Treatment involves intensive supportive care and effective antibiosis. However, before any antibiotics are given, a blood sample should be taken, in a sterile manner, so that the bacteria may be cultured and their antibiotic sensitivity determined. Until the results are available, a broad-spectrum *antibiotic should be given intravenously. *See also* toxaemia.

septic sternal bursitis A condition of poultry involving inflammation and abscessation of the breast. It is due to the invasion of breast blisters by *Staphylococcus aureus* bacteria, and tends to affect older heavier birds, which may have bruising of the sternum as a result of jumping from perches or through leg weakness and conformation.

septum (*pl.* **septa**) A partition of dividing wall within an anatomical structure. For example, the *inverventricular septum* separates the left and right ventricles of the heart.

sequela (*pl.* **sequelae**) Any disorder or pathological condition that results from a preceding disease or accident.

sequestration The process by which a fragment of dead tissue (*sequestrum*) becomes separated from surrounding tissue. It usually refers to a fragment of bone that undergoes necrosis and separates from adjacent living bone. The separation may be partial or complete, and the fragment may eventually be broken down, fibrosed, or extruded through the skin. Sequestration also occurs in the lung in diseases such as *contagious bovine pleuropneumonia: portions of the lung undergo necrosis and separate from the surrounding living tissue.

sequestrum (*pl.* **sequestra**) The fragment of dead tissue separated off during *sequestration.

ser- (sero-) *Prefix denoting* **1.** serum. **2.** serous membrane.

serine *See* amino acid.

seroconversion *Antibody production in response to immunization or infection.

serology The study of blood sera and their constituents. This includes the detection of specific *antibodies to obtain evidence of previous infection.

serosa *See* serous membrane.

serotonin (5-hydroxytryptamine) A derivative of the amino acid tryptophan that is widely distributed in tissues, particularly in blood platelets, the intestinal wall, and central nervous system. It has important pharmacological effects, including the stimulation of smooth muscle contraction, and functions as a *neurotransmitter.

serotype A category into which material is placed according to its serological activity, particularly in terms of the *antigens it contains or the antibodies whose production it elicits. Thus, bacteria of the same species may be subdivided into serotypes that produce slightly different antigens. The serotype of an infective organism is important when treatment or prophylaxis with a vaccine is being considered.

serous **1.** Relating to or resembling serum. **2.** Producing a fluid resembling serum.

serous membrane A smooth transparent membrane, consisting of *mesothelium and underlying fibrous connective tissue, that lines certain large body cavities. The *peritoneum of the abdomen, *pleura of the chest, and *pericardium of the heart are all serous membranes. Each consists of two layers; the *parietal layer* lines the walls of the cavity and the *visceral layer* covers the organs concerned. The two are continuous, forming a closed sac with the organ(s) outside the sac. The inner surface of the sac is moistened by fluid derived from blood serum; this allows frictionless movement of the organs within their cavities. *Compare* mucous membrane.

Sertoli cell *See* sustentacular cell.

Sertoli cell tumour A tumour arising from the *sustentacular (Sertoli) cells in the testis. It is one of the three common neoplasms of the canine testis (*see also* interstitial cell tumour; seminoma) and occurs at least ten times more frequently in dogs with a retained testicle. The affected testicle is usually palpably enlarged, while the other is atrophied. The tumours frequently produce oestrogens and the dog will show signs of feminization, including mammary gland development, penile atrophy, pendulous prepuce, and decreased libido. Lethargy and bilaterally symmetrical hair loss over the flanks are also common signs. Treatment is by castration and the prognosis is fair to good, with resolution of secondary signs in most cases. However, metastases occur in about 25% of animals. The tumour occurs rarely in other species.

serum The fluid that separates from clotted blood or *plasma that has been allowed to stand. It differs from plasma in lacking *coagulation factors.

serum sickness A disease caused by the formation in the blood of complexes between host antibody and foreign antigens in injected serum. Similar complex-mediated disease is also induced by certain drugs in hypersensitive individuals. The complexes cause inflammation in the joints, heart, lymphoid organs, kidney, skin, and arteries. In acute cases there may be fever. In addition, there may be an immediate *hypersensitivity reaction mediated by antibodies of the IgE class. Avoidance of immediate reactions to serum is achieved in most cases by a small preliminary injection of the serum. If there are no undesirable effects within 30 minutes, the full dose can be given. Complex-mediated sickness is best prevented by avoiding repeated exposure to the offending antigen, and by using routes of administration other than the intravenous. Where possible,

serum from the same species should be used. The active ingredients (usually immunoglobulin) may also be used in purified form to obviate the injection of large amounts of miscellaneous serum protein.

serum therapy Treatment with *serum to induce passive immunity (*see* immunity).

service period 1. The number of days from calving to successful service in a dairy cow. The optimum service period is 85 days in order to achieve a *calving index of 365 days, but in practice, to attain this optimum, it will be necessary to serve most cows before 85 days. **2.** The period that a bull spends with a group of *heifers or suckler cows (*see* suckler herd) and during which it could serve them.

sesamoid bone An oval nodule of bone that lies within a tendon and slides over another bony surface. The *patella and other bones near joints in the limbs are sesamoid bones. The *distal sesamoid bone* occurs in the deep digital flexor tendon at the joint between the middle and distal phalanges in the digits of the fore- and hindfeet (manus and pes). In the horse it is often termed the *navicular bone* and it subject to pathological changes resulting in lameness (*see* navicular disease).

sex chromosome A *chromosome that operates in the sex-determining mechanism. In female mammals and male birds there are two identical large sex chromosomes (called the *X chromosomes* in mammals and *W chromosomes* in birds), making them the *homogametic sex in each case. The other (*heterogametic) sex has one X or W chromosome and a much smaller one, termed the *Y chromosome* in mammals and the *Z chromosome* in birds. In mammals, at least, this small Y chromosome appears to carry few if any genes other than that which initiates development of a male gonad. The X and W chromosomes carry genes not directly associated with the control of sex, in the same way as the other chromosomes. In the heterogametic sex, the genes on the X or W chromosomes are thus *hemizygous. *See also* sex-linked.

sex hormone Any steroid hormone, produced mainly by the ovaries or testes, that is responsible for controlling sexual characteristics and reproductive function. *Oestrogens and *progesterone are the female sex hormones; *androgens are the male sex hormones.

sex inversion The condition whereby animals that are structurally and functionally sexually normal at birth later come to resemble the opposite sex. For example, dogs with certain testicular tumours, notably *Sertoli cell tumour, may become feminized.

sex-limited Expressed only in one of the sexes. The expression of the *alleles of sex-limited genes is dependent on some interaction between the allelic product and a sex hormone; in the absence of the appropriate hormone the allele has no effect. Most secondary sexual characteristics are so controlled.

sex-linked Describing genes that are carried on the *sex chromosomes, usually on the X or Z chromosomes. Sex linkage accounts for the tendency of certain inherited characteristics or diseases (e.g. *haemophilia) to occur far more frequently in one sex than the other. An abnormal recessive allele is *hemizygous in the *heterogametic sex and can thus express its deleterious effects. In the *homogametic sex its effects are likely to be masked by a normal dominant allele.

sex ratio The relative abundance of members of the two sexes in a population. In most organisms this ratio is 1:1 at birth, but in the majority of controlled breeding programmes it is artificially altered by removal of many of the males. This leads to a reduction in the *effective population size and greater genetic uniformity.

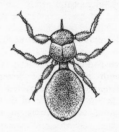

Sheep ked, *Melophagus ovinus*

sheep ked A small wingless *fly, *Melophagus ovinus*, that is a bloodsucking ectoparasite of sheep, on which the entire life cycle is spent (see illustration). The nearly mature larvae are laid in the fleece, and each develops into a pupa almost immediately. The adults are sometimes wrongly referred to as sheep ticks. Transmission is by direct contact between sheep. Sheep keds occur worldwide. Their irritating bite causes sheep to scratch themselves, damaging the fleece and resulting in sores that attract other flies. The faeces of the ked may also discolour the wool, and a severe infestation can cause anaemia. Sheep keds may also bite humans, especially during the shearing process. They are controlled by shearing or the use of dips containing a suitable *insecticide.

sheep nostril fly A large *fly, *Oestrus ovis*, also known as the nasal bot fly, whose larvae parasitize the nostrils, nasal passages, and sinuses of

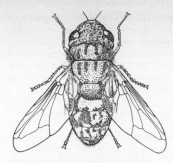

The sheep nostril fly, *Oestrus ovis*

sheep (see illustration). The short-lived adults have only rudimentary mouthparts; they are found in summer when females deposit their larvae in and around the host's nostrils. The larvae feed on mucous secretions, eventually migrating to the nasal passages and air sinuses causing irritation to the host and provoking copious mucous secretion and sneezing. Infested sheep push their noses into the ground or into the fleece of others in an attempt to relieve their distress, thereby interfering with their own feeding and causing weight loss. When fully grown, the larvae are sneezed out and pupate on the ground. Prevention entails painting an insect repellent, such as tar, around the nostrils or providing a salt lick smeared with tar. A suitable *insecticide will clear up existing larval infections.

sheep pox An infectious disease of sheep characterized by fever and generalized pocks, and caused by capripoxvirus (*see* poxvirus). Together with *goat pox it is the most economically significant animal pox disease. Sheep pox is enzootic in the Middle East, Central and North Africa, and Central Asia, and outbreaks have occurred in southern Europe in the 1980s. Transmission is by contact with an infected animal or via biting

flies; the incubation period is 8–12 days. The disease may be acute, mild, or symptomless, depending on the strain of virus and immunity of the animal. European breeds of sheep are susceptible to a highly acute (per-acute) form of the disease and may die before symptoms develop. In acute infections, fever is followed 24 hours later by a rash of skin lesions, which grow more prominent then, after 7 days, form scabs. There is also inflammation and discharge from the eyes and nose and inflammation of the lymph nodes. Mildly infected animals may only show single lesions. On post mortem, lesions may be found on the internal organs, particularly the lungs and lining of the abomasum. The virus may persist in the environment for many months. Control is by vaccination using an attenuated live vaccine. The sheep pox virus will infect goats, and many strains will infect cattle, causing symptoms similar to *lumpy-skin disease. Indeed, sheep pox, goat pox, and lumpy-skin disease may be caused by the same species of capripoxvirus. In the UK, sheep pox is a *notifiable disease.

sheep scab An intensely itchy skin disease affecting sheep and caused by the parasitic mite *Psoroptes communis* var. *ovis* (see illustration). The mites pierce the skin of their host to feed on tissue fluids. Very itchy moist papules develop followed by matting of the wool. Self-excoriation results in severe damage to the fleece, which may be shed from large areas of the body. The disease is most common in upland flocks grazed over large areas, where it is often difficult to ensure that all sheep are gathered for dipping with a suitable *acaricide to control the disease. Also, the disease may persist from year to year as latent infestations in relatively 'hidden' parts of the body, such as the perineum and base of the ears, where

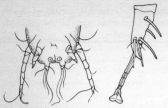

Posterior of male,   Distal end of leg
ventral view

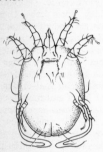

Female, ventral view

Sheep scab mite,
Psoroptes communis ovis

parasiticidal dressings may not penetrate. In the UK sheep scab is a *notifiable disease and annual dipping with an approved acaricide is compulsory.

Other mites of the genus *Psoroptes* produce *mange in goats, horses, cattle, and rabbits.

sheep tick *See* Ixodes.

Shigella A genus of rod-shaped non-motile aerobic or facultatively anaerobic Gram-negative *bacteria that cause bacillary dysentery (shigellosis) in humans and other primates. *Sh. flexneri*, *Sh. sonnei*, and *Sh. dysenteriae* affect humans, chimpanzees, and monkeys with occasional infection in dogs.

shigellosis Disease due to infection of the intestine with bacteria of the genus *Shigella*. *Sh. flexneri* and *Sh.*

sonnei sometimes cause a dysentery-like disease in captive apes and monkeys (*see* dysentery). The term 'shigellosis of foals' is sometimes used, incorrectly, to refer to *Actinobacillus equuli* infection of foals (*sleepy foal disease).

shipping fever *See* transit fever.

shivering (in horses) A condition, typically affecting the hindlimbs and tail (although occasional forelimb cases are recorded), characterized by apparently involuntary muscle twitching; the signs appear or are exacerbated when the horse is backed. The cause is unknown but a tentative link with previous respiratory disease has been suggested. The condition tends to be progressive and the prognosis is poor.

shock The condition associated with circulatory collapse, when the arterial blood pressure is too low to maintain an adequate supply of blood to the tissues. Clinical signs include acute depression, coldness, a weak rapid pulse, and fast breathing.
Shock may be due to a decrease in the volume of blood, as occurs after internal or external *haemorrhage, dehydration, burns, or severe vomiting or diarrhoea. It may be caused by reduced activity of the heart (*see* heart failure), or by widespread dilatation of the veins so that there is insufficient blood to fill them. This may be caused by the presence of bacteria or their toxins in the bloodstream (*septicaemic shock*), a severe allergic reaction (*anaphylactic shock*: *see* anaphylaxis), overdosage with drugs, such as certain anaesthetics, or acute stress. A combination of causes may be involved. Treatment depends on the cause. For example, any haemorrhage must be controlled and blood volume restored by *fluid replacement therapy or blood *transfusion.

shoeing The process of fitting shoes to a horse's feet to protect the feet from excessive wear and to give better grip on certain surfaces. The foot is prepared by removing horn that has grown since the last shoeing or, after a horse has been running at grass unshod, paring the hoof back to a normal shape. The foot must be made level and correctly balanced from toe to heel. The shoe is made from bar iron, fullered (*see* fullering) to countersink the heads of the nails; the nails are used to fix the shoe to the foot. Ready-made shoes are available in all sizes; these are satisfactory provided they are adjusted to fit the foot. Clips are drawn from the shoe – one at the toe of each front shoe and one each side of the toe in the hind shoes. The clips fit into a straight cut in the wall of the foot and prevent the shoe from sliding or twisting on the foot. The nails are driven through the shoe into the foot at the white line (the junction of the wall and the sole of the foot). Driven with their flat side towards the wall of the foot, they veer out through the wall. They should emerge higher at the toe than the quarters, and must be high enough to avoid splitting the wall but not so high that they endanger the sensitive laminae. The shoe is first nailed to the hoof by the toe nail, followed by the inside heel nail. Nails along either side are then fitted. After being driven home the nails are *clinched (or clenched) into a prepared bed. Every 4–6 weeks the shoes must be removed, the hoof reshaped, and either the existing shoes refitted or new ones fitted.

shotty eruption (sooty mange) A condition of pigs in which numerous *papules occur in the skin. The papules contain a black sebaceous material and elongated curled hairs. It is commonest on the belly and buttocks. The cause is unknown.

shoulder 1. The joint formed by the glenoid cavity of the *scapula and the head of the *humerus. It is a ball-and-socket type of joint but principally enables flexion and extension of the limb. **2.** The region of the forelimb surrounding the scapula.

shoulder gall A skin lesion occurring in the shoulder region of working horses, especially draught horses, caused by an ill-fitting collar. If the collar is too large it moves with each step of the animal, rubbing the skin and causing abrasions. If untreated, the abrasions provide sites for low-grade infection, which can result in the slow development of a mass of fibrous tissue resembling a tumour. This requires radical excision.

shoulder girdle (pectoral girdle) The assemblage of bones that connects the forelimb with the trunk. When fully developed, as in birds, it consists of the *scapula, *coracoid, and *clavicle. In the domestic mammals only the scapula is well developed, the coracoid having fused with it and the clavicle being present only as a rudiment in the brachiocephalic muscle. This arrangement allows wide-ranging movement during locomotion in quadrupeds.

shoulder slip *See* suprascapular paralysis.

sial- (sialo-) *Prefix denoting* **1.** saliva. **2.** a salivary gland.

sialic acid Acetylated *neuraminic acid. It is a component of some *glycoproteins, *gangliosides, and bacterial cell walls.

sialocele A soft fluctuating swelling of the jaw and upper neck in dogs due to the accumulation of saliva leaking from the damaged duct of a salivary gland, especially the *sublingual. The swelling most commonly develops high in the neck and between the rami of the mandible, and may on occasions burst to discharge rather viscid pale-brown fluid. A similar lesion may form below the tongue (*see* ranula). Treatment involves surgical removal of the affected sublingual gland – both monostomatic and polystomatic portions. The mandibular gland, which is surrounded by the same capsule as the monostomatic sublingual gland, is also excised. The swelling is opened ventrally to allow it to drain.

sialogogue An agent that increases the volume and fluidity of saliva. Cholinergic drugs (e.g. bethanecol, carbachol, pilocarpine, arecholine) and *anticholinesterases stimulate salivary secretion by acting at parasympathetic receptors in the salivary glands.

Siberian tick typhus (North Asian tick typus) *See* spotted fever.

side-bones A condition of horses in which the lateral cartilages of the foot ossify, i.e. they tend to lose their elasticity and become more like bone. Trauma, poor shoeing, or poor foot conformation may predispose to the condition. The degree of lameness varies and tends to be most marked during the ossification process, when some inflammation is present. Treatment is often not required, but can include grooving the hoof wall and corrective shoeing.

side-effect An unwanted effect produced by a drug in addition to its desired therapeutic effects. Side-effects are often undesirable and may be harmful.

sidero- *Prefix denoting* iron.

sideroblast A nucleated red cell containing iron-rich granules, probably of *ferritin or *haemosiderin. They are a normal feature of bone marrow. Their numbers decrease in iron deficiency and increase in cases of *lead poisoning.

siderocyte A mature red cell containing iron-rich granules. *See also* sideroblast.

sign An abnormality of function or behaviour that indicates disease. The term 'symptom' is often used synonymously but incorrectly: this is restricted to human medicine to mean an indication of disease noticed and communicated by the patient.

silage Material produced by the controlled fermentation of a high-moisture crop, such as grass, maize, or legumes, and used as an animal feedstuff, generally for ruminants. The moisture content is typically in the range 700–750 g/kg. The fermentation is controlled, either by encouraging the proliferation of lactic acid-producing bacteria naturally present on the crop, or by restricting fermentation by adding inorganic or organic acids or by wilting the crop before ensilage. Natural fermentation can be encouraged by adding soluble carbohydrates, cellulase enzymes, or selected strains of lactobacilli. It is essential that anaerobic conditions are established and maintained to prevent the build-up of clostridial bacteria and fungi, which results in unpalatable material of a generally lower nutritive value. This can be achieved by chopping the crop, adequate consolidation, and complete sealing of the silo. A recent innovation is *big bale silage*, in which big round bales of wilted grass are each sealed in an individual plastic bag or tightly wrapped in plastic film. Silage is less weather dependent than *hay, making it easier to achieve a high-quality product. Well-preserved silage should have a nutritive value comparable with that of the original material.

Badly preserved silage suffers from the breakdown of soluble nutrients and deamination of amino acids.

silent heat (silent ovulation) *See* suboestrus.

silicon A nonmetallic element occurring naturally in various rock and soil minerals, especially silica and silicates. Silicates, based on the SiO_4 group, appear to be necessary for proper bone growth. Symbol Si.

silicone Any of a group of polymeric compounds containing chains of silicon and oxygen atoms, with various organic groups linked to silicon atoms. *Methyl silicone* is a viscous liquid that is used as an *antizymotic to treat frothy bloat. It is administered orally or through an intraruminal cannula, causing an increase in surface tension and a decrease in foam stability. Other silicones are used as lubricants and coatings on needles and cannulas to produce a smooth surface and prevent the formation of blood clots.

sinistr- (sinistro-) *Prefix denoting* left or the left side.

sino- (sinu-) *Prefix denoting* **1.** a sinus. **2.** the sinus venosus.

sinoatrial node (SA node) The pacemaker of the heart: a minute mass of specialized cardiac muscle forming part of the *conducting system and situated in the wall of the right atrium near the entrance of the cranial vena cava. It contracts rhythmically, each contraction resulting in the spread of impulses through the atrial musculature to eventually reach the *atrioventricular node. Fibres of the autonomic nervous system supply the sinoatrial node and regulate the heart rate.

sinus 1. An air-filled cavity within a bone, especially in the skull (*see* paranasal sinus). **2.** Any wide channel containing blood, usually venous blood. *Venous sinuses* occur, for example, in the dura mater and drain blood from the brain. **3.** A pocket or bulge in a tubular organ, for example in blood vessels (*carotid sinus) or in the teat (*lactiferous sinus). **4.** An infected tract leading from a focus of infection to the surface of the skin or a hollow organ.

sinusitis Inflammation of the mucous membrane lining a sinus, usually a *paranasal sinus in the skull. It may result from extension of an abscess beneath a tooth or from infection in the nasal cavity (e.g. *rhinotracheitis). In horses sinusitis can be due to streptococcal infection, and the accumulation of pus in the sinus may cause severe pain and require surgical *drainage.

sinusoid A blood vessel resembling a large irregular blood capillary found in certain organs, such as the adrenal gland and the liver. They are more permeable than capillaries and blood flow can be slow or nonexistent within them.

sinus venosus A chamber of the embryonic heart that receives blood from several veins. In the adult heart it becomes part of the right atrium.

Siphunculina A genus of non-biting flies (*see* fly) including the eye fly of India, *S. funicola*, which feeds on secretions from the eye and spreads eye diseases, such as *conjunctivitis.

skeleton The rigid framework of connected *bones that gives form to the body, protects and supports its soft organs and tissues, and provides attachments for muscles and a system of levers essential for locomotion. The *axial skeleton* serves the head and

skin

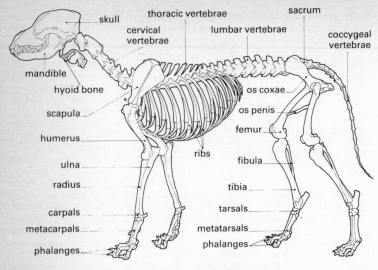

Skeleton of male dog

trunk; the *appendicular skeleton* serves the limbs. See illustration.

skin The outer covering of the body, consisting of an outer layer, the *epidermis, and an inner layer, the *dermis (see illustration). The skin may also bear a variety of specialized structures, such as *hair, *feathers, and scales. Beneath the dermis is a layer of fatty tissue. The skin has several functions. The epidermis protects the body from injury and from invasion by microorganisms. It also helps to prevent the body from becoming dehydrated. The combination of erectile hairs, *sweat glands, and blood capillaries in the skin form part of the temperature-regulating mechanism of the body. When the body is too hot, loss of heat is increased by sweating and by the dilatation of the capillaries. When the body is too cold the sweat glands are inactive, the capillaries contract, and a layer of air is trapped over the epidermis by the erected hairs. The skin also acts as an organ of excretion (by the secretion of sweat; *see* sweating) and as a sense organ (it contains receptors that are sensitive to heat, cold, touch, and pain). The layer of fat underneath the dermis can act as a reservoir of food and water.

skin graft The surgical transposition of skin from one area of the body surface to another. Two principal techniques are involved. With *sliding grafts* the skin alongside a defect is undermined and suitable incisions made to allow the freed portion of skin to be repositioned over the defect. This technique is very successful in animals. *Free grafts* are taken from elsewhere on the body; split-thickness grafts are used most commonly in humans, whereas full-thickness grafts are more often employed in animals. Both methods require careful preparation of the recipient site, and the graft must be held firmly in place and not disturbed until it has regained a blood supply. *See also* pedicle (def. 3).

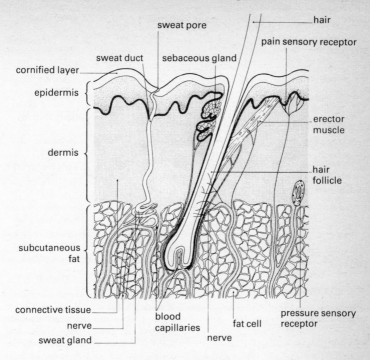

Section through the skin

skin tuberculosis A chronic nonfatal granulomatous skin disease of cattle, involving mainly the lower parts of the limbs. Firm rounded swellings develop, which may ulcerate or form cold abscesses. No agent has been isolated, but the lesions contain acid-fast bacteria, possibly a *Mycobacterium* species, and affected animals react to mammalian *tuberculin.

skull The skeleton of the head. It can be divided into the cranium, which encloses the brain in the cranial cavity, and the face, which includes the jaws. Rigid *joints connect virtually all the skull bones: *sutures connect the bones of the face and the bones forming the vault of the cranium;

synchondroses join the bones forming the base of the cranium. The exception is the *synovial joint (temperomandibular joint) whereby the lower jaw (mandible) articulates with the temporal bone of the cranium. See illustration.

Slaughterhouses Act (1974) (England and Wales) An Act of Parliament requiring that slaughterhouses and knackers' yards shall be licensed by the local authority. The Minister may make regulations for securing humane conditions of slaughter in slaughterhouses and knackers' yards and slaughtermen must hold a licence from the local authority.

Slaughterhouses (Hygiene) Regulations (1977)

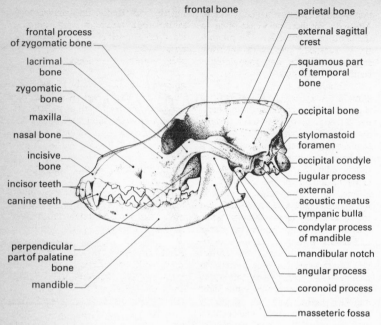

Skull of a dog (lateral view)

Labels (clockwise from top):
frontal bone · parietal bone · external sagittal crest · squamous part of temporal bone · occipital bone · stylomastoid foramen · occipital condyle · jugular process · external acoustic meatus · tympanic bulla · condylar process of mandible · mandibular notch · angular process · coronoid process · masseteric fossa · mandible · perpendicular part of palatine bone · canine teeth · incisor teeth · incisive bone · nasal bone · maxilla · zygomatic bone · lacrimal bone · frontal process of zygomatic bone

Slaughterhouses (Hygiene) Regulations (1977) (England and Wales) Statutes that lay down detailed requirements for construction, use, and hygienic practices in slaughterhouses. The Regulations also state the form of words to be used in the veterinary certificate accompanying injured animals sent for emergency slaughter (*see* casualty animal).

Slaughter of Poultry Act (1967) (England and Wales) An Act of Parliament that provides for the humane slaughter, for certain commercial purposes, of poultry.

sleep A state of natural reversible unconsciousness. In typical *deactivated sleep* there is absence of movement and a general reduction in muscle tone, although some muscles are more active, for instance in standing sleep in horses and in the perching behaviour of birds. Visceral functions, such as heart rate and blood pressure, are reduced. In higher mammals there also occur periods of *activated sleep*, associated with bursts of rapid eye movements (*REM sleep*), muscle twitching, and, in humans at least, dreaming. The exact purpose of sleep is not understood but it is necessary for health.

sleeper syndrome *See* Haemophilus septicaemia of cattle.

sleepy foal disease A bacterial disease, classically seen in foals between birth and 7 days of age. It is caused by **Actinobacillus equuli*, which produces a septicaemia and the formation of tiny abscesses in many organs. Affected foals become weak, often to the point of recumbency. The prognosis is guarded, even with intensive supportive therapy and the administration of antibiotics.

sling 1. A special bandage used to support a damaged limb during healing. In dogs, a sling is used to help maintain the position of a reduced (replaced) dislocated hip. The sling employed is a figure-of-eight bandage (often adhesive), applied so as to cause flexion of all the joints of the affected limb. It is kept in position for at least 4 days. **2.** A device used for restraining large animals while they recover from injury. In cattle and horses, a sling is employed occasionally to ensure that the animal remains standing for long periods. It consists of a broad sheet of strong canvas, which is passed under the animal's belly, held in place by leather straps in front and behind, and supported by metal hook-supports suspended from above. This gives the animal time to recover from an injury, such as a fall, where it is necessary to avoid the stress of rising from a lying position. It is important that no pressure is exerted on the body wall by the sling – it is a restraint rather than a support.

slink calf A premature or foetal *calf used for human food.

slipped tendon *See* perosis.

slough Dead tissue, such as skin, that separates from adjacent healthy tissue, usually following inflammation or infection.

slow virus One of a group of infective disease agents that resemble *viruses in some of their biological properties but whose physical properties (e.g. sensitivity to radiation) suggest that they may not contain

nucleic acid. Hence, they may not be viruses but rather a very unusual class of *proteins, and include the agent responsible for *scrapie in sheep. Other name: **prion**.

slurry A semiliquid mix of livestock dung and urine, usually containing very little or no bedding material. It is typically produced by cattle or pigs, especially ones housed on concrete or slatted floors.

small intestine *See* intestine.

smear A specimen of tissue or other material taken from a part of the body and smeared on a microscope slide for examination.

SMEDI An acronym describing reproductive failure in pigs – stillbirths (S), mummification (M), embryonic death (ED), and infertility (I). This syndrome is associated with infection of breeding sows with strains of the *enteroviruses and the *parvoviruses. *See* porcine parvovirus infection.

smegma The secretion of the glands of the *prepuce, which accumulates within the prepuce and has a white cheesy appearance.

smell *See* olfaction.

smooth muscle (involuntary muscle) Muscle that produces slow long-term contractions of which the individual is unaware. Smooth muscle occurs in hollow organs, such as the stomach, intestine, blood vessels, and bladder. It consists of spindle-shaped cells within a network of connective tissue (see illustration) and is under the control of the autonomic nervous system. *Compare* striated muscle.

snakebite poisoning A toxic state caused by *venom injected via the bite of certain snakes. The venom

snakeroot

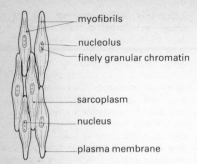

myofibrils
nucleolus
finely granular chromatin
sarcoplasm
nucleus
plasma membrane

Arrangement of smooth muscle cells

affects the nervous system and death is due to asphyxia. Treatment must be rapid and consists of the injection of a specific antiserum.

snakeroot (snakeweed) Any of various North American plants of which the roots or rhizomes have been used as a remedy for snakebite. They include white snakeroot, which contains a toxic alcohol (*see* white snakeroot poisoning), and members of the genus *Cicuta*, which may contain the toxic alkaloid cicutoxin (*see* hemlock water dropwort poisoning).

snare A loop of wire or rope that can be tightened as required. In surgery, snares may be used to remove growths, especially ones attached by a stalk to underlying tissue. Snares are also used in cases of difficult birth (*dystocia) due to foetal malpresentation; cord loops are placed around the limbs or head to correctly align the foetus for delivery.

sneeze A violent reflex expulsion of air through the nose and mouth provoked by irritation of the mucous membrane lining the nasal cavity.

sneezeweed poisoning *See* Helenium poisoning.

SNF *See* solids-not-fat.

snood (frontal process; nasal comb) A conical part of the wattle in turkeys that arises from the forehead and lies over the upper beak. It is highly vascular, contains much smooth muscle, and is extensible, measuring 1–10 cm. The risk of *cannibalism in intensively housed flocks is reduced by removing the snood (*desnooding) soon after the chicks hatch.

snow blindness Impaired sight due to excessive exposure to sunlight (especially ultraviolet light) reflected from lying snow. Animals, such as sheep, that wander on snow-covered land in brilliant sunlight are especially affected. However, it is important to distinguish this form of blindness from that due to *pregnancy toxaemia, which may be precipitated by a food shortage due to the snow cover.

soapwort poisoning A toxic condition due to the ingestion of *Saponaria officinalis*, a plant found in hedgerows and on waste ground. It contains githagenin, a saponin that causes gastroenteritis and, after absorption into the bloodstream, haemoglobinaemia and haemoglobinuria. Treatment is of the clinical signs.

socket (in anatomy) A hollow or depression into which another part fits, such as the cavity in the alveolar bone of the jaws into which the root of a tooth fits, or the cavity involved in a ball-and-socket type of synovial joint.

sodium A metallic element and one of the major minerals required in animal diets. Sodium ions (Na^+) are the principal cations in blood serum and other extracellular body fluids, but occur at relatively low concentrations inside cells. Their concentration is thus the main factor in determining the osmotic pressure and hence volume of body fluids, and also plays a role in maintaining the *acid-base balance. Moreover, the movement of sodium ions into and out of cells, closely linked with a counter-flow of potassium ions, is vital in maintaining the electrical potential of cells and the ability of nerve and muscle cells to transmit nerve impulses. Sodium is also required for the absorption of sugars and amino acids.

Sodium levels in blood are regulated by the kidneys under the influence of *corticosteroid hormones, notably *aldosterone. However, deficiency of sodium in the diet may lead to retarded growth, impaired egg production, and other clinical signs (*see* hyponatraemia). Excessive sodium in the blood (*hypernatraemia) also has various pathological consequences; the commonest cause is *salt poisoning.

sodium bicarbonate (sodium hydrogen carbonate; bicarbonate of soda) A white powder that is soluble in water, producing an alkaline solution. Sodium bicarbonate can be used as an *antacid, particularly in small animals to reduce stomach acidity and in ruminants after excessive carbohydrate feeding (carbohydrate overload) or in the treatment of ketosis. The rise in pH is temporary because carbon dioxide is released, and this can cause gastric distension stimulating further acid secretion. Sodium bicarbonate can also be used intravenously to counteract metabolic acidosis, or to increase urinary pH, particularly in carnivores. Possible indications for the latter are to increase the activity of aminoglycoside antibiotics, improve the solubility of excreted sulphonamides, and to prevent the formation of cystine or urate calculi (stones).

sodium chlorate poisoning A toxic condition of animals caused by ingestion of sodium chlorate. This can occur when fields, roadsides, or gardens are sprayed with sodium chlorate solution as a weedkiller. In wet weather the solution can collect in pools and its salty taste makes it attractive to all species. It causes purgation, abdominal pain, staggering, and discharge of tarry blood from the nostrils and anus due to the formation of methaemoglobin (*see* methaemoglobinaemia). As well as treatment of the clinical signs, intravenous injection of a 4% solution of methylene blue is recommended for treating cases among cattle and sheep; this reduces the methaemoglobin to haemoglobin.

sodium cromoglycate A *mast cell stabilizing agent used as a prophylactic to prevent allergic conditions in animals and humans. It is administered by inhalation using a nebulizer. Although it prevents mast cells discharging histamine when exposed to antigen the exact mode of action is unknown. Sodium cromoglycate is used in horses suffering from chronic obstructive pulmonary disease (allergic respiratory disease). The period of prophylaxis is said to depend on the number of consecutive days of treatment: a single treatment protects the animal for 3 days; treatment on 4 consecutive days gives protection for 20 days. The use of sodium cromoglycate to treat allergic intestinal diseases is being investigated. Tradename: **Cromovet Forte**.

sodium hydroxide (caustic soda) A white translucent solid, available as pellets, flakes, or sticks, which dissolve in water to produce a highly alkaline solution. The solution is caustic and irritant, and is used as a laboratory reagent and as a disinfectant. Concentrated solutions cause severe burns and any spillage on skin should be neutralized using an *acid and washed with copious amounts of water.

sodium iodide A water-soluble iodine salt with several uses in veterinary medicine. It can be injected intravenously or given orally in the treatment of iodine deficiency, found particularly in calves. It is also used as an antifungal agent, being applied locally or injected intravenously, and is used in the treatment of *actinobacillosis (wooden tongue). Sodium iodide also has *expectorant properties, increasing the secretion of fluid from bronchial glands. Signs of toxicity include laryngeal oedema, fever, cutaneous haemorrhages, increased salivation, sneezing, coughing, pulmonary oedema, gastrointestinal irritation, and depression.

sodium monofluoracetate poisoning See fluoracetate poisoning.

sodium nitrite A salt used orally as a *vasodilator to reduce systemic blood pressure, or injected as an antidote in the treatment of *cyanide poisoning. In the latter case, the nitrite converts haemoglobin to methaemoglobin, which combines with cyanide forming the harmless cyanmethaemoglobin. Nitrites can cause toxicity in animals. This is seen in animals grazed on highly fertilized land where the plants accumulate high levels of nitrates (see nitrate poisoning).

sodium salicylate See NSAID.

solanine poisoning A toxic condition due to the ingestion of plants containing the alkaloid solanine. The main sources of solanine for animals are the woody nightshade or bittersweet (Solanum dulcamara), the garden or black nightshade (Solanum nigrum), and the potato (Solanum tuberosum). The woody nightshade is to be distinguished from the *deadly nightshade, which contains different toxic substances. The woody nightshade commonly grows in hedgerows, has purple flowers with a yellow centre and shiny red berries. The black nightshade is a weed of cultivated land. Its flowers are white with a yellow centre and the shiny berries are black. Although properly harvested and stored potatoes are a staple food in temperate areas, tubers that have become green through exposure to light or have sprouted, the green berry-like fruits, and the stems and leaves of the potato plant all contain solanine. This is an irritant substance which on ingestion causes salivation, diarrhoea, tremors, staggering, convulsions, and death. Its haemolytic properties cause *haemoglobinuria. Cooking green or sprouted potatoes destroys the solanine.

solids-not-fat (SNF) The portion of the dry matter of *milk that is not *butterfat. It includes the nitrogen fraction (both protein and nonprotein nitrogen), lactose, minerals, enzymes, and water-soluble vitamins of the B complex and vitamin C. In the UK it is no longer reported since milk payment is now based on butterfat, protein, and lactose yields.

somat- Prefix denoting **1.** the body. **2.** somatic.

somatic 1. Relating to the nonreproductive parts of the body. A somatic mutation cannot be inherited. **2.** Relating to the body wall (i.e. excluding the viscera), e.g. somatic *mesoderm. Compare splanchnic.

somatomedin A protein hormone, produced by the liver in response to stimulation by *somatotrophin, that stimulates protein synthesis and promotes growth. It is biochemically similar to *insulin and has some actions similar to insulin; it is therefore sometimes said to have insulin-like activity (ILA) or is referred to as insulin-like growth factor (IGF).

somatopleure The body wall of the early embryo, which consists of a simple layer of ectoderm lined with mesoderm. The amnion is a continuation of this structure outside the embryo. *Compare* splanchnopleure.

somatostatin (growth-hormone-release inhibiting factor) A hormone, produced by the hypothalamus and some extraneural tissues, including the gastrointestinal tract and pancreas, that inhibits somatotrophin (growth hormone) release by the pituitary gland. Both growth-hormone releasing factor and somatostatin are controlled by complex neural mechanisms related to sleep rhythms, stress, neurotransmitters, blood glucose, and exercise.

somatotrophin (growth hormone) A hormone, synthesized and stored in the adenohypophysis, that promotes bone growth and stimulates protein synthesis (via *somatomedin). Its release is controlled by the opposing actions of growth-hormone releasing factor and *somatostatin. Production of growth hormone is greatest in early life. Excessive secretion of growth hormone results in gigantism before puberty and *acromegaly in adults. Lack of growth hormone in juveniles causes dwarfism.

Both human and bovine somatotrophin can now be synthesized using recombinant DNA techniques. Bovine somatotrophin has been found to increase the efficiency of milk production in lactating dairy cattle. It is given as a subcutaneous or intramuscular injection, starting at around the time of peak milk yield and continuing with daily injections throughout lactation. Increased milk production occurs within 2–3 days, accompanied by a slight increase in feed intake, giving an overall increase in the efficiency of feed utilization for milk production. There are no apparent effects on the long-term health of the cow but trials are being carried out. Somatotrophins are species specific and the bovine form has no activity and hence no side-effects in humans. Somatotrophins may, in the future, be used to increase production in various livestock species.

somite Any of the paired segmented divisions of the paraxial *mesoderm that develop in the early embryo. The somites develop into various structures associated with the body walls (i.e. excluding the viscera). Each somite soon becomes subdivided into *dermatome, *myotome, and *sclerotome.

sore A small *ulcer (less than 1 cm in diameter) in the skin or mucous membrane.

sorrel poisoning *See* oxalate poisoning.

sound 1. (in diagnosis) A noise arising in the body that is discernible at the body surface. Distinguishing between normal and abnormal sounds aids the diagnosis of pathological conditions. A routine clinical examination includes *auscultation of cardiac, respiratory, and, occasionally, gastrointestinal sounds. *See also* borborygmus; crepitation; murmur; rale; rhonchus. **2.** (in surgery) A blunt-ended instrument used to probe a body cavity or channel. Sounds may be used to detect the depth and direction of a sinus tract or to detect the presence of a foreign body or obstruction in the lumen of a tubular structure (e.g. in the oesophagus or urethra). In certain circumstances, sounds of increasing diameter may be employed to dilate a tubular organ that has undergone *stenosis (e.g. oesophagus or anus). **3.** To explore a cavity using a sound.

soursob poisoning A toxic condition due to ingestion of the sorrel, *Oxalis* *cernua.* Poisoning is due to the oxalic acid content of the plant (*see* oxalate poisoning).

sow An adult female pig used for breeding purposes, generally from the time of its second pregnancy.

Spanish fly A metallic-green beetle, the blister beetle (*Lytta vesicatoria*), in which the irritant and toxic chemical *cantharidin occurs. This causes blistering of the skin and was formerly used in veterinary medicine as a blistering agent. Blister beetles may occasionally be found in lucerne (alfalfa) hay. When eaten by horses acute enteritis and death may follow. Other blister beetles are *Paederus* and *Epicauta* spp.

sparganosis Disease due to infestation by plerocercoids (second larval stage) of tapeworms of the genus *Spirometra* (*see* sparganum). The genus is widespread in eastern Europe, the Far East, Madagascar, the USA, and Australia, and sparganosis occurs in a wide variety of vertebrates, including pigs and humans. Infestation follows ingestion of procercoid (first-stage) larvae in freshwater crustaceans, or sometimes by contact with carcasses of other vertebrates that already contain live plerocercoids. Infested pig carcasses are condemned, thus causing economic loss. In humans, the larvae cause inflammation, swelling, and fibrosis of tissues, usually beneath the skin or between the muscles but occasionally in the viscera and brain.

Sparganum The larvae of certain tapeworms, such as some species of *Spirometra*, that infect warm-blooded hosts, such as mice, carnivores, and humans, causing the disease *sparganosis. The generic name *Sparganum* is given to them because definite classification of the species is not possible from the larvae alone.

spasm A sustained involuntary muscular contraction. The causes are various and include the accumulation of toxic metabolites, such as lactic acid, in the muscle (*see* cramp), metabolic disorders, such as *hypomagnesaemia, and certain poisons, such as *lead and *mercury. An inherited congenital spasm occurs in Jersey cattle, probably due to a lesion in the cerebellum. Tetanus induces generalized and repeated muscular spasms, which eventually cause death from respiratory failure. *Compare* convulsions. *See also* Scottie cramp.

spasmodic Occurring in spasms or resembling a spasm.

spasmogenic An agent that increases the contractions of smooth muscle in the gastrointestinal tract. Gastrointestinal motility is under the control of the parasympathetic nervous system, and *parasympathomimetic compounds (e.g. carbachol and bethanechol) have a spasmogenic action. These drugs have been used to treat ruminal atony and intestinal impaction, but they have a powerful action and can cause gastric or intestinal rupture. The spasmogenic effect of an *enema helps to relieve constipation: the distension and irritation of the rectum and colon by the enema fluid increases intestinal contractions.

spasmolytic An agent that reduces involuntary muscle contractions, for example in the gastrointestinal tract. Spasmolytic drugs are used to decrease aberrant motility of the intestinal tract in the treatment of, for example, diarrhoea, spasmodic colic in horses, or following surgical correction of intestinal intussusception. Various types of drug can be used. *Parasympatholytic agents (e.g. atropine, homatropine, and hyoscine) decrease gastrointestinal motility but also reduce gastrointestinal secretions, with possible inspissation (thickening) of the intestinal contents and a predisposition to impaction. *Morphine initially produces increased motility followed by reduced motility and increased tone of sphincters; it is used at low concentrations with *kaolin to treat diarrhoea. *Pethidine and *butorphanol are used in the treatment of spasmodic colic in horses and have a painkilling and spasmolytic action of short duration. Other *opiates (e.g. diphenoxylate and loperamide) have good constipating effects and can be used in the treatment of diarrhoea.

spastic Describing a condition or individual characterized by *spasms. Certain breeds of cattle may suffer from a hereditary spastic paresis, which affects the gastrocnemius muscles in particular: the hock and stifle joints become forced into full extension so that the animal cannot walk properly. Another spastic syndrome known as 'crampy' or 'cramps' also occurs in cattle (*see* cramp). Both conditions are progressive and usually require euthanasia.

spastic paresis An inherited condition of cattle, controlled by a *recessive allele and characterized by the development of spastic lameness. It is a cause of great economic loss, and ranges from mild to , severe with the greatest incidence occurring in Holstein-Friesian and Aberdeen Angus breeds. There is some evidence to suggest that age of the dam and calving date may affect the appearance of the condition. The lower part of the thigh often forms an almost straight line with the leg and characteristically there is a straight pastern. Either one or both hindlimbs are extended backwards in a rigid convulsive-like stance for several minutes after getting up. Tremor follows this spastic state. When walking, the affected limb remains rigid causing the leg to be dragged and swung laterally. This impedes movement greatly, and sudden turning causes loss of balance. The tarsal region may become chronically inflamed due to excessive strain, but care should be taken in differentiating this feature from other causes of inflammation. Many cases have been traced to a few ancestral bulls, in particular ELSO-11-34, after which the condition is named in the USA (*Elsoheel*). Sires with this condition should not be used for breeding. Other names: **hereditary paralysis**; **period spasticity**; **spastic syndrome**.

spavin One of various conditions of the equine hock (*blood spavin, *bog spavin, or *bone spavin) or carpus (*knee spavin).

spaying Surgical removal of the ovaries, either alone (ovariectomy) or together with the uterus (*see* ovariohysterectomy). Female dogs (bitches) and cats (queens) are routinely spayed at about 6–8 months of age or after their first season on heat (oestrus). This renders them infertile, thus avoiding unwanted litters and the behavioural problems when in season. In the bitch spaying prevents *false pregnancy and the collection of pus in the uterus (pyometra). It may also decrease the risk of mammary gland tumours when performed before or after the first oestrus. After spaying, the animal often requires less food to maintain bodyweight and care must be taken to avoid obesity. This enhanced liveweight gain can be used to advantage in heifers used for beef production. In Africa and other areas of extensive beef production, it is routine to spay nonbreeding heifer calves to increase weight gain and prevent pregnancy. This is not common practice in the UK.

specific pathogen free (SPF) Describing an animal, usually a pig, that is removed from its dam just prior to term under sterile conditions, normally by hysterectomy. If the animal and its progeny from matings with similarly produced stock are reared and kept under sterile conditions, the stock are referred to as 'germ free'. This state is difficult to maintain in practice and, following initial rearing under sterile conditions, such animals are kept under carefully controlled conditions where strict standards of hygiene are enforced. Such commercial units are referred to as *minimal disease* (*MD*). Providing herd health is maintained, SPF stock are free of many of the enteric and respiratory infections which cause problems on intensive pig units.

speculum (*pl.* **specula**) An instrument for inserting into and holding open a body cavity to facilitate examination. Vaginal specula, such as Graves vaginal speculum, are used routinely in veterinary practice for examination of the vagina, urethral orifice, and cervix.

speedy cut An injury, occurring in the horse, due to the inside of a leg (fore or hind) being struck by the inside of the opposite foot. Shoes, especially badly fitting or neglected ones, increase the risk of serious injury. The injury can vary from a small scratch to a deep wound, which requires immediate treatment.

sperm *See* spermatozoon.

sperm- (spermi(o)- spermo-) *Prefix denoting* sperm or semen.

spermat- (spermato-) *Prefix denoting* **1.** sperm. **2.** organs or ducts associated with sperm.

spermatic cord The cord, consisting of the *ductus deferens, testicular blood vessels, nerves, *tunica vaginalis, cremaster muscle, and fascial coverings, that runs through the *inguinal canal in the ventral abdominal wall to the testis in the scrotum.

spermatid A male reproductive cell produced as an intermediate stage in the formation of spermatozoa (*see* spermatogenesis). They develop in the seminiferous tubules of the testis from spermatocytes and are transformed into spermatozoa without further cell division by a process called spermiogenesis, during which time they are attached to Sertoli cells.

spermatocele A cystlike accumulation of sperm behind an obstruction in the duct of the epididymis. It is known to occur in cattle, goats, and dogs. Formation of such a cyst may be the result of congenital malformation (aplasia), trauma, or post-infection scarring. Possible consequences include degeneration of the epididymal tube wall and testicular degeneration. If sperm leak and contact the supporting connective tissues, a granulomatous reaction may result (*see* granuloma).

spermatocyte A cell produced as an intermediate stage in the production of spermatozoa in the testis. *See* spermatogenesis.

spermatogenesis The process by which spermatozoa are produced in the testis. Male germ cells (*spermatogonia) line the inner wall of the seminiferous tubules, but although present in the embryo and foetus, do not start to produce spermatozoa until puberty. A single spermatogonium divides by mitosis to form *primary spermatocytes*, each of which undergoes the initial (reduction) division of meiosis to form two haploid *secondary spermatocytes*. Each of these undergoes the second meiotic division to form two spermatids, which in turn are transformed into mature spermatozoa without further cell division by a process known as *spermio-*

genesis. All these cell types are supported and nourished by adjacent Sertoli cells. The spermatozoa are finally released into the lumen of the tubule and carried to temporary storage in the duct of the epididymis, where they mature. The entire process takes several weeks to complete. In animals whose breeding activity is highly seasonal, such as deer and (possibly) sheep, spermatogenesis may be reduced or suspended out of the breeding season.

spermatogonium (*pl.* **spermatogonia**) A male germ cell found in the testis that gives rise to a sequence of cells culminating in the male gametes – spermatozoa. *See* spermatogenesis.

spermatozoa *See* spermatozoon.

spermatozoon (sperm) (*pl.* **spermatozoa**) A mature male gamete. Mammalian spermatozoa consist of a head, containing the nucleus and acrosome, and a whiplike tail for propulsion. They are produced in the seminiferous tubules of the testis (*see* spermatogenesis) and ejected in *semen at ejaculation. They swim towards the oviducts of the female, assisted by muscular contractions of the genital tract, and after a final maturation period lasting one to several hours, are capable of penetrating and fertilizing the ova. Spermatozoa can survive for varying periods in the female tract, depending on species: bovine and ovine, 24–48 hours; porcine, 24–42 hours; equine, 6 days; canine, 7 days. In birds sperm are stored in crypts within the vagina and retain their capacity for fertilization for up to 14 days.

spermaturia The presence of sperm in the urine. Reflux of sperm into the bladder occurs normally in some domestic animals, for example sheep and goats.

sperm count The concentration of spermatozoa in the ejaculate, expressed as number of spermatozoa per millilitre. Typical figures ($\times 10^6$/ml) are 1200–1800 for bulls, 2000–3000 for rams, and 250–350 for boars. *See also* semen.

spermiogenesis The process by which spermatids are transformed without further cell division into spermatozoa (*see* spermatogenesis). This is the final developmental stage to occur in the testis, after which the spermatozoa are wafted into the duct of the epididymis to mature.

spheno- *Prefix denoting* the sphenoid bone. Examples: *sphenomaxillary* (relating to the sphenoid and maxillary bones); *sphenopalatine* (relating to the sphenoid bone and palate).

sphenoid A bone of the base of the *skull. In domestic mammals it is divided into two parts, the *basisphenoid* and the *presphenoid*. Each consists of a *body* and a pair of *wings*.

spherocyte A red cell of abnormal shape, tending to a sphere. It is found characteristically in *canine autoimmune haemolytic anaemia.

sphincter A specialized ring of muscle that surrounds an orifice. Contractions of the sphincter partly or completely close the orifice. Sphincters occur, for example, around the *anus (*anal sphincter*) and at the opening between the stomach and duodenum (*pyloric sphincter*).

sphincterectomy The surgical removal of a sphincter. It is rarely performed.

sphincterotomy Surgical division of a sphincter muscle, usually performed to reduce the sphincter's efficiency, especially where it is overactive. The prime example is division of the muscle of the pyloric sphincter of the stomach to overcome pyloric *stenosis. Splitting of the sphincter of the teat in cows was employed when hand-milking was common since it made milking much easier. Splitting the anal sphincter has been employed in cases of anal stricture, but is liable to result in faecal incontinence.

sphingomyelin A *phospholipid that contains sphingosine, a fatty acid, phosphoric acid, and choline. Sphingomyelins are found in large amounts in brain and nerve tissue.

sphingosine A long-chain amino alcohol that is a constituent of sphingomyelin and cerebrosides.

sphygmo- *Prefix denoting* the pulse.

spica A special arrangement of bandaging, usually some variant of figure-of-eight, in which the turns cross one another so that the final pattern closely follows the contours of the underlying part to give support.

spider bite poisoning Toxicity due to spider venom. Certain species of spider are potentially harmful or even lethal to domestic pets and humans. For example, in parts of the American continent dogs are sometimes bitten by the black widow spider, *Latrodectus mactans*. The condition is painful and the venom causes dyspnoea and paralysis, often followed by death. A specific antiserum is available and the clinical signs should be treated appropriately.

spina bifida An inherited congenital abnormality in which the dorsal vertebral laminae are not fully closed (*see* vertebra); in some cases the spinal cord is exposed on the surface. This can occur at one or more vertebrae. It is thought to be controlled by an autosomal *recessive or *dominant allele of low penetrance and expres-

sivity. Where lesions are severe the condition is lethal. In less severe cases *paresis, paralysis, and incontinence will be shown. Other congenital disorders are frequently associated.

spinal anaesthesia A form of regional *analgesia achieved by the injection of a *local anaesthetic into the vertebral canal. In *subarachnoid analgesia* (*anaesthesia*) the injection is made into the cerebrospinal fluid. This affects both the spinal cord and nerve roots, and localization of the injected fluid is controlled by careful positioning of the subject. The technique is not widely used in animals because the results are difficult to control and it can produce a disastrous fall in blood pressure.

In *epidural analgesia* (*anaesthesia*) the injection is made into the space between the dura mater and the wall of the vertebral canal. Such injections tend to remain reasonably localized because of the epidural fat. The technique is used most commonly in cattle to facilitate obstetrical manipulation during calving. The injection site is at the caudal end of the vertebral canal, and the volume of anaesthetic injected determines the effects. A small volume will give analgesia of the tail, perineum, and vagina and cause cessation of straining. A large volume will produce approximately the same area of analgesia but will also cause the animal to lie down, without abolishing sensation in the legs. In horses, epidural analgesia requires special precautions because of the much greater tendency to lose control of the hindlimbs and hence risk of injury.

spinal column *See* vertebral column.

spinal cord (spinal medulla) The portion of the *central nervous system enclosed in the *vertebral canal, consisting of nerve cells and bundles

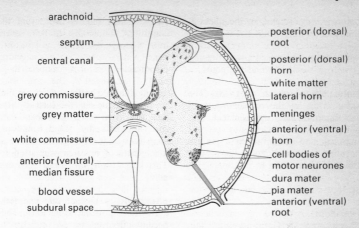

arachnoid

septum

central canal

grey commissure

grey matter

white commissure

anterior (ventral)
median fissure

blood vessel

subdural space

posterior (dorsal)
root

posterior (dorsal)
horn

white matter

lateral horn

meninges

anterior (ventral)
horn

cell bodies of
motor neurones

dura mater

pia mater

anterior (ventral)
root

Transverse section through the spinal cord

of nerve fibres connecting the various parts of the body with the brain. It has a narrow central canal surrounded by grey matter, which in turn is surrounded by white matter. The grey matter is subdivided into dorsal and ventral horns, with an additional lateral horn in the thoracic and cranial lumbar segments. The white matter is subdivided into dorsal, lateral, and ventral funiculi. The spinal cord has cervical and lumbar enlargements in those regions serving the limbs, and caudally tapers to a point as the *conus medullaris*. It terminates at the caudal lumbar or cranial sacral levels, depending on species. Beyond its termination it is continued as the *filum terminale*. The *spinal nerves arise from the spinal cord, the portion of cord associated with each pair of spinal nerves being termed a *spinal cord segment*. Surrounding the spinal cord are the three layers of membrane, the *meninges. See illustration.

spinal nerves The pairs of nerves that arise from the *spinal cord to be distributed to the body. A pair of spinal nerves emerges between each pair of adjacent vertebrae, through the intervertebral foramina; they are designated cervical, thoracic, lumbar, sacral, or coccygeal spinal nerves according to their origin. Each spinal nerve is attached to the spinal cord by two roots: a *dorsal root*, containing afferent (sensory) neurones, and a *ventral root*, containing efferent (motor) neurones. The dorsal root bears a prominent ganglion. The two roots unite just within the intervertebral foramen forming a mixed nerve. Beyond the intervertebral foramen the spinal nerve divides into a *dorsal ramus* and a *ventral ramus*, serving dorsal and ventral regions of the body respectively. *Compare* cranial nerves.

spindle A collection of fibres seen in a cell when it is dividing. The fibres radiate from the two ends (*poles*) and meet at the centre (the *equator*) giving a structure shaped like two cones placed base to base. It plays an important part in chromosome movement in *mitosis and *meiosis and is also involved in division of the cytoplasm.

spine 1. A sharp process of a bone. **2.** The *vertebral column.

spino- *Prefix denoting* **1.** the spine. **2.** the spinal cord.

spiral loop The coiled portion of the *colon in ruminants and the pig.

spiral organ (organ of Corti) The sense organ in the cochlear duct of the internal ear (*see* cochlea) that converts sound waves into nervous impulses and transmits these via the cochlear division of the *vestibulocochlear nerve to the brain.

spiramycin *See* macrolide antibiotics.

Spirillum A genus of aerobic or *microaerophilic Gram-negative *bacteria having rigid spiral cells. They are commonly found in both fresh and sea water and are generally nonpathogenic, except *S. minus*, which causes *rat-bite fever in humans. Rats act as natural reservoirs and carriers of infection.

spiro- *Prefix denoting* **1.** spiral. **2.** respiration.

Spirocerca A genus of parasitic *nematodes containing *S. lupi*, which infests dogs in tropical and subtropical regions. The adult worms are found in nodules or tumours in the aorta, oesophagus, and stomach; these tumours may occasionally become malignant and metastasize to produce secondary tumours in the lungs and elsewhere. Eggs are passed in the faeces and eaten by dung beetles, which may be eaten directly by dogs or by small mammals, amphibians, or birds, which may in turn be eaten by dogs. The larvae penetrate the stomach wall and migrate initially to the aorta and then to the oesophagus and other organs, causing haemorrhage, necrosis, and abscesses. In serious cases the parasite can cause blockage of the oesophagus and respiratory distress. Treatment with *diethylcarbamazine alleviates the clinical signs but will not kill all the worms; surgical removal of the lesions may be relevant.

spirochaete One of a group of long spiral Gram-negative *bacteria that have flexible cell walls and are motile but lack external flagella. Instead they have filaments or axial fibrils and move forwards by rapid rotations along their axis. The group includes three genera of veterinary importance: *Borrelia*, *Leptospira*, and *Treponema*.

spirochaetosis Disease due to infection with *spirochaete bacteria. The specific spirochaetoses of animals are *swine dysentery, *avian spirochaetosis, the various forms of *leptospirosis, and *rabbit syphilis. A spirochaete occurs as a secondary invader in some cases of *foot rot of sheep.

spironolactone A steroid that acts as an *aldosterone antagonist in the distal tubules of the kidney and therefore has a diuretic action. It decreases potassium loss and increases calcium excretion from the renal tubules. Administered orally, spironolactone is often used in combination with other diuretics to prevent *hypokalaemia. However, in advanced renal disease, very high levels of aldosterone are found and these can overcome the competitive antagonism of spironolactone.

splanch- (splanchno-) *Prefix denoting* the viscera.

splanchnic Relating to the viscera, e.g. splanchnic *mesoderm. *Compare* somatic (def. 2).

splanchnic nerves The series of nerves in the sympathetic part of the *autonomic nervous system that are distributed to the abdominal organs. They run from ganglia in the sympathetic trunk to enter the abdomen and branch profusely to form plexuses.

splanchnocranium The skeleton of the face and jaws. *See* skull.

splanchnopleure The wall of the embryonic gut, which consists of a simple layer of endoderm lined with mesoderm. The yolk sac is a continuation of this structure outside the embryo. *Compare* somatopleure.

splayleg An inherited (possibly *recessive) congenital predisposition to muscle underdevelopment (hypoplasia) in neonatal pigs and, rarely, calves. The condition is characterized by either the forelimbs or both fore- and hindlimbs being laterally or anteriorly splayed; the majority of animals are unable to stand or walk. This condition is noticed soon after birth when the young would normally be moving about, and lasts for up to 2 weeks after which the signs subside. There is some evidence to suggest that age of the dam may have some effect, with 1st and 7th and 8th litters showing a higher incidence; *choline deficiency in the sow may have some effect. However, addition of choline and methionine to the diet does not prevent the anomaly. Many affected piglets perform poorly. Other names: **myofibrillar hypoplasia**; **spraddle leg**.

spleen A large dark-red organ situated in the cranial part of the abdomen on the left of the stomach. It is enclosed within a fibrous capsule that extends into the spongy interior – the *splenic pulp* – to form a supportive framework. The pulp consists of *lymphoid tissue (*white pulp*) within a meshwork of *reticular fibres packed with red blood cells (*red pulp*). The spleen contains *phagocytes, which remove worn-out red blood cells and other particles from the bloodstream. It also acts as a reservoir for blood

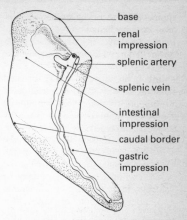

Spleen of the horse (visceral surface)

and, in the foetus, as a source of red blood cells. (See illustration.) Anatomical name: **lien**.

splen- (spleno-) *Prefix denoting* the spleen. Example: *splenorenal* (relating to the spleen and kidney).

splenectomy Surgical removal of the spleen. It is indicated in cases of neoplasm, especially haemangioma, which can result in gross intra-abdominal haemorrhage, and in cases of severe splenic trauma or splenic torsion.

splenitis Inflammation of the *spleen. The usual cause is blood-borne infection but the condition (which is rare) may arise from extension of local inflammation, penetrating foreign bodies (e.g. in *traumatic reticulitis in cattle), or parasites (e.g. *Strongylus infestation in horses).

splenium The most caudal part of the *corpus callosum in the brain.

splenomegaly Enlargement of the spleen. It occurs in various blood disorders or parasitisms, especially where there is destruction of red blood cells and consequent increased activity of

769

the reticuloendothelial system. Examples include *babesiosis, *septicaemia (with *anthrax in particular), and *heart failure. *See also* hypersplenism.

splint 1. (in surgery) A strip of rigid material, usually wood or metal, used to support or immobilize an injured limb. The splint is held in place by bandages arranged to give firm support without causing damage to the skin. Splints may be employed in the management of a fracture that can be reduced without operation, or may be valuable in protecting a vulnerable area after operation or injury, for example, a damaged tendon or ligament. **2.** (in equine anatomy) One of the second or fourth metacarpal or metatarsal bones in the horse's foot. They are firmly and closely attached to the corresponding third metacarpal or metatarsal (cannon) bone by a ligament (*see* metacarpus; metatarsus). **3.** (in equine orthopaedics) Damage within the ligament that attaches the splint bones. This may arise from poor conformation, poor shoeing, trauma, or malnutrition. Tearing of the ligament can lead to *periostitis and the development of fibrous tissue. The forelimbs are more frequently affected than the hindlimbs, and the second metacarpal bone is usually involved. Because the ligament tends to ossify with age, the condition is seen mainly in young horses. Heat, pain, and swelling may be evident, but radiography may be necessary to differentiate true splints from fractures of the splint bones. Recommended treatment regimes vary and include rest, ice-packs, nonsteroidal *anti-inflammatory drugs, and *corticosteroids. *Exostoses may develop, and if these interfere with the carpus or the suspensory ligament the new bone growth or the affected portion of the bone should be removed. The prognosis is generally favourable. Splints in older horses, unassociated with heat or swelling, are unlikely to cause lameness.

spondyl- (spondylo-) *Prefix denoting* a vertebra or the spine.

spondylitis Inflammation of the synovial joints of the vertebral column. This may lead to fusion of vertebrae (*see* ankylosis), producing rigidity of the spine. This process occurs in *spondylitis deformans*, which is common in ageing horses. In pigs and cattle *brucellosis may cause abscesses and necrosis in the vertebral joints, which then undergo ankylosis. In domestic fowls, spondylitis results from local infection of the 5th to 7th cervical vertebrae with *Staphylococcus aureus* bacteria or slipping of the 6th cervical vertebra in broilers. Affected birds show leg weakness due to pressure on the spinal cord.
Spondylitis can occur without evidence of inflammation: in this sense, the term is used to describe ankylosing proliferation of periosteal bone on vertebrae.

spondylolisthesis A condition of the vertebral column in which a vertebra is displaced with respect to an adjacent vertebra. *See also* kinky back.

spondylosis Degeneration of the intervertebral discs with the development of bony outgrowths (osteophytes) around the intervertebral joint. *Spondylosis deformans* is a chronic and progressive condition affecting older dogs. Clinical signs develop if the nerve roots from the spinal cord become compressed. Treatment involves *corticosteroid or analgesic therapy to reduce the pain and inflammation.

spongioblast A type of cell that forms in the early stages of development of the nervous system in the embryo, giving rise to *astrocytes and *oligodendrocytes.

sporadic Describing a disease that occurs only occasionally or in a few isolated places.

spore A small reproductive body produced by plants and microorganisms. Some kinds of spores function as dormant stages of the life cycle, enabling the organism to survive adverse conditions. Other spores are the means by which the organism can spread vegetatively. *See also* endospore.

sporicide An agent that destroys spores – the encapsulated reproductive cells of plants, fungi, and microorganisms that are very resistant to heat, water, and chemicals. Many spores can persist in tissues or in the environment for long periods, and only highly active disinfectants, such as halogenated compounds, strong acids, and strong alkalis, can kill them. Antimicrobial agents are generally ineffective.

sporidesmin Any of a group of very closely related *mycotoxins produced by the fungus *Pithomyces chartarum* and present in its spores. This widely distributed fungus lives as a saprophyte upon dead plant material, particularly on dead grass in pastures. Where conditions favour its rapid growth and sporulation, toxic spores contaminate the growing herbage; when ingested by grazing sheep or cattle these cause *facial eczema.

sporocyst A stage in the life cycle of a *fluke comprising a cyst that develops from the *miracidium larva within the intermediate host. It contains germinal cells that give rise either to daughter sporocysts or to the next larval stage, the *redia.

sporogony A type of multiple division in the life cycle of parasitic protozoa in which a zygote (formed by the fusion of gametes) divides into a number of *sporozoites. Sporogony is a feature of the *Apicomplexa.

sporotrichosis Infection by the fungus *Sporothrix schenkii* causing a chronic disease of humans and animals. This usually takes the form of subcutaneous nodules involving local lymphatic vessels, with subsequent ulceration and discharge of pus. Dissemination of infection to internal organs is rare and usually fatal. The fungus is primarily a saprophyte, growing on dead plant material or in the soil, and often contaminates vegetation and the coats of animals. Almost always infection enters through an injury to the skin, often on the legs and feet. Sporotrichosis occurs worldwide in humans, and has been reported in various animal species from a number of tropical and temperate countries, including the USA. Most reported animal infections have been in horses, mules, and donkeys, in which the disease must be distinguished from *epizootic lymphangitis; in contrast to the latter, sporotrichosis is not usually contagious. Although rare in cats, it seems readily transmitted by contact from cats to humans – an occurrence reported from several regions of the USA.

To establish the diagnosis it is usually necessary to isolate *S. schenkii* in culture from the lesions. A microscopic examination of impression smears or histology of a biopsy sample can sometimes give a more rapid result but, except in material from cats, the organism can be very difficult to find and to recognize. Intravenous and oral sodium or potassium iodides have been the treatments most often effective; *amphotericin B and ketoconazole have also been used, sometimes successfully.

Sporozoa *See* Apicomplexa.

sporozoite The form of a protozoan parasite produced by the process of *sporogony. Sporozoites are the normal infective stages for the vertebrate host and are produced within the *oocyst.

spotted fever Any of a group of principally human diseases caused by *rickettsial infections that can be transmitted between various wild and domesticated mammals, and from these to humans. The vectors are ticks, and the rickettsiae usually pass transovarially through successive generations of the tick. In the animal hosts, the infection is generally symptomless, but in humans fever and haemorrhagic rashes are characteristic. *Rocky Mountain spotted fever*, caused by *Rickettsia rickettsii*, occurs in both North and South America and is transmitted mainly by the American dog tick (*Dermacentor variabilis*) and the Rocky Mountain wood tick (*D. andersoni*), from various wild mammals and from domestic dogs; occasionally, febrile disease occurs in puppies. *Fièvre boutonneuse*, caused by *R. conorii*, occurs around the Mediterranean and the Black Sea, in Kenya, Central and South Africa, and parts of India; rats, and urban and wild dogs act as reservoirs of infection, the chief vector being the dog tick (*Rhipicephalus sanguineus*). In humans a button-like leg nodule marks the infected tick bite. *Siberian (North Asian) tick typhus*, caused by *R. sibirica*, is transmitted to humans from cattle, horses, dogs, and small wild mammals by ticks of various species. *R. australis* infects wild rats, bandicoots, dogs, and marsupials, and is transmitted by the scrub tick *Ixodes holocyclus*, causing *Queensland tick typhus* in Australia. *Rickettsialpox*, due to *R. akari*, occurs along the Atlantic coast of the USA, in the USSR, and in Korea, and is transmitted from house mice and rats by the mite *Allodermanyssus sanguineus*. *R.*

rhipicephalus is transmitted by the same ticks as *R. rickettsii* and infects dogs and other mammals, though not humans, in the USA. No disease of the spotted fever group occurs in the UK. All human spotted fevers respond to treatment with chloramphenicol or tetracyclines. *See also* typhus.

sprain Overstretching of all or part of a joint with damage to the joint capsule and ligaments and consequent local inflammation and swelling. Similar changes occur in tendons as a result of excessive stress. Immediate treatment involves support of the joint or tendon (e.g. with an elastic bandage) coupled with the application of ice packs to reduce the swelling. Recurrent or prolonged problems may need detailed investigation.

spring viraemia of carp An infectious disease of European carp caused by a *rhabdovirus and characterized by lethargy, abdominal swelling, prominent eyes (exophthalmia), and death. Mortality is highest in young fish at water temperatures in the range 10–22°C, but particularly at 16–17°C. On post mortem, haemorrhages can be found in the intestines and other abdominal organs. The only effective treatment is slaughter of all stock followed by thorough disinfection.

spurge poisoning A toxic condition arising from the ingestion of plants of the genus *Euphorbia*. The spurges contain acrid juices that cause blistering of the skin and severe gastrointestinal irritation, salivation, groaning, diarrhoea, convulsions, coma, and death. Treatment is of the clinical signs.

squalene An unsaturated hydrocarbon (a terpene), synthesized in the body, from which cholesterol is derived.

squama (*pl.* **squamae**) **1.** A thin plate of bone. **2.** A scale, such as any of the scales from the cornified layer of the *epidermis.

squamo- *Prefix denoting* **1.** the squamous portion of the temporal bone. **2.** squamous epithelium.

squamous cell carcinoma A malignant tumour of squamous epithelium, common in most domestic species, that affects the skin, mouth, and conjunctiva. In **cattle** and **cats** with white faces a solar-induced dermatitis is considered to be a precancerous state, and the tumour may affect the eyelids, external nares, and, in cats, the auricles (pinnae) of the ears. In **dogs** squamous cell carcinoma can arise at most sites on the skin but is more common in the digits, trunk, lips, and nose. Also, it is one of the three common malignant tumours (with *fibrosarcoma and malignant *melanoma) of the oral cavity in dogs. In subtropical areas, dogs that lie out in the sun have a higher incidence of this tumour on the hairless unpigmented areas of their ventral abdomen. The appearance of this tumour varies from a florid fungoid mass to an erosive and invasive lesion. Squamous cell carcinomas tend to be locally aggressive, invading neighbouring tissues; except for those involving the nail beds and tonsils, they rarely metastasize. Radical surgical excision may be curative, but cryosurgery and radiotherapy are also important in treatment.

squamous epithelium *See* epithelium.

squirrel corn *See* blood root poisoning.

stable A building in which animals, particularly horses, are housed. It may be a self-contained individual unit or contain several individual stalls, and is constructed typically of brick, concrete blocks, or wooden sections. The stable floor can be of concrete, bricks, or packed chalk or earth. The doorway must be high and wide enough to give easy access for the type of horse to be stabled, and each stable unit must be large enough to give the horse limited movement and allow it to lie down and stand. Wooden stalls must be protectively lined on the inside (to a height of 1.2 m). All windows must be guarded with mesh. Ideally stables should be fitted with automatic water bowls, a fixed manger or trough, and a hay rack or haynet. All stable fittings must be without projections that could injure the horse. *Bedding can be of straw or shavings.

stable cough *See* equine influenza.

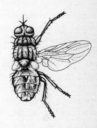

Stable fly, *Stomoxys calcitrans*

stable fly An ectoparasitic *fly, *Stomoxys calcitrans*, also known as the biting house fly (see illustration). Stable flies occur worldwide and are a serious livestock pest. The adults feed on the blood of a wide variety of hosts, including horses, sheep, cattle, and humans; they can often be seen on the lower legs and under the belly. Apart from their irritating bite they also transmit diseases, such as *equine infectious anaemia, *anthrax, and *surra and the nematode parasite of horses, *Habronema microstoma*. The eggs are laid in organic matter, often in soiled animal bedding or in horse manure, but never in cattle dung. Stable flies may be controlled by using a suitable *insecticide in barns, stables, and cowsheds, or applying it directly to livestock.

stadium (*pl.* **stadiums** or **stadia**) **1.** A stage in the course of a disease. **2.** A stage in the life history of an organism, especially the intervals between successive moults in insect development.

stag A male pig that has been castrated late in life.

staggers *See* hypomagnesaemia.

staggerweed poisoning *See* Helenium poisoning.

stain 1. A dye used to colour tissues and other specimens for microscopical examination. In an *acid stain* the colour is carried by an acid radical and the stain is taken up by parts of the specimen having a basic (alkaline) component. In a *basic stain* the colour, carried by a basic radical, is attracted to parts of the specimen having an acidic component. *Neutral stains* have neither acidic nor basic affinities. A *contrast stain* is used to give colour to parts of a tissue not affected by a previously applied stain. A *differential stain* allows different elements in a specimen to be distinguished by staining them in different colours. **2.** To treat a specimen for microscopical study with a stain.

standard livestock unit *See* stocking rate.

staphylococcal arthritis of poultry An arthritis or spondylitis of adult domestic fowls, turkeys, ducks, geese, and pheasants, caused by strains of the bacterium *Staphylococcus aureus*, sometimes following an initial septicaemia. When lesions develop on the feet, the condition is termed *bumblefoot.

Staphylococcus A genus of Gram-positive *bacteria widely distributed in nature and the commonest cause of localized infections. Spherical in shape and slightly less than 1 μm in diameter, they tend to occur in groups resembling a bunch of grapes. *S. epidermidis* is a normal commensal of the skin and mucous membranes of both humans and animals but it can cause disease following trauma, viral infections, or stress. *S. aureus* causes a disease of horses known as *botriomycosis; it also causes *mastitis and skin, eye, and urinary infections in all domestic animals. *Tick pyaemia, a disease of 2- to 5-week-old lambs occurring commonly in Britain, is also caused by *S. aureus* in association with heavy tick infestation and infection with the rickettsia of *tick-borne fever (*Cytoecetes phagocytophila*). Canine skin infections may involve both *S. aureus* and *S. intermedius*, while *S. hyicus* causes skin infections in pigs and cattle. In poultry and other birds *Staphylococcus* bacteria, chiefly *S. aureus*, cause conditions ranging from the more acute yolk sac infection (*see* omphalitis) and septicaemia, to chronic forms, such as *arthritis, *synovitis, *spondylitis, *bumblefoot, *septic sternal bursitis, and, possibly, *avian malignant oedema. *S. aureus* is usually found on the skin and upper respiratory tract of intensively kept poultry, infection being initiated by skin or mucosal damage.

staphyloma Protrusion of the iris through a rupture in the cornea of the *eye. It is often caused by injury. If the lesion is small, partial *iridectomy will remove the protrusion. Alternatively a cauterizing agent, such as silver nitrate, can be applied. An opacity of the cornea usually remains.

starch The form in which *carbohydrates are stored in many plants and a major dietary constituent. Starch consists of linked glucose units and occurs in two forms, α-*amylose* and *amylopectin*. In α-amylose the units are in the form of a long unbranched chain; in amylopectin they form a branched chain. *See also* amylase; dextrin.

stasis Stagnation or cessation of flow, for example of blood or lymph whose flow is obstructed or of the intestinal contents when onward movement (peristalsis) is hindered.

-stasis *Suffix denoting* stoppage of a flow of liquid; stagnation. Example: *haemostasis* (of blood).

State Boards of Veterinary Medicine (USA) Bodies empowered by state governments to examine, license, and regulate the activities of veterinarians. Veterinarians are licensed independently in each state, although some states may have reciprocity with others.

State Veterinary Service (UK) Part of the Ministry of Agriculture, Fisheries, and Food, consisting of three divisions: the Field Service, the regional *Veterinary Investigation Centres; and the Central Veterinary Laboratory at Weybridge. The Service is staffed by full-time Veterinary Officers and part-time Local Veterinary Inspectors. Functions of the Field Service include control of *notifiable diseases, meat hygiene, importation of livestock, and animal welfare. The State Veterinary Service is headed by the Chief Veterinary Officer. Head Office: Hook Rise South, Tolworth, Surbiton, KT6 7NF.

steaming up The practice of feeding dairy cows above their requirements during the 6–8 weeks before calving. The objective was to build up body reserves in preparation for lactation. The practice is no longer advised since it increases the risk of *milk fever and other metabolic disorders. Steaming up in mid-lactation is a similar but more efficient process in which body reserves are built up while the cow is still milking. However, the need for high levels of body reserves at calving is now questioned since it leads to low food intakes after calving and increased incidence of *fatty liver syndrome.

stearic acid *See* fatty acid.

steat- (steato-) *Prefix denoting* fat; fatty tissue.

steatitis A disorder of fat metabolism, also called yellow-fat disease, occurring in dogs, cats, and other fur-bearing animals. It is characterized by inflammation and yellow discoloration of the body fat. The cause is thought to be excess unsaturated fatty acids in the diet, possibly coupled with vitamin E deficiency, which results in fat-cell degeneration and the deposition of yellow pigment. Diets composed mainly of fish are incriminated. Affected animals, although apparently plump and 'well fed', become unwilling to move because of pain in the inflamed fat tissue. Fever and lack of appetite also occur. Vitamin E injections coupled with a balanced diet are the preferred treatment.

steatorrhoea The passage of abnormally increased amounts of fat in the faeces. The faeces appear yellow or clay-coloured, are foul-smelling, and stain red with *Sudan III stain. Steatorrhoea usually indicates disease of the pancreas or obstruction of the pancreatic duct, which interferes with the production or transport of fat-digesting enzymes. Biliary obstruction, which prevents the flow of bile, may have a similar effect in preventing fat digestion.

steer A castrated male ox, usually 6–24 months of age, that is used for meat production. *See* beef cattle; cattle husbandry.

stellate ganglion (cervicothoracic ganglion) A large star-shaped nerve *ganglion of the sympathetic trunk at the level of the first rib. It represents a fusion of the caudal cervical ganglion and one or more thoracic ganglia, and distributes sympathetic nerve fibres to the neck and thoracic organs.

steno- *Prefix denoting* 1. narrow. 2. constricted.

stenosis (*pl.* **stenoses**) The abnormal narrowing of a passage or opening. For example, *mitral stenosis* refers to the opening, guarded by the mitral (*bicuspid) valve, between the left atrium and left ventricle in the heart. Similarly, *tricuspid stenosis* refers to the opening between the right chambers. *Oesophageal stenosis* is narrowing of the oesophagus, due, for example, to tumours, inflammation, or scarring from injuries or surgery.

stent 1. A pad sutured over a wound after repair. They are used to relieve tension on the wound edges and to provide protection. However, they may harbour infection and can become wet, and should be removed if this occurs. 2. A splint left inside the lumen of a duct at operation to aid healing.

stephanofilariasis A disease of cattle caused by parasitic *nematodes of the genus *Stephanofilaria* and occurring in the USA and parts of Asia. The worms are transmitted by flies (*see* filariasis). It typically involves a chronic skin condition. In India *S. ammanensis* causes *dermatitis in the humps of cattle (*hump sore*) and also ulcers in the ears. In India and Indonesia *S. dedoesi* causes a form of der-

matitis known as cascado. Where cattle are in poor condition or in a very wet environment, 90% of the body may be affected. Lesions start as papules, which subsequently depilate, exude serum, and encrust. In Malaysia *S. kaeli* affects the legs of cattle. Treatment is by application to the skin of *organophosphorus compounds, e.g. trichlorophon, but recovery is often spontaneous with improved nutrition and housing.

Stephanurus A genus of parasitic *nematodes containing the kidney worm of pigs, *S. dentatus*, which is widespread in tropical regions. The adult worms are found in the perirenal fat, pelvis of the kidney, or on the ureter wall, residing in cysts from which canals lead to the lumen of the ureter. The eggs are passed out in the urine and the larvae become infective in 4–5 days. They can survive outside a host for 5 months, or, if ingested and carried by earthworms, for longer. Pigs are infested by ingesting the larvae or infested earthworms, or the larvae may penetrate the host's skin directly. They migrate to the liver via the portal vein. Initially they remain beneath the surface of the liver, but after 3 months they break through the liver capsule, enter the peritoneal cavity, and migrate to the perirenal area. Here they form fine canals leading into the ureters and encyst in adjacent renal tissue. Infestation causes retarded growth and emaciation, with hypertrophy of the liver. There is no effective treatment, and control demands good hygiene.

sterco- *Prefix denoting* faeces.

stercobilin A pigment derived from the breakdown of the haem constituent of *haemoglobin. It is mainly responsible for the colour of faeces.

stercolith A stone in the large intestine or rectum, especially one formed of dried compressed faeces. In dogs excessive consumption of bones may give rise to concretions in the faeces, which the animal is unable to void thus causing constipation. Enemas or suppositories coupled with digital breakdown of the concretion may be necessary.

stercoraceous Composed of or containing faeces.

stereoisomers Compounds having the same molecular formula but different three-dimensional arrangements of their atoms. The atomic structures of stereoisomers are mirror images of each other.

stereoscopic vision Perception of the shape, depth, and distance of an object as a result of having *binocular vision. The brain receives two distinct images from the eyes, which it interprets as a single three-dimensional image.

sterile 1. (of a living organism) Barren; unable to reproduce its kind (*see* infertility; sterility). **2.** (of inanimate objects) Completely free from bacteria, fungi, viruses, or other microorganisms that could cause infection (*see* sterilization).

sterility (barrenness) Failure to breed successfully, due either to *infertility, or because of a surgical operation (*see* castration; spaying).

sterilization 1. The process of rendering objects, wounds, etc. free from infective organisms. Surgical instruments and dressings are usually sterilized by steam under pressure in an *autoclave. This is much more effective than simply using boiling water, and may also have the advantage of incorporating a drying cycle. Commercially available pre-packaged disposable equipment is frequently sterilized by gamma radiation. Sterilization

using a hot-air oven is reliable but slow, and destructive of cloth materials. It is best employed for agents that cannot be sterilized by steam under pressure, such as powders, etc. Chemical *disinfectants and *antiseptics may be used to destroy bacteria and other microorganisms, for instance at an operation site (*see* asepsis). **2.** A surgical operation or other process that induces *sterility. *See* castration; spaying.

stern- (sterno-) *Prefix denoting* the sternum. Example: *sternocostal* (relating to the sternum and ribs).

sternebra (*pl.* **sternebrae**) One of the segments of the *sternum. They remain separate in some domestic species.

sternocephalic muscle A large muscle in the neck running from the sternum to the skull and, in cattle, also to the mandible.

sternum (*pl.* **sterna**) The bone lying in the ventral midline of the thoracic skeleton that articulates with the costal cartilages of the true ribs on either side. It consists of a series of segments (*sternebrae) joined by intervening cartilage. The cranial segment is termed the *manubrium*, and the caudalmost segment has a *xiphoid process, extended by the xiphoid cartilage. In birds the sternum is a single large bone; many species, including the domestic fowl, have evolved a large ventral *carina* or *keel* and lateral processes to provide attachment for the pectoral muscles – the principal muscles of flight.

steroid One of a group of *lipids derived from a saturated compound – cyclopentanoperhydrophenanthrene – which has a nucleus of three six-membered carbon rings and one five-membered carbon ring. A major group of steroid derivatives are the steroid alcohols (*sterols). Other steroids include the *bile acids, which aid digestion of fats in the intestine; the sex hormones (*androgens and *oestrogens); and the *corticosteroid hormones, produced by the adrenal cortex. *Vitamin D is also based on the steroid structure.

sterol Any of a group of *steroid-based alcohols having a hydrocarbon side-chain of 8–10 carbon atoms. Sterols exist either as free sterols or as esters of fatty acids. Animal sterols (*zoosterols*) include cholesterol and lanosterol. *See also* ergosterol.

stertor A snoring type of noisy inspiration. It may be heard in cases of laryngitis, swelling of the larynx, or paralysis of the vocal folds.

stethoscope An instrument used for listening to sounds from within the body, especially the thorax (*see* auscultation). It consists of two ear pieces connected via flexible tubes to a chest piece, which is usually bell-shaped or has a diaphragm, and is applied to the body. Recently developed models have electronic amplifier and filter systems built into the chest piece to enable more specific identification of abnormal sounds. A stethoscope is commonly used to listen to heart and respiratory sounds, and for the sounds of intestinal motility.

stick marks (meat inspection) A condition of bruising of the pig's skin caused by beating the animal with a stick. The marks are red wheals consisting of two red parallel lines closed at one end. They are commonest on the backs and buttocks and may be confused with *teeth marks.

stiff lamb disease *See* white muscle disease.

stifle (knee) 1. The complex joint in the hindlimb comprising the *femoro-*

tibial joint, formed by the condyles of the *femur and the *tibia, and the *femoropatellar joint*, formed by the *patella and the trochlea of the femur. Between the femoral and tibial condyles are located the lateral and medial *menisci (*see* meniscus). The joint is stabilized by many ligaments, of which the cranial and caudal *cruciate ligaments and the lateral and medial collateral ligaments are particularly important. The joint principally allows flexion and extension. **2.** The region of the hindlimb surrounding the stifle joint.

stigma (*pl.* **stigmata**) A mark on the skin, mucous membrane, or serosal surface. For example the point of rupture of an ovarian follicle is sometimes termed its stigma.

stilbenes A group of synthetic *oestrogens, derived from coal tar, including *diethylstilboestrol, *hexoestrol, and stilboestrol. They are not steroidal in structure and are less potent than natural oestrogens, but have a longer duration of action. They were formerly used as growth promoters, but their residues in meat were found to be oestrogenic and carcinogenic, prompting a ban on their use in food-producing animals. These drugs can still be used legally in some countries in the treatment of small animals, and are used in human medicine.

stilboestrol A *stilbene compound, formerly used as a growth promoter but now banned in food-producing animals. Its residues in meat have carcinogenic effects. Stilboestrol is still used in some countries in small animals for the treatment of hormonal alopecia, and adenomas, and prostatic hypertrophy, and to prevent conception after mismating in bitches.

stilet (stylet, stylus) 1. A slender probe. **2.** A wire placed in the lumen of a catheter to give it rigidity while the instrument is passed along a body canal (such as the urethra).

stillbirth The birth of dead offspring at full term of pregnancy. *See* abortion.

stimulant An agent that increases the activity of the central nervous system (CNS) and peripheral motor nerves. Such agents may act on the CNS causing general stimulation of the animal, or act at specific receptors in the peripheral nervous system. The amphetamines are *sympathomimetic drugs that cause respiratory and cardiovascular stimulation and increased alertness. These are *controlled drugs because of addiction in humans and depression on withdrawal. They have been used illegally to try to improve performance in greyhounds and racehorses. The *xanthines, particularly caffeine, have CNS stimulant properties, as does strychnine, which is a stimulant of the spinal cord (*see* strychnine poisoning).

Centrally acting stimulants, such as *picrotoxin, nikethamide, and *doxapram, are used as stimulants to try to reverse respiratory and circulatory collapse, especially in cases of anaesthetic overdosage and in neonates. The use of these drugs in life-threatening situations should be combined with supportive therapy, for example fluid replacement therapy and intermittent positive-pressure ventilation. Slight overdosage with CNS stimulants can precipitate clonic convulsions. The duration of action of stimulants is brief and repeated dosing causes CNS depression.

stimulus (*pl.* **stimuli**) Any agent that provokes a response, or particular form of activity, in a cell, tissue, or other structure, which is said to be *sensitive* to that stimulus.

stirk A young female ox (*heifer), usually aged 6–12 months, that is destined for meat production. In Scotland, the term can also refer to a young male ox.

stitch *See* suture.

St John's wort poisoning *See* photodynamic; photosensitization.

stocking density *See* floor space.

stocking rate The number of animals in a given area of land or *floor space. It is normally measured as the number of individuals or mass of animals per hectare. However, a more useful concept is *livestock units* (*LSUs*) per hectare; a *standard livestock unit* is the feed *energy allowance for the maintenance of a 600 kg Friesian dairy cow and the production of a 40 kg calf and 4500 litres of average quality milk. This is equivalent to about 48 000 MJ of *metabolizable energy per year. The energy allowances of all other stock can be divided by this figure to give their equivalent LSU, and tables are available of LSUs for different categories of livestock; examples are: cattle (12–24 months old) 0.54; ewes (60 kg) 0.09; lambs 0.04; sows with litters 0.44; laying hens 0.017. Output per animal usually falls as stocking rate increases, but the relationship between stocking rate and output per hectare is usually curvilinear, with a maximum output per hectare occurring at a stocking rate of about 3–5 LSU/ha.

stoma (*pl.* **stomata**) **1.** (in anatomy) The mouth or any mouthlike part. **2.** (in surgery) The artificial opening of a tube that has been brought to a surface.

stomach A distensible saclike organ in the cranial part of the abdomen that forms part of the *alimentary

stomach tube

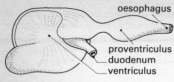

Stomach of the domestic fowl

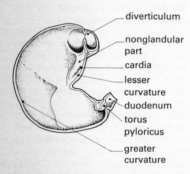

Section of stomach of the pig

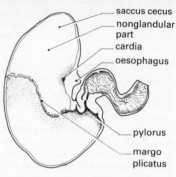

Section of stomach and part of duodenum of the horse

tract between the oesophagus and the duodenum. It communicates with the former through the cardia and with the latter through the pylorus. **Monogastric** species (e.g. horse, pig, dog, and cat) have a simple stomach whose shape is described in terms of greater and lesser curvatures and a cardiac part, a fundus, a body, and a pyloric part (see illustration). Glands in the mucosa produce *gastric juice, containing hydrochloric acid and the enzyme *pepsin, which contribute to chemical digestion. This, together with the churning action of the muscular layers of the stomach, reduces the food to a semiliquid partly digested mass that passes on to the duodenum.

Ruminants have a complex stomach consisting of four compartments – *reticulum, *rumen, *omasum, and *abomasum (see illustration). In the first three, bacterial fermentation of ingested food takes place, causing the breakdown of plant celluloses and hemicelluloses so enabling them to be

utilized by the animal. The abomasum is the equivalent of the stomach in monogastric species. In many species of **birds**, including the domestic fowl, the stomach consists of two parts: the *proventriculus, or glandular part, which produces gastric juice; and the *ventriculus (muscular part or gizzard), which has a mechanical grinding function. (See illustration.) Anatomical name: **gaster**.

stomach tube A rubber or plastic tube that can be passed into the stomach from outside the animal. It can be used for feeding, medication, removal of gas or liquid, or diagnosing and clearing a blockage of the oesophagus. Care must be taken to ensure that the tube passes down the oesophagus and not the trachea. In **dogs** a stomach tube can be passed through the mouth of a conscious dog to administer drugs or food. In cases of sudden distension of the stomach with gas, insertion of a stomach tube via the mouth allows gas to escape; this can be life-saving.

In **ruminants** a tube can be passed through the mouth in a conscious animal, although the use of a gag is advisable in adult cattle. It is useful for the relief of *bloat, allowing gas to escape from the rumen, or for fluid therapy, especially in young calves.

Horses A stomach tube can be passed up the nose and down the oesophagus to the stomach. The tube must be lubricated and care must be taken to push the tube up the lowermost nasal passage (ventral meatus) as this is the largest and leads most directly to the oesophagus, thereby minimizing the risk of a nosebleed. The tube should be advanced from the pharynx to the oesophagus when the horse swallows. As the tube passes down the neck it can be seen close to the jugular vein. It is an important route of medication (e.g. worming, liquid paraffin), is used to treat *choke (oesophageal blockage), and is used to prevent rupture of the stomach when excess liquid or gas are present. *Compare* probang.

stomat- (stomato-) *Prefix denoting* the mouth.

stomatitis Inflammation of the mucous membrane lining the mouth. It occurs as a major clinical sign in such diseases as *vesicular stomatitis and *foot-and-mouth disease. However trauma from barley awns or irritant poisons may also be causative factors. Nonspecific infection with various bacteria and fungi may be involved, especially in animals debilitated by vitamin deficiency or other conditions.

stomodeum (stomatodeum) (*pl.* **stomodea, stomatodea**) The ectoderm-lined depression that forms the primitive mouth cavity in the early embryo. At first it is separated from the foregut by the buccopharyngeal

membrane, but this breaks down at an early stage of development. *Compare* proctodeum.

-stomy (-ostomy) *Suffix denoting* a surgical opening into an organ or part.

straight A single feedstuff given to animals directly rather than being incorporated into a *compound feed. They may be processed before feeding, for example rolling barley. Straights do not normally provide all the *nutrient requirements of the animal. *Compare* concentrate.

strain 1. Excessive stretching or working of a muscle, resulting in pain and swelling of the muscle. 2. A group of organisms, such as a subgroup of a breed, obtained from a particular source or having special properties distinguishing them from other members of the same species.

strangles A contagious disease of horses characterized by fever, respiratory signs, and abscess formation in the lymph nodes of the head and caused by the Gram-positive bacterium *Streptococcus equi*. Young horses are particularly susceptible and following an initial high fever develop a nasal discharge and swelling of the throat region, which may obstruct breathing. The submaxillary lymph nodes become enlarged and develop abscesses; these may rupture below the jaw, discharging creamy yellow pus. Rarely, infection spreads to other body lymph nodes and becomes generalized, producing abscesses in other internal organs, such as the kidneys, lungs, spleen, and liver. Uncomplicated cases respond to treatment with *penicillin, although it may also be necessary to surgically drain the submaxillary abscesses. Horses with strangles may also be infected with other respiratory pathogens, such as *equine rhinopneumonitis virus. *Purpura haemorrhagica can be a consequence of strangles.

strangulated 1. Describing a passage or vessel (e.g. airway, intestine, or blood vessel) that is compressed or constricted so that flow through it is prevented. **2.** Describing a part of the body whose blood supply has been interrupted by compression of a blood vessel, for example a strangulated *hernia. This may lead to necrosis and gangrene of the affected part.

strangulation The closure of a passage. *See* strangulated.

strangury Difficult or painful urination (micturition). It is common in patients with urinary stones (*see* calculus), cystitis, or urethritis.

stratum (*pl.* **strata**) A layer of tissue or cells, such as any of the layers of the *epidermis of the skin (the *stratum corneum* is the outermost layer).

straw The dried stems and leaves of certain crop plants, usually cereals but also some legumes. Straw is extremely fibrous (*see* dietary fibre) and of very low nutritive value. Wheat and rye straws are used almost exclusively as *bedding, but barley and oat straws can be fed to cattle on store rations or, in limited quantities, used as a source of dietary fibre for dairy cows.

strawberry foot rot An unusual form of *dermatophilosis in sheep, reported only from Britain, in which inflammatory swellings appear on the lower parts of the limbs and develop thick crusts. Removal of the crusts leaves a raw area with bleeding points, resembling a strawberry.

'street' virus Describing strains of a virus, especially *rabies virus, occurring under natural rather than laboratory conditions.

Streptobacillus A genus of pleomorphic Gram-negative *bacteria that occur in chains, branching filaments, or club-shaped swellings. *S. moniliformis* inhabits the oropharynx of rats, in which it causes chronic abscesses of lymph nodes. Humans bitten by an infected rat may develop *rat-bite fever.

streptococcal meningitis A contagious disease of pigs characterized by fever, meningitis, and *polyarthritis and caused by the bacterium *Streptococcus suis* type 2. Pigs aged 3–12 weeks are the most susceptible, particularly at times of stress, such as at weaning, when litters are mixed, or when overcrowded; however, pigs of any age may be affected. The organism is distributed worldwide. The disease may be introduced by apparently healthy carrier pigs, but it is not always clear how infection enters a pig herd. Pigs can carry infection for at least a year, and it can persist in pigs being fed penicillin-medicated feed. The majority of pigs infected with the organism develop *arthritis; some show lameness within 24 hours of infection. Some of these animals also develop *meningitis although the factors that predispose to involvement of the central nervous system have not been determined. Pigs with meningitis develop a high fever, incoordination, vomiting, convulsions, and coma, followed by death. Death may occur before the development of any clinical signs.

The incidence of the disease can be reduced by avoiding stress (due to, for instance, overcrowding, poor ventilation, frequent introduction of new stock, and poor hygiene) and by using in-feed antibiotics, such as *penicillins, *tetracyclines, or *lincomycin. An 'all in–all out' management policy is recommended and pens should be thoroughly cleaned, for instance with a dilute solution of soap. Vaccines have been tried on an experimental basis but their success has been mixed. There is some evidence that humans can act as carriers of the bacterium and may rarely be affected by the disease.

Streptococcus suis type 1 causes outbreaks of meningitis affecting suckling pigs only. Meningitis due to other streptococci is sporadic only and does not spread.

Streptococcus A genus of spherical Gram-positive *bacteria occurring in chains or pairs. They are widely distributed in nature, being important pathogens but often found as normal commensals in the mouth, skin, and intestine of humans and other animals. They are also common contaminants of milk and milk products. S. *agalactiae* produces an acute or chronic mastitis in cows which is less common now than formerly. S. *dysgalactiae* causes an acute mastitis which is less common than that produced by S. *uberis* (one cause of the environmental form of the disease). S. *dysgalactiae* may also be involved, sometimes with other bacteria, in other forms of mastitis and also in *polyarthritis in lambs. S. *zooepidemicus* causes wound infections in horses, umbilical infection of foals, *endometritis in mares, acute and severe mastitis and arthritis in cows, and pleuritis, pericarditis, and pneumonia in sheep. S. *equizimilis* causes similar conditions to S. *zooepidemicus* in horses and frequently causes arthritis in piglets up to 6 weeks of age. S. *equi* causes *strangles in horses. S. *suis* (which can also occasionally affect man) causes septicaemia, arthritis, and meningitis in pigs, while S. *canis* has been associated with metritis and vaginitis in the bitch and conjunctivitis, lymphoadenitis, and localized abscesses in the cat.

streptodornase A largely obsolete term for a mixture of enzymes obtained from cultures of *Streptococcus*.

Streptomyces A genus of filamentous Gram-positive *bacteria that cause *mycetomas in animals, including humans.

streptomycin *See* aminoglycosides.

streptothricosis *See* streptotrichosis.

streptotrichosis An alternative and widely used name for the skin disease *dermatophilosis, especially as it occurs in cattle, horses, and goats. It is often incorrectly written as 'streptothricosis'. The name is derived from a now superceded classification of the causal organism (*Dermatophilus congolensis*) as a species of *Streptothrix*.

stress Any factor that threatens the health of an organism or has an adverse effect on its functioning. Such factors, or *stressors*, may occur in the external environment or arise within the body. They include insufficient or unsuitable food, excessive heat or cold or sudden changes in temperature, undue physical work or exercise, pain (e.g. due to disease or injury), overcrowding, or ill-treatment, such as rough handling. The signs of stress are various, and may include poor appetite or failure to eat, reduction or cessation of reproductive activity, poor growth, and reduced productivity. Odd behavioural patterns may emerge, including various vices. Animals can normally adapt to mild chronic stress, but severe stress may precipitate a breakdown in the body's internal homeostatic mechanisms. Individuals vary in their sensitivity to stress; certain strains of pig are especially susceptible, and may collapse and die from the *porcine stress syndrome.

stretch receptor A nerve ending that responds to stretch and transmits impulses to the central nervous system through sensory nerves. Stretch receptors occur in muscles (*see* muscle spindle), tendons (*see* tendon organ), and the lungs.

stretch reflex (myotatic reflex) The reflex contraction of a muscle in response to its being stretched.

stria (*pl.* **striae**) (in anatomy) A streak, line, or thin band. The *stria terminalis* is a white band that separates the thalamus from the ventricular surface of the caudate nucleus in the brain.

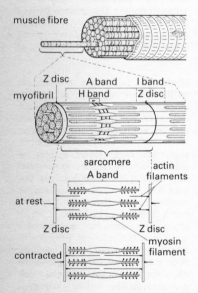

Structure of striated muscle

striated muscle A tissue comprising the bulk of the body's musculature. It is also known as *skeletal muscle*, because it is attached to the skeleton and is responsible for the movement of bones, and *voluntary muscle*, because it is under voluntary control.

Striated muscle is composed of parallel bundles of multinucleate fibres (each containing many *myofibrils*), which reveal cross-banding when viewed under the microscope. This effect is due to the alternation of *actin* and *myosin* protein filaments within each myofibril (see illustration). When muscle contraction takes place, the two sets of filaments slide past each other, so reducing the length of each unit (*sarcomere*) of the myofibril. The sliding is caused by a series of cyclic reactions resulting in a change in orientation of projections on the myosin filaments; each projection is first attached to an actin filament but contracts and releases it to become reattached at a different site.

stricture A narrowing of a tubular structure or duct. Strictures commonly result from inflammation and subsequent production of scar tissue, tumours, or pressure from adjacent organs. For example, an *oesophageal stricture* commonly follows traumatic injury or surgery; a *rectal stricture* can develop after ulcerative proctitis, which produces an annular scar in the rectum, preventing defecation and causing progressive distension of the abdomen.

stridor 1. A harsh vibrating sound heard during breathing when the airway is obstructed. *See also* sound. **2.** Stridor denticum: grinding of the teeth.

strike Infestation of the fleece of sheep by larvae of the *green-bottle fly. Female green-bottles are attracted by scent to wet soiled wool, where they lay their eggs, often around the rump and tail. The eggs hatch and develop rapidly into white-grey larvae, which reach a length of 1.5 cm within 3 days in favourable conditions. They then fall to the ground and penetrate the surface of the soil, where they pupate and turn into adults. Strike is extremely important in some sheep-raising areas of the world. Its incidence may be reduced by eliminating scouring (diarrhoea) in the flock and so preventing soiling of the hindquarters. Soiled areas of wool should be shorn. The flies may also lay their eggs on individuals of other species, especially recumbent debilitated animals, and in carcasses, which should be disposed of promptly.

stringhalt A condition of the horse in which the hock of one or both hindlimbs is jerked upwards while the animal is in motion (i.e. involuntary hyperflexion of the hock). This abnormal movement is often exacerbated by backing or turning. The cause is not known but involvement of the lateral digital extensor is suspected in some cases. The prognosis is variable but most horses show some improvement following surgical removal of a section of the lateral digital extensor tendon.

strip grazing (close folding) A system of allocating grass or root crops to grazing animals, particularly dairy cows, using an electric fence, which is moved daily to supply fresh herbage. Balancing the daily herbage allowance with the requirements of the herd ensures maximum utilization of grassland.

strobila (*pl.* **strobilae**) The body of a *tapeworm consisting of a chain of segments (*see* proglottis), which are differentiated in the neck region behind the head (*scolex).

stroke 1. A sudden attack of weakness caused by interruption to the blood supply to the brain. It may be due to thrombosis, embolism, or haemorrhage and can vary in severity. It is rare in domestic animals. **2.** Any sudden attack of a disorder, such as heat stroke (*see* heat exhaustion). *See also* lightning stroke.

stroma (*pl.* **stromata**) **1.** The supportive tissue of an organ, as opposed to the functional tissue (*parenchyma*). **2.** The spongy framework of protein strands within a red blood cell in which the blood pigment haemoglobin is packed.

strongylid A *nematode belonging to the family Strongylidae, which includes the genera *Oesophagostomum* and *Strongylus*. They are intestinal parasites possessing a characteristic mouth capsule with a crown of leaflets (leaf crown), and are closely related to the *hookworms.

Strongylus A genus of parasitic *nematodes, sometimes known as 'redworms', of which *S. equinus* and *S. vulgaris* occur in the large intestine of horses worldwide. Eggs are passed in the faeces and the larvae are found on vegetation or in the upper layers of the soil. They are ingested by the host and eventually mature in nodules on the walls of the large intestine or caecum. The larvae of *S. vulgaris* migrate through the intestinal wall, between the layers of the mesentery, and finally into one of the mesenteric arteries where they cause *equine verminous arteritis. Eventually they migrate back to the colon wall and into the lumen of the intestine. Affected animals can be treated with *pyrantel tartrate, fenbendazole (*see* benzimidazoles), or ivermectin.

strontium A yellow metallic element, absorption of which causes bone damage when its atoms displace calcium in bone. The radioactive isotope *strontium-90* is particularly harmful; present in fallout from nuclear explosions, it emits beta-rays and has a half-life of 28 years. Symbol Sr.

struck (Romney Marsh disease) An acute fatal *enterotoxaemia of young sheep, with enteritis and intestinal ulceration but rarely diarrhoea.

It is caused by multiplication in the intestine of the bacterium *Clostridium perfringens* type C and subsequent absorption of the bacterial toxin. The disease is recognized in Europe, the USA, and New Zealand; it is enzootic in the Romney Marsh area of Kent. Effective vaccines are available.

strychnine poisoning A toxic condition caused by ingestion of strychnine, an alkaloid obtained from the seeds of an Indian tree, *Strychnos nux-vomica*. Strychnine is used to poison moles, foxes, and other vermin and is therefore accessible to dogs and cats. It increases the reflex excitability of the spinal cord, and poisoned animals are restless, excited, and hypersensitive to light. They develop generalized muscular contractions and the pupils constrict. Death is due to cessation of breathing during a convulsion and is accompanied by evacuation of urine and faeces. Vomiting should be stimulated in affected dogs and the convulsions controlled by intravenous barbiturates. Excretion of strychnine is rapid so that the condition usually lasts no more than 6 hours. Hemlock water dropwort and cowbane contain alkaloids that produce toxic effects similar to strychnine. *See* hemlock water dropwort poisoning.

stud tail A condition of cats in which there is loss of hair and thickening of the skin at the base of the tail. It is caused by oversecretion of the large *sebaceous glands in that area, and is often accompanied by secondary bacterial infection. The condition is commonest in entire toms, but can also occur in females, or in neutered cats of either sex. Mild cases may not need any treatment, but if secondary infection is a problem, antibiotic therapy may be required, followed by the long-term use of a topical antiseptic and degreasing agent.

stumped-up toe A condition of the horse's foot in which the horn of the toe is pared away excessively to compensate for setting the shoe too far back on the foot. The bearing surface is reduced and there is a risk of damage to the thinned hoof wall and underlying sensitive laminae by the toe clip. Also, excessive paring exposes the horn tubes, causing evaporation from the horn and dry brittle feet. If the animal is on wet pasture, too much water will be absorbed and the feet will become soft and spongy.

stunting syndrome *See* runting and stunting syndrome.

sturdy *See* coenurosis.

stye Inflammation of a sebaceous gland in the eyelid. Though less common in domesticated animals than in humans the lesion causes pain and, if sufficiently large, irritates the cornea and distorts the shape of the eyelid. Acute inflammation may be treated topically with a suitable antibiotic, but an enlarged and chronically inflamed sebaceous gland may need surgical removal. Medical name: **hordeolum**. *See also* chalazion.

sub- *Prefix denoting* **1.** below; underlying. Examples: *sublingual* (below the tongue); *submandibular* (below the mandible). **2.** partial or slight.

subacute Describing a disease that progresses more rapidly than a *chronic condition but does not become *acute.

subarachnoid space The space between the pia mater and the arachnoid *meninges. It is filled with cerebrospinal fluid.

subscapularis muscle

subclavian artery The main artery supplying the forelimb. It arises from the brachiocephalic trunk or directly from the aorta. On entering the *axilla it becomes the *axillary artery*.

subclinical Describing a disease that has not reached the stage of showing clinical signs. Some diseases remain subclinical throughout their course; others progress to show clinical signs.

subcutaneous Beneath the skin. A *subcutaneous injection* is given beneath the skin. *Subcutaneous tissue* is loose connective tissue, often fatty, situated under the dermis.

subdural Below the dura mater (the outermost of the meninges); relating to the space between the dura mater and arachnoid.

subinvolution Failure of the return to normal size (*involution) of an organ following its enlargement. For example, subinvolution of the uterus after parturition delays conception and is an important economic problem in dairy cows.

sublingual gland One of the major *salivary glands, located below the tongue. In all domestic mammals except the horse there are two glands: the *monostomatic sublingual gland*, which has a single duct opening close to the duct of the mandibular gland; and the *polystomatic sublingual gland*, which has a number of ducts opening on the fold of mucous membrane under the tongue. The horse has only a polystomatic sublingual gland.

subluxation Partial *dislocation (luxation) of a joint or of the lens of the eye.

submaxillary gland *See* mandibular gland.

submucosa The layer of loose connective (*areolar) tissue underlying a mucous membrane; for example, in the wall of the intestine.

submucosal plexus A nerve plexus in the wall of the alimentary canal, formed by a network of fibres, many of them parasympathetic, which supply the gut mucosa and its glands.

suboestrus (silent heat) The phenomenon in which an animal ovulates normally but does not show the normal behavioural signs of *oestrus (heat) (although the male of the species may be able to detect oestrus). Suboestrus is most common at puberty and in the first oestrus following parturition; in both cases there is no *corpus luteum in the ovary and therefore no production of *progesterone. The progesterone normally acts to prime the nervous system so that it can respond fully to the *oestrogen produced during oestrus and thus enable the characteristic behaviour patterns.
Suboestrus may also be due to environmental and husbandry factors. For example in cows it is more common in winter, possibly resulting from a combination of short daylengths and low temperatures, although it has also been associated with specific nutrient deficiencies and obesity. Treatment involves the use of a *prostaglandin or *progestogen. In sows it is relatively common after weaning, when it is often associated with poor body condition; it can be treated by administering *gonadotrophins. Suboestrus in mares usually results from an inadequate environment, although other factors, such as anxiety, may be involved. *Compare* anoestrus.

subscapularis muscle A broad flat muscle lying in the subscapular fossa of the *scapula and inserting to the lesser tubercle of the humerus. It acts

787

as a strong medial collateral ligament to stabilize the shoulder joint.

substrate (in biochemistry) A molecule on which an *enzyme acts catalytically. The substrate binds to the active site of the enzyme, thus facilitating its conversion to another molecule. Most enzymes catalyse reactions involving more than one substrate, i.e. of the type: A + B = C + D.

subthalamus Part of the *diencephalon, situated between the thalamus and the midbrain.

succinylcholine *See* suxamethonium.

succus Any juice or secretion of animal or plant origin.

succus entericus A term formerly used for the enzyme-containing secretion produced by the intestinal mucosa. However, it is now recognized that most enzymatic activity involves enzymes linked to the brush border of the intestinal cells or within the cells themselves, and that these enzymes are not secreted into the lumen of the intestine to any significant degree. Secretion of water and electrolytes does occur in the *Lieberkühn's glands.

sucking A vice occurring among dairy cows where one cow sucks milk from another. This can result in considerable milk loss. Often the habit is acquired at an early age and animals exhibiting the vice are best sold. A cure is to fit the offending animal with a spiked nose plate; cows being sucked will not tolerate the spikes for long. *Navel sucking* is a common habit in young calves, and may persist after weaning. It can cause swelling of the umbilicus and lead to infections, such as *navel ill and joint ill. Calves should be provided with highly palatable dry food from the

outset, to divert their attention after the milk feed (*see* calf husbandry).

suckler herd A herd of cattle in which the calves are reared naturally by suckling their mothers, as opposed to rearing them artificially (*see* calf husbandry). The target performance is two calves per cow per year in lowland areas and one calf per cow per year in upland areas. The ideal suckler cow is hardy, fertile, and long-lived with good mothering ability and adequate milk yield yet with good beef characteristics. In the UK, the commonest suckler cows are the Hereford–Friesian cross and the Blue Grey (whitebred Shorthorn–Galloway cross). In harsher hill areas, purebred hill breeds, such as the Welsh Black or Galloway, are more suitable. Calves are born either in the autumn or spring and traditionally sold in the autumn sales at 6–12 months of age for finishing in lowland areas.

sucrase An enzyme that hydrolyses *sucrose to glucose and fructose. It is present in mucosal cells of the small intestine.

sucrose (cane sugar; beet sugar) A disaccharide comprising linked *glucose and *fructose residues.

suction The use of reduced pressure to remove unwanted fluids or other material through a tube for disposal. Suction may be supplied by a syringe, a vacuum pump, or by mouth. It is used to clear secretions from the airways of the newborn to aid breathing; to remove blood from the area of operation during surgery; and to remove air from the thorax following surgery or post-traumatic *pneumothorax.

Sudan stains A group of azo compounds used for staining fats. The group includes *Sudan I*, *Sudan II*,

Sudan III, Sudan IV, and *Sudan black.*

sudden death syndrome *See* acute death syndrome.

suffocation *See* asphyxia.

sugar Any *carbohydrate that dissolves in water, is usually crystalline, and has a sweet taste. Most sugars can be classified chemically as *monosaccharides or *disaccharides. Table sugar is virtually 100% pure *sucrose and contains no other nutrient; brown sugar is less highly refined sucrose. *See also* fructose; glucose; lactose.

sulcus (*pl.* **sulci**) A cleft or groove. The cerebral sulci are the many clefts or infoldings of the surface of the cerebral hemispheres. The raised outfolding on each side of a sulcus is termed a *gyrus.*

sulphadiazine *See* sulphonamides.

sulphadimidine *See* coccidiostat.

sulphadoxine *See* sulphonamides.

sulpha drugs *See* sulphonamides.

sulphamethoxypyridazine *See* sulphonamides.

sulphamethylphenazole *See* sulphonamides.

sulphaquinoxaline *See* coccidiostat.

sulphatroxazole *See* sulphonamides.

sulphonamides (sulpha drugs) A group of chemically similar antimicrobial agents, discovered before the antibiotics, with a broad spectrum of activity against Gram-positive and Gram-negative bacteria and activity against coccidia. They are not effective against *Pseudomonas*, mycoplas-

mas, or rickettsiae. Sulphonamides are *bacteriostatic, preventing nucleotide synthesis in bacteria, but not in mammals. The mode of action involves competitive inhibition of incorporation of p-aminobenzoic acid into the folic acid molecule. Many different sulphonamide compounds have been synthesized using different substituents on the nitrogen of the sulphonamide group. They are administered orally or by injection usually as the sodium or potassium salt, and distribute to all tissues but do not cross the blood–brain barrier as readily as other barriers. Excretion is via the urine; about 50–60% is excreted unchanged, about 30% as the acetyl metabolite, but these amounts vary considerably between compounds and species.

Sulphonamides are used in the treatment of bacterial infections, including respiratory conditions, foot rot, enteritis, skin infections, mastitis, and urinary tract infections. Most preparations are short-acting and once or twice daily administration is necessary; long-acting preparations (e.g. sulphamethoxypyridazine and sulphamethylphenazole) are available, with activity lasting several days. In poultry sulphonamides are incorporated in feed or water to treat coccidiosis, although they are effective only at a late stage in the infection when intestinal damage may have occurred. The sulphonamides and to a greater extent the acetyl metabolites can precipitate as crystals in the urine, which cause irritation. This is more apparent in acidic urine (found in carnivores). The problem is reduced by administering a mixture of three different sulphonamide compounds. In cattle, signs of toxicity can include a fall in milk yield and diarrhoea. Long-term oral administration, for instance as a coccidiostat in poultry, can induce a vitamin K deficiency with gastrointestinal haemorrhage. Rapid intravenous injection can cause collapse.

To reduce the toxicity of sulphonamides and improve their antibacterial efficacy they are used in combination with other drugs that also have a bacteriostatic action, mainly *trimethoprim. Trimethoprim acts synergistically with the sulphonamides, producing increased activity against Gram-negative organisms and a bactericidal action. Combinations of one part trimethoprim to five parts sulphonamide have the best activity, and the effective dose of sulphonamide is only about one tenth that required when used alone. Various combinations are available: sulphadiazine and trimethoprim (Tribrissen, Duphatrim), which is a short-acting suspension for intramuscular injection; sulphadoxine and trimethoprim (Trivetrin, Borgal), which is a solution for intravenous or intramuscular injection and has intermediate duration of action; and sulphatroxazole and trimethoprim (Leotrox), which is a longer-acting solution for intravenous use. These are available also as oral preparations for calves and small animals. Trimethoprim is destroyed rapidly in the rumen.

sulphur A nonmetallic element, occurring principally in the animal body as a constituent of the *amino acids cysteine, cystine, and methionine. As sulphate it is found as a component of certain polysaccharides, such as *heparin and *chondroitin sulphate. Dietary intake is normally in the form of sulphur-containing amino acids and any deficiency of the element is thus indicative of protein deficiency. Symbol S.

summer disease See avian monocytosis.

summer mastitis An acute suppurative *mastitis of dry (nonlactating) cows or heifers caused by the bacterium *Corynebacterium pyogenes. The pathogen is transmitted by flies during the summer months, entering via a teat canal. The affected quarters become swollen, firm, and painful, and may discharge externally. Other bacteria may be present: concurrent infection with the anaerobic Peptostreptococcus indolicus is responsible for the sweetish smell of the udder secretion and discharge. Failing antibiotic treatment, severe systemic illness and frequently death result from absorption of bacterial toxin produced in the udder. Prevention is by routine intramammary administration of a long-acting antibiotic depot at drying off.

summer sores See habronemiasis.

sunburn (solar dermatitis) Inflammation of the skin following prolonged exposure to the harmful rays in sunlight. The hair covering of most animals guards against sunburn. However, white pigs (particularly baby pigs) are prone to sunburn, as are the tips of the ears of white cats; in the latter, *squamous cell carcinoma may develop at the site of sunburn. The severity of the signs depends upon the brightness of the sunlight and duration of exposure. Signs can develop within several hours of exposure, with *erythema and *oedema; subsequent sloughing of the skin occurs in severe cases.

sunstroke See heat exhaustion.

super- Prefix denoting 1. above; overlying. 2. extreme or excessive.

superfecundation A pregnancy involving offspring sired by different males.

superficial (in anatomy) Situated at or close to a surface. Superficial blood vessels are those close to the surface of the skin.

superfoetation A pregnancy carrying offspring conceived at two different oestrous periods.

superinvolution (hyperinvolution) 1. Excessive shrinkage (involution) of the uterus after parturition to a size less than its prepregnant state. **2.** Excessive reduction in the size of any organ after it has attained an extremely large size.

superior (in anatomy) Situated uppermost in the body in relation to another structure or surface. In quadrupeds the use of the term is limited to certain structures in the head, e.g. lips and eyelids.

superovulation The artificial production of an abnormally large number of ova from an ovary. This is achieved by administering follicle-stimulating hormone (FSH) or pregnant mare's serum gonadotrophin (PMSG), which increases the number of follicles maturing and ovulating. Superovulation provides eggs and embryos for experimental work and for *embryo transplantation.

superpurgation Extreme and prolonged *purgation, which may be fatal. It can result from the excessive use of *purgatives, from eating unwholesome food, or following sudden overindulgence in food to which the animal is unaccustomed, for example when animals gain illicit access to lush pasture. Large volumes of liquid (often frothy) faeces are produced. The animal is very dull and weak and may show excessive thirst, although drinking can exacerbate the signs. Careful administration of fluids parenterally is necessary (*see* fluid replacement therapy), and sedation is often indicated.

supplement A composite package including all the *essential elements and *vitamins necessary to comple-

ment the feedstuffs in a *diet in order to meet the requirements of the animal. The supplement may also contain legally permitted levels of growth promoter and therapeutic agents under prescription. The term may also describe any feedstuff added at levels up to 50 g/kg to an existing diet to improve its nutritive value.

Supplementary Veterinary Register A list, maintained by the Royal College of Veterinary Surgeons, of *veterinary practitioners; they are permitted to perform limited forms of veterinary surgery. The list is now closed.

suppository A solid preparation of a medication designed for insertion into the lumen of an organ, particularly the uterus, vagina, rectum, or urethra. The suppository melts or dissolves when placed in the body, producing a highly localized therapeutic action.

suppression 1. The cessation or complete inhibition of any physiological activity. **2.** Treatment that removes the outward signs of an illness or prevents its progress.

suppuration The production or discharge of *pus.

supra- *Prefix denoting* above; over. Examples: *supraclavicular* (above the clavicle); *suprarenal* (above the kidney).

suprarenal glands *See* adrenal glands.

suprascapular paralysis (shoulder slip) A condition involving damage to the suprascapular nerve, which was formerly common in draught horses, particularly young horses used in ploughing. The damage results from collar pressure when the horse walks with one foot in the furrow. Consequent atrophy of the supraspinatus and infraspinatus muscles causes the spine of the scapula to project prominently. Also, the loss of muscle action leads to a degree of shoulder joint instability, so that it jerks outward at each step. There is some minor degree of difficulty in movement, but recovery is usual provided the animal is rested. Shoulder slip is now very uncommon because horses are seldom worked in collars.

supraspinatus muscle The muscle lying in the supraspinous fossa of the *scapula. It inserts to the greater tubercle of the humerus and acts to extend the shoulder joint.

supravital staining The application of a *stain to living tissue, particularly blood cells, removed from the body.

suramin A complex aromatic compound used as a *trypanocide. It is effective against Trypanosoma evansi, T. brucei, T. equinum, and T. equiperdum but has no activity against T. congolense, T. vivax, or T. simiae. The drug is available as a 10% solution for intravenous injection. There is no prophylactic effect and repeated doses at weekly intervals may be needed. When suramin is injected in combination with other trypanocides (e.g. homidium) the period of protection against infection is prolonged. Toxicity is common, with hepatotoxicity, renal toxicity, and damage to the spleen and adrenal glands. The drug's therapeutic index in horses is very low.

surfactant (surface-active agent) An agent, such as soap or detergent, that is added to a liquid to increase its spreading or wetting properties by reducing its surface tension. A phospholipid pulmonary surfactant is secreted by type II *pneumocytes in the alveoli of the lungs to prevent collapse of the alveoli during expiration.

surgery The branch of medicine that treats injuries, deformities, or disease by operation or manipulation. *See also* microsurgery.

surgical spirit *Methylated spirit with castor oil, diethyl phthalate, and methyl salicylate. It is used to sterilize skin, for instance before surgery, disinfect surgical instruments, etc.

surra A disease of horses, camels, and other animals caused by the protozoan parasite Trypanosoma evansi. The term also embraces the disease in South America caused by T. equinum, which is now regarded as a strain of T. evansi (*see* mal de Caderas). T. evansi is morphologically indistinguishable from T. brucei (*see* Trypanosoma) but is not tsetse-transmitted. It occurs in North Africa, the Middle East, Asia, the Far East, and in Central and South America and is transmitted by horse flies and, in South America, by vampire bats. The trypanosome does not undergo any biological development in these vectors. Surra is a severe and usually fatal disease in horses unless treated. It is also a very important disease of camels, especially in Sudan. The clinical syndrome is similar to other trypanosomiases (*see* trypanosomiasis) but oedema is a marked feature.

susceptibility Lack of resistance to disease. Many factors affect susceptibility, including genetic constitution, nutritional status, environment, and previous exposure to a disease. Methods, such as vaccination, may be used to increase resistance to specific diseases.

suspensory ligament A ligament that serves to support or suspend an organ in position. For example, the suspensory ligament of the ovary is a

swab

thickened cord in the cranial border of the broad ligament of the uterus.

sustentacular cells The elongated pyramid-shaped supporting cells of the seminiferous epithelium, which lines the seminiferous tubules of the *testis. They are believed to have a nutritive and protective function for the spermatogenic cells.

sutural bone (wormian bone) One of a number of small bones located within the *sutures of the skull.

suture 1. (in anatomy) An immovable *joint in which two bones are united by fibrous connective tissue. Sutures occur between the flat bones in the vault of the cranium and in the facial skeleton. 2. (in surgery) The closure of a wound or incision using material such as catgut or silk, to facilitate healing. The stitching must not be so tight as to obstruct blood supply to the tissue but must keep the two sides in apposition. The type of suture used varies between different tissues and types of incision or injury (see illustration). The *simple interrupted suture* is often used in skin, subcutaneous tissue, and muscle. If one stitch pulls through or becomes loose, the others in the line should hold. However, it is a time-consuming procedure. The *simple continuous suture* is often used in subcutaneous tissue and muscle. It is a speedy procedure but if one stitch loosens or pulls through, the whole line is at risk. A *mattress suture* may be used in skin or muscle and can provide improved holding power while maintaining good tissue apposition. Other suture patterns are used to repair hollow organs, such as the intestine or uterus; these include the *Lembert, Cushing, Connell*, and *Gambee* sutures. 3. The material used to sew up a wound or incision. There are two major categories. *Absorbable*

materials are used in most internal organs, muscle, and subcutaneous tissue. They include catgut, polyglycolic acid (Dexon), and polyglactin 910 (Vicryl). *Nonabsorbable materials* may be used in the skin and in other sites where prolonged suture action is required; these include silk, nylon, cotton, polypropylene (Prolene), polymerized caprolactam (Supramid, Vetafil), polyesters (Dacron, Mersilene, Ethibond), and stainless steel.

suxamethonium (succinylcholine) A depolarizing *muscle relaxant that induces paralysis. In avian species there is persistent stimulation at the neuromuscular junction causing spastic paralysis. The drug is administered intravenously and acts rapidly, causing muscle fasciculations after 20–30 seconds and paralysis for 5–10 minutes. There is some species variation in the length of action, depending on the rate at which the drug is metabolized. The muscle fasciculations are extremely painful and anaesthesia or analgesia should be induced before injecting suxamethonium with facilities for positive-pressure ventilation. Other side-effects include cardiac arrhythmias, hyperkalaemia, muscle damage, and myoglobinuria. There is no antidote, and *anticholinesterases prolong the action of depolarizing muscle relaxants.

swab 1. (in surgery) A pad of sterile absorbent material used to clear blood from the operative site and to apply pressure on small blood vessels to reduce bleeding. 2. (in bacteriology) A small cotton wad attached to a short stick inside a sterile container. The stick, attached to the top of the container, can be removed without direct handling and the swab used to sample tissue or fluid for bacteriological investigation. It is then replaced in the container without further contamination.

793

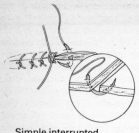

Simple interrupted

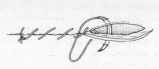

Simple continuous

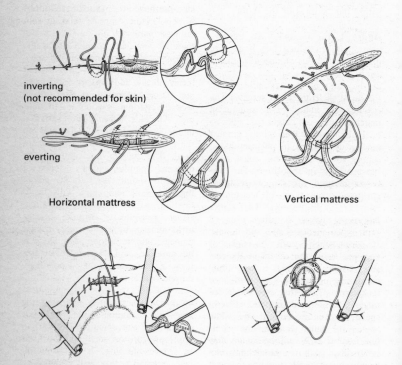

inverting
(not recommended for skin)

everting

Horizontal mattress

Vertical mattress

Lembert – an inversion suture for repairing hollow organs. The suture lies at an angle to the incision and may be interrupted or continuous.

Cushing – a continuous inversion suture used in similar situations as the Lembert. The needle passes parallel to the incision, first on one side then on the other.

Examples of suture patterns used in surgery

swallowing (deglutition) The process by which food is transferred from the mouth to the oesophagus, and thence to the stomach. The voluntary action of the tongue forces a *bolus of food into the pharynx. This is followed by an *involuntary* or *pharyngeal phase*, which is initiated reflexly by receptors, especially in the tonsillar region, and conveys the bolus through the pharynx. The entrance to the larynx is closed to prevent inhalation of food, and at the same time there is brief inhibition of breathing. The upper portion of the oesophagus relaxes as the bolus enters the oesophagus and is conveyed to the stomach by *peristalsis. This is the *oesophageal phase* of swallowing. The cardiac sphincter relaxes to permit entry to the stomach. The whole process is coordinated by centres in the medulla oblongata and pons in the brain.

swamp cancer *See* equine phycomycosis.

swamp fever *See* equine infectious anaemia.

swayback Colloquial name for a copper deficiency syndrome of lambs. Copper-deficient ewes give birth to lambs which show incoordination progressing eventually to paralysis, blindness, and death. The deficiency leads to dysmyelination of nerve tracts in the brain and spinal cord which explains the clinical signs. The copper deficiency is commonly complicated by excess molybdenum (*see* teart soils). Treatment is seldom practicable because the lesions are well established before birth, but pregnant ewes should be given copper supplements in areas where the disease occurs. Other name: **enzootic ataxia**. *See also* hypocuprosis.

sweat gland A simple coiled tubular *exocrine gland that lies in the dermis of the *skin. A long duct carries its secretion (sweat) to the surface of the skin. Sweat glands are widely distributed throughout the skin; those in the digital pads of carnivores and the frog of ungulates have a distinctive type of secretory cell. In the horse the glands are active and produce visible sweat, whereas in other species secretion is more sparse.

sweat gland tumour A skin tumour arising from a sweat gland, not uncommon in dogs and cats but rare in other species. They develop as a subcutaneous usually solitary mass on the head, neck, or body, tend to be invasive, and may metastasize to distant sites. Their potentially malignant nature means a guarded prognosis, and surgical resection should include a wide margin of normal skin. Irradiation and cytotoxic therapy may also be of use.

sweating The process, occurring in mammals, whereby sweat is secreted onto the skin by the *sweat glands. Excess body heat is used to evaporate the sweat, thereby cooling the skin surface. Sweat is a salty fluid containing small amounts of urea, and its value in temperature control is obviously determined by the amount produced, and hence by the density and distribution of the sweat glands. Birds have no sweat glands, evaporative cooling taking place largely from the respiratory tract. *See also* diaphoresis.

sweating sickness A disease of calves, thought to be a tick-borne *toxicosis, occurring in certain parts of Africa and southern India. Clinical signs include raised body temperature, pharyngitis, and a moist eczema with ulceration. Mortality varies but may reach 30–40%. Tick control is the only effective preventive measure. Exposed animals may develop immunity.

sweet itch A dermatitis of horses caused by *hypersensitivity to the bites of certain midges of the genus *Culicoides*. It occurs over the summer months and affected animals, mainly ponies, show recurrence of the condition in successive seasons. The condition has been reported from many different parts of the world and various local names are given for example, summer eczema, Kasen, and Queensland itch. The lesions are itchy papules formed along the middle of the back, with lateral spread in successive seasons. The itching (pruritus) causes the animal to rub affected areas and may result in thickening of the skin with loss of the mane and damage to the long hair of the tail; in severe cases the animal may be rendered unworkable. With the onset of cold weather in the late autumn, biting activity decreases and the lesions resolve so that an affected horse may appear normal in mid-winter. In the British Isles the active period of the disease is April to the end of November. Affected animals should be housed when the midges are most active – usually at daybreak or late evening, although activity may occur throughout daylight hours when conditions are mild, humid, and still. Alternatively, synthetic pyrethroid *insecticide should be applied to the entire dorsal midline at 6-day intervals. Other name: **summer seasonal recurrent dermatitis**.

swimming puppy syndrome A developmental abnormality found especially in dogs with short legs and wide chests, such as the English bulldog, basset hound, and Scottish terrier. Affected puppies develop a weakness of the limbs, apparent from about 2 weeks of age, so that they push themselves along the ground on their chest with swimming movements of the limbs rather than attempting to raise themselves up onto their legs. Soft bedding on which the puppies can gain a grip may help, and hobbles can be made out of sticky tape to stop the hindlimbs splaying. Some puppies gain in strength as they grow older, but when the deformities are severe the animal may have to be destroyed.

swine dysentery A severe dysentery of young weaners caused by the spirochaete bacterium *Treponema hyodysenteriae*. It is characterized by diarrhoea with mucus, blood, and/or fibrin in the faeces. Pigs over 2–3 weeks old can be affected, but those aged 8–14 weeks are especially susceptible. The pathogenesis is still not fully understood, but pen contact and oral dosing can experimentally transmit the disease. The spirochaetes invade the colonic mucosal epithelial cells, release toxins, and induce hypersecretion of mucus. Damage to the mucosa results in failure of fluid absorption, which causes the diarrhoea. In susceptible groups, the introduction of a carrier or affected pig can produce 90% morbidity and mortality of 30%.

Diagnosis is usually made on clinical and autopsy evidence, since isolation of the causal agent requires selective media. Treatment of individuals is by parenteral administration of antibiotics, such as tylosin and lincomycin, with fluid and electrolyte replacement. Medication of drinking water to in-contact animals is helpful. Control measures involve preventive antibiotic medication of feed; avoidance of overcrowding or transit stress; and general hygiene improvements. The feeding of medicated rations can complicate the picture in some intensive units where 'drug-delayed' or drug-resistant swine dysentery may occur. There is no effective vaccine to date.

swine erysipelas An infectious disease of pigs with either acute or chronic signs, caused by the bacterium *Erysipelothrix rhusiopathiae*, and distributed worldwide. Pigs aged under 12 months are most susceptible. The bacteria can survive in the environment for a considerable time and can replicate in the soil in warm conditions. In the *acute form* affected pigs develop a high fever and skin discoloration and may vomit; collapse and death follow in 2–3 days. Pigs affected with the *milder form* develop a fever and diamond-shaped areas of red discoloration on the skin (*see* diamonds); mortality is low. Pigs that have recovered from an infection, whether acute, mild, or inapparent, may develop *arthritis and vegetative *endocarditis resulting in mitral valve insufficiency and congestive heart failure. Control is by vaccination with a dead vaccine. Pigs suffering acute disease respond well to penicillin. Recovered pigs can carry the bacteria for a considerable time and be a source of infection for susceptible animals. There are a number of different strains of *E. rhusiopathiae* and immunity to one strain does not necessarily provide complete immunity to the disease. Variations in strain may also account for the appearance of disease in vaccinated pigs.

swine fever A disease of pigs caused by a *pestivirus and characterized by fever and haemorrhages in the skin and internal organs. It is enzootic in Central and South America, Africa, Asia, and parts of southern Europe. Although officially eradicated from northern European countries, swine fever continues to pose a threat, with recent outbreaks in Germany, Belgium, France, and the UK. The virus will cross the placenta of an infected pregnant sow, and, depending on the stage of gestation, can cause abortion, congenital abnormalities, and poor survival of newborn pigs, or persistently infected clinically normal piglets. Transmission can also occur by direct contact with infected pigs or their products, and new outbreaks are usually associated with the feeding of uncooked swill or the introduction into the herd of a persistently infected pig. The incubation period is 3–10 days, followed by fever, loss of appetite, and depression. After an initial constipation the affected pig has diarrhoea. Skin discoloration, particularly of the nipples, ears, and tail, severe conjunctivitis, and nervous signs are characteristic of the acute disease. Mortality in virgin outbreaks may approach 100%, but infection with milder strains of the virus causes a much lower mortality with fewer clinical signs in affected pigs. The post-mortem lesions seen in acute cases are mainly haemorrhagic: the internal lymph nodes resemble blood clots and areas of haemorrhage can be seen in the spleen, on the surface of the kidney, and on the lining of the large intestine and bladder. However, many of the milder strains of swine fever virus at present circulating in Europe cause chronic disease with few of the classical post-mortem lesions. Control in enzootic areas is by vaccination with a dead or attenuated vaccine, and by segregation of pigs joining an existing herd. Swine fever is a *notifiable disease in the UK, USA, and Canada (among other countries). Other name: **hog cholera**. *See also* African swine fever.

swine influenza A rapidly spreading respiratory disease of pigs characterized by fever, loss of appetite, coughing, and respiratory distress and caused by type A *influenzavirus. Although the virus is distributed worldwide, outbreaks of classical clinical disease are restricted to North America, and these usually occur only in the autumn, winter, and early spring. The strain of virus is closely related to strains that infect humans and may even have originated from humans. A vaccine does exist but is rarely used.

swine pox *See* pig pox.

swine vesicular disease (SVD) A contagious disease of pigs characterized by vesicles on the feet and caused by an *enterovirus. The disease was first identified in Italy in 1966 and was diagnosed in the UK in 1972. Infection usually occurs by ingestion but can enter existing cuts on the feet. Following an incubation period of 2–7 days, vesicles develop on the coronary bands of the feet, on the bulbs of the heel, between the toes, and occasionally on the snout. These rupture after 2–3 days, lameness develops, but if secondary infection is not severe, healing occurs in 2–3 weeks. Occasionally the horn of the feet is shed. Pigs kept on soft bedding may fail to develop obvious clinical signs. Because the lesions are indistinguishable from those found in *foot-and-mouth disease, the disease is notifiable in the UK (*see* notifiable disease). Although it has been eradicated from the UK there is constant surveillance by the Ministry of Agriculture because of the threat of reintroduction of the disease, particularly by the feeding of uncooked swill (garbage) to pigs. Humans are susceptible to infection with SVD virus.

swollen head syndrome A disease affecting broiler breeders and also possibly growing birds, thought to be caused by TRT virus (*see* turkey rhinotracheitis), and reported in South Africa, the Middle East, and Europe. Signs include head swelling, a drop in egg production lasting 2–2½ weeks, conjunctivitis, twitching of the head, and twisting of the neck. It appears to be exacerbated by poor site hygiene and clean-out, inadequate ventilation, and high stocking density.

symbiosis An intimate and obligatory association between two different species of organism (*symbionts*) in which there is mutual aid and benefit, for example the microorganisms in the rumen of ruminants. *Compare* commensal; mutualism; parasite.

symmetry (in anatomy) The state of opposite parts of an organ or parts at opposite sides of the body corresponding to each other.

sympathetic nervous system One of the two divisions of the *autonomic nervous system. Its fibres run in the thoracic and first few lumbar spinal nerves and reach the *sympathetic trunk. From here fibres run to supply the internal organs of the body in the thorax, abdomen, and pelvis, various glands in the head region and the skin, the eye, and blood vessels throughout the body. The system works in balance with the *parasympathetic nervous system, the actions of which it frequently opposes. See illustration.

sympathetic trunk The paired nerve trunk of the *sympathetic nervous system. It comprises two chains of ganglia, connected by lengthways fibres, lying either side of and closely ventrolateral to the bodies of the vertebrae and extending the whole length of the vertebral column. In the cervical region it is united in a common sheath with the vagus nerve, forming the *vagosympathetic trunk*. The ganglia are joined to the corresponding *spinal nerve by a *ramus communicans. Nerve fibres run from the trunk to supply various structures.

sympatholytic A drug that opposes the effects of the *sympathetic nervous system. Such drugs can act by blocking the alpha or beta receptors at the postganglionic neuroeffector synapses (*see* alpha blocker, beta blockers), or by interfering with the synthesis, storage, or release of catecholamines from the presynaptic vesicles (e.g. *reserpine, metaserpate, α-methyldopa, and α-methyl-m-tyro-

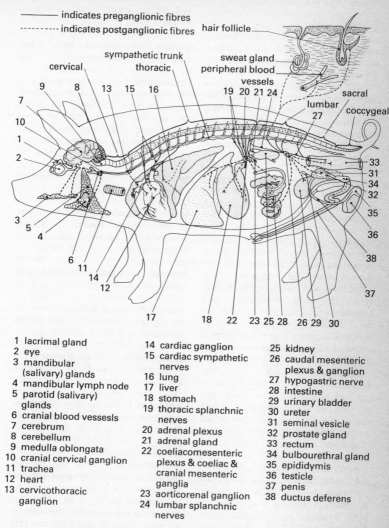

indicates preganglionic fibres
indicates postganglionic fibres

hair follicle

sympathetic trunk
thoracic

cervical

sweat gland
peripheral blood
vessels

9 8 13 15 16

19 20 21 24

sacral

7

lumbar
27

coccygeal

10

1

2

33
31
34
32

3

35

5

36

4

6

38

11

14

12

37

17

18 22 23 25 28

26 29 30

1 lacrimal gland
2 eye
3 mandibular
  (salivary) glands
4 mandibular lymph node
5 parotid (salivary)
  glands
6 cranial blood vessesls
7 cerebrum
8 cerebellum
9 medulla oblongata
10 cranial cervical ganglion
11 trachea
12 heart
13 cervicothoracic
   ganglion

14 cardiac ganglion
15 cardiac sympathetic
   nerves
16 lung
17 liver
18 stomach
19 thoracic splanchnic
   nerves
20 adrenal plexus
21 adrenal gland
22 coeliacomesenteric
   plexus & coeliac &
   cranial mesenteric
   ganglia
23 aorticorenal ganglion
24 lumbar splanchnic
   nerves

25 kidney
26 caudal mesenteric
   plexus & ganglion
27 hypogastric nerve
28 intestine
29 urinary bladder
30 ureter
31 seminal vesicle
32 prostate gland
33 rectum
34 bulbourethral gland
35 epididymis
36 testicle
37 penis
38 ductus deferens

Sympathetic division of the autonomic nervous system in a pig

sine). Many sympatholytics are used to lower blood pressure in human patients with hypertension.

sympathomimetic A drug that has the effect of stimulating the *sympathetic nervous system. Their actions are *adrenergic*, i.e. resembling those of *noradrenaline, and they can be divided into two groups depending on their precise mode of action. One group, including the catecholamines, act directly at the same sites as noradrenaline. The other group act indirectly by stimulating the release of noradrenaline at nerve endings. The catecholamines include the naturally occurring compounds *adrenaline, noradrenaline, and dopamine (*see* dopa) and the synthetic compound isoprenaline. Adrenaline acts at alpha (α) and beta (β) receptors, noradrenaline at α and β_1 receptors, and isoprenaline at β receptors. Other sympathomimetics act specifically at β_2 receptors, for example *clenbuterol, which is used in horses, and salbutamol, terbutaline, and orciprenaline, which are available for use in human medicine. The indirectly acting sympathomimetics include *ephedrine, amphetamine, and methylamphetamine. They cause the release of adrenaline and noradrenaline from neurones, producing marked stimulation of the central nervous system and peripheral sympathetic effects. These are *controlled drugs because of their addictive properties.

symphysis (*pl.* **symphyses**) A cartilaginous joint in which the bones are separated by fibrocartilage, which minimizes movement and makes the bony structure rigid. Examples are the *pelvic symphysis* (the midline joint between the bones of the pelvis) and the joints between the bodies of the vertebrae, which are separated by intervertebral discs. **2.** The line that marks the fusion of two bones that were separate at an early stage of development.

syn- (sym-) *Prefix denoting* union or fusion.

synapse The minute gap between the termination of the nerve fibre of one neurone and part of another. A *nerve impulse causes the release of a *neurotransmitter, which diffuses across the gap and triggers an electrical impulse in the next neurone. Some brain cells have more than 15 000 synapses. *See also* neuromuscular junction.

synchronous diaphragmatic flutter *See* exercise problems.

syncope (fainting) Temporary loss of consciousness due to insufficient flow of blood to the brain. This is commonly due to a sudden fall in blood pressure in cases of *shock. Recovery is typically prompt with no lasting ill-effects.

syncytium (*pl.* **syncytia**) A mass of *protoplasm containing several nuclei. Striated muscle fibres are syncytia.

syndesmosis (*pl.* **syndesmoses**) A *joint between two bones formed of much fibrous connective tissue.

syndrome A combination of clinical signs that characterize a particular disease.

synechia An adhesion between the iris and another part of the eye. An *anterior synechia* is between the iris and cornea; a *posterior synechia* is between the iris and lens. Inflammation of the iris (*iritis) is the immediate cause, and the adhesion prevents the proper movement of the iris in response to light. Moreover, drainage of fluid from the anterior chamber may be affected, resulting in *glaucoma. Iritis is relatively common in horses and cases involving synechia tend to be recurrent and progressive.

syneresis (in blood coagulation) The contracture of a blood clot, observed in the test tube and presumably occurring in the body, that forms part of the process whereby patency is restored to blood vessels occluded by a *thrombus. It is made possible by the extensive incorporation of *platelets within the clot and the activation of the contractile protein, thrombasthenin, contained in the platelets.

synergism 1. The interaction of two drugs or a drug and chemical to produce a combined effect greater than the sum of their individual effects. It can also occur where one drug in the combination has no effect at a particular site but increases the activity of the other drug. Examples of synergistic drug combinations are *penicillin/streptomycin, *sulphonamide/ *trimethoprim, and amoxycillin/clavulanate; in each case the activity of the antibacterial compounds is enhanced. **2.** The interaction of two or more muscles such that their combined effects are greater than the sum of their individual effects.

Syngamus A genus of parasitic *nematodes comprising the gapeworms, which are found in the trachea and bronchi of birds and mammals. *S. trachea* is a parasite of turkeys, pheasants, and young domestic fowls, causing the condition *gapes. The male is permanently attached to the vulva of the female by its copulatory bursa, giving the pair a forked appearance. Eggs are coughed up and then swallowed to be passed in the faeces. Infective larvae are swallowed by a bird directly, or they may be ingested by an invertebrate carrier host (e.g. earthworm), which in turn is eaten by a bird. See illustration.

synostosis (*pl.* **synostoses**) A bony union between two previously separate bones, for example between the epiphysis and the diaphysis of a long *bone.

synotia An inherited condition involving abnormal development of the ears, with fusion of the ears above the forehead. Deafness is invariably the consequence although gross alterations of the inner ear have not been found. Other deformities, namely *agnathia, *aglossia, and brachygnathia, are commonly associated, in which cases stillbirth is frequent.

synovia (synovial fluid) The thick colourless lubricating fluid that fills a joint, bursa, and a tendon sheath. It is secreted by the synovial membrane.

synovial joint A freely movable *joint.

synovial membrane (synovium) The membrane, composed of connective tissue, that forms the sac enclosing a freely movable joint (synovial joint). It secretes the lubricating synovial fluid. *See* joint.

synovioma A rare benign tumour

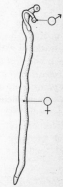

Syngamus trachea: gravid female showing attached male

arising from the synovium, i.e. the lining of a joint cavity. Its malignant counterpart is called a *synoviosarcoma*. These tumours present as an irregularly swollen joint with associated lameness. On radiography a solid mass of soft tissue is seen; in the case of the malignant form it may also invade the neighbouring bones. Surgical excision should be attempted but, in the case of malignant tumours, amputation of the affected limb may be more appropriate.

synoviosarcoma *See* synovioma.

synovitis Inflammation of the synovial membrane of a joint or bursa. A common cause is infection of the joint, resulting from either systemic infection carried by the bloodstream or by penetration of a foreign body. The lesion may be part of a more general inflammation of the joint (*see* arthritis). Similarly, a bursa may become infected, for instance with the bacterium *Brucella abortus* in the case of *fistulous withers. Treatment depends on the cause. *See also* tenosynovitis.

In **poultry** synovitis usually affects the leg joints, causing lameness. It can be due to bacteria, such as *Staphylococcus aureus* or *Escherichia coli*, or mycoplasma infection (*see* infectious synovitis of poultry). Bacterial synovitis is often associated with *osteomyelitis. The hock and feet are most frequently affected, becoming painful, hot, and swollen; there is pus in the joint. Birds are disinclined to walk and lose condition, but fatalities are rare. Joint infections often follow general bacterial infections, such as fowl *cholera and *pullorum disease.

syring- (syringo-) *Prefix denoting* a tube or long cavity, especially the central canal of the spinal cord.

syringe An instrument designed for the injection or withdrawal of fluids. The most widely used form is the hypodermic syringe, which consists of a piston (fitted with a sealing washer) in a tight-fitting tube that is attached to a hollow needle. These are available in presterilized sealed packs. An *enema syringe* (*Higginson's syringe*) consists of a rubber bulb with a tube connected at each end; one tube is placed in the appropriate site in the patient, the other into a container with the enema fluid. Special multidose syringes have been developed for the purpose of administering a set volume of fluid to large numbers of animals, for example anthelmintic dosing syringes.

syrinx (*pl.* **syrinxes** or **syringes**) The specialized organ responsible for voice production in birds. It is located where the trachea divides into the left and right primary bronchi (see illustration). In the angle between the two bronchi is a bar of bone, the *pessulus*. The gaps between the tracheal and bronchial cartilages are bridged by the *lateral* and *medial tympaniform membranes*, vibration of which produces the sounds.

systemic Relating to or affecting the body as a whole, rather than individual parts and organs.

systemic circulation The system of blood vessels that supplies all parts of the body except the lungs. It consists of the aorta and all its branches, carrying oxygenated blood to the capillaries in the tissues, and all the veins draining deoxygenated blood into the venae cavae. *Compare* pulmonary circulation.

systemic lupus erythematosus (SLE) An *autoimmune disease of unknown cause characterized by inflammation and destruction of a variety of tissues. SLE is frequently

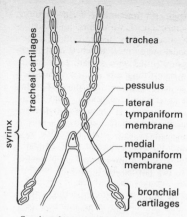

Section through the syrinx of the domestic fowl

reported in dogs and more rarely in other veterinary species. The clinical presentation is varied but a common feature is the presence of a number of autoantibodies, in particular antibodies to nucleic acid. The damage to tissues is mediated by the antibody, either by the activation of *complement or by the formation of antibody-antigen complexes, involving such antigens as nucleic acid or tissue protein.

*Canine autoimmune haemolytic anaemia, which also occurs in isolation, can form part of the SLE syndrome. The other common manifestations are platelet deficiency and inflammation in blood vessels, joints, skin, peripheral nervous system, meninges, and the thyroid. It seems that most canine autoimmune disorders may appear, in different combinations, as part of the SLE complex. The commonest presentation is of *haemolytic anaemia, lameness, nephritis, and platelet deficiency leading to *purpura. The signs may occur together or sequentially. Treatment is by *corticosteroids or, in resistant cases, by immunosuppressive drugs, such as azathioprine or *cyclophosphamide.

systole The period of the cardiac cycle during which the heart muscle is contracting. Contraction of the atria (*atrial systole*) precedes that of the ventricles (*ventricular systole*). *Compare* diastole.

T

tachy- *Prefix denoting* fast; rapid.

tachycardia An increase in the heart rate above normal. This is usually demonstrated by measuring the *pulse rate. Tachycardia occurs normally with exercise or excitement, or it may be due to illness, such as fever, septicaemia, toxaemia, circulatory failure, and hyperthyroidism. Adrenalin and adrenergic drugs also increase the heart rate. Tachycardia may be accompanied by *arrhythmia, especially when there are lesions of the myocardium. *Compare* bradycardia.

tachypnoea Unduly rapid breathing. It is distinguishable from normal increased breathing (*hyperpnoea) by being both rapid and shallow, and is caused by a failure of the normal breathing control mechanisms (*see* respiration), often an indication of underlying disease.

tactile Relating to or affecting the sense of touch.

taenia (*pl.* **taeniae**) A flat ribbon-like anatomical structure. The *taeniae coli* are the longitudinal ribbon-like muscles of the colon in the horse and the pig.

Taenia

Taenia A genus of *tapeworms that are intestinal parasites of dogs, cats, and humans. The adults can attain lengths of up to 1–1.5 m in dogs and 8 m in humans. Species parasitic in dogs include *T. pisiformis* (with intermediate hosts the rabbit and hare) and *T. hydatigena* (intermediate hosts include sheep, cattle, and pigs). Scavenging dogs, hounds, and farm dogs are thus particularly prone to infection. *T. multiceps*, another tapeworm of dogs, is smaller than other taeniids and is often placed in a different genus as *Multiceps multiceps*. The cat tapeworm, *T. taeniaeformis*, has a rodent as its intermediate host. The beef tapeworm, *T. saginata*, in which cattle are the intermediate hosts, infests humans when beef containing the tapeworm cysts is eaten raw or inadequately cooked. However, the cysts are killed by freezing and infected carcasses can be held in cold storage for 3 weeks. *T. solium*, in which pigs are the intermediate hosts, can also infest humans in a similar manner.

tail The caudal part of the vertebral volumn that extends beyond the trunk. In domestic mammals the tail skeleton comprises some or all of the coccygeal *vertebrae, which vary in form and number according to species and breed. Thus in dogs the tail may be straight or tightly curled. In apes and humans the tail is represented by the coccyx, which consists of several fused coccygeal vertebrae. In birds the tail feathers are supported by the pygostyle, which represents the fused caudal vertebrae. The tail is variously used for balance, display, and as a fly whisk; in birds the tail is essential for braking and other manoevres in flight.

tail-biting A vice occasionally encountered in intensive pig units, usually when young pigs from different litters are mixed at weaning. It is distinct from short-lived fighting, which invariably occurs at this time, and is more persistent and frequently attributable to only a few individuals in the group. Apart from being unsightly, the tail wound represents a route of infection into the body. Thus animal health, well-being, and carcass quality may all suffer. Both diet and environment have been implicated as causative agents. A cure is difficult and, on units where the problem is encountered, prevention is by removal of the tail shortly after birth.

tail sores A condition, primarily of intensively reared piglets, in which animals chew the tail tips of their companions, with resulting inflammation. Local *abscesses may form, and occasionally infection may spread to the spinal cord with serious results. Where tail sores are a serious problem, pig farmers may cut off the tip of the tail and 'corner' the teeth of baby pigs to prevent damage. Animals with long tails, such as greyhounds, may also suffer sore tail tips, for example if confined in cramped kennels.

Talfan See Teschen/Talfan.

talus (*pl.* **tali**) One of the tarsal bones. See tarsus.

tampan A soft tick of the genus *Argas*, also known as the fowl tick.

tamponade Abnormal pressure on a part of the body, for example, pressure on the heart due to the accumulation of excessive fluid in the *pericardium. This may be the result of haemorrhage following rupture of the heart wall (e.g. by a nail or piece of wire) or rupture of the base of the aorta (especially in horses). Death usually follows very rapidly. Also, oedemal fluid may accumulate in the pericardial sac to cause tamponade.

tannic acid A yellowish complex organic compound that can be prepared from acorns. In the past it was used as a constipating agent in the treatment of dysentery and diarrhoea. It has also been used as a burn dressing because of its ability to cause rapid vasoconstriction at mucosal surfaces, and is used as an antidote in alkaloid poisoning, converting the alkaloids to insoluble tannates. Ingestion of tannic acid causes necrosis of the gastric and intestinal mucosa and renal toxicity. When used as a burn dressing only a small area of skin should be treated because absorption of tannic acid causes hepatic necrosis. Treatment with oral calcium hydroxide may reduce toxicity, but once renal toxicity is advanced the prognosis is very poor.

tannin One of a group of complex organic chemicals found in many plants, notably oak leaves and acorns, tea, and coffee. They can cause toxicity in animals (*see* acorn poisoning). *See also* tannic acid.

tapetum (*pl.* **tapeta**) A specialized layer or membrane, especially the *tapetum lucidum* – the reflecting layer in the choroid behind the retina of the eye; it is present in domestic mammals other than the pig.

tapeworm (cestode) A flatworm (*see* Platyhelminthes) that is an endoparasite and belongs to the class Cestoda. The adults are found in the intestines and body cavity of vertebrates. Several genera are of veterinary significance, including *Dipylidium* (in dogs), *Moniezia* (in cattle and sheep), and *Taenia*, which includes the common dog and cat tapeworms as well as the two human tapeworms. Tapeworms typically have long ribbonlike bodies with no mouth or digestive system, absorbing nutrients from their host's gut through their body wall. The head (scolex) has suckers or sucking grooves and usually also a small anterior projection (rostellum) bearing hooks for attachment to the host. Behind the scolex is a short narrow neck, which gives rise to the body (strobila) composed of a chain of segments, each of which is called a *proglottis and contains a set of male and female reproductive organs. The mature posterior segments are gravid and contain fertilized eggs. Cross-fertilization between individuals in the same gut usually occurs otherwise they are self-fertilizing. The terminal gravid segments break off and pass out with the faeces. When the larval stage (*oncosphere) is eaten by a suitable intermediate host it develops into the infective form – e.g. *coenurus, *cysticercus, or *hydatid cyst. If the intermediate host is eaten by the final host, these larval stages develop into adult tapeworms.

Mild tapeworm infestation causes little or no harm to the host; however, pathological signs can range from general debility and poor growth to digestive troubles and inflammation of the intestine. The larvae are usually more damaging than the adults, causing diseases in their intermediate hosts, such as *cysticercosis, *hydatid disease, *coenurosis, and *sparganosis. Infestations of adult tapeworms can be treated with suitable *anthelmintics, given either orally or injected. Treatment should be on a regular basis where reinfestation is likely. In grazing animals infestations can be minimized by regular rotation of pastures and by grazing young stock on 'clean' pastures rather than those recently used by adults. *See also* Anoplocephala; Diphyllobothrium; Hymenolepis.

tapping 1. *See* aspiration; paracentesis. 2. The preparation of a hole drilled through bone so that it will take a screw.

tar Any of various black semisolid mixtures of hydrocarbons, obtained by distillation of coal, wood, or shale. *Stockholm tar* (*wood tar*) is used as a preservative on hoofs and horns to maintain moisture and prevent cracking and infection, and on sheep and other livestock as a fly repellant, especially on areas of blowfly strike or headfly strike in sheep. The phenolic content of tar products gives them a characteristic carbolic smell. Tar products are also used as wood preservatives, and toxicity in animals can result due to contact and licking of treated areas. Signs of toxicity are depression of the central nervous system, weakness, inappetence, increased respiratory rate, convulsions, and paralysis. Contact with road tar can cause irritation to the feet of small animals. Tar can be removed from the skin using solvent oils.

target cell An *erythrocyte that has its greatest opacity at the rim and the centre, thus resembling a sporting target. *See also* leptocyte.

target organ The specific organ or tissue upon which a hormone, drug, or other substance acts.

tarsal Relating to the *tarsus.

tarsorrhaphy An operation in which the upper and lower eyelids are sutured together, either completely or along part of their length. This may be performed as a temporary measure to afford protection to the eyeball, or it may be permanent, in which case the lid margins should be denuded of epithelium to ensure that healing takes place. In the management of prolapse of the eyeball in brachycephalic dogs, tarsorrhaphy of the temporal part of the palpebral fissure is described as *external canthoplasty*.

tarsus (*pl.* **tarsi**) **1.** The hock: the region of the hindlimb corresponding to the human ankle. The bones of the tarsus articulate proximally with the tibia and fibula and distally with the metatarsals. They basically comprise the talus and calcaneus proximally; the central tarsal in the middle; and tarsals 1, 2, 3, and 4 distally. This arrangement occurs in carnivores and the pig. In the horse tarsals 1 and 2 are usually fused, and in ruminants tarsals 2 and 3, the central tarsal, and tarsal 4 are fused. In birds such as the domestic fowl, the proximal tarsal bones fuse with the tibia forming the *tibiotarsus*, and the distal tarsal bones fuse with the metatarsals forming the *tarsometatarsus*. See illustration at pes. **2.** A plate of dense fibrous tissue that lies within and maintains the form of the upper and lower eyelids. It contains the *tarsal* (*meibomian*) *glands* – small sebaceous glands.

tartar (**dental calculus**) *Dental plaque that has become mineralized and hardened, mainly by deposition of calcium carbonate (in dogs) or phosphates (in horses). It is frequently present in mature dogs and cats, causing painful *gingivitis. Unless it is removed by scaling and polishing, it may lead to *periodontal disease.

taste The sense for determining the quality of substances by their effect on the *taste buds and consequent nerve impulses to the brain. Four primary sensations of taste are recognized: sour, salt, sweet, and bitter. Investigation in animals, either by behavioural experiments or direct recording from sensory nerve fibres, indicates that most domestic species are able to distinguish most of the primary sensations.

taste buds The sensory receptors concerned with the sense of *taste, located mainly in the tongue and elsewhere in the oral mucosa. Receptor cells and support cells are grouped around a taste pore to form a taste bud, which can respond to one of the four *taste sensations; those of each type tend to be localized in particular regions. Their specificity probably depends on the type of receptor in the membrane of the taste cells that will bring about depolarization and also the connections in the central nervous sytem of the sensory fibre from each cell. The receptor cells remain stimulated until saliva washes away the chemical.

tattooing A method of identifying individual animals by the use of numbered pins and indelible ink. A tattoo can be applied, for example, shortly after birth into the ear lobe of piglets. *See also* branding.

taurine (2-amino ethyl sulphonic acid) A component of *bile, in which it occurs combined with cholic acid to form taurocholic acid – a bile salt.

taurocholic acid *See* bile salts.

taxis (in surgery) The returning to a normal position of displaced bones, organs, or other parts by manipulation only, unaided by mechanical devices.

Taylorella A genus of nonmotile pleomorphic Gram-negative *bacteria comprising a single species, *T. equigenitalis* (formerly *Haemophilus equigenitalis*). It is a facultative anaerobe and causes the venereally transmitted disease *contagious equine metritis in mares.

tears The salty fluid secreted by the *lacrimal glands to keep the front of the eyeballs moist and clean. It contains the enzyme *lysozyme, which has antibacterial activity. Irritation of the eye causes excessive production of tears.

teart *See* molybdenosis.

teart soils Soils with a high concentration of molybdenum that limit the absorption of copper in grazing animals producing a condition known as teart in cattle (*see* molybdenosis).

teaser An animal, usually a vasectomized male, used for *oestrus detection in cattle, sheep, and pigs.

teat *See* papilla.

teat dipping The application of disinfectant by means of a cup or spray to a cow's teats after milking, to control *mastitis. The chemical used is usually an *iodophor or *hypochlorite.

teat necrosis Death of tissue in the teat skin, usually with ulceration. It commonly follows injury, such as treading with hoofs. Also teat chapping with necrosis may occur if the teats are exposed to frequent washing in cold windy conditions. *Bovine herpes mamillitis, caused by a herpesvirus, may result in extensive teat necrosis with sloughing. Treatment depends on establishing the cause. Emollient antiseptic ointments may be used to relieve chapping and prevent infection; iodophor solutions can serve as udder disinfectants. Care is needed to prevent teat lesions spreading inwards to cause *mastitis; if the teat orifice is affected, prophylaxis with antibiotics may be indicated.

tectospinal tract A tract of nerve fibres that runs from the *tectum of the midbrain to the cervical region of the spinal cord. It controls reflex movements of the head and neck in response to sudden visual or auditory stimuli.

tectum (*pl.* **tecta**) The roof of the midbrain, consisting of the paired rostral and caudal colliculi (*see* colliculus).

teeth marks (meat inspection) A condition of the pig's skin caused by fighting. It consists of irregular red scratches and bruising, mainly on the backs and around the ears, and may be confused with *stick marks. If bruising is severe, haematomas or *ear ballooning may occur.

tegmen (*pl.* **tegmina**) A structure that covers an organ or part of an organ. For example the *tegmen tympani* is the bony roof of the middle ear.

tegmentum (*pl.* **tegmenta**) The dorsal portion of the cerebral peduncle of the midbrain. It lies ventral to the tectum and contains the nuclei of the oculomotor and trochlear nerves, the red nucleus, and various ascending and descending pathways.

tel- (tele-, telo-) *Prefix denoting* **1.** end or ending. **2.** distance.

tela Any thin weblike tissue, particularly the *tela choroidea*, a folded double layer of *pia mater containing numerous small blood vessels that extends into several of the *ventricles of the brain.

telangiectasis (*pl.* **telangiectases**) A cluster of abnormally dilated blood capillary vessels. This may occur subcutaneously, visible as a reddened area, which may eventually undergo fibrosis and change to brown. However, the most common form of telangiectasis in veterinary medicine occurs in the liver of cattle. It is seen after slaughter or at post-mortem examination as irregular red areas, both on the surface and within the substance of the liver; sometimes many such lesions occur in the same liver. They have no clinical significance but are unsightly and make the liver unfit for human consumption.

telangitis Inflammation of the blood capillaries. The term is not commonly used. *See* angiitis.

telencephalon *See* cerebrum.

telocentric A chromosome in which the centromere is situated at either of its ends.

telodendron One of the branches into which the *axon of a neurone divides at its destination. Each telodendron finishes as a synaptic vesicle, which takes part in a *synapse or a *neuromuscular junction through the elaboration and release of transmitter substances.

telophase The final stage of *mitosis and of each of the divisions of *meiosis, in which the chromosomes at each end of the cell become long and thin and the nuclear membrane reforms around them. The cytoplasm then begins to divide.

temperate (virology) Describing a *bacteriophage that can enter the *prophage condition. Because such phages can carry bacterial genes, some (e.g. lambda phage and its derivatives) have been used in gene manipulation (*see* recombinant DNA).

temperature *See* body temperature.

temporal bone A bone of the *skull. It consists of the *petrous part*, which encloses the internal ear, the *tympanic part*, which surrounds the external acoustic meatus, and the *squamous part*, which forms part of the vault of the cranium.

temporalis A powerful muscle running from the skull to the coronoid process of the *mandible. It contracts to raise the mandible during mastication.

tenaculum 1. (in anatomy) A fibrous band of tissue that holds a part in place. **2.** (in surgery) A hooklike instrument used for fixing and restraining tissue during surgery.

tendinitis Inflammation of a tendon. It usually results from partial rupture of the tendon fibres during strenuous exercise, especially in horses; the flexor tendons of the forelegs are particularly prone. Common causes are overexercise without proper training, fast galloping on hard or rough ground, or improper shoeing. The inflammation results in lameness with local swelling and pain. The lesion eventually heals but may leave a permanent thickening and weakness. Treatment to reduce the swelling must be prompt and consists in applying cold packs to the affected area and administration of anti-inflammatory drugs. A period of rest is important to prevent the lesion progressing to a chronic stage.

tendon A tough fibrous structure, consisting of numerous parallel bundles of collagen fibres, that serves to attach a muscle to a bone or other structure. Tendons are inelastic but flexible; they assist in concentrating the pull of the muscle on its point of insertion. Some tendons are rounded cord-like structures and other are flattened bands or even sheet-like structures (aponeuroses). In certain cases tendons are surrounded by *synovial sheaths*; these are tubular double-layered sacs, lined with synovial membrane and containing synovial fluid. They surround the tendons at the *carpus and *tarsus, where they minimize friction and facilitate movement.

tendon organ (Golgi tendon organ) A *stretch receptor found within a tendon that responds to the tension or stretching of the tendon and relays impulses to the central nervous system. Like stretch receptors in muscle (*see* muscle spindle), tendon organs are part of the *proprioceptor system.

tenesmus Ineffectual but repeated efforts to defecate or urinate. Common causes are diarrhoea and constipation, especially if due to obstruction. Cattle undergo tenesmus when suffering from bloat or during parturition. Less commonly, tenesmus may be due to lesions of the central nervous system involving paralysis of the anus. Rabies or meningitis may cause undue straining.

teno- *Prefix denoting* a tendon.

tenoplasty The surgical correction of tendon defects. This may involve shortening a stretched tendon, attempting to lengthen a shortened tendon, or the reconstitution of a severed tendon.

tenosynovitis Inflammation of a tendon sheath. This commonly represents an extension of *tendinitis, but it may also be caused by penetrating foreign bodies that introduce purulent infection, or by the spread of infection from neighbouring structures. Resolution of the inflammation may result in fibrosis with adhesions, which give rise to long-term lameness. In horses tenosynovitis of the deep digital flexor tendon of the hock is known as *thorough-pin. Early treatment is vital to prevent long-term weakness. Nonsteroidal *anti-inflammatory drugs can be helpful, together with antibiotics to clear up any infection. Chronic lesions have a poor prognosis. *See also* viral tenosynovitis.

tenotomy The surgical sectioning of a tendon. It is not commonly employed in animals, although it has been used in cattle to overcome the effects of spastic paresis, i.e. overextension of the hock joint and dysfunction of the affected leg. The extensor tendons were cut above the hock to allow hock flexion, and many cases were thus improved.

tentorium A curved infolded sheet of *dura mater that dips inwards from the skull and separates the cerebellum caudally from the cerebral hemispheres cranially. The part closest to the skull may be ossified to form the *tentorium ossei.*

terat- (terato-) *Prefix denoting* a monster or congenital abnormality.

teratogen. An agent or process that interferes with development of the embryo or foetus to produce abnormal young. Known teratogens include certain drugs, some viruses, and ionizing radiation (e.g. X-rays).

teratoma A tumour composed of several tissue types and originating from a multipotential cell, i.e. a cell that has the ability to differentiate into many types of tissue. The most common sites for teratomas are the testis and ovary, where the composite mass may contain hair, bone, teeth-like structures, and multiple cysts. Testicular teratomas can occur in an undescended testis in stallions.

teres muscle One of two round muscles, *teres major* and *teres minor*, that act to flex the shoulder joint.

terpene Any of a group of unsaturated hydrocarbons containing multiples of 5 carbon atoms (usually 10 or 15), many of which are found in plant oils and resins and are responsible for the scent of these plants (e.g. mint). Larger terpenes include vitamin A, squalene, and the carotenoids.

Teschen/Talfan An infectious disease of pigs characterized by fever and nervous signs and caused by *enterovirus. In a fully susceptible herd, pigs of all ages may be affected, but usually where the herd is persistently infected, disease is seen in weaning pigs as the protection provided by maternal antibody wanes. Transmission is by breathing in virus particles carried by moisture droplets in the air or by ingestion of contaminated feed. Following an incubation period of up to 10 days the affected pig develops a fever with tremors, incoordination, paralysis, and convulsions. The majority of an affected litter may die. Teschen is the severe form and is a *notifiable disease in the UK, while Talfan is less severe and more sporadic. Live and dead vaccines are available to control the disease in continental Europe.

testicle *See* testis.

testis (*pl.* **testes**) Either of the pair of male gonads that produce spermatozoa and secrete the male sex hormones *androgens. The testis forms within the abdomen of the foetus but descends into the *scrotum in order to maintain a lower temperature that favours the production and storage of spermatozoa (*see* spermatogenesis). The substance of the testis is composed of long convoluted *seminiferous tubules lined by specialized seminiferous epithithelium, where the spermatozoa are formed. They pass from the tubules to the *rete testis and thence to the ductuli efferentes and the *epididymis to complete their maturation, ready for discharge at *ejaculation. The *interstitial cells produce androgens.

testosterone A steroid sex hormone (*see* androgen) produced by the interstitial cells of the testis. Little testosterone is produced prior to puberty in males, but after puberty, testosterone production causes development of the male secondary sexual characteristics. Preparations of testosterone are administered to control reproductive activity and for therapeutic purposes, especially in bitches. Natural testosterone is not effective if given orally but is used as an implant or oil-based injection. It is rapidly metabolized and excreted. Esters of testosterone (e.g. testosterone propionate) are used in oil and have a longer duration of action. Methyl testosterone is not degraded in the liver and is effective after oral administration. Methyl testosterone is used in bitches to suppress lactation during false pregnancy. Again in bitches, testosterone silicone rubber implants or oral mibolerone (an androgenic anabolic steroid) are used to suppress oestrus. Side-effects include clitoral enlargement and clitoral fossa discharge. The anabolic actions of testosterone are useful in therapy to stimulate appetite and increase weight gain, and compounds with similar anabolic activity but less androgenic properties (e.g. nandrolone) have been developed. Testosterone is ineffective in the treatment of infertility in male animals, and its efficacy in attempts to increase libido, improve spermatogenesis, and treat hormonal alopecia has not been proven.

tetan- (tetano-) *Prefix denoting* **1.** tetanus. **2.** tetany.

tetanolysin An *exotoxin produced by the bacterium *Clostridium tetani* that causes haemolysis and local tissue necrosis and is lethal to laboratory animals.

tetanospasmin A neurotoxin produced by the bacterium *Clostridium tetani*. It is a heat-stable and poorly absorbed protein that acts by binding specifically to gangliosides in nerve tissue, resulting in continuous stimulation and tetanic spasm of muscles.

tetanus An acute infectious disease affecting all domesticated species and humans caused by the toxins (teta-nospasmin, tetanolysin) of the bacterium *Clostridium tetani*. It has a worldwide distribution and a very high mortality rate.

Initial signs are usually stiffness and an unsteady gait; in ruminants *bloat is often seen. As the disease progresses the muscles of the jaw are affected and the animal is unable to eat and drools saliva. Other signs include high carriage of the tail and protrusion of the third eyelid. The disease lasts 5–10 days, and mild cases may recover if well nursed. Death is caused by convulsions and respiratory failure. The spores of *Cl. tetani* can survive for years in the soil and are found in animal faeces. Infection is usually via deep wounds that become contaminated with soil containing the spores. Treatment of infected animals with antitoxin is rarely effective, but antitoxin can be administered as a precautionary measure prior to castration, docking, etc., in areas where tetanus is common. Active immunization with toxoid (detoxified toxin) can provide longer-lasting protection. Prompt treatment of human cases with penicillin and antitoxin is usually effective.

tetany A condition marked by prolonged involuntary contraction of muscles. Tetany commonly occurs in the various forms of *hypocalcaemia or *hypomagnesaemia affecting animals at or near parturition, because of dietary factors or because of *hypoparathyroidism. It is also the principal sign of *tetanus, while certain poisons, such as strychnine or cyanide, induce tetanic spasms.

tetracyclines A group of closely related *antibiotics with a broad spectrum of activity. Chemically they are based on the tetracycline nucleus, and various substituent groups are introduced to produce chlortetracycline, demethylchlortetracycline, doxycycline, methacycline, minocycline, oxytetracycline, and tetracycline. They are bacteriostatic, with activity against Gram-positive and Gram-negative bacteria, mycoplasmas, rickettsiae, and chlamydias. Their activity against Gram-positive organisms is less than that of *penicillins. Tetracyclines inhibit protein synthesis in microorganisms by binding to ribosomes and preventing peptide binding. Microorganisms can develop side-resistance to other members of the group, and there may be cross-resistance with *chloramphenicol.

Tetracyclines chelate readily with calcium and magnesium ions and they should not be administered with milk or bone meal. Absorption from the gastrointestinal tract is incomplete but varies with the compound, and in adult ruminants they are extensively broken down in the rumen. Apart from oral administration, tetracyclines can be injected intravenously, intramuscularly, or subcutaneously. Solutions in water are highly alkaline and require a buffer. Polyvinylpyrrolidine is a commonly used alternative solvent. Local anaesthetics and buffering with magnesium may reduce the pain of injections. Tetracyclines are partly metabolized, and are also excreted in the urine, bile, and faeces. Because tetracyclines are bacteriostatic it is important to maintain the concentration of antibiotic throughout the treatment period; daily injections or oral administration every 12 hours (every 6 hours for tetracycline) give adequate concentrations. Oxytetracycline is available as a long-acting preparation for intramuscular injection and has activity for 3 days.

Tetracyclines are used in the treatment of systemic infections (e.g. respiratory disease) and are also used topically in the eye and on skin and hoofs (e.g. for foot rot). They are relatively nontoxic, but various side-effects have been noted. In young animals tetracycline-calcium chelates can be deposited in bones and teeth causing yellow staining. In ruminants gastric irritation may follow oral administration. Intravenous injection in cattle should be performed slowly to avoid anaphylactoid reactions (due to chelation of calcium), which may cause respiratory embarrassment and collapse. Injection of *adrenaline will suppress the anaphylaxis. In horses a condition called *colitis X (possibly due to *Clostridium perfringens* overgrowth in the gastrointestinal tract) has followed the use of tetracyclines. Abscesses or fibrous reactions at the site of injection are common.

tetrad (in genetics) **1.** The four cells resulting from meiosis after the second telophase. **2.** The four chromatids of a pair of homologous chromosomes in the first stage of meiosis.

Texas fever Formerly a very important cattle disease in the southern United States. The discovery by Smith and Kilborne in 1893 that it was caused by the protozoan parasite *Babesia bigemina* and was transmitted by ticks was a landmark in veterinary and medical history, being the first demonstration of the transmission of a disease by an arthropod. Subsequently the disease was eradicated from the USA. *See also* babesiosis.

TGE *See* transmissible gastroenteritis.

thalam- (thalamo-) *Prefix denoting* the thalamus. Example: *thalamolenticular* (relating to the thalamus and lenticular nucleus of the brain).

thalamus (*pl.* **thalami**) One of a pair of egg-shaped masses lying deep to each cerebral hemisphere either side of the third ventricle in the brain. It is a relay station for all information (except olfactory) being transmitted to the cerebral cortex. Conscious awareness of the sensations of temperature, pain, and touch probably begins in the thalamus.

theca (*pl.* **thecae**) A sheathlike surrounding tissue. For example, the *theca folliculi* is the outer wall of an *ovarian follicle.

Theileria A genus of protozoan parasites that parasitize the lymphocytes and red blood cells of sheep, cattle, and other grazing animals throughout the world, especially in tropical and subtropical regions. *Theileria* are transmitted by hard ticks, which pick up infection either as larvae or nymphs and transmit it as nymphs or adults. There is no transmission through the egg of the tick vector. Species affecting cattle do not naturally infect sheep, and vice versa. However, some African *Theileria* species may be shared between cattle and wild ungulates, such as buffalo or eland.

After transmission by the tick the parasite invades lymphocytes at the lymph nodes. It multiplies by stimulating replication of the host cells, growing and dividing in step with them. At this stage the parasites may be seen in lymphocytes in the circulation as well as in lymph nodes. In stained smears the multinucleate parasites form dark-blue masses (*Koch's bodies*) inside, and sometimes outside, cells. Further multiplication and division is followed by invasion of red blood cells, in which the parasites form oval or comma-shaped *piroplasms, 1–2 μm long. There may be multiple infection of a single red cell but the piroplasms do not form linked pairs like the parasites of the related genus *Babesia*. Examples of important *Theileria* species are *T. parva* (*see* corridor disease; East Coast fever), *T. annulata* (*see* Mediterranean fever), and *T. mutans* (*see* tzaneen disease).

theileriosis A disease of cattle and sheep caused by protozoan parasites of the genus *Theileria* and transmitted by ticks. The causal parasite multiplies in lymph nodes causing lymph-node enlargement, fever, and ultimately the destruction of lymphocytes leading to a fall in the number of white cells. Some *Theileria* species also replicate in red blood cells (e.g. *T. annulata* and *T. mutans*) and cause anaemia. The disease may be severe and fatal, especially *T. parva* infections (*see* East Coast fever), or mild. Animals that recover are immune to reinfection (though this immunity is species- and, in some cases, strain-specific) but may remain carriers of low-grade infection. Young animals derive immunity from their dams and may become infected without signs of severe disease. If susceptible animals are introduced to enzootic areas, serious disease outbreaks are likely. Prevention entails the use of *acaricides to control the tick vectors. A vaccine has been developed for *T. annulata*. Treatment of the disease by tetracycline antibiotics is possible for some species of parasite; parvaquone is effective for *T. parva* infections. *See also* corridor disease; Mediterranean fever; tzaneen disease.

Thelazia A genus of parasitic *nematodes found in the conjunctival sac and lacrimal ducts of the eye in various animals and occasionally in humans. *T. callipaeda* is found in dogs in the Far East; *T. californiensis* occurs in sheep, dogs, and deer in mountainous scrub regions in California. *T. rhodesi* infests cattle in eastern Siberia and can be spread by flies; *T. lacrymalis* affects horses worldwide. *T. gulosa* and *T. skrjabini* occur in the eyes of European cattle. *See* eye-worm.

theobromine *See* xanthine.

theophylline *See* xanthine.

therapeutic index A measure used to indicate the safety of a drug. It is found by dividing the drug's *LD_{50} by its *ED_{50}. A high therapeutic index should mean a good measure of safety. However, the calculation employs group means, and does not take into account variation of the lethal dose within a group. Hence some individuals may be killed by doses of the drug below the effective dose, even though the drug's index is relatively high.

theriogenology The study of the reproductive diseases of animals.

therm- (thermo-) *Prefix denoting* **1.** heat. **2.** temperature.

thermography A technique for measuring and recording the heat produced by different parts of the body. Images (*thermograms*) are obtained by using film sensitive to infrared radiation. The technique may be used to detect heat from inflamed damaged tissue before outward signs are discernable. It can also reveal areas of poor circulation, which produce less heat, or tumours, which may have an abnormally increased blood supply and hence appear as 'hot spots' on a thermogram.

thermolabile Heat-sensitive. The term is especially used in relation to the biological activity of a *protein.

thermometer An instrument for measuring temperature. In veterinary practice it is inserted into the rectum to determine the animal's *body temperature. Thermometers in routine clinical use contain mercury in a bulb at one end of a sealed glass tube. With increased temperature the mercury expands along the column, and the reading is taken from the height of the column. Resistance thermometers measure temperature according to

changes in electrical resistance of a metal wire or semiconductor.

thermotherapy The use of heat to alleviate pain and stiffness in joints and muscles and to promote an increase in circulation. *Diathermy provides a means of generating heat within the tissues themselves.

thiabendazole *See* benzimidazoles.

thiamin (thiamine) *See* vitamin B_1.

thiamylal *See* barbiturate.

thiazide diuretics (benzothiadiazines) A large group of *sulphonamide derivatives with a diuretic action. The principal members used in veterinary medicine are chlorothiazide, hydrochlorothiazide, and bendrofluazide, which are administered to reduce oedema. They are very weak carbonic anhydrase inhibitors and their main action is at the distal tubules in the kidneys, inhibiting the reabsorption of sodium and consequently of chloride. There is increased potassium excretion and the consequent risk of hypokalaemia. They can be administered orally or injected intramuscularly and are active for 12–24 hours. Urine volume is increased 2–3 times, but they are less potent than *frusemide. Thiazides have been found to decrease urine production in cases of *diabetes insipidus. Toxicity is rare. Hypokalaemia due to long-term therapy is treated with potassium chloride, given orally.

thigh The region of the hindlimb related to the *femur.

thin sow syndrome A syndrome in which lactating sows or those in early pregnancy lose weight dramatically and fail to regain weight. The result is emaciation, infertility, and death. The cause is thought to be a combination of low environmental temperature, parasitic infestation, and inadequate food intake. These are not uncommon problems in pig units.

thiopentone (*US* **thiopental**) *See* barbiturate.

thiophanate *See* benzimidazoles.

thiouracil An antithyroid drug used in the treatment of hyperthyroidism in dogs and cats. It acts by blocking the incorporation of iodine into thyroglobulin thus preventing formation of monoiodotyrosine and diiodotyrosine, the precursors of the thyroid hormones. Methylthiouracil is four times less active than propylthiouracil.

thiourea *See* ANTU.

third eyelid A fold of *conjunctiva around a T-shaped piece of cartilage at the medial (inner) angle of the eye. The cartilage is intimately related to the *gland of the third eyelid. During blinking the eye is pulled back into the orbit by the action of the retractor bulbi muscle. This results in increased pressure in the fat in the orbit, causing the third eyelid to move across the front of the eye.

thirst The desire to drink. Water intake is controlled by a group of neurones in the hypothalamus, which act as a 'thirst centre'. Increasing concentration of the body fluids and consequent intracellular dehydration triggers thirst. Moreover, reduced cardiac output, for example following a severe haemorrhage or in cardiac failure, also induces thirst. In animals, dryness of the mouth due to cessation of salivation does not induce drinking, except when they are also eating.

thorac- (thoraco-) *Prefix denoting* the thorax or chest.

thoracic Relating to the *thorax or chest.

thoracic duct One of the principal vessels of the *lymphatic system. It commences at the *cisterna chyli and runs cranially in the thorax close to the aorta and azygos vein, terminating in the great veins near the commencement of the cranial vena cava.

thoracocentesis *See* pleurocentesis.

thoracotomy Surgical opening of the chest cavity. For example, in dogs it may be performed for the management of diaphragmatic rupture; the removal of oesophageal foreign bodies or correction of other oesophageal defects; the closure of patent ductus arteriosus and correction of other cardiovascular defects; and the excision of lobes of a lung affected by neoplasm, bronchiectasis, or torsion.

thorax (*pl.* **thoraxes** or **thoraces**) The chest: the part of the body between the neck and the diaphragm. The skeleton of the thorax is formed by the sternum, ribs and costal cartilages, and the thoracic vertebrae. It encloses the lungs, heart, great vessels, oesophagus, and associated structures.

thornapple poisoning *See* deadly nightshade poisoning.

thorough-pin A condition of the hock (*see* tarsus) of the horse due to *tenosynovitis of the tarsal sheath enclosing the deep digital flexor tendon. The cause is assumed to be trauma. Lameness is rarely present.

threadworm *See* pinworm.

three-day sickness *See* ephemeral fever.

three-quarter shoe A type of horseshoe fitted when it is necessary to avoid pressure on one of the heels of the foot. The shoe makes contact with the front of the foot, one side, and across the frog, but is cut away from the affected side, thus relieving pressure on the heel and bar on that side and the area of sole between them.

threonine An *amino acid. See also essential amino acid.

threshold (in neurology) The point at which a stimulus begins to evoke a response, and therefore a measure of the sensitivity of a system under particular conditions.

-thrix Suffix denoting a hair or hair-like structure.

throat See pharynx.

thromb- (thrombo-) Prefix denoting 1. a blood clot (thrombus). 2. thrombosis. 3. blood platelets.

thrombin A blood *coagulation (clotting) factor formed by the action of factors Xa, Va, *platelet factor 3, and calcium on plasma *prothrombin. Thrombin promotes *fibrin and *plasmin formation, platelet aggregation, and the activation of *complement and of several other plasma proteins concerned with coagulation and *inflammation.

thrombocyte See platelet.

thrombocytopenia A reduction in the number of *platelets in the blood. The causes are various, including various *autoimmune diseases (see also systemic lupus erythematosus), *hypersplenism, intravascular blood clotting leading to the overconsumption of platelets, *myelofibrosis, *lymphosarcoma and other leukoses, *bracken poisoning, and synthetic *oestrogens or other drugs. The majority of drug-induced thrombo-cytopenias are probably immunologically mediated or result from bone marrow depression. Equine infectious anaemia and canine ehrlichiosis have also been reported in association with platelet loss (see haemolytic anaemia). Thrombocytopenia is most often reported in dogs. Signs do not usually appear until the platelet count has fallen from the normal of $200 \times 10^9/l$ to about $20 \times 10^9/l$. The animal may then be progressively subject to deficiency of blood clotting, haemorrhage, and bleeding into the skin (*purpura). Treatment consists in removal of any identifiable cause, and *corticosteroid therapy to counter autoantibody formation. Transfusions of fresh blood or fresh platelet-rich plasma may be given to offset acute deficiencies. Removal of the spleen is sometimes considered in refractory cases, but the benefit is not generally proven in animals.

thrombocytosis An excess of *platelets in the blood. This rare condition may occur as a primary bone-marrow disorder involving cancerous multiplication of the platelet-forming stem cells (megakaryocytes). Thrombocytosis is also occasionally found as a secondary change in other cancers, especially when bone marrow is involved, and in chronic inflammation and some immunological disorders.

thromboembolism The process whereby particles dislodge from a *thrombus and are carried freely by the circulation until they lodge in a narrowing vessel. At this point the separated particle (thromboembolus) may obstruct blood flow and will usually form the focus of a new thrombus. Where the original thrombus was infected with bacteria, as occurs in bacterial *endocarditis, the thromboemboli may also carry the infection to the new site of thrombus formation. Compare embolism. See also thrombophlebitis; thrombosis.

thrombolytic A drug that reduces blood clots (thrombi) within blood vessels. Such drugs activate tissue *plasminogen, thereby producing plasmin, which causes lysis of fibrinogen and fibrin and reduction of clots. They are used in human medicine to treat thromboembolism, and can be used in animals to remove vascular emboli, for instance caudal vena caval embolism in cats. Drugs available include streptokinase, which is obtained from beta haemolytic streptococci; urokinase, obtained from culture of human renal cells; and tissue type plasminogen activator, obtained using recombinant DNA techniques. These agents are used intravenously, and the animal should be checked for the development of widespread systemic haemorrhages. *Heparin can be used to treat disseminated intravascular coagulation, but increased risk of haemorrhage is a side-effect.

thrombophlebitis Inflammation of a vein in combination with blood-clot formation (*thrombosis). The cause is usually an infection derived from local injury, from a pre-existing tissue infection, or from a thromboembolus (see thromboembolism). Thrombophlebitis may also give rise to further infected thromboemboli, thus spreading the infection. This process is usually involved in *navel ill, an infection that starts at the umbilicus in the newborn but subsequently spreads and becomes generalized.

thromboplastin (thrombokinase) 1. Blood *coagulation Factor Xa. This generates *thrombin from its plasma precursor prothrombin and thereby plays an essential and central role in blood coagulation (clotting). **2.** Certain tissue extracts (notably brain and lung) that are rich in lipid and provide a potent source of activator of Factor X in the presence of Factor VII.

thrombopoiesis The production of *platelets in the bone marrow (see haemopoiesis).

thrombosis (pl. **thromboses**) The formation of a blood clot or *thrombus within the heart or blood vessels. The processes of thrombosis are the same as those of normal blood *coagulation, and, probably in all cases, begin following damage or inflammation in the blood-vessel lining (endothelium). This permits platelet adhesion to the damaged parts and the activation of *coagulation factors. Once the coagulation mechanism has effected a repair, its products are normally dispersed rapidly. For thrombosis to occur, two other factors are probably required – local alteration in blood flow and change in the composition of the blood.

Alterations in blood flow are usually either stasis, such as results in veins from general circulatory slowing or from some local obstruction (including a pre-existing thrombus), or turbulence, which is found near sites of damage or distortion in arteries and heart valves. Changes in blood composition include increased number and adhesiveness of platelets, both of which are likely to occur after trauma. Thrombi themselves produce such changes so that progressive growth or propagation of thrombi is seen, especially in veins. Thrombosis obstructs blood flow resulting in *infarction or venous congestion. There is also danger of *thromboembolism and thus of vascular damage, inflammation, infection, or thrombosis elsewhere. Thrombi are sometimes resolved by the normal processes of clot dispersal. They may also become organized, i.e. invaded by fibrous tissue and so rendered permanent. In some cases fresh blood vessels penetrate the thrombus, by a process known as recanalization, and restore circulatory function.

Several types of thrombosis occur in domestic animals. In **horses** thrombosis of the anterior mesenteric artery can follow initial damage of the artery by larvae of *Strongylus vulgaris*. Consequent restriction of blood flow to the intestines may result in *colic. Iliac thrombosis resulting in hindlimb lameness is probably caused by aberrant *Strongylus* larvae. In **dogs** and **cats** aortic thrombosis and thromboembolism may occur, usually presenting as a loss of hindlimb movement, often with coldness and absence of pulse in these limbs and sometimes with generalized shock. These signs are associated with the presence of a thrombus at the point of bifurcation of the dorsal aorta.

Bacterial *endocarditis occurs in many species but is most common in cattle, pigs, horses, dogs, cats, and lambs. The disease in these species is associated with specific bacterial infections and accompanied usually by *heart failure and sometimes by thromboembolism and *pyaemia with associated *arthritis.

thrombus (*pl.* **thrombi**) A solid clot formed in the vascular system from blood constituents during life. *See* coagulation; thrombosis.

thrush Oral *candidiasis.

thumps A colloquial name for the respiratory sign in pigs caused by migrating larvae of *Ascaris* nematodes.

thym- (thymo-) *Prefix denoting* the thymus.

thymectomy Surgical removal of the thymus gland.

thymic aplasia Absence or underdevelopment of the *thymus. This leads to a deficiency in cell-mediated immunity. It is seen in some inbred lines of dogs and cattle. The animals become runted and suffer high mortality after weaning.

thymidine A molecule containing thymine and the sugar deoxyribose. *See also* nucleoside.

thymine One of the nitrogen-containing bases (*see* pyrimidine) occurring in the nucleic acid DNA.

thymitis Inflammation of the *thymus gland. In domestic animals it is rare.

thymocyte A *lymphocyte in the *thymus.

thymoma A tumour, rare in animals, arising from the epithelial or lymphoid components of the thymus. They may be either benign or malignant, but this can be difficult to assess histologically. Clinical signs relate to the presence of a mass in the anterior part of the chest, i.e. dyspnoea and dysphagia. As in humans, there may be an association between thymomas and *myasthenia gravis.

thymus A bilobed organ located, in mammals, in the root of the neck and the mediastinum of the thorax; in birds it extends the length of the neck in a long strand. The mammalian thymus is encapsulated and divides into lobules, each consisting of cortex and medulla; the cortex contains many lymphocytes (*thymocytes*). The thymus is well-developed in the foetus and young animal, controlling the development of the immune system, particularly allergic responses, autoimmunity, and rejection of organ transplants. After puberty it undergoes marked involution, being largely replaced by fatty tissue.

thyro- *Prefix denoting* the thyroid gland. Example: *thyroglossal* (relating to the thyroid gland and tongue).

thyrocalcitonin *See* calcitonin.

thyroglobulin A protein in the thyroid gland from which the thyroid hormones (*thyroxine and *triiodothyronine) are synthesized.

thyroid cartilage The large shield-like cartilage of the *larynx, consisting of two broad plates that join ventrally to form a V-shaped structure.

thyroid gland An *endocrine gland, located near the larynx in most species, that produces the hormones *thyroxine and *triiodothyronine. It consists of two lobes joined by an isthmus (although the isthmus may be rudimentary or absent in horses and dogs). Each lobe contains a large number of closed follicles inside which is a jelly-like colloid, which contains the active secretory substances. Each follicle is surrounded by a network of blood capillaries and penetrated by fine lymphatic vessels. The thyroid is stimulated by *thyroid-stimulating hormone (TSH) to increase its uptake of iodine and the release of thyroid hormones. Chronically stimulated glands will undergo hypertrophy and hyperplasia to produce *goitres. Iodine deficiency commonly causes goitres, a result of continued TSH secretion without adequate hormone production. *See also* hyperthyroidism; hypothyroidism.

thyroid hormone *See* thyroxine; triiodothyronine.

thyroiditis Inflammation of the thyroid gland. A form of the disease caused by an autoimmune response, known as *lymphocytic thyroiditis* (akin to Hashimoto's disease in humans), occurs in Doberman Pinscher dogs. This appears to involve the produc-

tion of autoantibodies to *thyroglobulin. The clinical signs are of *hypothyroidism, and include obesity and coldness. The coat thins, becomes dry, and may progress to baldness. *Myxoedema may develop. In many cases the autoimmunity extends to other body tissues, including joints, muscles, and the liver, resulting in a complex clinical pattern. Treatment involves immunosuppressive drug therapy and hormonal supplementation with thyroxine.

thyroid-stimulating hormone (TSH; thyrotrophin) A hormone, synthesized and secreted by the adenohypophysis, that stimulates the thyroid gland to produce the hormones *thyroxine and *triiodothyronine. The production of TSH is itself controlled by negative feedback from the thyroid hormones.

thyrotoxicosis The syndrome due to excessive amounts of thyroid hormones in the bloodstream. *See* hyperthyroidism.

thyrotrophin *See* thyroid-stimulating hormone.

thyrotrophin-releasing hormone (TRH) A hormone, produced in the nuclei of the hypothalamus and released into the hypothalamo-hypophyseal portal system, that stimulates the synthesis and release of *thyroid-stimulating hormone and prolactin from the pituitary gland. Other name: **thyroid-stimulating-hormone releasing hormone (TSHRH)**.

thyroxine (T_4) The principal hormone produced by the *thyroid gland, formed from the conjugation of two tyrosyl residues and containing four iodine atoms, hence T_4. It is stored in the thyroid follicles in the form of *thyroglobulin*. Stimulation by *thyroid-stimulating hormone causes its conversion to thyroxine and

tiamulin

release. Like the other thyroid hormone, *triiodothyronine (T_3), thyroxine is essential for normal metabolism and physical development. Both stimulate the catabolism of carbohydrate, fat, and protein. Synthetic thyroxine is used orally to treat *hypothyroidism in small animals. Overdosage causes restlessness, sleeplessness, increased heart rate, weight loss, increased body temperature, and osteoporosis.

tiamulin An antibiotic with good activity against Gram-positive bacteria, mycoplasmas, and spirochaetes, especially *Treponema hyodysenteriae*, the causative agent in swine dysentery. Tiamulin is administered in feed or (as the hydrogen fumarate salt) in water to control mycoplasma infections in poultry and enzootic pneumonia and swine dysentery in pigs. Care should be taken when handling the drug, which is irritant to skin and mucous membranes. Tiamulin is incompatible with most *ionophores, such as monensin, and feed containing monensin should not be used during or immediately after tiamulin therapy. The tiamulin interferes with monensin metabolism causing severe depression and death.

tibia The larger of the two long bones of the lower hindlimb. Proximally it articulates with the femur at the *stifle joint, and in such species as the dog it forms proximal and distal joints with the *fibula (see illustration). In the horse the fibula is incompletely ossified and its lateral malleolus forms part of the tibia. In ruminants the lateral malleolus is present as a separate bone, which articulates with the tibia. Distally the tibia articulates with the proximal row of tarsal bones forming part of the tarsal joint (see tarsus). In birds it is fused with the proximal row of tarsal bones forming the *tibiotarsus*.

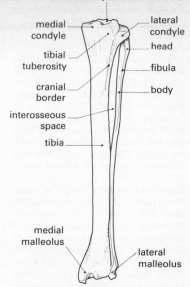

Left tibia and fibula of the dog
(cranial aspect)

tibial dyschondroplasia (focal osteodystrophy) A form of lameness affecting growing poultry, particularly meat birds, such as broilers, turkeys, and ducks. It results from a proliferation of uncalcified cartilage in the metaphysis at the head of the tibia. Subclinical cases can be found in a high proportion in a flock, while the highest incidence of lameness is seen in roaster (heavy broiler) flocks, where it perhaps reaches a few percent. Downgrading of carcasses often results. The causes are uncertain, but there may be a genetic factor, while lowered feed intake in early life can reduce the incidence sharply. *Compare* twisted leg.

tibial nerve One of the terminal divisions of the *sciatic nerve. It supplies muscles and skin in the caudal part of the hindleg and back of the hindfoot.

ticarcillin *See* penicillin.

tick A parasitic arachnid belonging to the order Acarina (*see* acarid), which also includes *mites. Ticks are all ectoparasites of birds or mammals, feeding on the blood of their hosts. Livestock, pets, and humans worldwide are liable to infestation. Ticks resemble mites but are larger, with mouthparts modified as boring and attachment organs. Their legs terminate in claws for attachment to the host. Ticks are divided into two families. The *hard ticks* (Ixodidae) include the *dog ticks and sheep ticks (*see* Ixodes). They have a protective hard shield (scutum) on their back and the mouthparts can be clearly seen from above. The females may become greatly enlarged when engorged with blood and the adults live permanently on the host. The larva, nymph, and adult are each usually found on different hosts (three-host ticks), although sometimes there are only one or two hosts. The *soft ticks* (Argasidae), which include the fowl tick (*see* Argas), have no dorsal scutum and the ventral mouthparts are not visible from above, except in the larva. The sexes are almost indistinguishable and they are generally nocturnal, the adults leaving the host after each meal.

Ticks are of considerable veterinary and economic importance. Their bites are painful and irritating resulting in loss of condition, and a heavy infestation can lead to anaemia. Some species transmit the rickettsiae that cause, for instance, Rocky Mountain fever, also bacterial and virus diseases, such as *tick pyaemia and *louping ill, as well as protozoan parasites, such as *Babesia* spp., which cause babesiosis and *Texas fever in cattle. Certain species are responsible for *tick paralysis, probably caused by a toxin in the tick's saliva. Treatment entails dipping, spraying, or shampooing animals with a solution of one of the many suitable *acaricides. These give a degree of residual protection preventing further infestation. However, resistance to a particular acaricide can develop. In the case of infestations of soft ticks, poultry and animal houses must be thoroughly cleaned and disinfected to ensure that all stages of the life cycle are eradicated.

tick-borne fever An infectious disease of sheep and cattle characterized by very high fever and leucopenia and caused by the rickettsia *Cytoecetes phagocytophila*. The disease occurs in temperate regions of Europe where the vector tick, *Ixodes ricinus*, is common, and outbreaks are related to the seasons of maximum tick-activity, i.e. summer and autumn. The disease has also been reported in Africa and India. In the tick the organism is not transmitted transovarially, but it survives during the long hibernation periods. The incubation period following infection varies from 4 to 7 days, after which the disease has a sudden febrile onset, with peak febrile reactions exceeding 41–42°C over 4–10 days and frequent relapses. During this period the rickettsiae are found in large numbers in the neutrophils and, to a lesser degree, in the monocytes. A severe reduction in circulating white blood cells and platelets occurs, initially due to reduced numbers of lymphocytes followed by a severe and prolonged reduction of neutrophils. Other signs of the disease are mild, but pregnant animals may abort and the milk yield of lactating animals is severely reduced. Furthermore, affected animals are susceptible to other infections: common sequelae include *tick pyaemia of lambs, abortions, *listeriosis, *pasteurellosis, and respiratory infections due to viruses or chlamydias. Diagnosis is based on the demonstration of the rickettsia within infected white blood cells using Giemsa-stained blood smears. Treatment of infected animals or prophylaxis of susceptible animals with oxytetracycline is effective. Control of ticks by regular dipping of livestock is also beneficial.

tick paralysis A form of flaccid *paralysis caused by a neurotoxin generated by certain ticks, such as the common wood tick (*Dermacentor variabilis*) in the USA and *Ixodes holocyclus* in Australia. It affects dogs, other domestic species, and humans. Progressive paralysis occurs with death due to respiratory paralysis. Treatment involves removal of the ticks; the use of hyperimmune serum is practised in Australia.

tick pyaemia A *pyaemia of lambs caused by *Staphylococcus aureus*. The acute form is characterized by death from toxaemia, the chronic form by multiple abscesses. The bacterium occurs harmlessly on the skin; during seasons of tick activity (e.g. spring and early summer in the UK) it is inoculated by biting ticks (e.g. *Ixodes ricinus*), although the ticks do not act as vectors (*compare* spotted fever). Prevention is by avoidance of tick-infested pasture or, where feasible, tick eradication. Other names: **tick-bite pyaemia; lamb pyaemia**.

tidal volume The volume of air inspired and expired with each normal breath.

tight junction *See* zonula occludens.

timber preservatives *See* phenol poisoning.

timolol A beta adrenergic antagonist (*see* beta blocker) used in the treatment of cardiovascular disease and glaucoma. Available as tablets for oral administration, it is given to decrease heart rate and reduce hypertension. Timolol is rapidly absorbed but is metabolized in the liver and excreted in the urine. The plasma half-life is 4 hours, and it is 5–10 times more potent than propranolol. It is also used as eye drops in the treatment of glaucoma, causing a fall in intraocular pressure and a reduction in the production of aqueous humour. The effect in the eye is maintained for approximately 8 hours.

tinea A Latin term for *ringworm, derived from a fanciful resemblance of the characteristic patchy hair loss to the effects of the clothes moth (*Tineola biselliella*). It is used more in human than veterinary medicine, and is often combined with a term for the region of the body affected, for example *tinea capitis* (head or scalp ringworm), *tinea barbae* (ringworm of the beard).

tip A half horseshoe worn to protect the hoof wall against splitting and to allow the full use of the frog. They are fitted to horses at grass and ponies in light work living at grass. Many farriers doubt their effectiveness.

tissue A collection of cells specialized to perform a particular function. The cells may be of the same type (e.g. in nervous tissue) or of different types (e.g. in connective tissue). Aggregations of tissues constitute organs.

tissue culture *See* cell culture.

tissue mite nodules A condition of the subcutaneous tissue of poultry, consisting of yellowish-white caseous and calcareous nodules, about 2 mm in diameter. It is caused by the flesh mite *Laminosioptes cysticola*.

titre (in immunology) The extent to which a solution of an *antibody can be diluted before it ceases to cause *agglutination of the matching *antigen in vitro. Since concentrated solutions of antibody can sustain more dilution than weak ones before their activity ceases, the titre is a measure of the original concentration of the antibody.

T-lymphocyte *See* lymphocyte.

toadstool poisoning A toxic condition caused by the ingestion of fruit bodies (basidiocarps) of certain fungi of the family Agaricaceae (agarics or toadstools). There are few dangerously poisonous toadstools and even fewer reports of animals (other than humans) being poisoned by them. The fungi involved have usually been species of *Amanita*, though sheep eating *Cortinarius speciosissimus* in the course of grazing have died with severe kidney damage. *Amanita verna* has caused losses among cattle grazing in woodland. *A. muscaria* and *A. pantherina* have both poisoned dogs and the latter cats also. The main toxin in both fungi is ibotenic acid. Neither contains muscarine in pharmacologically significant amounts and the use of the specific antidote for muscarine, atropine, is ill-advised since it potentiates the activity of ibotenic acid. Induced vomiting or stomach lavage may be helpful; treatment otherwise is symptomatic.

tocopherol *See* vitamin E.

togavirus A family of RNA *viruses having naked icosahedral *capsids and containing positive-stranded RNA. The main genera are the *alphaviruses, *flaviviruses, and *pestiviruses. The genus rubivirus (rubella) infects only humans.

tolerance 1. (in immunology) An acquired immunological state in which the subject becomes specifically unresponsive to a given *antigen. The prime example is the tolerance normally shown by the immune mechanisms to the body's own components. Breakdown of this self tolerance may cause *autoimmune disease. Self tolerance is evidently acquired during prenatal development, when the body is also uniquely susceptible to the development of tolerance to antigens in general.

The mechanisms of immunological tolerance are not fully understood. For example, clones of immature B-*lymphocytes or T-lymphocytes may be deleted or inactivated by contact with antigen. In contrast, suppressor T-lymphocyte activity may prevent the differentiation of B- or T-cells effective against the particular antigen. Alternatively, the presence of antibody or antigen-antibody complexes may block further contact of antigen with lymphocyte membranes and hence prevent lymphocyte activation.

High-zone tolerance is induced by high repeated doses of antigen. This corresponds to prenatal tolerance as outlined above. *Low-zone tolerance* is induced by small repeated doses of antigen. It is inducible in adults but can easily be broken, for instance by giving the antigen with an adjuvant.
2. (in pharmacology) The reduction or loss of the normal response to a drug or other substance that usually provokes a reaction in the body. *Drug tolerance* can develop after repeated administration: a given dose of drug produces a reduced effect or increasingly larger doses are required to produce the same effect. Tolerance can occur with a wide variety of drugs, including barbiturates, opiates, and anticholinergic drugs. The mechanisms of tolerance development also vary. For example there may be an increased rate of drug metabolism or a change in the sensitivity of the drug's receptors.

tolguacha

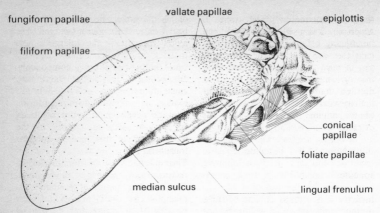

fungiform papillae

filiform papillae

vallate papillae

epiglottis

conical papillae

foliate papillae

median sulcus

lingual frenulum

Tongue of the dog

tolguacha Jimsonweed (thornapple). *See* deadly nightshade poisoning.

toluidine blue A *stain used in microscopy to demonstrate *basophilic substances in tissue specimens.

-tome *Suffix denoting* a cutting instrument. Example: *microtome* (instrument for cutting microscopical sections).

tomography The technique of using X-rays or ultrasound waves to produce an image of structures at a particular depth within the body, bringing them into sharp focus while deliberately blurring structures at other depths. The visual record of this technique is called a *tomogram*. *Computerized axial tomography* (*CAT*) is a sophisticated form used primarily in human medicine. X-ray scans of successive sections of the body are integrated by computer to give a complete image of an area.

-tomy (-otomy) *Suffix denoting* a surgical incision into an organ or part. Example: *gastrotomy* (into the stomach).

tone *See* tonus.

tongue A muscular organ attached to the floor of the mouth. It consists of an *apex*, a *body*, and a *root*. The muscles of the tongue attach to the mandible in front and behind, to the styloid process above, and the hyoid bone below. It is covered by mucous membrane, which is continuous with that of the mouth and pharynx. On the undersurface of the tongue a fold of mucous membrane, the *frenulum linguae*, connects the midline of the tongue to the floor of the mouth. The surface of the tongue is covered with minute projections – the *papillae*; these may be filiform, conical, fungiform, vallate, or foliate. *Taste buds are arranged around the papillae, especially the fungiform and circumvallate papillae. Filiform papillae are particularly large in the cat. The functions of the tongue include manipulation of food during mastication and swallowing, grooming, taste, and thermoregulation by panting. See illustration.

tongue worm *See* Linguatula serrata.

tonic 1. Relating to muscle tone. **2.** A preparation used to improve the functioning of a particular body system; they are classified accordingly – e.g. cardiac, digestive, vascular, uterine, or general. Tonics can be used during convalescence to try to improve the condition of an animal. Many contain a collection of plant extracts, vitamins, and oils. *Bitter tonics*, or *bitters*, are a collection of plant substances that stimulate gastric secretion and are used to improve appetite.

tonicity 1. *See* tonus. **2.** The effective osmotic pressure of a solution. *See* hypertonic; hypotonic; isotonic; osmosis.

tono- *Prefix denoting* **1.** tone or tension. **2.** pressure.

tonofibril A tiny fibre occurring in bundles in the cytoplasm of cells that lie in contact, as in epithelial tissue. Tonofibrils are concerned with maintaining contact between adjacent cells. *See* macula adherens; zonula adherens.

tonsil A clearly demarcated lymphatic nodule without a capsule, found in close association with a wet epithelium and usually surrounding a crypt in the epithelium. Tonsils have only efferent *lymphatics, but probably have functions similar to other lymphoid organs (*see* lymph node). The locations of tonsils include the caecum and oesophagus in birds, the soft palate and pharynx in most mammals, the epiglottis in the pig, and the root of the tongue in cattle.

tonsillitis Inflammation of the *tonsils. This is uncommon in most domestic species but fairly frequent in dogs, in which tonsillitis often occurs in conjunction with *rhinitis or *pharyngitis and affects the pharyngeal and/or palatine tonsils. Species

of *Streptococcus* or *Escherichia coli* bacteria are most commonly involved, although foreign bodies lodged in the tonsillar crypt may be the primary cause. The affected dog shows signs of discomfort or pain in the throat, coughing, retching, or difficulty in swallowing. The condition must be distinguished from tonsillar neoplasia. In the pig chronic abscesses of the tonsils are reported and a necrotic tonsillitis may also occur in cases of *swine fever. Treatment involves correcting any primary cause and administering antibiotics. Chronic tonsillitis may be treated by surgical excision of the tonsils (*tonsillectomy*).

tonus (tone) The normal state of partial contraction (tonicity) of a resting muscle, maintained by reflex activity.

tooth (*pl.* **teeth**) One of the hard structures in the mouth used for cutting and chewing food. Each tooth is embedded in a socket (alveolus) in the bone of the upper jaw (premaxilla and maxilla) or lower jaw (mandible), and is attached by the *periodontal membrane. On the basis of their position, form, and function, four types of teeth can be distinguished: *incisors, *canines, *premolars, and *molars. Their numbers vary in different species. Two sets of teeth occur during life: temporary and permanent (*see* dentition).

On the basis of their composition and growth pattern, the teeth of domestic mammals fall into two categories. *Brachydont teeth* include all those of carnivores, the incisors of ruminants, and the teeth of the pig other than the canines of the boar. They are short and stubby and cease to grow on the completion of eruption. The crown is covered by *enamel; this overlaps at the neck with the *cementum, which covers the root(s). Beneath the enamel and cementum is a thick layer of *dentine, which

toothache

enclose the *dental pulp. *Hypsodont teeth* include all those of the horse, the premolars and molars of ruminants, and the canines (tusks) of the boar. They continue to grow after eruption as they are worn down. Cementum covers the entire outer surface of the tooth and overlies both enamel and dentine. On the wearing (occlusal) surface the enamel and cementum invaginate into the dentine forming infundibula. Dentine and cementum wear more rapidly than enamel, leading to the formation of ridges on the surface.

toothache Pain due to inflammation, erosion, or other lesion of a tooth or its root cavity. Although tooth decay is relatively uncommon in domestic animals compared to humans, it may occur in dogs and cats and occasionally in horses. Also, abscesses may form at the tooth apex, often due to infection entering via a fractured tooth, or in the root cavity, following *periodontal disease (*see* alveolar abscess). Damage to the gums or irregularities of wear may also lead to toothache. Clinical signs include difficulty in eating, reluctance to drink cold water, and holding the head to one side. Food remains in the mouth, producing an unpleasant odour. The face or jaw may be swollen, especially if there is an abscess. Treatment depends on the cause.

topical Describing a drug that is applied directly to a certain part of the body, for example the skin or eye. The drug may have activity at the site or may be absorbed to act systemically. To penetrate intact skin, the compound must be lipid- and water-soluble. *Dimethylsulphoxide is used to increase the penetration of drugs through skin. Highly lipid-soluble compounds can remain in the sebum layer on the skin surface, a property exploited for many persistent insecticidal preparations. The

topical use of antibiotics may encourage the development of antibiotic-resistant strains in the normal skin flora.

topo- *Prefix denoting* place; position; location.

torsalo (macaw worm) fly A medium-sized *fly, *Dermatobia hominis*, found in Central and South America and also known as the tropical warble fly or human bot fly. The larvae are parasites of cattle and other domestic animals as well as humans. The eggs are laid on the body of a bloodsucking insect, usually a mosquito, and hatch when the mosquito feeds on a mammal. The larvae pierce the skin of their mammal host and form a painful tumour in which they grow and moult, finally leaving the host to pupate on the ground. Treatment may involve surgical removal of the larvae or dipping in washes containing a suitable *insecticide.

torsion Twisting. Abnormal twisting of a part, for example a loop of intestine or a spermatic cord, can impair blood and nerve supplies to the affected part and cause serious damage. *See also* volvulus.

touch The sense by which contact of the body with a foreign object is detected. *Mechanoreceptors in the skin are stimulated by external pressure to generate nerve impulses, which are conveyed by sensory nerve fibres to the central nervous system. In many animals, body hairs are important as touch receptors, particularly the long facial whiskers of cats and dogs. *See also* Pacinian corpuscle.

tourniquet A device to press upon an artery and prevent flow of blood through it. It may be applied in an emergency, usually around a limb, to reduce bleeding due to injury. Material, such as a bandage or cord, is passed around the limb and tightened by twisting it with a rigid bar. The time of application should be noted – tourniquets should be removed as soon as possible to prevent ischaemic tissue damage in the limb. More commonly, tourniquets are employed to reduce haemorrhage at an operation site. To achieve a bloodless site, an Eschmark rubber bandage is applied upward from the foot to above the operation site and fastened. Then the lower part is removed to expose the operation site. The tourniquet is slackened at the latter stage of the operation to permit bleeding points to be identified and ligated prior to wound closure or the application of a dressing.

tox- (toxi-, toxo-, toxic(o)-) *Prefix denoting* **1.** poisonous; toxic. **2.** toxins or poisoning.

toxaemia A clinical condition resulting from the dissemination of an antigenic or metabolic toxin through the bloodstream (toxic conditions due to the assimilation of plant, insect, or chemical poisons are excluded). Toxaemia invariably accompanies *septicaemia, as a result of the release of antigenic *exotoxins or *endotoxins from the circulating bacterial cells. It occurs, without septicaemia, in many localized infections, such as *pyometra, hyperacute *mastitis, *enterotoxaemia, and *tetanus, and also in *botulism, when preformed toxin has been ingested in the food. Toxaemia is not an essential feature of *bacteraemia, though it may be present when that condition arises from local infection with a toxigenic bacterium. Some helminth parasites liberate antigenic toxins, and toxaemia may accompany severe infestations.

Bacterial toxaemias are usually rapid in onset, with signs including varying degrees of shock, hypotension, hypoglycaemia, circulatory impairment,

*disseminated intravascular coagulation and haemorrhages, changes in the adrenal cortex, and either leucocytosis or leucopenia. In severe cases there is collapse and death; in milder ones malaise and depression. Pyrexia (fever) may occur but when shock is marked, hypothermia supervenes (*see also* endotoxaemia). Exotoxins of Gram-positive bacteria may give rise to specific neural or other signs that overshadow or replace the general toxaemia syndrome, as in tetanus (muscle spasm) and botulism (paralysis). Where there is infection, treatment includes appropriate antibiotics, and specific antitoxic sera if available; *fluid replacement therapy, incorporating electrolytes, glucose, and amino acids, is also given, usually with a *corticosteroid, such as dexamethazone. In acute toxaemic crises all of these are administered intravenously.

Metabolic toxaemias result from the incomplete elimination of endogenous body metabolites, as in *ketosis in cattle, *pregnancy toxaemia of sheep, hepatic dysfunction, jaundice, and uraemia. The signs vary and treatment is directed towards removal of the cause, together with supportive measures.

Toxascaris A genus of parasitic *nematodes containing *T. leonina*, which affects dogs. The adults are found in the intestine and have a life cycle similar to that of *Toxocara*.

toxic fat syndrome A condition of young domestic fowls caused by feed incorporating fat that, due to poor storage or processing, contains toxins. It principally affects chicks aged 2–6 weeks old. The signs are fluid in the abdomen (ascites), huddling and listlessness, heart abnormalities, and, occasionally, respiratory signs. Outbreaks are rare but when encountered usually result in high mortality, up to 100%. The toxins are stored in the birds' body fat and deaths occur even after the feed is changed. Badly affected flocks should be slaughtered; the carcasses cannot be processed for human consumption. Other names: **alimentary toxaemia**; **chick oedema**; **water belly**. *Compare* ascites.

toxicity the degree to which a substance is poisonous. *See also* LD$_{50}$.

Toxicodendron (Rhus) A genus of temperate or subtropical woody vines and shrubs, several members of which can cause reddened and itchy skin with blister formation following contact. The poisonous principle is 3-n-pentadecylcatechol, which is contained in the sap. The genus includes *T. radicans* (markweed, poison ivy, poison vine), *T. vernix* (poison elder, poison sumac), *T. quercifolia* (*quercifolium*) (eastern poison oak), and *T. diversilobum* (western poison oak). Only humans and closely related primates are generally susceptible.

toxicology The study of poisons and their effects on living organisms.

toxicosis The deleterious effects of a toxic substance. Toxicosis may be caused by the ingestion or inhalation of poisons in the environment (*see* poisoning) or by *toxins produced within the body by pathogenic organisms, especially bacteria.

toxin A poisonous substance, usually of biological origin and especially one produced by a bacterium. *See* endotoxin; enterotoxin; exotoxin.

Toxocara A genus of parasitic *nematodes that cause disease (*toxocariasis) in dogs (*T. canis*), cats (*T. cati*), cattle (*T. vitulorum*), and humans in temperate regions. Adult worms reside in the intestine and pass eggs in the faeces. Following ingestion the larvae migrate through

the body before settling in the intestine and developing into adults. Immunity in adult hosts keeps parasite numbers low and causes the larvae to lie dormant in the host tissues. However, in pregnant females the larvae are mobilized from the tissues and pass across the placenta to infest the foetuses, or after parturition may pass through mammary tissues into the milk to be ingested by sucking offspring.

toxocariasis Disease caused by parasitic *nematodes of the genus *Toxocara*; it principally affects dogs, cats, and cattle but may also occur in humans. Puppies are most at risk. Migration of the larvae through the lungs may cause coughing, while infestation of the intestine can lead to enteritis or even blockage of the bowel. Misplaced larvae can cause small grey lesions in the fundus of the eye. Severe infestation may cause death. Immunity in adults reduces the degree of infestation, hence disease is less apparent. Affected animals can be treated with *piperazine adipate; puppies can be treated from 1–2 weeks of age. Alternatives are *diethylcarbamazine and mebendazole (*see* benzimidazoles). Prophylactic use of these anthelmintics will control the disease.

Puppies can infect humans, especially children. *Toxocara* eggs may be accidentally ingested, for example in food or drink contaminated with the faeces of an infected pet. The larvae, which migrate around the body (i.e. *visceral larva migrans*), may cause a fever or rash. Larvae can also lodge in the retina of the eye, where they cause inflammation and granuloma. Diagnosis is confirmed by an *enzyme-linked immunosorbent assay (ELISA). There is no satisfactory treatment.

toxoid A preparation of purified *toxin with which an animal can be inoculated to stimulate the develop-

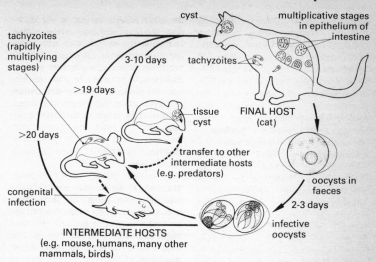

Life cycle of *Toxoplasma gondii*

ment of immunity to the toxin. When the animal subsequently encounters the toxin, for example in cases of *tetanus or *botulism, the toxin is quickly inactivated and clinical signs of disease are prevented.

Toxoplasma A genus of protozoa in the group *Apicomplexa containing one major species, *T. gondii*. This parasite can infect any warm-blooded animal and is probably the most common parasite in the world. *T. gondii* often undergoes a two host (predator/prey) life cycle, but this is not essential. Only cats (or other felids) can act as definitive hosts. In these, the parasite multiples in the intestine and produces resistant *oocysts, which are passed in faeces. These take 2–3 days to develop into the infective form, which can infect any animal ingesting them, including humans. In these intermediate hosts the parasite invades the body multiplying, at first rapidly, inside various cells of the body before forming tissue cysts in muscle and brain. Foetuses can become infected in utero

leading to either foetal abnormality or abortion, or congenital infection. Cats become infected by ingesting tissue cysts (in raw meat or prey). Moreover, any other carnivore can become infected by eating tissue cysts, and in these the parasite invades the tissues of the host. However, oocysts are only produced in cats or other felids. See illustration.

Infection is lifelong, the tissue cysts remaining viable but usually causing no harm. Moreover, the host is immune to any new infection. Cats develop a strong immunity after infection and produce oocysts for only one period of a week or so in their lives. During this time, however, a single cat may produce hundreds of millions of oocysts, which may persist in the environment for several months or longer. Most infections are benign or accompanied by only mild clinical signs, but in some cases severe disease occurs (*see* toxoplasmosis).

toxoplasmosis A disease caused by the protozoan parasite *Toxoplasma gondii*, of worldwide distribution and affecting many species, including humans. Infection during pregnancy can lead to foetal infection and abortion (especially common in sheep) or congenital abnormalities in humans). In nonpregnant animals the majority of infections are undiagnosed, but occasionally severe disease with involvement of liver or lungs occurs in dogs, cats, or others, perhaps in association with intercurrent immunosuppressive virus infections. Although the normal parasite life cycle in the cat results in the production of hundreds of millions of *oocysts, this is not associated with enteritis or disease. In nonpregnant humans infection is associated with flu-like symptoms and swollen lymph nodes. More severe signs occur in immunosuppressed individuals (e.g. AIDS patients).

In domestic animals, toxoplasmosis is of greatest importance as a cause of abortion in **sheep** and is particularly significant in Britain, Australia, and New Zealand. Abortions occur characteristically towards the end of pregnancy after infection during mid-pregnancy by the ingestion of oocysts from contaminated feed or pasture. Previous infection confers a strong lifelong immunity; sheep will abort only once in their life and subsequent pregnancies will be normal. Currently there is no means of controlling this disease; attempts can be made to increase flock immunity by retaining for breeding those ewes that have aborted or have been infected (as revealed by blood testing).

trabecula (*pl.* **trabeculae**) **1.** Any of the bands of tissue that pass from the outer part of an organ to its interior, dividing it into separate chambers. For example, trabeculae occur in the spleen. **2.** Any of the thin bars of bony tissue in spongy *bone.

trace element *See* essential element.

tracer A substance that is introduced into the body and whose progress can subsequently be followed to provide information about dispersion, metabolism, etc. Radioactive tracers give off radiation and can be detected by apparatus (*see* scintillascope) outside the body, thus enabling a permanent record to be made of the tracer's distribution.

trache- (tracheo-) *Prefix denoting* the trachea.

trachea (*pl.* **tracheae** or **tracheas**) The windpipe: the part of the airway extending caudally from the *larynx to where it divides into the left and right principal *bronchi. Its wall is supported by a series of tracheal cartilages.

tracheitis Inflammation of the mucosal lining of the trachea. The condition commonly involves inflammation of the adjacent airways, including the nasal passages, pharynx, and bronchi. Several specific diseases are involved, including infectious canine laryngotracheitis (*see* kennel cough), *avian infectious laryngotracheitis, feline viral rhinotracheitis (*see* cat flu), and *infectious bovine rhinotracheitis. Parasitic infestation may also cause tracheitis. Treatment depends on the cause.

tracheotomy (tracheostomy) A surgical operation in which an opening is made into the trachea through the neck. It is performed to relieve obstruction of the upper respiratory tract and may be indicated as an emergency procedure. Temporary tracheotomy is carried out by splitting one or two tracheal rings and inserting a tube to keep the site open. In horses, permanent tracheotomy is performed to allow animals affected by *laryngeal paralysis to undergo strenuous work. This involves the excision of parts of tracheal rings and the insertion of a special tracheotomy tube, which can be removed for cleansing and which has a cover to prevent foreign material being aspirated.

track leg Swelling of the inner aspect of the tibia, occurring usually in greyhounds. Repeated damage to the periosteum is caused by contact between the inside of the hindleg with the outside of the foreleg when the animal is at full speed. Mild cases may be treated as *sprains, but accumulations of fluid between the periosteum and the bone cortex may need *aspiration or more specialized treatment.

tract 1. A group of nerve fibres passing from one part of the central nervous system to another, forming a distinct pathway, e.g. the spinothalamic tract, pyramidal tract, and corticospinal tract. **2.** An organ or collection of organs providing for the passage of something, e.g. the digestive tract.

tranquillizer (ataractic; neuroleptic; psychotropic agent) Any of a group of drugs that depress conditioned responses in the central nervous system and, at high doses, produce some sedation and catalepsy. In veterinary medicine they are used to reduce an animal's awareness of its surroundings and facilitate handling. Tranquillizers may also be used with narcotic analgesics to produce *neuroleptanalgesia in the animal. Various groups of tranquillizers are available, including *phenothiazines, *butyrophenones, and benzodiazepines (e.g. *diazepam).

trans- *Prefix denoting* through or across.

transaminase *See* aminotransferase.

transamination A process involved in the metabolism of amino acids in which an amino group ($-NH_2$) is transferred from an amino acid to an α-keto acid, with the production of the corresponding keto acid and amino acid. The reaction is catalysed by enzymes (*see* aminotransferase), which require pyridoxal phosphate as a coenzyme.

transcription The process in which the information contained in the *genetic code is transferred from DNA to RNA: the first step in the manufacture of proteins in cells. *See* messenger RNA; translation.

transduction The transfer of DNA from one bacterium to another by means of a *bacteriophage (phage). Some bacterial DNA is incorporated into the phage. When the host bacterium is destroyed the phage infects another bacterium and introduces the DNA from its previous host, which may become incorporated into the new host's DNA.

transection 1. A cross-section of a piece of tissue. **2.** Cutting across the tissue of an organ (*see also* section).

transferase An enzyme that catalyses the transfer of a group (other than hydrogen) between a pair of substrates.

transferrin A *glycoprotein present in blood serum that transports iron around the body. Each transferrin molecule binds two atoms of ferrous iron. *See also* ferritin; haemosiderin.

transfer RNA A type of *RNA whose function is to attach the correct amino acid to the protein chain being synthesized at a *ribosome. *See also* translation.

transfusion The injection of a volume of blood or plasma obtained from a healthy animal (the *donor*) into the circulation of an animal (the *recipient*) whose blood is deficient in quantity or quality, through accident, disease, or surgery. Certain risks attend transfusion, principally the possibility that the recipient will mount an immunological reaction against the transfused blood cells and thus destroy them (*see* blood typing). Such *hypersensitivity reactions are manifested by anaphylactic shock, haemoglobinuria, jaundice, and sometimes by *disseminated intravascular coagulation. Hypersensitivity reactions may occur in response to plasma proteins or leucocytes as well as to blood-group antigens.

The risk of tranfusion reaction is largely obviated by selecting donors that match the recipient for the major blood groups. Where typing is not feasible cross-matching is a practical alternative (*see* blood typing). In veterinary medicine, untyped unmatched first transfusions between members of the same species are generally considered an acceptable risk in an emergency, since reactions in this situation are rare. However typing or cross-matching are desirable for first transfusions, and in horses they are accepted practice. It is especially important to protect breeding mares from incompatible transfusion, since this increases the risk of *equine autoimmune haemolytic anaemia affecting the newborn foal. In all cases, second transfusions carried out one or more days after the first carry a significant risk of immune reaction unless compatibility is ensured. The risk increases with the number of transfusions given. *Exchange transfusion* is a method of virtually replacing an animal's circulating blood volume with transfused blood. This is undertaken chiefly as a treatment for equine autoimmune haemolytic anaemia.

In some species, notably humans, individuals possess natural antibodies to blood group antigens dissimilar to their own. These antibodies are able to destroy red cells immediately on transfusion of incompatible blood, making blood typing mandatory for all human transfusions.

Donor plasma is sometimes transferred instead of whole blood. Although unable to replace oxygen-carrying capacity, plasma is a valuable means of restoring blood volume. It lacks the dangers associated with blood-group incompatibility and is easier to store than whole blood. Washed red cells are also used as an alternative to blood, particularly to treat equine autoimmune haemolytic anaemia.

transit erythema A condition seen in many pig carcasses, consisting of a red rash or red patches on the skin, mainly on the belly and hindlimbs. It is caused by the irritant action of urine or disinfectants coupled with constant friction from the floors of vehicles during transit.

transit fever (shipping fever) An acute infection of cattle characterized by fever, dyspnoea, and fibrinous pneumonia and typically associated with the stress of prolonged transportation. Infection with the bacteria *Pasteurella multocida* and/or *P. haemolytica* is widely regarded as the ultimate cause of shipping fever, but certain other organisms, such as *Corynebacterium* spp., mycoplasmas, and viruses, may be involved. Stress factors responsible for precipitating the disease include weaning, transportation, extremes of environmental temperature, irregular or inadequate feeding, and vaccinations. The disease varies in severity from acute to inapparent, but usually there is general depression with a very high fever, coughing, and a variable level of mucopurulent nasal discharge. Control measures should focus on reducing the stressing factors that may lead to the disease. Antibiotic treatment during incidents reduces the mortality, and a vaccine is available. Other names: **pneumonic pasteurellosis**; **shipping pneumonia**; **transit pneumonia**.

Transit of Animals (Road and Rail) Order (1975) (England and Wales) A Parliamentary Order providing for the welfare of cattle, sheep, pigs, goats, and horses being moved by road or rail. Standards of construction of vehicles are prescribed, as are certain conditions for the treatment of animals during carriage, such as forbidding overcrowding or inadequate ventilation and ensuring protection from the weather or escaping or falling from the vehicle.

transit tetany A condition of horses due to a low concentration of calcium in the blood (*hypocalcaemia) and characterized by tetany of all superficial muscles. This results in muscle tremors, a stilted gait, *trismus, rapid shallow breathing, and an anxious expression. Sweating may occur. It is usually associated with transportation, and lactating mares in oestrus are particularly susceptible. The prognosis is good if a calcium-phosphorus-magnesium solution is administered. The condition must be differentiated from true *tetanus: many of the signs are similar but there is no protrusion of the third eyelid in hypocalcaemia, and tetanus cases would not respond to the above therapy.

translation (in cell biology) The manufacture of proteins in a cell, which takes place at the ribosomes. The information for determining the correct sequence of amino acids in the protein is carried to the ribosomes by *messenger RNA, and the amino acids are brought to their correct position in the protein by *transfer RNA.

translocation (in genetics) A type of chromosome mutation in which part of a chromosome is transferred to

another part of the same chromosome or to a different chromosome. This changes the order of the genes on the chromosomes and can be associated with genetic disorders.

transmethylation The process whereby a methyl $(-CH_3)$ group is transferred to another molecule. *Methionine is the principal methyl donor in the body.

transmigration The act of passing through or across, for example the passage of blood cells through the intact walls of capillaries and venules (i.e. diapedesis).

transmissible gastroenteritis (TGE) A highly infectious disease of pigs characterized by severe diarrhoea, vomiting, and death in young piglets and caused by a *coronavirus. Following an incubation period of less than 24 hours piglets aged less than 10 days develop acute diarrhoea and die. Older piglets have a less severe form of disease but infection can predispose to other enteric infections and result in poor growth. Sows may lose their milk (*agalactia). Nervous signs may also be seen. TGE is usually introduced to a herd by a symptomless carrier of the virus. Recovered sows pass immunity to their piglets through their milk, and once the disease has entered a herd it is considered essential to allow it to spread to all pregnant sows thereby allowing them time to develop immunity and so protect their litters. There is no effective vaccine, and control is by keeping the herd closed or operating an 'all-in/all-out' policy. *See also* epidemic diarrhoea; vomiting/wasting disease.

transmissible venereal tumour (TVT) A tumour of dogs affecting mainly the external genitalia, transmitted during coitus, and thought to be caused by a virus. It is enzootic in certain parts of the world, particularly in tropical and subtropical regions. Clinically this tumour presents as erythematous vegetative lesions on the mucous membranes of the external genitalia. Occasionally it involves the oral cavity and the skin of the body. Most tumours regress spontaneously after about 6 months, but electrosurgical excision or cytotoxic chemotherapy can be used to treat it. Other name: **infective granuloma**.

transplantation The relocation of an organ or tissue taken from one part of the body to another part, or from one individual to another. *See* graft.

transudation The passage of a liquid through a membrane, especially of blood through the wall of a capillary vessel. The liquid is called the *transudate*. *See* exudation.

transverse (in anatomy) The plane situated at right angles to the long axis of the body of an organ.

transversus abdominis muscle The deepest of the sheets of muscle in the lateral abdominal wall. Its fibres run transversely and insert to the *linea alba by means of an *aponeurosis, which contributes to the internal sheath of the *rectus abdominis. The muscle acts to increase intra-abdominal pressure.

trapezius A large flat muscle in the back running from the cervical and thoracic vertebrae to the scapula.

trapezoid body A bundle of nerve fibres crossing transversely in the brainstem and forming part of the auditory pathways.

traumatic reticulitis A disease of cattle and to a lesser extent sheep, goats, and camels caused by penetration of the wall of the *reticulum by ingested sharp objects, such as pieces

of fencing or baling wire or nails. Infection is introduced to the abdominal cavity via the wound, causing *peritonitis. Deeper penetration can lead to perforation of the diaphragm, *pleurisy, or *pericarditis. The majority of cases involve only localized peritonitis, which produces abdominal pain, grunting, mild *bloat, loss of appetite and milk yield, and raised body temperature. Animals often stand with an arched back. The most effective method of treatment is removal of the foreign body via a surgical incision through the left flank and wall of the *rumen. Recovery rates are good.

travel sickness Vomiting induced by motion during transportation. Small animals, often particular individuals, seem especially susceptible, although the problem causes only temporary distress, to both the animal and its owner. Treatment involves giving an *antiemetic before the journey: *antihistamines, which have sedative side-effects, are also commonly recommended.

tread wounds A condition seen in turkey carcasses, consisting of severe wounds on the back and sides of the body. These are caused by the claws of the male turkey during mating. As a preventative measure, toe cutting is carried out in the males within 3 days of hatching.

trematode *See* fluke.

tremor A rhythmical alternating movement that may affect any part of the body. *Physiological tremor* occurs normally during sustained contraction of muscles, for example while maintaining the standing position. Various other types of tremor may occur as a result of neurological disease.

trenbolone acetate A synthetic steroidal growth promoter with weaker androgenic activity than testosterone but similar anabolic properties. It is thought to act directly on muscle cells, causing a decrease in muscle protein turnover and consequently a net increase in protein synthesis. Plasma concentrations of the thyroid hormone *thyroxine are reduced, lowering the metabolic rate to allow increased growth and better feed conversion efficiency. It is used as an implant in heifers and steers. In steers there is an increased effect if the drug is used in combination with an oestrogenic compound. Tissue residues are undetectable 60 days after implantation. Trenbolone acetate has been banned in the EEC as a growth promoter in food-producing animals because of consumer concern over residues in meat. It can still be used as an anabolic to promote protein synthesis, improve appetite, and increase calcium retention in various diseases (e.g. chronic kidney disease, pregnancy toxaemia) and to improve fracture healing. Tradenames: **Finaplix** (implant); **Finajet** (injectable).

trephine An instrument used to remove a disc of bone from the skull. It may be employed to gain access to the cranial cavity, but is more often used to facilitate drainage from chronically infected paranasal sinuses in the horse, or to give access to the roots of check teeth so that they can be removed by being punched out of their alveoli.

Treponema A genus of Gram-negative *spirochaete bacteria characterized by their sharp thin spirals and tapering ends. They are commonly found as saprophytes in the mouth, alimentary tract, and genitalia of animals, including humans, and some are important pathogens. *T. pallidum* is the cause of syphilis in humans, *T. hyodysenteriae* has been associated with *swine dysentery, and *T. cuniculi*

causes the venereally transmitted disease *rabbit syphilis.

triceps brachii muscle A large muscle in the back of the upper forelimb that extends the elbow joint. It consists of three principal heads of origin – *lateral*, *medial*, and *long*, and, in most species, an additional *accessory* head.

trich- (tricho-) *Prefix denoting* hair or hairlike structures.

trichiasis A condition in which the eyelashes turn inwards and cause irritation of the eyeball. It accompanies *entropion.

Trichinella A genus of minute parasitic *nematode worms. *T. spiralis* is an intestinal parasite of many mammals and birds, including pigs, dogs, and humans. Infestation is established following the ingestion of infested rats, imperfectly cooked infested pork, or raw swill or garbage containing infected pork. The female worms are ovoviviparous and discharge larvae which reach the lymphatic system of the intestine, and thence the diaphragm and skeletal muscles. Here they develop to the fourth-stage larvae and become surrounded by a fibrous cyst, which may calcify. When infested meat is eaten the cysts are digested and the larvae released to invade the duodenal and jejunal mucosae and develop into adults.

In humans the larvae cause disease (*trichinosis* or *trichiniasis*), which may involve enteric symptoms, such as diarrhoea and nausea, or, as larvae migrate around the body, fever, vertigo, delirium, and acute pains in the limbs. The larvae may cause muscle pain and stiffness. In all cases, treatment is with mebendazole, which is effective against both adults and larvae in the muscles.

trichlorophon *See* organophosphorus (OP) compounds.

trichobezoar *See* hair ball.

trichoepithelioma A benign tumour arising from the cells lining a hair follicle. They are uncommon tumours of the skin in dogs and cats and are rare in other species. Clinically they are moderately well demarcated and occur more commonly on the back. Following surgical excision the prognosis is good. *Compare* pilomatricoma.

Trichomonas A genus of *flagellate protozoan parasites that live in the urogenital or intestinal tracts of mammals and birds. Many species are harmless but a few cause disease. The pear-shaped organisms bear three, five, or more flagella. They do not form cysts and are transmitted directly between hosts in body secretions. *T. foetus* causes infertility and abortion in cattle and is venereally transmitted (*see* trichomoniasis).

trichomoniasis A disease caused by protozoa of the genus *Trichomonas*. There are several different species of *Trichomonas* causing disease in different animals. The most important is **bovine** trichomoniasis caused by *T. foetus* and of worldwide distribution. This is a nonfebrile venereally transmitted infection of the prepuce of the bull and the reproductive tract of the cow. While infected bulls remain asymptomatic and fertile, infection in cows causes infertility, early abortion, or possibly womb infection (*pyometra). The use of artificial insemination is associated with decreased incidence of infection. In **birds** some *Trichomonas* infections in the intestines may cause severe diarrhoea and mortality.

Trichophyton A genus of *dermatophyte fungi including about a dozen species that can infect animals. *T. verrucosum* chiefly causes *ringworm in cattle but occurs sporadically in other species (often as a result of contact with cattle), including horses, sheep, pigs, and humans. *T. equinum* is responsible for most ringworm in horses and is uncommon in other animals. *T. mentagrophytes* has the widest natural host range of the dermatophytes; besides humans it often affects dogs, occasionally cats, is the usual cause of porcine ringworm in Britain, and is sometimes prevalent in colonies of domesticated rodents, often with few clinical signs.

The asexually sporing state, identifiable as a *Trichophyton* species, is seen in normal laboratory cultures. However, sexual spore-forming ('perfect') states of some species have been observed and classified in the ascomyete genus *Arthroderma*.

trichosis Any abnormal growth or disease of hair. Poor nutrition, endocrine diseases, or congenital defects may result in abnormal hair growth, while certain pathogens, for example *dermatophytes, may destroy hair. Some toxic substances may actively interfere with hair growth and replacement, resulting in alopecia (baldness).

Trichostrongylus A genus of parasitic *nematodes that inhabit the stomach (abomasum) and intestine of ruminants, rabbits, hares, horses, and occasionally humans. They are small red-brown worms, about 5–8 mm long, and are fairly widespread in tropical regions. *T. axei* infects ruminants and horses; sheep and goats are infested by *T. colubriformis*, *T. vitrinus*, and *T. capricola*. They are mainly a problem in lambs, in which they can cause black scours and anaemia. In older sheep infestation remains at low levels. Eggs are passed in the faeces and production peaks soon after parturition, when lambs are beginning to graze. Infestation can be treated with benzimidazoles or ivermectin.

Trichuris A genus of parasitic *nematodes, commonly known as 'whipworms'. They are common parasites of vertebrates in moist warm countries worldwide, and are found in the caecum and large intestine of many animals, including cattle (*T. bovis*), sheep (*T. ovis, skrjabini*), pigs (*T. suis*), dogs (*T. vulpis*), and mice (*T. muris*). In lambs whipworms are found in the lower ileum. The life cycle is direct: the adults discharge eggs in the faeces and these do not hatch until swallowed by a host. Whipworms cause disease (*trichuriasis*) only if infestation is severe. In pigs heavy infestations can cause anaemia. Treatment is with dichlorvos in the feed, benzimidazoles or ivermectin. In humans, heavy infestation with *T. trichiura* may cause bloody diarrhoea, anaemia, weakness, and abdominal pain.

tricuspid valve (right atrioventricular valve) The valve in the heart between the right atrium and right ventricle. It consists of three flaps or *cusps that channel the flow of blood from the atrium to the ventricle and prevent backflow. *See* atrioventricular valve.

triflupromazine *See* phenothiazines.

trigeminal nerve The fifth *cranial nerve (V). It is the general sensory nerve for the head, consisting of three divisions: the *ophthalmic division* consists of fibres carrying general sensation from the eyeball, eyelids, and skin of the frontal region, including the horn in ruminants; the *maxillary division* serves the upper jaw region, including the teeth and the palates; and the *mandibular division* serves the lower jaw region, including the teeth and the tongue, and also contains motor fibres supplying the muscles of mastication.

trigeminal paralysis Muscular paralysis and/or loss of sensation due to a lesion of the *trigeminal nerve (fifth cranial nerve). The signs produced depend upon which division of the nerve is affected. A lesion of the mandibular division affects the muscles of mastication and results in inability to close the mouth, if both sides are affected, and sensory loss in the lower jaw region. In many cases, if the rest of the trigeminal nerve is unaffected, spontaneous recovery takes place in a few weeks. A lesion of the maxillary or ophthalmic divisions will cause a lack of sensory response in the areas which they supply.

triglyceride (triacylglycerol) A lipid consisting of three long-chain *fatty acids esterified to *glycerol. Triglycerides are the major constituents of fats and *oils and provide a concentrated food energy store in living organisms. In *simple triglycerides* all three fatty acids are identical; in *mixed triglycerides* two or three different fatty acids are present.

triiodothyronine (T_3) A hormone that is similar to but metabolically more active than *thyroxine (T_4) – the chief thyroid hormone. Most triiodothyronine is produced by the removal of an iodine atom from thyroxine (hence T_3) in the liver and kidney. *Reverse T_3 (rT_3)* is also produced by T_4 to T_3 conversion, but it has almost no biological activity. Inadequate energy intake favours the conversion to rT_3 rather than T_3 for survival. Synthetic T_3 (liothyronine) can be used orally to treat hypothyroidism.

trimethoprim A *bacteriostat with a broad spectrum of activity against Gram-positive and Gram-negative bacteria. It inhibits a bacterial enzyme, dihydrofolate reductase, involved in nucleotide synthesis. The drug's half-life is short, and it is broken down rapidly by microorganisms in the rumen. After absorption trimethoprim is excreted unchanged in the urine. In animals it is used in combination with *sulphonamides to potentiate the action of the sulphonamide and reduce toxicity, both compounds having activity at different points in the same metabolic pathway. In human medicine it is used alone to treat urinary tract infections.

triose A carbohydrate with three carbon units: for example, glyceraldehyde.

tripelennamine *See* antihistamine.

triploid Describing cells, tissues, or individuals in which there are three complete chromosome sets. *Compare* diploid; haploid.

trismus Spasm of the jaw muscles, keeping the jaws tightly closed. This is a characteristic sign of *tetanus (lockjaw).

trisomy The state in which a nucleus contains three copies of a certain chromosome instead of the normal two copies. *Compare* monosomy.

trocar (trochar) A sharp pointed solid instrument used to enter a body cavity or viscus. It is generally used inside a *cannula so that following penetration the trocar can be withdrawn leaving the cannula in place. Its most important veterinary use is for the relief of acute *bloat in ruminants, especially cattle, when the trocar is inserted into the rumen. It is also used to relieve caecal distension in horses.

trochanter Any of the three protuberances (*major*, *minor*, and *third*) for muscle attachment at the proximal end of the *femur.

trochlea (*pl.* **trochleas** or **trochleae**) An anatomical part having the structure or function of a pulley; for example the groove at the lower end of the *humerus or the fibrocartilaginous ring in the frontal bone (where it forms part of the orbit), through which the tendon of the dorsal oblique muscle passes.

trochlear nerve The fourth *cranial nerve (IV). It supplies the dorsal oblique muscle, one of the muscles responsible for moving the eyeball in its socket.

Trombicula A genus of *mites, widely distributed and known as harvest mites or bracken bugs. The adults and nymphs are free-living but the bright-red larvae, or chiggers, are ectoparasites of mammals, including humans. The larvae have bladelike mouthparts, feeding on lymph and skin tissues and causing intense irritation, *allergic dermatitis, and, in humans, scrub typhus. *See* trombiculosis.

trombiculosis Disease due to infestation with larvae (chiggers) of harvest mites. In the UK, the only parasitic species is *Neotrombicula autumnalis*. The orange larva is about 0.2 mm in diameter and has a round body with six long legs. It is active between April and November, particularly during warm days. All mammals and birds may become infested. The mites can attach themselves to any part of the body, particularly skin folds (e.g. between the toes or folds of the external ear). Larger domestic animals may be parasitized on the lower extremities. The larvae penetrate the epidermis and feed on tissue fluid, becoming engorged within 72 hours, when they measure about 0.5 mm in diameter. There may be sufficient mites on the skin to produce small orange patches. The mites cause irritation, and the animal may nibble or shake affected parts, which show soreness and redness, resulting in a localized moist *dermatitis. In humans, multiple small red papules may be found on the lower limbs or trunk. After feeding the mites drop to the ground to complete their life cycle in the soil as nonparasitic nymphs and adults. Control is difficult because of the harvest mite's very wide distribution, its life cycle, and the availability of numerous hosts. However, it is less common on clay soils, which engorged larvae have difficulty in penetrating. Affected skin should be dabbed with benzyl benzoate (diluted 50:50 with water for cats and used sparingly) or other safe insecticides. Related species of harvest mite are important disease vectors in warmer countries.

troph- (tropho-) *Prefix denoting* nourishment or nutrition.

trophoblast The tissue lying peripheral to the *embryonic disc that forms the wall of the *blastocyst. It is involved with the absorption of nutrients at an early stage of embryonic development, and later participates in forming the *foetal membranes.

-trophy *Suffix denoting* nourishment, development, or growth. Example: *dystrophy* (defective development).

-tropic *Suffix denoting* **1.** turning towards. **2.** having an affinity for; influencing.

tropocollagen The molecular unit of *collagen. It consists of a helix of three collagen molecules: this arrangement confers on the fibres structural stability and resistance to stretching.

truncus A *trunk. The *truncus arteriosus* is the main arterial trunk arising

from the embryonic heart. It develops into the aorta and the pulmonary trunk.

trunk 1. The main part of a blood vessel, lymph vessel, or nerve, from which branches arise. For example, the pulmonary trunk gives rise to the left and right pulmonary arteries. **2.** The body excluding the head and limbs.

trypanocide A drug used to prevent or treat *trypanosomiasis. They include *suramin, which is used in therapy, *homidium bromide and diminiazene, which have a prophylactic effect for a short period, and *quinapyramine and isometamidium, which produce a longer period of prophylaxis. These agents differ in their activity against the various species of trypanosomes, and some resistant trypanosome strains have evolved.

Trypanosoma A genus of flagellated *protozoa containing several important pathogens of animals, including humans, that cause *trypanosomiasis in tropical and subtropical regions. Trypanosomes are blood parasites that live free in the plasma. In Africa south of the Sahara, transmission is mainly by the *tsetse fly, in which the trypanosome undergoes a complex cycle of migration and development. Elsewhere transmission is by other biting insects, for example horse flies, bugs (*see* Chagas disease), and fleas. Moreover, some trypanosome species are transmitted by vampire bats (in South America) or venereally (*T. equiperdum*: *see* dourine). The form of trypanosome found in the bloodstream is elongated, $10-35\ \mu m$ long, with a central nucleus. From the posterior end a single flagellum arises and runs forward along the body, to which it is attached by an undulating membrane; this beats rapidly propelling the trypanosome. Trypanosomes may also parasitize extravascular tissue fluids in skin, lymph nodes, and the nervous system. They multiply by longitudinal division into two daughter organisms. Although infected animals respond to infection by producing antibodies, trypanosomes can vary their surface antigens to evade the host response (i.e. *antigenic variation). They therefore persist as chronic undulating infections in the blood, often with severe and fatal consequences.

Tsetse-transmitted trypanosomes of veterinary importance in Africa include *T. vivax* and *T. congolense*, which cause *nagana in cattle, *T. brucei* (horses, dogs, and cattle), and *T. simiae* in pigs. Species transmitted by other vectors include *T. evansi*, which is closely related to *T. brucei* and causes disease in horses and camels (*see* surra), and *T. vivax*, which causes disease in cattle in South America. In humans, subspecies of *T. brucei*, namely *T. b. gambiense* and *T. b. rhodesiense* cause sleeping sickness in West and East Africa respectively and are tsetse-fly transmitted. These subspecies can also infect wild and domesticated animals, usually without causing disease. However, such animals can constitute a reservoir of infection for humans, especially in East Africa. In South America, *T. cruzi* causes *Chagas disease in humans.

trypanosomiasis A disease of animals, including humans, caused by *protozoa of the genus *Trypanosoma* in tropical and subtropical regions. Trypanosomiasis is especially important in Africa south of the Sahara, where it is transmitted by *tsetse flies and effectively excludes cattle from vast areas (*see* nagana). Various disease syndromes are produced in different animals by different *Trypanosoma* species. The disease is generally characterized by fever, which may resolve or become intermittent, and by a chronic course with anaemia, wasting, swelling of lymph nodes, and perhaps localized oedema. The disease is frequently fatal in susceptible animals, sometimes after a period of months. In humans the disease is also characterized by parasite invasion of the central nervous system and the induction of a torpid state (hence 'sleeping sickness'), but this is unusual in animals.

Diagnosis is confirmed by the detection of trypanosomes in blood or tissue fluids, but this may be difficult due to the fluctuating and often very low numbers present. Because of this difficulty a great many different techniques have been developed to aid diagnosis. Drugs are available to treat or prevent infections but drug resistance can be a problem. No vaccine is currently available and the antigenic diversity of the parasite poses considerable technical difficulties in developing one. The control of tsetse-transmitted trypanosomiasis has largely depended on control of the vector fly by bush clearance or insecticide application to the fly's resting sites in trees and shrubs. Because of the tsetse's restricted flight range, areas can be cleared and kept tsetse-free in well-controlled eradication schemes. Certain breeds of cattle are genetically resistant to the disease (*trypanotolerant*) and are being increasingly utilized. *See also* Chagas disease; dourine; mal de Caderas; surra.

trypsin An endopeptidase enzyme (*see* peptidase) occurring in the small intestine. The inactive zymogen *trypsinogen* is secreted by the pancreas and converted to the active trypsin by the enzyme enterokinase, and by trypsin itself. Trypsin is important in the digestion of *protein, hydrolysing mainly *peptide bonds on the carboxyl side of the basic *amino acids arginine and lysine.

tryptophan An *amino acid. *See also* essential amino acid.

tsetse fly A large ectoparasitic *fly of the genus *Glossina* that has a forwardly projecting proboscis used for sucking the blood of reptiles, birds, and mammals. Tsetses transmit the protozoan blood parasites of the genus *Trypanosoma* that cause the disease *nagana in many types of domestic animals and sleeping sickness in humans. The female tsetse deposits a single mature larva, which has developed within her body, on soft soil. The larva pupates in the soil rapidly. Tsetse flies are found only in tropical Africa, their distribution being controlled by temperature, humidity, and vegetation. Each of the various species shows a preference for particular hosts and habitats. Nearly all species are active in the daytime and most feed close to trees, bushes, or thickets in which they rest after feeding, and where they breed. Control is difficult. Clearance or selective spraying with residual insecticides of the breeding grounds, particularly near human habitations, or the application of insecticides directly to cattle are the most effective methods against both pupae and adults. The destruction of game, which is a food source for tsetse, has also been successful but is rather drastic. The introduction into the population of insect parasites of the pupae and sterilized adult males has also been tried with limited success. A more recent innovation is the strategic placement of insecticide-coated screens baited with tsetse *pheromone.

TSH *See* thyroid-stimulating hormone.

tubercle 1. (in anatomy) A small rounded protuberance on a bone, for example, the greater and lesser tubercles at the proximal end of the *humerus, which are sites for muscle attachment. 2. (in pathology) A nodule of chronic inflammation that is a characteristic lesion of *tuberculosis. Wherever the causal bacteria settle (most commonly in the lungs) they induce a defensive reaction in the host tissue. Local cellular proliferation occurs with the production of large epithelioid cells, which tend to coalesce into multinucleate giant cells. This reaction becomes surrounded by fibrosis, while the centre undergoes *caseation with eventual calcification. Some tubercles may become grossly enlarged and burst, releasing their contents into the lung or blood vessels thus initiating further spread of infection.

tubercular Having small rounded swellings or nodules, not necessarily caused by tuberculosis.

tuberculin An extract of a *Mycobacterium* culture (normally *M. tuberculosis*, *M. bovis*, or *M. avium*) containing heat-stable tuberculoprotein, used in the *tuberculin test. *Old tuberculin* (*OT*, *Koch's OT*) was an early form of tuberculin of low specificity, devised by Robert Koch and made by heat concentration of a broth culture of *M. tuberculosis*. It has now been replaced by *PPD* (*purified protein derivative*) tuberculin, which has greater specificity. It is purified during manufacture by precipitating the tuberculoprotein with trichloracetic acid or other protein precipitant. The comparative intradermal test used in cattle employs 'mammalian PPD' (made from *M. tuberculosis* until 1975 in the UK but now made from *M. bovis*, which gives a more specific reaction) and 'avian PPD', made from *M. avium*.

tuberculin test A diagnostic test to detect clinical or subclinical *tuberculosis in living animals, involving a *hypersensitivity reaction to *tuberculin. Because of cross reactions

tuberculoid mastitis

between *Mycobacterium* species, including some of the atypical mycobacteria, tuberculin tests are not completely specific. In the *subcutaneous test*, a positive reaction is denoted by a rise in body temperature when tuberculin is injected subcutaneously. In the *single comparative intradermal test* (which is used for cattle in the UK), two injections, of mammalian and avian PPD tuberculin, are given intradermally at neighbouring sites in the neck region. About 70% of infected animals react to mammalian PPD with a skin thickening or swelling at the injection site. A reaction to mammalian PPD alone indicates infection with *M. bovis* or *M. tuberculosis*. A further reaction to avian PPD indicates a nonspecific *Mycobacterium* infection.

tuberculoid mastitis A form of sporadic usually chronic *mastitis of cows caused by *Mycobacterium smegmatis*, less frequently by *M. fortuitum* or *M. phlei*. These bacteria are present in the environment or in the animal's own natural body flora, and act as opportunist pathogens, gaining entrance to the udder, for instance through unhygienic application of intramammary medication, particularly with preparations having an oily base, which favours growth of the mycobacteria.

tuberculosis (TB) A chronic progressive disease affecting all groups of vertebrates, including domesticated animals and humans, caused by bacteria of the genus *Mycobacterium*. It is characterized by the formation of granulomatous lesions, which are frequently multiple and tend to be nodular in form (*see* tubercle). Bodily wasting is a regular feature of the condition; other signs vary according to the site of the lesions. *M. bovis* is the principal cause of tuberculosis in ruminants; *M. avium* infects birds (*see* avian tuberculosis); and *M. tuberculo-*

sis causes pulmonary and other forms of tuberculosis in humans. However, interspecies transmission of these agents occurs in warm-blooded animals; for example, both pigs and humans are susceptible to all three of the above *Mycobacterium* species. Other *Mycobacterium* species are occasionally isolated from tuberculosis-like disease: these may or may not have a causal role and are termed *atypical mycobacteria*; the disease conditions are sometimes described as 'tuberculoid' – for example, *M. kansasii* can cause tuberculoid lung disease in cattle (*see also* tuberculoid mastitis). Different species cause tuberculosis in fish, reptiles, and other cold-blooded animals. Diagnosis of both overt and subclinical forms of the disease in living animals is achieved by the *tuberculin test.

Tuberculosis in cattle causes great economic loss in countries where the disease is enzootic, through wasting, death (or compulsory slaughter) of stock, condemnation of meat and milk, and infection of calves. The most frequent form in adult animals is a chronic nodular (tubercular) bronchopneumonia (*see* pneumonia) with caseation and sometimes calcification; liver, kidney, and intestinal involvement is also common. The primary spread is via the lymphatic system, and lymph nodes draining affected organs are invariably enlarged. Later, spread via the bloodstream, metastatic lesions may form anywhere in the body, or *miliary tuberculosis may develop. Calves are infected congenitally or by suckling, and develop a rapidly fatal tuberculous *meningitis. Tuberculous mastitis results in infected milk, which if consumed raw causes disease of the lymph nodes in children and young adults, and sometimes serious disease in later life; pasteurization or ultraheat treatment of milk destroys the bacterium. Cattle tuberculosis has been eradicated from a number of countries by a programme of intensive tuberculin testing and slaughter of reactors. Where the disease is initially widespread, as it was in the UK before 1950, some form of *area eradication scheme is usual. After elimination from cattle, the infection may persist in wildlife reservoirs, such as badgers in southwest England, and possums.

A range of tuberculostatic drugs is available for treatment of the disease in humans (streptomycin, isoniazid, rifampicin, ethambutol, etc.), but treatment of animals is rarely attempted because it is lengthy, requires laboratory control, and places other animals and human contacts at risk. Vaccination of calves with *BCG gives a degree of protection but is not employed because it renders them positive to tuberculin testing.

In the UK, animals showing overt clinical signs of tuberculosis, particularly an indurated udder or other chronic udder disease, emaciation, or chronic cough, must be reported under the *notifiable diseases legislation. Reactors to the tuberculin test are covered by the controlled diseases legislation.

tuberose *See* tuberous.

tuberosity A large rounded protuberance of a bone, for example, the tuberosity at the proximal end of the *tibia.

tuberous (tuberose) Knobbed; having nodules or rounded swellings.

tubule (in anatomy) A small cylindrical hollow structure. *See also* renal tubule; seminiferous tubule.

tularaemia (rabbit fever) An infectious disease of rodents, lagomorphs (rabbits, etc.) and certain birds (e.g. partridges, quails, and pheasants) that can also affect domestic animals and humans. It is caused by the bacterium *Francisella tularensis* and is characterized by fever and tubercle-like nodule formations in the liver, spleen, and lymph nodes. In natural outbreaks of disease in wild rodents and lagomorphs, clinical signs are rarely observed; animals are usually found dead with typical pathological lesions of white necrotic foci scattered over visceral organs, such as the liver, spleen, and lymph nodes. In affected domestic animals, for example, sheep, some clinical signs, such as stiffness of joints, a rise in body temperature, laboured breathing, and diarrhoea, may be observed. In humans tularaemia has a sudden onset characterized by headaches, nausea, and fever. Dogs and other carnivores often become infected by consuming infected carcasses of rabbits and rodents. Humans may acquire infection from contamination of their skin when skinning pheasants, other wild birds, rabbits, etc. Infections may also be transmitted by ticks or flies. Diagnosis can be established by isolating the causal organisms from the nodules in visceral organs and lymph nodes. Humans can be effectively treated with chloramphenicol, streptomycin, or tetracyclines. Control measures may include the control of importation of dead or live wild rodents, lagomorphs, and birds, and reduction of their numbers when disease becomes enzootic.

tumbu fly A large African blowfly, *Cordylobia anthropophaga*, whose larvae are parasites of mammals, especially dogs and humans (*see* myiasis). The eggs are laid in the bedding or soiled clothing of the host, and the small spine-covered larvae burrow just under the skin forming a swelling or 'tumbu' with an opening to the exterior enabling the larva to breathe. Treatment entails placing a drop of oil or Vaseline over this breathing hole thus forcing the larva to emerge.

tumefaction The process in which a tissue becomes swollen and tense by accumulation within it of fluid under pressure.

tumour 1. A noninflammatory growth of tissue that is outside the normal control mechanisms of the body. Such growths can be classified as either *benign or malignant (*see* cancer). *Benign tumours* are usually slow growing and well defined; their cells resemble those of the tissue of origin and the effects on the host are minimal, resulting from direct mechanical interference or the production of hormones. *Malignant tumours* tend to grow relatively rapidly and invade the surrounding tissues; they also have the potential ability to spread to distant sites (metastasize). Their cells may appear very different from those of the tissue of origin, and the effect on the host is ultimately life-threatening.
2. Any abnormal swelling in or on the body. *Compare* cyst.

Tunga A genus of *fleas comprising *jiggers, also known as sand fleas or chigoes, found in tropical America and Africa.

tunica (*pl.* **tunicae**) A covering or layer of an organ or part; for example, a layer of the wall of a blood vessel (*see* adventitia, intima; media). The *tunica albuginea* is a fibrous membrane comprising one of the covering tissues of the ovary, penis, and testis. The *tunica vaginalis* is the extension of peritoneum which invests the testis and the spermatic cord.

turbinate bone *See* nasal concha.

turkey A large bird of the family Gallinaceae originating from Central America. A number of subspecies are recognized: *Meleagridis gallopavo gallopavo* was introduced from Mexico to Europe during the Spanish conquest and subsequently reintroduced into North America, where it was crossed with the local eastern subspecies, *M. g. silvestris*. This was probably the origin of the American bronze turkey, which became popular in Europe during the early 20th century. A large proportion of the turkeys now reared intensively for their meat are white-feathered hybrids whose genotypes are designed for specific markets. However, traditional nonwhite birds are still popular for the Christmas market. The double-breasted characteristic has benefited carcass lean meat yield but makes natural mating with a mature stag difficult. Hence *artificial insemination is widely practised.

turkey husbandry All aspects of the rearing and management of *turkeys. In Great Britain turkeys are traditionally reared for the Christmas market (and Thanksgiving market in North America), although there is now increasing nonseasonal demand for a variety of processed turkey products, causing a diversification in turkey husbandry systems. Various hybrid genotypes have been developed, with age at maturity being one of the principal selection criteria. Thus smaller types mature at 14 weeks of age at a liveweight of 5 kg whereas larger types mature at 24 weeks of age weighing 14 kg. The excessive fat content of females approaching maturity means that they are slaughtered earlier than males.
*Intensive husbandry systems produce birds throughout the year in controlled environments; careful management is required to prevent *cannibalism, which may be serious in turkeys, and to minimize disease e.g. *blackhead. Extensive systems of husbandry are limited to the production of the heavier birds for the Christmas market. Beyond about 8 weeks of age turkeys are quite hardy and consequently can be reared under fairly

rudimentary conditions, needing only shelter from wind and rain.

turkey rhinotracheitis (TRT) A viral infection of turkeys causing respiratory signs, production losses, and variable mortality. It arrived in Britain on the Norfolk coast in summer 1985 and has since become widespread. The cause has now been identified as a *pneumovirus. (*Swollen head syndrome in broiler breeders, first observed at about the same time, appears to be due to the same virus.) Rhinotracheitis can affect turkeys of all ages above about 1 week. Respiratory signs vary from mild to severe, and younger growing birds tend to be worst affected. Outbreaks spread through a flock within 24 hours, typically affecting nearly all birds. There is general inflammation of the upper respiratory tract, including the trachea, sinuses, and turbinates with some *conjunctivitis. The main signs are swollen sinuses, nasal discharge, snicking, coughing, head shaking, and some gaping or gasping, with general depression. Mortality can exceed 50%, and deaths can occur several weeks after the initial signs, due to secondary infections, such as *colisepticaemia. Long-term consequences in more severely affected flocks may include culling due to leg problems, and downgrading of carcasses.

In breeding birds, the disease is milder; there may be some mortality but the main signs are a sharp fall in feed consumption, with a drastic drop (up to 60%) in egg production soon after. Prolapse of the oviduct as a result of coughing in laying turkey hens is also important. Most flocks return to normal egg production in a few weeks, although there may be later problems with shell or poult quality. There is no reliable treatment. The severity of outbreaks may be reduced by attention to ventilation, stocking density, litter condition,

and hygiene. A vaccine is currently (1987) under development.

turkey X disease A form of *aflatoxicosis affecting turkeys and other birds. The term was originally applied to a mystery disease that killed 100 000 turkey poults in 1961. The cause was traced to an aflatoxin produced by the fungus *Aspergillus flavus* growing on mouldy groundnut (peanut) meal used in rations. Ducklings are also very sensitive to aflatoxicosis, and chicks show retarded growth.

turning sickness A clinical syndrome characterized by nervous signs, including circling and head pressing. It is an uncommon sequel to *Theileria infections. See also theileriosis.

turpentine, medicinal oil of An oily liquid extracted from pine resin. Oil of turpentine is used as an *antizymotic and antifoaming agent in the treatment of colic in horses and bloat in ruminants. It can taint meat and milk, and may be irritant, causing inflammation of the gastric mucosa and nephritis.

twin-lamb disease See pregnancy toxaemia.

twins Two individuals who are born at the same time and of the same parents. *Dizygotic twins* are the most frequent and develop from separate *zygotes. They are genetically no more alike than ordinary full siblings. Each embryo develops independently with its own separate set of foetal membranes, although in the cow, for example, these undergo fusion, which leads to exchange of blood between the foetuses (see freemartin). *Monozygotic twins* are derived from an initial single zygote and divide at a fairly early but variable stage of embryonic development, causing variation in the arrangement of the foetal membranes. They are of the same sex and genetically identical. *Fused (Siamese) twins* are monozygotic in origin and result from the incomplete division of a single embryo.

twisted leg A form of lameness in growing poultry, particularly broilers and turkeys, caused by outward twisting of the bones around the hock joint. The condition leads to suboptimal growth and downgrading of carcasses. It is usual to see a few cases in a flock. Occasionally it leads to *perosis. The causes are uncertain, but there may be a genetic factor and also a link with high energy intake during early life. *Compare*

tying-up syndrome *See* azoturia.

tying-up syndrome *See* azoturia.

tylosin *See* macrolide antibiotics.

tympan- (tympano-) *Prefix denoting* 1. the eardrum. 2. the middle ear.

tympanic membrane The ear drum: the membrane at the inner end of the external acoustic meatus that separates the external ear and middle ear. Its outer surface is concave and formed of skin continuous with that of the external acoustic meatus; its convex inner surface is formed of mucous membrane continuous with that of the tympanic cavity. Sound waves reaching the tympanic membrane cause it to vibrate; it transmits these vibrations to the *malleus, which is attached to its inner surface. *See* ear.

tympanites (tympany) Distension of the abdomen due to the accumulation of air or gas in the gastrointestinal tract or abdominal cavity. The abdomen is resonant (drumlike) on *percussion. This condition commonly occurs in cattle suffering from *bloat,

in which large amounts of gas become trapped in the rumen. Another form, which occurs in the horse, and sometimes also in pigs, is caused by gas generated in the large intestine. If the accumulation is due to an intestinal blockage, surgical intervention may be required.

tympanum (*pl.* **tympana** or **tympanums**) The middle *ear (tympanic cavity) and/or the eardrum (*tympanic membrane).

tympany *See* tympanites.

typhlitis Inflammation of the caecum. An important example occurs in *coccidiosis due to *Eimeria tenella* in domestic fowls, in which the protozoa initiate severe haemorrhagic typhlitis.

typhus Any of a group of principally human diseases caused by infection with *rickettsiae. Various animal species may act as reservoirs of infection, and thus represent a health hazard to humans. The various forms of typhus are characterized by a widespread rash, prolonged high fever, and delirium. They all respond to treatment with chloramphenicol or tetracyclines. *Murine typhus (endemic typhus)* is caused by *Rickettsia typhi*. The primary reservoir is rats (*Rattus rattus*, *R. norvegicus*), among which the agent is transmitted by the rat louse (*Polyplax spinulosus*) and the rat flea (*Xenopsylla cheopis*); the rickettsia also readily infects the human flea (*Pulex irritans*) and body louse (*Pediculus humanus*). Any of these vectors can transmit the infection to humans. *Epidemic typhus (classical typhus)*, caused by *R. prowazekii*, is almost exclusively human, being transmitted by body lice. However, it has recently been demonstrated in Southern flying squirrels (*Glaucomys volans*) in Florida, the louse vector being *Neohaematopinus sciuropteri*.

There are in addition several kinds of tick-borne typhus; *see* spotted fever.

tyrosine *See* amino acid.

Tyzzer's disease A disease occurring sporadically in foals, cats, rodents, and rhesus monkeys, caused by the bacterium *Bacillus piliformis* and characterized by a necrotizing hepatitis and colitis. In North America the bacterium is carried by wild muskrats. *Tetracycline is used to treat the disease in foals.

tzaneen disease A disease of cattle caused by the protozoan parasite *Theileria mutans*, which is widely distributed in Africa and is transmitted by hard ticks of the genus *Amblyomma*. *T. mutans* multiplies in red blood cells and lymph nodes causing anaemia with occasionally severe consequences. It may ocur in association with *East Coast fever caused by *T. parva*. Recovery from *T. mutans* does not confer immunity to *T. parva*.

U

ubiquinone (coenzyme Q) One of various benzoquinone derivatives with side chains of differing lengths that act as electron carriers in the mitochondria of cells (*see* electron transport chain).

udder *See* mammary gland.

UHT *See* ultrahigh temperature.

ulcer A break in the skin or mucous membrane that generally starts as an area of necrosis with unsuccessful repair involving regeneration from the surrounding epithelial cells coupled with the growth of granulation tissue from the floor of the ulcer. If the

cause of ulceration persists the erosion progressively deepens and perforates the submucosal layers. This may result in, for example, the rupture of an artery and serious haemorrhage, or penetration of the peritoneum and peritonitis. Ulcers are common lesions, and may be present without causing clinical signs. However, the complications caused by their progressive changes produce disease and possibly even death, especially with *gastric ulcers.

There are many causes of ulcer formation, including systemic disease (e.g. glanders, mucosal disease, orf, swine fever), local trauma and infection (e.g. pressure from a harness or collar), reduced blood flow (*ischaemia), and exposure to toxic or irritating substances (e.g. in food or due to the misapplication of drugs). Predisposing factors include old age, malnutrition, or other chronic debility. Treatment depends on the site and stage of the ulcer, but in all cases any underlying cause must be corrected. External ulcers may respond to topical application of a suitable antiseptic, possibly coupled with an antibiotic. *See also* eosinophilic granuloma complex.

ulcerative lymphangitis A chronic infectious disease of horses caused by *Corynebacterium pseudotuberculosis* (*C. ovis*) of a type slightly different from that found in ovine *caseous lymphadenitis. Corded suppurating swellings develop along subcutaneous lymph ducts, especially of the hindlimbs; the swellings burst and discharge a greenish pus. The condition may resemble cutaneous *glanders or *epizootic lymphangitis, and tends to recur for approximately 12 months before spontaneous resolution takes place. Some scarring of tissue remains. The same organism is also responsible for the subcutaneous abscessation affecting the ventral abdominal region of horses; this is treated surgically and with antibiotics.

ulna (*pl.* **ulnae** or **ulnas**) One of the bones of the lower forelimb (forearm). Typically, as in the dog, it forms proximal and distal *radioulnar joints* with the *radius. Proximally, with the radius, it joins with the humerus forming the *elbow joint. Distally it articulates with the proximal row of carpal bones (*see* carpus). In ruminants it is reduced in diameter but present along its whole length and fused to the radius. In horses the distal two-thirds is lost, and the proximal third is fused to the radius.

ulnar nerve One of the nerves of the forelimb. It originates in the *brachial plexus and supplies some of the muscles and skin in the back of the lower limb (forearm) and back of the foot.

ultra- *Prefix denoting* **1.** beyond. **2.** an extreme degree (e.g. of large or small size).

ultracentrifuge A *centrifuge that works at extremely high speeds of rotation: used for separating large molecules, such as proteins.

ultrafiltration Filtration under pressure. In the glomeruli of the *kidney, the blood is subjected to ultrafiltration to remove water, urea, and other waste material that go to make up urine.

ultrahigh temperature (UHT) A method of treating *milk to improve its storage qualities by heating it to 125–150°C for a few seconds. This kills most pathogens and other micro-organisms and produces *long-life* milk. The process may destroy some vitamins and immunoglobulins. *Compare* pasteurization.

ultramicroscope A microscope for examining particles suspended in a gas or liquid under intense illumination from one side. Light is scattered or reflected from the particles, which can be seen through the eyepiece as bright objects against a dark background.

ultramicrotome An instrument for cutting extremely thin sections of tissue (not more than 0.1 μm thick) for electron microscopy. *See also* microtome.

ultrasonics The study of the uses and properties of sound waves of very high frequency (*see* ultrasound).

ultrasonography The technique of obtaining a visual record of structures in the body using *ultrasonic waves (ultrasound). These waves are directed into the body and are reflected at different wavelengths by different tissues. Recording of the reflections enables visualization of body structures. The technique does not involve harmful radiation and is used routinely for pregnancy diagnosis. Also, structures not opaque to X-rays (e.g. soft tissues) can be visualized using ultrasound.

ultrasound (ultrasonic waves) Sound waves of extremely high frequency (above 20 000 Hz), inaudible to the human ear. Ultrasound scanning can be used to examine the structure of the inside of the body (*see* ultrasonography). The vibratory effect of these sound waves can also be used in the treatment of various disorders of deep tissues, and even to break up stones in the kidney or elsewhere. *See also* echography.

umbilical artery The paired artery that conveys deoxygenated blood from the foetus to its placenta. After birth the portion within the body becomes converted to the ligamentum teres of the urinary bladder.

umbilical cord The band of tissue connecting the foetus with its placenta. It is composed of the *umbilical arteries and vein(s) supported by mesenchyme (*Wharton's jelly), and includes the remnants of the *allantois and *yolk sac. It becomes ensheathed by the *amnion. After parturition the umbilical cord ruptures and the blood vessels retract, preventing haemorrhage from the umbilical stump.

umbilical vein The initially paired but later single vein that conveys oxygenated blood to the foetus from its placenta. After birth the portion within the body becomes converted to the ligamentum teres of the liver.

umbilicus (*pl.* **umbilici** or **umbilicuses**) The depression in the skin in the centre of the ventral abdominal wall overlying a fibrous scar. It is the site of attachment of the foetal *umbilical cord.

Uncinaria A genus of parasitic *nematodes containing the species *U. stenocephala*, a *hookworm found in dogs and foxes in Europe. It is closely related to the genus *Ancylostoma*. *See also* verminous dermatitis.

unconsciousness A condition in which an animal is unaware of its surroundings, as in *sleep, or is unresponsive to stimulation. An unnatural state of unconsciousness may be caused by factors that reduce brain activity, such as lack of oxygen, a blow on the head, poisoning, blood loss, or disease, or it can be produced deliberately by general *anaesthesia.

undecylenate A salt of undecylenic acid with antifungal properties, used in the topical treatment of ringworm and also as a fungistat in various topical preparations for the treatment of skin infections. Undecylenic acid has activity against a wide range of fungi,

including *Microsporum* spp. However, it is irritant to skin and therefore the zinc or copper salts are used.

undulant fever *See* brucellosis.

uni- *Prefix denoting* one.

unicellular Describing organisms or tissues that consist of a single cell. Unicellular organisms include the protozoa, most bacteria, and some fungi.

unilateral (in anatomy) Relating to or affecting one side of the body or one side of an organ or other part.

unipolar (in neurology) Describing a neurone that has one main process extending from the cell body. *Compare* bipolar; multipolar.

United States Department of Agriculture (USDA) The branch of the US federal government concerned with agriculture and related issues. It is headed by the Secretary of Agriculture. The two divisions most concerned with veterinary medicine are the Animal and Plant Health Inspection Service (APHIS) and the Food Safety and Inspection Service (FSIS). *Accredited veterinarians attached to the Veterinary Services of APHIS control reportable diseases and administer the eradicable disease programmes and interstate health certificates. The FSIS administers the inspection of all animals slaughtered for food in accordance with federal law. The Science and Education Administration manages the programme of research grants and contracts awarded by the USDA.

urachus (*pl.* **urachi**) The part of the *allantois that extends from the urinary bladder to the umbilicus in the foetus. It allows urine to pass into the cavity of the allantois. After birth the urachus normally closes and degenerates, but occasionally it remains patent, allowing the leakage of urine from the umbilicus.

uracil One of the nitrogen-containing bases (*see* pyrimidine) occurring in the nucleic acid RNA.

uraemia An abnormally high concentration of urea in the blood. Urea is normally excreted in the urine, hence both acute and chronic kidney disease lead to a progressive increase in blood urea levels. Uraemia can also occur in cattle and sheep fed urea, especially in the form of self-feed blocks or licks with a molasses base. Hungry animals may overindulge and suffer *urea poisoning. Urea itself is not especially toxic but it is rapidly broken down in the rumen to ammonia, which is much more toxic.

urataemia The presence of excessive amounts of urates (uric acid salts) in the blood. This may be associated with *gout in poultry and reptiles. In mammals its significance is poorly understood. *Compare* uraturia.

urate The salt of *uric acid.

uraturia The presence of excessive amounts of urates (uric acid salts) in the urine. This occurs particularly in Dalmatian dogs, which lack the ability to convert uric acid to allantoin in the liver. They tend to suffer from urinary stones (calculi) composed of ammonium urate. Prevention of recurrence involves feeding low-protein diets. In other animals uraturia occurs when liver failure disrupts uric acid metabolism and excess urates have to be excreted.

urea (carbamide) The main nitrogenous excretory end-product of most domestic animals. In pure form it is a white crystalline deliquescent solid, widely used as a cheap source of nonprotein nitrogen in feeds for rumi-

nants. Urea is suitable for its role in excretion because of its high solubility and, compared to ammonia (the immediate product of much nitrogen catabolism), its low toxicity. It is produced by a series of reactions – the *urea cycle* – involving the *amino acids ornithine, citrulline, and arginine. The two nitrogens of urea are derived from the amino acids aspartate and glutamate, and the whole process requires energy in the form of ATP. In birds and terrestrial reptiles, *uric acid is the principal excretory nitrogenous compound.

Urea added to ruminant diets is hydrolysed to ammonia and carbon dioxide by the urease enzymes of rumen microorganisms. High levels of urea in the diet can lead to ammonia toxicity (*see* urea poisoning). It is generally recommended that no more than one-third of dietary nitrogen should come from urea, that a rapidly fermentable source of carbohydrate (e.g. molasses) should be fed at the same time, and that urea should be fed in small and frequent amounts.

urea poisoning A toxic condition due to an excessive intake of urea and consequent rise in ammonia concentration in the blood. Urea should be introduced gradually to the feed, and initially it is dangerous to exceed a dose of 0.5 g/kg bodyweight, but animals slowly become tolerant to larger doses. Overdosage produces salivation, nystagmus, excitement, and diarrhoea.

urease An enzyme that catalyses the hydrolysis of urea to ammonia and carbon dioxide.

ureter Either of a pair of tubes that conduct urine from the kidney to the urinary bladder. The wall of each ureter contains a thick layer of smooth muscle, which contracts by peristalsis to force urine into the urinary bladder. This muscle layer lies between an outer fibrous layer and an inner mucous membrane; this latter contains glands in the horse.

ureter- (uretero-) *Prefix denoting* the ureter(s). Example: *ureterovaginal* (relating to the ureters and vagina).

ureteritis Inflammation of the ureter. It may be due to the lodgment of stones (calculi), but it is more usually the result of infection spreading from the renal pelvis, for example as in *pyelonephritis in cattle due to *Corynebacterium renale*. This involves progressive destruction of the renal pelvis with gross thickening and chronic inflammation of the adjacent ureter.

urethr- (urethro-) *Prefix denoting* the urethra.

urethra The tube that conducts urine from the urinary *bladder to the exterior. The female urethra is quite short and opens in the *vestibule of the vagina. The male urethra is longer, consists of a pelvic part and a spongy part, and receives the secretions of the male accessory glands (*prostate gland, *bulbourethral glands, and, when present, seminal vesicles) and spermatozoa from the ducti deferentes (*see* ductus deferens). The *pelvic part* runs initially through the *prostate gland; on the dorsal surface of the urethra is a ridge, the *urethral crest*, at the centre of which is a small elevation, the *colliculus seminalis*, where the ducti deferentes discharge. The *spongy part* is incorporated into the *penis, where it is surrounded by the *corpus spongiosum. In the ram the terminal part of the urethra projects beyond the penis as the *urethral processus*.

urethral obstruction Blockage of the urethra, usually due to lodgment of stones (calculi). This occurs especially in male animals with a urethral flex-

ure (e.g. ruminants and pigs). Surgery is often indicated for relief. *See also* feline urological syndrome; urolithiasis.

urethritis Inflammation of the urethra. This commonly follows ascending infection from the external orifice involving bacteria, such as *Escherichia coli*, *Staphylococcus aureus*, or *Proteus vulgaris*, and may accompany inflammation of the urinary bladder (*cystitis). Clinical signs include frequent urination or a tendency to dribble urine. Antibiotics may be used in treatment. Another cause is the lodgment of irritant stones (calculi) in the urethra. These may have to be removed surgically. Urethritis may occasionally result in an abscess, which bursts to the exterior forming a fistula and allowing urine to seep from beneath the penis.

urethrostomy The surgical creation of an opening into the urethra. It is usually performed to remove an obstruction caused by urinary calculi. In the **dog** this is generally carried out immediately behind the os penis directly in the midline, so as to avoid local cavernous tissue. The operation site is allowed to heal without suturing.
Where the obstruction occurs at a site not readily accessible, as in cattle, or where recurrent obstruction occurs, a permanent opening may be made just below the pelvis, by suturing the opened urethra into the skin.

uric acid A relatively insoluble *purine that is the principal nitrogenous excretory end-product in birds and terrestrial reptiles. It can be excreted in solid form and thus helps conserve water in these animal groups. In humans and other primates, uric acid is the end-product of purine catabolism; in other mammals it is oxidized to *allantoin* prior to excretion. Uric acid is a common

uridine

constituent of 'stones' or calculi (*see* calculus), while a defect in uric acid metabolism causes the disease *gout.

uridine A compound containing uracil and the sugar ribose. *See also* nucleoside.

urin- (urino-, uro-) *Prefix denoting* urine or the urinary system.

urinary bladder *See* bladder.

urinary calculi *See* urolithiasis.

urinary tract The entire system of ducts and channels that conduct urine from the kidneys to the exterior. It includes the ureters, the bladder, and the urethra.

urination *See* micturition.

urine The aqueous fluid formed by the excretory organs of animals for the removal of metabolic waste products. In higher animals it is produced by the *kidneys. Mammals temporarily store urine in the urinary *bladder, while in birds it is mixed with the faeces in the cloaca. Urine contains many of the body's waste products, being the main route by which the end-products of nitrogen metabolism – *urea, *uric acid, and *creatinine – are excreted. Sodium chloride and many other materials in trace amounts are usually present also. Biochemical analysis of urine is frequently undertaken for diagnostic purposes; for example, high levels of urinary glucose occur in *diabetes mellitus.

urinometer A hydrometer for measuring the specific gravity of urine.

urocele A cystic swelling in the scrotum containing urine that has escaped from a ruptured bladder or ureter. It is rarely reported in animals.

urogenital Of or relating to the organs and tissues concerned with excretion and reproduction, which are anatomically closely associated.

urolith A *calculus or concretion in the urinary tract. *See* urolithiasis.

urolithiasis 1. The formation of calculi (*see* calculus) or *gravel within the urinary system. Urinary calculi (*uroliths*) occur in most domestic species, most commonly within the urinary bladder. They can be composed of several different salts or be of mixed composition. In carnivores the most common urolith salt is magnesium ammonium phosphate (often termed *struvite*), which accounts for 50% of canine urolithiasis. Oxalate, urate, uric acid, and cystine uroliths are also found. In horses, calcium carbonate and calcium oxalate are the most common. In ruminants, triple phosphate and amorphous phosphates and oxalates occur.

The presence of crystals in the urine may, in certain cases, lead to calculus formation and possible urinary tract dysfunction. Bilirubin and phosphate crystals in carnivores, and carbonate crystals in horses and cattle may be considered normal components of urine. Their presence is dependent on urine pH. Urates are normally excreted by Dalmatian dogs. In severe liver disease metabolism is altered and ammonium biurates or tyrosine, not normally present in urine, may be detected. Oxalate crystals occur in large numbers in *ethylene glycol (antifreeze) poisoning, and drugs (e.g. sulphonamides) may also lead to crystal formation in the urine. Lambs and calves develop uroliths when fed large amounts of concentrates.

Bacterial infection, especially with *Staphylococcus* spp., may contribute to calculi formation. Desquamated epithelial cells may act as a *nidus for calculi formation, and pasture with plants containing high levels of oxalates or oestrogens may also predispose to calculi formation. Moreover, picornavirus, calicivirus, and feline herpesvirus have all been implicated in calculi formation. Irritation by urinary crystals is the cause of *feline urological syndrome (FUS), the most important cause of lower urinary tract disease in cats. Also, this may involve the formation of struvite calculi within a proteinaceous matrix; these obstruct the urethra. In dogs, a hereditary defect in amino acid transport mechanisms allows cystine calculi to form. Dalmatian dogs are prone to urate and uric acid gravel in the urinary tract.

The presence of uroliths may or may not cause clinical signs. Obstruction of the urethra generally occurs at the ischial arch, os penis, vermiform appendage, or sigmoid flexure, depending on the species involved; this results in *tenesmus, dysuria, and incontinence. Calculi in the bladder can cause erosion of the mucosa leading to irritation, haematuria, and dysuria. Acute renal failure may occur if obstruction of the tract is complete, with a rapid onset of uraemia. In all species there are signs of pain and discomfort; in horses this is described as *false colic*. Diagnosis is based on typical clinical signs together with radiographic evidence, often involving the use of contrast media. Treatment usually involves surgical intervention followed by prophylactic measures to prevent recurrence. Dietary changes, increased water intake, control of infections, and urine acidifiers may all be used to provide some protection. However, up to 30% of cases are likely to recur.
2. Disease caused by the presence of uroliths.

urticaria A raised reddened circumscribed area of oedema of the superficial layers of the skin, which is often itchy. The oedema may extend deeply into the dermis and subcutaneous tissue (i.e. *angioedema*). There are numerous causes of urticaria, including some drugs, antigen sensitivity (atopy), cold, and heat. The coat of most animals protects the skin from the irritating hairs of plants like the stinging nettle, which may produce urticaria in humans.

uter- (utero-) *Prefix denoting* the uterus.

uterine Of or relating to the uterus.

uterine tube In mammals, either of the pair of tubes that transport *oocytes from the ovary to the uterus. The ovarian end of the tube is expanded into a funnel-shaped *infundibulum* with finger-like projections (fimbriae); these surround the ovary and guide oocytes into the uterine tube. The main portion of the uterine tube, the *ampulla*, narrows to an *isthmus* before opening into the uterus at the *uterine ostium*. Fertilization of oocytes occurs in the ampulla towards the ovarian end of the uterine tube. *Compare* oviduct.

uterus (*pl.* **uteri** or **uteruses**) The part of the female reproductive system that, in most mammals, is specialized to allow the embryo to undergo *implantation so that nourishment, derived from the maternal blood, can be provided for the growing foetus (see illustration). In domestic mammals the uterus is *bicornuate*, with left and right horns leading from the single body; this is continuous caudally with the *cervix and *vagina. At the tip of each horn is the opening of the uterine tube, whence the embryo(s) enters the uterus. The form of the uterus varies with species and is related to the potential number of offspring. In the pig the uterine horns are long and narrow and the body is relatively small, whereas the horse has a large uterine body and short broad horns. Cows and sheep exhibit an

uterus masculinus

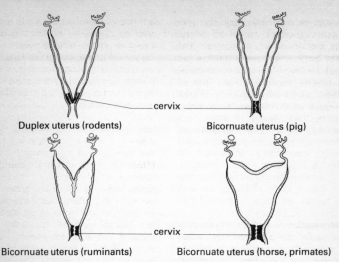

Duplex uterus (rodents)

Bicornuate uterus (pig)

Bicornuate uterus (ruminants)

Bicornuate uterus (horse, primates)

Simplified diagrams showing various forms of the uterus

intermediate form. Primitive mammals have two entirely separate uteri.

The uterine wall consists of the outer serosa (perimetrium), the middle muscularis (myometrium), and the inner mucosa (*endometrium). In ruminants the endometrium has rounded projections, *caruncles*, which form specialized regions of the *placenta. The uterus is attached to the abdominal and pelvic walls by the paired *broad ligaments which also carry blood vessels to the uterus. In **birds** the uterus is the part of the *oviduct that secretes the shell. See illustration.

uterus masculinus The vestige of the *paramesonephric duct system, which may occur in the male; it represents the uterus in the female.

utricle The larger of the two sacs of the membranous labyrinth of the internal *ear that lie within the vestibule. Its wall contains a *macula which helps in sensing the position of the head.

uvea (uveal tract) The vascular coat of the *eye.

uveitis Inflammation of the uveal tract (*see* uvea) of the eye, involving the iris, ciliary body, and choroid. It may be described as *anterior* or *posterior*, depending on the parts of the uveal tract involved; *panuveitis* affects the entire tract. Various causes exist, but trauma and intraocular parasites are the main ones. Some infectious diseases also result in inflammation of the eye, especially *toxoplasmosis in dogs and cats, *aspergillosis in poultry, and *strangles in horses. Glaucoma, cataract, and corneal opacity may be secondary complications.

*Periodic ophthalmia, affecting horses, is a form of uveitis thought to be due to *hypersensitivity to certain parasitic infections. In the dog, a granulomatous or plasmacytic panuveitis occurs rarely and is considered to be immune mediated because of its recurrent nature and response to corticosteroids, although no causal agents have been identified. In the cat, the coronavirus of *feline infectious peritonitis causes a recurrent diffuse uveitis with mixed inflammatory response. The optic nerve sheath is often infiltrated heavily by lymphocytic-plasmacytic cells, but affected cats often succumb to the more severe peritoneal/pleural involvement or are destroyed before eye lesions become more advanced. *See also* panophthalmitis.

V

vaccination A means of producing immunity to a disease by using a *vaccine to stimulate the formation of appropriate antibodies. The term originally referred to treatment with *vaccinia virus to protect against smallpox in humans. However, it is now used synonymously with *inoculation* as a method of *immunization against any disease. Vaccination is used to protect against many viral, bacterial, protozoan, and parasitic diseases. The vaccine is usually given by injection, but may be administered orally (e.g. lungworm vaccine in cattle). Vaccination may need to be repeated periodically to maintain protection (*see* booster). The use of serum derived from animals immune to specific diseases to protect others already exposed to disease may also be referred to as vaccination, although this form of protection is of only short duration and does not stimulate the animals' own immune systems against disease.

vaccine A living or dead preparation used to stimulate active immunity in animals. *Live vaccines* consist of living organisms, which replicate in the recipient animal. They comprise either attenuated strains (*see* attenuation) of a disease-producing organism, or a species of organism closely related to the disease-producing organism that causes the development of an immunity embracing the related organism. Lungworm vaccines for cattle are live vaccines produced from virulent organisms but irradiated so that they do not complete their life cycle. This stimulates immunity without producing clinical signs of disease. *Dead vaccines* are either purified, inactivated, and concentrated preparations of the disease-producing organism or purified preparations of bacterial toxins (*toxoids). Live vaccines produce a stronger and longer-lasting immunity than dead vaccines, but are susceptible to unintentional inactivation (e.g. by sunlight or high temperature) and can become contaminated with other pathogens during preparation. Most live vaccines are now produced in tissue culture and severely tested for safety. Dead vaccines are more stable than live vaccines but do not stimulate the complete range of host immune responses and are thus less effective. Also, care must be taken to ensure complete inactivation of the virulent organisms.

Vaccines have also been developed synthetically by joining peptides in specific sequences (*peptide vaccines*) to copy the antigenic sites present on certain viruses, such as *foot-and-mouth disease virus. *Vector vaccines* are engineered in the laboratory by taking the gene sequence that codes for the antigenic determinant of a disease-producing virus, such as *rabies virus, and inserting it into the genome of a larger virus, such as *vaccinia virus. Vaccination with this live recombinant vaccine stimulates immunity without any danger of causing the disease. *See also* vaccination.

vaccinia A usually mild infectious disease affecting a wide range of mammals, including humans, characterized by the formation of pustules and caused by an orthopoxvirus (*see* poxvirus). Vaccinia virus was used to protect humans against infection with smallpox until the worldwide eradication of this disease. The virus, however, spread into domestic and wild animal populations. It causes the development of small swellings, which become fluid-filled vesicles and eventually pustules. The pustules soon rupture and become scabs. These lesions on the teats of cows frequently develop secondary infections, which may result in *mastitis. The lesions of vaccinia are indistinguishable in cattle from those of *cowpox, and in buffaloes from those of *buffalopox. The vaccinia virus has been genetically engineered to include segments of the genetic material of other viruses. The recombinant virus can be used in vaccines to immunize animals against these other viruses.

vacuole A space within the cytoplasm of a cell, formed by infolding of the cell membrane, that contains material taken in by the cell. White blood cells form vacuoles when they surround and digest bacteria and other foreign material.

vagin- (vagino-) *Prefix denoting* the vagina.

vagina The tubular part of the female reproductive system connecting the cervix of the uterus to the *vestibule (which in turn opens at the vulva). It is lined by mucosa and has a well-developed muscular layer in its wall. The vagina receives the erect penis during *coitus, and is the site of semen deposition in the sow.

vaginitis Inflammation of the vagina. *See* infectious bovine pustulovaginitis; vulvovaginitis.

vago- *Prefix denoting* the vagus nerve.

vagotomy Surgical cutting of the *vagus nerve, either one one side

(unilateral) or on both sides (bilateral). This is not common practice in domestic species except in experimental surgery.

vagus nerve The tenth *cranial nerve (X), which supplies the muscles of the pharynx and larynx and carries parasympathetic fibres to the organs of the thorax and abdomen and sensory fibres from these same organs.

valgus Any condition in which a bone or part is displaced outwards or away from the midline to an abnormal degree (e.g. *valgus vara). *Compare* varus.

valgus vara ('knock knee') A deformity of the legs in which the feet are displaced outwards and the 'knees' (carpus or tarsus) move together. It is important in horses and may be congenital or acquired. Both the fore- and hindlimbs may be affected, most commonly due to a defect of the carpus or tarsus. Severe deviation from the upright (>4°) can cause lameness and the condition becomes progressive. Accurate diagnosis of the cause is vital for successful treatment, which may involve surgery.

valine An *amino acid. *See also* essential amino acid.

vallecula (*pl.* **valleculae**) A furrow or depression in an organ or other part. On the undersurface of the cerebellum a vallecula separates the two hemispheres.

valve A structure found in some tubular organs that directs the flow of fluid within them. Valves are important in the heart, veins, and lymphatic vessels. *See* atrioventricular valve; bicuspid valve; semilunar valve; tricuspid valve.

valvular disease Disease of the heart valves. The two main forms are: *val-*

vular insufficiency – incomplete closure of a valve, which allows backflow of blood; and *valvular stenosis* – narrowing of the opening guarded by a valve, which obstructs blood flow. In either case the myocardium hypertrophies to compensate. Eventually, congestive heart failure occurs. Identification of the nature and site of the lesion depends on interpreting the various heart murmurs heard on *auscultation.

valvulitis Inflammation of a valve, especially a heart valve.

varicocele Dilatation of the spermatic veins in the scrotum. The condition is of no clinical significance and does not influence fertility. Between one and two percent of rams are affected, and it occurs occasionally in stallions.

varus Any condition in which a bone or part is displaced inwards or towards the midline to an abnormal extent. *Compare* valgus.

vas (*pl.* **vasa**) A vessel or duct.

vas- (**vaso-**) *Prefix denoting* **1.** vessels, especially blood vessels. **2.** the vas deferens.

vasa vasorum The tiny arteries and veins that supply the walls of larger blood vessels.

vascular Relating to or supplied with blood vessels.

vascularization The development of blood vessels (usually capillaries) within a tissue.

vascular system *See* cardiovascular system.

vas deferens (*pl.* **vasa deferentia**) *See* ductus deferens.

vasectomy Surgical removal of a section from each *ductus deferens (vas deferens). The blood vessels and nerves to the testes are left functional so that the animal exhibits normal libido and sexual behaviour (including copulation), but conception cannot take place as the spermatozoa can no longer pass to the urethra for ejaculation. The operation involves an incision into the scrotum to expose the spermatic cord followed by the removal of a 3–5 cm section of each ductus deferens and *ligature of the cut ends. A period of several weeks is needed following surgery before the animal can be guaranteed sterile, in order to allow for clearance of spermatozoa in the remaining ducts.
The technique can be used as a form of *contraception, while vasectomized bulls, rams, and boars are often used as 'teasers' in *oestrus detection. The introduction of a vasectomized ram into a flock of ewes can result in the induction and synchronization of seasonal breeding. Similarly, vasectomized boars may be used to induce and synchronize puberty in gilts. *Compare* vasotomy.

vasoactive Affecting the diameter of blood vessels, especially arteries. Examples of vasoactive agents are pressure, carbon dioxide, and temperature. Some exert their effect directly, others via the *vasomotor centre in the brain.

vasoconstriction A decrease in the diameter of blood vessels, especially arteries. This results from activation of the *vasomotor centre in the brain, which brings about contraction of the muscular walls of the arteries through stimulation by the sympathetic nervous system; this produces an increase in blood pressure.

vasoconstrictor An agent that causes increased tone of the smooth muscle of blood vessels, thus causing

vasodilatation

vasoconstriction and increasing blood pressure. *Sympathomimetic compounds act as vasoconstrictors, for example adrenaline, noradrenaline, methoxamine, and metaraminol. These can be used in situations of severe life-threatening vasodilatation; for instance, adrenaline is used intravenously to counteract anaphylactic shock. They are also applied locally to prevent haemorrhage from small blood vessels at wounds and during surgery. Centrally acting *stimulants, such as amphetamines, also cause vasoconstriction of blood vessels. *Angiotensin II is a powerful natural vasoconstrictor, found in the membranes of blood vessels, lungs, and other organs. When released there is a rapid rise in blood pressure and release of adrenaline. Analogues of angiotensin II are available to control hypotension. These have been used in the treatment of circulatory collapse and heart failure. Fluid replacement therapy is now used as an alternative or in addition to some of these drugs.

vasodilatation An increase in the diameter of blood vessels, especially arteries. This results from activation of the *vasomotor centre in the brain, which brings about relaxation of the muscular walls of arteries through a reduction in the action of the *sympathetic nervous system; this produces a decrease in blood pressure.

vasodilator An agent that causes relaxation of smooth muscle in blood vessel walls, thus inducing vasodilatation and reducing blood pressure. Vasodilatation can be local or generalized. Vasodilatation at the site of inflammation is caused by the mediators of inflammation, notably histamine and prostaglandins. Smooth muscle tone in blood vessel walls is maintained by the sympathetic nervous system, and drugs with blocking activity at alpha adrenoceptors or ganglia act as vasodilators (*see* sym-

patholytic). Other drugs act centrally or directly on the smooth muscle in blood vessel walls. Vasodilators are used to control hypertension in man and treat circulatory and cardiac diseases. *See* hypotensive agent.

vasomotor centre A collection of nerve cells in the medulla oblongata of the brainstem that receives information from the *baroreceptors in the circulatory system and produces reflex changes in heart rate and the diameter of blood vessels so that blood pressure can be adjusted. These changes are mediated via the autonomic nervous system. The vasomotor centre also receives impulses from elsewhere in the brain so that emotional states (e.g. fear) may also affect heart rate and blood pressure.

vasomotor nerve Any nerve, usually belonging to the *autonomic nervous system, that controls the circulation of blood through blood vessels, either by its action on the muscle fibres within the vessel walls or by its action on the heart beat. The *vagus nerve slows the heart and reduces its output; sympathetic nerves increase the rate and output of the heart and increase blood pressure by causing the constriction of small blood vessels at the same time.

vasopressin (antidiuretic hormone; ADH) A hormone produced by specialized nuclei in the supraoptic and paraventricular regions of the *hypothalamus and stored and released in the neurohypophysis. It is released in response to elevated blood osmolarity and causes increased resorption of water at the distal tubules and collecting ducts in the kidneys. Deficiency of vasopressin results in *diabetes insipidus. Vasopressin tannate in oil (pitressin) and the synthetic analogue desmopressin can be used to treat diabetes insipidus in dogs.

858

vasopressor Stimulating the contraction of blood vessels, thereby increasing blood pressure.

vasotomy Surgical incision into the lumen of the *ductus deferens (vas deferens). *Compare* vasectomy.

vasovagal Relating to the action of impulses in the *vagus nerve on the circulation. The vagus reduces the rate at which the heart beats, and so lowers its output.

vector An animal, usually an insect, tick, or mite, that transmits parasitic microorganisms – and therefore the diseases they cause – from animal to animal or from infected animals to humans (or vice versa).

vegetation An abnormal outgrowth, fancied to resemble a vegetable growth. For example, vegetative thrombi are found on the membrane lining the heart valves in certain forms of *endocarditis.

vegetative 1. Relating to growth and nutrition rather than to reproduction. **2.** Functioning unconsciously.

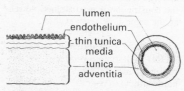

Transverse section through a vein

vein A blood vessel conveying blood towards the heart. All veins except the *pulmonary veins carry deoxygenated blood from the capillaries of the tissues to the *venae cavae. The walls of veins consist of three layers, but these are much thinner and less elastic than those of arteries (see illustration). Veins contain *valves that direct the flow of blood towards the heart.

veld sickness *See* heartwater.

velum (*pl.* **vela**) (in anatomy) A veil-like covering. The rostral and caudal *medullary vela* are two thin layers of tissue that form part of the roof of the fourth ventricle of the brain.

vena (*pl.* **venae**) *See* vein.

vena cava (*pl.* **venae cavae**) Either of the two main veins, conveying blood from the other veins to the right atrium of the heart. The *caudal vena cava*, formed by the union of the left and right common iliac veins, receives blood from the abdomen, pelvis, and hindlimbs. The *cranial vena cava*, formed by the union of left and right brachiocephalic veins, receives blood from the head, neck, thorax, and forelimbs.

vene- (veno-) *Prefix denoting* veins.

venereal disease Any infectious disease that is transmitted by coitus (sexual intercourse). The most important sexually transmitted diseases in domestic species are *brucellosis, *trichomoniasis, *campylobacteriosis of cattle, and infectious *vulvovaginitis of cattle. Dogs are susceptible to *transmissible venereal tumour (TVT), and various fibropapillomata may be transmitted in numerous species (*see* fibropapilloma). Only monkeys are prone to infection by syphilis and gonorrhoea, the venereal diseases of greatest significance to humans.

venereology The study of *venereal diseases.

veno- *Prefix. See* vene-.

venography (phlebography) *Radiography of a vein. *See* angiography.

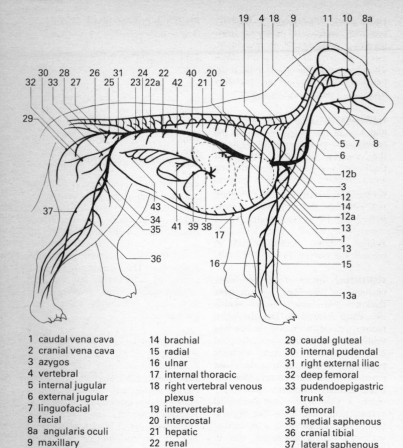

Venous system of the dog

1	caudal vena cava	14	brachial	29	caudal gluteal
2	cranial vena cava	15	radial	30	internal pudendal
3	azygos	16	ulnar	31	right external iliac
4	vertebral	17	internal thoracic	32	deep femoral
5	internal jugular	18	right vertebral venous	33	pudendoepigastric
6	external jugular		plexus		trunk
7	linguofacial	19	intervertebral	34	femoral
8	facial	20	intercostal	35	medial saphenous
8a	angularis oculi	21	hepatic	36	cranial tibial
9	maxillary	22	renal	37	lateral saphenous
10	superficial temporal	22a	testicular or ovarian	38	portal
11	dorsal sagittal sinus	23	deep circumflex iliac	39	gastroduodenal
12	axillary	24	common iliac	40	splenic
12a	axillobrachial	25	right internal iliac	41	caudal mesenteric
12b	omobrachial	26	median sacral	42	cranial mesenteric
13	cephalic	27	prostatic or vaginal	43	jejunal
13a	accessory cephalic	28	lateral caudal		

venom The toxic substance produced by snakes, scorpions, spiders, and other animals for injecting into their prey or enemies. Venom may contain certain factors that damage the tissues at the site of the bite and others that, after absorption, affect the nervous system and other tissues of the body. Their effects range from local pain and swelling to death. *See* snakebite poisoning; spider bite poisoning.

vent gleet (cloacitis) A formerly common condition of domestic fowls involving inflammation of the cloaca, associated with an unpleasant smell. The cause is unknown but it is believed to be contagious, probably involving venereal transmission.

ventilation 1. The passage of air into and out of the respiratory tract to enable gaseous exchange to occur in the *alveoli of the lungs. The air that reaches only as far as the conducting airways cannot take part in gaseous exchange and is known as *dead space ventilation*. *See also* breathing; respiration. **2.** *See* housing.

ventral Related to, situated at, or close to the undersurface of the body.

ventricle 1. Either of the two lower chambers of the *heart, which have thick muscular walls. The left ventricle, which is thicker than the right, receives blood from the pulmonary veins via the left atrium and pumps it into the aorta. The right ventricle pumps blood received from the venae cavae and coronary sinus (via the right atrium) into the pulmonary trunk. **2.** One of the four fluid-filled cavities within the brain (see illustration). The paired first and second ventricles (*lateral ventricles*), one in each cerebral hemisphere, communicate with the third ventricle in the midline between them. This in turn leads through a narrow channel, the *cerebral aqueduct*, to the fourth ventricle in the hindbrain. This is continuous with the spinal canal in the centre of the spinal cord, and also communicates, via its paired lateral apertures and single median aperture (when present), with the surrounding subarachnoid space. *Cerebrospinal fluid circulates through all the cavities; it is produced by the *choroid plexus of the ventricles. **3.** The paired cavity in the *larynx lying between

the vestibular folds and vocal folds. It is absent in ruminants.

ventricul- (ventriculo-) *Prefix denoting* a ventricle (of the brain or heart).

ventricular system The series of interconnected cavities within the brain. *See* ventricle.

ventriculus (*pl.* **ventriculi**) **1.** The stomach. **2.** Part of the avian stomach, otherwise termed the muscular part of the stomach or the gizzard. It has a thick muscular wall, which squeezes and grinds ingested food.

venule A minute vessel that drains blood from the capillaries. Many venules unite to form a vein.

vermicide An agent that destroys worms, especially parasitic worms. *See* anthelmintic.

vermifuge An agent that induces the expulsion of intestinal worms, either by killing them directly or by acting as a purgative. *See* anthelmintic.

verminous Describing a condition caused by parasitic worms; for example, *equine verminous arteritis.

verminous arteritis Inflammation of the arteries due to infestation with parasitic worms. *See* equine verminous arteritis.

verminous bronchitis (parasitic bronchitis) Inflammation of the bronchi due to infestation with parasitic worms. *See also* gapes; lungworm.

verminous dermatitis Inflammation of the skin by *nematodes. This may arise in three different ways. Firstly by migration of parasite larvae through the skin of the host to their final site in other tissues. For example, dogs exercised over ground

verminous ophthalmia

infested with larvae of the hookworm *Uncinaria stenocephala* may suffer dermatitis of the feet and ventral body surfaces as the larvae pass through the skin en route to the intestine, where they mature. In another example, larvae of *Onchocerca cervicalis* are deposited in the skin of horses by midges; these may produce serpentine tracts in the skin (creeping eruption) before finally passing to the ligamentum nuchae. Secondly, mature worms may pass to the skin from the internal organs so that infective larvae may be discharged. An example of this is the guinea worm (*Dracunculus medinensis*), which parasitizes humans in Africa and Asia. Thirdly, nonparasitic nematode larvae (e.g. *Pelodera strongyloidis*) present in filthy bedding may penetrate the skin of dogs, horses, cattle, and other animals via abrasions. Such larvae can probably only penetrate the skin of animals that have scratched themselves, due, for instance, to itching associated with ectoparasitism.

verminous ophthalmia Inflammation of the eye caused by parasitic worms. The best known examples are due to *Toxocara canis*, a common roundworm of dogs (*see* toxocariasis), and the various *eyeworms. See also* onchocerciasis; periodic ophthalmia.

vermis The middle region of the *cerebellum, lying between its two hemispheres.

vernier A device for obtaining accurate measurements of length, to 1/10, 1/100, or smaller fractions of a unit. It consists of a fixed graduated main scale against which a shorter vernier scale slides. The vernier scale is graduated into divisions equal to 9/10 of the smallest unit marked on the main scale. The vernier scale is often adjusted by means of a screw thread. A reading is taken by observing which of the markings on the scales coincide.

verruca *See* papilloma.

version The process of turning a foetus in the uterus during a difficult birth (*dystocia). *See also* presentation.

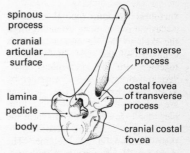

Thoracic vertebra of dog (cranial lateral aspect)

vertebra (*pl.* **vertebrae**) One of the bones of which the *vertebral column is composed. Each vertebra typically consists of a body (*centrum*) and a dorsal arch (*neural arch*) consisting of paired *pedicles* and a *lamina*. The body and arch together enclose the *vertebral foramen*, through which the spinal cord passes. The arch has a *spinous process* dorsally, paired *transverse processes* laterally, and paired cranial and caudal *articular processes*, which articulate with the adjacent vertebrae in the vertebral column. See illustration.

vertebral canal The cylindrical cavity within the *vertebral column formed by the series of vertebral foramina (*see* vertebra) and the interconnecting ligaments between adjacent vertebral arches. It accommodates the *spinal cord, the *meninges, and the *cauda equina.

Composition of the vertebral column in various species

Vertebrae	Horse	Ox	Sheep	Pig	Dog
Cervical	7	7	7	7	7
Thoracic	18	13	13	14–15	13
Lumbar	6	6	6–7	6–7	7
Sacral	5	5	4	4	3
Coccygeal	15–21	18–20	16–18	20–23	20–23

vertebral column (spinal column)
A flexible rod of bone extending from the skull to the tip of the tail. It is composed of the series of *vertebrae together with the intervening *intervertebral discs, all bound together by a series of ligaments. The vertebrae are designated cervical, thoracic, lumbar, sacral (fused together to form the sacrum), or coccygeal, according to their location in the column. The numbers of each type vary with species (see table). The vertebral column forms joints with the skull (atlantooccipital joints), with the ribs (costovertebral joints), and with the ossa coxarum (sacroiliac joints). In the domestic fowl the column is divided into cervical, thoracic, lumbosacral, and caudal regions. Three regions of fusion occur, forming the *notarium* (thoracic), *synsacrum* (lumbosacral), and *pygostyle* (caudal). *See also* vertebral canal.

vesicant An agent that is applied locally to the skin to cause severe and acute inflammation and blisters. Vesicants, such as mercuric iodide and cantharides, were formerly used as 'counterirritants' in the treatment of chronic inflammatory conditions (tendonitis, arthritis, bone splints, etc.) in horses. The induced inflammation was thought to improve the blood supply and drainage from the area and ultimately clear the site of chronic inflammation. However, it is now thought that any benefit was achieved by the ensuing enforced rest rather than by the vesicants. The use of vesicants is now considered to be harmful rather than beneficial.

vesicle 1. A small blister in the skin that is filled with clear fluid (serum). It may rupture to leave a raw surface, or undergo ulceration. Vesicles are characteristic of many diseases, including foot-and-mouth disease, orf, swine vesicular disease, and vesicular stomatitis. **2.** (in anatomy) Any small pocket, cavity, or bladder, especially one filled with fluid, such as the paired *seminal vesicles.

vesicular exanthema A disease of pigs and sea mammals caused by a *calicivirus and characterized in pigs by fever and vesicles on the snout, lips, tongue, and feet. The disease in pigs has only been reported from the western coast of North America. Following an incubation period of 2 days vesicles develop in the mouth, on the snout, and on the coronary bands of the feet. The affected pig is lame and salivates. Vesicular exanthema has not been diagnosed in pigs since 1956, but because the lesions are indistinguishable from those caused by *footand-mouth disease, vesicular exanthema remains a *notifiable disease.

vesicular stomatitis A disease affecting cattle, pigs, horses, sheep, goats, and many species of wild animals that is caused by *vesiculoviruses and is characterized by a fever and vesicles in the mouth. It is enzootic in parts of North and South America. The incubation period is 2–4 days followed by a fever and the development of vesicles in the mouth, although lesions may develop on the coronary band of the foot in pigs or on the teats in cattle. The affected animal salivates and has a reduced appetite. Transmission is by contact between infected and susceptible animals, and the virus probably enters the body through existing skin abrasions or via biting insects. The disease is rare in sheep and goats. Because the lesions of vesicular stomatitis are indistinguishable in cattle and pigs from those caused by *foot-and-mouth disease, the disease is notifiable (*see* notifiable disease). Humans are susceptible to infection with the virus, which causes a mild influenza-like disease.

vesiculitis Inflammation of a vesicle, especially the *seminal vesicle, or vesicle gland. This may occur as a result of infection with *Brucella abortus* or *B. ovis* by extension of lesions in the epididymis (*see* epididymitis). Occasionally, seminal fluid or sperm may penetrate the connective tissue of the seminal vesicle to form a spermatocele, which causes an inflammatory reaction and abscess.

vesiculopapular Describing a skin condition that has both *vesicles and *papules.

vesiculopustular Describing a skin condition that has both *vesicles and *pustules.

vesiculovirus A genus of the *rhabdovirus family. It contains the viruses responsible for *vesicular stomatitis in cattle, horses, pigs, and sheep.

vessel A tube conveying a body fluid, especially a blood vessel or a lymphatic vessel.

vestibular apparatus The semicircular canals, utricle, and saccule of the internal *ear.

vestibular fold A fold of mucous membrane in the lateral wall of the *larynx, just cranial to the *ventricle. It occurs in the horse and the dog.

vestibular glands The two pairs of mucus-secreting glands – *major* and *minor vestibular glands* – situated in the wall of the *vestibule between the vagina and vulva. Their secretions lubricate the genital tract.

vestibular nerve *See* vestibulocochlear nerve.

vestibular nuclei A group of paired nuclei in the medulla oblongata and pons of the brain. Comprising *rostral*, *caudal*, *lateral*, and *medial vestibular nuclei*, they make connections with the vestibular division of the *vestibulocochlear nerve, the cerebellum, the cranial nerves governing eye movements, and the spinal cord via the *vestibulospinal tracts*. They are important in coordinating muscular activity to maintain equilibrium and balance.

vestibule (in anatomy) A cavity situated at the entrance to a hollow organ. The vestibule of the *ear is the part of the bony labyrinth that accommodates the utricle and the saccule. The vestibule of the mouth is the cleft-like space between the lips and cheeks and the teeth and gums (*see* oral cavity). The vestibule of the *vagina extends from where the urethra opens at the caudal limit of the vagina to the vulva; in the cow and sow it includes the suburethral diverticulum. The vestibule of the *larynx is the region of the laryngeal cavity extending from the laryngeal inlet to the vocal folds.

vestibulocochlear nerve (acoustic nerve; auditory nerve) The eighth *cranial nerve (VIII), responsible for the transmission of nervous impulses from the internal ear to the brain. It has two divisions: the *vestibular division* carries impulses from the semicircular canals, utricle, and saccule, which are concerned with posture, movement, and balance; the *cochlear division* carries impulses from the *spiral organ in the cochlea and is the nerve associated with hearing.

vestigial Existing only in a rudimentary form. The term is applied to organs whose structure and function have diminished during the course of evolution until only a rudimentary structure exists.

veterinarian A graduate of a college of veterinary medicine who holds one of several recognized degrees. Veterinarians are usually licensed by a government agency or some body to whom authority has been delegated (e.g. *Royal College of Veterinary Surgeons, *State Boards of Veterinary Medicine). Licensed veterinarians are permitted to perform *veterinary surgery, as well as participate in animal disease control, meat inspection, veterinary research, and other activities in veterinary science. *See also* veterinary surgeon.

veterinary ethics *See* Guide to Professional Conduct.

Veterinary Investigation (VI) Centre (UK) Any of several regional centres, run as part of the *State Veterinary Service, that provide laboratory facilities and the expertise of full-time veterinary investigation officers for examining samples from farm animals submitted by veterinarians in practice and for investigating disease problems.

veterinary legislation *See* Legislation Affecting the Veterinary Profession in the United Kingdom.

veterinary nurse A person included in the List of Veterinary Nurses who has been trained and examined in accordance with the veterinary nursing byelaws of the *Royal College of Veterinary Surgeons (RCVS). They were formerly known as Registered Animal Nursing Auxiliaries (RANAs).

veterinary practitioner In the UK, a person who is permitted by the *Veterinary Surgeons Act (1966) to carry out limited forms of veterinary surgery and who is listed in the Supplementary Veterinary Register. This is a closed category of persons who although experienced in aspects of veterinary practice, qualified before 1948 and do not hold a university veterinary degree.

Veterinary Products Committee (UK) An advisory body established under the *Medicines Act (1968) to advise the Secretary of State for Agriculture on the safety, quality, and efficacy of veterinary medical products. The Committee also collects and investigates reports of adverse reactions to these products.

veterinary specialist A person with knowledge of a particular veterinary speciality. In the UK, the *Veterinary Surgeons Act (1966) does not provide for the status of a veterinary specialist or consultant. However, the *Royal College of Veterinary Surgeons examines for and awards fellowships, diplomas, and certificates in certain specialities.

veterinary student A person who is studying on a recognized university veterinary course. He or she may, as part of his or her clinical training, examine animals and, under varying degrees of direction and supervision of a *veterinary surgeon, treat and operate upon animals in accordance with the Veterinary Surgeons (Practice by Students) Regulations Order in Council (1981).

veterinary surgeon A licensed *veterinarian who provides medical and surgical treatment for animals in accordance with the legislation regulating the veterinary profession. In the UK the *Veterinary Surgeons Act (1966) requires that such a person must be registered with the *Royal College of Veterinary Surgeons, bearing either of the titles Member or Fellow of the Royal College of Veterinary Surgeons (MRCVS or FRCVS), or *veterinary practitioner. Registration and the title of MRCVS is granted for those holding a UK, EEC, or certain other recognized university veterinary degrees (*see* Register of Veterinary Surgeons). Temporary registration (without the title of MRCVS) is available for holders of other overseas veterinary qualifications, granting a limited right to practise. In the USA, veterinarians are licensed in each state by the *State Boards of Veterinary Medicine.

Veterinary Surgeons Act (1966) (UK) An Act of Parliament that regulates the veterinary profession in the UK. It establishes the *Royal College of Veterinary Surgeons (RCVS), provides for the recognition of *veterinary surgeons, and vests disciplinary control in the RCVS. The Act also defines *veterinary surgery and those who practise it.

veterinary surgery The art and science of veterinary medicine and surgery. In the UK this is defined by the *Veterinary Surgeons Act (1966) to include the diagnosis of diseases and injuries in animals, the giving of advice based on such diagnosis, and the medical and surgical treatment of animals. In general, veterinary surgery must be performed by a *veterinary surgeon or a *veterinary practitioner registered with the *Royal College of Veterinary Surgeons under the Veterinary Surgeons Act (1966) whether the animal is domesticated or wild and whether or not a fee is charged. The Act applies to all species except fish (and possibly amphibians) and invertebrates. Specific exceptions in the Act permit any person to provide first aid for an animal in an emergency; for example, this may be performed by the owner of an animal, a member of the owner's family, or an employee. Certain animal husbandry and other procedures may be performed by non-veterinarians or by students in restricted circumstances (*see* veterinary student).

veterinary technician US term for a *veterinary nurse.

Veterinary Written Direction (VWD) *See* Medicines (Medicated Animal Feeding Stuffs) Regulations (1985).

Vibrio A genus of aerobic or facultatively anaerobic rod-shaped or curved *bacteria, some of which require added salt for growth. Commonly found as saprophytes in surface and sea water, some species are pathogenic to humans, for example *V. cholerae*, which causes human cholera.

Vibrio fetus *See* Campylobacter.

vibrionic abortion *See* campylobacteriosis of sheep; campylobacteriosis of cattle.

vibrissa (*pl.* **vibrissae**) A stiff coarse hair, especially one of the stiff hairs that lie just inside the nostrils.

vices Any of various behavioural disturbances, which may result in economic loss, injury, or death. In poultry they include *feather pecking, *cannibalism, and *egg-eating; examples in horses are *crib-biting and *wind-sucking. Others are sucking (in cattle) and tail-biting (in pigs).

villus (*pl.* **villi**) One of many short finger-like processes that project from the surface of some membranes. Numerous *intestinal villi* project from the circular folds in the small *intestine. Each contains a network of blood capillaries and a *lacteal. Their function is to absorb the products of digestion and they greatly increase the surface area over which this can occur. *Chorionic villi* are projections from the outer surface of the *chorion in the placenta, where they provide an extensive area for the exchange of oxygen, carbon dioxide, nutrients, and waste products between the maternal and foetal circulations. *Arachnoid villi* are fine processes projecting from the *arachnoid into the venous sinuses of the dura mater to allow cerebrospinal fluid to pass into the venous system.

vincristine A cytotoxic alkaloid, extracted from the periwinkle plant, used as an antitumour agent. In cells it binds to the spindle protein tubulin, disrupting the mitotic process and preventing cell division. It also affects the formation of microtubules, which are necessary for intracellular transport. Vincristine is most toxic to rapidly dividing cells, and is administered orally in the *chemotherapy of lymphosarcoma and mastocytoma in dogs, usually in combination with other agents (such as *cyclophosphamide, cytosine arabinoside, and prednisolone). The tumour is not usually completely destroyed but the survival time of the patient is extended. Side-effects include bone marrow depression, gastrointestinal disturbances, and peripheral neuropathy.

vinculum (*pl.* **vincula**) A connecting band of tissue. The *vincula tendinum* are threadlike bands of synovial membrane that carry blood vessels to the flexor tendons of the digits.

viraemia The presence of infectious virus particles in the circulating blood. Viruses may be either free in the plasma or associated with the white or red blood cells. Many viruses are disseminated throughout the body by the circulating blood, usually following an initial stage of replication at the site of entry into the host. As the infected host starts to develop an immune response to the virus, free viruses in the circulating plasma are usually reduced and eventually eliminated. However, some viruses, such as *bluetongue virus, can remain in the red blood cells for the lifetime of the infected cells (up to 120 days). Other viruses may infect the white cells responsible for the development of the immune response, while yet others fail to stimulate the development of an effective immune response in the host.

viral arthritis *See* viral tenosynovitis.

viral haemorrhagic septicaemia An infectious disease of salmon and trout characterized by lethargy, prominent eyes (exophthalmia), haemorrhages on the gills, and death. It is caused by a *rhabdovirus, which is present in Europe but absent from North America and Japan. Disease is typically seen in intensively farmed fish in late autumn, winter, and early spring when water temperatures are lowest, particularly when below 8°C. Young fish are most severely affected and mortality may reach 80%, although all age groups are susceptible. Following an incubation period of 5–20 days, affected fish become

viral hepatitis

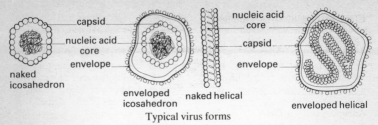

Typical virus forms

lethargic and many die; others survive longer, developing exophthalmia, gill haemorrhages, and a dark skin. Raising the water temperature above 15°C can reduce the mortality, although the virus will persist in the fish. It is a *notifiable disease in the UK. *Compare* infectious haematopoietic necrosis.

viral hepatitis *See* canine viral hepatitis.

viral tenosynovitis (viral arthritis) A disease of young broilers characterized by inflammation of the tendon sheaths of the hindlimbs. Caused by a *reovirus infection, the disease generally affects birds from 5 weeks old and causes leg weakness and unthriftiness. The virus is probably often present without clinical signs appearing. However, in extreme cases up to 50% of a flock may show signs; other infections may occur concurrently. Vaccines are used in a number of countries.

virion The infective particle of a *virus. It consists of a protein shell (capsid), which is commonly icosahedral or helical in shape. The capsid encloses the viral nucleic acid and is itself enclosed by an *envelope in some virus families (see table at virus).

virology The scientific study of *viruses.

virulence The disease-producing (pathogenic) ability of a microorganism. *See also* attenuation.

virulent (virology) Describing a virus that interacts with a host cell so as to cause the death of the cell and the release of many progeny *virions. *Compare* latency; temperate.

virus A noncellular infective agent that reproduces only in an appropriate host cell, outside of which it is totally inert. Viruses can infect animal, plant, or bacterial cells (*see* bacteriophage) and many are important agents of disease; they differ in their host range. The infective particle (*virion) consists of a core of nucleic acid (either DNA or RNA) surrounded by a protein shell (capsid); some bear an outer *envelope (see illustration). After entering a suitable cell, the virus utilizes the cell's *ribosomes and other apparatus to produce many thousands of progeny virions. These are released when the host cell disintegrates. The most common virus–cell interaction is this *virulent or lytic type. However, viruses can enter other types of interaction with their host, for example *latency. *Oncogenic viruses are capable of transforming host cells into a cancerous state.

Viruses are classified into families and genera: eleven families of RNA viruses and seven DNA virus families have so far been distinguished (see table), largely on the criteria of virion

Classification of virus families

Virus family	Nucleic acid type	Molecular weight ($\times 10^6$) of nucleic acid*	Capsid	Envelope
Adenovirus	dsDNA	25	icosahedral	–
Arenavirus	ssRNA(–)	2–3 ($\times 3$)	coil	+
Bunyavirus	ssRNA(–)	3,2,0.5	helical	+
Calicivirus	ssRNA(+)	2.7	icosahedral	–
Coronavirus	ssRNA(+)	6	helical	+
Hepadnavirus	ss/dsDNA	1.5		
Herpesvirus	dsDNA	100–150	icosahedral	+
Iridovirus	dsDNA	200	'brick'	+
Orthomyxovirus	ssRNA(–)	0.2–1 ($\times 8$)	helical	+
Papovavirus	dsDNA	3–10	icosahedral	–
Paramyxovirus	ssRNA(–/+)	5–7	helical	+
Parvovirus	ssDNA(–/+)	1.5		–
Picornavirus	ssRNA(+)	2.5	icosahedral	–
Poxvirus	dsDNA	200	'brick'	+
Reovirus	dsRNA	0.3–2.7 ($\times 10$)	icosahedral	–
Retrovirus	ssRNA(+)	3 ($\times 2$)	icosahedral	+
Rhabdovirus	ssRNA(–)	4	helical	+
Togavirus	ssRNA(+)	4	icosahedral	–

* Some families have segmented genomes in which the viral nucleic acid is in a number of pieces (shown in brackets) rather than a single molecule. The retroviruses have two copies of a ssRNA molecule, i.e. these viruses are diploid.

structure and mode of replication. The nucleic acid may be double- (ds) or single-stranded (ss), and viruses with single-stranded RNA may be positive- (+) or *negative-strand (–) viruses, depending on whether or not the RNA codes directly for viral proteins. In some, the viral nucleic acid is in a number of pieces instead of a single molecule.

*Vaccines can provide good protection against viral diseases, and *antiviral agents may have limited usefulness in treatment. Antibiotics are ineffective against viruses.

virus encephalitis *See* encephalitis.

virus pneumonia *See* calf pneumonia.

viscera (*sing.* **viscus**) The organs within the body cavities, especially the organs of the abdominal cavities (stomach, intestines, etc.).

visceral gout *See* gout.

visceral larva migrans *See* toxocariasis.

viscus *See* viscera.

visna *See* maedi/visna.

visual purple *See* rhodopsin.

vital centre Any of the collections of nerve cells in the brain that act as governing centres for different vital body functions – such as breathing, heart rate, blood pressure, temperature control etc. – making reflex adjustments according to the body's needs. Most lie in the hypothalamus and brainstem.

vitamin One of a group of organic compounds, distinct from *essential amino acids and *essential fatty acids, that are required in small amounts for normal growth, production, reproduction, and maintenance of animals. When an animal cannot synthesize a particular vitamin, either at all or not in quantities sufficient to meet its requirements, that vitamin must be supplied in the diet. Fourteen vitamins are generally recognized: the *fat-soluble vitamins* A (retinol), D (calciferols), E (tocopherols), and K (quinones, menaphthones); and the *water-soluble vitamins* C (ascorbic acid) and the B-complex – B_1 (aneurin, thiamin), B_2 (riboflavin), B_6 (pyridoxine), B_{12} (cyanocobalamin), biotin, choline, folic acid (folacin), nicotinic acid (nicotinamide, niacin), and pantothenic acid. Other compounds, for example carnitine, inositol, orotic acid, pangamic acid, para-aminobenzoic acid, ubiquinones, and vitamin U (or S-methylmethionine sulphonium salts), have not been proven as essential to vertebrates and

are not generally accepted as vitamins.

Foods may serve as a source of a vitamin itself or of its precursors (*provitamins*), which are chemically changed to the active form of the vitamin in the body. Some vitamins are synthesized by microorganisms, including those in the intestines of animals. However, this source can be unreliable, and if synthesis is mainly in the large intestine coprophagia (ingestion of faeces) may be required for the animal to benefit. In ruminants microbial synthesis of the B-complex vitamins and vitamin K in the rumen is generally adequate to meet requirements, although synthesis of thiamin and vitamin B_{12} may be insufficient in certain conditions. Milk-fed preruminants which do not have a fully functional reticulorumen, require dietary sources of all vitamins. Many vitamins are destroyed by oxidation, a process that is accelerated by light and heat (e.g. in the processing and storage of diets) and by acids, alkalis, and certain metals (such as iron), which are found in vitamin/mineral premixes and in diets. The dietary requirements of a vitamin are affected by the nature of the diet and the animals' health and metabolic or productive states.

Deficiency of a vitamin may cause disease, the clinical signs of which depend partly on the vitamin's metabolic role. *Avitaminosis*, i.e. a total lack of a particular vitamin, is usually caused by feeding very unbalanced diets and is very uncommon. Partial lack of a particular vitamin (i.e. *hypovitaminosis*) is more common but often causes only nonspecific signs of deficiency, for example poor appetite, low growth and productivity, poor reproductive efficiency, and increased susceptibility to infection. Diagnoses of avitaminoses and hypovitaminoses can be assisted by laboratory tests, although some mild hypovitaminoses are most easily diagnosed by determining the responses of the animals to supplementation with the particular vitamin. Treatment of hypovitaminoses may be either by parenteral supplementation or, more commonly, by supplementation of the diet and/or changing the composition of the diet. However, excessive intakes of a vitamin may also cause disease (*see* hypervitaminosis).

vitamin A (retinol) A fat-soluble *vitamin that is required for the formation of visual pigments (e.g. *rhodopsin) and for the normal metabolic functions of many cells and tissues, especially epithelial tissues and bones. Good sources include liver, fish-liver oils, milk fat, colostrum, and eggs. Some plant carotenoid pigments, for example β-*carotene, can act as provitamins A and can be converted to vitamin A in the gut and liver of most animal species, except cats. The efficiency of this conversion is low and variable. Carrots and green grasses are good sources of provitamins A, but most cereals, except maize (corn), contain very little. Well-preserved grass silages and green grass hays are moderate sources of the provitamins. Liver stores of vitamin A are variable but can be adequate for several months in, for example, grazing animals. Vitamin A is easily destroyed by heat, air, moisture, sunlight, and some metallic ions. There is controversy about whether or not β-carotene itself is required by fish and cattle. In cattle it is claimed to be required for normal oestrus, ovulation, and conception rates. Maize silages and straws have lower contents of β-carotene than grass silages.

Vitamin A deficiency In cattle deficiencies are most likely in animals given large quantities of cereals, for example barley beef, and in store cattle and the calves of dams fed poor-quality feeds, such as straw, poor hay, or root crops, for several months.

Similarly, cereal-based diets for pigs and poultry also require vitamin A supplementation, as do cat diets comprising solely plant-derived foods. Also, dogs and cats given meat diets that exclude liver may become deficient.

Deficiency signs are many and varied, and include decreased ability to see in dim light (*night blindness), poor appetite, and decreased productivity. There may be *osteodystrophies, causing shortening and thickening of bones and failure of foramina to widen, which may cause, for example, blindness, deafness, and paralysis. There may be increased pressure of the cerebrospinal fluid, and degeneration and keratinization of epithelial structures, causing a wide variety of signs, including papilloedema (swelling of the optic nerve), incoordination, deafness, blindness, convulsions, *xerophthalmia, *keratitis, and conjunctivitis. Impairment of epithelial structures in the gastrointestinal, respiratory, urinary, and reproductive tracts may cause increased incidences of enteritis, pneumonia, urinary calculi, and infertility respectively. The signs of infertility include abortions, stillbirths, foetal malformations, weak neonates, high incidence of retained placenta, decreased ovarian size with low conception rates and abnormalities of oestrous cycles, and testicular atrophy. In fish, eye lesions are common signs of vitamin A deficiency. For diagnosis and treatment *see* vitamin.

Hypervitaminosis A occurs most commonly in domestic cats fed for several months on diets either containing large quantities of fish-liver oils or based mainly on liver. Signs include cervical spondylosis, lameness, gingivitis, weight loss, and poor ungroomed hair coat.

vitamin B₁ (thiamin; thiamine) A *vitamin of the B-complex that, as the diphosphate ester, is an essential coenzyme in carbohydrate metabolism, for example in glycolysis and the *Krebs cycle. It is synthesized by most plants and microorganisms, including the microorganisms in the reticulorumen and large intestine of animals. Good natural sources are liver, eggs, milk, yeast, the pericarp and germ of cereal grains, and many green plants. Vitamin B₁ is destroyed by heat, moisture, and alkaline conditions, and large losses may result from various food preservation methods, including pelleting, extruding, canning, gamma irradiation, and additions of sodium metabisulphite and sulphur dioxide. Losses of 10% per month may be expected in stored foods. The vitamin is destroyed by certain antagonists, including amprolium (a drug used in the control of coccidiosis) and thiaminase enzymes, which are found in raw fish, ferns (bracken), moulds, and bacteria (including some bacteria found in the gut of animals). Thiaminases are destroyed by cooking.

Vitamin B₁ deficiency This is uncommon in pigs and poultry given cereal-based diets. However, deficiencies in these species, as well as in humans and other animals, including fish, usually occur because of the vitamin's destruction during food processing or by thiaminases in the diet or in the gut. Initial signs of deficiency may include anorexia, weight loss, diarrhoea, muscular weakness, and cramps; later there may be signs of paralysis, such as incoordination, blindness, nystagmus, circling, altered sensitivity to stimuli, hypothermia, opisthotonus, spasm, and convulsions. However, the onset of signs may be rapid and include those of paralysis, followed a few hours later by coma and death. In some cases, especially humans, pigs, and poultry, there may be abnormal cardiac rhythms and heart failure. Specific deficiency disorders include *polyneuritis (in poultry), *cerebrocortical necrosis (or polioencephalomalacia) (in cattle and sheep), brain rot and blind staggers (in ruminants), *chastek paralysis (in fur-bearing animals), and *beri-beri (in humans). For diagnosis and treatment see vitamin. Other names: **aneurin**; **aneurine**.

vitamin B₂ (riboflavin) A *vitamin of the B-complex that is a constituent of the flavoprotein coenzymes *FMN (flavin mononucleotide) and *FAD (flavin dinucleotide), which are essential to the transfer of hydrogen in the metabolism of carbohydrates, fats, and amino acids, and in cellular respiration. It is synthesized by most green plants and microorganisms, including those in the gut of animals. Good natural sources include liver, milk, yeast, animal protein meals, wheat bran, soya-bean meal, and groundnut (peanut) meal. Cereals are poor sources. The vitamin has good stability to heat but is rapidly destroyed by light and alkaline solutions. It may be antagonized metabolically by mycotoxins.

Vitamin B₂ deficiency The requirements of non-milk-fed ruminants are met by microbial synthesis of the vitamin in the reticulorumen. In monogastric animals and milk-fed ruminants deficiencies are likely with inadequately supplemented cereal-based diets. Initial signs are loss of appetite, poor growth, and low productivity; later there is diarrhoea, inflammation of mucosae, dermatitis, paralysis, and, especially in fish, dogs, and cats, eye lesions, including conjunctivitis, cataracts, and vascularization and opacity of the cornea. In pigs there may be increased incidences of anoestrus and stillbirths. Poultry may show decreased hatchability of eggs, with embryos and/or hatched chicks showing characteristic coiling or 'clubbing' of the down feathers and degeneration of peripheral nerves causing the chicks to walk on their hocks with toes curled inwards (*curled toe paralysis). For diagnosis and treatment see vitamin. Other name: **lactoflavin**.

vitamin B$_6$ (pyridoxine; pyridoxamine; pyridoxal) A *vitamin of the B-complex that is required for the synthesis of pyridoxal phosphate, a coenzyme essential to many metabolic processes involving amino acids, including the synthesis of *serotonin, *haemoglobin, and *globulins. The vitamin is synthesized by most plants and microorganisms, including microorganisms in the reticulorumen and large intestine of animals. Good natural sources are liver, eggs, milk, yeast, wheat bran, maize (corn) gluten, soya-bean meal, cottonseed meal, and fish meals. Cereals and green plants contain moderate amounts. Pyridoxine, pyridoxamine, and pyridoxal are different forms of vitamin B$_6$ with similar activity. They are destroyed by heat and light.

Vitamin B$_6$ deficiency This is uncommon because of the vitamin's wide distribution. Ruminants obtain adequate supplies from microbial synthesis in the gut. Monogastric animals and milk-fed ruminants may rely on coprophagia (ingestion of faeces) to utilize microbial synthesis in the large intestine. Requirements are increased by high dietary protein levels and by the antagonists *diethylstilboestrol and the *sulphonamides. Initial signs of deficiency are loss of appetite, poor growth, and low productivity; later there is diarrhoea, hyperkeratosis (often with secondary infection), anaemia, lymphocytopenia, and disturbances of nerve function, producing some weakness, incoordination, increased irritability, and convulsions. Poultry may show decreased hatchability of eggs with increased embryonic mortalities, while in cats there may be renal tubular damage. Some species of fish exhibit greenish-blue discoloration of the skin. For diagnosis and treatment see vitamin.

vitamin B$_{12}$ (cyanocobalamin) A *vitamin of the B-complex that, with *folic acid, is required as a cofactor in the enzymatic transfer of one-carbon groups in the metabolism of, for example, propionate, nucleic acids, fats, and methionine. It contains the element *cobalt and has several physiologically inactive analogues. Natural synthesis of the vitamin is performed only by microorganisms, including those found in the reticulorumen and intestine. Plant-derived foods contain little or no vitamin B$_{12}$, and its content in animal protein feeds varies greatly with methods of processing. Good natural sources are fish meals, liver, kidney, eggs, and milk. The vitamin is moderately stable in the presence of moisture but is affected by heat, light, oxidizing agents, acids, and alkalis. In most animals its absorption from the gut is greatly enhanced by glycoprotein carriers (*intrinsic factors), which are secreted by the gastric and/or duodenal mucosae.

Vitamin B$_{12}$ deficiency This is uncommon in monogastric animals and milk-fed ruminants but is common in ruminants given cobalt-deficient diets or grazing pastures with cobalt-deficient soil. Animals fed exclusively on plant foods and kept on floors uncontaminated with faeces may also develop deficiency. Normal body reserves of the vitamin are usually sufficient to prevent deficiency for several weeks. Young animals are more susceptible to deficiencies than adults. Initial signs are loss of appetite and poor growth; later there is anaemia, leucopenia, dermatitis, and neurological impairment. Poultry exhibit increased embryonic deaths in the week before hatching; pigs suffer decreased reproductive performance. Deficiency signs in ruminants include poor growth, weight loss, low milk yields, and a preference for roughage instead of concentrates. There may be increased incidences of *ketosis in cattle, of *pregnancy toxaemia in ewes, and of mortality in lambs. Sub-clinical cobalt deficiencies that cause poor growth rates are important economically. For diagnosis and treatment see vitamin.

Pharmacologically, vitamin B_{12} has been used as an appetite stimulant. Other names: **cobalamin**; **hydroxycobalamine**; **animal protein factor**.

vitamin C (ascorbic acid) A water-soluble *vitamin required for metabolic oxidation-reduction reactions, transport of iron, synthesis of corticosteroids, and formation of intercellular substances and collagen in connective tissues, bone, cartilage, and dentine. In most vertebrates it is synthesized from glucose in quantities sufficient to meet normal requirements; exceptions include humans, other primates, guinea pigs, some species of fish, and possibly very young animals, such as newborn calves and newly hatched chicks. Good natural sources include fresh green plants, citrus fruits, liver, and kidney. It has low stability and considerable losses may occur in the processing and storage of food.

Vitamin C deficiency The signs are similar to those of scurvy in humans and include decreased appetite and growth; weakness, swellings, and haemorrhages in gums, joints, and serosal surfaces; and increased susceptibility to infections. In all species it may be important for resistance to *stress. However, the benefits of additional vitamin C in conditions of stress, and in hypertrophic *osteodystrophy in dogs, are uncertain. Deficiency in fish causes poor appetite and lethargy, skeletal deformities, abnormal cartilages in the eyes, gills, and fins, and internal haemorrhages. For diagnosis and treatment see vitamin.

vitamin D (calciferol; cholecalciferol) A fat-soluble *vitamin

that is required, with parathyrin, calcitonin, and calcium-binding protein, for the incorporation and maintenance of calcium and phosphate in bones, teeth, and eggshells. It stimulates the absorption of calcium and phosphate from the intestine and their reabsorption from the renal tubules. Good natural sources include liver, fish-liver oils, kidney, milk, eggs, and sun-cured hay. However, most plant and animal tissues contain only the vitamin D precursors *ergosterol* and *dehydrocholesterol*, respectively. Animals absorb these and secrete them onto their skin, where the precursors are converted by ultraviolet light to *ergocalciferol* (*vitamin D_2*) and *cholecalciferol* (*vitamin D_3*). These are reabsorbed and metabolized to active forms. In mammals, but not in birds, vitamin D_3 has similar activity to vitamin D_2. The precursors and vitamins are destroyed by light, moisture, heavy metals, and pelleting of diets. Some *mycotoxins may interfere with vitamin D metabolism.

Vitamin D deficiency This is likely to occur in animals kept (indoors or outdoors) in the more northerly or southerly latitudes and/or in industrial haze. Animals normally have sufficient stores of the vitamin to prevent deficiency for several weeks. Requirements increase with growth rates, and are least if both the absolute quantities and the ratios of calcium to phosphate in diets are optimal. Certain foods, including fresh green cereals and yeast in diets of mammals, and raw liver and isolated soya-bean protein in diets of poultry, may greatly increase vitamin D requirements. Deficiency signs include poor appetite, apathy, muscular weakness, stunted growth, poor dentition, and *rickets (in young animals) and *osteomalacia (in adults). Poultry may also have low egg productivity and low hatchability of eggs, with increased proportions of thin, soft, or cracked eggshells. In cattle deficiency may cause poor irregular oestrus, with delayed onset of oestrus after calving. For diagnosis and treatment *see* vitamin.

Large doses of vitamin D or, preferably, its metabolite 1,25-dihydroxycholecalciferol, may be used to prevent *milk fever. Excessive intakes may cause toxicity, with signs including metastatic calcification and *osteodystrophies.

vitamin E (α-tocopherol) A fat-soluble *vitamin required in the body principally as a biological antioxidant to prevent the formation of peroxides, which can damage cells, especially the phospholipids of cell membranes. Vitamin E is thus essential for the maintenance of cellular and organelle membranes, and also for normal reproduction, muscular function, and blood capillary integrity. Any peroxides that do form are normally inactivated by the selenium-containing enzyme, glutathione peroxidase. Hence, vitamin E and selenium (Se) have complementary metabolic roles, and deficiency of either or both may produce similar clinical signs.

There are several naturally occurring forms of vitamin E, including various tocopherols and tocotrienols. However, the biological activity of forms other than α-tocopherol is low. Good sources include milk, colostrum, animal fats, green plants, green fodders, well-preserved anaerobic silages, alfalfa, and wheat bran. Whole dry wheat and barley grains are moderate sources. Natural vitamin E is readily oxidized in the presence of heat, air, and moisture, although the acetate ester is more stable. Large losses occur as a result of hay-making, the storage of feeds (especially if stored moist), food processing, and the presence of alkalis and polyunsaturated fats/fatty acids (PUFAs). With high-fat diets, synthetic antioxidants are valuable in preserving vitamin E. Dietary requirements are increased as the dietary fat content increases, and with the presence of mycotoxins. Absorption of the vitamin from the intestine is facilitated by the presence of digestible fats, and unlike vitamins A and D, vitamin E is not preferentially stored in the liver.

Vitamin E deficiency The clinical signs of deficiency are many and varied. In **ruminants** and **foals** the most common manifestation of vitamin E/Se deficiencies is nutritional *muscular dystrophy (*see* white muscle disease). The highest incidence is at turnout in the spring, when grass has a high PUFA content and animals experience a sudden increase in muscular activity. Especially susceptible are lambs and calves born to dams fed diets based on straw, root crops, and poor-quality hays, silages, and cereal grains. Other signs of deficiency in ruminants may include poor growth and infertility, and, in cattle, diarrhoea, *paralytic myoglobinuria, and increased incidences of retained placenta and *downer cows.

In **poultry**, **pigs**, **cats**, and **mink** deficiencies of vitamin E may be either primary, for example due to inadequately supplemented diets (especially if the diets are based on maize (corn), soya-bean meal, or moist cereal grains), or secondary, due to a high fat content in the diet, especially if the fats are oxidized (rancid) or of a high PUFA content. In poultry common signs of deficiency include low hatchability of eggs, *encephalomalacia (crazy chick disease) in chicks less than 3 weeks old, and *exudative diathesis. Less common signs in poultry include pancreatic fibrosis, perosis, and necrosis of the gizzard and pectoral muscles. In pigs deficiency signs include hepatic necrosis (hepatosis dietetica) and cardiac degeneration and haemorrhages (*mulberry heart disease). Cats, mink, and other fur-bearing animals may suffer *steatitis (yellow fat disease). In several species deficiency causes increased erythrocyte fragility, and in **fish** signs include anaemia, myopathies, and exudative diathesis. For diagnosis and treatment *see* vitamin.

vitamin K A fat-soluble *vitamin required for the synthesis of prothrombin and coagulation factors VIII, IX, and X, which are essential for the normal coagulation (clotting) of blood. It may also be required for cellular respiration and electron transport. There are three groups of compounds with vitamin K activity: *phylloquinones* (*naphthoquinones* or *vitamin K₁*), which are synthesized by most green plants; *prenylmenaquinones* (*vitamin K₂*), which are synthesized by many bacteria, including those found in the intestine and reticulorumen; and *menaphthones* (*vitamin K₃*), which are synthetic forms, slightly soluble in water. Good natural sources of vitamin K include most green leafy plants, especially lucerne, cabbage, and kale. Most animal products, except egg yolk and fish meals, are poor sources. The intestinal absorption of the K_1 and K_2 forms are dependent on the presence of digestible fat and bile salts. It is antagonized by sulphaquinoxaline, *warfarin, and coumarin derivatives, for example *dicoumarol, which is found in spoiled feeds, especially spoiled sweet clover and sweet vernal. The vitamin is destroyed by sunlight, alkalis, acids, high humidity, irradiation, and food processing, for example drying and steam pelleting.
Vitamin K deficiency This is uncommon and usually secondary to the ingestion of antagonists, to decreased intestinal synthesis following antibiotic administration, or to increased requirements arising from chronic haemorrhage, for example in intestinal coccidiosis. Primary deficiencies may occur in recently hatched poultry and in newborn piglets if the diets of the adult females are deficient. There is very little storage of vitamin K in the liver or in other tissues and signs of deficiency may occur after only 1–2 weeks of a deficient diet. Signs of deficiency are those of *anaemia and of delayed clotting time, and include haemorrhaging at body orifices, bruising, haematomas, and lameness due to haemorrhages in joints and over bony prominences. There may be increased haemorrhaging following surgical operations, and in piglets at birth there may be increased bleeding from the navel. In poultry, mortality from coccidiosis may be increased. For diagnosis and treatment *see* vitamin. Other name: **coagulation factor**.

vitreous humour (vitreous body) The transparent jelly-like material that fills the chamber behind the lens of the *eye.

viviparous Describing an animal in which the developing embryo(s) are nourished within the mother's body via an intimate connection with maternal tissues, usually through a placenta. Their foetal development culminates in the birth of live young. Viviparity is the state occurring in most mammals. *Compare* oviparous; ovoviviparous.

vocal cords *See* vocal folds.

vocal folds The true vocal cords: the pair of mucous-membrane folds on the lateral wall of the *larynx. Each is wrapped around a *vocal ligament, and its edge forms part of the *glottis. Changes in the position of the vocal folds govern the shape of the glottis and are important in phonation.

vocal ligaments The pair of fibroelastic cords extending from the vocal processes of the arytenoid cartilages to the thyroid cartilage in the *larynx. Each is enclosed within a *vocal fold. Alterations in the tension of the vocal ligaments determine the pitch of sound during phonation.

voice The sound produced within the *larynx of mammals or the *syrinx of birds.

volar Relating to the back of the fore- or hindfoot; i.e. the area corresponding to the palm or sole. *See also* palmar.

volatile fatty acid (VFA) A short-chain *fatty acid containing between one and 8–10 carbon atoms. VFAs, particularly acetic, *propionic, and *butyric acids, are the principal end-products (with methane and carbon dioxide) of the fermentation of carbohydrates by microorganisms in the gut of animals, most notably in the rumen of ruminants and in the caecum and large intestine of horses. They are absorbed into the bloodstream and used as a source of energy by the animals. The amounts and proportions of the acids produced vary with the nature of the diet. Much smaller quantities of pentanoic acid (C5) and branched-chain VFAs, such as isobutanoic and isopentanoic acids, are produced by the microbial *deamination of *amino acids in the rumen.

voluntary food intake (VFI) The amount of food consumed under ideal *ad lib conditions. It is influenced by the age of an animal and the nutrient density of the diet. In nonruminants a diet with a lower nutrient density will tend to promote a higher VFI as the animal attempts to maintain a constant nutrient intake. In ruminants, however, diets with a low nutrient density tend to be bulky and contain a lot of dietary fibre. Hence the physical capacity of the gut, particularly the rumen, becomes a limiting factor and so VFI increases with nutrient density until physical capacity of the gut is no longer limiting.

Physiological control mechanisms then prevail as in nonruminants, and VFI decreases with further increase in nutrient density. Imbalances in dietary nutrients will tend to reduce VFI.

voluntary muscle *See* striated muscle.

volvulus Twisting of part of the gastrointestinal tract, especially a loop of intestine (bowel) on its mesentery. It occurs most frequently in horses, being commonest in the small intestine. It causes acute abdominal pain and shock, especially in cases where the twist strangulates the blood supply causing ischaemic necrosis and gangrene of the intestine. There is also obstruction of the intestine. Prompt surgical removal of the affected portion of intestine may be successful in resolving the problem.

vomer A thin plate of bone that contributes to the bony part of the nasal septum.

vomeronasal organ (Jacobson's organ) One of a pair of blind tubular diverticula lying on the floor of the nasal cavity close to the nasal septum. Each communicates with the *incisive duct*, which in most species opens on the roof of the oral cavity on the *incisive papilla*. It is believed to be an accessory organ of olfaction, particularly, in carnivores, to determine the flavour of food in the mouth.

vomiting (emesis) Violent expulsion of the stomach contents via the mouth. The vomiting reflex is initiated by a centre in the brain, which stimulates forceful contractions of the abdominal and diaphragmatic musculature and simultaneously opens the cardiac sphincter of the stomach. The reflex may be triggered by irritation of the stomach mucosa, for example due to disease or toxic substances, or by stomach distension following intestinal obstruction. The appearance of the vomit may give a clue to the cause of the problem. For example, altered blood, resembling coffee grounds, indicates gastric haemorrhage, while mucus suggests catarrhal inflammation.

Some animals, for example rodents and ruminants, are unable to vomit and cannot easily expel ingested poisons. In species capable of vomiting, *emetics can be administered to stimulate vomiting in an emergency, for example after an animal has accidentally swallowed a poison. Conversely, excessive and persistent vomiting may need treating with *antiemetic drugs or *demulcents, which are designed to protect the irritated gastric mucosa. Persistent vomiting leads to dehydration and severe loss of electrolytes from the body fluids. Such cases may need supportive therapy in the form of intravenous infusion of fluid and salts. Vomiting may also occur during transportation (see travel sickness).

vomiting/wasting disease (of piglets) A disease of pigs under 3 weeks of age characterized by vomiting, nervous signs, and poor growth and caused by a *coronavirus. The virus causes *encephalomyelitis and manifests itself in three distinct syndromes, all of which may appear in the same litter. Some piglets persistently vomit, while others may become depressed or hyperexcitable, while a third group merely fail to thrive, remaining as runts. Older pigs become infected but do not show clinical disease. Recovered sows pass immunity to the disease to their litters through their milk. Other name: **haemagglutinating encephalomyelitis of piglets**. *See also* epidemic diarrhoea; transmissible gastroenteritis.

von Willebrand's disease A generally mild inherited bleeding disorder described in dogs and pigs and characterized by a functional deficiency of *von Willebrand factor*, an essential plasma cofactor for the normal adhesion of *platelets to damaged blood vessels. The clinical signs are highly variable: severe cases show spontaneous mucosal haemorrhage whereas in milder cases abnormal bleeding occurs only after injury or surgery. There are reports that the condition is exacerbated by stress and concurrent disease, and that the severity diminishes with age and repeated pregnancies in affected females. Bleeding episodes are managed by infusion of plasma or whole blood. Other name: **pseudohaemophilia**.

vulva (*pl.* **vulvas** or **vulvae**) The external female genital organs, formed by the *vulva lips* surrounding the *vulvar cleft*.

vulvitis Inflammation of the vulva, often in conjunction with vaginitis (see vulvovaginitis). An ulcerative vulvitis occurs in ewes, which is thought to be spread venereally from rams with an enzootic form of inflammation of the penis and its sheath. The cause is not fully understood.

vulvovaginitis Inflammation of the vulva (vulvitis) and vagina (vaginitis). A herpesvirus, similar to that causing *infectious bovine rhinotracheitis (IBR), causes *infectious bovine pustulovaginitis (IPV) in cows and balanoposthitis (see balanitis) in bulls: bulls destined for AI use should therefore not be given live IBR vaccine. Another form of bovine vulvovaginitis is caused by *Mycoplasma* species. Mycotoxic vulvovaginitis (oestrogenism) of sows is caused by the ingestion of grain spoiled by the fungus *Fusarium roseum*, which releases an oestrogen producing vulval tumefaction and catarrhal vaginitis.

W

walkabout disease See Kimberley horse disease.

walking dandruff *See* Cheyletiella.

wall eye A condition of the horse's eye in which the iris is unpigmented, giving the effect of a pale ring around the pupil.

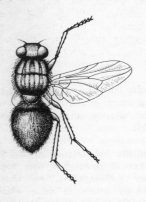

The warble fly, *Hypoderma bovis*

warble fly One of several species of *fly belonging to the genus *Hypoderma* that parasitize cattle, especially *H. bovis* and *H. lineatum*, which are found in the northern hemisphere, the latter being more common in warmer climates (see illustration). *H. bovis* is relatively large (about 30 mm long) with a softly hairy body tinged with yellow behind the head, at the waist, and at the tip of the abdomen. *H. lineatum* is smaller with hairier legs. In the UK the adult flies are on the wing from May until August and lay their eggs on the legs of cattle. The eggs hatch to form larvae which bore through the skin and migrate to the spine and oesophagus. Here they lie dormant from December to February

before continuing their migration to the skin of the back, appearing there from March to July. The tissues around each larva become swollen creating the characteristic lump (warble) in the skin with a small hole through which the larva breathes. Economic loss is caused by the damage to hides, while badly affected carcasses may be declared unfit for human consumption.

Treatment with systemic *insecticides in the autumn is effective in eliminating the migrating larvae, although it is dangerous to treat after November. In the spring, after the larvae have emerged on the back, treatment with contact insecticides is also effective but does not prevent damage to the hide. Warble fly infestation is a *notifiable disease in the UK, where it has been almost eradicated.

warfarin A *coumarin derivative and anticoagulant, structurally similar to *dicoumarol, that is used as a rodenticide and in the treatment of *navicular disease in horses. It acts as a competitive antagonist of *vitamin K, which is necessary for the formation of blood *coagulation factors I, II, VII, IX, and X in the liver. Without these factors prothrombin is not converted to thrombin and blood does not clot. Warfarin is odourless and tasteless, and is absorbed after ingestion (or oral administration). In rodenticides it is incorporated with a suitable bait. After ingestion, 24–48 hours may elapse before levels of coagulation factors fall and clinical signs of toxicity develop, depending on the dose (*see* warfarin poisoning). Rodents typically consume repeated small doses of baited warfarin before succumbing. However, some rats can metabolize the anticoagulant rapidly, thus preventing toxicity. Warfarin has been used in combination with calciferol (vitamin D_2), which causes calcification of arteries and increases the tendency to haemorrhage.

In the treatment of navicular disease, warfarin is administered orally to reduce coagulation in peripheral blood vessels. Blood clotting time must be monitored to prevent accumulation of the drug and toxicity. Concurrent administration of other highly protein-bound drugs (e.g. phenylbutazone) can increase the free circulating levels of warfarin and precipitate toxicity.

warfarin poisoning A toxic condition caused by ingestion of warfarin. Warfarin and other *coumarin derivatives affect the blood coagulation mechanism so that blood will not clot. Rodents are particularly susceptible to the long-term ingestion of these poisons, hence they are widely used as rodenticides. However, other animal species which gain repeated access to warfarin become lame due to subcutaneous haemorrhages, particularly on the bony prominences. Wounds show persistent bleeding and the animals become blind, paralysed, and die from respiratory distress. Treatment consists of daily injections of vitamin K and also blood transfusion in anaemic animals.

wart See papilloma.

washing See bathing.

water belly See ascites; toxic fat syndrome.

water dropwort poisoning See hemlock water dropwort poisoning.

waterhammer pulse A *pulse characterized by a good forcible beat but followed by an immediate collapse of the artery. It indicates aortic valve incompetence.

water hemlock poisoning See hemlock water dropwort poisoning.

water requirements The water needed by animals for optimum health and performance. Water is supplied directly from drinking water, from water present in food, and from water formed by metabolic processes in the body. The contribution of each and hence water requirement is often difficult to estimate, being influenced by animal species, type of production, and environmental conditions. Ideally, clean water should be available freely and continuously. Productivity can be seriously affected if the supply is restricted, especially in dairy cows and laying poultry whose water requirements increase at higher environmental temperatures. Also, feeds with high dry-matter content increase the amount of water voluntarily consumed, as do high dietary levels of salt.

High water intake may be associated with a specific *nutrient deficiency; for example, suboptimal dietary levels of *essential fatty acids for rapidly growing pigs are associated with dry cracked skin, which results in excessive water loss through evaporation. Various enteric disorders involving diarrhoea lead to rapid water loss and possible death through dehydration, and in other diseases, e.g. kidney failure, diabetes mellitus, etc., water requirements can be greatly increased.

W chromosome See sex chromosome.

weal See wheal.

weaner A young pig, usually between weaning age and the time of its entry into the fattening or rearing herd.

weaning The process of transferring young mammals from a liquid diet to solid food. The time of weaning depends on the species and the type of production system. Piglets are weaned at between 21 and 42 days old; lambs from approximately 56 days onwards. Suckler calves destined for beef production are weaned when several months old, compared to 3–10 weeks for artificially reared calves (*see* calf husbandry). Weaning is traumatic for the young animal and often causes a growth check. If not performed satisfactorily, serious health problems may arise, for example post-weaning diarrhoea.

Weaning of a **foal** usually takes place in the autumn when the foal is 4½–7 months old and used to eating concentrates. The break with the mare can either be sudden and total –by taking the mare out of earshot and leaving the foal with other foals – or the mare and foal can be separated at night but turned out together during the day. This second method allows the foal some milk during the day. Suitable feeds for weaned foals are rolled or crushed and bruised oats, crushed linseed cake, bran, carrots, and hay.

Young **puppies** and **kittens** normally develop the ability to lap liquids, such as milk substitutes, from about 4 weeks onwards, and cereal can be mixed in over the next couple of weeks to gradually thicken the food. By 6 weeks of age most puppies and kittens are able to eat and digest either finely minced meat with moistened biscuit, or a proprietary food designed for their consumption. Most young puppies and kittens will continue to suckle from their mother, mainly for comfort, and the weaning process will only be completed when the mother rejects the approaches from her young, or they are separated. It is generally accepted that the ideal time for complete weaning is at about 8 weeks of age.

The adverse effects of weaning can be minimized in various ways. The gradual introduction of solid food prior to weaning is essential, particularly in pigs. Housing is also an important factor, especially in animals weaned relatively early. Thus pigs, which are born in a relatively immature state, require weaner houses with good insulation and heating.

weatings *Offals from the milling of wheat, sometimes referred to as middlings. They have a lower fibre content than *bran, and may be classed as coarse or fine, depending upon their nature.

weaving A vice of highly bred horses in which the head and neck sway repetitively from side to side. In extreme cases the weight is transferred from one forefoot to the other. Anxiety and excitement precipitate temporary weaving in young horses. Established cases can be controlled by a top stable door designed to restrict head and neck movement. Stabling in an inside stable facing into a building is also a good corrective measure. Regular exercise will help prevent the habit or reduce its manifestation.

wedge osteotomy Surgical realignment of a bone achieved by the excision of a wedge-shaped portion from the site of a defect. It is sometimes performed to correct deviation at the distal ends of the radius and ulna of young dogs following trauma and damage to the growth plate. In horses wedge osteotomy was formerly employed to correct deviation of the distal radius, which occurred in young animals, but it has largely been superseded by periosteal stripping, on the convex side of the defect, which produces good results without bone section. A special variety of wedge osteotomy is performed below the neck and greater trochanter of the femur to produce altered weight bearing and better function in an arthritic hip joint.

weedkiller poisoning *See* paraquat poisoning; sodium chlorate poisoning.

weighing methods Techniques for determining the liveweight of animals. The chosen method depends primarily on the size of the animal. Small animals, such as lambs or piglets, can be weighed using a simple hand-held balance. Adult pigs and sheep or calves can be weighed in a weigh crate with a dial pointer or electronic load cells. Large cattle are usually weighed in a larger version of the weigh crate that incorporates a *crush and has either a dial indicator, beam balance, or electronic readout. For very accurate weighing of large cattle an electronic weighbridge can be used. However, the normal fluctuations in liveweight seen in adult cattle (up to 30 kg in one day) due to gut fill, drinking water, milking, and defecation make such accurate weighing pointless. Various weighbands are available for all classes of stock allowing estimation of liveweight from chest girth. These are not very accurate but are useful for comparing individuals.

Weil's disease *See* leptospirosis.

welfare codes (UK) Codes of recommendations for the welfare of livestock. Such codes have been published for cattle, pigs, sheep, domestic fowls, and turkeys under the Agriculture (Miscellaneous Provisions) Act (1968), which followed the report of the *Brambell Committee. If a person is prosecuted under the Act for causing unnecessary suffering to livestock on agricultural land, his or her failure to follow the provisions of the codes may be used in evidence.

Wesselbron disease A mosquito-borne disease of sheep and cattle caused by a *flavivirus and characterized by fever, abortion, and death of newborn lambs. The disease is prevalent in Central and Southern Africa. The post-mortem lesions of *jaundice and *hepatitis can cause confusion with *Nairobi sheep disease.

western duck disease *See* botulism.

wetting agent (surfactant) A substance, usually a detergent, that allows an aqueous solution to wet a surface, for example the inner surface of narrow tubing. The surfactant action of phospholipids, lecithin, and phosphatidyl glycerol appears to be necessary for inflation of the alveoli in newborn animals.

Wharton's jelly The loose jelly-like *mesenchyme surrounding the umbilical vessels within the *umbilical cord.

wheal (weal) A sharply-defined raised area of the skin, usually at least 1 cm in diameter, resulting from an underlying accumulation of fluid (*oedema). They may be caused by allergy, hypersensitivity to insect bites, or sharp blows to the skin, but typically disappear quickly.

whey The liquid residue remaining when milk has been treated with rennet to precipitate casein in cheese making. Although of lower nutritive value than milk, it is nevertheless a useful feedstuff for pigs. It is fed usually in liquid form as it tends to form compacted material when dried. High levels of lactose in whey can be associated with scouring.

whipworm *See* Trichuris.

whistling (in horses) *See* roaring.

white blood cell (white blood corpuscle) *See* leucocyte.

white comb *See* favus.

white heifer disease A disorder in female cattle involving the malformation during embryonic development of parts of the *paramesonephric duct system. In female embryos this normally develops into the uterine tubes, uterus, and vagina. The condition is common in white Shorthorn cattle, in which there is a genetic link between arrested development of the paramesonephric duct system and coat pigmentation. However, the condition can occur in most breeds of cattle and pigs. Severity of the disorder ranges from simply an *imperforate hymen to rudimentary development or complete absence of the vagina, cervix, or uterus. Affected animals are often sterile or have reduced fertility. In addition inhibition of drainage from the uterus may give rise to distended segments of tubular genitalia with the associated risk of infection. Early diagnosis in heifer calves and culling where necessary are paramount in intensive farming situations.

white line In the horse, the line of lighter-coloured and softer horn at the junction between the wall and the sole of the *hoof.

white matter Nerve tissue of the central nervous system that is paler in colour than the associated *grey matter because it contains more nerve fibres and thus larger amounts of the insulating material *myelin. In the brain the white matter lies within the grey matter of the cerebral cortex and cerebellar cortex and surrounds the nuclei of grey matter in the brainstem. In the spinal cord it lies around the X-shaped central core of grey matter.

white muscle disease (nutritional muscular dystrophy) A form of *muscular dystrophy caused by *selenium and/or *vitamin E deficiency and affecting cattle, sheep, goats, foals, and, to a lesser extent, pigs. The disease may be acute or subacute. In **cattle,** the acute form occurs mainly in calves recently turned out

to pasture. Sudden death without any warning signs is usual, due to heart muscle degeneration. In subacute disease, which also usually affects recently turned out calves, the signs are stiffness, muscular weakness, and trembling. The muscles are hard and swollen and there may be laboured breathing. In severe cases the shoulder blades protrude above the line of the back. The skeletal muscles are principally involved and at postmortem examination appear white, as if boiled, hence the name.

In **sheep,** in which the disease is also known as *stiff lamb disease,* the clinical signs are identical to those seen in cattle. Lambs born to selenium-deficient ewes may die suddenly within 2–3 days of birth. Chronic cases move stiffly and may become paralysed before death. **Goats** are similarly affected. In **pigs,** subacute white muscle disease is less common than in ruminants. However, the related acute condition, known as *mulberry heart disease, causes sporadic sudden deaths among fast-growing pigs. Treatment and prevention is as for selenium and vitamin E deficiencies.

white scours *See* enteric colibacillosis of calves.

white snakeroot poisoning A toxic condition caused by consumption of the perennial herbaceous plant *Eupatorium rugosum* (white snakeroot), which occurs primarily in the eastern USA. It contains a toxic fat-soluble complex benzyl alcohol (tremetol); repeated exposure to small amounts leads to a build-up of toxic concentrations in the body, and the toxic principle is excreted in the animal's milk. The clinical signs are weakness, trembling, constipation, paresis, coma, and death. Treatment is symptomatic.

whorl A distinct local formation in a horse's coat in which flattened hair

Wild Free-Roaming Horses and Burros Act

radiates from a central point, where the skin is visible. Whorls can be single, double, or in lines, and may occur either side of the crest, on the underside of the neck or front of the chest, under the jaw, and at or above the point of the stifle. Their distribution in an individual horse (together with the horse's white markings) is recorded on silhouettes showing different aspects of the horse. These are used as means of identification for registration and export purposes.

Wild Free-Roaming Horses and Burros Act (USA) A federal Act designed to protect free-roaming horses and burros (donkeys) on public lands. It prohibits the removal of these animals or their use without prior permission of the Secretary of the Interior.

Wildlife and Countryside Act (1981) (England and Wales) An Act of Parliament that gives statutory protection to certain species of indigenous birds, wild animals, and their habitats.

Wilm's tumour *See* nephroblastoma.

wind gall (wind puff) A condition of the *fetlock of the horse due to *tenosynovitis of the sheath of the digital flexor tendons. The cause is assumed to be trauma. Lameness is rarely present.

windpipe *see* trachea.

wind-sucking A vice of horses, often associated with *crib-biting, consisting of air-swallowing (aerophagia) – air is forced down the oesophagus, accompanied by a gulping noise. It may be due to boredom and/or learned behaviour, and can lead to weight loss and a tendency for recurrent *colic.
Apart from measures to counter any associated crib-biting, other options include removal of the neck strap muscles and/or associated nerves (*Forsell's operation* and *modified Forsell's operation*) and *buccostomy. The prognosis for curing the habit is guarded.

winter dysentery A highly contagious *enteritis of cattle that is of uncertain aetiology; the bacterium *Campylobacter fetus* subsp. *jejuni* and enteroviruses of low pathogenicity have been isolated. It occurs widely during the winter months in Canada and the northern states of the USA, mainly in housed adult cows. A bloody watery diarrhoea is characteristic. Most cases recover spontaneously in 24–36 hours.

withers The region of the back of a horse overlying the top of the scapulae (shoulder blades).

wobbler A condition, particularly of horses and dogs, in which instability of the cervical vertebrae causes abnormalities of the spinal cord in that region and consequent locomotor difficulties. In mild cases, the hindlimbs only are affected, but all four legs can be involved. Affected animals tend to be large (e.g. Doberman pinschers, Great Danes, well-grown horses) and the condition usually becomes apparent in the young adult. Signs include ataxia, apparent weakness, reluctance or inability to back or turn, and neck pain. Diagnosis requires radiography, with or without *myelography; flexion of the neck for radiography can help in obtaining diagnostic plates. Cervical spinal cord function in horses can be assessed by the *slap-test* for laryngeal adduction. The prognosis is guarded, especially if clinical signs are severe, but good results have been obtained in dogs by surgical stabilization of the affected vertebrae. This is feasible in horses but the probable suboptimal result is less acceptable in this species. The possibility of an inherited component to the condition is under debate.

wooden tongue *See* actinobacillosis.

wood preservatives *See* phenol poisoning.

Wood's light An ultraviolet light (sometimes called *black light*), with a wavelength of about 365 nm, used in human and veterinary dermatology to excite fluorescence characteristic of certain fungal infections; notable examples in animals are certain types of *ringworm. Parts of individual hairs or nails (but not skin scales) that have been invaded by certain species of *Microsporum* become brightly fluorescent with a characteristic apple-green hue under Wood's light. This is so in nearly all infections by *M. canis* and *M. equinum*, but less frequently with *M. gypseum*. Fluorescence that is associated with *Trichophyton* infections is rare in animals, although some (e.g. *T. simii*) may fluoresce.

Fluorescence aids the location of infected material in samples under examination in the laboratory. But its greatest value is in examining the whole animal. Often in daylight there is no visible sign of a lesion, although infection is suspected. This is particularly so with cats: many of those transmitting *M. canis* infection to humans show only scattered fluorescent hairs and no obvious lesion. A well-darkened room is essential for effective examination, and it is essential to differentiate between the green fluorescence produced in ringworm, the blue-white fluorescence of many fabric fibres, and some fluorescent topical medications. Absence of green fluorescence does not exclude a diagnosis of ringworm; scrapings from any skin lesions should still be examined by microscopy and culture and brush samples taken from suspected asymptomatic carriers.

woody nightshade (bittersweet) poisoning *See* solanine poisoning.

wool *See* fleece; hair.

wool balls *See* hair ball.

wool rot *See* lumpy wool.

wormer A drug used to remove helminth parasites from animals. *See* anthelmintic.

wormian bone *See* sutural bone.

wound A break or division in any tissue, caused by injury or surgical operation. Bruises, grazes, tears, cuts, punctures, and burns are all examples of wounds. Treatment depends on the location and extent of the wound, whether it is noninfected or septic, open (i.e. draining freely) or closed, etc.

X

xanthaemia *See* carotenaemia.

xanthine 1. A *purine that is an intermediate compound in the oxidative degradation of *adenine and *guanine to *uric acid. The molybdenum-containing enzyme *xanthine oxidase* oxidizes xanthine to uric acid, and also hypoxanthine to xanthine. Elevated uric acid levels in blood can be treated with allopurinol, an inhibitor of xanthine oxidase (*see* gout). **2.** Any of a group of derivatives of xanthine, some of which are used in the treatment of respiratory diseases and heart disease. The group includes the naturally occurring methylxanthine alkaloids caffeine, theophylline, and theobromine, as well as the synthetic analogues of theophylline (e.g. aminophylline and etamiphylline). They act by inhibiting the enzyme phosphodiesterase, which degrades cyclic *AMP, thereby increasing intracellular concentrations of cyclic AMP. This leads to stimulation of the central nervous system (CNS) with increased motor activity, respiratory stimulation, and increased vasomotor tone. Caffeine is more potent than the others as a CNS stimulant. Xanthines act on the cardiovascular system, increasing the rate and force of cardiac contraction. There is peripheral vasodilatation but increased vasomotor activity from the CNS may counteract this, and a possible overall increase in blood pressure may result. Transient diuresis (lasting 1–2 days) also occurs. The order of potency (on the heart and as diuretics) is: theophylline, theobromine, caffeine. Etamiphylline does not cause an increase in heart rate and produces an overall fall in blood pressure. Xanthines also cause relaxation of bronchial smooth muscle, especially theophylline, and stimulate glycogenolysis in skeletal muscle, especially caffeine.

The main drugs used therapeutically are theophylline, aminophylline, and etamiphylline. They are absorbed from the gastrointestinal tract after oral administration or can be injected. In respiratory diseases they improve bronchodilation and remove pulmonary oedema. They can also be used alone or in combination with *cardiac glycosides to treat congestive cardiac failure. Overdosage with xanthines causes gastrointestinal disturbances, with vomiting and diarrhoea, and in some cases there is CNS stimulation, tachycardia, and cardiac arrhythmias. Caffeine and theobromine have been used to try to improve the performance of racing horses and dogs. This is illegal and care should be taken to ensure that feed given to such animals does not contain natural xanthine alkaloids.

xantho- *Prefix denoting* yellow colour.

xanthophyll A yellow pigment found in green leaves. An example of a xanthophyll is *lutein*.

xanthosis A yellow-brown discoloration of the skeletal and heart muscles of dairy cattle (especially Ayrshires) due to deposition of the purine derivative *xanthine. Although when the muscle is examined histologically, pigment granules can be seen within the muscle fibres, there are no obvious pathological effects. The condition may be due to an inherited deficiency of the enzyme xanthine oxidase. In affected animals xanthine may be excreted in the urine (xanthinuria).

X chromosome *See* sex chromosome.

xenograft A graft transferred between members of different species. *Compare* allograft. *See also* histocompatibility.

Xenopsylla A genus of mainly tropical and subtropical *fleas. The rat flea, *Xenopsylla cheopis*, found throughout the world, can transmit plague and murine typhus to humans.

xero- *Prefix denoting* a dry condition.

xerophthalmia Dryness of the conjunctiva of the eye, usually due to a deficiency of tears. It results in mucopurulent inflammation and ulceration. Xerophthalmia is a sign of *vitamin A deficiency in calves and pigs, and is a common disorder in dogs after distemper infection. Another possibility is obstruction of the tear duct (*see* lacrimal apparatus), which may be a hereditary defect. Surgical reconstruction of the duct can be attempted, or even transplantation of the parotid duct, but euthanasia may be required. In simple and early cases topical ther-

xylose

apy with 'artificial tears' is an option, or *pilocarpine may be used to stimulate tear production.

xerosis Abnormal dryness of the skin, mucous membranes, or the conjunctiva. In the latter case it is due not to decreased production of tears (*see* xerophthalmia) but to changes in the membrane.

xerostomia Dryness of the mouth due to a diminished flow of saliva. Decreased salivary secretion can be caused by certain drugs (e.g. atropine) or by extreme dehydration (e.g. due to fever or water deprivation). It can occur secondarily to such conditions as severe diarrhoea, nephritis, or diabetes mellitus.

xiphoid process The caudal extension of the most caudal sternebra of the *sternum. It may be further extended by the *xiphoid cartilage*.

X-rays Electromagnetic radiation of extremely short wavelength (beyond ultraviolet but longer than gamma radiation). They are produced by an X-ray tube, in which a beam of high-energy electrons strikes a metal target. The radiation is used diagnostically to visualize internal body structures (*see* radiography) and in certain forms of *radiotherapy. However, great care must be exercised to avoid unnecessary exposure of both personnel and patients to X-rays because of their potentially harmful effects. The primary beam should be as small as possible and only the structures to be investigated should be in this beam. All personnel should be protected by lead screens or lead clothing. In veterinary practice sedation or general anaesthesia should be considered whenever manual restraint of the patient is likely to be unsatisfactory or entail risk.

xylazine A sedative used in the chemical restraint of animals. It is chemically unlike other tranquillizers and acts as an α_2 adrenergic agonist, blocking transmission of impulses in the central nervous system by acting at presynaptic sites. This drug is potent in ruminants and is used mainly for the restraint of cattle. It can be injected intramuscularly or intravenously. In cattle and sheep there is a dose-related response, varying from mild to deep sedation with analgesia and muscle relaxation. Xylazine is often used with local anaesthetics for restraint during surgical procedures in cattle to avoid the risks associated with general anaesthesia. The duration of action is 30–60 minutes with rapid recovery. In horses much higher doses of xylazine are required to produce sedation, but it is very effective and widely used. In dogs, cats, and horses xylazine is used as a premedicant prior to anaesthesia or in conjunction with *ketamine to improve muscle relaxation. In cats, and occasionally in dogs, vomiting is seen after administration. Other side-effects include vagal bradycardia (in horses, dogs, and cats), with dropped beats – these can be prevented by using *atropine; respiratory depression; salivation (in cattle and horses); urine retention (in cattle); ruminal tympany; and abortion in late pregnancy in cattle. Tradename: **Rompun.** *Detomidine* is a similar drug used as a sedative in horses. It has a longer duration of action than xylazine. Tradename: **Domosedan.**

xylene (dimethylbenzene) A liquid used for increasing the transparency of tissues prepared for microscopic examination after they have been dehydrated.

xylose A pentose sugar (i.e. one with five carbon atoms). It is used to assess small intestinal function in suspected cases of *malabsorption.

Y

Y chromosome *See* sex chromosome.

yeast Any of a large and ubiquitous group of *fungi whose sole or predominant growth form is unicellular, with new cells arising asexually from mature ones, usually as detachable outgrowths produced by a process of budding. *Dimorphic fungi have both a yeast phase and a mycelial phase (*see* mycelium). Diseases of veterinary importance caused by yeasts include *candidiasis, *mycotic mastitis, and *cryptococcosis.

yellow fat disease *See* steatitis.

yellow fatted sheep A genetic disorder of some sheep, in which the yellow pigments of grass and other herbage, *carotene and *xanthophyll, cannot be broken down, resulting in the animals having bright-yellow body fat. It is important to distinguish the condition from *jaundice. A similar condition occurs in some rabbits.

yellow jessamine poisoning A toxic condition resulting from the ingestion of yellow jessamine (*Gelsemium sempervirens*), a woody evergreen vine occurring primarily in the southern USA. It is also known as the Carolina jessamine or evening trumpet flower. It contains toxic alkaloids, related to strychnine, that cause weakness, incoordination, convulsions, coma, and death. Treatment is symptomatic to control the convulsions and respiratory paralysis.

yellow lamb disease A rapidly fatal *enterotoxaemia of nursing lambs caused by the bacterium *Clostridium perfringens type A, seen in California and Oregon. Exotoxin absorbed from the gut causes massive intravascular haemolysis; the name of the disease refers to the resulting jaundice.

yelt An infrequently used term for a young female pig. *See* gilt.

Yersinia A genus of aerobic or facultatively anaerobic pleomorphic Gram-negative bacteria. The three known species are parasites of animals. *Y. pestis* causes human bubonic plague and also infects rats, which serve as reservoirs of infection for humans. It does not affect other animals. *Y. enterocolitica* is widespread in nature and causes enteric infections in humans and some animals. *Y. pseudotuberculosis* causes a disease similar to human plague in rodents but can also infect other domestic animals (*see* pseudotuberculosis).

yersiniosis Disease caused by bacteria of the genus *Yersinia.

yew poisoning A toxic condition caused by the ingestion of leaves of the English yew (*Taxus baccata*), an evergreen tree, or related species, including the American yew (*T. canadensis*), Japanese yew (*T. cuspidata*), and Western yew (*T. brevifolia*). The leaves are eaten by grazing animals when their normal food is scarce, for example in winter, or when they inadvertently gain access to gardens or churchyards where the trees are growing. The leaves contain 1% of the alkaloid taxine, which slows and then stops the heart. Horses die rapidly after the ingestion of 100–200 g of yew leaves, but cattle seem to be more resistant and *rumenotomy is recommended to remove ingested yew and prevent absorption of toxic amounts of the alkaloid.

yolk (deutoplasm) A substance, rich in protein and fat, that is laid down within the egg cell as nourishment for the embryo. It is nearly absent from mammalian egg cells but is abundant in the avian *egg.

yolk sac One of the *foetal membranes, formed of endoderm lined with mesoderm, that lies ventral to the embryo. Its cavity forms the *archenteron (primitive gut) and eventually the definitive embryonic gut, with which it continues to communicate through the narrow vitellointestinal duct passing through the *umbilicus. It probably assists in transporting nutrients to the early embryo and is one of the earliest sites of blood cell formation. The endoderm of the yolk sac is the site of origin of the primordial germ cells, which become the *oogonia and *spermatogonia.

yolk sac infection *See* omphalitis.

Z

Z chromosome *See* sex chromosome.

zein The principal protein of maize (corn). It is deficient in the *essential amino acids lysine and tryptophan.

zeranol A nonsteroidal growth promoter used in cattle to improve feed conversion efficiency. It has mild oestrogenic properties, and is thought to act as an anabolic by stimulating the pituitary to increase production of somatotrophin (growth hormone). It causes increased nitrogen retention, increased muscle and bone growth, mobilization of fat, elevated blood glucose and insulin, and an increase in the size of the adrenal glands. Heifers, steers, and bulls can be implanted; the effects last 90–120 days. In heifers on a high plane of nutrition there may be slight mam-

mary development. Zeranol has been used in conjunction with other anabolic compounds, such as *trenbolone acetate. Residues of zeranol are undetectable in tissues 70 days after implantation. However, the use of zeranol as an implant in food-producing animals is to be banned in the EEC because of concern about residues in meat. Tradename: **Ralgro**.

zero grazing A system of feeding grass to cattle that are housed permanently in yards or paddocks instead of being allowed access to pasture. Zero grazing enables full utilization of grass, allowing higher stocking rates, and avoids the problems of poaching and fouling of pasture. However, the system demands reliable machinery to cut and collect the grass and the machines may damage the pasture and cause soil compaction. Also no opportunity is given for selective grazing of the more nutritious parts of the grass.

zinc A metallic element that is a trace element (*see* essential element) required in the diet for animals. It is a component of some enzymes (e.g. carboxypeptidase) and a cofactor for many others. In chicks, deficiency in the diet causes poor growth, 'frizzled' feathers, skin lesions, and bone abnormalities ('swollen hock syndrome'). In pigs, zinc deficiency is associated with impaired growth, depressed appetite, and skin lesions (*see* parakeratosis). The bran and germ of cereal grains are good sources of the element.

zinc phosphide poisoning A toxic condition caused by ingestion of zinc phosphide, which is used as a rodenticide. Carelessly laid bait is liable to be eaten by all species, especially poultry, and an intake of more than 30 mg/kg bodyweight will lead to abdominal pain followed by coma and death. Ingestion of the poison is confirmed by the detection of phosphine in the gut contents. Use of zinc phosphide has been largely superseded by *warfarin compounds.

zona pellucida The thick membrane that develops around the mammalian oocyte within the *ovarian follicle. It is penetrated by a spermatozoon at fertilization and then persists around the conceptus, thus preventing expansion of the conceptus until it reaches the cavity of the uterus.

zonula adherens An intercellular junction that surrounds epithelial cells in a belt-like fashion. The adjacent cell membranes are thickened and filaments converge to this region from the cytoplasm. See junctional complex.

zonula occludens (tight junction) An intercellular junction that occurs principally between columnar epithelial cells. The outer laminae of adjacent cell membranes are fused, forming a barrier that prevents the passage of substances into the intercellular space. See junctional complex.

zonule (zonula) (in anatomy) A small band or zone. The ciliary zonule is the zone of attachment of the lens of the *eye to the ciliary processes by the zonular fibres.

Zoo Licensing Act (1981) (England and Wales) An Act of Parliament under which zoos are subject to licensing. The Act defines a zoo as an establishment where wild animals are kept for exhibition to the public; it does not include circuses or pet shops. The local authority may grant an initial licence for four years and subsequent licences for six years.

zoonosis (pl. zoonoses) Any infectious disease that is naturally transmissible between vertebrates and humans. The World Health Organization lists about 150 zoonoses of significance. Some are fatal, such as anthrax and rabies, others are less severe, for instance cowpox, or may cause recurring symptoms, such as brucellosis in humans. Still others involve complex life cycles, for example Japanese B *encephalitis. Zoonoses are of obvious significance to farmers, veterinary surgeons, and others working with livestock. Also, intimate contact with domestic pets may infect humans with parasites such as Toxocara canis (see toxocariasis) and *Echinococcus. Children are especially at risk.

zygomatic arch (zygoma) The bar of bone extending from the orbit of the *skull to the ear.

zygomatic bone Either of a pair of bones of the *zygomatic arch.

zygomatic gland A *salivary gland lying below the orbit in carnivores. It represents a condensation of the small dorsal buccal glands of other species.

zygomycosis Any disease caused by infection with a *fungus belonging to the class Zygomycetes; a type of *phycomycosis. The term therefore includes the various forms of *mucormycosis and also (usually) the subcutaneous infections *conidiobolomycosis and basidiobolomycosis (although the latter conditions are sometimes grouped together as *entomophthoromycoses).

zygote The structure formed after fertilization of the ovum but before the commencement of *cleavage that restores the diploid number of chromosomes.

zygotene The second stage of the first prophase of *meiosis, in which the homologous chromosomes form pairs (bivalents).